Surgery of the
MUSCULOSKELETAL
SYSTEM

SECOND EDITION

Section Editors

Richard I. Burton, M.D.   Professor and Chairman, Department of Orthopaedics, University of Rochester School of Medicine and Dentistry, Rochester, New York
  Section 2: The Hand

Robert H. Cofield, M.D.   Professor of Orthopedic Surgery, Department of Orthopedics, Mayo Medical School; Consultant in Orthopedic Surgery, Mayo Clinic, Rochester, Minnesota
  Section 3: The Shoulder, Arm, and Elbow

Henry R. Cowell, M.D., Ph.D.   Lecturer, Harvard Medical School, Boston, Massachusetts
  Section 9: The Foot

Charles H. Epps, Jr., M.D.   Professor of Orthopaedic Surgery, Department of Surgery, and Dean, Howard University College of Medicine, Washington, D.C.
  Section 12: Amputations

C. McCollister Evarts, M.D.   Senior Vice President for Health Affairs, Dean, Pennsylvania State University College of Medicine, and Professor of Orthopaedic Surgery, Department of Surgery, The Milton S. Hershey Medical Center, Hershey, Pennsylvania
  Section 1: Musculoskeletal Surgery — Introduction
  Section 6: The Hip

Donald B. Kettelkamp, M.D.   Executive Director, The American Board of Orthopaedic Surgery, Inc., Chicago, Illinois
  Section 7: The Knee

Gerald S. Laros, M.D.   Professor and Chairman, Department of Orthopaedic Surgery, Texas Tech University Health Sciences Center School of Medicine, Lubbock, Texas
  Section 5: The Pelvis and Proximal Femur

Robert E. Leach, M.D.   Professor and Chairman, Department of Orthopaedic Surgery, Boston University Medical School, Boston, Massachusetts
  Section 8: The Tibia and Ankle

Henry J. Mankin, M.D.   Edith M. Ashley Professor of Orthopaedic Surgery, Harvard Medical School; Orthopaedist-in-Chief, Massachusetts General Hospital, Boston, Massachusetts
  Section 11: Bone and Soft Tissue Tumors

Carl L. Nelson, M.D.   Professor of Adult Reconstructive Surgery and Chairman, Department of Orthopaedic Surgery, University of Arkansas for Medical Sciences, Little Rock, Arkansas
  Section 10: Infections

Thomas E. Whitesides, Jr., M.D.   Professor, Department of Orthopaedics, Emory University School of Medicine, Emory University Clinic, Atlanta, Georgia
  Section 4: The Spine

Surgery of the
MUSCULOSKELETAL SYSTEM

SECOND EDITION

Edited by

C. McCollister Evarts, M.D.

Senior Vice President for Health Affairs
Dean, Pennsylvania State University College of Medicine
Professor of Orthopaedic Surgery
Department of Surgery
The Milton S. Hershey Medical Center
Hershey, Pennsylvania

Churchill Livingstone
New York, Edinburgh, London, Melbourne

Library of Congress Cataloging in Publication Data

Surgery of the musculoskeletal system/edited by C. McCollister
   Evarts. — 2nd ed.
        p.   cm.
      Includes bibliographical references.
      ISBN 0-443-08516-1 (set)
      1. Orthopedic surgery.   I. Evarts, C. McCollister, date
      [DNLM: 1. Orthopedics.   WE 168 S961]
RD731.S87   1990
617.4'7—dc20
DNLM/DLC
for Library of Congress   89-23856
                                                           CIP

Distributed in the United Kingdom by Churchill Livingstone, Robert Stevenson House, 1–3 Baxter's Place, Leith Walk, Edinburgh EH1 3AF, and by associated companies, branches, and representatives throughout the world.

Accurate indications, adverse reactions, and dosage schedules for drugs are provided in this book, but it is possible that they may change. The reader is urged to review the package information data of the manufacturers of the medications mentioned.

The Publishers have made every effort to trace the copyright holders for borrowed material. If they have inadvertently overlooked any, they will be pleased to make the necessary arrangements at the first opportunity.

Acquisitions Editor: *Robert A. Hurley*
Assistant Editor: *Leslie Burgess*
Copy Editor: *Ann Ruzycka*
Production Designer: *Angela Cirnigliaro*
Production Supervisor: *Sharon Tuder*

Printed in the United States of America

First published in 1990

*To past, present,
and future orthopaedic residents*

Contributors

John P. Albright, M.D.
Professor and Director, Sports Medicine Services, Department of Orthopaedic Surgery, University of Iowa College of Medicine, Iowa City, Iowa

Ian J. Alexander, M.D.
Foot Service, Department of Orthopaedic Surgery, Cleveland Clinic Foundation, Cleveland, Ohio

William C. Allen, M.D.
Professor and Chief, Division of Orthopaedic Surgery, Department of Surgery, University of Missouri — Columbia School of Medicine, University of Missouri Health Sciences Center, Columbia, Missouri

Harlan C. Amstutz, M.D.
Professor and Chief of Orthopaedic Surgery, Department of Surgery, University of California, Los Angeles, UCLA School of Medicine, Los Angeles, California

Allan W. Bach, M.D.
Clinical Associate Professor, Department of Orthopaedics, University of Washington School of Medicine, Seattle, Washington

Alan R. Baker, M.D.
Senior Investigator, Surgery Branch, National Cancer Institute, National Institutes of Health, Bethesda, Maryland

Robert W. Beasley, M.D., F.A.C.S.
Professor of Plastic Surgery, Department of Surgery, New York University School of Medicine; Director of Hand Surgery Services, New York University Medical Center and Bellevue Hospital Center, New York, New York

Robert D. Beckenbaugh, M.D.
Associate Professor of Orthopedic Surgery, Department of Orthopedics, Mayo Medical School; Consultant in Orthopedic Surgery and Surgery of the Hand, Mayo Clinic, Rochester, Minnesota

Douglas A. Becker, M.D.
Instructor in Orthopedic Surgery, Department of Orthopedics, Mayo Medical School; Senior Associate Consultant in Orthopedic Surgery, Mayo Clinic, Rochester, Minnesota

Edna J. Becker, M.D.
Associate Professor, Department of Radiology, University of Toronto Faculty of Medicine; Senior Radiologist, Toronto General Hospital, Toronto, Ontario, Canada

Stephen K. Benirschke, M.D.
Assistant Professor, Department of Orthopaedics, University of Washington School of Medicine, Seattle, Washington

James B. Bennett, M.D.
Chief, Hand and Upper Extremity Surgery Section, Division of Orthopaedic Surgery, Department of Surgery, Baylor College of Medicine; Consultant in Hand and Upper Extremity Surgery, Shriners Hospital for Crippled Children; Consultant in Hand and Upper Extremity Surgery, Institute for Rehabilitation and Research, Houston, Texas

A.G. Björkengren, M.D.
Assistant Professor, Department of Radiology, University Hospital, Lund, Sweden

Craig E. Blum, M.D.
Clinical Assistant Professor, Department of Orthopaedics, State University of New York at Buffalo School of Medicine and Biomedical Sciences, Buffalo, New York

Oheneba Boachie-Adjei, M.D.
Assistant Professor, Department of Orthopaedic Surgery, University of Minnesota Medical School—Minneapolis; Attending Staff, University of Minnesota Hospital, Abbott-Northwestern Hospital, and Minneapolis Children's Hospital, Minneapolis, Minnesota

George P. Bogumill, Ph.D., M.D.
Professor of Orthopaedic Surgery, Department of Surgery, Georgetown University School of Medicine, Washington, D.C.; Clinical Professor, Department of Surgery, Uniformed Services University of the Health Sciences F. Edward Hébert School of Medicine, Bethesda, Maryland; Adjunct Associate Professor, Department of Orthopaedic Surgery, George Washington University School of Medicine and Health Sciences, Washington, D.C.; Consultant in Orthopaedic and Hand Surgery, Walter Reed Army Medical Center, Washington, D.C.; Consultant, Veterans Administration Hospital, Washington, D.C.

Henry H. Bohlman, M.D.
Professor, Department of Orthopaedic Surgery, Case Western Reserve University School of Medicine; Chief, Acute Spinal Cord Injury Service, Veterans Administration Medical Center; Chief, The Reconstructive and Traumatic Spine Surgery Center, University Hospital, Cleveland, Ohio

Brett Bolhofner, M.D.
Assistant Clinical Professor, Department of Orthopaedic Surgery, University of South Florida College of Medicine, Tampa, Florida

Robert B. Bourne, M.D.
Professor of Orthopaedic Surgery, Department of Surgery, University of Western Ontario Faculty of Medicine; University Hospital, London, Ontario, Canada

David S. Bradford, M.D.
Professor, Department of Orthopaedic Surgery, University of Minnesota Medical School—Minneapolis; Director, Spine Service and Twin Cities Scoliosis Center; Attending Staff, University of Minnesota Hospital, Abbott-Northwestern Hospital, and Minneapolis Children's Hospital, Minneapolis, Minnesota

Malcolm A. Brahms, M.D.
Assistant Clinical Professor, Department of Orthopaedic Surgery, Case Western Reserve University School of Medicine; Visiting Orthopaedic Surgeon, Mount Sinai Hospital, Cleveland, Ohio

Richard A. Brand, M.D.
Professor, Departments of Orthopaedic Surgery and Biomedical Engineering, University of Iowa College of Medicine, Iowa City, Iowa

Mark P. Broderson, M.D.
McFarland Clinic, Ames, Iowa

Peter J. Brooks, M.D. F.R.C.S.(C)
Lecturer, Department of Surgery, University of Toronto Faculty of Medicine; Orthopaedic Surgeon, Mt. Sinai Hospital and Toronto General Hospital, Toronto, Ontario, Canada

Bruce Browner, M.D.
Professor and Chairman, Division of Orthopaedic Surgery, Department of Surgery, University of Texas Medical School at Houston, University of Texas Health Science Center at Houston, Houston, Texas

Richard S. Bryan, M.D.
Emeritus Professor of Orthopedic Surgery, Department of Orthopedics, Mayo Medical School; Consultant in Orthopedic Surgery, Mayo Clinic, Rochester, Minnesota

Robert W. Bucholz, M.D.
Professor of Orthopaedic Surgery, Department of Surgery, University of Texas Southwestern Medical Center at Dallas Southwestern Medical School, Dallas, Texas

William P. Bunnell, M.D.
Professor and Chairman, Department of Orthopaedic Surgery, Loma Linda University School of Medicine, Loma Linda, California; Former Director of Orthopaedics, Alfred I. DuPont Institute, Wilmington, Delaware

Ernest M. Burgess, M.D.
Clinical Professor of Orthopaedic Surgery, Department of Orthopaedics, and Director and Principal Investigator, Prosthetics Research Study, University of Washington School of Medicine; Director, Special Teams for Amputation Mobility, Prosthetic/Orthotic Program, Veterans Administration Medical Center, Seattle, Washington

Barry W. Burkhardt, M.D.
West-End Orthopaedic Clinic, Richmond, Virginia

Albert H. Burstein, Ph.D.
Professor of Applied Biomechanics, Department of Surgery, Cornell University Medical College; Director, Department of Biomechanics, The Hospital for Special Surgery, New York, New York

Richard I. Burton, M.D.
Professor and Chairman, Department of Orthopaedics, University of Rochester School of Medicine and Dentistry, Rochester, New York

Jason Calhoun, M.D., M.Eng.
Assistant Professor of Orthopaedic Surgery, Department of Surgery, University of Texas Medical School at Galveston, Galveston, Texas

Mario Campanacci, M.D.
Professor, Department of Orthopaedics, University of Bologna; Chief, Orthopaedic Service, Istituto Rizzoli, Bologna, Italy

Richard B. Caspari, M.D.
Clinical Associate Professor of Orthopaedic Surgery, Department of Surgery, Virginia Commonwealth University Medical College of Virginia School of Medicine; Tuckahoe Orthopaedic Associates; Director, Orthopaedic Research of Virginia, Richmond, Virginia

Donald P.K. Chan, M.D., B.S., F.A.C.S.
Professor and Chief, Section of Surgery of the Spine, Department of Orthopaedics, University of Rochester School of Medicine and Dentistry, Rochester, New York

Kwan-Ho Chan, M.D., F.R.C.S.(C)
Associate Orthopaedic Surgeon, Chedoke-McMaster Hospital, Hamilton, Ontario, Canada

Edmond Y.S. Chao, Ph.D.
Professor, Department of Bioengineering, Mayo Medical School; Consultant in Biomechanical Research, Mayo Clinic, Rochester, Minnesota

Michael W. Chapman, M.D.
Professor and Chairman, Department of Orthopaedics, University of California, Davis, School of Medicine, Davis, California

George Cierny III, M.D.
Associate Professor of Orthopaedic Surgery, Department of Surgery, Emory University School of Medicine; Veterans Administration Medical Center, Atlanta, Georgia

Mack L. Clayton, M.D.
Clinical Professor, Department of Surgery, University of Colorado School of Medicine, University of Colorado Health Sciences Center, Denver, Colorado

Frank W. Clippinger, M.D.
Professor of Orthopaedic Surgery, Department of Surgery, and Director, Rehabilitation Center, Duke University School of Medicine, Duke University Medical Center, Durham, North Carolina

Robert H. Cofield, M.D.
Professor of Orthopedic Surgery, Department of Orthopedics, Mayo Medical School; Consultant in Orthopedic Surgery, Mayo Clinic, Rochester, Minnesota

David N. Collins, M.D.
Assistant Professor of Adult Reconstructive Surgery, Department of Orthopaedic Surgery, University of Arkansas for Medical Sciences; Acting Chief of Orthopaedic Surgery, John L. McClellan Veterans Administration Hospital, Little Rock, Arkansas

Thomas Comfort, M.D.
Assistant Professor, Department of Orthopaedic Surgery, University of Minnesota Medical School—Minneapolis, Minneapolis, Minnesota

William P. Cooney III, M.D.
Professor of Orthopedic Surgery, Department of Orthopedics, Mayo Medical School; Consultant in Orthopedic Surgery, Mayo Clinic, Rochester, Minnesota

Charles N. Cornell, M.D.
Assistant Professor of Orthopaedics, Orthopaedic Surgery, and Traumatology, Department of Surgery, Cornell University Medical College; Assistant Attending, Orthopaedic Surgery and Traumatology, New York Hospital; Assistant Attending, Orthopaedic Surgery and Traumatology, The Hospital for Special Surgery, New York, New York

Mark B. Coventry, M.D., M.S.
Emeritus Professor of Orthopedic Surgery, Department of Orthopedics, Mayo Medical School; Emeritus Consultant in Orthopedic Surgery, Mayo Clinic, Rochester, Minnesota

Henry R. Cowell, M.D., Ph.D.
  Lecturer, Harvard Medical School, Boston, Massachusetts
Andrea Cracchiolo III, M.D.
  Professor of Orthopaedic Surgery, Department of Surgery, University of California, Los Angeles, UCLA School of Medicine, Los Angeles, California
Edward V. Craig, M.D.
  Assistant Professor, Department of Orthopaedic Surgery, University of Minnesota Medical School — Minneapolis; Consultant, Department of Orthopaedic Surgery, Veterans Administration Hospital, Minneapolis, Minnesota
Robin Davidson, M.D.
  Associate Professor of Neurosurgery, Department of Surgery, University of Massachusetts Medical School, Worchester, Massachusetts
Genevieve M. de Bese, B.A., M.A.
  Consultant, Prosthetics Laboratory, New York University Medical Center, New York, New York
Kenneth E. DeHaven, M.D.
  Professor and Head, Section of Athletic Medicine, Department of Orthopaedics, University of Rochester School of Medicine and Dentistry, Rochester, New York
Sanjay S. Desai, M.D.
  Resident in Orthopaedic Surgery, Combined Orthopaedic Residency, University of Massachusetts Medical School, Worcester, Massachusetts
Dennis P. Devito, M.D.
  Assistant Clinical Professor, Department of Orthopaedics and Rehabilitation, Vanderbilt University School of Medicine, Nashville, Tennessee
William M. Deyerle, M.D.
  Clinical Professor of Orthopaedic Surgery, Department of Surgery, Virginia Commonwealth University Medical College of Virginia School of Medicine; Richmond Orthopaedic Clinic, Richmond, Virginia
James H. Dobyns, M.D.
  Professor of Orthopedic Surgery, Department of Orthopedics, Mayo Medical School; Consultant in Orthopedic Surgery and Surgery of the Hand, Mayo Clinic, Rochester, Minnesota
David M. Drvaric, M.D.
  Assistant Professor, Department of Orthopaedics, Brown University Program in Medicine; Assistant Surgeon, Division of Pediatric Orthopaedics, Department of Orthopaedics, Rhode Island Hospital, Providence, Rhode Island
Paul Dubravcik, M.D., F.R.C.S.(C)†
  Former Associate Professor, Department of Surgery, McGill University Faculty of Medicine; Former Chief of Orthopaedics, Reddy Memorial Hospital, Montreal, Quebec, Canada
Edward J. Dunn, M.D.
  Professor of Orthopaedic Surgery, Department of Orthopaedics, University of Massachusetts Medical School; Chief of Orthopaedic Surgery, Worcester Memorial Hospital, Worcester, Massachusetts
Harold K. Dunn, M.D.
  Professor and Chairman, Division of Orthopaedic Surgery, Department of Orthopaedics, University of Utah School of Medicine, Salt Lake City, Utah

---

† Deceased

Charles C. Edwards, M.D.
Associate Professor of Orthopaedic Surgery, Department of Orthopaedics, University of Maryland School of Medicine; University of Maryland Hospital, Baltimore, Maryland

Frank J. Eismont, M.D.
Professor and Chief of Spine Surgery, Department of Orthopaedics and Rehabilitation, University of Miami School of Medicine, Miami, Florida

John A. Elstrom, M.D.
Clinical Assistant Professor, Department of Orthopaedic Surgery, University of Illinois, Abraham Lincoln School of Medicine, Chicago, Illinois; Attending Orthopaedic Surgeon, Department of Orthopaedic Surgery, Northern Illinois Medical Center, McHenry, Illinois

William F. Enneking, M.D.
Distinguished Service Professor and Eugene L. Jewett Professor of Orthopaedics and Pathology, University of Florida College of Medicine, Gainesville, Florida

Charles H. Epps, Jr., M.D.
Professor of Orthopaedic Surgery, Department of Surgery, and Dean, Howard University College of Medicine, Washington, D.C.

Richard P. Evans, M.D.
Attending Orthopaedic Surgeon, Presbyterian-St. Luke's Hospitals, Denver, Colorado

C. McCollister Evarts, M.D.
Senior Vice President for Health Affairs, Dean, Pennsylvania State University College of Medicine, and Professor of Orthopaedic Surgery, Department of Surgery, The Milton S. Hershey Medical Center, Hershey, Pennsylvania

Michael C. Fajgenbaum, M.D.
Instructor, Department of Orthopaedics, University of Florida College of Medicine, Gainesville, Florida

Donald C. Ferlic, M.D.
Assistant Clinical Professor of Orthopaedic Surgery, Department of Orthopaedics, University of Colorado School of Medicine, University of Colorado Health Sciences Center, Denver, Colorado

J. William Fielding, M.D., F.R.C.S.(C)
Clinical Professor, Department of Orthopaedic Surgery, College of Physicians and Surgeons of Columbia University; Director, Department of Orthopaedic Surgery, St. Luke's-Roosevelt Hospital Center, New York, New York

Henry A. Finn, M.D.
Assistant Professor of Orthopaedics and Reconstructive Surgery, Department of Surgery, University of Chicago, Pritzker School of Medicine; Director of Orthopaedic Oncology, Michael Reese Hospital and Medical Center, Chicago, Illinois

Adrian E. Flatt, M.D., M.Chir., F.R.C.S.
Chief, Department of Orthopaedics, Baylor University Medical Center, Dallas, Texas

William P. Fortune, M.D.
Professor, Department of Orthopaedic Surgery, George Washington University School of Medicine and Health Sciences, George Washington University Medical Center, Washington, D.C.

Bruce K. Foster, M.B., B.S., F.R.A.C.S.
Lecturer, Department of Paediatrics, Adelaide University, North Adelaide; Deputy Director, Department of Orthopaedic Surgery, Adelaide Children's Hospital, North Adelaide; Visiting Specialist, Flinders Medical Center, Bedford Park, South Australia, Australia

Frank J. Frassica, M.D.
Special Fellow in Orthopedic Oncology, Mayo Graduate School of Medicine; Assistant Professor of Orthopedic Surgery, Department of Orthopedics, Mayo Medical School, Rochester, Minnesota

Jorge O. Galante, M.D.
The William A. Hark, M.D. – Susanne G. Swift Professor and Chairman, Department of Orthopaedic Surgery, Rush Medical College of Rush University, Rush-Presbyterian-St. Luke's Medical Center, Chicago, Illinois

Mark C. Gebhardt, M.D.
Assistant Professor, Department of Orthopaedic Surgery, Harvard Medical School; Assistant Orthopaedic Surgeon, Massachusetts General Hospital and The Children's Hospital, Boston, Massachusetts

William Giles, M.D.
Orthopaedic Surgeon, South Mississippi Orthopaedic Specialists, Hattiesburg, Mississippi

Dale B. Glasser, M.S.
Research Associate, Orthopaedic Surgery, Memorial Hospital for Cancer and Allied Diseases and The Hospital for Special Surgery, New York, New York

Victor M. Goldberg, M.D.
Professor and Vice Chairman, Department of Orthopaedics, Case Western Reserve University School of Medicine, Cleveland, Ohio

J. Leonard Goldner, M.D.
James B. Duke Professor and Chief Emeritus, Division of Orthopaedic Surgery, Department of Surgery, Duke University Medical Center, Durham, North Carolina

David P. Green, M.D.
Clinical Professor, Department of Orthopaedics, University of Texas Health Science Center at San Antonio, Texas

Harry J.L. Griffiths, M.D.
Professor, Departments of Radiology and Orthopaedic Surgery, University of Minnesota Medical School — Minneapolis; Senior Radiologist and Head, Musculoskeletal Radiology and MRI, University of Minnesota Hospital, Minneapolis, Minnesota

Allan E. Gross, M.D., F.R.C.S.(C)
Professor and Chairman, Division of Orthopaedic Surgery, Department of Surgery, University of Toronto Faculty of Medicine, Toronto, Ontario, Canada

Gary S. Gruen, M.D.
Clinical Fellow, Department of Orthopaedic Surgery, University of Pittsburgh School of Medicine, Pittsburgh, Pennsylvania

Ramon B. Gustilo, M.D.
Professor, Department of Orthopaedic Surgery, University of Minnesota Medical School — Minneapolis; Chairman, Department of Orthopaedic Surgery, Hennepin County Medical Center, Minneapolis, Minnesota

Ray J. Haddad, Jr., M.D.
Lee C. Schlesinger Professor and Chairman, Department of Orthopaedics, Tulane University School of Medicine, New Orleans, Louisiana

Gregory A. Hanks, M.D.
Assistant Professor of Orthopaedic Surgery, Department of Surgery, Pennsylvania State University College of Medicine, The Milton S. Hershey Medical Center, Hershey, Pennsylvania

Sigvard T. Hansen, Jr., M.D.
Professor, Department of Orthopaedics, University of Washington School of Medicine, Seattle, Washington

Richard J. Hawkins, M.D.
Professor of Orthopaedic Surgery, Department of Surgery, University of Western Ontario Faculty of Medicine; Consultant, University and St. Joseph's Hospitals, London, Ontario, Canada

John H. Healey, M.D.
Assistant Professor of Orthopaedic Surgery, Department of Surgery, Cornell University Medical College; Assistant Attending Orthopaedic Surgeon, The Hospital for Special Surgery; Assistant Attending, Orthopaedic Surgery, Memorial Sloan-Kettering Cancer Center, New York, New York

David A. Heck, M.D.
Associate Professor, Department of Orthopaedic Surgery, Indiana University School of Medicine; Chief of Orthopaedics, Richard L. Roudebush Veterans Administration Medical Center, Indianapolis, Indiana

James D. Heckman, M.D.
Professor and Chairman, Department of Orthopaedics, University of Texas Medical School at San Antonio, University of Texas Health Science Center, San Antonio, Texas

Jan Eric Henstorf, M.D.
Attending Physician, Washington Hospital; Member, Fremont Orthopaedic Medical Group, Fremont, California

James H. Herndon, M.D.
David Silver Professor and Chairman, Department of Orthopaedic Surgery, University of Pittsburgh School of Medicine; Chief, Department of Orthopaedics and Rehabilitation, Presbyterian-University Hospital, Pittsburgh, Pennsylvania

Marcia L. Hixson, M.D.
Assistant Professor, Section of Hand Surgery, Department of Orthopaedic Surgery, University of Arkansas for Medical Sciences, Little Rock, Arkansas

Mason Hohl, M.D.
Clinical Professor of Orthopaedics, Department of Surgery, University of California, Los Angeles, UCLA School of Medicine, Los Angeles, California; Consultant in Orthopaedic Surgery, Veterans Administration Medical Center, West Los Angeles, California

Roger W. Hood, M.D.
Chief of Orthopaedic Surgery, Humana Hospital, Overland Park, Kansas

John D. Hsu, M.D., C.M., F.A.C.S.
Clinical Professor, Department of Orthopaedics, University of Southern California School of Medicine, Los Angeles, California; Chairman, Department of Surgery, Rancho Los Amigos Medical Center, Downey, California

Louis C.S. Hsu, F.R.C.S.E., F.A.C.S.
Reader in Orthopaedic Surgery, University of Hong Kong; Medical Director, Duchess of Kent Children's Hospital, Hong Kong

Leonard F. Hubbard, M.D.
Garden City Medical Park, Cranston, Rhode Island

David S. Hungerford, M.D.
Professor, Department of Orthopaedic Surgery, The Johns Hopkins University School of Medicine; Chief, Division of Arthritis Surgery, The Good Samaritan Hospital, Baltimore, Maryland

Kamal Ibrahim, M.D., F.R.C.S.(C)
Clinical Associate Professor, Department of Orthopaedics and Rehabilitation, Loyola University of Chicago Stritch School of Medicine; Chief, Section of Pediatric Orthopaedics and Scoliosis, Loyola University Medical Center, Maywood, Illinois

John N. Insall, M.D.
Professor of Orthopaedic Surgery, Department of Surgery, Cornell University Medical College; Chief, Knee Service, and Attending Orthopaedic Surgeon, The Hospital for Special Surgery; Attending Orthopaedic Surgeon, New York Hospital, New York, New York

Michael E. Jabaley, M.D.
Clinical Professor of Orthopaedic and Plastic Surgery, Department of Surgery, University of Mississippi Medical Center, Jackson, Mississippi

Hans Jaberg, M.D.
Orthopaedic Surgeon in Praxis, Berne, Switzerland

James O. Johnston, M.D.
Professor of Orthopaedic Oncology, Department of Orthopaedic Surgery, The University of California, San Francisco, School of Medicine, San Francisco, California

Alexander Kalenak, M.D.
Professor of Orthopaedic Surgery, Department of Surgery, Pennsylvania State University College of Medicine, The Milton S. Hershey Medical Center, Hershey, Pennsylvania

Herbert Kaufer, M.D.
Professor of Orthopaedic Surgery, Department of Surgery, The University of Michigan Medical School, Ann Arbor, Michigan

Patrick J. Kelly, M.D.
Professor of Orthopedic Surgery, Department of Orthopedics, Mayo Medical School; Consultant in Orthopedic Surgery, Mayo Clinic, Rochester, Minnesota

Donald B. Kettelkamp, M.D.
Executive Director, The American Board of Orthopaedic Surgery, Inc., Chicago, Illinois

Douglas J. Kilgus, M.D.
Assistant Professor of Orthopaedic Surgery, Department of Surgery, University of California, Los Angeles, UCLA School of Medicine, Los Angeles, California; Attending Orthopaedic Surgeon, UCLA Medical Center, Los Angeles, California; Staff Orthopaedic Surgeon and Chief, Joint Replacement Service, Veterans Administration Medical Center, West Los Angeles, California; Consulting Attending Orthopaedic Surgeon, Harbor/UCLA Medical Center, Torrance, California

Scott H. Kitchel, M.D.
Spine Consultant, Orthopaedic and Fracture Clinic, Eugene, Oregon; Staff Orthopaedic Surgeon, Shriners Hospital for Crippled Children, Portland, Oregon

Robert J. Krushell, M.D.
Clinical Instructor, Harvard University Medical School; Attending Surgeon, Brigham and Women's Hospital, Boston, Massachusetts

Joseph M. Lane, M.D.
Professor of Orthopaedic Surgery, Department of Surgery, Cornell University Medical College; Chief, Metabolic Bone Disease Unit, and Chief, Department of Orthopaedic Surgery, Memorial Sloan-Kettering Cancer Center, New York, New York

Thomas A. Lange, M.D.
Associate Clinical Professor, Department of Surgery, University of Minnesota Medical School—Minneapolis, Minneapolis, Minnesota; Chairman, Department of Orthopaedics, St. Paul-Ramsey Medical Center, St. Paul, Minnesota

L. Lee Lankford, M.D.
Clinical Professor of Orthopaedic Surgery, Department of Surgery, University of Texas Southwestern Medical Center at Dallas Southwestern Medical School; Teaching Staff, Department of Orthopaedics, Baylor University Medical Center; Founding Director, Parkland Memorial Hospital Hand Service, Dallas, Texas

Gerald S. Laros, M.D.
Professor and Chairman, Department of Orthopaedic Surgery, Texas Tech University Health Sciences Center School of Medicine, Lubbock, Texas

Robert E. Leach, M.D.
Professor and Chairman, Department of Orthopaedic Surgery, Boston University Medical School, Boston, Massachusetts

Robert D. Leffert, M.D.
Associate Professor, Department of Orthopaedic Surgery, Harvard Medical School; Chief, Surgical Upper Extremity Rehabilitation Unit and the Department of Rehabilitation Medicine, Massachusetts General Hospital, Boston, Massachusetts

Dennis W. Lennox, M.D.
Clinical Assistant Professor, Department of Orthopaedic Surgery, The Johns Hopkins University School of Medicine; Chief, Division of Hip and Knee Reconstructive Surgery, Union Memorial Hospital, Baltimore, Maryland

John C.Y. Leong, F.R.C.S., F.R.C.S.E., F.R.A.C.S
Professor and Head, Department of Orthopaedic Surgery, University of Hong Kong; Chief of Orthopaedic Surgery, Queen Mary Hospital and Duchess of Kent Children's Hospital, Hong Kong

Alan M. Levine, M.D.
Associate Professor of Orthopaedic Surgery, Department of Orthopaedics, University of Maryland School Medicine; University of Maryland Hospital, Baltimore, Maryland

David W. Lhowe, M.D.
Instructor, Department of Orthopaedic Surgery, Harvard Medical School; Assistant in Orthopaedics, Massachusetts General Hospital, Boston, Massachusetts

Ronald L. Linscheid, M.D.
Professor of Orthopedic Surgery, Department of Orthopedics, Mayo Medical School; Consultant in Orthopedic Surgery of the Hand, Mayo Clinic, Rochester, Minnesota

Graham Lister, M.B., F.R.C.S., F.A.C.S.
Professor and Chief of Plastic Surgery, Department of Surgery, University of Utah School of Medicine, Salt Lake City, Utah

J. William Littler, M.D.
Senior Attending Surgeon, St. Luke's-Roosevelt Hospital Center, New York, New York

G. Dean MacEwen, M.D.
Professor and Chairman, Section of Pediatric Orthopaedics, Department of Orthopaedics, Louisiana State University School of Medicine in New Orleans; Chairman, Department of Orthopaedics, Children's Hospital, New Orleans, Louisiana; Former Medical Director, Alfred I. DuPont Institute, Wilmington, Delaware

Robert P. Mack, M.D.
Denver Orthopaedic Clinic; Attending Surgeon, St. Joseph's Hospital, Denver, Colorado

Ian Macnab, F.R.C.S., F.R.C.S.(C)
Emeritus Professor, Department of Surgery, University of Toronto Faculty of Medicine, Toronto, Ontario, Canada

Jon T. Mader, M.D.
Associate Professor of Infectious Diseases, Department of Medicine, Member, Marine Biomedical Institute, and Chief, Division of Marine Medicine, University of Texas Medical School at Galveston, Galveston, Texas

John T. Makley, M.D.
Professor, Departments of Orthopaedics and Pathology, Case Western Reserve University School of Medicine; Director, Musculoskeletal Tumor Center, Department of Orthopaedics, University Hospital of Cleveland, Cleveland, Ohio

Martin M. Malawer, M.D., F.A.C.S.
Associate Professor of Orthopaedic Surgery and Orthopaedic Oncology, George Washington University School of Medicine and Health Sciences, Children's Hospital National Medical Center, Washington, D.C.; Consultant in Orthopaedic Oncology, Surgery Branch, National Center Institute, National Institutes of Health, Bethesda, Maryland

Henry J. Mankin, M.D.
Edith M. Ashley Professor of Orthopaedic Surgery, Harvard Medical School; Orthopaedist-in-Chief, Massachusetts General Hospital, Boston, Massachusetts

Roger A. Mann, M.D.
Chief, Foot Surgery, Samuel Merritt Hospital; Director, Foot Fellowship; Private Practice, Orthopaedic Surgery, Oakland, California

Kenneth E. Marks, M.D.
Head, Section of Musculoskeletal Oncology, Department of Orthopaedic Surgery, Cleveland Clinic Foundation, Cleveland, Ohio

John C. Marshall, M.D., F.R.C.S.(C)
Assistant Professor, Department of Surgery, Dalhousie University Faculty of Medicine; Attending Surgeon, Victoria General Hospital, Halifax, Nova Scotia, Canada

Frederick A. Matsen III, M.D.
Professor and Chairman, Department of Orthopaedics, and Chief, Shoulder and Elbow Service, University of Washington School of Medicine, Seattle, Washington

Joel M. Matta, M.D.
Associate Professor, Department of Orthopaedics, University of Southern California School of Medicine, Los Angeles, California

Larry S. Matthews, M.D.
Professor of Orthopaedic Surgery, Department of Surgery, The University of Michigan Medical School, Ann Arbor, Michigan

Andrew A. McBeath, M.D.
Fredrick J. Gaenslen Professor and Chairman, Division of Orthopaedic Surgery, Department of Surgery, University of Wisconsin Medical School; University of Wisconsin Hospital and Clinics, Madison, Wisconsin

Newton C. McCollough III, M.D.
Clinical Professor, Department of Orthopaedics and Rehabilitation, University of South Florida College of Medicine; Director of Medical Affairs, Shriners Hospital, Tampa, Florida

Donald E. McCollum, M.D.
Professor of Orthopaedic Surgery, Department of Surgery, Duke University School of Medicine, Duke University Medical Center, Durham, North Carolina

Robert M. McCormack, M.D.
Emeritus Professor of Plastic Surgery, Department of Surgery, University of Rochester School of Medicine and Dentistry, Rochester, New York

Jessop McDonnell, M.D.
Medical Director, Tacoma Osteoporosis Center, Tacoma, Washington; Consultant in Orthopaedic Oncology, Madigan Army Medical Center, Madigan, Washington; Staff Orthopaedic Surgeon, St. Joseph Hospital and Multicare Medical Center, Tacoma, Washington

Gorden B. McFarland, M.D.
Clinical Professor of Orthopaedic Surgery, Department of Orthopaedics, Louisiana State University School of Medicine in New Orleans; Associate Chairman, Department of Orthopaedic Surgery, The Ochsner Clinic, New Orleans, Louisiana

Robert M. McFarlane, M.D.
Professor and Chief of Plastic Surgery, Department of Surgery, The University of Western Ontario Faculty of Medicine, London, Ontario, Canada

Michael H. McGuire, M.D.
Associate Professor and Chief of Orthopaedic Surgery, Department of Surgery, Creighton University School of Medicine, Omaha, Nebraska

Martin C. McHenry, M.D.
Chairman, Department of Infectious Diseases, Cleveland Clinic Foundation, Cleveland, Ohio

Jonathan L. Meakins, M. D., D.S.C., F.R.C.S.(C), F.A.C.S.
Professor, Departments of Surgery and Microbiology, McGill University Faculty of Medicine; Senior Surgeon, Royal Victoria Hospital, Montreal, Quebec, Canada

Dana C. Mears, M.D., Ph.D.
Associate Professor, Department of Orthopaedic Surgery, University of Pittsburgh School of Medicine; Staff, Presbyterian-University Hospital and Children's Hospital of Pittsburgh, Pittsburgh, Pennsylvania

Viktor E. Meyer, M.D.
Professor and Director of Plastic Surgery, Department of Surgery, University of Zurich, Medical School, Zurich, Switzerland

Jo Miller, M.D., F.R.C.S.(C)
Senior Orthopaedic Surgeon, The Montreal General Hospital, Montreal, Quebec, Canada

Richard J. Miller, M.D.
Associate Professor, Department of Orthopaedics, University of Rochester School of Medicine and Dentistry, Rochester, New York

Wallace E. Miller, M.D.
Professor Emeritus, Department of Orthopaedic Surgery and Rehabilitation, University of Miami School of Medicine, Miami, Ohio

Eugene R. Mindell, M.D.
Professor of Orthopaedic Surgery, Department of Surgery, State University of New York at Buffalo School of Medicine and Biomedical Sciences, Buffalo, New York

Erik A. Moberg, M.D., Ph.D.
Professor Emeritus and Former Head, Orthopaedic and Hand Surgery, Sahlgrenksa Hospital, Göteborg, Sweden

Richard J. Montgomery, M.B., B.S., F.R.C.S.
Senior Registrar in Orthopaedic Surgery, Northern Regional Health Facility, Newcastle upon Tyne, England

Michael M. Moore, M.D.
Hand Surgery Consultants; Arkansas Hand Microsurgery Center, Little Rock, Arkansas

Tillman M. Moore, M.D.
Emeritus Professor of Clinical Orthopaedics, University of Southern California School of Medicine, Los Angeles, California

Bernard F. Morrey, M.D.
Professor of Orthopedic Surgery, Department of Orthopedics, Mayo Medical School; Chairman, Department of Orthopedics, Mayo Clinic, Rochester, Minnesota

Maurice E. Müller, M.D.
Emeritus Professor of Orthopaedic Surgery, University of Berne Faculty of Medicine, Berne, Switzerland

David G. Murray, M.D.
Professor, Department of Orthopaedic Surgery, State University of New York Health Science Center at Syracuse, College of Medicine, Upstate Medical Center, Syracuse, New York

James F. Murray, M.D., F.R.C.S.(C)
Professor Emeritus, Department of Surgery, University of Toronto Faculty of Medicine; Department of Plastic Surgery, Sunnybrook Medical Centre; Consultant in Hand Surgery, Workman's Compensation Board, Toronto, Ontario, Canada

John A. Murray, M.D.
Professor of Orthopaedics, Department of Surgery, University of Texas Medical School at Houston; Chief, Orthopaedic Service, M.D. Anderson Cancer Center, Houston, Texas

George Muschler, M.D.
Assistant Attending Surgeon, Cleveland Clinic Foundation, Cleveland, Ohio

James R. Neff, M.D.
Professor of Orthopaedic Surgery and Pathology, University of Kansas Medical Center School of Medicine, Kansas City, Kansas

Carl L. Nelson, M.D.
Professor of Adult Reconstructive Surgery and Chairman, Department of Orthopaedic Surgery, University of Arkansas for Medical Sciences, Little Rock, Arkansas

James A. Nunley, M.D.
Associate Professor of Orthopaedic Surgery, Department of Surgery, Duke University School of Medicine, Duke University Medical Center, Durham, North Carolina

James W. Ogilvie, M.D.
Assistant Professor, Department of Orthopaedic Surgery, University of Minnesota Medical School — Minneapolis; Abbott-Northwestern Hospital, Twin Cities Scoliosis Center, Minneapolis, Minnesota

George E. Omer, Jr., M.D., M.S., F.A.C.S.
Professor and Chairman, Department of Orthopaedics and Rehabilitation, Professor and Co-Chief, Division of Hand Surgery, Department of Surgery, Professor, Department of Anatomy, and Medical Director, Physical Therapy Program, University of New Mexico School of Medicine, Albuquerque, New Mexico

Manohar M. Panjabi, Dr. Tech., Ph.D., B.E.
Professor of Orthopaedics and Rehabilitation and Director of Biomechanic Research, Department of Orthopaedics and Rehabilitation Medicine, Yale University School of Medicine New Haven, Connecticut

Arsen M. Pankovich, M.D.
Clinical Professor, Department of Orthopaedic Surgery, New York University School of Medicine; Attending Orthopaedic Surgeon, Hospital for Joint Diseases Orthopaedic Institute, New York, New York; Director of Orthopaedic Surgery, Booth Memorial Hospital, Flushing, New York

Vincent D. Pellegrini, Jr., M.D.
Assistant Professor, Department of Orthopaedics, University of Rochester School of Medicine and Dentistry, Rochester, New York

Paul M. Pellicci, M.D.
Associate Professor of Orthopaedic Surgery, Department of Surgery, Cornell University Medical College; Associate Attending Surgeon, The Hospital for Special Surgery, New York, New York

William Petty, M.D.
Professor and Chairman, Department of Orthopaedics, University of Florida College of Medicine, Gainesville, Florida

Douglas J. Pritchard, M.D.
Professor and Head, Section of Orthopedic Oncology, Department of Orthopedics, Mayo Medical School; Consultant in Orthopedic Surgery, Mayo Clinic, Rochester, Minnesota

James A. Rand, M.D.
Assistant Professor of Orthopedic Surgery, Department of Surgery, Mayo Medical School; Consultant in Orthopedic Surgery, Mayo Clinic, Rochester, Minnesota

George Reading, M.D.
Associate Professor of Plastic Surgery, Department of Surgery, University of Rochester School of Medicine and Dentistry, Rochester, New York

John M. Roberts, M.D.
Professor and Acting Chairman, Department of Orthopaedics, and Professor, Department of Pediatrics, Brown University Program in Medicine; Surgeon-in-Chief, Department of Orthopaedics, and Surgeon-in-Charge, Division of Pediatric Orthopaedics, Rhode Island Hospital, Providence, Rhode Island

Andrew E. Rosenberg, M.D.
Assistant Professor, Department of Pathology, Harvard Medical School; Visiting Pathologist, Massachusetts General Hospital, Boston, Massachusetts

Richard H. Rothman, M.D., Ph.D.
James Edwards Professor and Chairman, Department of Orthopaedic Surgery, Jefferson Medical College of Thomas Jefferson University, Philadelphia, Pennsylvania

Stephen L.G. Rothman, M.D.
Consultant Radiologist, Rancho Los Amigos Medical Center, Downey, California; Rothman-Chafetz Medical Group, Long Beach, California

Clinton T. Rubin, Ph.D.
Associate Professor of Orthopaedic Surgery, Department of Orthopaedics, State University of New York at Stony Brook Health Sciences Center School of Medicine, Stony Brook, New York

Eduardo A. Salvati, M.D.
Professor of Orthopaedic Surgery, Department of Surgery, Cornell University Medical College; Associate Attending Surgeon, The Hospital for Special Surgery, New York, New York

Robert L. Samilson, M.D.†
Former Clinical Professor, Department of Orthopaedic Surgery, University of California, San Francisco, School of Medicine, San Francisco, California

Roy Sanders, M.D.
Assistant Professor, Department of Orthopaedic Surgery, University of South Florida College of Medicine, Tampa, Florida

Anthony A. Schepsis, M.D.
Assistant Professor, Department of Orthopaedic Surgery, Boston University Medical School; Team Physician, Intercollegiate Athletic Program, Boston University, Boston, Massachusetts

Alan L. Schiller, M.D.
Professor, Department of Pathology, Mount Sinai School of Medicine of the City University of New York; Chief of Pathology, Mount Sinai Medical Center, New York, New York

David J. Schurman, M.D.
Professor of Orthopaedic Surgery, Department of Surgery, Stanford University School of Medicine, Stanford, California

Wayne J. Sebastianelli, M.D.
Assistant Professor, Department of Orthopaedics, University of Rochester School of Medicine and Dentistry, Rochester, New York

David Segal, M.D.
Professor, Department of Orthopaedics, Hadassah University School of Medicine; Director, Hadassah Hospital, Jerusalem, Israel

Frank H. Sim, M.D.
Professor of Orthopedic Surgery, Department of Surgery, Mayo Medical School; Consultant in Orthopedic Surgery, Mayo Clinic, Rochester, Minnesota

Edward H. Simmons, M.D., M.S.(Tor)
Professor of Orthopaedic Surgery, Department of Orthopaedics, State University of New York at Buffalo School of Medicine and Biomedical Sciences; Head, Department of Orthopaedics, Buffalo General Hospital, Buffalo, New York

Michael A. Simon, M.D.
Professor of Orthopaedic Surgery and Rehabilitation Medicine, Department of Surgery, University of Chicago, Pritzker School of Medicine, Chicago, Illinois

Clement B. Sledge, M.D.
Professor and Chairman, Department of Orthopaedic Surgery, Harvard Medical School; Brigham and Women's Hospital, Boston, Massachusetts

---

† Deceased

Robert F. Spetzler, M.D.
Professor and Chairman, Section of Neurosurgery, Department of Surgery, University of Arizona College of Medicine, Tucson, Arizona; Director and Chairman of Neurological Surgery, Barrow Neurological Institute, Phoenix, Arizona

Phillip Spiegel, M.D.
Professor and Chairman, Department of Orthopaedic Surgery, University of South Florida College of Medicine, Tampa, Florida

Dempsey S. Springfield, M.D.
Associate Professor, Department of Orthopaedic Surgery, Harvard Medical School; Visiting Orthopaedic Surgeon, Massachusetts General Hospital, Boston, Massachusetts

E. Shannon Stauffer, M.D.
Professor and Chairman, Division of Orthopaedics and Rehabilitation, Department of Surgery, Southern Illinois University School of Medicine, Springfield, Illinois

Richard N. Stauffer, M.D.
Professor of Orthopedic Surgery, Department of Orthopedics, Mayo Medical School; Consultant in Orthopedic Surgery, Mayo Clinic, Rochester, Minnesota

Sharon Stevenson, D.V.M., Ph.D.
Assistant Professor, Department of Orthopaedics, Case Western Reserve University School of Medicine, Cleveland, Ohio

Frank E. Stinchfield, M.D.
Professor and Chairman Emeritus, Department of Orthopaedic Surgery, College of Physicians and Surgeons of Columbia University, Columbia-Presbyterian Medical Center, New York, New York

James W. Strickland, M.D.
Clinical Professor, Department of Orthopaedic Surgery, Indiana University School of Medicine; Chief, Section of Hand Surgery, St. Vincent Hospital, Indianapolis, Indiana

Dale R. Sumner, Jr., Ph.D.
Assistant Professor, Department of Orthopaedic Surgery, Rush Medical College of Rush University, Rush-Presbyterian-St. Luke's Medical Center, Chicago, Illinois

Steven C. Thomas, M.D.
Resident, Department of Orthopaedics, University of Washington School of Medicine, Seattle, Washington

William W. Tomford, M.D.
Assistant Professor, Department of Orthopaedic Surgery, Harvard Medical School; Associate Orthopaedic Surgeon and Director, Bone Bank, Massachusetts General Hospital, Boston, Massachusetts

Hugh S. Tullos, M.D.
Head, Division of Orthopaedic Surgery, Department of Surgery, Baylor College of Medicine, Houston, Texas

James R. Urbaniak, M.D.
Professor and Chief, Division of Orthopaedic Surgery, Department of Surgery, Duke University School of Medicine, Duke University Medical Center, Durham, North Carolina

Jack Vander Schilden, M.D.
Assistant Professor and Head, Section of Sports Medicine, Department of Orthopaedic Surgery, University of Arkansas for Medical Sciences, Little Rock, Arkansas

Luke Vaughan, M.D.
Head, Section of Orthopaedic Oncology, Division of Orthopaedic Surgery, Scripps Clinic and Research Foundation, La Jolla, California

F. William Wagner, Jr., M.D.
Clinical Professor of Orthopaedic Surgery, Department of Orthopaedics, University of Southern California School of Medicine, Los Angeles, California; Chief Consultant, Ortho-Diabetes Service, Rancho Los Amigos Medical Center, Downey, California; Chief, Foot and Ankle Service, Los Angeles County — USC Medical Center, Los Angeles, California

Russel F. Warren, M.D.
Associate Professor of Orthopaedic Surgery, Department of Surgery, Cornell University Medical College; Director of Sports Medicine, The Hospital for Special Surgery, New York, New York

Andrew J. Weiland, M.D.
Professor, Departments of Orthopaedic Surgery, Plastic Surgery, and Emergency Medicine, The Johns Hopkins University School of Medicine, Baltimore, Maryland

Augustus A. White III, M.D.
Professor, Department of Orthopaedic Surgery, Harvard Medical School; Orthopaedic Surgeon-in-Chief, Beth Israel Hospital, Boston, Massachusetts

Thomas E. Whitesides, Jr., M.D.
Professor, Department of Orthopaedics, Emory University School of Medicine; Emory University Clinic, Atlanta, Georgia

Sam W. Wiesel, M.D.
Professor, Department of Orthopaedic Surgery, George Washington University School of Medicine and Health Sciences, George Washington University Medical Center, Washington, D.C.

Alan H. Wilde, M.D.
Chairman, Department of Orthopaedic Surgery, Cleveland Clinic Foundation, Cleveland, Ohio

E.F. Shaw Wilgis, M.D.
Associate Professor of Orthopaedic Surgery and Plastic Surgery, Department of Surgery, The Johns Hopkins University School of Medicine; Chief, Division of Hand Surgery, Union Memorial Hospital, Baltimore, Maryland

Philip D. Wilson, Jr., M.D.
Professor of Orthopaedic Surgery, Department of Surgery, Cornell University Medical College; Surgeon-in-Chief, The Hospital for Special Surgery, New York, New York

Leon L. Wiltse, M.D.
Clinical Professor, Department of Orthopaedics, University of California, Irvine, School of Medicine, Irvine, California; Orthopaedic Staff, Long Beach Memorial Hospital; California Spine Surgery Medical Group, Long Beach, California

Russell E. Windsor, M.D.
Assistant Professor of Orthopaedic Surgery, Department of Surgery, Cornell University Medical College; Assistant Chief, Knee Service, and Assistant Attending Orthopaedic Surgeon, The Hospital for Special Surgery; Assisting Orthopaedic Surgeon, New York Hospital, New York, New York

Robert B. Winter, M.D.
Clinical Professor, Department of Orthopaedic Surgery, University of Minnesota School of Medicine—Minneapolis, Minneapolis, Minnesota; Chief of Spine Service, Gillette Children's Hospital, St. Paul, Minnesota; Minnesota Spine Center, Minneapolis, Minnesota

Donald Wiss, M.D.
Assistant Professor of Orthopaedic Surgery, Department of Orthopaedics, University of Southern California School of Medicine, Los Angeles, California

Timothy M. Wright, Ph.D.
Associate Professor of Applied Biomechanics, Department of Surgery, Cornell University Medical College; Associate Director, Department of Biomechanics, The Hospital for Special Surgery, New York, New York

Isadore G. Yablon, M.D.
Professor and Director of Research, Department of Orthopaedic Surgery, Boston University School of Medicine; Senior Attending Surgeon, University Hospital, Boston, Massachusetts

Michael J. Yaremchuk, M.D.
Assistant Professor, Department of Plastic Surgery, Harvard Medical School; Staff Plastic Surgeon, Massachusetts General Hospital, Boston, Massachusetts

David J. Zukor, M.D., F.R.C.S.(C)
Assistant Professor, Department of Surgery, McGill University; Orthopaedic Surgeon, Royal Victoria Hospital, Montreal, Quebec, Canada

Preface to the Second Edition

Many advances have been made in the surgical treatment of the musculoskeletal system during the 6 years since this book was first published in 1983. Refinements of surgical procedures have occurred and new ideas have been introduced. It is the intent of the second edition to capture these changes. To do so, we have added new chapters, combined some previous chapters, and revised every chapter to include an up-to-date presentation of its topic. There are 27 new authors, and once again we have turned to those who are leaders—both present and future—in their fields. They were asked to participate based upon their expertise and their ability to write authoritatively on each topic. Greater attention has been given to the description and illustration of surgical procedures. We have also reorganized the format of the book; the larger pages and consecutive numbering are designed to make the book easier to use, and to make finding a specific subject a simple task. In addition, the sections, while still based on anatomy, have been reorganized so that the information needed about any area is found in that section. For example, tumors and amputations of the hand are now found in the hand section, rather than in two other sections of the book.

Topics presented for the first time in this edition include bone ingrowth, osteoporosis, and diagnostic imaging. Arthroscopy coverage is expanded to include new chapters on the shoulder and knee, and an overview of the topic. Shoulder and elbow fractures are discussed, as are fractures of the talus, os calcis, and foot. Chapters on surgical exposure of the shoulder and hip join a much-expanded one on exposure of the spine.

One field that has really come of age is joint replacement. To reflect this, new chapters on knee arthroplasty and hip arthroplasty join Stinchfield's review of the subject, and Müller has updated his chapters on hip techniques.

Also new is a chapter on the biomechanics of the knee—a crucial thing for the orthopaedist to understand when making a surgical judgement.

Compartment syndromes of the lower leg are covered in a new chapter, and chapters on osteomyelitis, prevention of sepsis, antimicrobial treatment, immune responses, and management of traumatic defects have been added to the section on infections. The tumor section has new chapters on tumors of the foot, extra-abdominal desmoid tumors, and hip reconstruction in metastatic disease.

The purpose of the text remains the same: "to present in one source the information needed to assess, plan, and perform a surgical procedure on the musculoskeletal system of the adult." As with any text of this magnitude, much work and many hours have gone into the writing and production of these five volumes. It is my hope that the text will help all who use it improve the quality of patient care.

C. McCollister Evarts, M.D.

Preface to the First Edition

The past decade has seen a remarkable proliferation in basic and applied research in disorders of the musculoskeletal system. Interdisciplinary efforts have resulted in new discoveries and advances, many of which have been applied to the clinical practice of orthopaedics. In a relatively short period, new surgical procedures, including those involving ligamentous reconstruction of the knee, total joint reconstruction, replantation of the digits, vascularized bone grafts, instrumentation of the spine, and whole bone grafts for tumor surgery, have been developed and refined by the orthopaedic surgeon. Moreover, those procedures that have been in use for some time have also benefited from the information developed during this period of intense scientific activity.

The purpose of this book is to present in one source the information needed to assess, plan, and perform a surgical procedure on the musculoskeletal system of the adult. As pediatric musculoskeletal problems have been well covered in several other works, the discussions here are confined to the adult musculoskeletal system. The text is divided into twelve sections that cover problems both of specific regions and those not localized to one region, such as infections and tumors. Each section has an editor who is a recognized authority on his section's subject and who is particularly conversant in the current research and clinical practice. The section editors and I have selected the contributing authors on the basis of their expertise and experience with the particular clinical problems they were asked to discuss. In their chapters the authors examine a specific problem rather than survey a general topic and present their first-hand experience with the treatment of the disorder.

Each chapter is organized so that the material is presented in a uniform manner, as follows: general statement of the problem; indications and contraindications for the surgical procedure; detailed description of the operative technique; and discussion of the postoperative management of the patient. Each author has been encouraged to state his preferred method of treatment and his reasons for favoring one procedure over another. The book, although not designed as an atlas, has many illustrations, which should aid the reader in diagnosis and treatment. In addition, each chapter ends with a comprehensive list of references.

The reader will note that this work includes contributions from an impressive group of authors. These surgeons were asked to participate without regard to their institutional affiliation or geographical location; rather, it was our intention to have contributors who could write authoritatively on the assigned topic, drawing on their broad range of experience.

Much work and many hours have gone into the making of this book. It is the hope of those who have participated in its preparation that the book will ultimately result in the improvement of the quality and results of patient care.

C. McCollister Evarts, M.D.

Acknowledgments

Many individuals have contributed their time and talent to the preparation of the second edition of *Surgery of the Musculoskeletal System.* The book represents the combined efforts of a large number of persons — section editors, authors, artists, photographers, secretaries, publishers, and others — all of whom have been generous with their expertise.

The second edition could not have been created without the section editors. Without question, as with the first edition, they make this book possible.

I would like to thank all of the authors, as they gave much of themselves and their time in preparation of the various chapters.

At Churchill Livingstone, Leslie Burgess, Assistant Editor, has been most helpful as the editorial coordinator for the text; Robert Hurley, Vice President and Editor-in-Chief, and Toni Tracy, President, have lent their expertise and support in keeping the project moving toward its final goal.

Contents

VOLUME 3

VOLUME 5

Section 10:   INFECTIONS
Carl L. Nelson, Section Editor

Section 7

THE KNEE

Donald B. Kettelkamp

Section Editor

Introduction

Donald B. Kettelkamp

The field of surgery of the knee has been rapidly changing over the past fifteen years through the basic and clinical research of many individuals. The framework upon which the current approach and techniques are based rests on a knowledge of functional anatomy, applied biomechanics, and materials. The importance of applied basic science to current and future developments of knee reconstruction is emphasized in this edition with the addition of chapters on knee biomechanics and implant fixation.

The chapters in this section that deal with the management of injuries and their sequelae deserve special comment. This area has undergone significant advances in the past few years. Repair of peripheral tears of the menisci and minimal meniscectomy with arthroscopic surgery or as part of a more extensive open procedure have a sound biomechanical basis. The rapid advances in arthroscopic technique hold the promises of less morbidity and faster convalescence for those with less severe injuries. The methods of late reconstruction of ligament injuries, based on detailed anatomy, dynamic stability, the properties of maturing collagenous structures, and developing ligament substitutes, deserve careful study and judicious application. An improved classification of plateau fractures and better fixation will improve the results of these often difficult fractures. A better understanding of the functional biomechanics of the patellofemoral articulation and the long-term results of realignment procedures have altered the surgical techniques applicable to patellofemoral problems.

Unlike most of the other procedures discussed in this section, the management of musculotendinous maladies and bursal lesions has changed relatively little, although the frequency of operative procedures in both areas has decreased as newer methods of treatment have evolved.

Composite bone-cartilage grafts have a long history; however, there is renewed interest in their use because of difficulties with large prosthetic implants after tumor resection. With improved preservative methods, a better understanding of immune and healing responses, and a growing realization of the limitations of implant replacement, the composite graft may be the solution for difficult — although infrequent — reconstructive problems. Proximal tibial osteotomy for unicompartmental degenerative arthritis has a firm biomechanical basis and new potential with the advent of the barrel-vault technique and more rigid methods of internal fixation. Long-term follow-up studies of both proximal tibial osteotomy and implant replacement have sharpened the indications for the respective procedures.

Prosthetic knee placement, rivaled only by arthroscopic surgery, has undergone more change in design, fixation, indication, technique, result studies, and salvage methods than any other area of knee surgery since the first edition of this book. This entire section has been reorganized and revised. Chapter 120 deals with primary knee arthroplasty and Chapter 121 with revision knee arthroplasty. The authors of these chapters have presented the indications and techniques, including those for correction of deformity, for primary and salvage situations. In addition, Chapter 122 deals with arthrodesis of the knee, a procedure that with the advent of joint arthroplasty perhaps has greater application and certainly presents greater technical difficulty.

As the largest and most complicated joint in the body, the knee provides a fertile field for the application of basic and applied research. The answers as we know them at this time are presented in the following chapters.

Biomechanics of the Knee

111

David A. Heck
David G. Murray

Biomechanics is the discipline of fundamental orthopaedic science, which is commonly approached with great trepidation by orthopaedists. It incorporates the engineering disciplines of physics and mathematics with those of biology. The orthopaedist possesses a knowledge of anatomy, biology, and physiology. Biomechanics can complement that knowledge by giving added understanding about the function of the knee, its underlying pathology, and the procedures designed to improve or restore its function.

BIOMECHANICS OF THE KNEE

Evolution has developed the knee into a complex structure that is capable of withstanding loads of many times body weight, preserving the second greatest range of motion of any joint in the lower extremity while maintaining stability. The knee, being physically located between the two longest levers of the body, is the most frequently injured major joint in the body among active persons. It is the second most commonly replaced major joint in the body.[33] Replacement is required most frequently in patients who suffer from the wear and tear of osteoarthritis. Deciphering the complexities of three-dimensional motion and forces requires a grasp of the mechanical engineering disciplines of statics and dynamics.

KINETICS

Kinetics is the branch of mechanics that deals with the study of bodies in motion and of the forces that cause those motions. In general, because of practical and ethical considerations, it has been necessary to calculate the in vivo loads from noninvasive measurements using force plates. The resulting motions (kinematics) have been measured as independent quantities from both invasive (pin) and noninvasive surface techniques.

Kinematics

The orthopaedic surgeon will find that basic knowledge of knee kinematics is necessary to understand the functioning of the knee in its varied normal and abnormal conditions. Furthermore, this knowledge can help the surgeon select appropriate surgical procedures, braces, and prosthetic systems to permit maximal restoration of function and implant longevity.[3] Studies of the mechanics of knee joint motions date back to Da Vinci (ca. 1500 A.D.), who grossly delineated the relationship of knee motion with the function of the muscles of the thigh.[59] Knowledge of the influence of musculature on knee motion was further expanded during the mid-1800s by the Weber brothers, who investigated the function of the intraarticular and periarticular structures. This was followed by the contributions of Meyer, who described and analyzed the screw movement of the knee joint based on the asymmetry of the femoral condyles.[8]

To fully describe the relative motions of two rigid bodies in space, information on a minimum of six independent parameters must be defined. Several different coordinate systems could be used to convey this information. The most commonly used system is the three-dimensional cartesian coordinate system with the independent axes X, Y, and Z. These axes are mutually perpendicular and follow the right-hand rule. This means that the crossproduct of the positive unit vectors (directions) x and y will result in the positive z-unit vector. Three rotations and three translations about these axes comprise the necessary 6 degrees of freedom.

Motion of any two rigid bodies can be then divided into information on constraints, or stops, to motion as well as individual unrestrained motions. For example, a simple hinge permits rotation about the center of the hinge pin. No rotation about the long axis or in the plane of the hinge flanges is allowed (Fig. 111-1). It does not permit translation in any direction. Therefore a simple hinge is described as having 1 degree of freedom with five constraints.

In describing the motions at the knee joint, Grood and Suntay[26] proposed the use of two cartesian coordinate systems linked by six clinically relevant independent motions. The first coordinate system is that of the femur and the second that of the tibia.

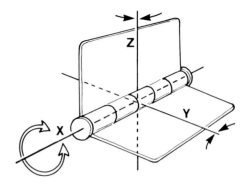

Fig. 111-1. Simple hinge joint with a single degree of freedom motion.

The origin of the femoral mechanical axis (the Z axis) has been defined as the line that connects the center of the femoral head to the posterior surface of the distal femur midway between the medial and lateral condyles.[45] The frontal plane contains this line and is parallel to the most posterior points of the femoral condyles. This correlates anatomically with the medial and lateral epicondyles. The Y axis is specified as the cross product of the Z axis and the posterior condylar line such that the anterior direction is positive. The X axis is the intersection of the frontal and the transverse plane, which contains the posterior condylar line. The X axis is positive laterally for the right knee and medially for the left, in compliance with the right-hand rule. All reference planes are mutually perpendicular (Fig. 111-2A,B).

The tibial frame is defined similarly. The tibial anatomic axis (Z axis) is that line connecting the center of the ankle joint distally with that of the midpoint between the tibial intercondylar eminences proximally. The Y axis is again defined as being positive in the anterior direction. It is specified as being the crossproduct of the anatomic axis with that of a line connecting the centers of the tibial plateaus. The X axis is again defined as being positive in a lateral direction for the right knee and in a medial direction for the left (Fig. 111-3A,B).

Obviously, these definitions are approximations, given the known geometric variability of individual knees and the nonorthogonality of the joint line with respect to the femoral head. (The transverse plane of the distal femur is in an average of three degrees of varus with respect to the center of the femoral head.[34,44,64]) Nevertheless, this coordinate

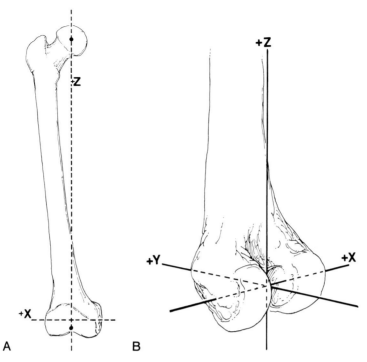

Fig. 111-2. **(A)** Frontal plane view of the femoral reference frame mechanical axes. **(B)** Posterior oblique view of the femoral reference frame mechanical axes.

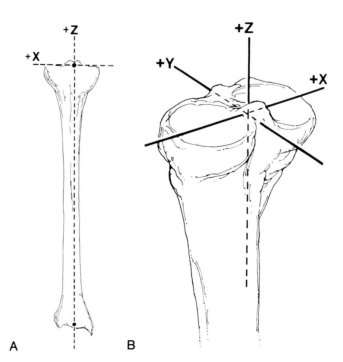

Fig. 111-3. **(A)** Frontal plane view of the tibial reference frame mechanical axes. **(B)** Posterior, superior, oblique view of the tibial reference frame mechanical axes.

system is the most generally accepted system for expressing knee-joint motion. It serves as a baseline for future developments in the objective assessment of knee motion.

The linkage between the two defined coordinate systems is as follows: sagittal plane rotation corresponds to flexion/extension and translation to anterior/posterior drawer. In the transverse plane, rotation is internal or external in direction, and translation is either medial or lateral. To complete the description, the coronal plane rotation is the same as abduction/adduction, and translation is axial compression or distraction (Fig. 111-4).

LaFortune[39] measured these motions in a similar reference frame, using pins rigidly fixed to the femur and tibia in five normal adult subjects. The data can be summarized as follows:

1. In the sagittal plane during level gait, rotation (sagittal flexion) at heel strike averages 2 degrees. In early stance phase, the knee flexes to 20 degrees. It then extends and finally flexes, reaching a maximum of 60 degrees during swing phase. Medial to lateral translation (x axis)

occurs from an initial neutral position at heel strike proceeding to medial displacement, oscillating toward lateral displacement, and returning in a medial direction just before toe off. Stance phase translation averages 4 mm. During the swing phase, maximal medial translation of 6 mm occurs.

2. Rotation in the transverse plane (screw home) closely parallels sagittal flexion of the knee. The tibia is in relative external rotation at heel strike. The tibia then proceeds into internal rotation with flexion during early stance to an average of 4 degrees. In swing phase extension, the tibia again goes into external rotation relative to the femur. The average total motion is 9 degrees. This correlates well with the intracortical pin data of Levens, who found an average motion of 8.7 degrees in their 12 subjects.[41] Axial translation (compression/distraction or z axis) also closely parallels sagittal rotation. This translation represents predominantly the varying radii of curvatures of the femoral condyles and averages 3 mm.

3. Rotation in the coronal plane is limited. The

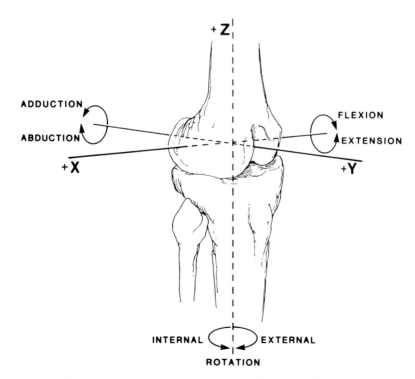

Fig. 111-4. Representative mechanical linkage of the knee.

knee is in slight abduction at heel strike, which then generally increased to 6 degrees in swing phase. Overall coronal rotation averages only approximately 5 degrees. Anteroposterior translation (y axis) is approximately 5 mm during the stance phase. Posterior translation of the tibia with respect to the femur increases to approximately 15 mm in the swing phase. Overall translation closely parallels the magnitude of sagittal flexion.

On first inspection, several of these motions, especially translations of only 4 to 6 mm in the sagittal and transverse planes, might appear to be insignificant.[14] However, one should be aware that the significance of these numbers come in determining what effect this might have in the normally conforming/constraining geometry of an intact knee. Anatomically, this is a result of the combined effects of the joint articular surface and the menisci. Burstein[12] showed that the more congruent the surfaces are, the greater the change in contact point. A simple shift of 2 mm in tibial position will result in changes of 8 to 10 mm in femorotibial contact. Furthermore, in abnormal states, such as in ligament deficiency or prosthetic replacement, marked contact point abnormalities may occur. The most extreme case is of course dislocation of the femorotibial articulation in which noncontact with the articular surface of either plateau can occur. Clearly, a full understanding of all 6 degree-of-freedom motions and their constraints is necessary for a full definition of the function of a normal knee.

According to other authorities using surface-mounted external monitoring systems, other activities of daily living, such as stair climbing, require a mean of 87 degrees of flexion. Descending stairs requires an average of 91 degrees.[2] Activities such as getting out of a chair require approximately 105 degrees of rotation. Lifting objects requires 117 degrees of flexion.[40,65]

Patellar Kinematics

Less information is available on three-dimensional patellofemoral motion. Feress et al.[21] studied the in vivo patellofemoral motion in a series of four patients after proximal tibial osteotomy using a roentgen stereophotogrammetric technique. Reider et al.[58] performed a cadaveric in vitro experiment on 20 knees. A static quadriceps load of 22.5 nts was applied. LaFortune[39] attempted in vivo assessment but had difficulty with the patellar reference frame stability.

It is generally understood that patellar motion is similarly complex requiring comparable 6 degree-of-freedom assessment.[36] Using the same femoral and tibial reference systems as above, an additional patellofemoral linkage frame must be defined. Using Reider's general relationships, the patella undergoes mediolateral (Y-axis) translation. The "predominant" pattern of motion, when moving from 90 degrees of flexion to maximal extension, is as follows:

1. In sagittal rotation, the patella qualitatively follows that of the femoral trochlear surface. Translation was found to average 14 mm in a medial (-x) direction with increasing extension.
2. In transverse rotation (patellar tilt) the patella tilted medially 12 degrees. Translation (Z axis) closely parallels the flexion angle with proximal motion with increasing extension.
3. In coronal rotation the patella rotated six degrees inward (Clockwise on the right and Counterclockwise on the left). In translation (Y axis) the patellar moves anterior, ascending the intercondylar notch, with increasing extension. This anterior/posterior motion results in the patella transmitting a posteriorly directed force on the tibia below 74 degrees of flexion. With further extension the extensor mechanism results in anteriorly directed forces which are resisted by the anterior cruciate ligament.[69]

Significant variability in patellar motion is characteristic of these and other experiments. Further understanding and correlation of the source of these variables with clinical phenomena is necessary.

Forces

The other half of the understanding of knee kinematics is that of the forces experienced in the major articulations of the joint. The forces experienced by both the femorotibial and patellofemoral articulations have been calculated on theoretical grounds from indirect measurements. These forces are dependent on variations in anatomy and activity. The peak force in the femorotibial articulation approximates three times body weight for level gait.[49,50,68] Other activities such as getting out of a chair result in forces of 2.45 times body weight. Simple use of the chair arms reduced this to 1.46 times body weight.[63] High-level or impact activities would be expected to give correspondingly increased forces of up to 24 times body weight, but these are more difficult to quantify.[13,66,70]

The femorotibial load is distributed unequally between the medial and lateral compartments of the knee. Quantitation of this distribution is dependent on limb alignment, local surface geometry, ligamentous tension, muscular attachment, muscular activity, and inertial effects associated with the speed of gait. Inertial effects are small.[9] Three-dimensional evaluation of compartmental loading in the cadaver has demonstrated that the medial compartment bears three times the average lateral compartmental load.[68] Gait evaluation has shown that significant variability is present. Subjects can alter the load distribution through the knee and "compensate for insufficiency of the limb."[27,35] Nevertheless, static limb or joint malalignment, which can induce altered compartmental joint loading due to certain acquired defects at long-term follow-up, is associated with premature joint failure.[29,38] High adductor moments have also been correlated with premature clinical failure after osteotomy for osteoarthritis.[56]

The patellofemoral joint in level gait is subject to forces of 0.5 times body weight.[59] This low force level is due to the relatively small amount of flexion needed for level gait. Getting out of a chair results in forces of 2.4 times body weight. The use of the chair arms causes a dramatic reduction in patellofemoral force to 0.72 times body weight. However, with bent knee activities such as stair climbing, the patellofemoral joint experiences a peak force of 3.3 times body weight. The patellofemoral joint may experience up to 17 times body weight during certain sporting activities.[66]

Contact Area

Determination of articular cartilage load (force per unit area) requires a knowledge of both the applied force and the contact area between the surfaces in question. It is generally believed that excessive articular cartilage stress over time will lead to premature osteoarthritis. This can occur as a function of global malalignment, local malalignment, meniscectomy, or the presence of an intra-articular loose body, or by kinematic abnormality secondary to ligament deficiency. Multiple investigators have measured ex vivo joint contact areas using a variety of techniques in an attempt to quantify the articular cartilage load.[23,38,46,61,62,71]

Recently, one group attempted to measure cartilage stress directly using a piezoelectric strain-gauge technique.[10] Brown and Shaw found surface stresses to be lower than previously calculated. However, regardless of the specific method of load determination, it has been consistently identified that meniscectomy reduces the cartilage contact area and increases cartilage contact stress. Furthermore, clinical correlation of quantitative surface stress is required in order to establish its relationship with the development of osteoarthritis.

PROSTHETIC BIOMECHANICS

Kinetics

A full reproduction of the normal motions of the knee requires a delicate balance among the articular surface, the menisci, and the ligamentous structures. Since this is difficult to achieve, prosthetic replacement is a compromise. If the articular surfaces are highly constraining and minimal disruption has occurred in the surrounding ligamentous and capsular envelope, marked increases in both residual ligament tensions and bone prosthesis interface stresses will be seen.[42,44] This constellation of events is probably best represented by early attempts at total knee arthroplasty in which single-axis single-degree-of-freedom prostheses, such as the Waldius or Shiers components, were used. Clinical experiences with loosening, premature device failure, and restricted range of motion were all evident. This is not to say, however, that a prosthesis should be designed without constraint. The ICLH prosthesis, as originally conceived, had no constraint to medially or laterally directed forces. This resulted in translational instability in the transverse plane.[24] Excessive unconstrained tibial rotation also may be associated with patellofemoral disorders.[11,37,51]

Implant Selection

Selection of an individual implant is therefore dependent on the initial patient status. Patients with relatively minimal degrees of deformity and generally intact supporting ligamentous structures will be best served through the use of a minimally constrained prosthesis. Preservation of the cruciate ligaments, especially the posterior cruciate, will assist in deceleration functions such as descending stairs.[2,19,67]

One must be wary, however, of the preservation of the posterior cruciate ligament when using prostheses with a high level of surface constraint. This combination can cause rocking of the femorotibial articulation, increased wear, increased bone prosthesis interface stresses, and excessive ligamentous stresses. These phenomena are particularly associated with an excessively constraining elevated flange along the posterior aspect of the tibial surface.[42] However, total elimination of articular surface constraint is neither necessary nor perhaps even desirable.

When sacrificing the anterior cruciate ligament, some provision for sagittal plane stability is necessary. Several solutions exist: (1) reliance on extracapsular scar tissue formation, (2) the use of a posterior polyethylene tibial component flange, (3) the use of an elevated posterior cam, (4) alteration in the anatomic tibial plateau angle (the use of a neutral plane rather than one of 10 degrees of posterior inclination), (5) ligamentous substitution, or (6) some combination of these. The optimum solution, if one exists, has not yet been established and will most likely be dependent on a variety of individual patient and surgical parameters.

In patients who have greater degrees of deformity, especially those with flexion contractures of greater than 30 degrees, it is often necessary to resect the posterior cruciate ligament in order to obtain full extension. In these circumstances and in those patients with greater than 25 degrees of varus or valgus deformity, a more constrained prosthesis to compensate for the lack of soft tissue support is frequently required. In cases of maximal ligament and bone deficiency, as in tumor surgery or certain revision procedures, it is necessary to proceed to more highly constrained prostheses such as the total condylar III,[7] a rotating hinge design, or even to a custom fusion prosthesis.[15] Prostheses with such increased articular constraint require more degrees of activity reduction to minimize excessive stress at the bone prosthesis interface and within the device itself, which can lead to premature clinical failure.

FEMORAL COMPONENT DESIGN

Femoral component design should incorporate a central patellar groove with lateral condylar buttressing to prevent patellar subluxation. The condylar radii should vary anatomically in the sagittal plane to duplicate normal kinematics. However, the exact curvature of the runners in the frontal plane is open to question. Relatively flat condylar surfaces result in improved surface load distribution on unconstrained polyethylene tibial surfaces. This design feature also improves stability to varus and valgus forces through the maximization of the contact moment arm.[1] However, especially when ligament insufficiency exists, flattening of these surfaces can increase the potential for loading at the prosthetic edges. This flattening, through a "teetering" effect, will result in increased interface bony stresses and tibial polyethylene surface wear.[6] The use of a central stem in a primary femoral arthroplasty is generally not necessary for load transmission but may assist in establishing the proper alignment. Revision prostheses will frequently require the use of central stems in order to transfer load more proximally when there is insufficient bone stock or ligamentous support.

TIBIAL COMPONENT DESIGN

Because total knee replacement failures have occurred most commonly on the tibial side, special attention must be directed at this component in order to reduce failure.[20] The tibial component must offer a low-friction surface to articulate with the femoral component. The most satisfactory materials to date for this low-friction surface have been ultrahigh-molecular-weight polyethylene contacting cobalt chrome molybdenum. In addition, the tibial component surface should be capable of being contoured to present variable degrees of constraint to accommodate the existing ligamentous status. Relatively thin layers of polyethylene, which are not supported, should not be used, as they have been associated with cold flow, breakage, loosening, and tibial subsidence.[5] Thick layers of polyethylene or a metal backing can distribute the load over a broad area. This mechanical solution under the best of circumstances still cannot duplicate the normal coefficients of friction.

To minimize bony resection, metal backing of the polyethylene surface appears to be the most rational approach. Furthermore, because of its thermal conductivity, metal backing can decrease peak temperatures during the insertion of components with methyl methacrylate cement.[47]

Adding carbon fibers to ultrahigh-molecular-weight polyethylene in an attempt to reinforce it has been investigated extensively. Indeed, the ultimate strength and stiffness of this composite structure are increased. However, fatigue resistance is decreased.[17] Furthermore, the increased stiffness results in a decreased contact area and increased surface stress. Since most failures begin at, or close to, the articulating surface, it seems unlikely that this approach will help address the concerns of wear in total knee arthroplasty.[5,52] The use of other composite types of polyethylene, however, may reduce surface contact stress while allowing for anatomic bone strain distribution.[57,58]

The use of a single central tibial stem is the best way to obtain satisfactory bony fixation.[44] This requires resection of only the relatively weak intercondylar bone and decreases peak interface stress.[25] It is quite clear, however, that none of the currently available prostheses or prosthetic approaches is capable of anatomically redistributing the load across the proximal tibial surface.[22,52,53] Optimization of load transfer requires maximization of proximal tibial contact.[4] Peripheral cortical contact, when using metallic tibial trays, appears to have minimal benefit.[16] Practically, the achieve-

ment of precise cortical contact is difficult with the variability in tibial bone resection and the presence of tibial anthropometric differences, even if performed on a custom basis.

The role of cemented porous-backed tibial components is controversial. The predominant mode of loosening does not occur at the prosthesis–cement interface but rather at the bone–cement interface. Relatively rough surfaces indeed allow improvement in cement strength because of a local reinforcement effect. A three-dimensional interlock between the cement and the prosthetic surface will allow improved tensile and shear stress transmission with the advantageous reduction of peak loads.

The technology used to apply the porous surface is still in evolution. Fatigue failure of the underlying tibial component resulting from the alteration in grain size as a function of sintering is a major concern. In addition, the introduction of numerous notches at every point of application of the bead or wire is alarming because of its deleterious effect on fatigue performance.[48] Finally, problems of surface delamination and breakage (loose beads and wires) need to be resolved.[28,29]

Optimal parameters for tibial component design in the biologic ingrowth mode are currently ill-defined. Experimentally, it appears likely that a combination of smooth stems and porous plateaus will prove satisfactory. Whether the use of a single central stem, of multiple stems, or of screws is the most satisfactory will require further investigation. Finally, it is unclear as to what the optimal biologic ingrowth tissue is. An organized fibrous tissue has been demonstrated to have the potential for comparable biomechanical performance to that of ingrowth by cancellous bone if the initial biomechanical environment is satisfactory.[30,31]

PATELLAR COMPONENT DESIGN

Relatively little information is available on the ideal patellar component design. Currently three general shapes are available. A trapezoidal component is used in some knee designs to prevent dislocation of the patella. However, this design constrains the femoral component runners to a nonanatomic grooved design. It appears that, with appropriate lateral soft tissue release and adequate femorotibial rotational constraint, this high degree of patellar articular constraint is unnecessary.

A dome-shaped or an offset dome-shaped component is the most commonly used configuration. Technically, it is easy to insert because rotational alignment requires minimal attention. It is axisymmetric about its apex and therefore can be used in the right or left knee. This is advantageous, as an abbreviated inventory of components is possible. The eccentric dome-shaped patella offers the theoretical advantages of improved tracking combined with the practical advantage of a lower level of surgical precision. However, these designs have the theoretical disadvantage of concentrating load in relatively small areas of articulation. This should predispose to polyethylene failure, especially when the thickness is borderline and when metal backing is present.[60]

An anatomically designed prosthesis that may minimize the problems of polyethylene failure and provide adequate levels of constraint to patellar subluxation or dislocation. Surgical precision is necessary during insertion to be certain that proper rotational alignment is present, as improper alignment will result in increased surface and interface stresses.

Patellar component fixation to bone is probably best accomplished through the use of multiple small stems rather than a single central stem. This allows for greater rotational stability at the bone–prosthesis interface and minimizes problems with patellar fracture associated with single large central posts.

EX VIVO MACHINE TESTING

Murray and co-workers tested the variable axis total condylar, stabilocondylar, spherocentric, and Noiles implants to failure in a knee simulator. The variable axis with no constraint to rotation and the Noiles hinge prosthesis survived 10 million cycles

without failure. The total condylar sustained plastic cold-flow at 8 million cycles. The tibial component of the stabilocondylar became loose at 6.0 million cycles. Data are not currently available for the commonly used resurfacing implants.

The wear characteristics of implants are relatively poorly understood as they relate to changes in stiffness and area of contact over time. Hillberry and co-workers[18,32] at Purdue University have tested the Insall-Burstein, multiradius, geopatellar/geometric, RMC, cruciate condylar, spherocentric, and anametric knees in a knee simulator. The stiffness varied with the number of simulated steps, and the area of contact gradually increased between 0 and 100,000 steps. Misalignment was found to result in altered wear, increased shear stress at the bone-cement interface, and instability at the articulating surfaces.[1]

REFERENCES

1. Abarotin VA: In vitro measurement of forces in prosthetic knees. Masters thesis, Purdue University, W Lafayette, IN, 1984
2. Andriacchi TP, Galante JO, Fermier RW: The influence of total knee-replacement design on walking and stair-climbing. J Bone Joint Surg 64A:1328, 1982
3. Andry N: Orthopaedia: or, the Art of Correcting and Preventing Deformities in Children. Classics of Medicine Library, Birmingham, AL, 1980
4. Bargren JH, Day WH, Freeman MAR, Swanson SAV: Mechanical tests on the tibial components of non-hinged knee prostheses. J Bone Joint Surg 60B:256, 1978
5. Bartel DL, Bicknell VL, Wright TM: Analysis of stresses causing surface damage in metal-backed plastic components for total knee replacement. Orthop Res Soc 9:104, 1984
6. Bartel DL, Bicknell VL, Wright TM: The effect of conformity, thickness, and material on stresses in ultra-high molecular weight components for total joint replacement. J Bone Joint Surg 68A:1041, 1986
7. Bartel DL, Burstein AH, Santavicca EA, Insall JN,: Performance of the tibial component in total knee replacement. J Bone Joint Surg 64A:1026, 1982

8. Bick EM: Source Book of Orthopaedics. Williams & Wilkins, Baltimore, 1948

9. Bresler B, Frankel JP: The forces and moments in the leg during level walking. Transactions of the American Society of Mechanical Engineers, 48A:62, 1950

10. Brown TD, Shaw DT: in vitro contact stress distribution on the femoral condyles. J Orthop Res 2:190, 1984

11. Buchanan JR, Bowman LS, Shearer A, et al: Clinical evaluation of the variable axis total knee replacement. Presented at the Forty-ninth Annual Meeting, Final Program, American Academy of Orthopaedic Surgeons, New Orleans, 1982

12. Burstein AH: Biomechanics of the knee. p. 21. In Insall JN (ed): Surgery of the Knee. Churchill Livingstone, New York, 1984

13. Cavanagh PR, LaFortune MA: Ground reaction forces in distance running. J Biomech 13:397, 1980

14. Chao EYS: Justification of triaxial goniometer for the measurement of joint rotation. J Biomech 13:989, 1980

15. Chao EYS, Sim FH: Tumor prosthesis design: a system approach. p. 335. In Chao EYS, Ivins JC (eds): Tumor Prosthesis for Bone and Joint Reconstruction. Thieme-Stratton, New York, 1983

16. Cheal EJ, Hayes WC, Lee CH, Miller J: Stress analysis of a condylar knee tibial component: influence of metaphyseal shell properties and cement injection depth. J Orthop Res 3:424, 1985

17. Connelly GM, Rimnac CM, Wright TM, et al: Fatigue crack propagation behavior of ultrahigh molecular weight polyethylene. J Orthop Res 2:119, 1984

18. Cullom CD: Force and displacement characteristics of total knee prostheses. Masters thesis, Purdue University, Lafayette, IN, 1982

19. Draganich LF, Anderson GBJ, Andriacchi TP, Galante JO: The influence of the cruciate ligaments on femoral-tibial contact movement during knee flexion. p. 29. In Transactions of the Thirtieth Annual Meeting, Orthopaedic Research Society, Atlanta, 1984

20. Ducheyne P, Kagan A II, Lacey JA: Failure of total knee arthroplasty due to loosening and deformation of the tibial component. J Bone Joint Surg 60A:384, 1978

21. Feress SA, Lippert FG, Hou CY, Takamoto T: Patellar tracking patterns measurement by analytical X-ray photogrammetry. J Biomech 12:639, 1979

22. Fortna JH, Hillberry BM, Heck DA: A comparison of finite element analysis and clinical results for a unicompartmental tibial prosthesis. p. 400. In Transactions of the Thirty-third Meeting of the Orthopaedic Research Society, San Francisco, 1987

23. Fukubayashi T, Kurosawa H: The contact area and pressure distribution pattern of the knee: a study of normal and osteoarthrotic knee joints. Acta Orthop Scand 51:871, 1980

24. Goldberg VM, Henderson BT: The Freeman-Swanson ICLH total knee arthroplasty: complications and problems. J Bone Joint Surg 62A:1338, 1980

25. Goldstein SA, Wilson DL, Sonstegard DA, Matthews LS: The mechanical properties of human tibial trabecular bone as a function of metaphyseal location. J Biomech 16:965, 1983

26. Grood ES, Suntay WJ: A joint coordinate system for the clinical description of three-dimensional motions: application to the knee. J Biomed Eng 105:136, 1983

27. Harrington IJ: Static and dynamic loading patterns in knee joints with deformities. J Bone Joint Surg 65A:247, 1983

28. Heck DA, Chao EY, Kelly PJ: The biomechanical performance of a conical coupling in porous-coated modular prosthesis design. Orthop Res Soc 9:342, 1984

29. Heck DA, Chao EY, Sim FH, et al: A roentgenographic analysis of patients with titanium fibermetal segmental bone and joint prostheses. Clin Orthop 204:266, 1986

30. Heck DA, Nakajima I, Kelly PJ, Chao EY: The effect of load alteration on the biological and biomechanical performance of a titanium fibermetal segmental prosthesis. J Bone Joint Surg 68A: 118 1986

31. Heck DA, Nakajima I, Kelly PJ, Chao EYS: The effect of load alteration on the biological and biomechanical performance of a titanium fibermetal segmental prosthesis. J Bone Joint Surg 68A:118, 1987

32. Hersch JF: Laboratory evaluation of knee prostheses. Masters thesis, Purdue University, W Lafayette, IN, 1980

33. Holbrook TL, Grazier K, Kelsey JL, Stauffer RN: The Frequency of Occurrence, Impact and Cost of Selected Musculoskeletal Conditions in the United States. American Academy of Orthopaedic Surgeons, Chicago, 1984

34. Hungerford DS, Krackow KA, Kenna RV: Alignment in total knee arthroplasty. p. 9. In Dorr LD (ed): The Knee. Papers of the First Scientific Meeting of the Knee Society. University Park Press, Baltimore, 1985

35. Johnson F, Leitl S, Waugh W: The distribution of load across the knee: a comparison of static and dynamic measurements. J Bone Joint Surg 62B:346, 1980

36. Kaltwasser P, Uematsu O, Walker PS: The patello-femoral joint in total knee replacement. p. 292. Transactions of the Thirty-third Annual Meeting of the Orthopaedic Research Society, San Francisco, 1987

37. Kettelkamp DB: Surgery of the Knee. American Academy of Orthopaedic Surgeons, Instructional Course Lectures, CV Mosby, 1984

38. Kettelkamp DB, Jacobs AW: Tibiofemoral contact area—determination and implications. J Bone Joint Surg 54A:349, 1972

39. LaFortune MA: The use of intra-cortical pins to measure the motion of the knee joint during walking. Doctoral thesis, Pennsylvania State University, University Park, 1984

40. Laubenthal KN, Smidt GL, Kettelkamp DB: A quantitative analysis of knee motion during activities of daily living. Phys Ther 52:32, 1972

41. Levens AS, Berkeley CE, Inman VT, Blosser JA: Transverse rotation of the segments of the lower extremity in locomotion. J Bone Joint Surg 30A:859, 1948

42. Lew WD, Lewis JL: The effect of knee-prosthesis geometry on cruciate ligament mechanics during flexion. J Bone Joint Surg 64A:734, 1982

43. Lewis JL, Askew MJ, Jaycos DP: A comparative evaluation of tibial component designs of total knee prosthesis. J Bone Joint Surg 64A:129, 1982

44. Lewis JL, Lew WD: A method for locating an optimal "fixed" axis of rotation for the human knee joint. J Biomed Eng 100:187, 1978

45. Maquet P: Biomécanique du genou et gonarthrose. Rev Med Liege 24:170, 1969

46. Maquet PG, Van De Berg AJ, Simonet JC: Femoro-tibial weight-bearing areas. J Bone Joint Surg 57A:766, 1975

47. Mjoberg B, Pettersson H, Rosenqvist R, Rydholm A: Bone cement, thermal injury and radiolucent zone. Acta Orthop Scand 55:597, 1984

48. Mooz A: Mechanical properties of a surgical grade titanium alloy. Masters thesis, University of Toronto, 1980

49. Morrison JB: Bioengineering analysis of force actions transmitted by the knee joint. Biomed Eng 164, 1968

50. Morrison JB: The mechanics of the knee joint in relation to normal walking. J Biomech 3:51, 1970

51. Murray DG, Webster DA: The variable-axis knee prosthesis. J Bone Joint Surg 63A:687, 1981

52. Murrish DE: Finite element analysis of the tibia with and without knee prostheses. Masters thesis, Purdue University, Lafayette, IN, 1984

53. Murrish DE, Hillberry BM, Heck DA: Strain distribution in the proximal tibia with and without tibial prostheses: a FEM study. p. 122. In Transactions of the Thirty-first Annual Meeting, Orthopaedic Research Society, 1985

54. O'Malley CD, Saunders JBdCM: Leonardo da Vinci on the Human Body. Henry Schuman, New York, 1952

55. Parsons JR, Alexander H, Weiss AB: Absorbable polymer-filamentous carbon composites: a new concept in orthopaedic biomaterials. p. 873. In Szycher M (ed): Biocompatible Polymers, Metals, and Composites. Technomic Publishing, 1983

56. Prodromos CC, Andriacchi TP, Galante JO: A relationship between gait and clinical changes following high tibial osteotomy. J Bone Joint Surg 67A:1188, 1985

57. Ranawat CS, Chitranjan S: The patellofemoral joint in total condylar knee arthroplasty: pros and cons based on five- to ten-year follow-up observations. Clin Orthop 205:93, 1986

58. Reider B, Marshall JL, King B: Patellar tracking. Clin Orthop 157:143, 1981

59. Reilly DT, Martens M: Experimental analysis of the quadriceps muscle force and patello-femoral joint reaction force for various activities. Acta Orthop Scand 43:126, 1972

60. Schaff JA: Stability tests and clinical correlation of laboratory tested knee prostheses. Masters thesis, Purdue University, W Lafayette, IN, 1983

61. Seedhom BB: Transmission of the load in the knee joint with special reference to the role of the menisci. I. Anatomy, analysis and apparatus. Engin Med 8:207, 1979

62. Seedhom BB, Hargreaves DJ: Transmission of the load in the knee joint with special reference to the role of the menisci. II. Engin Med 8:220, 1979

63. Seedhom BB, Terayama K: Knee forces during the activity of getting out of a chair with and without the aid of arms. Biomed Eng 11:278, 1976

64. Shaw JA, Murray DG: The longitudinal axis of the knee and the role of the cruciate ligaments in controlling transverse rotation. J Bone Joint Surg 56A:1603, 1974

65. Sledge CB, Walker PS: Total knee replacement in rheumatoid arthritis. p. 697. In Insall JN (ed): Surgery of the Knee. Churchill Livingstone, New York, 1984

66. Smith AJ: A study of the forces on the body in athletic activities with particular reference to jumping. Doctoral thesis, Leeds University, Great Britain, 1972

67. Soudry MJ, Walker PS, Reilly D, Sledge CB: Interface forces of tibial component: the effect of PCL

sacrifice and conformity. p. 37. In Transactions of the Twenty-ninth Annual Meeting, Orthopaedic Research Society, Anaheim, 1983

68. Tansey HH III: A three-dimensional kinematic and force analysis of the human tibio-femoral joint during normal walking. Masters thesis, Purdue University, W Lafayette, IN, 1976

69. Van Eijden TMGJ, DeBoer W, Weijs WA: The orientation of the distal part of the quadriceps femoris muscle as a function of the knee flexion-extension angle. J Biomech 18:803, 1985

70. Wahrenberg H, Lindbeck L, Ekholm J: Dynamic load in the human knee joint during voluntary active impact to the lower leg. Scand J Rehab Med 10(10):93, 1978

71. Walker PS, Hajek JV: The load-bearing area in the knee joint. J Biomech 5:581, 1972

Acute Ligament Injuries and Dislocations

112

Kenneth E. DeHaven

Acute ligamentous injuries to the knees are among the most common injuries sustained by the musculoskeletal system. Athletic trauma is a frequent cause, but vehicular and occupational injuries as well as falls in the home often produce these injuries. Even minor ligamentous injury to the knee caused disability; more serious injuries are capable of producing chronic disabilities, including functional instability, meniscus tears, loose-body formation, and degenerative arthritis. Proper diagnosis and management of these injuries is extremely important if the early and long-term disabilities are to be minimized.

According to standard nomenclature, ligamentous injuries are classified as sprains. They are further classified as first degree, second degree, or third degree, according to severity. A third-degree injury indicates complete disruption of that particular ligament, a first degree injury indicates a mild injury involving only a few of the fibers, and a second-degree injury indicates a moderate amount of injury involving more of the fibers but with the basic integrity of the ligament remaining intact. The clinical diagnosis is based on a mechanism of injury that applies tensile stress to the ligament, tenderness over the injured portion of the ligament

(if the ligament is palpable), and the integrity of the ligament as determined by clinical stress testing. Grade I injuries have no demonstrable laxity, grade II injuries may show mild but insignificant laxity, and grade III injuries demonstrate significant laxity.

Since O'Donoghue demonstrated the superiority of primary surgical repair of torn knee ligaments as compared with nonoperative treatment,[16,17] primary surgical repair of torn knee ligaments has become the recognized standard of orthopaedic care unless contraindications exist to override the indications for primary repair. Spontaneous healing does occur with collateral ligament injuries, but with the elongation that occurs prior to rupture the spontaneous healing often occurs in the elongated position, leading to chronic instability. Complete tears of the anterior and posterior cruciate ligaments, however, are not capable of spontaneous healing, since they fall away from their normal anatomic positions. Primary surgical treatment of third-degree ligamentous injuries of the knee provides the opportunity to replace the ligamentous fibers into their normal anatomic positions and with normal or near-normal length and tension relationships, so that there is less chance of residual instability. Furthermore, where primary repair alone does not give highly predictable results, augmentation or even primary reconstructive procedures can be added to primary repair to optimize the ultimate functional result. The time required for ligamentous healing appears to be the same whether the injury is treated surgically or nonsurgically.

Primary repair of torn collateral ligaments should ideally be carried out within the first 72 hours following injury, and certainly within the first 7 days following injury. After 7 days the early spontaneous healing process makes accurate dissection of the torn ligament very difficult, and the edematous tissues do not hold sutures or staples well. Similarly, primary repair of torn anterior or posterior cruciate ligaments ideally should be carried out within the first 72 hours of injury, but since primary spontaneous healing does not occur, repairable injuries to the cruciate ligaments remain repairable for up to 14 to 21 days.

Contraindications to primary ligamentous repair include life-threatening associated injuries to the head and neck, thoracic or abdominal contents, active sepsis, or associated vascular compromise. Acute vascular compromise obviously takes precedence over ligamentous repair, but frequently the ligaments can be repaired within the same operation once arterial and venous repair has been satisfactorily accomplished.

MEDIAL INJURIES

General Statement

The medial stabilizing structures are known collectively as the medial collateral ligament system. These structures include the superficial medial collateral ligament, the deep medial collateral ligament (or deep capsular ligament), the posterior oblique ligament, and the posterior medial capsule. These structures can be torn in various locations and combinations depending on the nature and direction of the stresses imposed. The usual mechanism of injury involves a direct blow to the lateral aspect of the knee or thigh with the foot fixed to the ground. Frequently there is also an element of external tibial rotation as these medial stresses are being applied.

Precise localization of the areas of maximum tenderness and soft-tissue puffiness over the anatomic landmarks of the medial collateral ligament system (Fig. 112-1A,B) is of great help in identifying the damaged portions. Significant laxity to medial or valgus stress makes the diagnosis a third degree injury. Significant medial laxity demonstrated with the knee in full extension indicates an extremely severe injury involving not only the medial collateral ligament system but also the posterior capsule and the posterior cruciate ligament, and possibly also the anterior cruciate ligament. Less severe third-degree injuries show no laxity with the knee in full extension but will demonstrate significant laxity when the knee is tested at 30 degrees of flexion. This position relaxes the cruciate ligaments and the posterior capsule and allows a more isolated evaluation of the medial collateral ligament system. All tests for knee ligament stability should be carried out in every knee to look for other associated injuries.

Nonoperative Management

In recent years, there has been an increasing trend toward nonoperative functional treatment of isolated tears of the medial collateral ligament. Several reports have documented satisfactory results and decreased recovery time as compared with surgical repair.[9] (Andrews JR: personal communication, 1987). Indications are strict: valgus laxity when tested at 20 to 30 degrees of flexion but not in full extension, and negative Lachman and anterior drawer signs. This indicates injury confined to the medial collateral ligament with an intact anterior cruciate ligament. Examination under anesthesia and arthroscopy are usually recommended to confirm the isolated nature of the medial collateral ligament injury. Treatment guidelines include protection in a hinged-splint or knee brace and early range of motion and rehabilitation of the musculature. Functional rehabilitation follows, with protective bracing recommended when returning to strenuous activity.

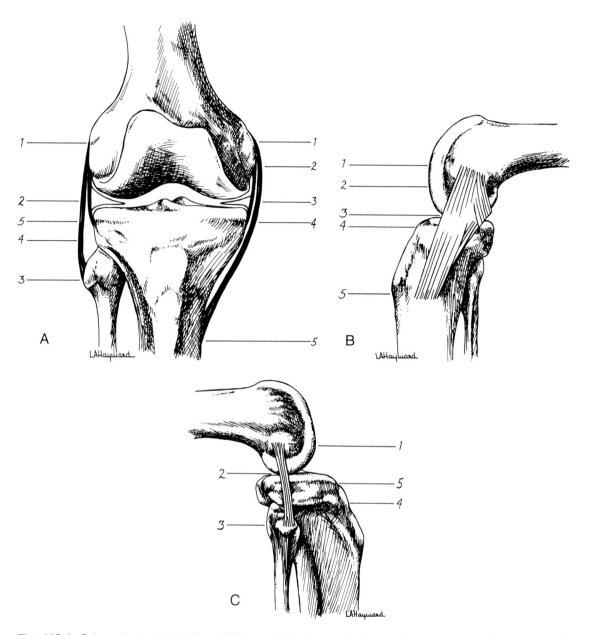

Fig. 112-1. Schematic representation of the anatomic landmarks for medial and lateral collateral ligament injuries. **(A)** Frontal view. Medial side: (1) Attachment of superficial medial collateral ligament at the medial femoral epicondyle, (2) attachment of the deep (capsular) layer of the medial collateral ligament on the femur, (3) joint line level, (4) level of attachment of the deep (capsular) layer of the medial collateral ligament to the tibia, and (5) attachment of the superficial medial collateral ligament to the tibia. Lateral side: (1) proximal attachment of lateral collateral ligament system to a collateral femoral epicondyle, (2) joint line level, (3) attachment of fibular collateral ligament and biceps tendon to the fibular head, (4) level of Gerdy's tubercle, where iliotibial band attaches to the tibia, and (5) site of attachment of the deep (capsular) layer to the tibia. **(B)** Medial ligamentous landmarks. (1) Attachment of superficial medial collateral ligament to medial femoral epicondyle, (2) attachment of the deep (capsular) layer of the medial collateral ligament of the femur, (3) joint line level, (4) level of attachment of the deep (capsular) layer to the tibia, and (5) attachment of the superficial medial collateral ligament to the tibia. **(C)** Landmarks of lateral side structures. (1) Proximal attachment site at lateral femoral epicondyle, (2) joint line level, (3) distal attachment of fibular collateral ligament and biceps tendon at the fibular head, (4) Gerdy's tubercle where iliotibial band attaches to the tibia, and (5) level of attachment of the deep (capsular) layer of the tibia.

Indications

In general, nonoperative treatment is indicated for isolated medial collateral injuries, and surgical treatment for grade III medial side injuries associated with tears of the anterior or posterior cruciate ligaments or with a repairable meniscal tear. In addition, there are occasional isolated medial collateral ligament tears with marked acute laxity, even though the anterior cruciate ligament is intact. For these exceptional cases, especially in high-performance athletes, the results of surgical repair have been superior to nonoperative treatment in my experience, and justify the risks of surgery and increased recovery time.

Methods of Treatment

The treatment options are nonoperative or primary surgical treatment consisting of either primary repair alone or primary repair with augmentation using such structures as the pes anserinus, semimembranosus, medial gastrocnemius, and adductor longus.

Author's Preferred Method

The preferred method of treatment is direct primary repair. Augmentation of the primary repair with pes anserinus transfer is considered when there is a medial collateral and anterior cruciate ligament tear with marked anteromedial rotatory instability. Augmentation with the modified pes anserinus transfer is carried out when there is a shredded jointline tear of the medial collateral ligament with an associated anterior cruciate ligament tear.

Surgical Technique

The medial aspect of the knee is exposed through a medial utility approach under tourniquet control. The medial collateral ligament system is then exposed by incising the overlying medial retinaculum from the adductor tubercule to the superior border of the pes anserinus. The exposure is facilitated by converting this incision into an L or a T proximally (Fig. 112-2A). The pathology is then identified (the surgeon should recall where the pinpoint locations of maximal tenderness and soft tissue puffiness were found on the preoperative clinical examination). The superficial portion of the medial collateral ligament may be torn at or near its femoral attachment, at or near the joint line, or well distal to the joint line at or beneath the pes anserinus. The deep capsular ligament can be torn in the meniscofemoral or meniscotibial interval. The posterior oblique ligament may be torn from the femur, across the joint line, or from its tibial attachment (Fig. 112-2B). The posterior capsule may be torn from the tibia.

Once the areas of disruption have been adequately identified and exposed, the repair is made as anatomically as possible, layer by layer, beginning with the deepest structures. If the posterior capsule has been torn from the tibia, it is repaired with sutures brought forward through drill holes placed from anterior to posterior through the tibia after the method of O'Donoghue, so that when the sutures are tied anteriorly over the surface of the tibia the posterior capsule will be repositioned (Fig. 112-2C). If the tear has occurred along the rim of the meniscus, the rim is included in the repair to save the meniscus, which should be removed only if there is a major tear extending into its substance. Any tear in the deep (capsular) portion of the medial collateral ligament is next repaired with direct, plicating sutures to restore normal tension in the deep capsular layer (Fig. 112-2D).

Careful attention is paid to restoring the normal tension and attachments of the posterior oblique ligament; if it has been torn from the tibia, it should be repaired back to a prepared bony bed with plicating sutures brought up through the fibers of the semimembranosus tendon and then passed back through these fibers so that when the stitch is tied the posterior oblique ligament is pulled back into normal position and tension (Fig. 112-2E). At each step of repair the knee should be tested for stability. Complete stability should be obtained at the time of surgical repair, since the stability will never be better than it is on the operating table.

Attention is then turned to the superficial portion of the medial collateral ligament, which is similarly repaired depending upon the site of the lesion. If the tear is distal, at or below the level of the

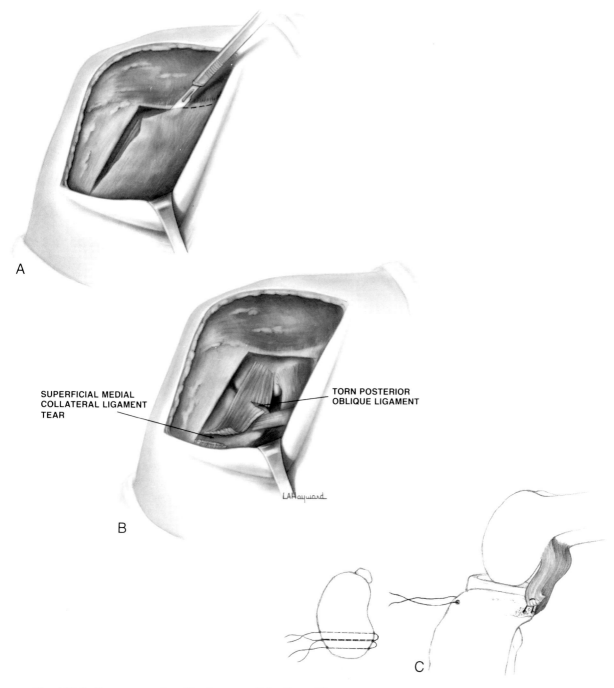

SUPERFICIAL MEDIAL
COLLATERAL LIGAMENT
TEAR

TORN POSTERIOR
OBLIQUE LIGAMENT

Fig. 112-2. Exposure and repair of torn medial collateral ligament. **(A)** Initial exposure through a medial utility approach, with initial incision through the retinacular layer being coverted to an L proximally. **(B)** The exposed medial collateral ligament, demonstrating a tear of the superficial medial collateral ligament near the tibial attachment, and the posterior oblique ligament from the tibia, with an underlying tear of the deep capsular portion in the meniscotibial interval (not shown). **(C)** Schematic representation of repair of the posteromedial capsule to the tibia using sutures passed through drill holes from anterior to posterior through the proximal tibia. *(Figure continues.)*

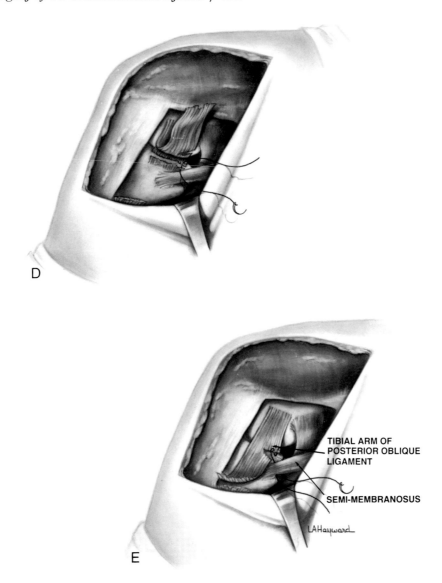

Fig. 112-2 *(Continued).* **(D)** The deep (capsular portion of the medial collateral ligament is shown torn in the meniscotibial interval, being repaired with direct, plicating sutures. **(E)** The tibial arm of the posterior oblique ligament is being repaired back to a prepared bony bed with a plicating suture passed through the Sharpey's fibers of the semimembranosus tendon. *(Figure continues.)*

pes anserinus, it can be fixed with a barbed staple or with sutures passed through drill holes (Fig. 112-2F). If the tear is more proximal, repair with plicating sutures is preferred.

Once the primary repair of the medial structures has been completed, augmentation can be considered if there is reason to doubt the adequacy of the repaired tissues. A standard pes anserinus transfer can be considered for combined medial collateral ligament and anterior cruciate ligament tears (see Ch. 113). The modified pes anserinus transfer (see Ch. 113) is often carried out when the medial collateral ligament structures have been torn in a shredded fashion along the joint line in association with a tear of the anterior cruciate ligament. If either or both of the cruciate ligaments are torn in

Indications

The indication for surgical repair is the presence of significant lateral laxity, especially in the relatively young and active individual who is going to place significant demands upon the knee. With varus alignment, even those with low demands may have functional instability with significant laxity, however. Associated injuries to menisci, cruciate ligaments, or articular surfaces should also be treated.

Treatment Options

The treatment options are nonoperative treatment utilizing a cast or cast brace for 6 to 8 weeks, followed by comprehensive rehabilitation (see under Rehabilitation), or primary surgical treat-ment, which consists of direct repair or repair with augmentation utilizing the iliotibial band (MacIntosh, Ellison, or Andrews procedures) or biceps femoris transfer.

Author's Preferred Method

The preferred method of treatment is acute primary repair of all of the torn structures. Augmentation utilizing the iliotibial band (modified Andrews tenodesis) considered with the combination of lateral collateral and anterior cruciate ligament tears.

Surgical Technique

The lateral aspect of the knee is exposed through a utility approach under tourniquet control. Hemostasis is secured throughout the procedure. Preop-

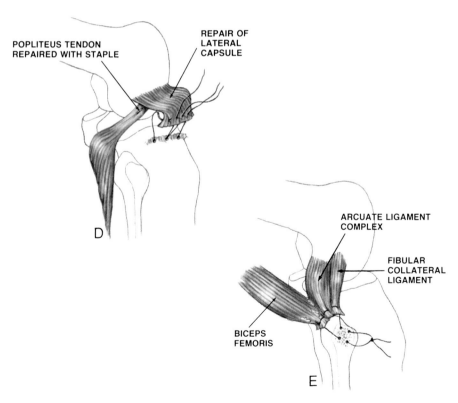

Fig. 112-3 *(Continued).* **(D)** The avulsed popliteus tendon can be reattached to the femur with a barbed staple, and the deep lateral capsule is best repaired back to the tibia with sutures passed through drill holes or Sharpey's fibers attachments. **(E)** The avulsed distal attachments of the fibular collateral ligament, arcuate ligament complex, and biceps femorus are repaired back to the fibular head with sutures passed through drill holes. *(Figure continues.)*

erative localization of points of maximum tenderness and soft tissue puffiness helps direct the surgical exposure to the structures that are disrupted (Fig. 112-3A). The iliotibial band is frequently torn near its attachment to Gerdy's tubercle. The lateral capsule is generally torn from the tibia and the lateral collateral ligament and the biceps tendon torn from the fibular head. The popliteus tendon may be avulsed from the lateral femur, and the arcuate ligament complex may be torn proximally from the femur, distally from the tibia, or anyplace in between. The posterior lateral capsule may also be torn. Careful exploration and protection of the peroneal nerve should always be carried out, particularly if there is a peroneal palsy; the nerve is usually found to be intact but edematous and hemorrhagic. Peroneal nerve function normally recovers, but it may take 12 to 18 months.

A layer-by-layer repair is carried out starting with the deepest structures. If the posterolateral capsule is torn, it is repaired with sutures that pass through drill holes made from anterior to posterior through the tibia after the method of O'Donoghue, so that when those sutures are tied anteriorly over the tibial surface, the posterior capsule is pulled back into its normal position (Fig. 112-3B,C). Every effort should be made to retain the lateral meniscus unless there is a significant tear into its substance. Any ligamentous structures that are torn from the rim of the meniscus can be repaired with direct suture.

The posterolateral stabilizing structures should be repaired next in sequence, after any defect in the posterior capsule is repaired. The popliteus tendon can be reattached to the femur with a small staple (Fig. 112-3D). The biceps femoris and fibular collateral ligament are sutured to the fibular head through drill holes (Fig. 112-3E), and the ar-

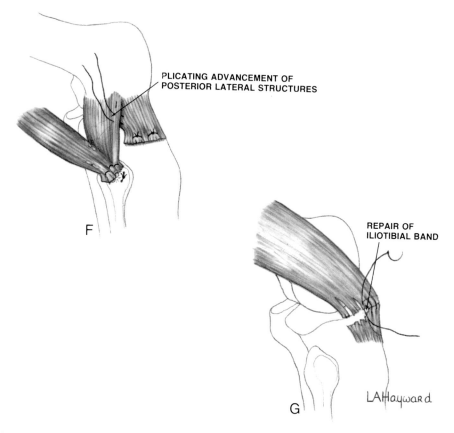

Fig. 112-3 *(Continued).* **(F)** The interval between the anterior and posterior structures is closed with plicating sutures. **(G)** The iliotibial band is repaired. (From Goldstein[7] with permission.)

cuate ligament complex is appropriately sutured. Next in sequence is repair of the deep lateral capsule, which can be attached to the tibia with sutures passed through Sharpey's fibers of the normal attachment, or through drill holes. The interval between the anterior and posterior structures can then be closed with plicating sutures (Fig. 112-3F); the iliotibial band is repaired last (Fig. 112-3G).

If the anterior or posterior cruciate ligaments are torn in conjunction with the lateral collateral ligament complex, they are repaired according to the techniques described later in this chapter. The modified Andrews iliotibial band tenodesis (described under Augmentation Procedures for the anterior cruciate ligament) would be considered for the combined lateral collateral and anterior cruciate tears.

After all structures have been repaired, the tourniquet is released and further hemostasis is secured. After thorough irrigation with saline and antibiotic solution, the wound is closed in layers over suction drainage. Prophylactic antibiotics are routinely used as described for repair of medial tears. Postoperatively the knee is immobilized in either a long-leg cast or a hinged-knee splint in 60 degrees of flexion with the tibia in neutral rotation. In the combination injury of lateral collateral and anterior or posterior cruciate ligament tears the position is 45 degrees of flexion with the tibia in neutral rotation.

Further aftercare and rehabilitation, complications, and results are discussed in separate sections later in this chapter.

ANTERIOR CRUCIATE LIGAMENT INJURIES

General Statement

Few topics are more enigmatic and controversial than acute tears of the anterior cruciate ligament. Many surgeons feel that there is no such thing as an isolated tear of the anterior cruciate ligament. Certainly the anterior cruciate ligament cannot be torn without significant interstitial damage also occur-

ring to other ligamentous structures about the knee, in particular to the secondary restraints that function along with the anterior cruciate ligament to provide stability against anterior displacement of the tibia. However, it is clinically useful to consider "isolated" tears of the anterior cruciate ligament, in which the anterior cruciate ligament is completely torn, with no associated meniscus tear and with no other ligamentous structure being completely torn. It is important to remember, though, that in most instances, anterior cruciate ligament tears are accompanied by tears of one or both menisci and also frequently occur with tears of the medial or lateral collateral ligaments.

The mechanism of injury is usually a twisting or cutting stress applied to the weight-bearing extremity in varying degrees of flexion and rotation. Nearly 50 percent of the time there is a history of contact being made against the lateral aspect of the thigh or knee. Another classically described mechanism involves internal rotation of the femur on the fixed tibia. Hyperextension and hyperflexion mechanisms can also damage the anterior cruciate ligament.

The diagnosis of acute tear of the anterior cruciate ligament is based on the typical history of a significant injury with a mechanism as described above, with the patient frequently hearing or appreciating a "pop" in the knee, followed by immediate disability because of pain and the early onset of hemarthrosis (within 2 to 6 hours) even if there has been application of ice and compression.

Physical examination will demonstrate the hemarthrosis and the lack of full extension, and often there will be posteromedial and/or posterolateral joint-line tenderness indicative of possible associated meniscus tears. Acute "isolated" tears frequently will not demonstrate a classic anterior drawer sign, and because of this the diagnosis may be missed.[5] More sophisticated tests for rotatory instability, such as the lateral pivot-shift sign[6] or the flexion-rotation drawer test,[14] are much more reliable (85 to 95 percent) but require patient relaxation, and they usually cannot be demonstrated in the acute situation because of pain and guarding. The most reliable clinical test is the Lachman sign, in which the anterior drawer maneuver is performed near full extension rather than at 90 degrees.[19] Diagnostic adjuncts of arthrography and particularly arthroscopy can be of great help in delineating the full extent of the pathology.[5,14]

Indications

There is great controversy regarding surgical treatment of acute tears of the anterior cruciate ligament. Because of tenuous vascularity, many surgeons feel that primary repair has such minimal chance of success that it should not be undertaken. Also, it has been observed that some individuals can function quite well, even in athletics, without an anterior cruciate ligament.

However, the sequelae of chronic anterior cruciate ligament insufficiency can be so devastating that increasing attention is being focused on primary treatment of the acute injury, particularly in relatively young active individuals who are placing significant demands on the knee. Other considerations include the degree of laxity and any associated injuries, such as meniscal tears and osteochondral fractures.

Treatment Options

Anterior cruciate ligament injuries can be treated nonoperatively, but if significant associated meniscus injuries have occurred, the meniscal lesions should be treated surgically, followed by a period of protection with the knee in a cast brace. This procedure permits healing of the interstitially damaged secondary restraints, which should be followed by a rehabilitation program similar to cases undergoing surgical treatment.

Surgical options include primary repair of the anterior cruciate ligament with fatpad coverage to help facilitate the vascular response, or primary repair with augmentation. Intra-articular augmentation can be performed with the patellar tendon, semitendinosus, or iliotibial band. Extra-articular static augmentation can be performed with utilization of the iliotibial band laterally or capsular plication medially, and/or dynamic augmentation can be undertaken with biceps femoris transfer laterally and pes anserinus transfer medially.

A third treatment option would be primary intra-articular reconstruction of the anterior cruciate ligament with no effort at primary repair of the ligament stump.

Author's Preferred Method

In the active young patient with an acute complete tear of the anterior cruciate ligament, I prefer to carry out anatomic repair of the anterior cruciate ligament stump back to bone whenever possible. The rationale is that this provides the only opportunity to achieve a fiber arrangement and broad attachment zone resembling the normal ligament, as contrasted with primary substitution with autogenous tissue grafting, which essentially produces a point to point rope with parallel fiber arrangement. Some type of augmentation is also carried out in addition to primary repair in every case. Augmentation procedures can be classified as static or dynamic, intraarticular or extraarticular, and high strength (initial tensile strength equal or greater than the ACL) or low strength (initial strength 50 to 75 percent ACL strength).

Anterior cruciate ligament stumps are classified into three categories: (1) a stump ideal for primary repair is of good tissue quality and more than 90 percent of the ligament is of sufficient length to be repairable back to its anatomic attachment site to bone; (2) a stump considered to be marginal for primary repair has 50 to 80 percent of the ligament of good tissue quality and repairable to bone; (3) a poor stump is a true mid-third "mop-end" disruption of the ligament. The surgical approach depends upon what type of stump is present. In cases with an ideal stump, primary repair is carried out with lateral extraarticular augmentation but no intraarticular augmentation. Cases with a marginal stump are treated with primary repair and intraarticular augmentation with a low-strength graft along with an extraarticular lateral augmentation. In cases with a poor stump, primary substitution is carried out with a high-strength intraarticular graft as well as extraarticular lateral augmentation. The ligament stumps are also used as much as possible in the procedure.

Primary Repair with Extra-articular Augmentation

The knee is exposed through an anteromedial parapatellar approach, taking care to avoid the VMO, and the patella is not dislocated. If the ligament is torn near or at the femoral attachment (the

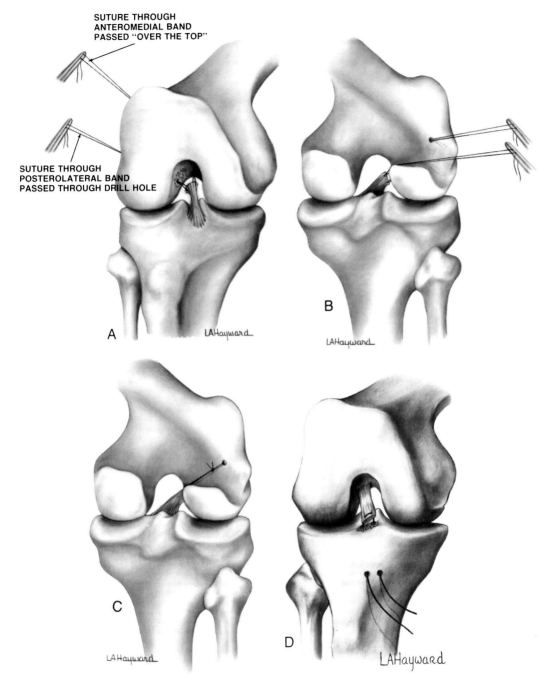

SUTURE THROUGH
ANTEROMEDIAL BAND
PASSED "OVER THE TOP"

SUTURE THROUGH
POSTEROLATERAL BAND
PASSED THROUGH DRILL HOLE

Fig. 112-4. Repair of the anterior cruciate ligament. A suture is placed in the anteromedial band and passed out through the posterior capsule adjacent to the lateral femoral condyle and "over the top," while the second suture is placed through the posterolateral portion of the ligament and passed through a drill hole in the lateral femoral condyle. The exit site for the sutures is exposed through a separate lateral incision. When the sutures are pulled tight, the anterior cruciate ligament is anatomically repositioned with a broad contact area of the femur, as seen on an anterior view **(A)** and a posterolateral view **(B)**. The repair sutures are then tied to each other over the external surface of the lateral femoral condyle **(C)**. The anterior cruciate ligament is repaired back to the tibia, with the repair suture being passed through drill holes and tied over the anterior surface of the tibia **(D)**. **(D** from Goldstein,[7] with permission).

most common situation), it is repaired with a two-suture technique: one suture is placed through the anteromedial band portion of the ligament, while a second suture is placed in the posterolateral portion of the ligament. The posterior portion of the lateral femoral condyle is freshened in the posterior lateral aspect of the intercondylar notch, with the surgeon taking care not to detach any remaining proximal fibers of anterior cruciate ligament still attached to the femur.

The lateral aspect of the knee is then exposed through a lateral utility approach if biceps femoris transfer is to be performed. If it is not, a straight lateral incision is used to expose the lateral femoral epicondylar region for passage of the repair sutures. A fiber-splitting incision is made through the iliotibial band beginning at the lateral femoral epicondyle and proceeding proximally for 6 cm. The vastus lateralis is retracted anteriorly, and the lateral intramuscular septum is followed to the linea aspera. A small hole is then carefully made in the lateral intramuscular septum at the linea aspera to provide access to the over-the-top space, as described by MacIntosh.[11]

Attention is then returned to the anteromedial exposure, and a single drill hole is placed through the posterior portion of the lateral femoral condyle to exit laterally anterior to the lateral intramuscular septum, in the area previously exposed. The suture in the anteromedial band portion of the anterior cruciate ligament is passed back through the posterior capsule and over the top of the lateral femoral condyle, as described by MacIntosh.[11] The second suture is passed through the drill hole in the lateral femoral condyle. (Fig. 112-4A,B), and the two sutures are tied together over the external surface of the lateral femur with the knee in approximately 30 degrees of flexion (Fig. 112-4C). This technique consistently repositions the anterior cruciate ligament in an anatomic position. A lobe of the fat pad is then sutured over the repaired ligament to help provide vascularity.

In the relatively few cases in which the ligament has been torn from the tibial attachment, the entire repair can be carried out through the anteromedial incision by passing two drill holes from the anterior surface of the tibia to the proximal surface in the area of the normal attachment of the anterior cruciate ligament. The repair sutures are placed in the ligament stump, passed through the drill holes (Fig. 112-4D), and tied over the anterior surface of the tibia with the anterior cruciate ligament stump pulled back into its normal position. A lobe of the fat pad is sutured to the repaired ligament to help enhance vascularity.

No intra-articular augmentation is performed, but extraarticular lateral augmentation is routinely performed. For many years, I performed dynamic lateral augmentation using anterior transfer of the superficial portion of the biceps tendon with generally satisfactory results, but more recently a static procedure similar to the iliotibial band tenodesis described by Andrews (see Ch. 113) has been performed with better early results. Treatment by primary repair and extraarticular augmentation has been suitable for approximately 15 to 20 percent of the acute ACL patients I have operated on in the past 2 years.

Extra-articular dynamic lateral augmentation can be provided by anterior transfer of the superficial portion (long head) of the biceps femoris. The biceps tendon is carefully dissected where it divides to pass superficially and deep to the fibular collateral ligament. The tendon fibers superficial to the fibular collateral ligament are carefully released from their attachment to the anterior border of the fibula. Care is taken not to disturb the fibers inserting into the posterior border of the fibular collateral ligament and deep to the fibular collateral ligament, since they help reinforce the posterolateral capsule. Once the correct plane has been established distally, the dissection is carried proximally well up into the muscle belly of the biceps femoris, with the surgeon taking care not to include the muscle fibers that ultimately insert into the fibular collateral ligament and the posterolateral capsule (Fig. 112-5A). A vertical incision is made through the origin of the anterior tibial muscle just anterior to the fibula, and a large periosteal elevator is utilized to prepare a subperiosteal bed beneath the origin of the anterior tibial muscle. The mobilized biceps tendon is then attached to the prepared anterolateral surface of the tibia by placing plicating sutures through the strong fascia adjacent to the patellar tendon that then pass beneath the anterior tibial muscle belly and, when pulled tight, bury the tendon in the prepared subperiosteal bed (Fig. 112-5B).

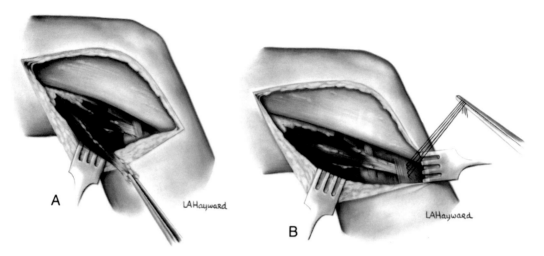

Fig. 112-5. Dynamic lateral augmentation for anterior cruciate ligament repair using the superficial portion of the biceps femorus. The superficial portion of the biceps femorus is carefully dissected and released from the fibular head **(A)**, with care taken not to disturb the deep portion of the biceps insertion. The mobilized superficial biceps is then reattached to the anterolateral surface of the tibia beneath Gerdy's tubercle **(B)**.

Primary Repair with Low-Strength Intra-articular Augmentation

When a marginal stump is encountered, it is usually the anterior portion of the ligament that is suitable for repair, with the posterior 10 to 40 percent of the ligament being torn in midsubstance. The vast majority are torn from the femur. The repairable portion of the ligament is reattached to the femur using the two-suture technique described above but is augmented by a low-strength intraarticular graft using the Puddu-Perugia semitendinosis technique.[17] The semitendinosis is detached distally with a small piece of bone, and released from its various expansions into the pes anserinus and distally into the calf to permit sufficient advancement into the wound (Fig. 112-6A). The muscle-tendon junction is not disturbed. The tendon is then passed beneath the remainder of the pes anserinus and through a 6-mm tibial tunnel that begins at the anterior border of the medial collateral ligament and exits adjacent to the middle of the ACL attachment on the tibia (Fig. 112-6B). The tendon graft then passes through the joint with the ACL stump and into the same 6-mm posterior femoral tunnel used to pass the posterior repair stitch from the ACL stump. In this way, the semitendinosis is anatomically replacing the posterior por-

tion of the ACL. In the unusual instance in which the anterior portion of the ligament is torn midsubstance and the posterior two-thirds is reparable to bone, the semitendinosis is brought into the joint at the anterior margin of the ACL attachment to the tibia and is carried over the top to replace the anterior portion of the ligament. Lateral extraarticular augmentation is also carried out by means of the Andrews iliotibial band tenodesis. Primary repair with low-strength intraarticular augmentation has been done in approximately 50 percent of acute ACL repairs that I have performed over the past 2 years.

In a patient with wide open epiphyses, where it is considered undesirable to place bone tunnels across the epiphyseal plates, the two-suture primary repair can be carried out as described and augmented by Bergfeld's "tomato stick" augmentation using a 6- to 8-mm strip of the central third of the patellar tendon taken without bone from the patella, laid over the anterior surface of the tibia, incorporated into the ACL stump, and then carried over the top (Bergfeld JA: Personal communication, 1985). This provides an augmented repair without violating either epiphyseal plate.

If augmented anterior cruciate ligament repair alone has been carried out, the knee is placed in a hinged splint with the hinges locked at 45 degrees

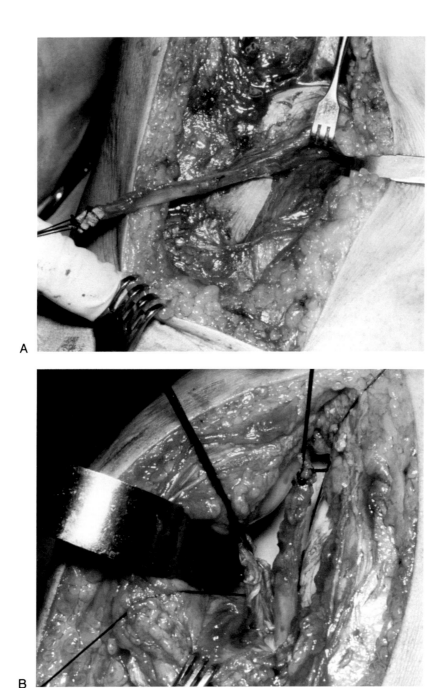

Fig. 112-6. (A). The semitendinosis has been detached from its tibial insertion with a small piece of bone, and expansions to the remainder of the pes anserinus and calf fascia are released to permit advancement into the wound. **(B.)** The semitendinosis augmentation graft has been passed through the tibial tunnel exiting just adjacent to the middle zone of ACL attachment to the tibia. The anterior ACL repair suture is pulling the ACL stump slightly anteriorly, while the lead suture for the semitendinosis is pulling it slightly posteriorly.

with the foot free. For cases with combined MCL or LCL and ACL repairs, the position is also 45 degrees flexion, with the foot free to assume neutral position.

Further aftercare and rehabilitation, complications, and results are discussed in later in this chapter.

POSTERIOR CRUCIATE LIGAMENT INJURIES

General Statement

Posterior cruciate ligament tears do not occur as frequently as anterior cruciate ligament injuries, but prompt recognition and treatment is extremely important because of the vitally important role of the posterior cruciate ligament in normal knee function. The most common mechanisms of injury for the posterior cruciate ligament are hyperextension and posterior stress applied to the proximal tibia with the knee in flexion ("dashboard knee"). The posterior cruciate ligament can also be torn by continuation of severe valgus or varus stresses in conjunction with tears of the medial or lateral collateral ligaments.

The diagnosis of posterior cruciate ligament tears in conjunction with medial or lateral collateral ligament tears is demonstrated by significant straight medial or lateral opening with the knee in full extension, as emphasized by Hughston.[7] The posterior drawer sign may not be prominent in such injuries. In isolated tears of the posterior cruciate ligament (taken in the same context as isolated tears of the anterior cruciate ligament) the posterior drawer sign is usually positive, but it is frequently misinterpreted as a positive anterior drawer sign. Occasionally, the posterior cruciate ligament will be torn from the tibia along with a piece of bone, which can be seen radiographically.

Indications

While there is a great controversy over repair of anterior cruciate ligament tears, there is very little controversy regarding the indications for primary surgical treatment of PCL tears in combination with other ligament tears such as MCL, LCL, or posterolateral. Treatment of acute "isolated" PCL tears is more controversial however, with nonoperative treatment frequently recommended for all except those associated with bone avulsion from the tibia.[1,18] But Clancy et al.[4] has documented severe medial compartment degenerative changes in some cases of untreated isolated PCL tears that occurred over a short period of time without having functional instability. There is no reliable way to identify those patients who will not do satisfactorily with nonoperative treatment of isolated PCL rupture.

Treatment Options

If nonoperative treatment is elected, protection of the interstitially damaged secondary restraints should be adequate in a hinged-knee splint with the hinges set to permit motion from 0 to 30 degrees for 6 weeks, followed by vigorous rehabilitation similar to operated cases.

For cases undergoing surgical treatment, the options are primary repair, primary repair with augmentation, and primary reconstruction without any attempt at primary repair.

Author's Preferred Method

The method of treatment I recommend is acute primary repair with augmentation for combined PCL ruptures and also for isolated tears in high-demand persons with severe laxity (3+). When more than 60 percent of the ligament can be repaired back to bone, the semitendinosis tendon is used for augmentation (Lindemann technique).[10] If less than 60 percent is suitable for repair to bone, primary substitution is carried out using a free patella tendon graft (Clancy) (see Ch. 113), which incorporates repair of as much of the PCL stump as possible. Use of the medial gastrocnemius tendon (Hughston technique — see Ch. 113) can also be considered for augmentation or substitution.

Surgical Technique

If the posterior cruciate ligament is torn from the tibia with a piece of bone, which can be recognized radiographically, the repair is carried out with the patient in the prone position; the lesion is exposed through a classic posterior approach. The bony fragment is repositioned and fixed with a screw. If there has been significant elongation of the posterior cruciate ligament, the bony fragment should not be replaced anatomically but should be fixed in a more distal position so that the posterior cruciate ligament is under adequate tension.

Posterior cruciate ligament tears without a bone fragment are exposed initially through an anteromedial approach. If the ligament is torn from its femoral attachment, direct repair can be carried out with sutures that are passed through drill holes

placed in the femoral condyle through the anterior incision and that are then tied over the external surface of the femur (Fig. 112-7A,B).

If the ligament is torn from the tibial attachment, the repair is carried out through a combined anteromedial and posteromedial approach. The ligament is delivered into the anterior incision, and repair sutures placed in the distal stump of the ligament. A standard posteromedial incision is then made and carried through the deep fascia to expose the underlying posteromedial capsule. The capsular incision is made in the soft spot just posterior to and parallel with the obliquely oriented fibers of the

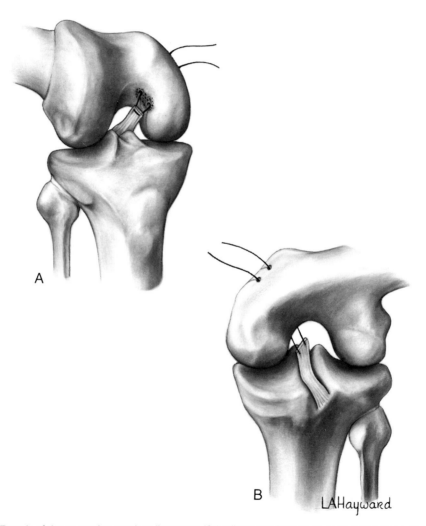

Fig. 112-7. Repair of the posterior cruciate ligament. If the ligament is torn at or near the femoral attachment, it can be repaired directly with repair sutures passed through drill holes in the medial femoral condyle **(A,B)**. *(Figure continues.)*

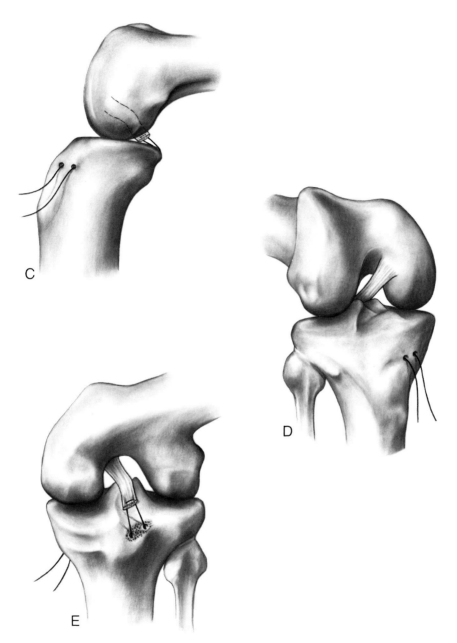

Fig. 112-7 *(Continued)*. If torn at or near the tibial attachment, the repair is made through a combined anterior medial and posterior medial approach, with the repair sutures passed from posterior to anterior through drill holes placed in the proximal tibia which exit posteriorly at the normal site of attachment of the posterior cruciate ligament **(C–E)**. (From Goldstein,[7] with permission.)

trailing edge of the medial collateral ligament (tibial arm of the posterior oblique ligament). This permits access with the tip of the finger to the posterior attachment site of the posterior cruciate ligament. This normal attachment site is on the posterior surface of the tibia just below the joint-line level. This region is freshened with a periosteal elevator and/or curette, and drill holes are placed from anterior to posterior through the tibia in such a way that they exit posteriorly at the normal attachment of the posterior cruciate ligament. The previously placed repair sutures are then passed posteriorly and brought from posterior to anterior through the drill holes, so that when they are pulled tight and tied over the anterior surface of the tibia the posterior cruciate ligament will be pulled into its normal position and brought into contact with the posterior aspect of the tibia under satisfactory tension (Fig. 112-7C–E).

If the posterior cruciate ligament is torn in its middle third, primary substitution using patella tendon free graft (Clancy) is preferred (see Ch. 113).

If the medial or lateral collateral ligament complexes or the anterior cruciate ligament has been torn in combination with the posterior cruciate ligament, primary repair of those structures should be carried out as discussed under the appropriate sections in this chapter.

Because of the difficulty in maintaining the proper position of the tibia in relation to the femur while posterior cruciate ligament tears are healing, I recommend the use of a skeletal fixation pin to prevent tibial drop-back during the first 8 to 12 weeks. In the past, a large tibial-femoral transarticular pin was used that had the disadvantage of preventing motion. More recently, the Grammont technique of olecranization of the patella has been used. Once all the repair sutures, bone tunnels, and augmentation grafts have been placed but not yet fixed, the tibia is appropriately reduced relative to the femur at 90 degrees of flexion. A heavy smooth Steinmann pin is placed from superior to inferior through the patella, passed posterior to the patella tendon, and into the tibia posterior to the tibial tubercle. This prevents tibial drop-back and permits gentle motion from 10 to 90 degrees without undue stress to the pin. Once the fixation pin has been placed and checked by intraoperative radio-

graphs, the repair sutures and augmentation grafts are secured. Just enough of the fixation pin is left protruding from the superior pole of the patella (but not through the skin) to permit removal under local anesthesia 8 to 12 weeks following surgery.

When the olecranization pin has been used, the knee is placed in a hinged-knee splint with the hinges locked at 45 degrees. Passive and gentle active motion in the hinged splint from 10 to 90 degrees is begun at 2 weeks and continued until the pin is removed. If the olecranization pin is not used, I recommend immobilization at or near the fully extended position to minimize the tendency for tibial drop-back. Prophylactic antibiotics are routinely used.

Further aftercare, rehabilitation, complications, and results are discussed under separate sections later in this chapter.

DISLOCATION OF THE KNEE

General Statement

Dislocation of the knee represents a special type of ligamentous injury, usually accompanied by more severe and multiple ligamentous injuries to the knee and frequently associated neurovascular injury, particularly to the popliteal artery and the common peroneal nerve.

The clinical diagnosis is usually obvious from the marked deformity; it is confirmed by routine roentgenograms. Classification is based on the position of the tibia in relation to the femur, with five basic categories: medial, lateral, anterior, posterior, and rotatory. The rotatory category is further subdivided into anteromedial, posteromedial, anterolateral, and posterolateral. In general, at least two or more major ligamentous structures will be torn with any dislocation. However, assessment of the ligamentous damage should be made only after the dislocation has been reduced, since attempts to examine for ligament integrity with the knee in the dislocated position will be misleading.

Often knee dislocations will spontaneously reduce and will have a deceptively benign appearance, since there will be no deformity and radiographs may be negative. However, if there is significant medial or lateral laxity when testing is done with the knee in full extension, the collateral ligament complex, both cruciates, and a portion of the posterior capsule have been torn; this situation must be considered to represent a dislocation with spontaneous reduction.

Of critical importance in assessment of any dislocation of the knee (whether spontaneous reduction has occurred or not) is careful evaluation of the neurovascular status. The reported incidence of vascular injury accompanying dislocation of the knee is 30 to 50 percent. The most frequently reported lesion is intimal damage to the popliteal artery, and the findings initially may be very subtle. One cannot be content with a warm, pink foot with adequate capillary refill and palpable dorsalis pedis and posterior tibial pulse, since all of these findings can be present in the presence of a significant popliteal artery injury. The key to the diagnosis is that the distal pulses in the suspect limb normally are equal to those of the opposite side; any diminution in the differential pulse pressure indicates probable damage to the popliteal artery, and oscillometry and/or arteriography are indicated. Vascular surgery consultation is advisable. Failure to recognize and treat injury to the popliteal artery is associated with devastating complications, including the necessity of amputation. Careful clinical evaluation for associated neurologic injury to rule out damage to the peroneal or posterior tibial nerves must be done.

Indications

Dislocation of the knee is a orthopaedic emergency. The essential priorities are as follows. First, the dislocation must be reduced, which may relieve neurovascular compromise; second, if it is a compound dislocation, prompt debridement and reduction in the operating room is indicated; third, when there has been damage to the popliteal artery, prompt vascular repair is essential in an effort to preserve the limb. While routine arteriography should not be considered mandatory, it also cannot be criticized. My preference is to first perform oscillometry (Doppler); if there is any diminution of the pulse pressure compared to the other limb, then proceed with arteriography without delay.

If the dislocation is not compound and if there is no vascular compromise, closed reduction followed by close observation in the hospital for several days is indicated to be certain that vascular compromise does not ensue from subintimal damage causing gradual occlusion. If this does not occur, then repair of the torn ligaments is indicated as discussed in the appropriate sections of this chapter. At surgical repair, any involved nerve should be explored to be certain that it has not been completely divided. The usual finding is that the nerve is in continuity but is edematous and hemorrhagic.

Contraindications

Only the most desperate life-threatening situation would override the priority indications of reduction of the dislocation, debridement of the open wound, and repair of vascular injury. Repair of the ligamentous injuries per se should not be carried out if the face of life-threatening associated injuries or with an open dislocation. With successful repair of the vascular injury, an individual judgment will have to be made regarding advisability of attempting ligamentous repair at the same time. Even when acute surgical treatment of the ligament injuries is not considered appropriate, use of the olecranization pin (as described in conjunction with PCL repair) to prevent tibial drop-back greatly facilitates nonoperative management of the ligament injuries.

Treatment Options

The options regarding treatment of the ligamentous injuries are nonoperative treatment in a cast or cast brace (following reduction of the dislocation) for 6 to 8 weeks, followed by a rehabilitation program, or surgical repair of the torn ligaments as either primary, delayed primary, or late reconstruction.

Author's Preferred Method

In a closed injury in which vascular compromise has not occurred or in which it has been adequately repaired, primary or delayed primary repair of all torn ligaments is recommended. The techniques are the same as those described for individual ligaments in this chapter. For compound dislocations, initial debridement is carried out without ligamentous repair, which can then be considered 1 to 2 weeks later if there is no evidence of active sepsis.

When vascular or other overriding associated injuries make primary or delayed primary repair of the torn ligaments inadvisable, nonoperative treatment is carried out with the expectation that late reconstructive procedures will be performed if residual laxity and functional instability are present. Use of the olecranization pin (as described in the PCL section) can be considered to prevent tibial drop-back and permit early motion for nonoperative as well as operative cases.

The details of surgical technique, aftercare, rehabilitation, complications, and results are discussed in separate sections of this chapter.

AFTERCARE OF ACUTE LIGAMENT INJURIES

General Considerations

There are time constraints to ligament healing; they are not documented for man, but according to primate studies by Noyes[13] and Clancy et al.[3] it is reasonable to project that maximum tensile strength in a healed ligament does not occur until 9 to 12 months following the injury. At the same time, it is known that joint motion is necessary for normal nutrition of articular cartilage and that active joint function helps decrease muscle atrophy and stimulate collagen healing in laboratory animals.

The following aftercare program allows as much function as possible for the benefit of the articular cartilage and muscles and the stimulation of collagen healing, yet attempts to avoid mechanical overloads to the healing ligaments that could compromise ultimate stability.

Postoperative Protection

For the first 1 to 2 weeks after surgery, the knee is held in a hinged-knee splint with the hinges locked at 45 degrees, except for isolated PCL cases in which the olecranization pin has not been used. For these cases, the hinges are locked at 0 degrees. Tibial rotation is not fixed but is permitted to assume its neutral position. "Global" isometric exercises are carried out, with the quadriceps and hamstrings contracted at the same time. Once muscular control of the leg has been demonstrated, the patient is allowed to ambulate on crutches with no more than touchdown weight bearing.

Approximately 1 to 2 weeks following surgery the hinges on the splint are adjusted to permit limited motion. Collateral ligament cases without cruciate involvement are started on active motion between 20 and 90 degrees. For cases involving ACL surgery, active motion is begun from 45 to 90 degrees along with intermittent passive extension. Following PCL surgery the routine is active motion from 0 to 30 degrees with intermittent passive flexion.

Eight weeks following surgery the hinged splint is removed and a protective brace is applied. Prefabricated noncustom braces are selected since custom-molded braces fitted at this time would be unlikely to fit properly later when optimal fit is more important. If there is any tendency toward distal swelling below the brace, a shortleg elastic stocking is worn. The brace is worn at all times the patient is ambulating (even with crutches) but is removed for sleeping, bathing, and at other times during quiet sitting, to give the skin a rest. Ambulation is continued on crutches with touch-down weight bearing but with every effort to achieve a normal gait pattern. Once crutches have been discontinued, the brace is worn for all ambulation until 4 to 5 months following surgery.

Rehabilitation Program

The rehabilitation program is divided into an early phase, from the time of surgery through the first 16 weeks, an intermediate phase, from 16 weeks through 24 weeks, and an advanced phase, from 6 months through 12 months following surgery.

Early Phase

From the day of surgery through the first 8 weeks, the patient walks on crutches with touchdown weight bearing and does isometric exercises. If the anterior cruciate ligament has been involved in the injury, the isometrics are global, so that the quadriceps and hamstrings are contracted simultaneously. Straight-leg exercises are performed in the splint unless anterior cruciate ligament repair has been carried out. General exercises for the opposite leg and upper body are carried out. Limited motion is begun at 1 to 2 weeks as outlined above.

Between 8 and 12 weeks following surgery, the hinged splint is discontinued and a noncustom brace applied. More vigorous active range-of-motion exercises are initiated. Patient-controlled passive exercises emphasizing flexion and extension are started. Progressive-resistance exercises (PRE) are also initiated at this time. The general guidelines are that the patient do these exercises one leg at a time, three sets of 10 repetitions, once daily, using an exercise machine or weight boot, with stretching exercises for individual muscle groups before and after the exercises. The basic program uses isotonic or variable resistance quadriceps, hamstring, and hip-abduction exercises.

Several important modifications are made for specific injuries. For ACL cases, quadriceps PRE are limited to the arc from 90 to 45 degrees for the first six months following surgery. Whenever this routine causes patellofemoral pain, it is further modified to an isometric technique at 45 degrees flexion. Another specific modification is for PCL cases, in which quadriceps PRE are performed between 30 degrees and full extension, and hamstring PRE is avoided altogether during the early phase of rehabilitation. For combined ACL/PCL cases, isometric quadriceps PRE are performed at the 45-degree position. These modifications are to prevent potentially deleterious stresses to healing tissues from forceful quadriceps contraction between 0 and 30 degrees (anterior stress) and hamstring contraction and/or quadriceps contraction at flexion angles greater than 60 degrees (posterior stress).

Weight bearing progresses gradually according to the level of quadriceps strength. Minimal weight bearing is permitted until the patient is lifting 4.5 kg (10 pounds). For 4.5 to 7 kg (10 to 15 pounds) of lifting strength, weight bearing is increased to 75 percent as tolerated within the limits of pain. Once the patient is lifting 7 kg (15 pounds), full weight bearing is permitted, but the patient continues to ambulate in the knee brace.

From 12 to 16 weeks following surgery, the progressive-resistance exercises and range-of-motion exercises are continued and the patient continues ambulating in the brace. General conditioning is begun with swimming and the use of a stationary bicycle or rowing machine.

Intermediate Phase

After 4 months, it usually is no longer necessary for the patient to ambulate in the brace. A graduated running program is initiated at approximately 5 months if there is a nearly full range of motion, pain-free ambulation without effusion, and a minimum of 13.5 kg (30 pounds) strength with the quadriceps progressive-resistance exercises. The general guidelines for the running program are that it be disciplined, with straight-ahead running only and emphasizing form. No hard starts, stops, or "cutting" maneuvers (sudden changes of direction) are permitted, and no other running or jumping activities are to be performed. The knee brace is worn during running workouts. The running program progresses according to the strength level in the quadriceps progressive-resistance exercise program. The general guidelines for athletes are as follows: 13.5 kg (30 pounds), jogging; 18 kg (40 pounds), half-speed running; 22.5 kg (50 pounds), three-quarters-speed running; and 27 kg (60 pounds), full-speed running. These figures can be adjusted up or down depending on individual size and functional demands. General conditioning is continued with swimming, stationary-bicycle exercising, and regular cycling.

Advanced Phase

If the graduated running program described above has been successfully completed, the patient is now permitted to add starts and stops, right and left cutting maneuvers, figure-eight running (continuing to wear the brace for all running activities). These activities are all initiated at half speed but gradually progress to three-quarters and then full speed. Once the patient can successfully execute all of these activities, jumping activities are added.

Competitive Athletics

After the patient has regained the ability to sprint, start and stop, cut, and jump, normal preparticipation drills and activities for return to competitive athletics can be carried out during the remainder of the time up to 12 months following surgery. At 12 months, if the patient is functionally capable and has met or surpassed all of the functional criteria, return to competitive contact and jumping sports is permitted. Continued use of the brace for these activities is encouraged.

If the patient is a nonathlete or a recreational athlete, there is no change in the early care through the time of ambulation without crutches. The progressive-resistance exercises, however, are carried on only to the 13.5-kg (30-pound) level for nonathletes and to the 13.5- to 27.5-kg (30- to 50-pound) level for recreational athletes depending on the level of demand. However, the overall time constraints for return to vigorous activity remain the same.

COMPLICATIONS

While many complications can occur in association with surgery to repair ligamentous injuries to the knee, careful attention to detail by the surgeon can prevent or minimize these complications, and early recognition and management of complications that do occur will help minimize the sequelae.

Sepsis

Deep infection can jeopardize both the repair and the articular cartilage of the joint. Infection is best prevented by a combination of sound surgical technique and prophylactic antibiotics. Factors of

surgical technique that deserve emphasis include (1) avoiding operation through an area of skin abrasion or superficial infection, (2) anatomic exposure along recognized tissue planes, (3) avoiding prolonged operating time, and (4) frequent irrigation of the surgical wound with saline and antibiotic solutions.

I recommend routine use of prophylactic systemic antibiotics. Effective tissue levels of antibiotics should be present prior to the inflation of the pneumatic tourniquet. My recommended regimen is 1 gram of a cephalosporin as an intravenous push at the time of induction of anesthesia (well before inflation of the tourniquet) followed by another 1 gram in the intravenous solution once the tourniquet is released. Antibiotic coverage is continued by 1 gram intravenously every 6 hours for the first 24–48 hours postoperatively. If there is a history of sensitivity to penicillin or the cephalosporins, I recommend that clindamycin be used, 300 mg every 8 hours for the first 24 to 48 hours, postoperatively.

The patient should be monitored very closely during the postoperative period for any signs of temperature elevation and/or inordinate pain in the incisional area. If sepsis does develop, aggressive early diagnosis and treatment will minimize its impact on the overall result. If there is any question, the wound should be inspected; if there is erythema, warmth, swelling, and/or undue tenderness, the skin sutures should be removed so that specimens can be obtained for adequate culture and sensitivity tests, and drainage should be initiated. Adequate local wound care plus administration of appropriate antibiotics should suffice for a superficial wound infection. If deep infection is present, wide incision of the wound for irrigation and debridement in the operating room is recommended, including intraarticular drainage and irrigation, followed by loose closure of the wound over suction-irrigation tubes for 48 to 72 hours.

Thromboembolic Complications

Major ligamentous repair in otherwise healthy individuals seems to be associated with a low incidence of deep venous thrombosis, clinically evident thrombophlebitis, or pulmonary embolism.

However, it must be emphasized that adequate incidence studies have not been carried out, and the incidence of deep venous thrombosis may be much higher than is clinically appreciated. Certainly, cases of deep venous thrombosis and/or pulmonary embolism are encountered in healthy young individuals; if this type of surgery is being carried out on older patients or those with previous history of thromboembolic disease, the risk becomes much greater.

No prophylactic measures are employed for routine procedures performed on young healthy patients. If there is a positive history or other indication of increased risk of thromboembolic disease, prophylaxis with warfarin is carried out as described in the chapter on thromboembolism (see Ch. 5).

The surgeon needs a high index of suspicion to make prompt diagnosis of thrombophlebitis or pulmonary embolism. The measures for clinical detection and management of these entities are discussed elsewhere in this book.

Vascular Complications

Significant vascular complications in the involved extremity can occur from unrecognized trauma associated with the primary injury, from inadvertent surgical trauma, or from compressive vascular compromise due to postoperative circumferential casts or dressings. As discussed under Dislocations, significant vascular trauma must be suspected with any recognized dislocation and with any combination injury involving either of the collateral ligaments and both cruciate ligaments. Vascular evaluation, including arteriography, is recommended if there is any suspicion of associated vascular injury.

Inadvertent surgical trauma to the posterior neurovascular structures should be avoidable under most circumstances, but it has been reported. Thus it must be recognized if it occurs, and appropriate repair must be carried out to avoid the grim sequelae of a ischemic lower extremity.

Circumferential casts or tight compressive dressings must be utilized with great caution to prevent compressive vascular occlusion to the extremity. Releasing the tourniquet to obtain hemo-stasis prior to closure will help minimize this complication, but the patient must be monitored closely for evidence of vascular compression. Monitor color, temperature and sensation in the toes, along with the patient's ability to actively and passively flex and extend the toes without undue pain. Inordinate postoperative pain is a symptom of excessive compression by a circumferential cast or dressing, even if the neurovascular status of the toes seems adequate. Early splitting of the cast or compressive dressing all the way to the skin is recommended if there is any question that vascular compromise may be developing because of compressive forces.

Neurologic Complications

Like vascular complications, neurologic complications can stem from unrecognized trauma at the time of the initial injury (particularly of the peroneal nerve), surgical trauma, or compressive neuropathy from circumferential casts or dressings or from direct pressure. Careful evaluation of the patient's motor and sensory status should be carried out as part of the initial evaluation of the injury preoperatively, and motor and sensory status must be closely monitored postoperatively.

Limitation of Motion

Significant limitation of either extension or flexion following repair of ligamentous injuries to the knee will seriously compromise the functional result. Recognition of limited motion is no problem; prevention and management are the key issues.

An anatomic repair that is isometric throughout a full range of motion is the first step in preventing the complication of limited motion. Early initiation of active and passive motion (within the limits imposed by specific procedures) utilizing commercially available hinged splints has proven to be helpful adjunct to the patient's regaining functional motion in the early postoperative period. During the rehabilitation program, particularly during the early and intermediate phases, the range of motion should be closely followed and measured to ensure that the patient is making progress in regaining both extension and flexion.

The goal for return of extension is always neutral extension (0 degrees). While lack of 5 degrees (or even up to 10 degrees) is often compatible with a good functional result, it is not desirable because of increased compressive forces imposed upon the articular surfaces. An extension deficit of more than 10 degrees is even more of a complication because it causes the patient to limp when walking, and also becomes disabling for running activities as well. Stability is usually not a problem for patients lacking full extension, but they are predictably very unhappy with their result if the deficit is 10 degrees or greater.

Prompt return of full extension or even hyperextension with minimal effort and within the first 3 months following surgery usually is a poor prognostic sign as it is frequently associated with residual laxity. The more desired and usual course is that the amount of extension (and flexion to be discussed below) to be regained is not fully realized until 4 to 6 months postoperatively, and sometimes even longer.

Similarly, rapid return of full flexion soon after termination of the postoperative immobilization also is generally associated with residual laxity. A slight limitation of full flexion seldom causes any significant functional disability. Flexion also should be gradually regained with a certain amount of effort 4 to 6 months (and occasionally longer) postoperatively. Adequacy of return of flexion should always be determined by the measured flexion in the opposite (and, it is hoped, normal) knee, since there is such a wide variation in normal flexion from patient to patient. For one patient, 125 degrees may be full flexion, while 145 degrees is a significant limitation for someone who flexes to 165 degrees. Severe limitation of flexion results in significant disability for activities of daily living, and limitations of greater than 5 degrees are associated with decreased running speed for athletes.

The key to avoiding significant limitations of either extension or flexion in the patient is institution of carefully controlled (by the patient) passive stretching exercises in the early postoperative period (1 to 16 weeks), when the adhesions are relatively soft and can be stretched relatively easily. It is essential that the patient be followed at frequent intervals during this important period and that the range of motion be measured with a goniometer so

that the surgeon can be certain that it is increasing. As long as it is increasing satisfactorily, nothing but continued effort of the same type should be necessary to ensure that the patient regains adequate range of motion. However, if the patient tends to reach a plateau and stops progressing, additional measures, such as daily supervised physical therapy or dynamic splints or even serial casting or gentle manipulation under anesthesia should be considered early (4 to 6 months) rather than later. As time progresses, the adhesions become stronger and increased motion becomes impossible to achieve or requires forceful manipulation under anesthesia which risks further complications — rupture of the ligamentous repair or of the extensor mechanism or intraarticular or periarticular fracture.

The causes of arthrofibrosis remain obscure, but in my experience there is a significant risk when acute ligament surgery that includes intraarticular work is carried out in patients over the age of 25. For these patients, the indications for surgical intervention should be carefully considered, and aggressive early motion instituted. While I do not routinely use continuous passive motion for ligament surgery, it is begun 48 hours postoperatively whenever acute ligament surgery is performed on patients over 35, followed by active and passive motion in the hinged splint. It is not yet known whether this will decrease the incidence of arthrofibrosis in these patients, but early results are encouraging. Reflex sympathetic dystrophy is also associated with increased risk of arthrofibrosis.

Reflex Sympathetic Dystrophy

Reflex sympathetic dystrophy (RSD) or reflex sympathetic imbalance (RSI) (cases with incomplete expression of the syndrome) can be another serious complication of the injury and/or surgical treatment. The key to recognition is inordinate postoperative pain that is found not to be due to neurovascular compression, sepsis or thromboembolism. Acute RSD or RSI is also usually associated with hypersensitivity to even light touch and cool or cold temperature of the extremity. Aggressive early treatment with prolonged lumbar sympathetic blockade achieved by constant infusion through an epidural catheter for 3 to 5 days is preferred. Concomitant pain control with analgesics, TENS, and use of CPM is also recommended.

For subacute or chronic RSD or RSI, clinical suspicion should be confirmed by a trial outpatient sympathetic block. A positive response will confirm the diagnosis and may also be therapeutic by temporarily breaking the cycle of sympathetic overactivity, permitting more conventional physiotherapy to succeed. Brief improvement with relapse should be managed with prolonged blockade as an inpatient followed by the other measures.

Residual Laxity and Instability

Residual laxity with functional instability is a disappointing complication of primary repair of ligamentous injuries of the knee. Several factors can have a negative influence on the ultimate result. Certainly the nature and extent of injury and the presence of associated injuries are important factors. A shredded joint-line tear of the medial collateral ligament, especially when associated with anterior and/or posterior cruciate ligament tears, does not have the same prognosis as a tear of the collateral ligament at or near its bony attachment with the cruciate ligaments intact. The importance of an adequate repair is obvious, and careful preoperative examination for all of the various types of ligamentous laxity as well as careful and thorough surgical exploration are necessary to recognize and therefore repair all areas of significant damage. The timing of the repair can also affect the ultimate result; the basic principle is the earlier the better, and repair should be carried out within the first 72 hours of injury if at all possible. The upper limits for adequate repair is approximately 7 days for collateral ligaments and 3 weeks for cruciate ligaments.

When the ligamentous tissues have been severely attenuated or damaged, making primary repair tenuous, augmentation should be carried out; the lack of appropriate augmentation can compromise the ultimate result. Inadequate rehabilitation of the injured extremity can significantly jeopardize the functional result of an otherwise optimal repair. Deep sepsis can be associated with residual laxity of the repaired ligaments.

Recognition and management of residual laxity with functional instability is the subject of Chapter 113.

RESULTS

It has been recommended by Hughston[9] and others that results of ligamentous as well as other types of surgery of the knee be analyzed according to subjective and objective criteria. Among important subjective parameters are pain, swelling, stiffness, giving way, and assessment of knee function in stressful activities including running, cutting maneuvers, and jumping. Among important objective parameters are range of motion, muscular strength, effusion, localized tenderness, stability, and degenerative articular changes. Whenever results have been analyzed according to these criteria, the subjective results are invariably superior to the objective results.

The ultimate result of functional stability with no more than mild discomfort, a functional range of motion, and no more than 1 + laxity (on a 4 + scale) should be anticipated for medial and lateral collateral ligament repairs 90 percent of the time. For anterior cruciate ligament tears, objective stability of negative to 1 + for the Lachman, anterior drawer, and anteromedial rotatory instability tests as well as negative to trace + lateral pivot shift represent a satisfactory result and should be expected in 85 percent of cases. Posterior cruciate ligament tears frequently end up with static laxity to anteroposterior testing in the 1 to 2 + range, which is usually a combination of anterior and posterior displacement, but with hard, firm endpoints. An anteroposterior displacement of zero to trace with the tibia in internal rotation is a consistent and important difference between repaired and unrepaired posterior cruciate ligament tears. Functional stability without subsequent development of meniscus tears or increasing laxity is also consistent with a satisfactory primary repair even with the mild residual laxity as described above. Various combined injuries yield results that obviously are related to the number of structures damaged and to the severity of damage.

In general, the results of primary repair of ligamentous injury to the knee are superior to the results of late reconstruction. The reasons for this superiority include the fact that one has the opportunity to restore the anatomy of the torn ligament or ligaments and to do so at a time when the articular surfaces are still intact, when those secondary restraints that have not been completely torn may not be significantly stretched or attenuated,[2] and when, one hopes, the menisci either are still intact or are torn in such a way that they can be repaired and retained. By contrast, at the time of ligamentous reconstruction the secondary restraints have usually been stretched, one or both menisci may well be torn, and degenerative articular changes are usually present. Accordingly, the patient's best chance of ending up with as normal a knee as possible is for the surgeon to repair the acutely injured knee unless there are existing contraindications.

REFERENCES

1. Bergfeld JA, Parolie J: Non-operative treatment of isolated PCL injuries in the athlete. Am J Sports Med (14)1:35, 1986
2. Butler DE, Noyes FR, Grood ES: Ligamentous restraints to anterior-posterior drawer in the human knee: A biomechanical study. J Bone Surg 62A:259, 1980
3. Clancy WG, Jr, Narechania RG, Rosenberg TD, et al: Anterior and posterior cruciate ligament reconstruction in rhesus monkeys. A histological, microangiographic and biomechanical analysis. J Bone Joint Surg 63A:1270, 1981
4. Clancy WG Jr, Shelbourne KD, Zoellner GB, et al: Treatment of knee joint instability secondary to rupture of the posterior cruciate ligament. Report of a new procedure. J Bone Joint Surg 65A:310, 1983
5. DeHaven KE: Diagnosis of acute knee injuries with hemarthrosis. Am J Sports Med 8:9, 1980
6. Galway RD, Beauprey A, MacIntosh DL: Pivot shift: a clinical sign of anterior cruciate ligament insufficiency. J Bone Joint Surg 54B:763, 1972
7. Goldstein LA, Dickerson RC: Atlas of Orthopaedic Surgery. 2nd Ed. CV Mosby, St. Louis, 1981
8. Hughston JC, Andrews JR, Cross MJ, et al: Classification of knee ligament instabilities. I. The medial compartment and cruciate ligaments. J Bone Joint Surg 58A:159, 1976
9. Indelicato PA: Non-operative treatment of complete tears of the medial collateral ligament of the knee. J Bone Joint Surg 65A:322, 1983
10. Lindemann K: Uber Der Platischer Ersatz Der Kreuzbander Durch Gestielte Schnenver Pflanzung. Z Orthop 79:316, 1950
11. MacIntosh DL, Tregunning RJ: A follow-up study of "over-the-top" repair of acute tears of the anterior cruciate ligament. J Bone Joint Surg 59B:511, 1976
12. Marshall JL, Warren RF, Wickiewicz TL, et al: The anterior cruciate ligament: a technique of repair and reconstruction. Clin Orthop 143:97, 1979
13. Noyes FR: Functional properties of knee ligaments and alterations induced by immobilization. A correlative biomechanical and histological study in primates. Clin Orthop 123:210, 1977
14. Noyes FR, Bassett RW, Grood ES, et al: Arthroscopy in acute traumatic hemarthrosis of the knee. Incidence of anterior cruciate tears and other injuries. J Bone Joint Surg 62A:687, 1980
15. O'Donoghue DH: Surgical treatment of fresh injuries. J Bone Joint Surg 32A:721, 1950
16. O'Donoghue DH: An analysis of end results of surgical treatment of major injuries to the ligaments of the knee. J Bone Joint Surg 37A:1, 1955
17. Perugia L, Puddu G, Mariani PP, Ferretti A: Atlante Di Chirugia Ortopedica. Vol. 2: La Ricostruzione Del Legamento Crociato Anteriore Con 1 Tendini Del Semitendinoso E Del Gracile. Pfizer Italiana S.p.A., Rome, 1985
18. Torg J, Barton T, Das M: Posterior cruciate insufficiency. A review of the literature. Sports Med 1:419, 1984
19. Torg JS, Conrad W, Kalen V: Clinical diagnosis of anterior cruciate ligament instability in the athlete. Am J Sports Med 4:84, 1976

Knee Ligament Reconstruction 113

William C. Allen
Jan Eric Henstorf

Knee ligament instability is defined as an abnormal rotational and/or translational movement of the tibial plateaus in relationship to the femoral condyles, occurring about one or more axes or in one or more planes of motion and resulting in a functional deficit. The key to evaluation and treatment of ligament instability is interpretation of the term *functional deficit*. Although two patients may have essentially the same degree of ligament instability, the functional impairment in each case is not necessarily the same because of different demands placed on the knee by each individual. Therefore, the plan for treatment in each case may be totally different.

Stability is provided by a combination of static and dynamic forces working together harmoniously. Static support is a function of the ligaments, capsule, menisci, and bony contour of the joint, while dynamic support is a function of the surrounding musculature and the stability provided by the forces of compression during weight bearing. Knee stability, even with normal ligaments, is at best a rather tenuous situation without the dynamic support of the various muscles of the thigh and calf that protect the static elements. Static structures define the limits of motion, while the musculotendinous units control motion through voluntary and kinesthetic mechanisms, creating appropriate motion and simultaneously serving as an energy-absorbing mechanism for extrinsic and intrinsic forces that might otherwise injure the static structures.

The capsule and ligaments surrounding the knee joint form a flexible dynamic cup embracing the femoral condyles, providing not only stability in the frontal and sagittal planes but rotational stability in the horizontal plane as well. The collagen fibers of the capsule and ligaments have a tendency to assume a triangular or V-shaped configuration.[91] Examples are the oblique popliteal ligament of the posterior capsule, the popliteal tendon, and the tibiocollateral ligament with the associated posterior oblique ligament and deep capsular ligament. A triangular configuration of collagen fibers provides the knee with rotational stability because some fibers are always oriented in a direction opposite to the direction of rotation.

The knee joint is the largest, most complex joint

in the human body. Although its location permits easy access for examination, the diagnosis of various knee problems is often quite difficult. The proper evaluation of knee problems depends on (1) a thorough understanding of functional anatomy, (2) a systematic and orderly examination, and (3) an understanding of the various pathologic entities that may affect the joint. This chapter deals with the various types of knee chronic ligament instabilities and the approaches to treatment.

6. Densely scarred lax ligaments are better tightened by reattaching them to bone in lieu of ligament-reefing procedures.
7. The menisci should be spared when possible. Partial meniscectomy, when feasible, is preferable to total meniscectomy.[57,115]
8. Reconstructed ligaments must have an adequate period of time for healing and require 8 to 12 months of protection to prevent subsequent stretching from repetitive overloading.[38,39,98,103]

GENERAL PRINCIPLES

Certain general principles have proved efficacious when applied to both acute ligament repair (within 2 weeks of injury) and reconstructive procedures (2 months or longer after injury):

1. Prognostically, acute ligament repair usually provides the best result,[107,110,112] although techniques developed more recently have enhanced the prognosis for reconstructive procedures.
2. Correct diagnosis of the type of instability is essential for selecting the proper surgical procedure.
3. An isolated ligament injury probably does not exist in the knee because of the involved interdependence of the ligaments. Initially, an acute injury may appear to be limited to one structure, when, in fact, other structures are also involved subclinically, either acutely, with interstitial damage that is not readily apparent, or secondarily, deteriorating from repetitive forces applied to either a normal ligament or a previously damaged one.[64]
4. Repositioning of appropriate musculotendinous units can provide dynamic reinforcement to prevent overloading of repaired or reconstructed static structures.[20,71,105,114,122,124,125,133]
5. Restoration of normal joint kinematics and ligament strength is the goal of knee ligament surgery. The possibility of creating abnormal joint kinematics or excessive force within the ligaments must be considered when techniques for reconstruction involve repositioning of the ligament insertion sites.[9]

INDICATIONS

The primary indication for knee ligament reconstruction is a significant functional disability due to instability. Reconstructive procedures are usually reserved for younger, more vigorous patients who are totally dissatisfied with the restrictions placed on their activity level. Generally, a decision to proceed with surgery should be preceded by a course of conservative treatment with a minimum period of 3 months for muscle rehabilitation and a trial of functional bracing. If conservative means fail, surgical reconstruction may be considered, but the patient should be informed that knee function will never be 100 percent normal. Even if the results following reconstruction are quite good, the patient must always exercise caution, particularly under strenuous conditions in which he or she does not have absolute control of knee function, such as contact sports or heavy labor on rough, uneven surfaces. We personally encourage patients postoperatively to continue wearing a brace during vigorous activity, even though during their normal activities they do not demonstrate or experience any sign of functional ligament instability.

The efficacy of reconstructive ligamentous surgery as a prophylaxis against late degenerative changes is as yet unclear.[29,31,40,68,69,80,81,86] It is not, in our opinion, an indication for surgery. Although animal experimentation has demonstrated that ligamentous laxity will lead to early degenerative changes, as suggested by most retrospective studies, this has not been a consistent finding in clinical practice. Many knees that are structurally stable exhibit considerable degenerative changes, while others with various degrees of laxity hold up surprisingly well. Many variables exist, such as the damage to the articular cartilage at the time of the original injury, the stress and use to which the knee is put, and the immeasurable constitution factors that determine an individual's joint wear.

CONTRAINDICATIONS

Knee ligament reconstructions should not be performed in patients who (1) do not have a significant functional handicap; (2) can be managed by conservative means (functional bracing, muscle rehabilitation, or an acceptable change in life-style); or (3) are not willing to follow the rigid postoperative rehabilitation routine required. Careful consideration must be given to those who have had previous wound infections, multiple knee surgeries, or thrombophlebitis or to those who have significant degenerative joint changes. Age and general health are additional considerations. If the patient is unwilling to accept the uncertainty of the long-term results, surgery should not be contemplated.

CLASSIFICATION OF KNEE INSTABILITIES

The success of any operation depends on an accurate diagnosis. Because of the interplay of all the supporting structures of the knee and their contributions as both primary and secondary stabilizers, degrees of combined instabilities exist in the knee in most situations. A complete understanding of the variety of chronic instabilities occurring in the knee is therefore both desirable and practical for the clinical evaluation and determination of treatment.

The classification of ligament instability is divided into one-plane, rotatory, and combined instabilities.[22,48,49,61,93] The classification relates to the abnormal translation of the tibia on the femur, which impairs the functional use of the knee.

One-Plane Instability

There are four types of one-plane (or straight) instability that involve no rotation of the tibia with respect to the femur.

Medial Instability

Medial instability in full extension usually involves laxity of the deep capsular ligament, the posterior oblique ligament, the tibial collateral ligament, the medial half of the posterior capsule, often the anterior cruciate, and/or occasionally the posterior cruciate ligament (Fig. 113-1); instability in full extension denotes a serious laxity

Medial instability in 30 degrees of flexion usually implies laxity of the tibial collateral ligament, the posterior oblique ligament, and the deep capsular ligament

Lateral Instability

Lateral instability in full extension is caused by tears of the fibular collateral ligament, the arcuate complex, the posterolateral capsule, the posterior cruciate ligament, and occasionally the anterior cruciate (Fig. 113-2); again, instability in full extension implies a serious laxity

Lateral instability in 30 degrees of flexion relaxes the cruciates and the posterior lateral capsule and suggests instability in the collateral ligament system

Posterior Instability

This type of instability occurs when the posterior cruciate is torn, and there is laxity or a tear of both the posterior oblique ligament and the arcuate complex (Fig. 113-3). It is manifested by a positive posterior drawer test in which both tibial condyles subluxate posteriorly an equal amount with no rotation.

Anterior Instability

This type of instability occurs when the anterior cruciate ligament is torn (Fig. 113-4). It is demonstrated by a positive anterior drawer sign in which

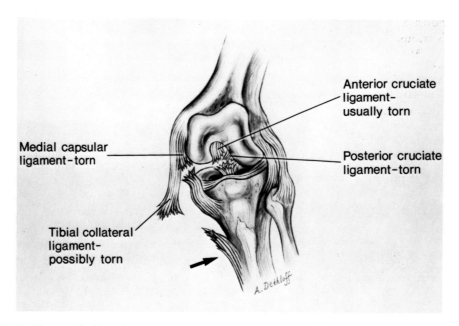

Fig. 113-1. Positive test for chronic medial (valgus) instability. The test is positive in 30 degrees of flexion if the tibial collateral ligament, posterior oblique ligament, and deep capsular ligament are ruptured. If positive in full extension, rupture of the anterior and/or posterior cruciate ligaments is also present.

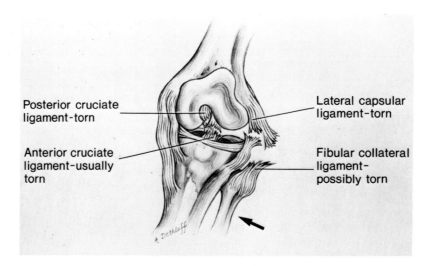

Fig. 113-2. Positive test for chronic lateral (varus) instability. The test is positive in 30 degrees of flexion if the lateral collateral ligament and the lateral capsule are ruptured. If positive in full extension, injury to the arcuate complex, the posterior capsule, the posterior cruciate ligament, and occasionally the anterior cruciate ligament, is also present.

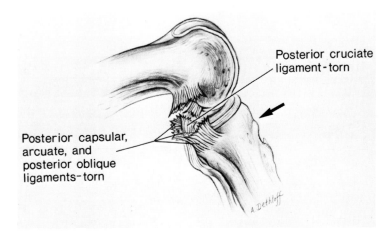

Posterior cruciate
ligament-torn

Posterior capsular,
arcuate, and
posterior oblique
ligaments-torn

Fig. 113-3. Positive test for chronic posterior instability. The test is positive if the posterior cruciate ligament and both the arcuate complex and posterior oblique ligaments are torn.

both tibial condyles subluxate anteriorly an equal amount with no rotation. When both anteromedial and anterolateral rotatory instability are present in combination and sometimes when there is only anterolateral rotatory instability, there may be an apparent, but not a true, straight anterior instability. Absence of or a tear of the posterior horn of the menisci accentuates this instability. The stabilizing effect of the menisci can be partially negated by testing the knee in near full extension.

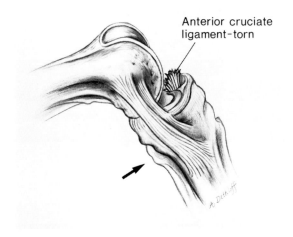

Anterior cruciate
ligament-torn

Fig. 113-4. Positive test for chronic anterior instability. The test is positive if the anterior cruciate ligament is torn. When combined with other ligament injuries, a rotatory component is also present.

Rotatory Instability

There are four patterns of rotatory instability of the tibia relative to the femur.

Anteromedial Rotatory Instability

This problem is characterized by the ability of the medial tibial plateau to rotate excessively anteriorly with respect to the femur (Fig. 113-5). It implies laxity of the posterior oblique and capsular ligaments and often the tibial collateral ligament. It is accentuated with anterior cruciate ligament rupture and by a rupture or tear of the posterior horn of the medial meniscus. In this situation, the abduction stress test is positive with the knee at 30 degrees of flexion, as is the anterior drawer test with the tibia in external rotation.

Anterolateral Rotatory Instability

Anterior rotatory instability is characterized by an abnormal anterior displacement or subluxation of the lateral tibial plateau in relationship to the lateral femoral condyle[61,62] (Fig. 113-6). It is caused by injury to the anterior cruciate ligament, the lateral capsule, and some, or all, elements of the arcuate complex (arcuate ligament, fibular collateral ligament, and popliteus). This is perhaps the most common type of instability encountered in the knee.

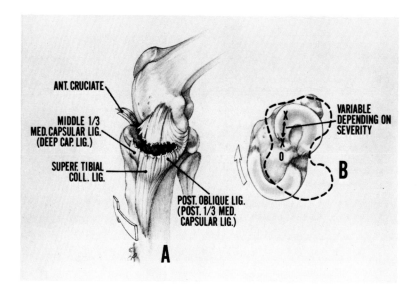

Fig. 113-5. Positive test for anteromedial rotatory instability. **(A)** The structures listed may be torn or stretched in various degrees of severity. **(B)** The excessive anterior rotation of the medial tibial plateau on the medial femoral condyle is allowed because of the relaxed medial structures allowing the axis of rotation to shift from the central location *(O)* laterally *(X)*. (Modified from Larson,[72a] with permission.)

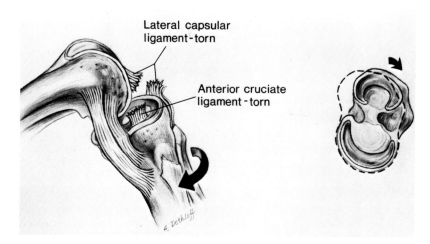

Fig. 113-6. Positive test for anterolateral rotatory instability. **(A)** The structures involved include the anterior cruciate ligament, the lateral capsule and some or all components of the arcuate complex. **(B)** The lateral tibial plateau rotates anteriorly as the center of rotation shifts medially and anteriorly.

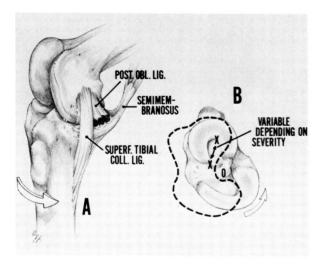

Fig. 113-7. Positive test for posteromedial rotatory instability. **(A)** The structures noted may be stretched or torn. **(B)** The shift of the axis of rotation from its normal position *(O)* to the posterolateral condyle *(X)* permits excessive motion of the medial tibial plateau posteriorly. (Modified from Larson,[72a] with permission.)

Posteromedial Rotatory Instability

Posteromedial rotatory instability is characterized by the ability of the medial tibial plateau to rotate in a posterior direction with respect to the femur (Fig. 113-7). It implies laxity of the medial capsular, posterior oblique, and tibial collateral lig-

aments, as well as the anterior cruciate ligament. It frequently involves either stretching or tearing of the semimembranosus tendon complex.

Posterolateral Rotatory Instability

Posterolateral rotatory instability is characterized by the posterior rotatory subluxation of the lateral tibial plateau relative to the lateral femoral condyle (Fig. 113-8). It results from injury to the lateral capsule, arcuate ligament, popliteus, and lateral half of the posterior capsule. Posterior cruciate ligament incompetency is often present, and injury to the lateral gastrocnemius tendon, biceps femoris, iliotibial tract, fibular collateral ligament, and anterior cruciate may also be associated.

Combined Instability

Various combinations of the various types of rotatory instability may occur. A complete evaluation of the patient in a stepwise fashion will reveal each instability pattern in the complex. Each may need to be addressed in any reconstructive effort.

The range of severity of instability is best thought of as a spectrum of functional deficits. There may be clinically detectable laxity with no functional impairment as far as the patient is concerned. At the other end of the spectrum is a totally unstable knee that is almost useless for function.

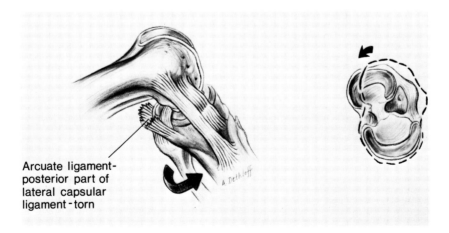

Arcuate ligament-
posterior part of
lateral capsular
ligament - torn

Fig. 113-8. Positive test for posterolateral rotatory instability. The structures involved include the lateral capsule, arcuate ligament, popliteus tendon, and the lateral half of the posterior capsule.

Between these extremes is the knee with an early ligament laxity that, because of abnormal motion, produces stretching to the other supporting tissues and progressively becomes functionally inadequate.

SPECIFIC INJURY PATTERNS

Of the possible types of chronic instabilities described in the preceding classification system, most are uncommon. In this section we will discuss the more common instability patterns, their pathomechanics, diagnosis, treatment options, surgical techniques available, and our preferred method and postoperative management.

Anterior Instabilities

Chronic Medial Instability

Chronic medial instability is manifested as an uncertainty of support on the inner side of the knee when a valgus thrust is applied to the weight-bearing leg (see Fig. 113-1). A directional change opposite that of the weight-bearing leg produces the sensation in the subject of inadequate support for this maneuver. A greater sense of insecurity is brought on when the subject "cuts" (changes direction suddenly) to the opposite direction of the planted foot while running.[123]

An instability described by MacIntosh and colleagues,[35,36,78] termed *the pivot shift,* involves the anterior subluxation of the lateral tibial plateau associated with a posterior subluxation of the lateral femoral condyle. This sudden event, often described as "my knee went out," should be differentiated from the more subtle anteromedial instability described above. Anterolateral instability produces one of the more common types of functional disability. It may occur due to increasing incompetence of the anterior cruciate ligament associated with medial ligament laxity.[73] Since anterolateral rotation of the lateral tibial plateau is its mechanism, it is classified with the lateral instabilities and is discussed in that section of this chapter.

Pathomechanics

Appreciation of the normal anatomy of the medial side of the knee is required to understand the abnormal mechanics of chronic medial instabilities (Fig. 113-9). The structural support of the medial side of the knee can be considered to a half-sleeve divided into three layers. The sleeve covers the area from the medial side of the patella and the patellar tendon around to the beginning of the posterior capsule behind the medial femoral condyle. Functionally, this sleeve has both dynamic and static components. Both components work in unison to stabilize and guide the knee through its normal arc of motion. The dynamic stabilizers are (1) the vastus medialis obliquus (VMO), (2) the pes anserinus group of muscles (sartorius, gracilis, and semitendinosus), (3) the semimembranosus muscle, and (4) the medial head of the gastrocnemius. The quadriceps mechanism, by its coaptation of the articular surfaces and the increase in surface resistance, acts in concert with the tibial collateral ligament to improve the efficiency of these structures.[137] The muscular layer is the most superficial of the three layers and is composed of the muscle groups mentioned above.

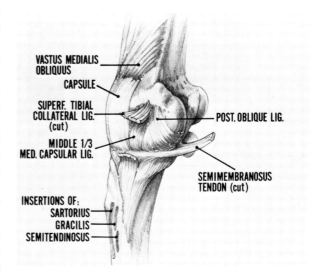

Fig. 113-9. The medial supporting structures of the knee. The three supporting layers are muscular, ligamentous, and capsular (see text). (Modified from Slocum,[123a] with permission.)

The static components constitute the next two layers of functional support. The middle layer, or ligamentous layer, consists of the superficial tibial collateral ligament. The fibers of the posterior trailing edge of this ligament coalesce with the posterior third of the deep capsular ligament to form the posterior oblique ligament, one of the chief stabilizers that prevents excessive anterior and outward rotation of the medial tibial plateau.[50]

The third layer of the medial side of the knee is the capsular layer. This consists of the medial capsule divided into anterior, middle, and posterior thirds. The middle third of the capsular ligament is sometimes referred to as the deep tibial collateral ligament. The medial capsular ligament is intimately attached to the medial meniscus; it is divided by the meniscus into a meniscotibial portion and a meniscofemoral portion. The clinical significance of such a division is that if the capsular ligament ruptures through either of these portions, it can be reapproximated, and healing can be expected to occur.[115] Rupture into the body of the meniscus, particularly central to its outer one-third, leaves insufficient blood supply to support repair.

The posterior capsule, the cruciate ligaments, the medial meniscus, and the bony contour of the femoral condyles and tibial plateaus also contribute to the static stability of the knee.

Palmer[112] wrote of the interplay and the primary and secondary contributions of various knee components toward stabilization. Noyes and co-workers[15,103,104] measured and further defined the resistance of the various ligaments toward planes of motion and classified them into primary or secondary stabilizers in a particular plane of motion.

The axis of rotation of the knee is located in the notch just in front of the femoral attachment of the posterior cruciate ligament[93,123] (see Fig. 113-5). This axis shifts slightly posteroanteriorly with knee flexion-extension. When the knee is fully extended, it is in the "screwed-home" position, with essentially no rotation allowed.

When ligamentous laxity has occurred, which allows anteromedial rotatory instability, the axis of rotation shifts laterally and anteriorly. Posteromedial rotatory instability is allowed when the axis shifts laterally and posteriorly due to relaxed medial supporting tissues[22,93] (see Fig. 113-7).

Two studies relate to the pathomechanics of medial ligamentous injury. Noyes et al.[103] showed the tibial collateral ligament to be the primary stabilizer preventing excessive external rotation of the tibia (Table 113-1). The anterior cruciate ligament was shown to be a secondary stabilizer. The tibial collateral ligament was also shown to be the primary stabilizer against valgus instability with the knee in approximately twenty degrees of flexion. In cadaveric studies using a stress machine, Kennedy and Fowler[63] demonstrated that with the knee in 90 degrees of flexion and with a progressive external rotation force, a tear occurred first in the medial capsular ligament. This led to an anteromedial instability without a valgus instability. If this external rotation force continued past 45 degrees with the addition of a valgus force, rupture of both the medial capsular layer and the tibial collateral ligament occurred, producing a combined valgus and anteromedial rotatory instability. Once the tibial collateral ligament was torn, additional force caused a tear of the anterior cruciate ligament with an increase in the instability in both valgus and rotation. Thus, the initiation injury to produce medial instability is an external rotatory force applied to a flexed knee with enhancement by a valgus force. Depending on the amount of flexion and rotation and valgus stress, a variety of injuries can occur to the medial structures, leading to functional deficits.[8]

Table 113-1. Contributions of Various Supporting Structures Preventing Valgus and External Tibial Rotation

	%
Valgus stability	
Primary	
Medial collateral ligament	80
Secondary	
Cruciates	15
Medial capsule	5
Drawer test in external rotation	
Primary—two major stabilizers	
Medial collateral ligament	58–40[a]
Anterior cruciate	35–50[a]
Secondary	
Medial capsule	Minimal

[a] With ↑ drawer, more contribution of anterior cruciate.
(Adapted from Noyes,[103] with permission.)

Several basic premises need to be considered when evaluating these ligamentous injuries. There is no true isolated ligamentous injury. Because of the integrated nature of the ligaments providing stability to the knee, an isolated tear of a single ligament is a theoretical impossibility. This has been demonstrated by Kennedy et al.[64] A loss of ligament tensile strength and functional competence can occur by stretching without actual visual disruption.[82,100] The term plastic deformation has been used to describe this situation.

Continued stress to secondary stabilizers from abnormal instability will cause the remaining intact ligaments to become incompetent due to abnormal stretching. Patients with chronic instabilities commonly present with a combination of instability patterns secondary to this abnormal motion.[54,73] This can be seen in chronic anteromedial rotatory instability, which produces increasing stresses to the anterior cruciate ligament. Ultimate stretching of the anterior cruciate leads to its insufficiency, producing both anteromedial and anterolateral rotatory instability.[97]

The development of associated instabilities can lead to subsequent pathologic changes. Chronic insufficiency of the anterior cruciate ligament places increased functional demands on the articular cartilage and menisci, leading to their ultimate degeneration.[29,31,80,81,86,93] Meniscal tears secondary to instability can occur.[123] Meniscectomy increases the instability, since the meniscus was helping to block the rotatory abnormality in its action as a secondary restraint.[122,135] It has been shown in animal studies that ligamentous injuries can lead to late degenerative changes of the joint.[69,80,81,111] This has also been noted in routine arthroscopic examination after major ligamentous injuries and surgical repair, when progressive cartilage deterioration occurred despite any initial symptoms. It was Noyes' opinion that the decreased functional stability allowed excessive wear.[103]

Diagnosis and Clinical Evaluation

The evaluation of patients with knee instability should have three major aims. The first is to evaluate the functional deficit. This can be done by both history and physical examination using functional tests. Functional deficits should be considered in patients who have instabilities limiting their ability to perform their work or sport. The desire of many to be physically active at all ages makes improvement of a disability to a higher functional level a worthwhile goal. The second aim is to define the type of instability accurately, be it one-plane, rotatory, or combined. Proper determination of the instability present will suggest the correct surgical procedure for its elimination. The third aim is to determine the patient's motivation for the prolonged rehabilitation program necessitated by ligamentous reconstructive surgery. The possibility that the patient may require bracing after the reconstructive procedure must also be explained. Unless a patient is highly motivated to undertake a 6- to 12-month rehabilitation program, knee ligamentous reconstruction procedures have little to offer.

The patient's history is important in defining the instability and functional deficits. It is helpful for the surgeon to ascertain the mechanism of the original injury. The usual occurrence is a valgus external rotation force to a flexed knee on the weight-bearing leg, as is commonly seen in football injuries, and that produces an anteromedial rotatory instability. Posteromedial rotatory instability usually occurs from a hyperextension valgus force. Chronic medial instability patterns usually present with a history of the knee "giving way" as the patient attempts to change direction, going away from the weight-bearing knee with this knee in some flexion. Pain is present in some cases on both the medial and the posteromedial sides of the knee. Symptoms of internal derangement, as well as those of patellar instability and chondromalacia, degenerative joint disease, and other instability patterns, may also be present.

Physical examination should assess both the general health of the patient and the general ligamentous laxity, with the surgeon paying particular attention to the opposite knee, if it is uninjured and normal. Specific instability tests can then be applied to the involved knee.

The first test is the valgus stress test, done at 0 degrees of extension (Fig. 113-10). If the test is positive (medial opening occurs), a relatively major instability involving all the medial structures of the knee, and often the cruciates, is present. A valgus stress test done at 30 degrees of flexion assesses the

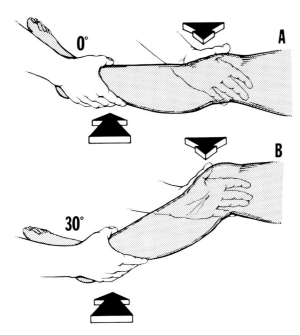

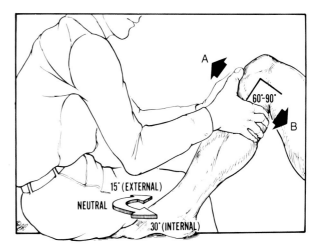

Fig. 113-11. (A) Testing of anteroposterior instability. (B) Testing for rotatory instability (see Fig. 113-5). (Modified from Larson,[72a] with permission.)

Fig. 113-10. AB stress test done with the patient lying flat and muscles relaxed, first with the knee at 0 degrees extension **(A)** (see Fig. 113-3), then with knee flexed 30 degrees **(B)** (see Fig. 113-5). (Modified from Larson,[72a] with permission.)

integrity of the medial capsular and tibial collateral ligaments, as well as the posterior oblique ligament. A variant of the abduction stress test can be performed with the knee in 30 degrees of flexion with the tibia held in external rotation. As the valgus stress is applied, the anteromedial portion of the tibial plateau will tend to rotate forward.

The anterior drawer test is done in internal, neutral, and external rotation of the tibia, with the knee flexed at 60 to 90 degrees and the foot stabilized to the examining table[122] (Fig. 113-11). The results are graded as trace, 1+ (0 to 5 mm), 2+ (6 to 10 mm), or 3+ (more than 10 mm). When the lower leg is placed in 30 degrees of internal rotation, tightening of the iliotibial tract and the posterior capsular ligaments occurs; the anterior drawer tests the integrity of these structures. If there is no laxity, competency of the lateral structures is present. In neutral rotation, anterior displacement of both tibial condyles equally implies anterior cruciate laxity. One may note that the lateral tibial plateau does come forward slightly more than the

medial with pure anterior cruciate laxity. Finally, in 15 degrees of external rotation, a positive drawer sign, increased over that in neutral, represents anteromedial rotatory instability. The more positive the anterior drawer test, the greater the involvement of the medial supporting structures. An anterior cruciate rupture is usually indicated by a marked anterior drawer test.

The valgus stress test at 0 degrees of flexion will demonstrate posterior medial corner sagging, if posteromedial rotary instability is present. For a positive sign, the displacement of the posteromedial corner should be greater than 2 to 4 mm. One must be careful to assess exactly what is happening by palpating the posteromedial corner of the tibia and watching for rotation and displacement of the tibial tubercle (Fig. 113-7). Hughston et al.[48] noted that if a posterior cruciate rupture is present, no rotatory instability is demonstrable, since the axis about which the knee rotates is lost.

Functional testing can be carried out to evaluate the stability of the knee during certain maneuvers.

> *Leaning hop test:* This test is done by asking the patient to hop up and down on the involved extremity, with the other leg held abducted at 30 degrees. Rotation one way and then the other while the patient is hopping accentuates the sensation of inadequate support. In the

more pronounced cases of instability, the patient will be hesitant or refuse to attempt the test. In the less severe instabilities, conscious muscle support allows the performance of the test without difficulty. This test may also show an asymmetry of push-off, indicating weakness in the involved leg.

Jogging in place: Particularly at a rapid pace, this may produce a feeling of instability. The patient is also observed for any asymmetry of leg action, which can be produced by decreased knee flexion, weakness, or uncertainty of support of the involved leg.

Squatting: With the feet rotated internally and externally, squatting tests for meniscal impingement. This test, as well as the other tests for meniscal entrapment, should be performed to evaluate meniscal stability.

Patellar evaluation: A patellar evaluation for increased mobility, facet tenderness, crepitation, or signs of degenerative changes should be made.

This clinical assessment, along with the other tests for a complete knee evaluation, should lead to a determination of the functional problem and the type of instability present.

Ancillary testing, such as stress radiographs, arthrography, or arthroscopy, may also be indicated prior to commitment to a particular rationale of treatment. Arthroscopy is often done at the time of planned surgical reconstruction, since, in most cases, the decision as to whether surgical intervention will be required can be made prior to this evaluation. Arthroscopy allows a better appreciation of any meniscal pathology and provides an inspection of the joint surfaces that may help in prognostication of the results of the operative procedure.

Treatment Modalities

Chronic knee instability is best prevented by an acute and adequate surgical repair of disrupted tissues. This was proved by O'Donoghue[107,108] in a clinical study of results after an acute injury with early repair, as compared with results for knees that had a later reconstructive procedure.

When chronic medial instability has been manifested as a functional problem, the available alternatives should be considered.[112] In those cases with a minor instability, a proper program of muscle-strengthening exercises may provide the support necessary for improved functional use. A brace may be accepted by some as an adequate alternative to a surgical procedure; in others, it may not provide adequate stabilization, or it may prove too inconvenient to be acceptable. Surgical intervention to modify the instability and lessen the functional deficit may be the modality with the greatest chance of achieving the objective of allowing the patient a more reasonable activity level.

Surgical correction of instabilities has been in use since the time of Hey Groves in 1917.[44,45] Palmer,[112] O'Donoghue,[109,110] Hughston et al.,[48] Nicholas,[93] Kennedy and co-workers,[61,63,64] MacIntosh,[78] and Slocum and co-workers[122-124] have all been responsible for development of an understanding of instability patterns and their mechanism and surgical treatment.

Surgical Procedures

The surgical procedures available can be categorized as static, dynamic, or combined. Historically, the static methods of reconstruction were the first to be used (Fig. 113-12). Hey Groves,[45] McMurray,[89] Blair,[11] and Hauser[41] described tethering operations for laxity of the tibial collateral ligament. Tightening by distal or proximal advancement of the collateral and capsular ligaments was described by Mauck[85] and by O'Donoghue.[110] Substitutive procedures using fascia were described by Milch[90] and by Bosworth and Bosworth.[12] A review of the literature will provide many other examples.[132]

The dynamic procedures (Fig. 113-13) include the pes anserinus transfer described by Slocum and Larson and co-workers.[122,125] This procedure transfers the distal two-thirds of the pes attachment proximally just beneath the metaphyseal flare of the tibia. The moment arm for flexion is diminished, while that of internal rotation is enhanced[54,105] (Fig. 113-14). A dynamic resistance to excess external rotation of the tibia that occurs with anteromedial rotatory instability is produced. Also, a dynamic sling is provided on the medial side to decrease valgus instability. The effects of this dynamic transfer have been investigated by Noyes and Sonstegard[105] and Perry et al.[114] and found to be kinetically sound.

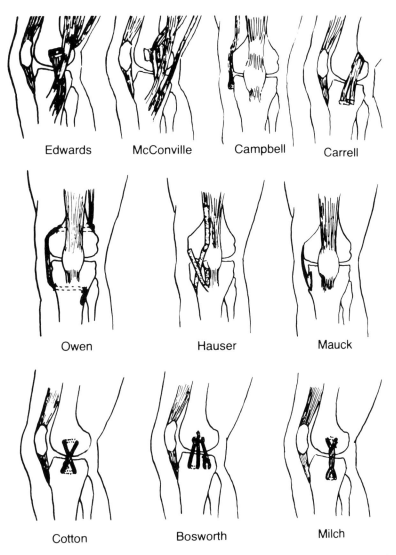

Edwards   McConville   Campbell   Carrell

Owen   Hauser   Mauck

Cotton   Bosworth   Milch

Fig. 113-12. Drawings of some of the procedures used in reconstruction of the tibial collateral ligament. (From Umansky,[132] with permission.)

Transfer of the semimembranosus provides a dynamic reinforcement of the posterior medial corner of the knee, particularly the posterior oblique ligament.[124] This transfer is accomplished by advancing the conjoined semimembranosus tendon superiorly and anteriorly, allowing it to rotate on its direct attachment at the posterior tibial tubercle. This is laced into the tightened posterior oblique ligament as this latter structure is imbricated in closure.

The vastus medialis obliquus can be advanced downward to reinforce the anteromedial capsule and retinaculum dynamically. Such a transfer also provides for dynamic support of the tibial collateral ligament by overlying its proximal insertion. Because of its action on the medial retinaculum, vastus medialis advancement provides a dynamic action to prevent lateral patellar instability.

The sartorial tendon has also been transferred superiorly and anteriorly in alignment with the tib-

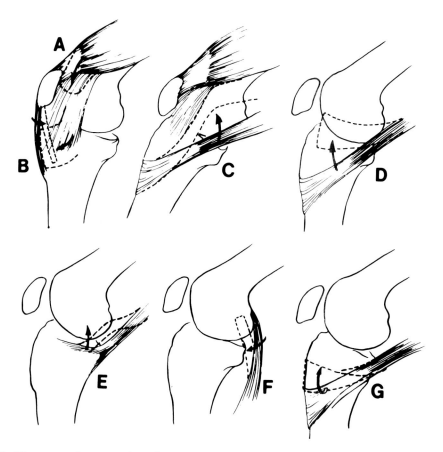

Fig. 113-13. Diagrammatic summation of procedures that can be used for the medial side of the knee for dynamic reinforcement of repaired tissue. **(A)** Distal advancement of vastus medialis obliquus. **(B)** Split patellar tendon and anterior advancement of the anterior medial capsule. **(C)** Advancement of sartorius. **(D)** Pes anserine transfer as a patch over deficient tissue. **(E)** Anterior proximal advancement of the semimembranosus. **(F)** Medial anterior reattachment of the medial half of the tendinous medial head of the gastrocnemius. **(G)** Pes anserinus transplant. (From Larson,[70] with permission.)

ial collateral ligament to provide a dynamic backup.[70] The distal attachment of the sartorius is left attached to the tibia; the tendinous and musculotendinous area is mobilized and reattached to the underlying tissue as described. The distal tendinous edge of the vastus medialis obliquus muscle is used for the superior anchoring sutures. This transfer is used when the ligamentous medial structures are severely attenuated and additional reinforcement is necessary. The maximum moment arm of the transferred muscle resists valgus-producing forces. Uses of the semitendinosus tendon in a similar manner has also been described.[126]

Other procedures[71] used include the following:

1. Anterior advancement of the medial head of the gastrocnemius with posterior capsular repair when markedly attenuated tissues are present in the posteromedial aspect of the knee
2. Splitting of the patellar tendon with tightening of the anteromedial retinaculum and capsule and transfer of the medial portion of the patellar tendon more medially
3. The 5-1 procedure described by Nicholas,[93] which is a combination of several static and dynamic procedures

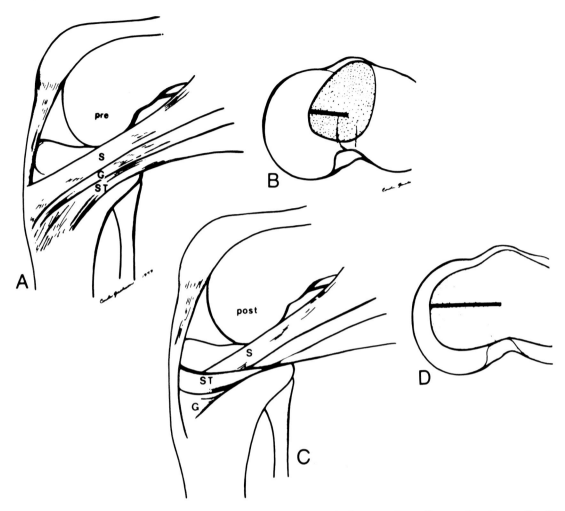

Fig. 113-14. **(A)** Relative position of the pes anserinus tendons before pesplasty. *S,* sartorius; *G,* gracilis; *ST,* semitendinosus. The semitendinosus has the largest moment arm for flexion, while the moment arm for internal rotation is quite short **(B)**. Following proximal transfer of the semitendinosus and gracilis into the tibial metaphyseal flare **(C)**, the moment arm for flexion is diminished, while that for internal rotation is lengthened **(D)**. (From James,[54] with permission.)

Ancillary procedures that may be considered in specific situations include the following:

1. *High tibial osteotomy.*[125] When degenerative changes are present in the medial joint compartment with osteoarthritis and joint-space narrowing significant enough to produce symptoms, unloading of this compartment by a high tibial osteotomy may provide an alteration of joint mechanics to allow for better function.
2. *Tibial tubercle transfer.*[124] When marked patellar instability exists with medial instability, tibial tubercle transplantation medially or split patellar tendon transfer, as described above, may be indicated.

The goal of the surgical procedure is to stabilize the knee to prevent excess valgus opening and anteromedial rotation of the tibia. Combinations of the procedures are often used. There can be no "cookbook" approach to reconstructive surgery of the knee. The various combinations of instability, associated conditions in the knee, and individual considerations involving each patient, require that surgical approaches to improvement of knee function be individualized. The simplest surgical exercise that will achieve improved functional use is most desirable.

Authors' Preferred Technique

Although several patterns of medial instability are described in the classification scheme presented earlier in this chapter, most of those resulting in surgical intervention are of the anteromedial rotatory instability type, with lesser or greater amounts of anterior instability. If the injury is longstanding, anterolateral rotatory instability may also be present with the development of a pivot shift phenomenon. If the latter has developed, a lateral reconstruction, as described later in this chapter, may be required in addition to the medial repair.

Generally, the procedure is preceded by diagnostic arthroscopy to confirm the preoperative assessment and to inspect the menisci. The menisci should be repaired and saved whenever possible.[115] The patient is positioned in the supine position, with the knee flexed initially at approximately 45 degrees of flexion. The incision starts on the medial side of the distal thigh, approximately 6 cm above the joint line. It extends distally along the border of the medial hamstring tendons to the level of the joint line. From there, it continues anteriorly to the medial side of the patella, parallel with the joint line. Just medial to the patella, it again curves distally to follow the medial border of the patellar tendon to approximately 2 cm distal to the tibial tubercle (Fig. 113-15). The incision can be modified to consider previous scars.

The anterior and posterior skin flaps are developed to the level of the medial patellar retinaculum, with all subcutaneous tissues left on the flaps to ensure survival.

This incision permits complete visualization of the medial half of the knee, from the patella to the posteromedial corner. This facilitates intra-articular repair and augmentation of either the anterior or posterior cruciates, with excellent exposure of the distal hamstrings when pesplasty or distal advancement are done, as well as exposing the distal quadriceps and patellar tendons for harvesting graft tissue.

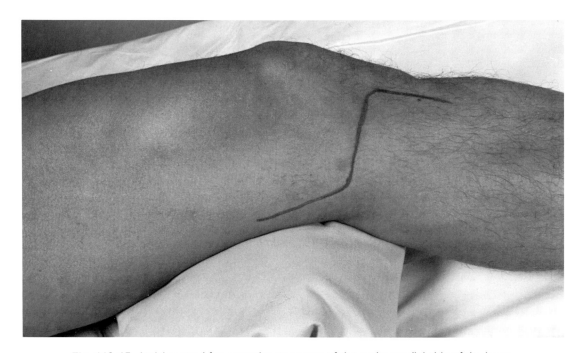

Fig. 113-15. Incision used for extensive exposure of the entire medial side of the knee.

The joint can be opened through a median parapatellar incision through the medial retinaculum for any intra-articular repairs required. Tears of the menisci are dealt with by removal of the torn tissue with preservation of as much of a stable symmetric rim as possible. Tears of the meniscus on the periphery can be repaired with a ligamentous repair if the body of the meniscus is intact. Generally, the anterior cruciate will show partial or complete rupture or a significant stretch injury. The age, activity level, and condition of the joint must be taken into account when one is making this assessment. A long protection phase and rehabilitation period to allow for revascularization and maturation of intra-articular anterior cruciate substitutes are necessary. The repair and augmentation of the anterior or posterior cruciates are presented under those sections of this chapter and is not repeated here. We find that repair and augmentation of the anterior cruciate ligament is usually necessary and should be undertaken at this point.

Occasionally, an anteromedial rotatory pattern will be present without a significant valgus or anterior instability. In this situation, there has often been a tear of the medial capsular ligament with mild stretching of the tibial collateral ligament. A dynamic constraint to excessive external rotation of the tibia, which may occur when the patient "cuts" (changes directions suddenly) to the opposite direction while running, can be provided by a pes anserine transplant (Fig. 113-16). The lower two-thirds of the pes anserine attachment is detached from its tibial attachment and reflected proximally, where it is attached to the medial edge of the patellar tendon. The site of the attachment should allow the reflected tendons to lie on the distal edge of the metaphyseal flare of the tibia. Care in mobilizing the pes anserinous lower border must be taken so as not to injure or entrap the sartorial branch of the saphenous nerve, which penetrates the interval between the lower edge of the sartorius and gracilis at the musculotendinous junction of the sartorius.

The most common technical errors in doing the procedure are (1) failure to include the semitendinosus tendon in the transplant, (2) improper positioning of the transplant, either proximally or distally, (3) laxity of the transplant due to inadequate anterior advancement, (4) injury to the sartorial

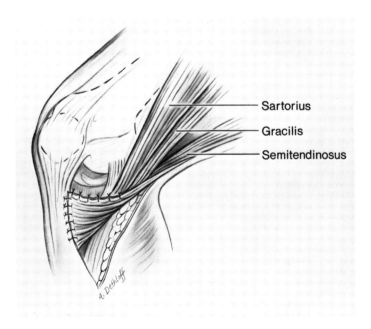

Sartorius

Gracilis

Semitendinosus

Fig. 113-16. The distal two-thirds of the pes insertion is elevated from the tibia and folded proximally and medially. It is then sewn to the metaphyseal flair medial to the patellar tendon.

branch of the saphenous nerve, and (5) hematoma formation due to failure to provide hemostasis or suction drainage at the operative site.

When there is a significant valgus component to the instability, the procedures required depend on the severity of the rotational instability and the valgus instability. In less severe cases, a pes anserine transplant is combined with a reefing of the posterior oblique ligament. The latter procedure is accomplished by incising the fascia overlying the posteromedial corner of the knee from the vastus medialis above to the sartorius below. This exposes the posterior portion of the medial capsule and the anteromedial limb of the semimembranosus muscle. The posterior oblique ligament is formed by the confluence of the trailing edge of the tibial collateral ligament, fascia from the anteromedial limb of the semimembranosus, and the posterior third of the medial capsular ligament. There is a relatively thin area lying just posterior to the trailing edge of the tibial collateral ligament, which can be defined by palpation. The incision into the posterior joint is made in this area. It extends from the medial femoral epicondyle slightly obliquely posteriorly and downward to the posterior capsule and tendon of

the semimembranosus. The entrance into the posterior joint allows inspection for any meniscal pathology of the posterior horn. The posterior capsule should also be evaluated for any deficiency or laxity that may require repair (Fig. 113-17).

The surgeon begins closure of the rent produced in the posterior oblique ligament by pulling the anterior margin posteriorly and distally with a mattress suture, bringing the anterior margin beneath the posterior flap (Fig. 113-18A). The anterior margin can thus be tightened by 1 to 2 cm by continuing the sutures proximally until the incision is closed. The posterior flap is then double-breasted over the closure and is advanced anteriorly and sutured with individual mattress sutures (Fig. 113-18B). In providing this closure, the surgeon should extend the knee to make certain that no restriction to extension has been produced by too tight a closure. Reefing of the posteromedial corner in this manner tightens the medial capsular sleeve and helps reduce the valgus and anteromedial rotatory instabilities.

When there is deficiency of the tissues of the posteromedial corner, or associated posteromedial rotatory instability is present, the closure is rein-

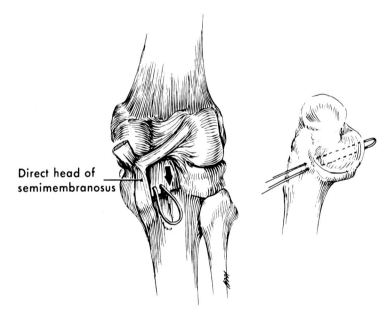

Direct head of
semimembranosus

Fig. 113-17. The posterior capsule should be repaired if it is torn. When it is detached from the posterior tibia, it can be reattached through drill holes in the proximal tibia placed lateral to the direct head of semimembranosus. (From Slocum,[124] with permission.)

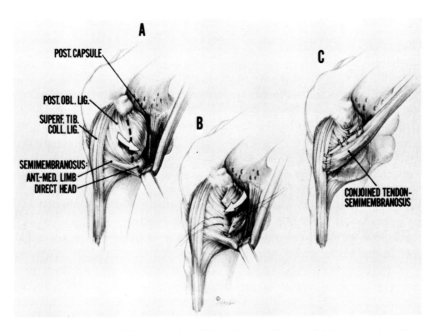

Fig. 113-18. **(A)** The anterior edge of the posterior oblique ligament is brought downward and backward toward the junction of the posterior capsule and the direct head of the semimembranosus. The sutures are continued proximally, tightening this area. **(B)** The posterior edge is then advanced over the tightened posterior oblique ligament to doubly reinforce this area. **(C)** The conjoined tendon and anteromedial limb of the semimembranosus can be advanced anteriorly to reinforce and dynamically augment the repair.

forced and dynamically augmented by anterior and proximal advancement of the conjoined and anteromedial limbs of the semimembranosus (Fig. 113-18C). This tendinous area is mobilized by incising the overlying tendon sheath. The conjoined tendon is then sutured over the repaired posteromedial corner. The anteromedial tendon is released from its tibial insertion beneath the posterior edge of the tibial collateral ligament and reattached superficially to this ligament in line with the conjoined tendon, so as to provide a direct line of pull with the muscle fibers. When marked valgus instability is present, a sartorial advancement is done to provide dynamic reinforcement to the inadequate tibial collateral ligament (Fig. 113-19). The sartorius muscle is mobilized, leaving its distal attachment intact. As the tendinous portion is mobilized, care is taken to protect the sartorial branch of the saphenous nerve from injury or entrapment. The tendinous portion of the sartorius is advanced anteriorly to alignment with the tibial collateral ligament. The most proximal suture for fixation is through the tendinous distal edge of the

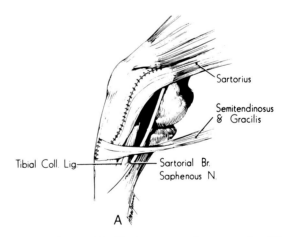

Fig. 113-19. **(A)** Modified pes anserinus transfer. The semitendinosus and gracilis have been reflected proximally and attached to the medial edge of the patellar tendon, as in the usual pes anserine transfer. The sartorius has been advanced anteriorly in line with the tibial collateral ligament. The distal insertion of the sartorius is left attached. Care is taken in mobilizing the muscle to protect the sartorial branch of the saphenous nerve. (See Fig. 113-14.) (From Larson,[70] with permission.)

vastus medialis obliquus, rotating the sartorius to the desired position of alignment. (When the muscle belly of the sartorius, rather than the tendinous portion, is approximated at this point, the under surface of the sartorius muscle will usually demonstrate an extension of tendinous or fascial tissue which will provide better fixation for the suture.) The sutures are continued distally along the anterior edge of the sartorius, attaching it to the tibial collateral ligament.

At this point, the wounds are copiously irrigated, the medial patellar retinacular tissue is repaired, and the wound is closed in the usual fashion over suction drains. The knee is placed in a removable hinged cast brace while in the operating room, with the hinges locked in 30 degrees of flexion.

Postoperative Management

The revascularization and strengthening of the anterior cruciate reconstruction is the rate-limiting step in the postoperative management of chronic medial instability. Following the section on chronic anterior instability is a description of our rehabilitation protocol for anterior cruciate reconstructions. As this is a part of most reconstruction for chronic medial instability, the same protocol is used. That protocol is not repeated here.

Chronic Anterolateral Rotatory Instability

Anterolateral rotatory instability (ALRI) is characterized by abnormal anterior displacement or subluxation of the lateral tibial plateau in relationship to the lateral femoral condyle[60,61] (see Fig. 113-6). This, perhaps, has become the most common type of instability encountered in the knee.

This type of rotational instability was brought dramatically to our attention in 1972 by Galway and MacIntosh and associates.[35,36,77] They described a form of lateral instability which they termed *the pivot shift*. Hey Groves,[45] in 1920, described the symptoms of anterior cruciate injury as "a moving forward of the tibia when weight is placed on the leg and the foot is put forward." He further stated that "sometimes this forward slipping of the tibia occurs abruptly with a jerk." Palmer,[112] in his treatise, On the Injuries to the Ligaments of the Knee Joint, in 1939, mentions a very similar phenomenon that quite likely was the same as that described by Hey Groves. He described "the active drawer" in which a patient could effect a sagittal displacement in the knee joint by using his or her muscles. It would therefore appear that this form of lateral instability, which we term ALRI, was actually recognized years ago but, as with many theories and findings related to ligament instability, it was neglected over the years.

Pathomechanics

The structural support of the lateral side of the knee (Fig. 113-20) can again be considered a half-sleeve divided into three layers, as we described for the medial side of the knee. This time the sleeve covers the area from the lateral side of the patellar tendon and the lateral side of the patella around to the beginning of the posterior capsule behind the lateral femoral condyle. This sleeve has both dynamic and static components. The dynamic components are (1) the vastus lateralis, (2) the iliotibial band, (3) the biceps femoris, (4) the popliteus, and (5) the lateral head of the gastrocnemius. The muscular layer is the most superficial layer of the sleeve. The static components constitute the middle and deep layers of functional support. The middle, or ligamentous, layer is made up of the fibular collateral ligament. The deep layer consists of the lateral capsule divided into anterior, middle, and posterior thirds. The anterior third of the capsular ligament has no attachment to the femur; rather, it blends into the lateral extension of the quadriceps mechanism (retinaculum). The posterior third includes both capsular and noncapsular ligaments, forming a single functional unit termed *the arcuate complex.* The components of this complex are the fibular collateral ligament (actually a portion of the middle layer), the arcuate ligament, and the tendoaponeurotic unit formed by the popliteal muscle.

The posterior capsule, the cruciate ligaments, the lateral meniscus, and the bony contour of the femoral condyles and tibial plateaus also contribute to the static stability of the knee.

The structures involved in producing instability include primarily the anterior cruciate ligament and the posterolateral capsule. Some or all of the elements of the arcuate complex (arcuate ligament), fibular collateral ligament, and popliteus) may also be involved.

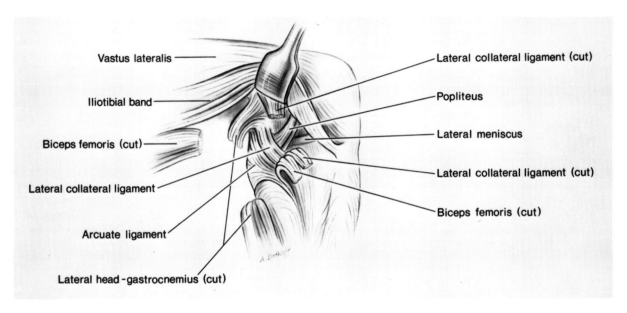

Fig. 113-20. Lateral supporting structures of the knee. The retractor holds the vastus lateralis and iliotibial band anteriorly so that the deep lateral structures can be seen as identified.

Several studies have been conducted to elucidate the pathology of ALRI.[30,49,53,96,134] These studies implicate the anterior cruciate ligament and the lateral capsule primarily. Usually, a mild valgus and anteromedial rotatory instability accompanies ALRI.

Chronically, this form of instability occurs during the weight-bearing phase when the patient pivots or twists toward the involved extremity in running or, in many instances, just walking. When the foot and leg are fixed, a cross-cut maneuver, in which the patient's body rotates toward the involved extremity, creates external femoral rotation while the tibia remains relatively fixed. This is usually initiated with the knee near full extension but proceeding into flexion. As the knee flexes, a valgus rotation force is created. With an incompetent or absent anterior cruciate ligament (as well as involvement of the lateral supporting structures), the femoral condyle is allowed to roll posteriorly down over the convex surface of the lateral tibial plateau.[87] The combination of weight bearing and tightening of the iliotibial tract will momentarily impinge the femoral condyle in this more posterior-than-usual position. Initially, the iliotibial tract[59] is positioned anterior to the transverse

centers of rotation; but, as knee flexion increases, the iliotibial tract glides posterior to the instant centers. At about 30 to 40 degrees of flexion, it abruptly reduces the lateral plateau in relation to the femoral condyle with a sudden snapping or popping sensation, thus, leading to the pivot-shift episode. This term actually describes the pivoting motion and the relative shifting of the lateral plateau and femoral condyle.

Strong opinions have developed about the pathology and mechanism involved in ALRI of the pivot-shift type. Some observers feel that the snapping sensation is caused entirely by the lateral femoral condyle snapping down off the posterior horn of the lateral meniscus during the moment of reduction.[24,26,30] Theoretically, when the anteriorly subluxated tibial plateau assumes its most maximum anterior position, the femoral condyle has displaced up over the posterior horn of the meniscus. When reduction occurs, the jumping or snapping phenomenon is created by the lateral condyle popping off the posterior horn.

It is important to note that the iliotibial tract must be intact to create the snapping phenomena described by MacIntosh, but it does not necessarily mean that ALRI is not present simply because the pivot-shift phenomenon is absent. If the iliotibial tract is no longer intact for one reason or another, the lateral tibial plateau may still subluxate anteriorly in relation to the lateral femoral condyle with routine drawer testing and even with some form of the MacIntosh test, but there is no sudden jerking or snapping sensation.

Diagnosis and Clinical Evaluation

The symptoms associated with this particular type of instability are (1) lateral pain, (2) "giving way," and (3) a snapping or popping sensation usually associated with a sudden deceleration and pivoting toward the involved extremity. Walking or running straight ahead is usually tolerated well, but a misstep or a sudden change in direction creates a feeling of instability. Initially, there may be some swelling and quite severe pain with the episodes but, as the condition becomes more chronic, the residual symptoms from each episode generally become less significant, with perhaps no swelling and only very transient pain.

The past history will usually include a traumatic incident to the knee, at which time the patient may have experienced a popping or giving-way sensation followed by acute swelling. Not infrequently, meniscectomy has been carried out on many of

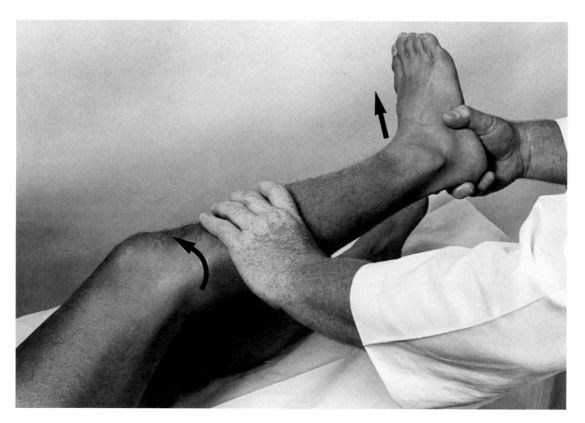

Fig. 113-21. The MacIntosh test is performed with the patient lying supine with the right lower extremity supported at the heel by the examiner's right hand. The examiner's left hand is placed laterally over the proximal tibia just distal to the knee. The more proximal hand applies a valgus force and internally rotates the tibia as the knee is moved from a position of full extension (a position of reduction) into flexion. At about 30 to 40 degrees of flexion, a sudden "jumping" sensation is noted as the lateral tibial plateau, which has smoothly subluxated anteriorly in relation to the femoral condyle, quite suddenly reduces. Palpation of the joint line, as this test is carried out, will demonstrate anterior displacement of the tibial plateau, and at the moment of reduction there is audible, visible, and palpable jumping sensation.

these people, once they have developed chronic symptoms. The symptoms are mistaken for meniscal impingement syndrome with the failure to detect an associated ALRI.

Functional tests of running in place, hopping, squatting, and "duck waddling" (walking in a crouched position) will sometimes create apprehension or will be difficult to perform. Palpation along the lateral joint line, while varus force is applied to the knee as the knee is moved through a range of motion, will often indicate crepitation secondary to lateral joint wear and may cause pain as well. Mild to moderate medial instability, characterized by slight valgus instability and mild anteromedial rotary instability (AMRI), is usually present.

The routine drawer sign (see Fig. 113-11) is often unremarkable, with perhaps no more than a trace to 1+ anterior drawer (1+, 0 to 5 mm; 2+, 6 to 10 mm; 3+, more than 10 mm) with the tibia in neutral position and external rotation. Occasionally, the drawer sign is positive with internal tibial rotation, which indicates abnormal anterior displacement of the lateral tibial plateau. If the iliotibial tract has remained intact, no instability in this position will be demonstrable. The anterior drawer

sign performed with the tibia in neutral position will sometimes demonstrate greater anterior subluxation of the lateral tibial plateau than the medial tibial plateau, if the displacement is observed quite closely. It is not unusual for tibial displacement to be a one-plane instability with both plateaus subluxating anteriorly, particularly with severe instability.

There are several specific tests to demonstrate the pivot-shift phenomenon. MacIntosh[35,36,77] was the first to describe the test that has become a routine part of most knee examinations (Fig. 113-21). Slocum,[16,121] Hughston et al.,[48] Losse et al.,[75] Noyes et al.[99] (Fig. 113-22), and James[53] have described variations to test for ALRI.

All the tests demonstrate ALRI and are quite reliable when performed properly; in some instances, however, one may be more sensitive than another. Therefore, all the techniques should be utilized if there is a high index of suspicion from the patient's history for ALRI. False-positive results may occur in patients exhibiting bilateral genu recurvatum.

Some patients can demonstrate an active anterior drawer sign. It is usually best demonstrated by the patient sitting with the knee flexed 90 degrees

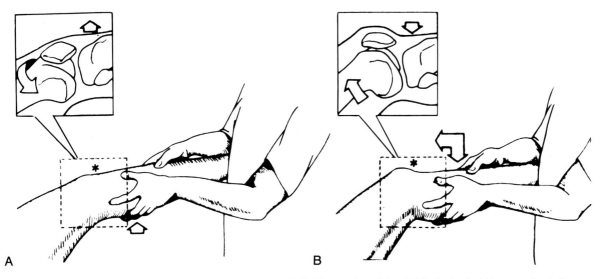

A   B

Fig. 113-22. Noyes's flexion-rotation drawer test. **(A)** Subluxated position. With the leg held in neutral rotation, the weight of the thigh causes the femur to drop posteriorly and, more importantly, to rotate externally, producing anterior subluxation of the lateral plateau. **(B)** Reduced position. Gentle flexion and a downward push on the leg (as in the posterior drawer test) reduces the subluxation. This test assesses the function of the anterior cruciate ligament in the control of both translation and rotation. (From Noyes, with permission.[99])

and the foot planted firmly on the floor. In this position, the voluntary anterior drawer sign appears to be produced either by contraction of the gastrocnemius muscles or by the popliteal muscle, which subluxes the lateral plateau anteriorly and internally rotates the tibia. Other patients can actively demonstrate anterolateral rotary instability by standing with partial weight on the involved extremity and moving the knee back and forth from extension to flexion while simultaneously applying slight valgus stress to the knee. A disassociation between the lateral femoral condyle and the lateral plateau can easily be seen.

One must be aware that, occasionally, posterolateral rotary instability (PLRI) can elicit a phenomenon that may be confused with a positive pivot shift test for ALRI.[51,75] This condition should be suspected if the patient walks with the tibia rotated internally or, if during the test for anterolateral rotary instability, it is observed that, as the knee is flexed from a position of complete extension, the tibia suddenly externally rotates in relation to the femoral condyle while valgus stress is being applied to the leg. This usually can be verified by placing the knee in the standard position for the drawer test, applying a posterior force to the proximal tibia, and observing that the lateral plateau drops more posteriorly than does the medial tibial plateau, indicating PLRI. Slocum (personal communication) has described a specific test for PLRI.

The examiner must also keep in mind that ALRI may be combined with other forms of rotational instability. A combination of ALRI and AMRI (anteromedial rotary instability) is the most frequent but, occasionally, a combination of ALRI and PLRI is encountered.

In summary, ALRI of the knee should be suspected when (1) there is a history of an acute injury to the knee followed by rapid swelling and perhaps accompanied by a popping and giving-way sensation at the time of injury; (2) there are progressive symptoms of instability characterized by the knee "going out," particularly with twisting, turning, or "cutting" maneuvers; (3) the patient can demonstrate a voluntary anterior drawer sign; or (4) one or more of the tests for ALRI is positive.

Standard radiographs may be helpful in diagnosing ALRI when a small fleck of bone is noted supe-

rior and posterior to Gerdy's tubercle, representing an avulsion of the meniscotibial portion of the middle third of the lateral capsule.[56,140] Likewise, an arthrogram may raise the incidence of suspicion when the anterior cruciate ligament is poorly outlined on the lateral anterior stress view. One must keep in mind, however, that, if the overlying synovium is intact, the cruciate ligament may be severely damaged without appearing to be so. A lateral anterior stress film will often demonstrate anterior subluxation of the tibia. Arthroscopy[99] is useful in its ability to demonstrate injury to the anterior cruciate ligament in acute cases or, perhaps, total absence of the cruciate in chronic situations. Patients unable to relax adequately during the course of routine examination may have grossly positive tests for ALRI under anesthesia. Computed tomography (CT) has been used to study the cruciate ligaments (Karpf M, personal communication). Results have correlated very well with cruciate function in diagnosing injury and for evaluating reconstruction.

Treatment Modalities

Reconstructive procedures for ALRI are directed at preventing anterior subluxation of the lateral tibial plateau in relationship to the lateral femoral condyle. The role of the iliotibial tract in producing the lateral privot-shift phenomenon is crucial to an understanding of reconstructive procedures for this type of instability. The basic technique for extra-articular reconstruction is to restrain a portion of the iliotibial tract posteriorly and distally behind the transverse centers of rotation. Most current procedures use a strip of iliotibial tract released either distally or proximally, which is then placed under the fibular collateral ligament such that it remains behind or posterior to the transverse centers of rotation at all times. Thus, it acts as a check rein against anterior subluxation of the lateral plateau. In this position, it can act as either a dynamic or a static element, depending on the technique used. Repositioning of a portion of the iliotibial tract posteriorly changes the orientation of this portion of the iliotibial tract, so that it will somewhat parallel the course of the anterior cruciate ligament. In essence, it may be thought of as an extra-articular cruciate ligament reconstruction but as one with a longer moment arm for resisting rotation due to its peripheral position.

Although ALRI is primarily a result of incompetency or absence of the anterior cruciate ligament, simple replacement of the anterior cruciate ligament alone is generally insufficient for stabilizing against rotational instability, since the cruciate is a midline structure for stabilization, predominantly in the sagittal plane and is not well located to resist rotational instabilities.

This section discusses only the peripheral reconstructive procedures for anterolateral rotary instability. These may be combined with some form of anterior cruciate reconstruction. Specific techniques for anterior cruciate ligament reconstruction are discussed later in this chapter and are not repeated here.

Surgical Procedures

Procedures Releasing a Strip of Iliotibial Tract Distally

Ellison Procedure Ellison[25,26] published a description of his procedure for ALRI, now commonly referred to in North America as the Ellison procedure. A very similar technique was reported by Nakajima et al.[92] from Japan the same year. The Ellison procedure is a distal transfer of a strip of iliotibial tract after it has been displaced under the proximal portion of the fibular collateral ligament. The insertion of the strip of iliotibial tract is released, along with a small button of bone from Gerdy's tubercle. It is about 1.5 cm in width distally and considerably widened proximally. The broad base preserves maximum blood supply and is also an attempt to preserve the dynamic pull of the tensor fascia lata and part of the gluteus maximus (Fig. 113-23A). Using blunt and sharp dissection where necessary, the anterior and posterior margins of the iliotibial tract are then freed to the patella superiorly and to the insertion of the iliotibial tract inferiorly (Fig. 113-23B). A curved hemostat is passed beneath the fibular collateral ligament from anterior to posterior by blunt dissection and is kept proximal near the insertion of the fibular collateral ligament on the lateral femoral condyle (Fig. 113-23C). The middle third of the lateral capsular ligament and arcuate ligament is imbricated under the fibular collateral ligament to re-

move the laxity in these structures. The biceps tendon is released distally, passed through the lateral aponeurotic portion of the lateral head of the gastrocnemius and posterior capsule and then under the distal portion of fibular collateral ligament, and is sutured to it. The distal end of the tendon is brought back over the ligament and sutured to the capsule of the proximal tibiofibular joint and the insertion of the arcuate ligament (Fig. 113-23D). The lateral head of the gastrocnemius is sutured to the distal half of the fibular collateral ligament. This creates a supplementary restraining force and further reinforces the posterior lateral corner. The strip of iliotibial tract is passed beneath the fibular collateral ligament, pulled distally, and reattached just anterior to Gerdy's tubercle in a shallow trough made to accept the bone block (Fig. 113-23E). The distal portion of the button of bone usually lies just under the lateral border of the tibial tubercle, which may have to be elevated slightly. The strength and stability of the transfer is tested by extending the knee. As the knee passes into extension, the proximal insertion of the lateral collateral ligament serves as a cam to prevent anterior movement of the strip of iliotibial tract, which, in turn, prevents anterior subluxation of the lateral tibial plateau. If the knee can be passed into less than 30 degrees of flexion, the transplant is too loose and should be advanced more anteriorly.

Ellison emphasizes that the defect in the iliotibial tract must be closed and that it is also important to note that the transferred strip of iliotibial tract is not secured to the fibular collateral ligament (Fig. 113-23F).

Postoperatively, the knee is immobilized in a long-leg cast at 60 degrees of flexion for a minimum of 6 weeks, followed by a posterior splint for 1 week, during which time hydrotherapy and gentle range-of-motion exercises are conducted. Full extension is not encouraged for a minimum of 12 weeks, and hyperextension is avoided. Major emphasis is placed on hamstring strength until it is brought to par with the quadriceps before quadriceps exercises are begun. This maximizes the posterior stabilizing effect of the hamstrings and minimizes the anterior displacing effect of the quadriceps during the early healing phase. A Lenox Hill derotation knee brace is used during the early months of convalescence.

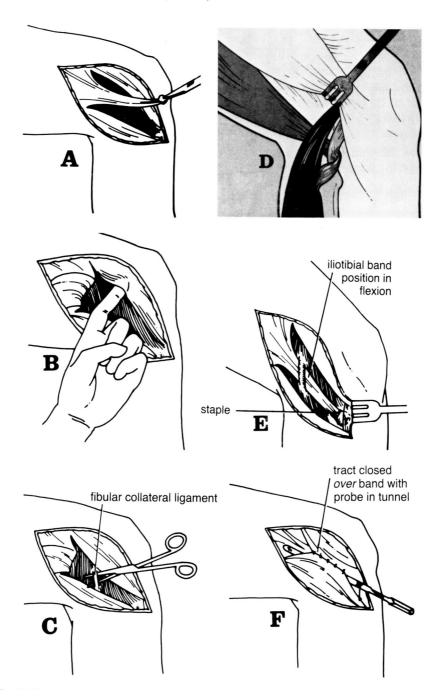

Fig. 113-23. (A) The insertion of the iliotibial band is released along with a button of bone, and a fascial strip is developed and broadened proximally. **(B)** The anterior and posterior margins of the iliotibial band are undermined. **(C)** A tunnel is created proximally under the fibular collateral ligament. **(D)** The biceps has been released, passed beneath the tendinous portion of the lateral head of the gastrocnemius and behind the distal portion of the fibular collateral ligament, and then sutured to the capsule of the proximal posterior tibiofibular syndesmosis and the insertion of the arcuate ligament. **(E)** The transplant is passed beneath the fibular collateral ligament, stapled into a bone trough, and sutured to the lateral fibers of the patellar tendon. **(F)** The iliotibial tract has been closed, except where its margins diverse proximally. (A, B, D, E, F from Ellison[25]; C from Ellison,[26] with permission.)

Ellison believes that the procedure has the following advantages: (1) the broad proximal base and proximal continuity of the transplant minimize vascular loss, (2) bone-to-bone fixation distally is the optimum anchorage of the transplant and permits immediate testing to verify proper position, (3) the lateral approach permits easy access for other operative procedures, (4) the procedure is rapid and technically easy, and (5) the biceps transfer adds dynamic support.

Johnson Procedure   Johnson and Pope[57] describes a procedure for advancing the lateral capsular ligament complex for control of ALRI (Fig. 113-24). His impression, based on clinical observations and laboratory studies on cadaver specimens, is that the integrity of the lateral capsular ligament is a primary element in stabilizing the knee against ALRI. Dissections demonstrated a distinct bony attachment of the lateral capsular ligament immedi-

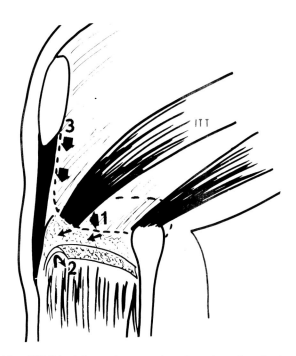

Fig. 113-24. Johnson's procedure for advancing the lateral capsular ligament complex for control of ALRI. (1) The released insertions of the iliotibial tract *(ITT)* and the lateral capsule are advanced and reattached on the tibia. (2) The retracted attachment of the anterior compartment muscles is then brought proximally to overlap the advanced structures. (3) Also shown is the line of capsular incision.

ately superior and somewhat posterior to Gerdy's tubercle. This bony attachment was found to be a direct continuation of the arcuate ligament coming from its attachment in the posterior intercondylar notch. On the basis of these observations, an operation was designed using the capsular ligament complex in a lateral extraarticular procedure.

Initially, a capsular incision is made parallel to the lateral aspect of the patellar tendon, and approximately 6 mm (¼ inch) of the lateral attachment of the patellar tendon insertion is elevated. The incision is carried proximally up to an area at the lateral tip of the patella. Through this incision, the capsule and overlying retinaculum are separated from the underlying synovium proximally as far as the superior aspect of the iliotibial tract is identified, and an incision is made from posterior to anterior as far forward as Gerdy's tubercle. The attachments of the lateral and anterior compartment muscles are released proximally from the tibia and retracted distally. An incision is made into the joint anterolaterally, and a blunt retractor (or joker) is placed under the meniscus and along the lateral gutter. The bony attachment of the lateral capsular ligament is then elevated parallel to the joint line and taking care not to violate the joint surface. The surgeon then skives off the capsular insertion at about 30 degrees tangential to the joint. The soft tissue dissection is carried to the most extreme posterior tibial corner in an effort to completely free the tissues and demonstrate continuity of the arcuate ligament, which is advanced in the horizontal plane by the procedure. With the knee at 90 degrees of flexion and the foot externally rotated, the bone released with the lateral capsular ligament is attached to a new bone bed in the area where Gerdy's tubercle was elevated. The bone that was released from Gerdy's tubercle is advanced anteriorly and inferiorly on the tibia in the same anatomic relationship. Both reinsertions are secured with towel clips and then transfixed with screws in their new bone beds. The screws are covered by suturing the fascia of the anterior compartment muscles to the lateral aspect of the patellar tendon.

Postoperatively, the patient is placed in a cylinder cast with the knee in 90 degrees of flexion. The cast is changed at 1 week and removed 6 weeks postoperatively. Approximately 3 additional weeks are required for the knee to gain adequate extension before weight bearing is begun. During that time, the patient is instructed in isometric quadriceps exercises, with emphasis placed on isometric straight leg raising and hamstring exercises. Three months are required for reduction of soft tissue swelling, and at least one year is needed for maturation of the fibrous tissues.

The primary objective of this operation is to control rotary instability for everyday activities. Patients are instructed that they are vulnerable to further injury and that acceleration-deceleration sports increase the chances of injury.

Johnson believes that the advantage to this procedure is that it does not disrupt the interconnections among the multiple contributors to the lateral capsular ligamentous complex. It corrects vertical laxity between the lateral aspect of the femur and the lateral aspect of the tibia, via the iliotibial tract. It also advances the arcuate ligament in the horizontal plane, which resists the rotational component of ALRI.

Procedures Releasing a Strip of Iliotibial Tract Proximally

Losee Procedure Losee et al.[75] described a "sling and reef" procedure, in which a strip of iliotibial tract, 2.5 cm in width and 15 cm in length, is created laterally, leaving it attached distally at Gerdy's tubercle and releasing it proximally. A tunnel is created through the lateral femoral condyle, with the location of the tunnel determined by positioning the strip of iliotibial tract at various loci on the condyle just anterior to the fibular collateral ligament insertion, in order to determine the point that represents the center of rotation for the arc, traversed by Gerdy's tubercle as the knee is flexed and extended. The tunnel exits posteriorly through the insertion of the lateral head in the gastrocnemius tendon. The strip of iliotibial tract is attached to a Gallie needle and threaded through that tunnel from anterior to posterior (Fig. 113-25A). Correct placement of the tunnel is verified by applying tension to the transferred portion and then noting, by passing the knee through a range of motion, whether or not it eliminates anterior subluxation of the tibial plateau. If it is found that the tunnel is improperly positioned and anterior subluxation of the plateau is not eliminated, the strip may be re-

positioned by passing it more horizontally beneath the proximal portion of the fibular collateral ligament and then through the tendinous head of the lateral gastrocnemius.

When the strip has been positioned properly through the tunnel, it is sutured to the periosteum at the entrance and exit of the tunnel or, if it has been passed beneath the fibular collateral ligament, it is sutured to the ligament. The strip is then passed through the tendon of the origin of the lateral head of the gastrocnemius, entering at a point 1 cm distal and 0.5 cm medial to the posterior opening of the tunnel, and then passed horizontally and laterally so that it encircles at least a 1-cm strip of the gastrocnemius tendon at its origin. A second reefing stitch is then passed through the gastrocnemius, starting 1.5 cm medial and 0.5 cm distal to the point of emergence of the previous reefing stitch. The strip is then directed distally and laterally so that it passes through the substance of the arcuate ligament posterior to the fibular collateral ligament and just above the level of the joint line. It is next passed beneath the fibular collateral ligament just distal to the joint line. Tension is placed on the strip to observe whether it pulls the gastrocnemius and posterior lateral structures into close approximation with the fibular collateral ligament. The strip is then pulled posteriorly around the fibular collateral ligament, the tibia is externally rotated with the knee flexed 45 degrees, and the anteriorly displaced gastrocnemius tendon and posterolateral part of the capsule are sutured to the fibular collateral ligament as tension is maintained on the strip of iliotibial tract. The strip is also carefully sutured to the fibular collateral ligament. The remaining portion of the strip is brought anteriorly and sutured to Gerdy's tubercle; any excess is used to reinforce the reconstruction (Fig. 113-25B). The defect in the iliotibial tract is closed if, such can be done easily. Leaving the defect open does not compromise the results of the reconstruction and leaves an asymptomatic muscle hernia.

Postoperatively, a long leg cast is applied with the knee flexed 30 to 45 degrees and the tibia in slight external rotation. After 7 weeks, the cast is replaced by a long-leg brace with a pelvic band or quadrilateral socket and free knee and ankle joints, with the foot maintained in 10 degrees external rotation; the brace is worn for 3 months. Partial

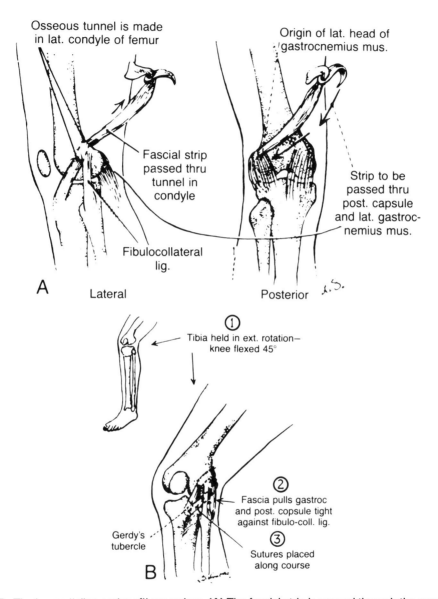

Fig. 113-25. The Losee "sling and reef" procedure. **(A)** The fascial strip is passed through the condylar tunnel (left) and exits through the lateral head of the gastrocnemius. **(B)** After reefing stitches are placed in the gastrocnemius tendon, the fascial strip passes forward through the arcuate ligament and under the fibular collateral ligament. The assistant holds the tibia in external rotation with the knee flexed 45 degrees (1). Tension is applied, and the posterolateral structures are secured to the fibular collateral ligament (2). The remainder of the strip is sutured to Gerdy's tubercle (3). (From Losee,[75] with permission.)

weight bearing with crutches is allowed until full knee extension is regained. Exercises are done in the cast and brace, concentrating on the quadriceps and biceps.

Arnold Procedure   Arnold et al.[7] used another modification with a strip of iliotibial tract that is left attached to Gerdy's tubercle. The iliotibial band is exposed, and a 15- to 18-cm strip, 2 cm in width, is freed proximally and dissected distally to the attachment at Gerdy's tubercle. A tunnel is made under the more proximal portion of the fibular collateral ligament near its insertion on the lateral condyle. The strip of fascia is passed beneath the ligament from anterior to posterior, looped back on itself, brought distally, and secured to an area of denuded bone just distal to Gerdy's tubercle with a large staple or boat nail, while the tibia is held externally rotated (Fig. 113-26). Any remaining strip is turned back on itself over the staple and sutured in position. Additional sutures are placed through the strip, where it passes about the fibular collat-

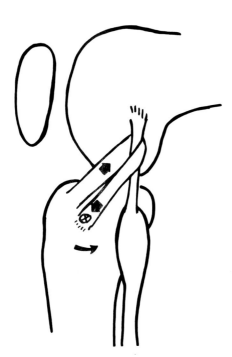

Fig. 113-26. Modification proposed by Arnold et al.[7] The strip of iliotibial tract is passed around the proximal portion of the fibular collateral ligament and brought back to be attached just distal to Gerdy's tubercle while the leg is externally rotated.

eral ligament. The reconstruction is then tested to see whether the instability has been eliminated. The defect in the iliotibial band need not necessarily be repaired, and its presence has apparently made no significant difference postoperatively.

Postoperatively, a long leg cast is applied with the knee flexed 60 degrees and the tibia externally rotated. Sutures are removed at 10 days, and the knee is then extended to 30 degrees for 3 weeks. Quadriceps, gastrocnemius, hamstring, and gluteal medius exercises are prescribed. The cast is removed and full knee extension achieved over the next 2 to 6 weeks, with gradual stretching. Total rehabilitation requires 6 to 9 months before the patient can return to full activities.

This procedure uses a strip of iliotibial tract as a check rein with a tenodesing effect. It is technically uncomplicated and uses the advantages of a peripheral restraint.

Andrews Procedures   Andrews[6] prefers a lateral extra-articular reconstruction using the iliotibial tract to stabilize the lateral tibial plateau by creating two "isometric" bundles, with one being tight in flexion and the other tight in extension. The iliotibial tract is incised longitudinally 2.5 to 3 cm anterior to its posterior border, and the posterior portion is retracted inferiorly. An area on the femur, just proximal to the lateral femoral condyle, is denuded of periosteum and soft tissue, and the area is "fish-scaled" with an osteotome. Two points in this area closely corresponding to the two major intra-articular attachments[107] of the anterior cruciate ligament are selected (Fig. 113-27A). The first and lowest is at the most distal end of the linea aspera, where the femoral condyle begins its flare just anterior to the posterior cortex. It corresponds to the intra-articular attachment of the anteromedial bundle of the anterior cruciate ligament. The second is 1 cm anterior and 0.5 cm distal to the first and corresponds to the attachment of the posterolateral bundle. Steinmann pins, with an eye in each end, are passed transversely across the femur parallel to each other through the points established on the femur.

Two #5 nonabsorbable sutures are woven into the iliotibial tract parallel to each other, running proximally from Gerdy's tubercle to the level of the drill holes. When properly placed, they create two

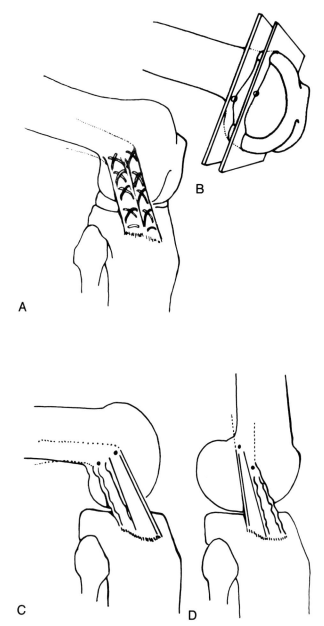

bundles that will be secured proximally to the femur via the drill holes (Fig. 113-27B). The sutures forming the anterior bundle are pulled through the anterior hole in the femur, and the sutures from the posterior bundle are pulled through the posterior hole to exit medially in the area of the adductor tubercle. Tension is applied to the sutures, and the bundles are observed as the knee is passed through a range of motion. If the points of attachment have been properly positioned, a full range of motion is available, with the posterior bundle becoming tight in extension and the anterior bundle tight in flexion, creating a tenodesis effect on the lateral tibial plateau (Fig. 113-27C,D). Anterolateral rotary instability should be eliminated. It is essential that the attachment points be properly positioned and tension within the bundles appropriately maintained. This sometimes has to be accomplished by trial and error, with repositioning of the drill holes and/or the sutures forming the bundles. Once proper position and tension are achieved, the sutures are tied to each other medially.

Postoperatively, a cylinder cast with the knee flexed 30 degrees is worn for 6 weeks. If medial reconstructive procedures are done, the knee is flexed 60 degrees. Progressive resistance quadriceps and hamstring exercises are done throughout the postoperative period, as well as bicycling. The patient is kept non-weight bearing on crutches for approximately 3 months and is cautioned against regaining extension too rapidly or applying weight too soon.

This procedure follows the principle of using a portion of the iliotibial tract to stabilize the lateral plateau. The iliotibial tract does not have to be completely released, and its blood supply is probably minimally interfered with. This is a relatively noninvasive procedure and one that uses bone fixation. It does, however, require exact attachment of the two bundles in order to achieve appropriate tension.

Authors' Preferred Technique

We begin with a diagnostic arthroscopy to confirm our preoperative impressions and examine the menisci. This helps tailor the specific operation to the individual patient. In our experience, nearly all

Fig. 113-27. Andrews lateral extra-articular reconstruction. **(A)** The placement of the drill holes in the femur closely corresponds in a transverse plane to the two femoral points of attachment of the anterior cruciate ligament. **(B)** Two sutures are woven into the iliotibial tract, creating two bundles extending from Gerdy's tubercle to the level of the drill holes in the femur. With correct placement of the drill holes and the creation of two bundles, there will be an isometric reconstruction in which the anterior bundle is taut in flexion **(C)**, and the posterior bundle is taut in extension **(D)**. (Courtesy of J.R. Andrews.)

patients with chronic anterolateral rotatory instability have ruptured the anterior cruciate ligament, with injury to both the lateral capsule and the arcuate ligament. We prefer making an incision that permits access to the joint, for anterior cruciate repair and augmentation, as well as to the posterolateral corner of the joint. As usual, the menisci are repaired, whenever possible, and trimmed as necessary.

The patient is placed in the supine position with the leg over a bolster to achieve 45 degrees of flexion of the knee. A gentle S-shaped curvilinear incision is made to the lateral side of the knee (Fig. 113-28), beginning 6 cm proximal to the joint line along the anterior border of the biceps femoris and gently sloping anteriorly to cross the joint line at approximately a 30-degree angle, meeting the joint line at a point 2 cm lateral to the patella. From here, the incision is extended distally, just lateral to, and parallel with, the patellar tendon, ending 2 cm distal to the tibial tubercle.

Anterior and posterior skin flaps are elevated superficial to the iliotibial band and lateral patellar retinaculum, as well as over the distal quadriceps and anterior surface of the patella, with all subcutaneous tissue maintained on the flaps to ensure viability. The iliotibial band is used in an Ellison pro-

cedure to stabilize the posterolateral corner of the knee.

Beginning 4 or 5 cm above Gerdy's tubercle, a straight incision is made along the anterior border of the iliotibial band distal to and around the tubercle. Using a sharp osteotome, the insertion of the iliotibial band is then released by raising a button of bone, about 1.5 cm in diameter, from Gerdy's tubercle. This is turned up and a strip of fascia about 1.5 cm in width, and, incorporating the iliotibial band, is shaped with scissors. The actual width will vary with the size of the patient. This fascial strip is then broadened superiorly and inferiorly such that the proximally attached base resembles a long-necked Ehrlenmeyer flask (Fig. 113-23A). This broad-based shape preserves the maximum blood supply to the fascia, the dynamic pull of the tensor fascia latae, and part of the gluteus maximus. The strip of iliotibial band can be tucked underneath the subcutaneous tissues proximally, if other surgery is to be done.

Using blunt and sharp dissection when necessary, the anterior and posterior margins of the iliotibial tract are then freed to the patella superiorly and to the insertion of the iliotibial tract inferiorly (Fig. 113-23B). This step is essential for proper closure; with minimum care, it is easily accom-

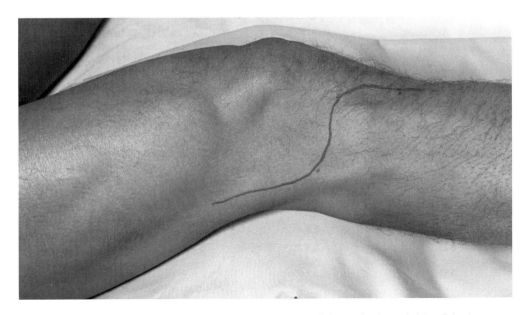

Fig. 113-28. The incision used for extensive exposure of the entire lateral side of the knee.

plished. Too-broad undermining posteriorly produces a partial biceps release. Therefore, the dissection should not be so extensive as to lose this inferior anchorage of the fascial layer. The anterior margin of the fascia can be retracted, and a lateral anterior parapatellar incision can be made for arthrotomy.

An inspection of the joint is made and meniscal trimming is performed, as necessary. We then repair and augment the anterior cruciate as described under Chronic Anterior Cruciate Instability. Once the anterior cruciate repair is complete, the parapatellar incision is closed over a suction drain.

The knee is gently flexed to 90 degrees, and a varus force is applied by the assistant (being careful not to stress the intra-articular repair), to tighten and create a better definition of the fibular collateral ligament.

A curved hemostat is passed beneath the ligament from anterior to posterior, either by blunt dissection or with superficial vertical incisions paralleling the two borders of the ligament (see Fig. 113-23C). This dissection remains superficial to the joint space. The jaws of the hemostat previously passed beneath the lateral collateral ligament are spread to obtain adequate space beneath the collateral ligament to pass the button of bone from Gerdy's tubercle, with its attached iliotibial band, from back to front.

It is important to carry the dissection of the fibular collateral ligament proximally as far as its bone insertion on the lateral femoral condyle. If the tunnel beneath the fibular collateral ligament is not proximal, the transplant will angulate on loose soft tissue rather than on bone and will erode away the tissue. The middle third capsular ligament and the arcuate ligament are then plicated beneath the fibular collateral with multiple horizontal mattress sutures. The transfer is then passed from posterior to anterior beneath the fibular collateral ligament.

Additional bone is removed from the proximal end of the tibia in the area of Gerdy's tubercle, or slightly anterior to it, as close to the joint line as is possible with safety. This creates a shallow trough in the direct line of the pull of the transplant. With the knee in 90 degrees of flexion and the lateral tibial condyle firmly held in the posterior, externally rotated, reduced position, a staple is placed just behind the button of bone removed from

Gerdy's tubercle, anchoring the transplant, bone to bone, in the trough (Fig. 113-23E). Additional sutures are taken to bone and periosteum at the approximate level of the lateral fibers of the patellar tendon. The most distal portion of the bone button is usually just under the lateral border of the patellar tendon. With the knee in 90 degrees of flexion, there should be a straight line of pull from the staple along the transferred iliotibial band, with no kinking of the band as it passes beneath the lateral collateral ligament.

The effectiveness of the transfer is immediately tested to be certain that all instability has been corrected. As the tibia moves toward extension, the proximal lateral collateral ligament insertion serves as an ever-tightening check rein, or cam, to prevent anterior movement of the tibia on the femur. This is the rationale of the procedure. If the knee can be extended to more than 30 degrees of flexion, however, the transplant is too loose and should be advanced further in the bone trough and anchored further anteriorly. This point is crucial.

The border of the patellar tendon and the periosteum from the distal end of the bone trough are sutured over the end of the transplant to provide coverage of the staple area and additional fixation of the transplant itself. When this is completed, and with the knee flexed 90 degrees, closure of the iliotibial tract over the transplant is begun at the midportion of the tract defect, over a probe (Fig. 113-23F). Two or three sutures are taken proximally and distally to this area, after which the knee is partially extended to complete the closure. As shown, the tract is closed directly over the transplant but is not sutured to it in any way.

It is essential to close the iliotibial tract completely over the transplant, except for the wide proximal base. If adequate release of the anterior and posterior margins of the tract has been carried out, full closure invariably can be achieved. Extending the knee to the limit of the transfer (about 30 degrees of flexion) is helpful. By obtaining a complete closure, a sleeve for the transplant is created, allowing it freedom to slide under both the collateral ligament and the repaired iliotibial tract. If the iliotibial tract is not repaired, varus instability will result.

Any sutures placed into the iliotibial band transfer will interfere with the excursion of the transplant jeopardizing or eliminating any dynamic function. The remainder of the wound is closed in the usual fashion. Following a sterile dressing, the leg is placed in a removable cast brace with the knee hinges locked in 60 degrees of flexion.

Postoperative Management

The postoperative rehabilitation for chronic anterolateral rotatory instability is similar to that for anterior cruciate reconstruction, in that the anterior cruciate is generally repaired in **ALRI** and the anterior cruciate repair revascularization process is the rate limiting factor in the rehabilitation process. With **ALRI**, however, the knee is braced initially in 60 degrees of flexion at surgery to permit healing of the iliotibial band transfer. Range of motion is delayed until the fourth week, at which time the hinges are progressively advanced at the rate of 5 degrees/week to allow more extension. The remainder of the program is the same as described in the postoperative management section of anterior cruciate reconstruction.

Chronic Anterior Cruciate Instability

In chronic cases of anterior cruciate ligament instability, patients have a primary complaint of recurrent giving way[31,48,86] (see Fig. 113-4). These episodes may or may not be accompanied by joint effusion. Frequently, an effusion is present with the initial episode but, with repeated episodes, swelling becomes less frequent. Straight ahead walking or running may be well tolerated, but pivoting, twisting, deceleration, or sudden changes in direction involving rotation on the involved extremity ("cutting") elicit instability. Not infrequently, these symptoms are interpreted as a meniscal lesion,[116] with episodic impingement of a meniscal fragment leading to meniscectomy, only to find that the symptoms have not abated postoperatively when the patient resumes normal activities.

Pathomechanics

The cruciate ligaments are complex structures, both architecturally and functionally.[3,4,34,39,88] They are located intra-articularly but extra synovially. The anterior cruciate ligament arises from the tibia anteriorly. It courses posteriorly, superiorly, and laterally to insert onto the lateral femoral condyle in a crescentic fashion, posterior and high in the notch near the articular margin of the lateral femoral condyle. The orientation of the femoral insertion site changes dramatically in relation to the tibial insertion as the knee passes from flexion to extension, creating a reciprocal tightening within the various portions of the ligament at all degrees of knee flexion.[136] Both cruciate ligaments play a role in stabilizing the medial and lateral sides of the knee statically, but biomechanically they are not positioned as effectively as are the collateral ligaments for resisting rotatory and/or varus–valgus-producing forces.

The midline position of the cruciates primarily provides anteroposterior stability in the sagittal plane. Functionally, the anterior cruciate ligament cannot be totally isolated from other ligamentous structures about the knee, but it is the primary stabilizer for the tibia against anterior subluxation and hyperextension. There have been instances at surgery in which the anterior cruciate ligament has been noted to be totally ruptured or even absent without a significant anterior drawer sign, because of stability provided by the intact collateral structures, which are secondary restraints against the anterior drawer.[15,100,103] In this situation, subsequent anterior instability is likely to develop as the collateral structures become stretched from overloading in the face of an incompetent anterior cruciate ligament. The antithesis of this situation is anterior instability with an ostensibly intact anterior cruciate ligament. The explanation for this phenomenon is that an anterior cruciate ligament may be functionally incompetent because of severe interstitial damage to its structure that is not apparent on gross examination. Kennedy et al.[67] pointed out that such a failed ligament may appear to be visibly intact, but that tests performed on specimens stressed just to the point of failure demonstrated very little difference in strength from those that had been taken to actual visible rupture. Such a failed ligament may appear to be intact but is functionally incompetent, posing a definite diagnostic and therapeutic problem in some instances.[22] In the past, some observers have concluded that the anterior cruciate ligament is not the primary stabilizer against anterior instability.

However, one must not be deluded into assuming that an anterior cruciate ligament is functioning normally when it is observed to be ostensibly intact at arthroscopy or arthrotomy.

Diagnosis and Clinical Evaluation

The most significant findings on physical examination are a positive anterior drawer sign[86,104] with the tibia in neutral or external rotation (see Fig. 113-11), a positive Lachman sign[128] (Fig. 113-29), a positive flexion-rotation drawer test,[102] or a positive test for anterolateral rotary instability. These diagnostic procedures are previously discussed under Chronic Medial Instability and Chronic Anterolateral Rotatory Instability.

Treatment Modalities

Immobilization will not result in healing of the anterior cruciate ligament once a chronic instability pattern develops. If the patient is experiencing a significant functional deficit that is not amenable to functional bracing, surgical intervention is appropriate.

Several structures[10] have been used for anterior cruciate reconstruction in both acute and chronic cases. The most common are (1) a portion of the patellar tendon,[3,4,5,58,116] (2) a strip of fascia,[12,109] (3) a semitendinosus[17,126] or gracillis[88] tendon, or (4) a meniscus.[19,74,127]

Current biomechanical testing of the various tissues suggests that a portion of the patellar tendon is the most appropriate material.[14,101] Several different procedures are currently being employed, most of which have demonstrated a reasonable degree of success. Few, if any, of these procedures are new. Most are simply modifications of previous methods.

Intra-articular placement of tendinous or fascial structures in the past has been somewhat discouraging, owing to eventual attenuation and disruption.[111] However, there are factors involved

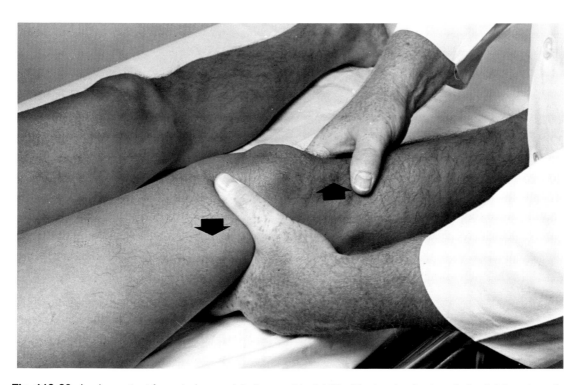

Fig. 113-29. Lachman test for anterior cruciate ligament instability. The involved extremity is slightly externally rotated. One hand firmly grasps the femur distally; the other grasps the proximal tibia, with the thumb on the anteromedial joint margin. An anteriorly directed lifting force is applied to the tibia; with anterior cruciate instability, anterior subluxation of the tibia can be felt and seen.

in tissue survival that justify reconsidering intra-articular anterior cruciate reconstruction. These factors are as follows:

1. Replacement of a cruciate ligament alone for complex instability has often resulted in subsequent return of the instability. This is because there was no consideration for simultaneous collateral ligament reconstruction.[54] In the latter instance, with significant instability (2+ or greater), anterior cruciate reconstruction should be combined with collateral reconstruction and appropriate muscle transfers for additional reinforcement in an attempt to prevent overloading of the new structure.

2. The replaced anterior cruciate ligament has often been improperly positioned. Thus, it is subject to abnormal forces.[37] Its complex architecture is impossible to duplicate surgically, but the actual positioning can be controlled, and it is essential that the new structure follow as closely as possible the course of the original ligament. Any deviation from the desired position will create eccentric forces tending to stretch the ligament out with time and to disrupt joint kinematics. Perhaps the most common mistake is placing the femoral insertion site too far anteriorly on the lateral femoral condyle, rather than high and posterior near the articular margin where the normal insertion is located.

3. Tissues placed intra-articularly for cruciate substitution usually are rendered avascular and must revascularize.[2-5,37] Covering the new structure with surrounding soft tissue, such as a flap of anterior fat pad, provides a source of more adequate blood supply for survival. Some newer techniques involve retaining a pedicle of fat pad still attached to a portion of patellar tendon and used for the substitute in an attempt to preserve its blood supply. Recent studies indicate that the initial nutrition of a newly substituted cruciate ligament is provided in part by diffusion from surrounding synovial fluid. Manske[79] conducted experiments that confirmed the contention that tendon nutrition can occur by diffusion rather than by direct circulation. More recently, Ginsberg et al.[38] explored this thesis and found, in the dog, that a patellar tendon left attached to the tibia, but isolated

from the synovium with a Jones-type anterior cruciate substitution, did not receive a significant blood supply from the tibial insertion site. They concluded, therefore that direct blood flow therefore did not contribute to nutrition, but that synovial diffusion may play a significant role in sustenance of the graft intra-articularly until revascularization.

Alm[2] studied survival of portions of patellar tendon used to reconstruct anterior cruciate ligaments in humans. Biopsies were taken from patients, with the shortest interval between surgery and biopsy being 3 months and the longest 5½ years. The transplanted tissue was viable on microscopic examination. Transplants which were tight, limiting instability to a minimal degree, were histologically similar to normal anterior cruciate ligaments; however, in joints that were still unstable, the transplants were less well organized histologically and had degenerated.

Leaving soft tissue present in the notch as a source of blood supply and covering the new ligamentous structure with a flap of anterior fat pad for additional coverage and source of blood supply, enhances the chance of survival.

4. Passing the reconstructed anterior cruciate ligament through a drill hole in the lateral femoral condyle. This technique has been frequently used for securing the proximal end. Positioning is somewhat of a problem from a technical standpoint, and the entrance to the tunnel serves as an area to concentrate shear forces.[46]

The angle by which the ligament approaches the tunnel in the condyle constantly changes, and this motion may abrade the ligament on the bony margins of the tunnel entrance, if the tunnel is not adequately radiused or beveled at its edge, resulting in failure of the reconstructed ligament.

Since the insertion site of the anterior cruciate ligament is high and posterior on the femoral condyle, some prefer to pass the new structure through the notch and across the former insertion site of the ligament, proceed "over the top" of the lateral femoral condyle, and secure the new ligament extra-articularly.[78] This avoids passing the new ligament over any sharp edges of bone, while allowing it to assume an essentially normal course. Technically, it is very easy to position the ligament properly, and this eliminates placing a femoral tunnel. We feel that the benefits of intraosseus attachment outweigh the difficulties encountered in placing and beveling a femoral tunnel. If the knee is maximally flexed during placement, the intraarticular enterance to the femoral tunnel can be created properly at the original site of insertion of the cruciate.

A tibial tunnel is made for the new structure. A concentration of forces at the tunnel exit is not present because the angle of approach of the ligament to the tibia remains relatively constant regardless of the knee position, avoiding subsequent abrasion and attenuation of the ligament at this point. This does not negate the fact that the tunnel exit on the tibia must be properly positioned in order for the new ligament to function without undue tension being placed upon it.

5. An adequate period of time must be allowed for the reconstructed ligament to mature, remodel, and revascularize.[4,111] This means that the new ligament must be protected from abnormal forces for several months. Eight to 12 months of protection is required for complete maturation. During this period of time the patient's activities must be carefully monitored.
6. A well-supervised rehabilitation program is essential. This period will allow for restoration of muscle bulk, strength, and endurance, to protect the knee from abnormal forces and reestablish kinesthetic mechanisms.

Although the results of the various procedures to be described are encouraging, an enthusiastic approach to anterior cruciate reconstruction must be tempered with caution. Patients should be selected carefully and the procedure thoroughly discussed with them, as well as the uncertainty of long-term results.[29] Follow-up visits in excess of 5 years are sorely lacking. Will the various procedures stand the test of time with continued stability and improved function; or, will subsequent deterioration and instability ensue? The patient must make the final decision as to whether to proceed with reconstruction after an honest appraisal has been presented by the surgeon.

Surgical Procedures

The procedures described should be preceded by examination of the knee with the patient under anesthesia. We suggest a diagnostic arthroscopy. If arthroscopy has not been performed, a thorough joint assessment should be carried out visually at arthrotomy.

Procedures Using a Portion of the Patellar Tendon

Marshall Procedure Marshall and associates[83,84] describe a technique modified after MacIntosh[76,78] that uses a central portion of the quadriceps tendon, soft tissue from the anterior aspect of the patella, and a central strip of patellar tendon left attached at the tibial tubercle (Fig. 113-30A). The quadriceps tendon portion of the graft is split longitudinally. One-half of the graft is folded distally over the thinned-out prepatellar soft tissue, which is then tubed about the folded-over portion of the quadriceps tendon, reinforcing the weak area of the graft. A tunnel is placed through the anterior aspect of the tibia, exiting at the old cruciate insertion site intra-articularly. The graft is passed through the tunnel, across the joint, and over the top of the lateral femoral condyle in a subperiosteal groove or, if preferred, through an appropriately placed tunnel in the lateral femoral condyle (Fig. 113-30B). The proximal end of the graft is stapled to the lateral femoral condyle, and stumps of the cruciate ligament and fat pad are sutured to the graft.

Postoperatively, soft bulky dressings are used for the first 5 to 6 days, after which time a cylinder cast is applied for an additional 5 weeks with the knee flexed 20 degrees. Progressive weight bearing is allowed to full weight bearing by 3 to 4 weeks. Following cast removal, a cast-brace or limited-motion, steel-hinged elastic knee brace with extension stops is worn for 8 weeks, during which time range-of-motion exercises are started. When flexion to 90 degrees is achieved, slow isotonic quadriceps and hamstring exercises are instituted, supplemented by gastrocnemius and abduction exercises.

The patient then progresses to power and endurance work with a gradual return to activities starting at about 3½ to 4 months postoperatively. Rehabilitation is continued for at least 12 to 18 months.

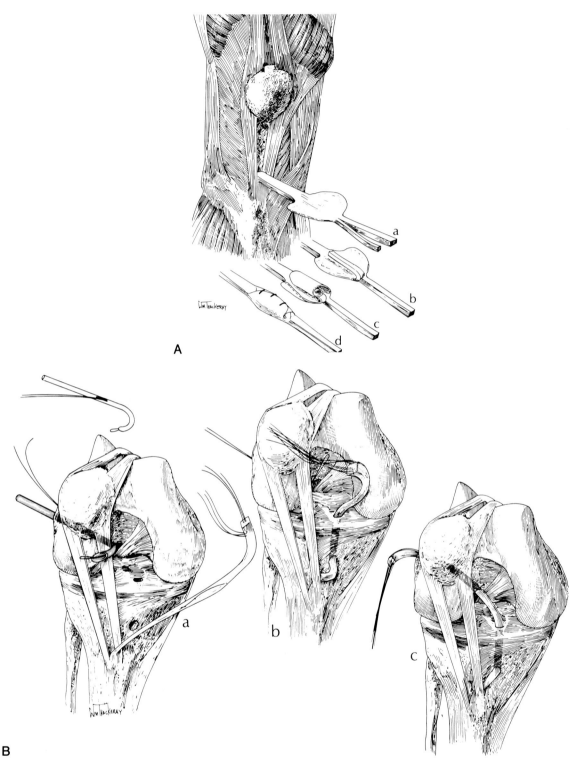

Fig. 113-30. Marshall procedure for reconstruction of the anterior cruciate ligament. **(A)** The graft is formed from a portion of the quadriceps tendon, prepatellar soft tissue, and central portion of the patellar tendon. **(B)** The tibial tunnel properly positioned and the graft sutures in the end *(a);* a ligature passer is inserted over the top of the lateral femoral condyle. Then the graft is passed into the joint through the tibial tunnel *(b).* Finally, the graft is positioned over the top of the lateral femoral condyle *(c).* (From Marshall,[83] with permission.)

Kennedy Procedure Kennedy et al.[66] used this technique with a modified attachment of the proximal portion of the graft. Instead of making a lateral incision for proximal attachment of the graft, the lateral condyle is approached through the defect in the quadriceps tendon. The surgeon recovers the graft emerging through the lateral intermuscular septum and secures it on the anterolateral surface of the femur to the periosteum. A specially designed curved introducer has been fashioned to facilitate this modification. The defect in the patellar tendon is closed with interrupted sutures.

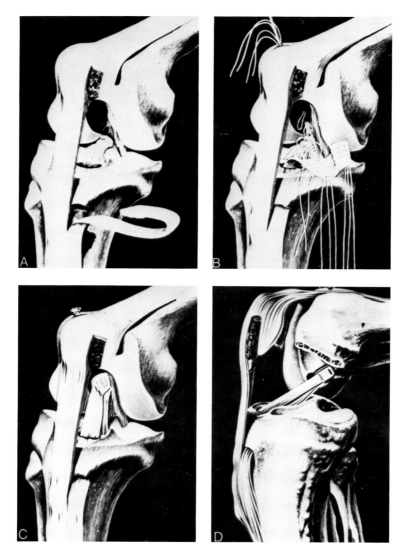

Fig. 113-31. Eriksson procedure. **(A)** The medial third of the patellar tendon, with a superficial layer of bone from the patella, is released. A tunnel is made from just above the tibial tubercle into the knee joint just anterior to the anterior cruciate insertion site. A rawbone bed is prepared high and posterior on the medial aspect of the lateral femoral condyle. **(B)** Four or five nonabsorbable 2-0 sutures are put through the ligament flap and bone. Two drill holes are made through the lateral femoral condyle and exit in the bone bed, one anterior and the other posterior. A ligature passer is inserted through the more posterior drill hole. **(C)** Anterior sutures are passed through the anterior hole and posterior through the posterior hole. Each pair, starting with the most distal, is drawn tight and tied laterally. **(D)** Sagittal view showing the flap in proper position. (From Eriksson,[27] with permission.)

The advantage of this particular procedure is that it uses a substantial piece of tissue of adequate length for cruciate substitution and can take advantage of the over-the-top route, which technically makes it easier to approximate the femoral insertion site of the ligament. A disadvantage is the weakened portion of the graft in the area of the prepatellar tissue.

Eriksson Procedure Eriksson[27,28] described a technique by Brostrom et al.[13] that was a modification of the original Jones[58] anterior cruciate reconstruction utilizing a portion of patellar tendon (Fig. 113-31). The medial third of the patellar tendon, with a thin layer of bone from the anteromedial aspect of the patella, is released, leaving the tendon attached distally. A tunnel is created through the anterior aspect of the tibia, exiting at the normal anterior cruciate insertion site intraarticularly. The flap is then fed through the tunnel into the joint and is attached to the medial aspect of the lateral femoral condyle at the old anterior cruciate insertion site. This is accomplished via four or five sutures passed through the flap, starting proximally in the bone block and proceeding distally into the tendon substance.

The sutures are tied laterally through a separate incision over the lateral femoral condyle, one pair at a time, starting with the most distal and proceeding proximally, creating more even tension on the new ligament. This technique has the advantage of using substantial tissue for reconstruction, but it is technically demanding. Eriksson has not been troubled with the flap being too short, but others have encountered this problem. Drez[23] modified this procedure by including a portion of the quadriceps tendon for additional length (Fig. 113-32). The proximal end of the flap is passed into an appropriately placed condylar tunnel, and sutures are tied over a plastic button, laterally. In addition, a pes anserinus plasty and biceps advancement are done to provide dynamic reinforcement.

Reconstruction of the Anterior Cruciate Ligament Using a Portion of the Iliotibial Tract

O'Donoghue Procedure In 1963, O'Donoghue[108] described a procedure as a modification of Hey Groves'[45] original method. This procedure has more recently been modified by Henning.[43] A tapering portion of fascia lata is released. This portion measures approximately 35 cm (14 inches) in length, 7.5 cm (3 inches) in width at its proximal end, and 2.5 cm (1 inch) in width where it crosses the joint. The strip is released from Gerdy's tubercle, but left attached where its expansion extends down as fascia over the anterior compartment muscles of the leg. A tunnel is created through the proximal tibia from anterolateral to exit intra-articularly on the tibia near the old cruciate insertion site. Another tunnel is made posteriorly in the lateral femoral condyle, again entering at the anterior cruciate insertion site and exiting laterally on the epicondylar ridge just above the flare of the lateral condyle.

The strip of iliotibial tract is passed through the tibial tunnel, across the joint, and out through the femoral canal, with the thickest and strongest portion of the strip placed intraarticularly to serve as the reconstructed anterior cruciate ligament (Fig. 113-33A). The structure is drawn tight and secured at the exit from the femoral canal with a staple and suture, while the remaining 20 to 25 cm (8 to 10 inches) of the graft is then used to close the lateral defect. The wider portion of the graft is folded over, creating two or three layers, pulled distally, and secured to the proximal tibia with a staple and then pulled back on itself and sutured in position to reestablish the integrity of the lateral structures (Fig. 113-33B). The intra-articular portion of the graft is covered with fat pad to provide a source of revascularization.

Henning Procedure Henning[43] modified this procedure primarily in the method of obtaining a graft by completely releasing the iliotibial tract at Gerdy's tubercle, by more complete fat pad coverage of the intra-articular portion of the graft, and by passing the proximal end of the graft over the top of the lateral femoral condyle rather than through a bony tunnel. Fat pad coverage is accomplished by using that portion of the fat pad that will easily reach the intercondylar notch area and by creating a tunnel through it so that the graft is completely encompassed by fat pad. Thus, the graft is passed through the tibial tunnel, through the fat pad, and over the top of the lateral femoral condyle subperiosteally and secured to the lateral collateral ligament insertion site.

Postoperatively, splints are applied and isomet-

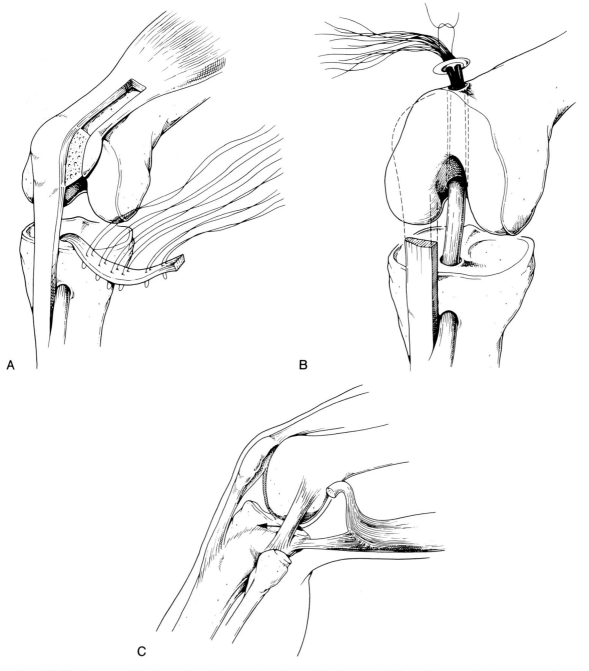

Fig. 113-32. Drez modification of the Eriksson technique. **(A)** The medial third of the patellar tendon, patellar bone, and a portion of the quadriceps tendon have been released and passed through a tibial tunnel, and a series of sutures has been placed through the proximal portion of the new ligament. **(B)** The new ligament has been fed into a lateral femoral condylar tunnel, with the sutures being tied over a button laterally. **(C)** The superficial portion of the biceps tendon is released, passed under the distal portion of the fibular collateral ligament, and advanced onto the tibia anterior to the fibular collateral ligament. (From Drez,[23] with permission.)

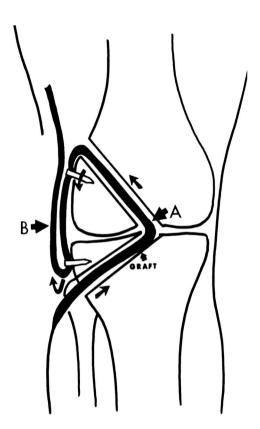

Fig. 113-33. O'Donoghue technique for replacing the anterior cruciate ligament with a strip of iliotibial tract, showing **(A)** the intraarticular portion of the graft, and **(B)** the lateral repair with folded over fascia. (From O'Donoghue,[109] with permission.)

ric exercises started as soon as tolerated. At 2 weeks, a long-leg cast with walking heel is applied; partial weight bearing is allowed during the next 4 weeks. The cast is then replaced with a splint worn for 2 additional weeks with progressive full weight bearing. Immobilization is discontinued, and gentle range of motion and strengthening exercises are started, with return to sports allowed when range of motion and strength are comparable to those of the normal side.

This procedure uses tissue of adequate length and places the heaviest portion of the graft intra-articularly. The lateral portion of the procedure, in essence, may accomplish that which more recent methods do for the ALRI, which was present perhaps in some of O'Donoghue's cases but that was not specifically described as ALRI.

Nicholas-Insall Procedures   Both Nicholas[94] and Insall[52] and their groups described a similar technique of transferring the distal portion of the iliotibial band, along with a block of bone from Gerdy's tubercle, intra-articularly to substitute for the anterior cruciate ligament. Gerdy's tubercle is released with a bone block approximately 2 cm (¾ inches) wide and 15 cm (6 inches) of attached iliotibial band broadened proximally (Fig. 113-34A). A defect is made in the posterior capsule proximally and adjacent to the lateral femoral condyle sufficiently large to accept the bone block and strip of iliotibial band. The bone block and strip, which is tubed (Fig. 113-34B), are passed through the defect in the posterior capsule, and through the intercondylar notch, and then brought forward to be attached into a new bony bed on the anteromedial tibial margin just in front of the tibial spine (Fig. 113-34C,D). The piece of bone on the iliotibial band is turned down over the new bed and secured with a cancellous lag screw (Fig. 113-34E). The iliotibial band defect is closed proximally but not distally.

Some of the problems encountered are (1) difficult passage of the transfer through the notch, (2) inadequate length of the transferred tissue, (3) fragmentation of the bone block, and, perhaps, (4) difficulty in fixing the bone block anteriorly on the tibia. If inadequate length is present, more proximal release of the iliotibial strip may solve the problem. Additional length may be gained with prolonged tension. Also, releasing the tourniquet may help. Scott et al.[120] recently showed better results when the posterior limb dissection, used to create the transfer, is limited to 4 cm from Gerdy's tubercle proximally, and the tibial bone block is attached within the notch and not over the anterior surface when the transfer is tight. This procedure is recommended for patients with combined instabilities requiring constant bracing preoperatively and should be done in conjunction with supplemental collateral reconstructive procedures.

Postoperatively, a cast is applied in extension if the knee is stable, or at 30 degrees of flexion if it is not stable in extension or if capsular repairs have been done. Within 1 to 2 weeks, the cast is changed and as much extension as possible is accomplished. Insall uses a bulky Jones dressing for 1 to 2 weeks and begins motion and weight bearing at 2 to 3

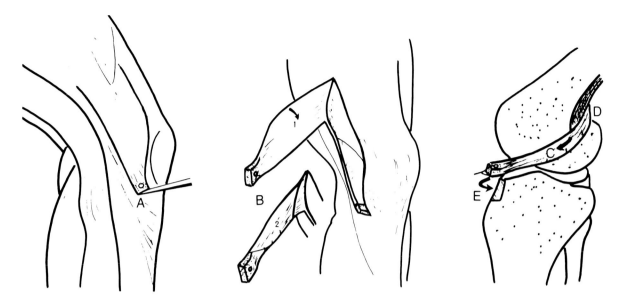

Fig. 113-34. Nicholas–Insall technique of transferring the distal portion of the iliotibial band along with a block of bone to substitute for the anterior cruciate ligament. **(A)** The iliotibial tract strip is released at Gerdy's tubercle with the attached bone block. **(B)** The strip of iliotibial tract is tubed. **(C)** The course of the new anterior cruciate ligament is shown. **(D)** The strip of iliotibial tract is passed through the posterior capsule into the intercondylar notch. **(E)** The pre-drilled bone block is attached with a screw into a new bed on the anteromedial lip of the tibia. (From Sisk,[120a] with permission. Courtesy of Dr. J. Insall.)

weeks. A well-supervised rehabilitation program is followed from that point.

The advantages of this procedure are (1) the relative technical simplicity, (2) the use of tissue that has adequate strength, (3) fascia lata has been found to survive quite well intra-articularly, and (4) bony fixation enhances the strength of the repair.

Zarins-Rowe Procedure   Zarins and Rowe[141] devised a technique combining intra-articular and extra-articular procedures for anterolateral rotary instability and anterior cruciate replacement (Fig. 113-35A). The semitendinosus tendon is identified and dissected free proximally to the musculotendinous junction, as far as possible. A 6-mm (¼-inch) drill hole is made in the anteromedial aspect of the tibia, exiting at the old anterior cruciate site intraarticularly. A 24 cm × 2.5-cm strip of iliotibial tract is dissected free from proximal to distal, leaving it attached at Gerdy's tubercle. The fibular collateral ligament, underlying lateral capsule, arcuate ligament, lateral head of the gastrocnemius, and intermuscular septum are exposed.

The semitendinosus tendon is passed through the tibial drill hole into the joint and exits through the posterior capsule adjacent to the lateral femoral condyle. It crosses over the top of the lateral femoral condyle and above the insertion of the lateral intermuscular septum. It is brought down across the posterolateral capsule and under the fibular collateral ligament and is secured to the firm attachment of the iliotibial strip (Fig. 113-35B). The iliotibial strip is passed in the opposite direction, under the fibular collateral ligament proximally, up across the posterolateral capsule, above the insertion of the lateral intermuscular septum, over the lateral femoral condyle, and into the joint to exit through the tibial tunnel, where it is secured to the attachment of the semitendinosus tendon. The fibular collateral ligament is not sutured to the underlying structures, but the semitendinosus tendon and iliotibial tract strip are sutured to the arcuate ligament just posterior to the fibular collateral ligament. The iliotibial tract defect is not closed laterally.

Postoperatively, sutures are removed at 1 week,

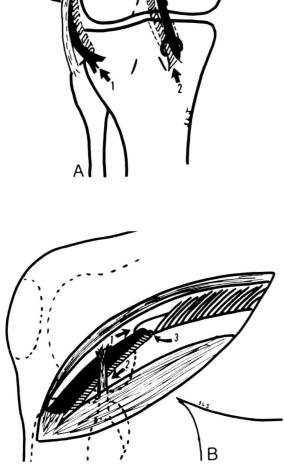

Fig. 113-35. Zahrins and Rowe technique for simultaneous intra- and extraarticular reconstruction. **(A)** Anterior schematic illustration. A strip of iliotibial tract (1) passes under the fibular collateral ligament (3), over the intermuscular septum and lateral femoral condyle, through the intercondylar notch, and out a tibial tunnel to be attached to the semitendinosus. The semitendinosus (2) passes in the opposite direction. **(B)** Laterally, the strip of iliotibial tract (1) passes under the fibular collateral ligament and over the intermuscular septum (3), and the semitendinosus (2) passes in the opposite direction.

and a hinged cast is applied with a posterior strap, preventing extension past fifty degrees of flexion. Partial weight bearing with crutches is allowed. The cast is removed at 7 weeks and a knee brace applied. Crutches are discontinued 3 months postoperatively. A rehabilitation program follows, with swimming at 3 months and running at 6 months. The patient can engage in full activities at 1 year.

The advantage of this procedure is that it combines intra- and extra-articular procedures, using the two transfers for additional strength. The extensor mechanism is not compromised, and Zarins and Rowe believe that the reconstruction is isometric to the knee position. A disadvantage is perhaps a thinner portion of the iliotibial tract being used intraarticularly, but this is reinforced with the semitendinosus.

Cho-Horne Procedure   Cho[17] and Horne and Parsons[46] described semitendinosus replacement of the anterior cruciate ligament (Fig. 113-36). James[53a] described the following technique in the previous edition of this book, which is a modification of the above-mentioned authors' procedure. The semitendinosus tendon is released at its musculotendinous junction as high as possible, and the semitendinosus muscle is anastomosed to the musculotendinous junction of the gracilis. A suture is placed in the end of the cut semitendinosus tendon. A tibial tunnel is drilled with a 5-mm drill, starting 2 cm proximal to the insertion of the semitendinosus and exiting intra-articularly at the insertion site of the old anterior cruciate ligament but somewhat medially, so that the new structure will avoid the lateral femoral condyle. Through a lateral approach, a second tunnel is made with a 5-mm drill bit starting 1 cm anterior and proximal to the insertion of the fibular collateral ligament on the lateral femoral condyle and exiting at the junction of the lateral femoral condyle and intercondylar notch just above the cruciate insertion on the lateral femoral condyle. Soft tissues are cleared off the lateral femoral condyle intra-articularly, and a defect is created in the posterior capsule by pushing a large tendon passer or forceps through it high in the notch area and posteriorly while palpating the progress of the instrument from posterior. A distally based flap of fat pad is created for attachment to the semitendinosus tendon.

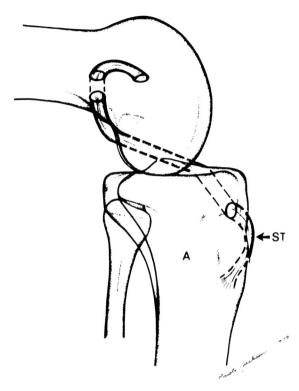

Fig. 113-36. Semitendinosus replacement for the anterior cruciate. The tendon *(ST)* passes through a tibial tunnel, across the intercondylar notch, through the posterior capsule, over the top of the lateral femoral condyle, and through a tunnel in the lateral femoral epicondyle. (From James,[54] with permission.)

The semitendinosus tendon is passed through the tibial tunnel and into the joint and then posterior to exit through the capsular defect, where it is recovered in the popliteal space posterolaterally. It is then passed from posterior to anterior through the condylar tunnel, and its position is checked by applying tension to the tendon as the knee is passed through a full range of motion. The tendon is observed to see if it pulls back into the tunnel, particularly with knee extension. If more than 5 mm of motion is noted, the tendon is improperly positioned. This can usually be corrected by enlarging the exit of the tibial tunnel posteriorly with a curette and allowing the tendon to displace more posteriorly in relationship to the tibia. Once the tendon has been properly positioned, it is secured by applying tension with the knee flexed 30 degrees, attaching the end of the semitendinosus to the insertion of the intermuscular septum, or the insertion of the fibular collateral ligament with the previously placed suture in the free end. This is often combined with an extra-articular tenodesing type of procedure, using a strip of iliotibial band; both structures may be passed through the tunnel in the lateral femoral condyle simply by enlarging it sufficiently.

Postoperatively, the knee is immobilized in a long-leg cast at 30 to 40 degrees of flexion for 3 weeks. A limited-hinge cylinder cast[42] is applied, permitting motion from 30 to 60 degrees for the next 7 weeks. Touch weight bearing only is allowed. Motion within the limits of the hinge is allowed along with straight-leg raising and hip abduction exercises. Electrical muscle stimulation is started the first day postoperatively and, if a portable unit is available, continued throughout the period of cast immobilization.

The advantages of this procedure are that it is relatively easy technically and takes advantage of the over-the-top route. Disadvantages are that the semitendinosus tendon is not as strong as the normal cruciate ligament and that, occasionally, it may be very small, precluding its use. If the patient has had previous ligament surgery medially, the semitendinosus may have already been incorporated in a pes plasty and may therefore be unavailable.

Several synthetic devices to replace or augment human ligaments have recently been developed.[1] Some are meant to replace the native ligament permanently, others augment autogenous repairs and permit earlier return of function while autogenous tissues are revascularizing. Some serve as scaffolds onto which neoligaments grow out of native collagen. No long-term results are available as yet for these devices. Although some studies show promising results, their use is not discussed here.

Authors' Preferred Technique

The technique described here is a modification of the Marshall procedure[83,84] previously described. We have found that isolated injury of the anterior cruciate ligament rarely is present in chronic situations. We therefore describe it as a separate entity, as a matter of convenience and to prevent repeating this description in each of the various instabilities of which it is a part.

Generally, chronic anterior cruciate ligament instability will be found in combination with either medial or lateral instabilities. As a result, the incision used will depend on the associated conditions. Generally, either the lateral or medial curvilinear incisions described under Chronic Medial Instability and Chronic Anterolateral Rotatory Instability (see Figs. 113-15, 113-28) should be used.

If the anterior cruciate ligament is an isolated injury, a midline incision can be used that starts approximately 8 cm above the superior pole of the patella, extending in the midline to 2 cm distal to the tibial tubercle. A median parapatellar incision is made into the knee joint, leaving approximately 1.5 cm of retinacular tissue around the edge of the patella for later closure. A 1.5-cm strip of the middle portion of the distal quadriceps tendon, 5 cm in length, is isolated (Fig. 113-37A). This is harvested in continuity with the anterior prepatellar soft tissue and periosteum, as for a Marshall procedure,[92] being careful not to slip over the edge of the patella and disrupt the retinacular attachments. At the inferior pole of the patella, the graft is continued to include the medial third of the patellar tendon to the level of the tibial tuberosity. The graft is left attached distally; 5 mm of the quadriceps portion of the graft is isolated longitudinally (Fig. 113-37AA) and turned down over the periosteal surface of the prepatellar soft tissue portion of the graft (Fig. 113-37AB). The ovoid prepatellar tissue is then folded over and tubed about the strip of quadriceps tendon. (Fig. 113-37AC,D) This is secured with multiple interrupted sutures. This fold over of quadriceps tendon and tubing of the patellar tissue adds reinforcement to the graft, where it is thin in the midportion.

A Steinmann pin is drilled into the anterior tibia just medial to the graft attachment at the tibial tuberosity. It is directed to exit within the midportion of the stump of the anterior cruciate ligament, remaining on the superior surface of the tibia. The anterior cruciate ligament stump is then separated into medial and lateral halves in a longitudinal fashion surrounding the pin (Fig. 113-37B). A cannulated drill bit, ⅜ inch in size, is then used to create a tunnel through the tibia for the graft. A second Steinmann pin is placed in the notch on the medial side of the posterior portion of the lateral condyle

of the femur, again, within the midsubstance of the femoral attachment of the anterior cruciate ligament. Marshall recommended using a small drill and starting from the lateral surface of the femur, drilling into the notch to prevent the drill point from slipping off of the condyle during drilling. We have not found this to be a problem when using a Steinmann pin as a guide for the cannulated drill with the knee in maximal flexion and believe that it is the position of the intra-articular portion of the hole that is most important to place properly. Once again, the stump of the anterior cruciate is split into medial and lateral halves longitudinally surrounding the pin. This pin is used to guide the cannulated ⅜-inch drill to create a tunnel in the femur.

After the tunnel in the femur is completed, a curette is used to bevel the entrance to the bone tunnels to prevent abrasion injury to the graft. Some workers[78,83] believe that an over-the-top technique, as proposed by McIntosh, is a better procedure, in that the graft does not enter a bone tunnel in the femur and is not at risk of abrasion injury. We believe that the benefits of a properly placed and radiused bone tunnel as well as the bony ingrowth provided outweigh the risks. If the knee is maximally flexed, exact placement is not difficult.

Exposure of the lateral femoral cortex can usually be obtained by dissecting laterally, superficial to the fascia latta, around to the lateral side of the thigh to the lateral intermuscular septum and, subsequently, to the lateral femoral cortex at the exit of the femoral bone tunnel. Occasionally, the cortex can be reached by subperiosteal dissection through the gap in the quadriceps tendon from the harvested proximal portion of the graft.

After both bone tunnels are made and the graft has been tubed, a heavy permanent suture is placed in a Bunnell fashion through the proximal portion of the graft to allow for passage of the graft through the bone tunnels. The graft is then placed from anterior to posterior through the tibial tunnel into the notch (Fig. 113-37C). Subsequently, it is passed in a retrograde fashion through the femoral tunnel and out over the lateral surface of the femur (Fig. 113-37D). At this point, the lateral surface of the femur is decorticated just superior to the tunnel exit with an osteotome or rasp. The leg is posi-

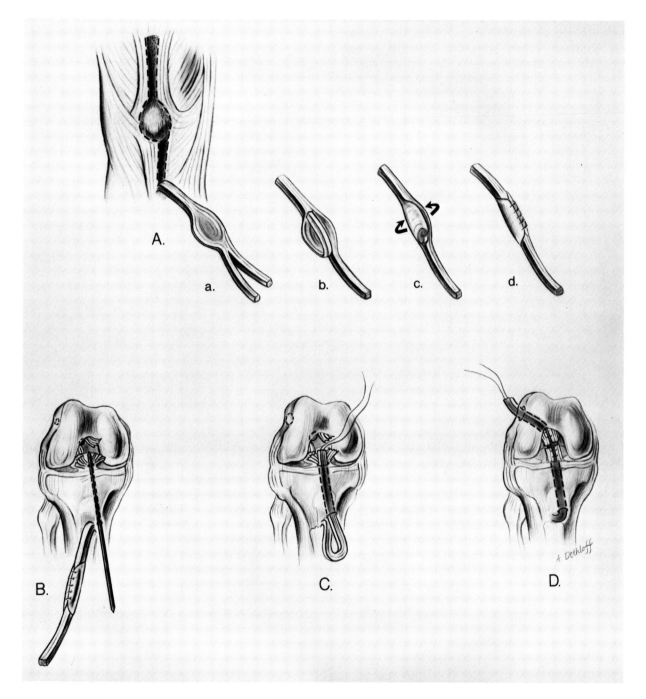

Fig. 113-37. Authors' preferred technique. **(A)** A graft is formed from a portion of the quadriceps tendon, prepatellar soft tissue, and the medial third of the patellar tendon. **(B)** The ruptured ACL is split into medial and lateral halves. A Steinmann pin is placed as a guide from the media tibial tubercle into the substance of the divided ACL. **(C)** The graft is then passed through the tibial tunnel. **(D)** Finally, the graft is passed through the femoral tunnel, drawn tight, and stapled to the lateral femoral cortex in a cancellous bone bed.

tioned in 60 degrees of flexion, and the graft is pulled taut as the assistant applies a posterior force on the tibia. The graft is placed into the decorticated bone bed superior to the exit hole on the lateral femur and is secured with a medium-size barbed staple. It is then folded back over the staple and sewn to itself with absorbable sutures.

After the graft is firmly attached, the longitudinal halves of the anterior cruciate ligament, if present, are used along with fat pad to enclose the graft as it passes through the notch. This works particularly well with acute ruptures when the anterior cruciate has a midsubstance tear and has not become so scarred as to prevent reapproximation of the ends over the graft.

The defects in the quadriceps tendon and patellar tendon are repaired with interrupted absorbable sutures. The wound is then closed in the usual fashion over suction drains, taking care to close the medial patellar retinaculum tightly. The patient is placed in a removable hinged cast brace in the operating room with the hinges locked in 30 degrees of flexion.

Postoperative Management

Postoperative care and rehabilitation are as important as the surgical reconstructive procedure. The best care is to prevent problems from arising. Noyes et al.[103] showed that revascularization can take as long as four months. It is imperative that the patient understand that the rehabilitation period is long and that it should be followed carefully, if a good result is expected.

The patient is placed in a removable hinged cast brace while in the operating room with the hinges locked in 30 degrees of flexion. Prophylactic antibiotics are given starting just before surgery and continuing until after removal of the drains.

On the second postoperative day, the patient is sent to the physical therapy suite for crutch ambulation training with touch-weight-bearing instructions. Discharge from the hospital usually follows within 1 or 2 days. The sutures are removed at the end of the second week. The hinges are then reset to permit range of motion from 30 to 45 degrees of flexion. Passive range-of-motion exercises are started with cautions to the patient not to contract

the quadriceps muscle. Contralateral straight-leg raising and ankle exercises are encouraged.

At 4 weeks, hip abduction, adduction, and extension exercises are started. Active range of motion of the hamstring muscle only, and not of the quadriceps, is also begun.

At the 6-week visit, partial weight bearing is instituted and is advanced as tolerated to full weight bearing by 8 weeks. In addition, range of motion is increased by adding 5 degrees of extension and 10 degrees of flexion to the limits of the hinges at weekly intervals.

By 8 weeks, the range-of-motion limits should be from 15 to 60 degrees of flexion. Once this point is reached, the brace can be removed while the patient uses crutches to protect against full weight bearing and the risk of forced full extension. The brace is worn when the crutches are not used. Exercises are added to include hamstring isotonics, hip flexion in the sitting position, wall slides for knee flexion, and quadriceps setting exercises with the knee in 45 degrees of flexion.

At 12 weeks, the patient is allowed to swim and bicycle within the available range of motion. A custom-fitted anterior cruciate ligament brace is ordered if adequate girth has returned to the thigh.

By 16 weeks, the patient is allowed to use full extension, if possible. Light swimming and cycling are continued. Toe raises, step-ups, and quadriceps eccentrics are added. The patient is allowed to jog on a minitramp in the physical therapy suite and progress to light jogging on the treadmill, while supervised.

At 24 weeks, the anterior cruciate brace is being worn full time. Swimming and cycling are continued. Except while in the therapy department, the patient is still not allowed to run or jump.

At 9 months, the patient can start running if deficits are 25 percent or less (compared with the contralateral side, by Cybex testing) and if there is an adequate range of motion and no swelling.

Activities are gradually increased and exercises are continued until 1 year, at which time strength and redevelopment of athletic skills are encouraged. The knee should be taped and the custom brace worn for strenuous exercise. For routine daily activities, the brace should be discontinued. The patient is counseled to avoid high-risk activities, which could reinjure the knee.

Modification of the Authors' Preferred Technique

Recently, the authors have modified their preferred choice and have begun harvesting a free graft of patellar tendon with a 2.5-cm piece of bone attached to either end.[68a] Using the arthroscope[118a] and appropriate instruments, an adequate notchplasty is done. After that, tibial and femoral guides are used intra-articularly so that a Steinmann pin can be placed across the tibia into the distal stump of the anterior cruciate, and a second Steinmann pin is placed across the lateral aspect of the femur into the proximal attachment area of the cruciate. A suture is then pulled through these two holes and grasped at both ends. The knee is then moved through a range of motion. If the suture length does not change more than 0.3 mm then the placement of the Steinmann pins is felt to be correct — or isometric.

The Steinmann pins are then replaced in the holes and over-drilled to the desired diameter of the graft. The inner aspect of the graft tunnels is bevelled using a file. The graft material is then attached to a suture and pulled across the joint into place, with the bony ends of the graft left remaining at one end in the tibial tunnel and at the other end in the femoral tunnel. The graft is pulled snug and fixed in place by putting a large screw into the bony tunnels of both the femur and the tibia, producing an interference type fixation.

For those familiar with the use of the arthroscope, the procedure can be done without opening the knee. This has both advantages and disadvantages, and only time will tell as to whether or not the arthroscopically assisted anterior cruciate ligament augmentation procedure described above will be significantly better than open techniques.

Following placement of the graft and fixation with the interference screws, the wounds are closed in a routine manner and the patient placed into a hinged brace in the operating room.

Postoperative Management

Because of the good fixation of the graft with the interference screws, early mobilization can be begun. The hinges on the brace are opened so that the patient can begin both active and passive range of motion through a protected range of approximately 30 degrees, extending from 15 degrees of flexion to 45 degrees of flexion.

The patient's leg is protected with the brace for a total period of 6 weeks. The brace is opened at 2 weeks to allow 60 degrees of flexion with 180 degrees of extension. At 4 weeks, the brace is opened to allow for normal amounts of flexion and extension. Active extension exercises are not part of the rehabilitation protocol until at least 4 months after the operation. At 6 weeks, the brace is discarded and exercises continued. At 8 weeks, cycling and light swimming are begun. From 16 weeks on, the protocol for rehabilitation is the same as that in the previous section.

Posterior Instabilities

The discussion in this section deals with posterior instabilities consisting of one-plane posterior instability and posterolateral rotary instability (PLRI). Posteromedial rotary instability is an entity that is but rarely encountered.

One-plane posterior instability and PLRI are frequently dealt with simultaneously in the unstable knee. One-plane posterior instability is described as an instability in which the tibia subluxates posteriorly with the knee in a semiflexed position, implying injury to the posterior cruciate ligament, as well as to the secondary collateral restraints. Posterolateral rotary instability occurs with the lateral tibial plateau subluxating posteriorly in relation to the lateral femoral condyle, implying more direct injury to the posterolateral structures, which may include the arcuate complex (fibular collateral ligament, popliteus, and arcuate ligament), perhaps the biceps tendon, and, in some instances, even the anterior cruciate ligament, as well as stretching or complete rupture of the posterior cruciate ligament. In this instance, however, the posteromedial supporting structures have remained intact, acting as a pivot point. Both types of instability can be severely debilitating, and both may require posterior cruciate reconstruction, as well as peripheral stabilizing procedures.

Chronic Posterolateral Rotatory Instability

Posterolateral rotatory instability is a particularly distressing and disabling type of rotary instability, in which the lateral tibial plateau rotates or subluxes posteriorly in relation to the lateral femoral condyle (see Fig. 113-8).

Pathomechanics

Pathologically, this entity is primarily a lesion involving the lateral capsule, arcuate ligament, popliteus, and lateral half of the posterior capsule. Posterior cruciate ligament incompetency is often present, and injury to the lateral gastrocnemius tendon, biceps femoris, iliotibial tract, fibular collateral ligament, and anterior cruciate ligament may be associated. The mechanism of injury appears to be either hyperextension and varus or forceful external rotation of the tibia with the knee in a flexed position.

Diagnosis and Clinical Evaluation

Symptomatically, patients complain that their knee hyperextends or feels unstable in extension and gives way. Posterolateral pain is common, and often there is anteromedial joint line pain as well from soft tissue impingement due to abnormal tibial rotation. Frequently, the symptoms appear out of proportion to clinical findings, with only a mild degree of posterolateral rotary instability.

Physical examination indicates a positive posterior drawer sign with the lateral plateau subluxating posteriorly when a posterior force is applied to the proximal tibia (Fig. 113-38). A positive external rotation-recurvatum test[51] may be found, characterized by excessive external rotation of the tibia with recurvatum and an apparent increased tibia varum (Fig. 113-39). This test is performed with the patient supine and the extremity supported at the heel. External rotation-recurvatum may also be demonstrated by having the patient walk and noting a back knee with weight bearing, along with a varus thrust at the knee. In cases in which the lateral stabilizing structures have been severely disrupted, varus instability will be present, but this is not a common finding. The initial examination may suggest a one-plane posterior instability but, on closer scrutiny, it will be noted that the posteromedial aspect of the tibia remains relatively stable, while the lateral tibial plateau displaces posteriorly.

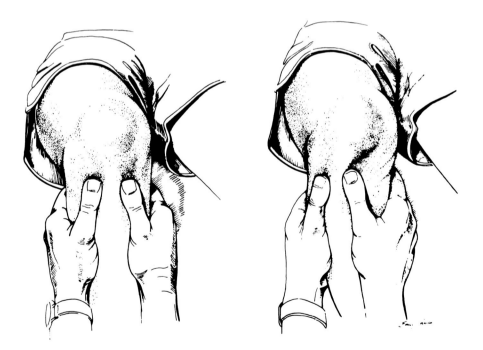

Fig. 113-38. Posterior drawer sign with posterior lateral rotary instability. The lateral tibial plateau rotates posteriorly while the medial plateau remains reduced. (From Hughston,[51] with permission.)

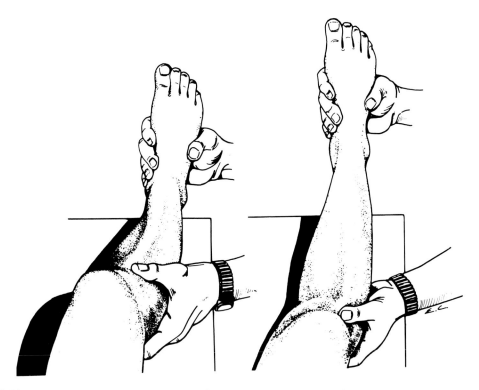

Fig. 113-39. External rotation-recurvatum test. The knee is initially slightly flexed and then slowly extended. A positive test will demonstrate external tibial rotation and recurvatum. (From Hughston,[51] with permission.)

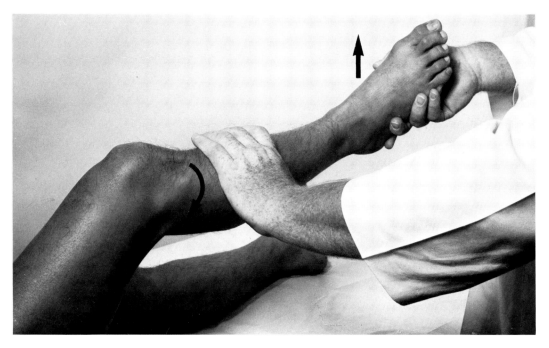

Fig. 113-40. Slocum test for posterolateral rotary instability (see text).

Slocum (personal communication) uses a test for PLRI of the knee that is somewhat similar to the MacIntosh test for pivot shift with ALRI. This test is performed by placing the patient supine on the examining table with the involved extremity elevated, supporting the patient's heel with the tibia in neutral rotation and the knee in full extension (Fig. 113-40). The surgeon's opposite hand is placed over the posterolateral aspect of the patient's proximal leg, forcing the knee into valgus and compressing the lateral joint surfaces. The tibia is then externally rotated as the knee is flexed. A palpable and occasional audible "thud" occurs as the knee passes into flexion and posterolateral subluxation of the tibial plateau occurs. This test may also be performed by extending the patient's knee from the fully flexed position again, with the tibia held in external rotation and a valgus force applied to the knee. As the knee passes into extension, a sudden reduction of the lateral plateau is palpable as it moves anteriorly to a reduced position. This test is particularly applicable in the more subtle forms of PLRI and must not be confused with the pivot-shift type of test for ALRI.

Standard radiographs are of little help in the diagnosis of PLRI, but a lateral stress view with posterior force applied to the proximal leg will often demonstrate posterior displacement of the lateral plateau. The displacement may be enhanced if the stress view is also done with the tibia externally rotated. Arthroscopy will help assess the status of intra-articular structures. Examination with the patient under anesthesia is particularly helpful with patients who are unable to relax.

Treatment Modalities

Most methods in the literature recommend transfer of the bony attachment of the lateral collateral ligament and/or popliteal tendon anteriorly and proximally on the lateral femoral condyle. In the event of posterior cruciate insufficiency or disruption, this may be combined with posterior cruciate reconstruction as well.

Surgical Procedures

Slocum et al.[124] described a repair for posterolateral rotary instability consisting of (1) a fascial reefing, (2) lateral gastrocnemius advancement, (3)

biceps femoris plasty, and (4) pes anserinus transfer (Fig. 113-41). The posterolateral reefing procedure may be carried out with a strip of fascia used as a suture or with heavy suture material. The posterolateral reefing tightens the lower portion of the posterior capsule and arcuate ligament to the lateral capsule and fibular collateral ligament. The gastrocnemius tendon, with the attached posterior capsule, is released from its insertion above the lateral femoral condyle and brought forward just anterior to the superior attachment of the fibular collateral ligament, where it is attached to the lateral femoral condyle. This effectively tightens the upper portion of the posterior capsule and oblique popliteal ligament and also provides muscular support for the posterolateral aspect of the knee. A biceps femoris transplant is accomplished by re-

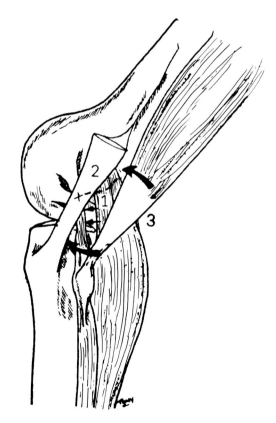

Fig. 113-41. Slocum reconstruction for posterolateral rotary instability. (1) Lateral gastrocnemius advancement. The posterior border of the iliotibial tract (2) is the attachment site for the biceps femoris transfer (3). (From Slocum,[124] with permission.)

leasing the posterior three-fourths of its attachment on the fibula and its insertion on the anterolateral aspect of the tibia and then rotating it upward, where it is attached along the trailing edge of the iliotibial tract. The biceps femoris transplant diminishes external tibial rotation normally induced by biceps contraction, yet provides active support to the lateral side of the knee. Care needs to be taken in mobilizing the biceps tendon to avoid traction on the peroneal nerve. Medially, a pes anserinus transplant is accomplished to help stabilize the tibia against abnormal external rotation.

Trillat[131] reports quite good success, with 10 of 11 athletes returning to sports following this reconstructive procedure for posterolateral rotary instability. Through a utilitarian lateral approach, the iliotibial tract is cut transversely near its insertion at Gerdy's tubercle (Fig. 113-42A). A lateral meniscectomy is routine. The popliteus tendon and fibular collateral ligament are exposed, and their insertion on the lateral femoral condyle is released en masse along with a small button of bone (Fig. 113-42B). The popliteal area on the posterior surface of the tibia is inspected. If the capsule has been detached or stretched, a new bed is prepared on the posterior aspect of the tibia, drill holes are made anteroposteriorly through the proximal tibia, and sutures are passed to secure the posterior capsule in its new bed. The insertions of the popliteal tendon and fibular collateral ligament are advanced anteriorly and proximally on the femur. The iliotibial tract is then repaired through drill holes placed on the lateral aspect of the tibia.

Trillat points out that severe lesions of the popliteal muscle are the cause for failures in this type of reconstruction. Also, gross lesions of the posterior cruciate will compromise the reconstruction. In those situations in which the posterior cruciate is irreparably damaged, Trillat has resorted to a prosthetic cruciate ligament for reconstruction.

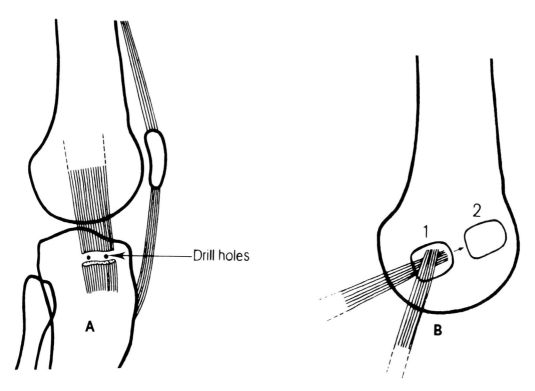

Fig. 113-42. Trillat's procedure. **(A)** The iliotibial tract is cut transversely, and drill holes are placed for reattachment. **(B)** Anterior and proximal transfer of the popliteal and fibular collateral insertion (1), arcuate ligament, lateral head of the gastrocnemius, and underlying posterior capsule (2). (From Trillat,[131] with permission.)

Authors' Preferred Technique

To eliminate posterolateral rotatory instability biomechanically, something must be done on the posterolateral aspect of the knee to restore the integrity of the structures that have a sufficient moment arm for resisting external tibial rotation. Our usual approach, which involves both static and dynamic structures, involves replacement or reconstruction of the posterior cruciate ligament and en masse advancement anteriorly and proximally of the arcuate complex. This approach not only provides stability for one-plane posterior subluxation of the tibia by replacing the posterior cruciate ligament, but also reconstructs more laterally positioned structures which have a better mechanical advantage to resist external tibial rotation.

In our experience, posterolateral rotatory instability usually involves injury to the posterior cruciate ligament, as well as to the posterolateral corner. As a rule, the posterior cruciate must be reconstructed. Our preferred procedure for the posterior cruciate reconstruction is described in the following section on chronic posterior cruciate instability in this chapter and is not duplicated here.

Diagnostic arthroscopy is initially carried out to establish the status of the menisci and joint surfaces. The procedure is performed through an S-shaped curvilinear incision, as shown in Figure 113-28.

The leg is positioned in 45 degrees of flexion over a bolster. The incision begins 6 cm above the joint line along the anterior border of the biceps femoris and extends gently distally, curving anterior toward the superior pole of the patella to meet the joint line 2 cm lateral to the patella. From here, the incision follows the lateral border of the patella 2 cm laterally to a point 2 cm distal to the patellar tendon attachment on the tibial tubercle. This exposes the anterior retinaculum, iliotibial band, and biceps femoris tendon. The iliotibial tract is incised longitudinally from Gerdy's tubercle to 5 cm proximal to the lateral femoral condyle. The margins are retracted, and dissection is carried out to expose the vastus lateralis, intermuscular septum, lateral gastrocnemius tendon, arcuate ligament, and popliteal tendon. The surgeon mobilizes the arcuate complex en masse with an osteotome by re-

leasing the popliteal tendon and fibular collateral insertion site with a 3- to 4-mm-thick button of bone, continuing posteriorly around the condyle and releasing the arcuate ligament insertion along with the gastrocnemius and underlying posterior capsule, leaving a very thin wafer of bone on these structures. Thus, the entire arcuate complex, lateral portion of the posterior capsule, and gastrocnemius tendon are totally mobilized in preparation for anterior and proximal advancement.

A new bone bed is fashioned anteriorly and proximally over the lateral femoral condyle to accept the small button of bone with attached popliteus tendon and fibular collateral ligament. These are advanced to the new bone bed and are secured with a cancellous bone screw and ligament washer (Fig. 113-43). This also advances the arcuate ligament and gastrocnemius tendon along with the posterior capsule. These latter structures are secured in their new position with heavy interrupted sutures.

The iliotibial tract is repaired, and the wound is closed in the usual fashion over suction drains. The patient is placed in a removable hinged cast brace at the termination of the procedure, with the hinges locked in 30 degrees of flexion.

Postoperative Management

Postoperative management of chronic posterolateral rotatory instability is identical to that for posterior cruciate ligament reconstruction.

Chronic Posterior Cruciate Instability

The symptoms and the degree of disability are quite variable in chronic cases (see Fig. 113-3). Function may range from very mild, or essentially no impairment, to severe disability with the patient requiring crutches or bracing to walk. Pain, giving way, stiffness, and swelling are the more common complaints. Giving-way episodes are more likely to occur when the patient is walking downhill or downstairs, wearing high-heeled shoes, or stopping suddenly with the knee flexed. Giving way in these situations is associated with forward subluxation of the femoral condyles on the tibial plateaus. The knee may feel more stable when kept in full extension and, consequently, patients may relate that they walk or run stiff-legged.

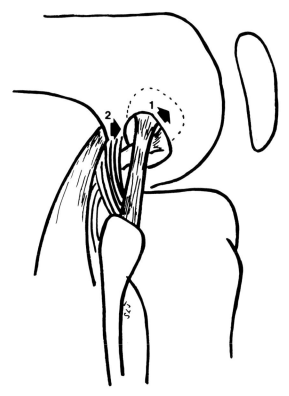

Fig. 113-43. Author's preferred technique. Proximal advancement of the posterior lateral structures. (1) The insertions of the fibular collateral ligament and popliteus tendon are moved proximally and anteriorly. (2) The insertions of the arcuate ligament and lateral head of the gastronemius with the underlying posterior capsule are advanced anteriorly on the femoral condyle.

Pathomechanics

A description of the mechanism of injury, if available, is particularly important and may help the examiner in determining whether a posterior cruciate ligament injury is likely to have occurred acutely. Kennedy and co-workers[62,65] have documented a more frequent occurrence of posterior cruciate ligament injuries than had been considered previously. A review of ligament repair and reconstructive procedures at their facility revealed one posterior cruciate ligament surgery for every six anterior cruciate ligament surgeries. Most posterior cruciate injuries were incurred in athletic activities or vehicular accidents. The mechanism of injury was a direct blow to the tibia with the knee flexed, a hyperextension injury, or a valgus side-swipe type of injury. Four groups were identified based on the ligament combination involved. Group I patients had essentially isolated posterior cruciate tears. Group II patients had associated anterior cruciate ligament injuries, in addition to the posterior cruciate. Group III patients had associated major medial or lateral collateral ligament disruptions but had intact anterior cruciates. Group IV, the largest group of patients, had associated anterior cruciate injury along with major disruption of either the medial or lateral collateral ligaments in conjunction with the posterior cruciate. These injuries probably could be considered dislocations.

The degree of degenerative changes correlated well with the number of associated ligament injuries and degree of instability: 58 percent of group IV patients developed significant degenerative changes, at an average follow-up of 44.6 months. The study suggests that cases with isolated posterior cruciate injury or those in which there is additional ligament injury without severe instability may be managed conservatively with considerably less chance of degenerative changes ensuing.

Another study giving some insight into the natural history of posterior cruciate instabilities is by Degenhardt and Hughston,[21] in which 92 patients with chronic posterior cruciate instability were evaluated. Forty others failed to respond to conservative treatment and underwent posterior cruciate reconstruction, and 52 were managed conservatively. Again, the results correlated closely with the degree of instability and the number of additional ligaments involved. Those patients requiring surgery had greater instability with a larger number of additional ligaments involved.

Diagnosis and Clinical Evaluation

The most salient physical findings are a wasting of the quadriceps, posterior sag sign, recurvatum, and a positive posterior drawer sign. One must also examine the knee for additional instabilities indicative of collateral or anterior cruciate ligament damage.

In performing the routine drawer test, with the hip flexed 45 degrees and the knee at 90 degrees, the starting position of the tibia must be ascertained in relationship to the femoral condyles.

With chronic posterior cruciate instability, the tibia may sag posteriorly when the knee is positioned for examination. With forward pressure applied to the posteriorly displaced tibia, it moves forward in what is often misinterpreted as a positive anterior drawer sign when, in actuality, the tibia is simply being reduced to its normal relationship with the femur. This trap may be avoided by positioning both knees for the drawer test and then observing from the side to see whether a posterior sag or displacement of the tibia is present relative to the normal side. Lesser degrees of posterior sag or subluxation can be determined by palpating the relationship of the femoral condyles to the anterior lip of the plateaus. If the femoral condyles are prominent, a posterior subluxation is suggested.

A new test for posterior instability was presented at the interim meeting of the AOSSM in San Francisco in February 1987 by Whipple.[138] For this simple test, the patient is placed in the prone position with the knee flexed to 45 degrees, gently stabilized by one finger on the anterior surface of the distal tibia at the level of the ankle. Gentle pressure is placed on the tibial tuberosity, directed in a posterior direction. When instability is present, a posterior drawer will occur. If a rotational component is present, the foot will rotate toward the side of the instability. If the knee is flexed to 90 degrees, the test becomes more specific for the posterior cruciate ligament. In this position, the posterior oblique ligament, the arcuate complex, and the posterior capsule are relaxed. This test is very sensitive in discriminating a true straight posterior instability from a posterior rotatory instability. In addition, it prevents misinterpretation of the reduction of a posterior sag as being an anterior instability.

Radiographs may show an avulsion fragment, usually at the insertion of the posterior cruciate ligament on the proximal tibia.[129,130] Arthroscopic examination can also be of benefit, particularly to determine the status of the remainder of the joint in relationship to meniscal lesions, degenerative changes, and possible osteochondral fractures. It is possible to view the posterior cruciate ligament from either a posteromedial portal or anteriorly with a 70-degree angled scope passed into the posterior aspect of the notch, where one can peer around the anterior cruciate ligament.

Single- or double-contrast arthrographic stress views will usually outline the cruciate ligaments quite clearly if they are intact. Lateral radiograph stress views also help determine cruciate stability by revealing excessive posterior displacement of the tibial plateaus in relationship to the femoral condyles.

Treatment Modalities

The decision for reconstruction may be made on the basis of the natural history of posterior cruciate ligament injuries and, most importantly, of the functional deficit in the individual patient. Patients with a mild (1+) degree of posterior instability (1+, 0 to 5 mm; 2+, 6 to 10 mm; 3+, over 10 mm) need not necessarily have surgical reconstruction, since this degree of instability is consistent with a satisfactory degree of functional activity in many instances. A trial of conservative therapy with a vigorous rehabilitation program is warranted in these situations. Posterior cruciate ligament instability associated with additional ligamentous insufficiencies of a significant degree are more likely to create functional deficits with subsequent degenerative changes than are lesser degrees of involvement. It should be kept in mind, however, that even the best of posterior cruciate ligament reconstructions will probably not result in anything better than a 1+ residual instability. Therefore, there seems to be little need to proceed with reconstructive procedures unless the patient has at least a 2+ posterior drawer sign associated with a significant degree of functional deficit. Patients with acute mild or only suspected posterior cruciate ligament injuries should be monitored for a number of months following the initial injury. It is not uncommon for a posterior drawer sign to be absent at the time of acute injury, only to progress with attrition of secondary supporting structures. These patients may develop functional instability of a significant degree in spite of early protection. Patients should be advised at the time of injury that, although there appears to be no immediate surgical indication, continued evaluation will be necessary and posterior instability of a significant degree may ensue.

Posterior cruciate reconstruction is generally not indicated for the elderly or relatively sedentary type of person, unless there is a significant functional impairment. Severe degenerative arthritic changes, a history of previous sepsis, knees that have had one or more previous reconstructive procedures, and patients with debilitating diseases certainly have a reduced prognosis for a good result. Because of the nature of the trauma involved, posterior cruciate ligament injuries are often associated with multiple injuries that may result in residual impairment or altered neuromuscular function in the extremity. These patients must be carefully evaluated before one embarks on extensive reconstructive procedures. Often, it is difficult to determine whether disability in the involved lower extremity is secondary to ligamentous instability of the knee or due to altered function from other problems, particularly neuromuscular deficiencies.

Surgical Procedures

Reconstruction of the posterior cruciate has long posed a difficult problem for the orthopaedist. Since this ligament is the strongest ligament and is the primary static stabilizer of the knee against posterior tibial subluxation,[15] it is not surprising that many of the results using local tissues as a substitute have been less than satisfactory. Numerous procedures have been described in the literature,[32,44,45,95,130] but many without significant follow-up studies.

Meniscus Substitution A meniscus that would otherwise be removed may be used as a posterior cruciate substitute[74,127] as a free graft with one end anchored into a tibial tunnel and the other into a medial femoral condyle tunnel. The meniscus must be basically intact, however, and not severely damaged in order to function as a graft. We feel that if a meniscus is in an adequate condition to be used as a graft, it should be repaired rather than sacrificed. This type of reconstruction is, therefore, presented for historical reasons only.

Hughston et al.[47] report that they used the meniscus for posterior cruciate reconstruction in some 10 or 11 chronic cases until 1973, but then discontinued its use because they believed that the "traumatic reaction of acute injury" from tissue healing in the joint, which was necessary for proper survival of this type of graft, was lacking in the chronic situation.

Patellar Tendon Free Graft Clancy et al.[18] and Karpf (personal communication) have used free grafts consisting of a portion of the patellar tendon with attached tibial tubercle and patellar bone blocks. The graft is harvested as described for anterior cruciate reconstruction and is secured in appropriately placed tibial and medial femoral condylar tunnels (Fig. 113-44). The graft is passed through the tibial tunnel from anterior to posterior and redirected into the intercondylar notch through the posterior capsule. The patellar bone block is then placed in the medial femoral condylar

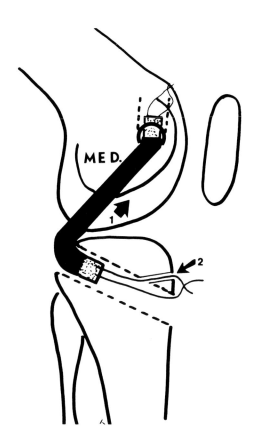

Fig. 113-44. Clancy/Karpf free graft secured in femoral condylar tunnels. The central third of the patellar tendon with attached patellar and tibial tubercle bone blocks is used for a posterior cruciate reconstruction. (1) The intraarticular portion of the graft. (2) A method for securing the graft by placing a small drill hole obliquely near the tunnel exit. One suture passes out through the larger tunnel exit and the other through the drill hole, to be tied together over a bony bridge.

tunnel. Both bone blocks should remain within the tunnels and not protrude into the joint.

The advantages of this procedure are that (1) it uses a structure of adequate strength, (2) studies have shown that a free graft does revascularize, (3) the approach avoids important neurovascular structures in the popliteal area, and (4) follow-up evaluation to date suggests satisfactory results.

Prosthetic Posterior Cruciate Replacement James and others have had an encouraging degree of success with prosthetic posterior cruciate reconstructions when combined with simultaneous intra-articular transfer of the medial head of the gastrocnemius to substitute for the posterior cruciate ligament[55,139] (Fig. 113-45). The prosthetic ligament serves as a temporary splint for several

months while the newly positioned gastrocnemius tendon replacement and associated extra-articular ligament reconstructions have a chance to mature. The prosthetic ligament may be easily removed when it ruptures, leaving the transferred gastrocnemius tendon to function as the permanent posterior cruciate ligament. These devices have not been released for general use but are being used at some of the major knee centers.

Authors' Preferred Technique

Our preferred technique for posterior cruciate reconstruction uses the medial tendon of the gastrocnemius, as originally described by Hughston[47] (Fig. 113-46). This is a heavy structure, readily available and technically not difficult to transfer for posterior cruciate substitution. It quite likely maintains some vascular supply from the muscle belly following transfer, and no functional deficit has been detected as a result of the transfer.

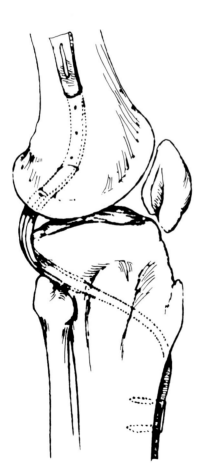

Fig. 113-45. Prosthetic posterior cruciate ligament used as a temporary splint to protect additional soft tissue reconstructive procedures. (From James,[55] with permission.)

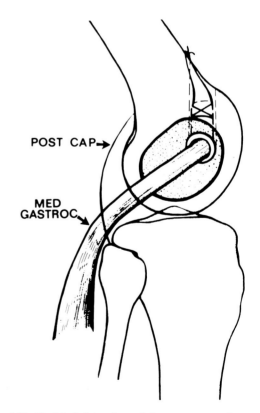

POST CAP→

MED GASTROC

Fig. 113-46. Medial tendon of the gastrocnemius transferred to substitute for the posterior cruciate ligament. (From James,[54] with permission.)

(ed): Musculoskeletal Disorders, Regional Examination and Differential Diagnosis. JB Lippincott, Philadelphia, 1977

53a. James SL: Knee ligament reconstruction. p. 7:31. In Evarts CM (ed): Surgery of the Musculoskeletal System. 1st Ed. Churchill Livingstone, New York, 1983

54. James SL: Biomechanics of knee ligament reconstruction. Clin Orthop 146:96, 1980

55. James SL, Woods GW, Homsy CA, et al: Cruciate ligament stents in reconstruction of the unstable knee. Clin Orthop 143:90, 1979

56. Johnson LL: Lateral capsular complex: Anatomical and surgical procedures. Am J Sports Med 7:156, 1979

57. Johnson RJ, Pope MH: Functional anatomy of the meniscus. p. 3. In Evarts CM (ed): Symposium on Reconstructive Surgery of the Knee. CV Mosby, St. Louis, 1978

58. Jones KC: Reconstruction of the anterior cruciate ligament. J Bone Joint Surg 45A:925, 1963

59. Kaplan EB: The iliotibial tract. Clinical and morphological significance. J Bone Joint Surg 40A:817, 1958

60. Kennedy JC: Classification of knee joint instability resulting from ligament damage. p. 33. In Schultz KP, Krahl H, Stein WH (eds): Late Reconstruction of Injured Ligaments of the Knee. Springer-Verlag, Berlin, 1978

61. Kennedy JC: The Injured Adolescent Knee. Williams & Wilkins, Baltimore, 1979

62. Kennedy JC: Natural history of the unoperated posterior cruciate. Presented at the Semiannual Meeting of the American Orthopaedics Society for Sports Medicine, Atlanta, Feb 1980

63. Kennedy JC, Fowler PJ: Medial and anterior instability of the knee. J Bone Joint Surg 53A:1257, 1971

64. Kennedy JC, Hawkins RJ, Willis RB, et al: Tension studies of the human knee ligaments. J Bone Joint Surg 58A:350, 1976

65. Kennedy JC, Roth JH, Walker DM: Posterior cruciate ligament injuries. Orthop Dig 7:19, 1979

66. Kennedy JC, Roth JH, Mendenhall HV, et al: Presidential address. Intra-articular replacement in the anterior cruciate ligament-deficient knee. Am J Sports Med 8:1, 1980

67. Kennedy JC, Stewart R, Walker DM: Anterolateral rotary instability of the knee joint. J Bone Joint Surg 60A:1031, 1978

68. Kennedy JC, Weinberg HW, Wilson AS: The anatomy and function of the anterior cruciate ligament as determined by clinical and morphological studies. J Bone Joint Surg 56A:223, 1974

68a. Lambert KL, Cunningham RR: Anatomic substitution of the ruptured ACL using a vascularized patellar tendon graft with interference fit fixation. p. 401. In Feagin J (ed): The Cruciate Ligaments. Churchill Livingstone, New York, 1988

69. Lane JM, Chisena E, Black J: Experimental knee instability: Early mechanical property changes in articular cartilage in a rabbit model. Clin Orthop 140:262, 1979

70. Larson RL: Dislocations and ligamentous injuries to the knee. p. 1182. In Rockwood CA, Green DP (eds): Fractures. JB Lippincott, Philadelphia, 1975

71. Larson RL: Combined instabilities: Combinations of surgical procedures. p. 207. In Evarts CM (ed): Symposium on Reconstructive Surgery of the Knee. CV Mosby, St. Louis, 1978

72. Larson RL: Complications of dislocations and ligamentous injuries (of the knee). p. 495. In Epps CH Jr (ed): Complications in Orthopaedic Surgery. Vol. 2. JB Lippincott, Philadelphia, 1978

72a. Larson RL: Knee injuries in sports. Hosp Med 14(2):Feb., 1978

73. Larson RL: Combined instabilities of the knee. Clin Orthop 147:68, 1980

74. Lindstrom N: Cruciate ligament plastics with meniscus. Acta Orthop Scand 29:150, 1959

75. Losee RE, Johnson TR, Southwick WO: Anterior subluxation of the lateral tibial plateau. A diagnostic test and operative repair. J Bone Joint Surg 60A:1015, 1978

76. MacIntosh D: MacIntosh "over the top" reconstruction. p. 979. In Edmonson AS, Crenshaw AH (eds): Campbell's Operative Orthopedics. CV Mosby, St. Louis, 1980

77. MacIntosh DL: The lateral pivot shift. Symposium on Treatment of Injuries of the Knee, ACS Clinitapes, C72-OR3, 1973

78. MacIntosh DL: Acute tears of the anterior cruciate ligament. "Over-the-top" repair. Presented at the American Academy of Orthopaedic Surgeons Annual Meeting, Dallas, 1974

79. Manske PR, Bridwell K, Lesker PA: Nutrient pathways to flexor tendons of chickens using tritiated preline. J Hand Surg 3:352, 1978

80. Marshall JL: Periarticular osteophytes. Initiation and formation in the knee of the dog. Clin Orthop 62:37, 1969

81. Marshall JL, Olsson SE: Instability of the knee. A long-term experimental study in dogs. J Bone Joint Surg 53A:1561, 1971

82. Marshall JL, Wang JB, Furman W, et al: The anterior drawer sign: What is it? Am J Sports Med 3:152, 1975

83. Marshall JL, Warren RF, Wickiewicz TL, et al: The

anterior cruciate ligament: A technique of repair and reconstruction. Clin Orthop 143:97, 1979

84. Marshall JL, Warren RF, Wickiewicz TL, et al: Reconstruction of functioning anterior cruciate ligament. Preliminary report using quadriceps tendon. Orthop Rev 8:45, 1979

85. Mauck HP: A new operative procedure for instability of the knee. J Bone Joint Surg 18:984, 1936

86. McDaniel WJ, Dameron TB: Untreated ruptures of the anterior cruciate ligament. A follow up study. J Bone Joint Surg 62A:696, 1980

87. McLeod WD, Moshi A, Andrews JR, et al: Tibial plateau topography. Am J Sports Med 5:13, 1977

88. McMaster JH, Weinert CR Jr, Scranton P Jr: Diagnosis and treatment of isolated anterior cruciate ligament tears. A preliminary report on reconstruction with the gracilis tendon. J Trauma 14:230, 1974

89. McMurray TP: The operative treatment of the ruptured internal lateral ligament of the knee. J Bone Joint Surg 6:377, 1919

90. Milch H: Fascial reconstruction of the tibial collateral ligament. Surgery 10:811, 1941

91. Muller W: Functional anatomy related to rotary stability of the knee joint. p. 39. In Chapchal G (ed): Injuries of the Ligaments and Their Repair. PSG, Littleton, MA, 1977

92. Nakajima H, Kando M, Kurosawa H, et al: Insufficiency of the anterior cruciate ligament. Arch Orthop Traum Surg 95:233, 1979

93. Nicholas JA: The five-one reconstruction for anteromedial instability of the knee. Indications, technique, and results in fifty-two patients. J Bone Joint Surg 55A:899, 1973

94. Nicholas JA, Minkoff J: Iliotibial band transfer through the intercondylar notch for combined anterior stability (TTPT procedure). Am J Sports Med 6:341, 1978

95. Noesberger B, Riesen H, Fernandez D, et al: Possibilities of treatment of posterior knee laxity. In Chapchal G (ed): Injuries of the Ligaments and Their Repair. PSG, Littleton, MA, 1977

96. Norwood LA, Andrews JR, Meisterling RC, et al: Acute anterolateral rotary instability of the knee. J Bone J Surg 61A:704, 1979

97. Norwood LA, Cross MJ: Anterior cruciate ligament: Functional anatomy of its bundles in rotatory instabilities. Am J Sports Med 7:23, 1979

98. Noyes FR: Functional properties of knee ligaments and alterations induced by immobilization. A correlative, biomechanical and histological study in primates. Clin Orthop 123:210, 1977

99. Noyes FR, Bassett RW, Grood ES, et al: Arthros-

copy in acute traumatic hemarthrosis of the knee. Incidence of anterior cruciate tears and other injuries. J Bone Joint Surg 62A:687, 1980

100. Noyes FR, DeLucas JL, Torrik PJ: Biomechanics of anterior cruciate ligament failure: An analysis of strain-rate sensitivity and mechanisms of failure in primates. J Bone Joint Surg 56A:236, 1979

101. Noyes FR, Grood ES: The strength of the anterior cruciate ligament in humans and rhesus monkeys. Age-related and species-related changes. J Bone Joint Surg 58A:1074, 1976

102. Noyes FR, Grood ES, Butler DL: The knee ligaments. Presented at the Western Orthopedics Association Meeting, Oregon Chapter, Gleneden Beach, OR, Nov 1978

103. Noyes FR, Grood ES, Butler DL, et al: Clinical biomechanics of the knee ligament restraints and functional stability. In Funk J (ed): Symposium on the Athlete's Knee: Surgical Repair and Reconstruction. CV Mosby, St. Louis, 1979

104. Noyes FR, Grood ES, Butler DL, et al: Clinical laxity tests and functional stability of the knee: Biomechanical concepts. Clin Orthop 146:84, 1980

105. Noyes FR, Sonstegard DA: Biomechanical function of the pes anserinus at the knee and the effects of its transplantation. J Bone Joint Surg 55A:1225, 1973

106. Ocha J, Fowler TJ, Gilliatt RW: Anatomical changes in peripheral nerves compressed by a pneumatic tourniquet. J Anesthesiol 113:433, 1972

107. O'Donoghue DH: Surgical treatment of fresh injuries to the major ligaments of the knee. J Bone Joint Surg 32A:721, 1950

108. O'Donoghue DH: An analysis of the end results of surgical treatment of major injuries to the ligaments of the knee. J Bone Joint Surg 37A:1, 1955

109. O'Donoghue DH: A method for replacement of the anterior cruciate ligament of the knee. J Bone Joint Surg 45A:905, 1963

110. O'Donoghue DH: Reconstruction for medial instability of the knee. Technique and results in sixty cases. J Bone Joint Surg 55A:941, 1973

111. O'Donoghue DH, Frank GR, Jeter GL, et al: Repair and reconstruction of the anterior cruciate ligament in dogs. J Bone Joint Surg 53A:710, 1971

112. Palmer I: On the injuries to the ligaments of the knee joint. Acta Chir Scand 81(suppl 53):3, 1938

113. Parker HG: Chronic anteromedial instability of the knee. Clin Orthop 142:123, 1979

114. Perry J, Fox JM, Boitano MA, et al: Functional evaluation of the pes anserinus transfer by electromyography and gait analysis. J Bone Joint Surg 62A:973, 1980

115. Price CT, Allen WC: Ligament repair in the knee with preservation of the meniscus. J Bone Joint Surg 60A:61, 1978

116. Reider B, Marshall JL: The anterior cruciate; guardian of the meniscus. Orthop Rev 7(5):83, 1979

117. Reifor HJ: Use and value of the patellar ligament in reconstruction of the cruciate ligaments. In Chapchal G (ed): Injuries of the Ligaments and Their Repair. PSG, Littleton, MA, 1977

118. Rorabeck CH, Kennedy JC: Tourniquet-induced nerve ischemia complicating knee ligament surgery. Am J Sports Med 8:98, 1980

118a. Rosenberg TD, Paulos LE, Abbott PJ: Arthroscopic cruciate repair and reconstruction: An overview and descriptions of technique. p. 409. In Feagin J (ed): The Cruciate Ligaments. Churchhill Livingstone, New York, 1988

119. Saunders KC, Louis DL, Weingarden SI, et al: Effect of tourniquet time on postoperative quadriceps function. Clin Orthop 143:194, 1979

120. Scott N, Pierce F, Marino M: Intra-articular transfer of the iliotibial tract. Two to seven year follow up results. J Bone Joint Surg 67A:532, 1985

120a. Sisk TD: Traumatic affections of joints — knee. p. 884. In Edmonson AS, Crenshaw AH (eds): Campbell's Operative Orthopaedics. 6th Ed. CV Mosby, St. Louis, 1980

121. Slocum DB, James SL, Larson RL, et al: Clinical test for anterolateral rotary instability of the knee. Clin Orthop 118:63, 1976

122. Slocum DB, Larson RL: Pes anserinus transplant. A simple surgical procedure for control of rotatory instability of the knee. J Bone Joint Surg 50A:226, 1968

123. Slocum DB, Larson RL: Rotatory instability of the knee. Its pathogenesis and a clinical test to determine its presence. J Bone Joint Surg 50A:211, 1968

123a. Slocum DB, Larson RL, James SL: Late reconstruction procedures used to stabilize the knee. Orthop Clin North Am 4:679, 1973

124. Slocum DB, Larson RL, James SL: Late reconstruction of ligamentous injuries of the medial compartment of the knee. Clin Orthop 100:23, 1974

125. Slocum DB, Larson RL, James SL: Pes anserinus transplant. Impressions after a decade of experience. Am J Sports Med 2:123, 1974

126. Tatsuzawa Y, Asai H, Hori J: Dynamic tenodesis of the semitendinosus tendon for medial instability of the knee. Technique and follow up of sixty three cases. J Bone Joint Surg 58B:261, 1976 (abstr)

127. Tillberg B: The later repair of torn cruciate ligaments using menisci. J Bone Joint Surg 59B:15, 1977

128. Torg JS, Conrad W, Allen VKP: Clinical diagnosis of anterior cruciate instability in the athlete. Am J Sports Med 4:84, 1976

129. Torisu T: Isolated avulsion fracture of the tibial attachment of the posterior cruciate ligament. J Bone Joint Surg 59A:68, 1977

130. Trickey EL: Rupture of the posterior cruciate ligament of the knee. J Bone Joint Surg 50B:334, 1968

131. Trillat A: Posterolateral instability. p. 99. In Schulitz KP, Krahl H, Stein WH (eds): Late Reconstruction of Injured Ligaments of the Knee. Springer-Verlag, Berlin, 1978

132. Umansky AL: The Milch fasciodesis for the reconstruction of the tibial collateral ligament. J Bone Joint Surg 34A:202, 1952

133. Unverforth LJ, Olex MI, Ketterer WF: A clinical follow up of pes anserine transfer for chronic anteromedial rotatory instability of the knee. Clin Orthop 134:149, 1978

134. Van Reus JG, Box RA: The lateral pivot-shift phenomenon of the knee. In Chapchal G (ed): Injuries of the ligaments and Their Repair. PSG, Littleton, MA, 1977

135. Wang C, Walker PS: Rotatory laxity of the human knee joint. J Bone Joint Surg 56A:161, 1974

136. Wang CJ, Walker PS, Wolf B: The effect of flexion and rotation on the length patterns of the ligaments of the knee. J Biomech 6:587, 1973

137. White AA, Raphael IG: The effect of quadriceps loads and knee positions on strain measurements of the tibial collateral ligament. Acta Orthop Scand 43:176, 1972

138. Whipple TL: My test for posterior rotary instability. Presented at the Interim Meeting of the American Orthopaedic Society for Sports Medicine, San Francisco, 1987

139. Woods GW, Homsy CA, Prewitt et al: Proplast leader for use in cruciate ligament reconstruction. Am J Sports Med 7:314-319, 1979

140. Woods GW, Stanley RF, Tullos HS: Lateral capsular sign: X-ray clue to a significant knee instability. Am J Sports Med 7:27, 1979

141. Zarins B, Rowe CR: Anterior cruciate ligament reconstruction using semitendinosus tendon and iliotibial tract. Presented at the Annual Meeting of the American Academy of Orthopaedic Surgeons, Atlanta, Jan 1980

Arthroscopy of the Knee

114

Alexander Kalenak
Gregory A. Hanks
Wayne J. Sebastianelli

HISTORY

Endoscopy of the knee was spawned in the wake of endoscopy of the urinary bladder. Joyce[191] dates the history of cystoscopy back to Bozzini of Frankfurt-am-Main, who in 1805 devised a *Lichtleiter*, which reflected light from a candle into the bladder. Nitze in 1876 devised the first instrument to introduce light directly into the bladder through a lens system, thus providing better visualization, as well as to provide a flow of water to protect the tissues.

In 1918 Takagi of Tokyo used a cystoscope to examine the knee joint of a cadaver. He redesigned the instrument and in 1931 produced a 3.5-mm-diameter arthroscope. With this instrument he performed what was probably the first arthroscopic surgical procedure in a joint distended with fluid.[306]

While Takagi was working in Japan, others around the world were also working on the technique and instrumentation. Bircher,[23,24] Kreuscher,[202] Finkelstein and Mayer,[108] and Burman et al.[30,31] were early pioneers in arthroscopic techniques. Their work, however, was not appreciated and therefore languished. Masaki Watanabe, a pupil of Takagi, tenaciously pursued the development of arthroscopy. In 1957 he and his associates published an *Atlas of Arthroscopy,* based on extensive experience in performing arthroscopy of the knee in Japan.[316] It was Watanabe's work that caught the attention of several investigators from the North American continent. Watanabe was a mentor and inspiration to several aspiring arthroscopic surgeons. Jackson of Toronto learned the technique in 1964 and reintroduced the concept to North America. Casscells[47] was the first to publish a paper in the United States demonstrating the accuracy of arthroscopy, and this was followed by a paper by Robert Jackson and I. Abe in 1972.[173]

Arthroscopy had been used primarily as a diagnostic procedure up until that time and was looked upon with skepticism by some and disdain by others. Persistence by pioneers of the procedure proved that arthroscopy was not merely a fad but had significant diagnostic value and furthermore was also potentially of significant therapeutic value. Richard O'Connor,[260] another disciple of Watanabe, established and popularized meniscectomy as a routine operation in the late 1970s. Lanny Johnson[184] popularized the use of the Needlescope and added valuable substance to the technique, performance, and instrumentation of arthroscopic surgery. Metcalf,[233,234] McGinty,[224-229] Casscells,[50,51,53] and others[177,324] added new and improved techniques and developed educational programs to satisfy the demand for knowledge of arthroscopic surgery. In 1978 in response to an American Academy of Orthopaedic Surgeons (AAOS) questionnaire, 50 percent of the AAOS membership stated they were using arthroscopic techniques. In a similar study by Johnson[186] in 1983, 98 percent of the respondents stated they were using arthroscopic techniques.

Because of the burgeoning interest in arthroscopy, there were significant technical advances in the 1970s. The advent of a fiberoptic lens and lighting system provided a dramatic improvement in visualization. Using instrumentation borrowed from other surgical specialties, investigators in Japan and the United States simultaneously began to perform surgical procedures. The advent of a hand-held television camera coupled to the arthroscope and monitor turned everyone into a member of the surgical team.[177,291] Arthroscopy began the move from a diagnostic tool to a therapeutic modality. Performance of the simplest surgical procedures, such as removal of loose bodies, gave way to the performance of more complex procedures, such as partial meniscectomy, articular cartilage shaving, synovectomy, resection of osteophytes and plicae, lateral retinacular release, and cruciate ligament repair and reconstruction.

What started out as a simple diagnostic procedure had grown by 1980 into a bona fide surgical discipline with significant therapeutic implications.

GENERAL PRINCIPLES

The general principles used in the performance of arthroscopic surgery are the same as those applicable to the performance of any surgical proce-

dure. Aseptic technique, gentle handling of tissue, retraction, exposure, hemostasis, etc., should be learned as part of an orthopaedic surgery training program. The practicing orthopaedic surgeon wishing to perform arthroscopic surgery should seek additional training in a fellowship program or in courses designed to teach basic and advanced surgical techniques.

In order to perform arthroscopy, a certain amount of native talent and psychomotor skills are prerequisites. The technique of arthroscopic surgery can be learned, and the skills necessary to perform those techniques can be refined and improved. Dexterity and a sense of spatial orientation to master the technique of *triangulation* are required. The surgeon must master the bimanual psychomotor skill of maneuvering two or more objects simultaneously in a confined space. A telescope and surgical instrument are introduced from separate anterior portals and aimed in such a way that the tip of the surgical instrument is introduced into the visual field. Placing the surgical instrument in a second portal offers improved mobility, a more advantageous angle of attack with the instrument, and less clashing and crowding of instruments. Triangulation represented a significant change from the side-by-side technique of O'Connor and his operating arthroscope, an arrangement that placed the instrument directly in the visual field but markedly restricted the area in which surgical work could be performed. The technique of triangulation described by Metcalf and others forever changed arthroscopy by transforming an often frustrating and disappointing surgical exercise into a gratifying, expeditious, and successful operative procedure.

Arthroscopic surgical procedures should be performed in the setting of a hospital or surgical center. Most procedures can be performed on an outpatient basis, with the patient going home the same day. Overnight stays occasionally become necessary because of anesthetic complications such as nausea, vomiting, and orthostatic hypotension. The decreased morbidity of arthroscopic surgery is a feature attractive to both patients and the surgeon. Small incisions and decreased bleeding and swelling result in less pain and limitation of motion. Patients respond favorably to early ambulation and going home the same day. The risk of thrombophlebitis is much less in patients who are mobilized immediately. The risk of infection is minimized owing to the copious volume of irrigating fluid used during the procedure.

INSTRUMENTATION AND OPERATING ROOM SETUP

Instruments

A multitude of arthroscopic instruments are available. This was not always so; initially, instrumentation was borrowed from other surgical disciplines. Endoscopes were borrowed from urology and gynecology, probes from neurosurgery and basket forceps from otorhinolaryngology and gynecology. Some worked well, but most required modification. Newer instruments were designed specifically for arthroscopic surgical procedures of the knee and this instrumentation continues to be modified and improved.

The telescope instrumentation incorporates a lens system and lighting system into one unit. Watanabe's early telescopes were fitted with an incandescent light bulb at the tip. Breakage was a serious complication. Fiberoptic light transmitted directly along side the lens system eliminated this problem and provided light bright enough to visualize dark recesses and to take photographs and make videotape records. A hand held video camera that clamps onto the eye piece is standard procedure. This provides a picture on a monitor viewed by the entire surgical team, who then become helpful and valuable assistants. The former practice of direct visualization through an operating arthroscope was not conducive to a helpful, cooperative and educational environment. The practice of direct visualization through the arthroscope did not permit other members of the team to view, appreciate and assist in the performance of arthroscopic surgical procedures. It is impractical and counterproductive but it may be necessary in a situation where the technical equipment (camera and monitor) become inoperative.

A myriad of instruments are available on the market. Irrigation and power systems and surgical instruments should be tested in order to make an intelligent decision. The arthroscope most often utilized is a 30-degree forward/oblique viewing telescope. Arthroscopes are available that permit forward/oblique viewing at various angles (10, 70, 90 degrees, etc.) The greater angle of obliquity permits viewing tissue closer to the lens system but out of the direct line of vision. It permits the surgeon to view "around a corner," for example, around the corner of a condyle of the femur into the posterior compartment. There is some distortion of the visual field with greater degrees of obliquity. It is best to become familiar with the 30-degree forward/oblique arthroscope and to use this primarily for all diagnostic and surgical work, using the other for special viewing.

The basic instrumentation on the scrub nurse's back table consists of a #11 scalpel, probe, soft tissue basket rongeurs, scissors, and grasping forceps (Fig. 114-1). Many other instruments can be added to this basic set; they include instruments that cut to the right and to the left and at various angles and motorized equipment such as shavers, abrasion instruments, and rongeurs to cut and suck out pieces simultaneously. Each instrument should be tried and tested to determine whether or not it fills a need in the surgeon's armamentarium.

The irrigation system is provided by two 4,000-ml bags of Ringer's lactate, set on a pole approximately 8 to 10 feet above the floor. This usually provides enough pressure to keep the joint distended. Some surgeons prefer to use commercially available pumps that provide continuous distention. A potential complication from using pumps is the extravasation of tissue fluid into the subcutaneous tissue spaces and muscle planes, which may cause entrapment and compression of neurovascular structures.

Preparation, Anesthesia, and Patient Positioning

Preparation and draping of the leg are done in a routine fashion. The leg is scrubbed with surgical soap and prepared with antiseptic solution from the ankle joint to the tourniquet (if used). The foot

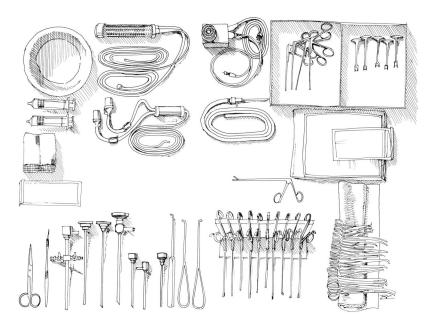

Fig. 114-1. Basic instrumentation. The first row contains scalpel, obturator-sheath-telescope systems, probes, and a tray of rongeurs, scissors, and grasping forceps. The second row contains the irrigation-suction system, video camera, motorized cutting system, and miscellaneous equipment.

is wrapped in a sterile sheet and covered with a stocking impervious to fluid. Waterproof tape seals the proximal portion of the stocking. Commercially available waterproof drapes ensure a watertight seal about the thigh. A floor pad or drainage device keeps the area free of large puddles of irrigating fluid. A "lily pad" with a trough around the perimeter, to which is attached a suction device, is one such product that will keep a relatively puddle-free area (Fig. 114-2).

The use of a tourniquet is at the discretion of the surgeon. Under general anesthesia there is no problem with local pressure tolerance, and a bloodless field is ensured. Pressure from the tourniquet will not be tolerated well if local anesthesia is used. A combination of epinephrine with a local anesthetic agent can provide a relatively bloodless field and eliminate the need for a tourniquet.

Many patients prefer general anesthesia because of anxiety and the inability to relax and cooperate. Spinal or epidural anesthesia is also successful with patients who are able to tolerate lying motionless on a table for 1 to 2 hours at a time. Local anesthesia can work well with patients for whom relaxation is no problem; 2 percent lidocaine and 0.5 percent

bupivacaine are used as local anesthetic agents, along with epinephrine for control of bleeding at the portal sites. The local anesthetic is instilled while the patient is in the anesthesia waiting area, 20 to 30 minutes before the start of the procedure; 5 to 10 ml of the combined local agents is used at each portal site and 20 to 25 ml is instilled directly into the knee joint cavity.

The positioning of the patient is important. The knee of the opposite extremity can be flexed by dropping the foot of the table to the 90-degree position. This provides free flexion and extension of the knee joint to be operated on and permits varus and valgus stresses to be placed across the knee joint and the thigh, which is clamped in the leg holder (Fig. 114-3). The leg holder is a device that firmly grasps the thigh and provides a buttress against which to apply a varus or valgus load to open up the lateral or medial side of the knee joint. The leg holder is a hindrance in using the superolateral portal for operative intervention, such as retrieval of a loose body, resection of a plica, or visualization of the patellofemoral articulation. The leg holder device, however, is very helpful if the surgeon is operating without an assistant.

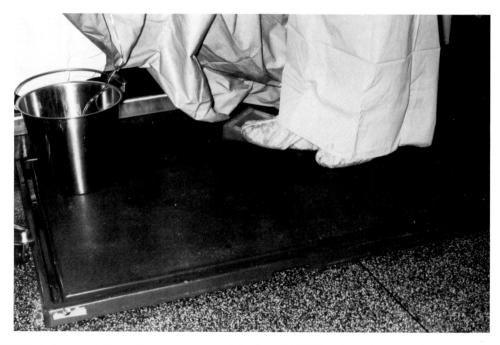

Fig. 114-2. A floor pad that collects and drains irrigating fluid falling from the operating area maintains a puddle-free environment.

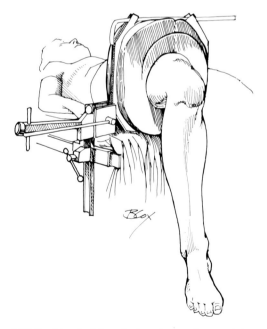

Fig. 114-3. A leg-holding device clamped around the thigh permits full flexion and extension and aids in applying a varus or valgus load to open the lateral or medial compartment.

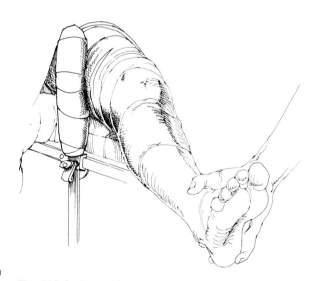

Fig. 114-4. A post clamped to the table runner bar provides a buttress that aids in applying valgus load for opening the medial compartment.

A simple post located on the lateral side of the extremity at or near the tourniquet can provide a buttress against which the medial side of the knee can be opened with valgus stress (Fig. 114-4). The post is placed in a standard clamp that attaches to the runner at the side of the table, leaving the femur, thigh, and knee joint free to rotate internally and externally. This is of some help in visualizing the medial compartment with varying degrees of flexion, extension, and rotation. The lateral side of the knee joint is opened to permit visualization by placing a varus load on the knee. The hip is flexed, abducted, and externally rotated, and the knee joint is flexed approximately 45 to 60 degrees. This is commonly called the "figure four" position (Fig. 114-5). The telescope should be switched from the lateral portal to the medial portal if there is any difficulty in visualizing the contents of the lateral compartment in that position. The ankle and foot rest on the opposite extremity, and additional varus stress can be placed at the knee joint by the assistant.

Portal Technique

Many portals have been described. The most important principle to follow is that portals should provide a straight tract that permits easy entrance and exit for the surgical instruments. False passages that hinder the penetration of the instruments into the knee joint are a waste of valuable operating time and a source of frustration to the surgeon. Four basic portals permit one to perform almost all arthroscopic surgical procedures. An imaginary longitudinal line and a transverse line drawn across the front of the knee, intersecting through the center of the patella, will divide the front of the knee into four quadrants (superolateral, superomedial, inferolateral, and inferomedial). Each quadrant is the site of a basic portal (Fig. 114-6).

The superolateral or superomedial portal can be used for irrigation outflow. The inferolateral portal is used for visualization and inflow of irrigation fluid through the sheath of the arthroscope. This inflow helps to push tissue away from the lens and light source. The inferomedial portal is used for surgical instrumentation. Probes are used for ex-

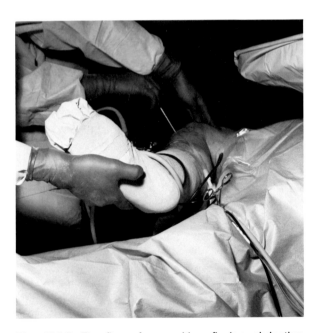

Fig. 114-5. The figure-four position: flexion, abduction, and external rotation of the hip, with the knee flexed 45 to 60 degrees and subjected to a varus load. The lateral compartment with the lateral meniscus can be visualized in its entirety.

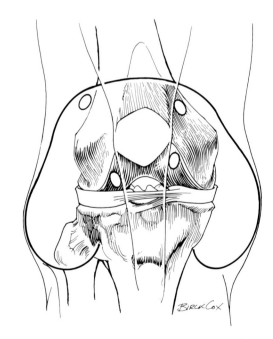

Fig. 114-6. The four basic portals: superolateral, superomedial, inferolateral, and inferomedial. Many accessory portals are utilized for special tasks.

ploration, and a variety of rongeurs, grasping forceps, knives, scissors, etc. can be used through this "operating portal." Both inferomedial and inferolateral portals can be interchanged for visualization and surgical instrumentation. The superolateral portal provides the best visualization for patella tracking and is also used to inspect the anterior aspect of the knee joint, especially the fat pad area, and when operating on a plica. The placement of the inferomedial and inferolateral portals is critical. They should be positioned in the center of the sulcus created by the femoral condyle, tibial plateau and meniscus, and the patella and patella tendon.

With the knee positioned at 45 to 60 degrees of flexion, an incision approximately 5 mm in length is made with a #11 scalpel blade and is oriented transversely or longitudinally. The tract is made with one incision through the skin, subcutaneous tissue, retinaculum, and fat pad, with care taken to avoid the articular surface of the femur. It is important that only one incision be made. Multiple thrusts with the knife blade may create "false" tracts, which may be dead ends for instrumentation. After the incision is made, a blunt obturator is inserted into the tract to ensure easy ingress and egress. The blunt obturator and arthroscope sheath are directed toward the intercondylar notch until they are passed through the superior part of the fat pad or into the interval between the fat pad and the patella, at which point the knee is extended and the obturator is directed beneath the patella and into the suprapatellar pouch. The telescope is inserted and the knee joint distended with approximately 100 ml of Ringer's lactate. The bulge produced in the suprapatellar pouch facilitates the making of the superolateral portal or superomedial portal. The knife is used to incise the skin, and a sharp obturator and sheath are inserted into the suprapatellar pouch. The outflow irrigation tubing is attached at that site.

A systematic examination is performed, first exploring the suprapatellar pouch, the lateral gutter, and the medial gutter. The patellofemoral articulation, joint surfaces, and positioning are noted. The medial compartment and fat pad are explored next, as well as the articular surfaces of femur and tibia. The medial meniscus is explored in its entirety (superior and inferior surfaces), starting with the ante-

rior horn, middle third, and then the posterior horn with the aid of applied valgus stress. The peripheral attachment in the posterior compartment is visualized by passing the telescope through the intercondylar notch, utilizing the channel between the posterior cruciate ligament and the femoral condyle. The details of this technique will be described in a subsequent section.

The anterior and posterior cruciate ligaments are visualized in the intercondylar notch and palpated with a probe. Integrity of the ligament is assessed by applying anterior and posterior drawer tests to the tibia while visualizing and probing the ligament. The lateral femoral condyle is visualized at the notch and at its intersection with the lateral tibial plateau. While maintaining that field in view, the knee is placed in the figure-four position, a varus load is applied, and the lateral meniscus is explored in its entirety.

The posteromedial portal and posterolateral portal as described by Metcalf may be necessary in order to retrieve loose bodies, perform synovectomy, and determine whether or not a peripheral meniscus tear exists in either the posteromedial or posterolateral compartments. Details of the technique follow in the section Diagnostic Examination of the Knee by Compartment.

INDICATIONS AND CONTRAINDICATIONS

The indications for performing arthroscopic surgical procedures are quite simple. Arthroscopy of the knee joint should be performed for the diagnosis and treatment of conditions that adversely affect the function of the knee joint and adversely affect the normal daily activities, work activities, or recreational activities of the patient.

There are few contraindications. The presence of sepsis or local infection at the operative sites should preclude an operation. Surgery should be avoided in the presence of a coagulopathy or some other serious systemic disorder. Ankylosis of the knee is a relative contraindication depending upon the amount of fibrosis that is present and the de-

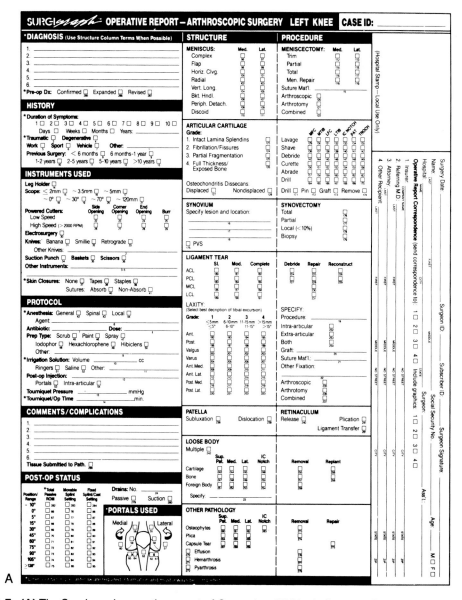

Fig. 114-7.   (A) The Surgi-graph operative report of Caspari and Whipple for recording operation information in detail. *(Figure continues.)*

gree of useful range of motion that can be obtained at surgery.

Many conditions of the knee lend themselves to arthroscopic surgical treatment, meniscus trauma and degeneration being the most common. Entities that may be treated include meniscus disorders, loose bodies, ligament injury, osteochondritis dessicans, patellofemoral disorders, synovial diseases, crystalline arthropathies, osteoarthritis, and tibial plateau or tibial eminence fractures.

DOCUMENTATION

There are many ways to document arthroscopic surgical findings other than the traditional handwritten note on the patient's chart and the formal dictated operative note. The operative note should be written in a systematic fashion with use of descriptive terms that are readily understood

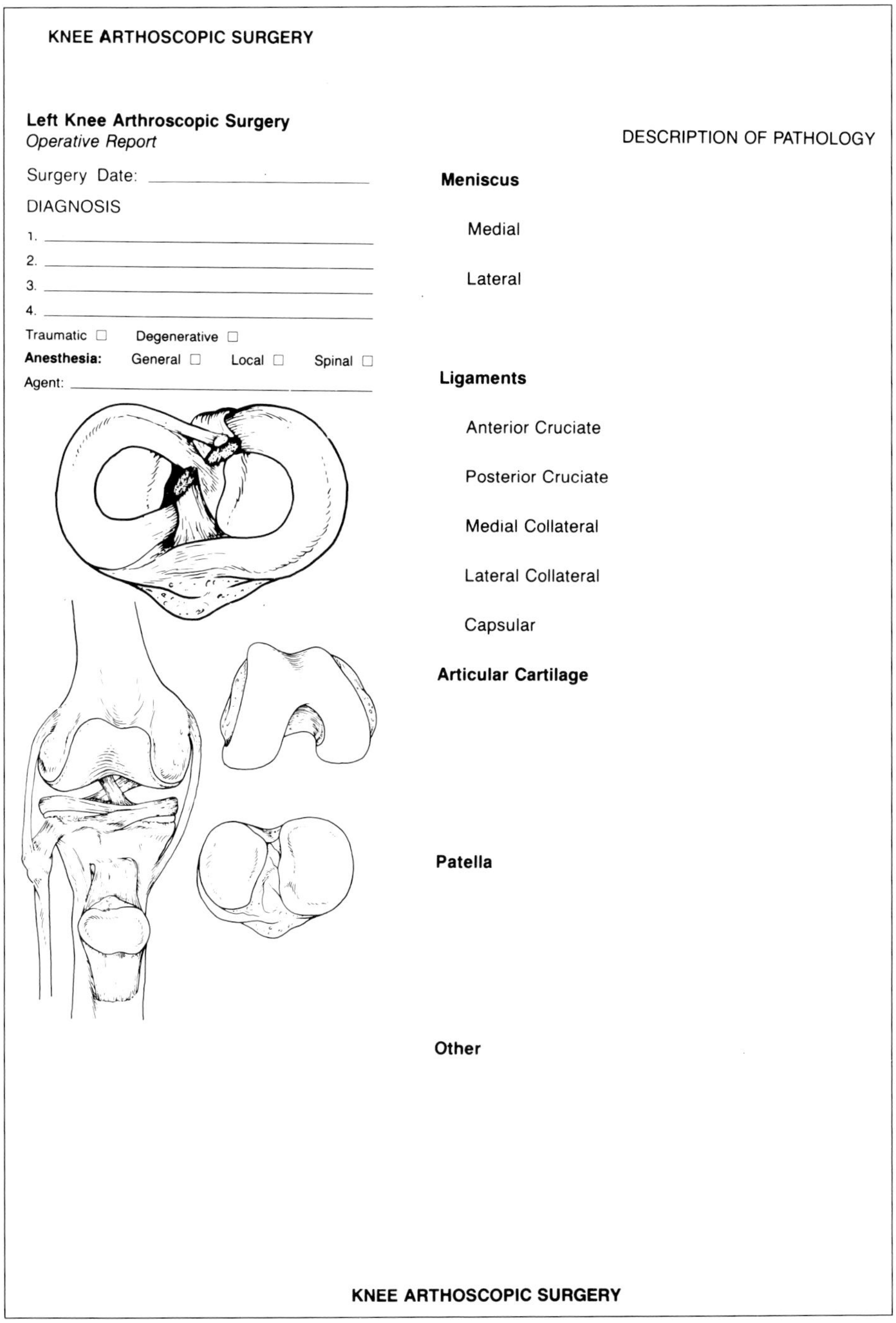

KNEE ARTHOSCOPIC SURGERY

Left Knee Arthroscopic Surgery
Operative Report

DESCRIPTION OF PATHOLOGY

Surgery Date: _____

DIAGNOSIS

Meniscus

1. _____

Medial

2. _____

3. _____

Lateral

4. _____

Traumatic ☐   Degenerative ☐

Anesthesia: General ☐   Local ☐   Spinal ☐

Agent: _____

Ligaments

Anterior Cruciate

Posterior Cruciate

Medial Collateral

Lateral Collateral

Capsular

Articular Cartilage

Patella

Other

KNEE ARTHOSCOPIC SURGERY

B

Fig. 114-7 *(Continued).* **(B)** A simplified graphic operative report for recording surgical data.

and interpreted and unmistakably clear to the reader. A drawing (freehand or preprinted) helps to depict the exact pathologic findings, and 35-mm slides, television tapes, and the new video printer photography all help to further document the pa-thology. In cases of unusual pathologic entities, in medical legal cases, and for patient education, doc-umentation by still photography or video taping can be helpful and instructive.

Surgical record and data forms that can be stored

in a computer have been developed by Johnson, by Caspari and Whipple (Fig. 114-7A), and by others. At the very least, a simplified graphic operative report should be included in all patient records (Fig. 114-7B).

REHABILITATION

Rehabilitation training is started the day the patient appears in the office and a decision is made for surgery. The patient is counseled in regard to the operation, postoperative care, and the details of the rehabilitation process. Instruction is given in simple resistive exercises for the quadriceps and hamstring muscles (straight leg lifts as well as standard progressive resistive exercises using weights). Postoperative rehabilitation is performed on a daily basis either in the patient's home or in a physical therapy facility. The patient is encouraged to walk immediately unless there are articular surface lesions, for which the patient should be non-weight bearing, or if meniscal or ligamentous repair has been performed. Range-of-motion exercises and strengthening exercises are prescribed from the outset. Electrical stimulation of the muscles is encouraged until there is active voluntary contraction of the quadriceps and straight leg lifting exercises can be performed easily. Weights are added to the straight leg lifting exercises when the patient can perform 30 repetitions easily. Isokinetic exercises with minimal resistance are started as soon as tolerated.

COMPLICATIONS

As with any surgery, complications do occur, but their incidence is low.[89,210] It is incumbent upon the surgeon to be aware of complications and to be prepared to deal with them forthrightly and expeditiously. Intraoperative complications include meniscus and articular cartilage injury, instrument breakage, sprain of collateral ligaments, bleeding, extravasation of irrigating fluid, and tourniquet pain. Postoperative complications most commonly encountered are hemarthrosis and effusion. The risks of thrombophlebitis and pulmonary embolism are minimal because of early ambulation and range-of-motion exercises. The incidence of infection is low because of the generous volumes of irrigation fluid that are used. Fistula formation and synovial herniation are rare complications as well as neuropraxia involving the infrapatellar branch of the saphenous nerve (Fig. 114-8).

DIAGNOSTIC EXAMINATION OF THE KNEE BY COMPARTMENT

In order to ensure that no injury or pathologic process is overlooked, every compartment and surface should be examined carefully and completely.[70,100,125,127,130,131] Systematic visualization is of utmost importance. The same methodical sequence of examination should be followed in each and every case; failure to do so may lead to inaccurate diagnosis and to intra-articular pathology remaining unrecognized.[120,121,164,169,171, 173–175,184,185,217,225,227,265]

For the purpose of arthroscopy the basic anatomy of the knee can be divided into six compartments and two gutters. These anatomic zones include the suprapatellar pouch and patellofemoral joint, lateral gutter, medial gutter, medial compartment, intercondylar notch, lateral compartment, and posteromedial and posterolateral compartments. Complete visualization of all these compartments will require at least three portals and several basic maneuvers, which will be discussed.

Suprapatellar Pouch and Patellofemoral Joint

Maximum distention is required for optimal visualization of this compartment. The knee is kept in full extension. Synovial hypertrophy may obscure visualization and require repositioning of the arthroscope in order to obtain maximum visibility.

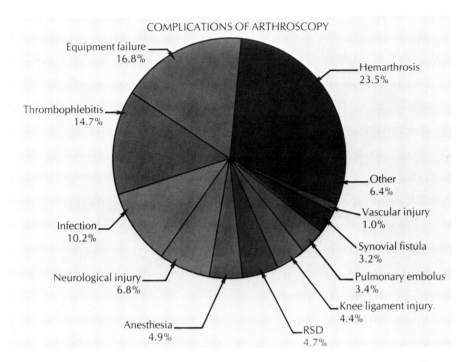

Fig. 114-8. Graphic representation of percentage complications from arthroscopic surgery. (Courtesy Arthroscopy Association of North America and Committee Chairman Jesse DeLee, MD.)

The systematic inspection should begin in the depths of the pouch and at one of its lateral margins. Maneuvering the arthroscope by advancing, angulating, or rotating the lens alters the visual field. After viewing the entire length and breadth of the compartment for loose bodies, plica, etc., the arthroscope can be rotated in order to visualize the undersurface of the extensor mechanism, which normally has a thin synovial covering. The uninvolved hand is used to compress the compartment from the outside. This bimanual examination aids visualization and also may dislodge loose bodies. The arthroscope is slowly withdrawn until the articular margins of the femoral sulcus and patella are visualized. With maximum distention, the patella tends to ride somewhat superior, anterior, and lateral to the depths of the femoral sulcus. By looking from lateral to medial, one can see across the patellofemoral joint. Angling the lens somewhat anteriorly allows visualization of the articular surface of the patella. If a diffuse synovitis that interferes with visualization is present, synovial fronds may be removed by a motorized shaver system. Patellofe-

moral tracking or docking can be viewed and the relationship of the patella and the sulcus to the knee observed at full extension and at 20, 45, and 90 degrees of flexion. Docking and tracking from the medial aspect of the patellofemoral joint can be observed by rotating and angulating the arthroscope toward the medial facet. The maneuvers of rotation, angulation, advancement, and withdrawal of the arthroscope are crucial to complete visualization of the compartment.

Lateral Gutter

After completing the inspection of the suprapatellar pouch and patellofemoral joint, the arthroscope is placed near the proximal end of the lateral gutter. The arthroscope is rotated for lateral and posterior viewing, following the contour of the articular margin of the lateral femoral condyle. The arthroscope will figuratively fall into the lateral gutter. Maximum distention of the joint at this point allows the best visualization. The distal end of the lateral gutter is at the junction of the periphery of the lateral meniscus and the popliteus hiatus with its tendon. The intra-articular portion of the tendon can be followed as it traverses inferiorly, medially, and posteriorly down to the popliteus hiatus. This area is palpated to detach any loose bodies hidden in the popliteus tendon sheath. It may be necessary to remove hypertrophic synovial tissue in order to provide a clear field. The arthroscope is then maneuvered back into the gutter, over the lateral femoral condyle, across the sulcus of the femur, and into the medial gutter.

Medial Gutter

According to Patel, a medial synovial plica can be identified in approximately 40 percent of cases, running from the medial wall of the gutter to the fat pad distal to the patella.[264] This synovial fold will often be nonpathologic (i.e., small and pliable). However, fibrosis or a thickened band of tissue may prevent the arthroscope from easily sliding into the medial gutter. This band can be responsible for anterior knee pain, a popping sensation, and chondromalacic changes on the medial femoral condyle. In order to disengage the plica and pass the arthroscope into the medial gutter, the arthroscope must be partially withdrawn. Maximum extension of the knee and distention of the pouch are necessary to view the gutter in its entirety. The arthroscope should be rotated to view slightly inferiorly and medially, following the margin of the articular surface of the medial femoral condyle. Bimanual examination should be performed to dislodge any possible intra-articular loose bodies. Upon reaching the inferior aspect of the articular margin of the medial femoral condyle, the fat pad and the anterior half of the meniscus are visualized with the coronary ligament attachment. At this point, flexing the knee to approximately 30 degrees and applying a slight valgus stress on the knee permits visualization of the medial compartment.

Medial Compartment

Once the arthroscope has been placed in the medial compartment, maximum distention is no longer necessary. The outflow cannula should be opened. A probe is inserted through the anteromedial portal and used to retract the fat pad and palpate the meniscus surfaces and margins. The free margin, or "airplane" edge, of the medial meniscus is visualized, along with the entire anterior horn. Valgus stress and knee flexion of approximately 30 degrees permit the arthroscope to be placed between the articular margins of the medial femoral condyle and the medial tibial plateau. The lens is rotated so that the middle third and posterior horn of the meniscus can be visualized. A normal meniscus can have a slightly wrinkled appearance. The superior and inferior surfaces as well as the peripheral attachment of the meniscus are probed to reveal any substance or peripheral tears. A peripheral detachment is suspected if the meniscus can be displaced partially or completely into the anterior compartment. Further extension of the knee at this point while maintaining valgus stress will often allow the arthroscope to advance further posteriorly, providing a better view of the posterior horn. Excessive force applied to the instruments may damage articular cartilage or cause instrument breakage.

Intercondylar Notch

For visualization of the intercondylar notch, the leg is allowed to hang over the side of the table with the knee flexed approximately 70 to 90 degrees. The arthroscope is maneuvered centrally to the intercondylar notch. Ligamentum mucosum veils or fibrous bands and an abundance of synovial fat pad tissue may be encountered. The ligamentum mucosum originates from the superior margin of the notch just slightly lateral to the midline. It traverses distally and anteriorly to attach to the retropatellar fat pad. Usually it is small and is easily bypassed, but in posttraumatic or inflammatory conditions it can be hypertrophied and quite fibrous. This can impede passage of the arthroscope or other instruments across the intercondylar notch. If necessary for maneuvering instruments or for better visualization, this pathologic ligamentum can be resected with an intra-articular shaver or retracted with a probe.

Finding and following the articular margins of the intercondylar notch will provide orientation when visualizing the contents of the intercondylar notch. Posterior to the ligamentum mucosum, the anterior cruciate ligament extends from the area anterior to the tibial spine to the lateral femoral condyle; it inserts into the lateral wall of the intercondylar notch, high and posterior, at the junction of the roof and wall of the notch. Flexing the knee between 45 and 90 degrees will allow the entire course of the ligament to be visualized. The vascularity and substance should be noted with the probe. Advancing and often pistoning the arthroscope posteriorly and slightly medial to the anterior cruciate ligament will allow visualization of the femoral origin of the posterior cruciate ligament with its overlying synovial tissue. The substance of this ligament should also be palpated with a probe.

After inspecting and probing the substance of the cruciate ligaments, tension can be tested under direct visualization by performing anterior and posterior drawer and Lachman's tests.

Lateral Compartment

The arthroscope is maneuvered laterally in order to visualize the articular margin of the lateral femoral condyle at the intercondylar notch. A probe can be helpful in retracting the fat pad. While maintaining this field of view on the television monitor (the lateral femoral condyle at the notch and its intersection with the lateral tibial plateau), the examiner flexes the knee approximately 70 degrees, and the assistant changes the position of the leg from the side of the table to the figure-four position on top of the table. This automatically places a varus stress on the lateral compartment and creates enough free space for the arthroscope to explore the lateral compartment. The posterior horn of the lateral meniscus is visualized and inspected. Because the lateral meniscus is quite mobile, the inferior and superior surfaces can be inspected much more easily than the medial meniscus. Further varus stress can be applied by having the assistant lift the foot off the operating table. Systematic visualization from posterior to anterior should be carried out, together with probing and inspection of the tibial and femoral surfaces of the meniscus. The popliteus hiatus is located at the junction of the posterior horn and middle third and is easily visual-

ized. The mobility of the meniscus at this point should also be studied carefully. The probe should be placed in the hiatus and the mobility of the lateral meniscus assessed. Not only the free margin of the meniscus but also the coronary ligamentous attachment throughout its course can be seen well. The articular surfaces of both the tibia and the femur can be completely visualized by varying the amount of flexion of the knee. Rotating the lens while performing this maneuver will offer several perspectives of the articular surfaces in this compartment.

If visualization of the lateral compartment is difficult owing to synovial inflammatory conditions, redundant tissue should be removed using an intra-articular shaver. If visibility is still poor, switching the arthroscope to the anteromedial portal may be helpful. The probe can be placed through the anterolateral portal and used as a retractor of the fat pad and ligamentum mucosum. Occasionally the anterior horn attachment of the lateral meniscus, particularly if involved with a pathologic tear, can obstruct the field of vision. Inspection from a superolateral portal may be necessary to gain access to this lesion. Orientation can be confusing in the lateral compartment unless one remembers that while the leg is in the figure-four position, the joint line is actually oriented almost perpendicular to the floor. The camera should be rotated so that the image of the plateau on the monitor remains parallel to the floor.

Posteromedial Compartment

The posteromedial compartment should be inspected routinely to search for peripheral tears of the posterior horn of the medial meniscus and for loose bodies.[123,124,216] The anterolateral portal is used to guide the arthroscope under direct visualization through the intercondylar channel created by the posterior cruciate ligament and the lateral wall of the medial femoral condyle. The entire posteromedial compartment can be visualized. If the telescope can not be inserted through this channel under direct visualization, it may be inserted blindly. The telescope is replaced by a blunt obturator, and the assembly is gently passed over the medial femoral condyle and maneuvered through the intercondylar notch between the posterior cruciate ligament and the wall of the notch. By extending the knee from the 90-degree position, the assembly can be inserted over the tibial spine, through the channel, and into the posteromedial compartment. Replacement of the obturator with the 30-degree telescope and maximum distention of the joint permit visualization of the "white cliffs of Dover" (the drop-off point of the coronary ligaments). This unique view of the coronary ligament attachment of the posterior horn of the medial meniscus can be further assessed by changing to a 70-degree arthroscope. Manual pressure applied at the posteromedial corner can ensure that no loose bodies are present. Rotation of the lens through a nearly complete circle will allow one to visualize the synovium and capsular reflection of the entire posteromedial compartment. Slow withdrawal of the arthroscope (after changing to a 30-degree lens) with the visual projection oriented inferolaterally brings into view the posterior cruciate ligament insertion into the tibial sulcus. The tip of the posterior horn of the medial meniscus can also be visualized.

A separate posteromedial or posterolateral portal can be utilized for probing, grasping, or even operating on appropriate lesions such as loose bodies, hypertrophic synovitis, etc. This technique has been described by Metcalf et al.[234] The knee is positioned at 90 degrees of flexion, either over the side of the table or in the figure-four position. The "soft-spot" of the posteromedial or posterolateral corner is palpated and may be seen to bulge with a bolus of irrigating fluid. A small skin incision is made over the soft spot. The sharp obturator and sheath are inserted through the bulging area at the moment of maximum distention and into the posteromedial or posterolateral compartment. The sheath is maneuvered through 360 degrees to ensure a clear tract for access of surgical instruments. If need be, this portal can be used for visualization, and surgical instruments can be inserted through the anteromedial or anterolateral portal and through the intercondylar notch.

Posterolateral Compartment

The technique for entering the posterolateral compartment is similar to that used to enter the posteromedial compartment. The blunt obturator and sheath are gently guided over the tibial eminence and maneuvered against the lateral wall of the intercondylar notch past the anterior cruciate ligament into the posterolateral compartment. The periphery of the posterior horn of the lateral meniscus is visualized. The arthroscope is directed inferiorly and laterally, and with this view the normal white cliffs of Dover (coronary ligament attachment), as well as the popliteus tendon and the popliteal hiatus, are inspected for injury. Bimanual examination again should be performed to locate loose bodies. The lens should be rotated through a complete circle with both the 30- and 70-degree instruments to obtain a complete examination of the compartment. Maximum distention is important during the examination of the posterior compartments.

A separate posterolateral portal can be created by the technique described by Metcalf.[234] A thorough diagnostic evaluation of both the posteromedial and posterolateral compartments can be performed, however, without the creation of these portals. While viewing through the intercondylar notch, a curved O'Donoghue probe, placed through the standard anterior portals and gently manipulated posteriorly around the condyle on the superior aspect of the meniscus, aids in retraction of redundant synovium in the posterior compartment, thereby providing better visualization of the coronary ligament attachment of the meniscus.

TREATMENT OF MENISCAL TEARS

Widespread application of arthroscopic surgical technique has revolutionized treatment of meniscus tears.[20,42,75,141,269] With these techniques it is possible to remove the affected portion of the meniscus expeditiously through tiny incisions and with minimal postoperative morbidity. This significant reduction in morbidity has allowed more rapid return to normal daily activities.[41,89,128,133,142,210,228,249,296] In addition to these short-term advantages, partial meniscectomy may provide a long-term significant benefit by reducing the incidence of degenerative joint changes that commonly occur following a total meniscectomy.[69,228,248] Biomechanical studies of stress distributions by Radin et al.[275] and others have shown that preservation of at least a meniscal rim is beneficial in preventing increase in articular cartilage contact forces.[201]

The basic techniques of arthroscopic surgery have been described previously in the section on principles.[78,185,186,234,233,302,325] The arthroscope is inserted through one portal and the operating instruments are inserted through a second portal and manipulated into the field of vision in a process called triangulation.[84] A polypuncture technique described by Whipple and Bassett[317] requires insertion of the arthroscope through a central portal, with two additional medial or lateral portals on either side of the arthroscope used for insertion of surgical instruments.

Meniscal tears occur in four basic patterns (as described by O'Connor) or in combinations of these patterns.[260,261,264] The four basic patterns include vertical longitudinal, horizontal, oblique (flap), and radial tears (Fig. 114-9). Variations of these include complex tears and degenerative tears (Figs. 114-10, 114-11).

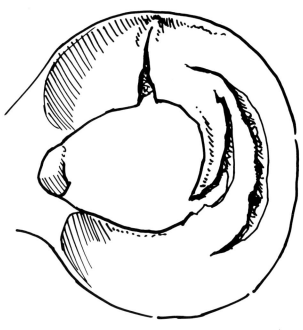

Fig. 114-10. Complex tear—a meniscal tear comprising several tear patterns.

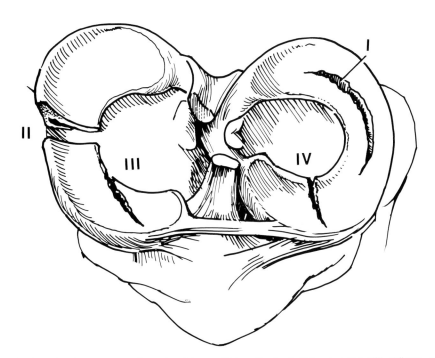

Fig. 114-9. The four basic patterns of meniscal tears: (I) longitudinal, (II) horizontal, (III) oblique, and (IV) radial.

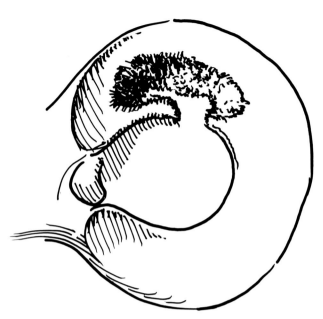

Fig. 114-11. Degenerative tear. Note that the posterior horn of the meniscus is worn out and the remaining edge is shaggy and irregular.

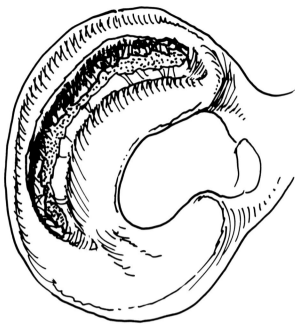

Fig. 114-12. A longitudinal tear. When this tear is long, it is called a "bucket handle" tear, and the fragment can displace centrally.

A longitudinal tear (parallel to the long edge of the meniscus) represents a splitting of the circumferential fibers. In this pattern the innermost fragment is unstable and can be displaced (Fig. 114-12). The peripheral rim, if not involved with a second tear, will be stable. Tears can be complete, through the entire body of the meniscus, or incomplete, involving a partial tear of either the superior or inferior fibers (Fig. 114-13). It is important to accurately locate peripheral longitudinal tears (either at the meniscal-capsular junction or in the peripheral third of the meniscus) (Fig. 114-14). These tears have the potential to heal because of a blood supply, as shown by Arnoczky, and are ideal candidates for meniscus repair, as described in a subsequent section. The classic bucket handle tear is a vertical longitudinal tear that extends through a significant portion of the meniscus and has a displaced central fragment. If this tear is located in the peripheral portion, it is still amenable to repair.

Horizontal tears can occur alone but are more commonly seen in association with either a vertical longitudinal, a flap, or a degenerative tear.[294] This tear pattern occurs on a plane parallel to the superior and inferior surface of the meniscus. It is often seen in the older age group and is thought to be possibly due to loss of elasticity in the meniscal fibers. Horizontal tears occur most commonly in

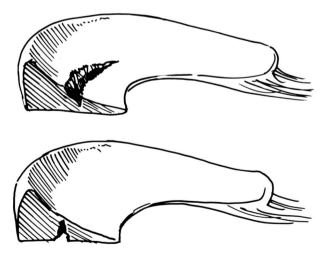

Fig. 114-13. Incomplete superior and inferior longitudinal tears.

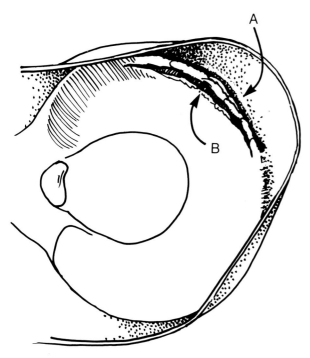

Fig. 114-14. Peripheral tears. **(A)** Meniscocapsular tear. **(B)** Peripheral longitudinal tear.

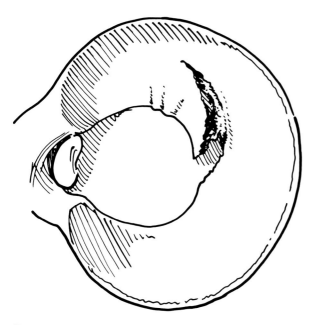

Fig. 114-15. Oblique tear.

the posterior horn of the medial meniscus and the middle third of the lateral meniscus. They often become evident only after resection of a flap or radial tear.

The third basic tear pattern is the oblique tear. This is a full-thickness vertical tear through the body of the meniscus, one portion of which exits on the inner edge of the meniscus (Fig. 114-15). It may represent a variation of the vertical longitudinal tear, with a continuation of the tear propagating obliquely to the inner margin of the meniscus, producing a loose fragment. A flap tear is a variation of an oblique tear that has a horizontal cleavage component in addition to the vertically oriented tear. The significance and treatment of this tear and of the oblique tear are identical (Fig. 114-16).

The fourth tear pattern is a radial tear, which is a vertical transverse tear most commonly located in the middle third of the lateral meniscus. These tears extend from the inner edge toward the periphery in varying lengths (Fig. 114-17). When a radial tear is complete, it extends to the meniscal synovial junction and essentially divides the meniscus completely into an anterior and posterior portion. Fortunately, most radial tears do not extend to the periphery but leave the meniscus with a small intact peripheral rim.

Variations of the four basic patterns include complex and degenerative tears. A complex tear occurs when there are several tear types in different locations or an extension of one tear type into another (Fig. 114-10). Many different variations can be seen, such as an oblique tear with an associated horizontal cleavage tear and possibly an additional radial tear. Following resection of a presumed simple tear, the remaining meniscus must be thoroughly inspected to diagnose and treat any additional tear pattern.

The degenerative tear is a chronic tear involving several tear patterns. The degenerative meniscus appears discolored and fibrillated and has shaggy, irregular torn surfaces (Fig. 114-11). It is often associated with arthritis of the articular cartilage. It is seen most commonly in the posterior horn of the medial meniscus and less frequently in the posterior horn or junction of the middle and posterior third of the lateral meniscus.

There are three basic types of meniscal resec-

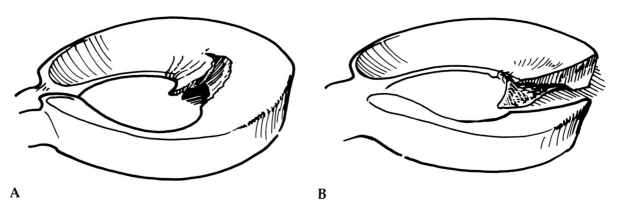

A   B

Fig. 114-16. Flap tears. **(A)** Superior flap tear involving the superior half of the meniscus in a horizontal cleavage split. **(B)** Inferior flap tear involving the inferior half of the meniscus.

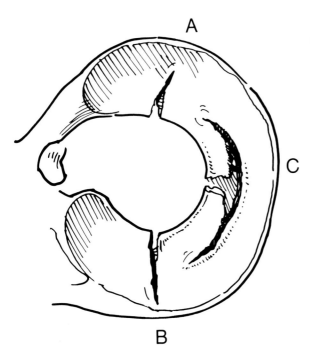

Fig. 114-17. Radial tears. **(A)** An incomplete radial tear involves part of the width of the meniscus. **(B)** A complete radial tear extends to the periphery. **(C)** An incomplete tear extending posteriorly or anteriorly is called a "parrot beak" tear.

tion, namely partial, subtotal, and total meniscectomy[261,283,294] (Fig. 114-18). A partial meniscectomy removes the torn portion of the meniscus as well as smaller amount of normal meniscus adjacent to the tear in order to produce a contoured smooth surface in the remaining intact meniscus (Fig. 114-19). Any loose or mobile fragments are excised, leaving a stable peripheral rim of remaining meniscus (Fig. 114-20). This is commonly used for vertical longitudinal and oblique tears, as well as for most radial and some degenerative tears. A partial meniscectomy is preferred over a subtotal or a total meniscectomy. A disrupted peripheral meniscal rim alters the normal transmission of force circumferentially.

A subtotal meniscectomy differs from a partial meniscectomy in that the peripheral rim is also affected, and a portion of the periphery is resected as well. This is often necessary in complex or degenerative tears or in radial tears that extend to the meniscal synovial junction (Fig. 114-21). Total meniscectomy involves removal of the complete meniscus. This is only necessary in very severe complex tears involving multiple segments of the meniscus and extending to the periphery. In the past total meniscectomy was necessary for peripheral detachments or large vertical longitudinal tears. These tears lend themselves to repair. Total meniscectomy should be avoided except for the most severely damaged meniscus.[129] Preservation

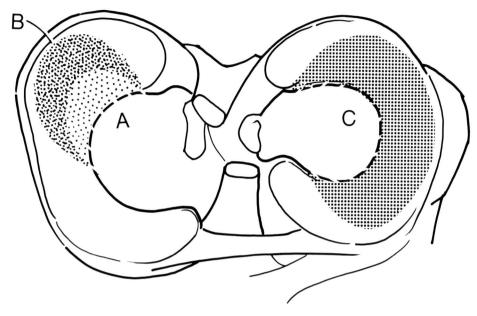

Fig. 114-18. Type of meniscal excision. **(A)** Partial meniscectomy. **(B)** Subtotal meniscectomy. **(C)** Total meniscectomy.

of meniscus tissue can minimize the degenerative articular changes that occur in a high percentage of patients following total meniscectomy.

Techniques for the Excision of Tears

The most common tear patterns of the medial meniscus are longitudinal tears (including peripheral and bucket handle tears), oblique tears, and flap tears arising from horizontal cleavage tears. Radial tears are more frequently found in the lateral meniscus. Excision of medial meniscal tears are performed by placing the leg in approximately 10 to 20 degrees of flexion and applying valgus stress to the knee either with the surgeon's body or by an assistant. Application of this valgus stress is facilitated by using either a leg-holding device (Fig. 114-3) or a post placed against the midthigh area on the side of the operating table (Fig. 114-4).

Proper treatment of longitudinal tears requires clear understanding of the type and extent of the tear (Fig. 114-22). Acute complete or incomplete tears within the peripheral third of the meniscus that are less than 1 cm in length can be treated by immobilization of the knee for 4 weeks. Complete acute tears in the peripheral third of the meniscus measuring more than 1 cm in length should be treated by meniscus repair (techniques for repairing a torn meniscus will be discussed in a subsequent section). A longitudinal tear in the periphery that has an additional complex tear pattern or is associated with marked deformity of the meniscus should be treated by partial meniscectomy. A chronic peripheral tear measuring less than 1 cm in length can be treated by preparation of the meniscus bed, sharp debridement (with shaver or scalpel) of the capsular-meniscus margins, and repair of the meniscus. Chronic tears in the vascular portions that measure more than 1 cm can be treated by meniscal repair after discussing the options with the patient. If the meniscus is not in good condition, the tear is best treated by partial meniscectomy. The decision as to whether or not to proceed

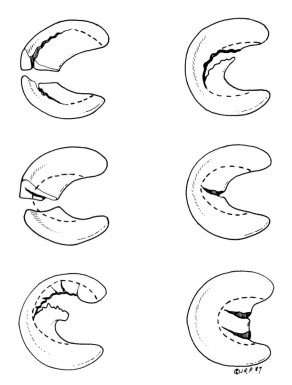

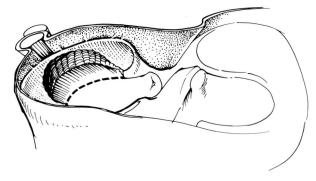

Fig. 114-20. A rim closing the popliteus hiatus was left intact.

Fig. 114-19. Classification of meniscal tears, with proposed partial meniscectomy shown in dotted lines. Top left: bucket handle. Top right: flap. Middle left: horizontal. Middle right: radial. Bottom left: degenerative flap. Bottom right: radial tears in discoid meniscus. (From Rosenberg,[283] with permission.)

with a meniscus repair in a chronic tear can be difficult. In general, a meniscus repair should be considered seriously in any young or active patient, whereas a partial meniscectomy would be the most appropriate treatment for an older or relatively inactive patient.

The technique for resection of a bucket handle tear or a longitudinal vertical tear of the medial meniscus involves placing the arthroscope in the anterolateral portal while placing a valgus stress on the knee.[186,261,294,301] The fragment is first resected at its anterior axilla with a basket roungeur or scissors or an arthroscopic scalpel inserted through the contralateral portal (Figs. 114-23, 114-24). An accessory portal is then made 1 to 2 mm superior to the inferior medial portal or from an additional

central portal. A grasping instrument is inserted, and the free anterior end of the meniscus is grasped. Tension is placed on the torn segment, displacing it into the intercondylar notch (Fig. 114-25). The posterior segment is then detached using a cutting instrument placed through the orig-

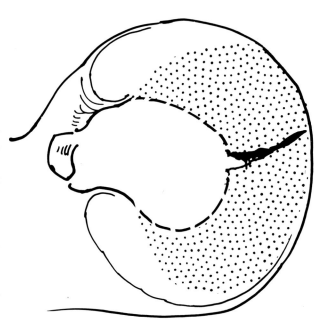

Fig. 114-21. A radial tear extending to the periphery. When this occurs a large portion of the meniscus should be removed.

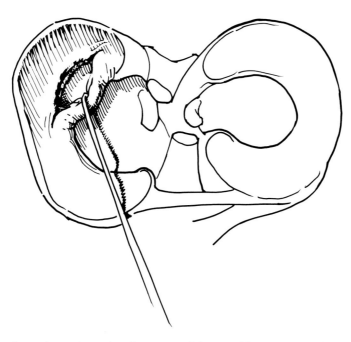

Fig. 114-22. The use of a probe to determine the extent of the tear. The entire inner fragment should be freely displaceable beneath the medial femoral condyle before excision is planned.

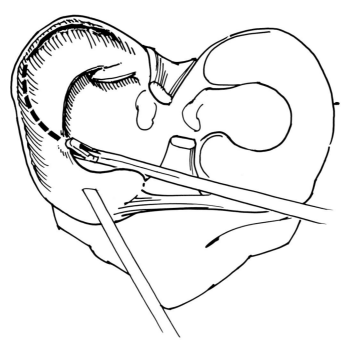

Fig. 114-23. Arthroscopic excision. The excision is begun by making an oblique cut across the middle third of the meniscus, with the cutting instrument coming across from the lateral compartment, while viewing arthroscopically through the medial portal.

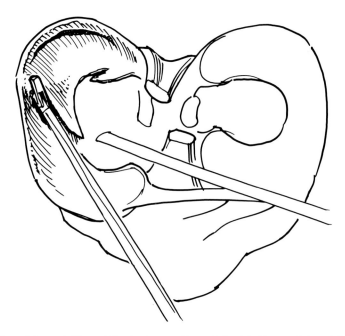

Fig. 114-24. Completion of the cut. The cutting instrument is switched to the medial portal and the arthroscope to the lateral portal.

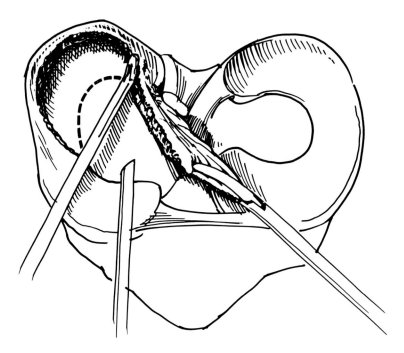

Fig. 114-25. The posterior attachment is being divided by the cutting instrument brought through an accessory medial portal, with the arthroscope brought through the anterior medial portal. The grasping instrument applies traction to the fragment from the lateral portal.

inal inferior medial portal. The amputation can be completed by using a Smillie-type knife, a basket rongeur, or scissors. The torn segment is then removed, and any remaining tip of meniscus is resected with a rongeur. Irregular edges or flaps of a body of the meniscus are carefully resected to fashion a contoured balance rim. This is followed by shaving and vacuuming with a motorized suction-cutter device. The goal with any excision is to preserve as large a peripheral rim as possible. It is important to remember that the operating instrument may need to be rotated 90 degrees, 180 degrees, or more in order to accomplish the resection at hand. If one size or configuration of instrument does not accomplish the task expeditiously, another instrument should be tried.

An alternative technique for resection of irreparable longitudinal tears involves partial resection of the posterior attachment, followed by resection of the anterior attachment[73] (Figs. 114-26, 114-27). The arthroscope is placed in the infero-lateral portal, and either a knife, scissors, or basket forceps is inserted into the inferomedial portal. The posterior attachment is incised to within 1 mm of the axilla of the tear. This 1-mm bridge is left intact until removal of the torn segment. The anterior attachment is then divided with a cutting instrument. Angled scissors or angled forceps are useful in making the cut in the oblique direction. By making the excision in an oblique manner, the anterior portion of the meniscal tear can be balanced and contoured while the torn segment is being excised. In some instances it may be necessary to switch the arthroscope and operating portals for division of the anterior segment. After resection of the anterior segment, the fragment is grasped and removed. Traction placed on the torn segment with a grasping instrument is usually sufficient to detach the 1-mm bridge of meniscal tissue. If not, the remaining posterior attachment will need to be incised. Any additional fragments are then removed as needed to obtain a well-balanced

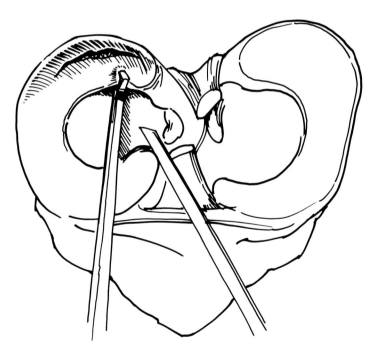

Fig. 114-26. Cutting of the posterior extremity of the fragment. The arthroscope is used through the lateral portal and a hook scissors through the medial portal.

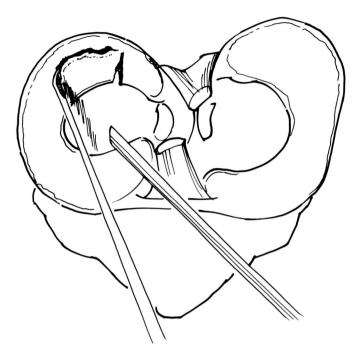

Fig. 114-27. Division of the anterior attachment of the fragment with a retrograde knife. The arthroscope remains in the lateral portal.

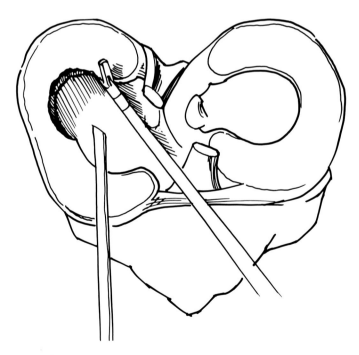

Fig. 114-28. Trimming the rim of the meniscus by using the arthroscope through the medial portal and basket forceps through a lateral portal. The fragment has been removed.

contoured edge (Fig. 114-28). Thorough inspection of the remaining meniscus is necessary to detect any additional tears or loose flaps.

Horizontal cleavage tears are treated by partial meniscectomy, usually performed by piecemeal excision, with preservation of as large a peripheral rim as possible.[283,294] It is often difficult to detect the depth of the horizontal tear by the first inspection. An attempt at en bloc excision of a segment may remove salvageable meniscus tissue. Piecemeal excision may be tedious and time-consuming, but this technique will avoid unnecessary resection of salvageable meniscal tissue. It is not necessary to excise the entire superior and inferior leaf of the torn segment if the tear extends into the peripheral third of the meniscus. Sharp debridement with a shaver into the cleavage extending into the periphery will stimulate bleeding and proliferation of primitive mesenchymal cells. This healing tissue will bind the two leaves together. It is crucial that the leaves that remain be in the peripheral third of the meniscus and be no more than 1 mm or so in width.

The technique of resection of an oblique or flap tear is similar to that described for resection of a longitudinal vertical or a bucket handle tear.[139,283,294] However, one segment of this tear exits on the inner rim of the meniscus, and thus only one segment of the tear needs to be resected (Figs. 114-29 to 114-31). A small portion of the adjacent remaining meniscus is resected to obtain a nicely balanced stable rim. It is crucial to perform a thorough inspection of the inferior, as well as the superior, surface of the torn meniscus to be sure that an additional flap has not become lodged between the tibial plateau and the meniscus or between the femoral condyle and the meniscus.

Radial tears are most commonly seen in the lateral meniscus and are treated by saucerization or contouring (Fig. 114-19) of a small amount of the adjacent meniscus on either side of the tear, angling the resection at approximately a 45-degree angle toward the apex of the tear.[283,294] If a radial tear transects the whole meniscus, a much wider resection is necessary (Fig. 114-21). Alternatively, a repair of a tear extruding into the peripheral third

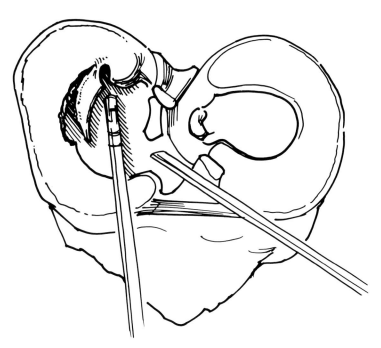

Fig. 114-29. Large posterior oblique tear. The posterior attachment of the fragment is divided first, leaving few fibers still attached.

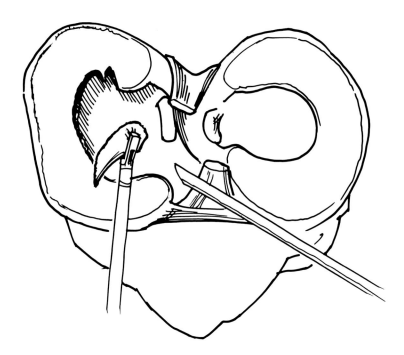

Fig. 114-30. Second stage of oblique tear resection. With the diagnostic arthroscope positioned inferolaterally, the pituitary rongeur is used through the inferomedial portal to grasp the fragment and remove it.

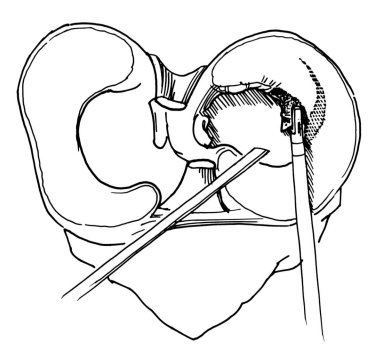

Fig. 114-31. Removal of the inferior flap by using a diagnostic scope inferolaterally and a basket forceps inferomedially. The flap is removed piecemeal, and the posterior horn is trimmed.

could be attempted (the technique will be described in a subsequent section).

Degenerative tears characterized by multiple small, irregular edges in abnormal-appearing meniscus tissues are most often found in the posterior horn of the medial meniscus.[261,283] The tissue is best removed piecemeal by using a basket rongeur. All torn and irregular flaps must be removed, but a peripheral rim should be preserved whenever possible. Following resection of a complex or degenerative tear, it is important to reinspect the posterior compartment to detect and remove any displaced fragments or loose bodies that may have floated into the posterior compartment. The posteromedial or posterolateral accessory portal is occasionally needed for removing any posterior fragments.

Lateral meniscus tears are seen less frequently than tears of the medial meniscus.[261,294] Shahriaree and O'Connor[294] state that this is due to the observation that the lateral meniscus normally has more mobility than the medial meniscus and therefore may be relieved of some of the stress and strain and hence be less vulnerable to injury. The location and pattern of tears in the lateral meniscus differ from those seen in the medial meniscus: whereas tears of the medial meniscus are usually in the posterior horn, tears in the lateral meniscus are more frequently seen in the middle third. Radial tears are the most common tears seen in the lateral meniscus.

Technique for excision of lateral meniscus tears requires opening or distracting the lateral compartment by placing the leg in the figure-four position, a technique discussed in connection with basic principles. The leg can be placed in varying (20 to 90) degrees of flexion, and a varus stress can be placed on the knee to aid in visualization of the menicus, condyle, and plateau. The pattern and extent of the tear, as well as the condition of the meniscal tissue, should be accurately assessed to determine whether meniscal repair or excision is indicated. The selection criteria for meniscus repair are identical to those previously discussed for medial meniscus tears and will be further discussed in the section on meniscus repair.

The diagnostic examination as well as many partial lateral meniscectomies can be performed while viewing from the anterolateral portal and using the anteromedial portal for insertion of cutting and grasping instruments. The portals can be interchanged to improve the angle of attack of the surgical instruments when necessary. Excision of the individual types of the lateral meniscus tears is performed similarly to the excisions described for medial meniscal tears.[283,294]

Postoperatively the patient is encouraged to move the knee through the range of motion that is comfortable. Early partial weight bearing with crutches is permitted and increased as tolerated. Ice bags are applied to the knee and changed every 2 hours. Straight leg lifting exercises are encouraged to prevent muscle atrophy. Most patients regain nearly full range of motion and are ambulatory, with full weight bearing, within 7 to 10 days. Additional strengthening exercises are then prescribed for the quadriceps and hamstring musculature. Return to sporting activities is permitted when adequate return of strength, motion, and painless running activities have been demonstrated.

The goal of meniscal surgery should always be preservation of as much meniscus as possible. Meniscus repair should be considered whenever a tear is located in the peripheral third of the meniscus. When the body of the meniscus has sustained significant damage and is degenerated, a partial or subtotal meniscectomy will be necessary. When a meniscal tear is excised, the remaining portion must be well balanced, with contoured edges to prevent any recurrent clicking, catching, or locking sensations. When properly performed, techniques for partial meniscectomy provide dramatic relief of symptoms after a relatively short phase of recovery and rehabilitation.

Discoid Lateral Meniscus

Meniscal problems in children may be due to a discoid lateral meniscus. Young[322] was the first to describe such a meniscus in a cadaver specimen in 1889. The clinical snapping syndrome or click associated with a discoid meniscus was reported by Kroiss in 1910.[203] The incidence of a discoid meniscus in meniscectomies has been estimated as 2.4 percent of 1,219 menisci reported by Nathan[243] and 4.2 percent of 8,000 meniscectomies reported by Smillie.[298] A discoid medial meniscus is much less common, the highest reported incidence being 0.3 percent.[91,278] A large study of 14,731 menisci by Dickason et al.[91] revealed discoid menisci to be present in 0.12 percent medially and 1.5 percent laterally.

The classic clinical finding termed *snapping knee* was thought to be pathognomonic of a discoid lateral meniscus.[194,203] Asymptomatic discoid menisci, however, have been observed during arthroscopic examination for unrelated disease in patients of all ages.[91,92] Symptomatic tears of discoid menisci have been reported in children, adolescents, and less commonly in adults.[21,194,243] The clinical presentation is sometimes uncertain because an accurate history of onset of symptoms or mechanism of injury is often lacking. The symptoms can include intermittent or persistent pain, effusions, buckling, locking, snapping, or limited range of motion.[194,243] The most consistent physical findings are palpable clicking, joint line tenderness, restricted range of motion, and occasionally effusions.[194,243]

Although radiographic changes have been reported, routine radiographs are most often normal. Some reported abnormalities include lateral joint widening, hypoplastic or flattened lateral femoral condyle, elevation of the fibular head, and hypoplasia of the lateral tibial spine.[243,278] The radiographs are useful in the diagnostic workup to rule out other causes of knee pain such as osteoid osteoma, osteomyelitis, fractures, and other lesions. Arthrography has been helpful in some cases but it is not generally recommended. Persistent symptoms suggestive of a meniscal lesion warrant arthroscopy as a diagnostic as well as a therapeutic tool.

The classification described by Watanabe[285,315] is widely accepted in both the adult and pediatric literature. The discoid lateral meniscus is classified into three types: (1) complete, (2) incomplete and, (3) Wrisberg ligament (Fig. 114-32). The complete discoid meniscus has meniscal tissue extending to the base of the lateral tibial spine. In the incomplete type the inner edge of the meniscus extends at a variable distance somewhere between the base of the lateral tibial spine and the normal position of a normal lateral meniscus. Both the complete and incomplete types have an intact meniscotibial ligament attaching the posterior horn to the tibial plateau. In the Wrisberg ligament type, however, the meniscotibial ligament is congenitally absent posteriorly and the discoid meniscus is attached posteriorly only by the meniscofemoral (Wrisberg) ligament. The arthroscopic appearance of a discoid meniscus may be somewhat confusing because in a complete type it may appear that there is no lateral meniscus at all. If this is encountered, one must

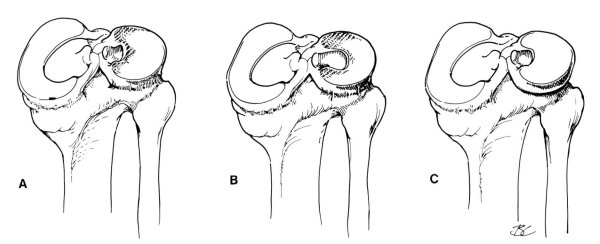

Fig. 114-32. The Watanabe classification of the discoid lateral meniscus. A posterior view showing: **(A)** complete type; **(B)** incomplete type; **(C)** Wrisberg-ligament type. Note the absence of the meniscotibial ligament to the posterior horn of the meniscus.

carefully inspect the base of the tibial eminence and search for the inner edge of the discoid meniscus. A discoid meniscus associated with a meniscal tear can be a challenging arthroscopic finding because the abundance of meniscal tissue can obscure visualization. Piecemeal excision of the torn portion may be necessary to obtain adequate visualization.

No treatment is required for asymptomatic discoid menisci or for patients with occasional lateral snapping but without locking or joint effusion.[92,285] In the past, complete or incomplete types that were symptomatic were treated by an open lateral meniscectomy.[194,243] Kurosaka et al.[204] presented good subjective long-term results in more than 90 percent of patients following total meniscectomy but demonstrated moderate to severe radiographic degenerative changes in 70 percent. Fujikawa et al.,[114] Ikeuchi,[165] Dickhaut,[92] Metcalf,[233] and Rosenberg et al.[283] have advocated central partial meniscectomy or saucerization for symptomatic complete or incomplete types (Fig. 114-33). Long-term studies are needed to determine the salutary effect of this technique.

Partial meniscectomy of the central portion of the discoid meniscus is one of the more challenging arthroscopic procedures. Excision should start by resecting the anterior portion with a side-cutting basket forceps or other suitable instrument (Fig. 114-33). The incision is then continued through the middle third by using scissors or a curved meniscal blade inserted from the inferomedial portal while viewing from the inferolateral portal. A second inferomedial portal is made superior to the first portal, and a grasping forceps is inserted. The central meniscal tissue is grasped and retracted into the intercondylar notch to improve the visualization of the posterior portion. The posterior discoid fragment is excised with a basket forceps or scissors. It may be necessary to switch the arthroscope to the inferomedial portal and to use the basket forceps in the inferolateral portal for removal of this posterior portion. The meniscus is then contoured so that the remaining width nearly approximates the width of a normal lateral meniscus. The remaining rim, however, will be thicker than the normal meniscus. In some cases it may be necessary to remove additional meniscus tissue in a piecemeal fashion in order to create a balanced rim. The

posterior horn must then be carefully probed and inspected to be sure that the meniscal tibial ligament is present and to determine whether or not an unstable posterior horn (i.e., a Wrisberg ligament type) is present. If so, the problem of an unstable posterior horn must be addressed. Until recently all authors had recommended total meniscectomy for this type. In 1982 Ikeuchi[165] reported performance of a central partial meniscectomy and a meniscus repair on one patient, but no follow-up data were available. Rosenberg et al.[285] in 1987 reported successful arthroscopic peripheral attachment after central partial meniscectomy of a Wrisberg ligament type of discoid lateral meniscus (Fig. 114-34). This technique warrants further investigation, but it should be performed only by those who have considerable experience with arthroscopic meniscal repair.

Postoperative care and rehabilitation are the same as for any partial meniscectomy.

Meniscus Repair

In the past, treatment options for a peripheral, meniscus tear were nonoperative treatment, subtotal or total meniscectomy. In 1948 Fairbanks[102] reported the radiographic degenerative changes found in postmeniscectomy knees: femoral condyle flattening, ridging on the anteroposterior (AP) view, and narrowing of the joint space. Jackson[168] in 1968 reviewed 640 knees following simple meniscectomy; he found a marked increase in degenerative changes and thought the articular stresses approached three times normal. In 1974 Johnson and Kettelkamp,[188] in a long-term follow-up of 99 meniscectomies, showed a 39 percent incidence of degenerative changes on radiographs, compared with 6 percent in the contralateral knee.

It became clear that meniscectomy was not an innocuous procedure, and it was reasonable to suggest that if an injured meniscus could be salvaged, even partially, the outcome of meniscal injuries and meniscectomies might improve.[48,68,76,128,201,275,311] In 1936 King[198] reported that torn menisci in dogs could be repaired with success. At that time he described the vascularity of the peripheral portion of the meniscus. It was al-

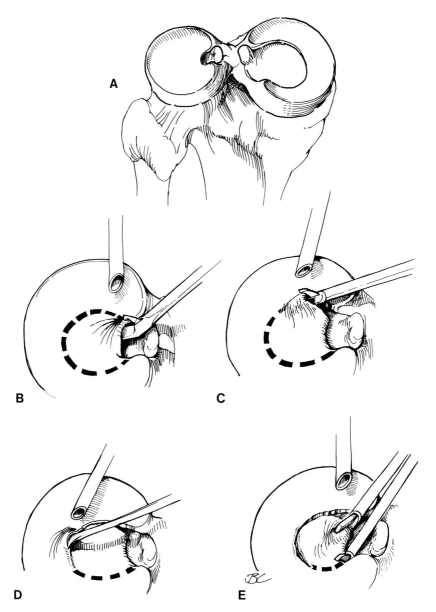

Fig. 114-33. Diagram of the technique for central partial meniscectomy of the discoid meniscus. The anterior aspect of the meniscus is shown on top and the posterior aspect on the bottom of each figure. Note that the posterior meniscotibial ligaments are intact. **(A)** Complete type of discoid meniscus. **(B)** The proposed amount of resection is indicated by the dotted line. **(C)** Resection of the anterior segment. **(D)** Resection of the middle portion. **(E)** The segment is grasped as the posterior attachment is released.

most 50 years before this work was elaborated by Arnosczky et al.[10,13,14] and later by Day et al.,[79] who confirmed that between 10 percent and 30 percent of the peripheral meniscus has a vascular supply. Embryology of the human meniscus revealed that

early in its development the meniscus has vessels throughout its entire substance and the inner portion gradually becomes avascular. Because of a network of blood supply, the peripheral portion of the meniscus has the potential to heal. Initial labora-

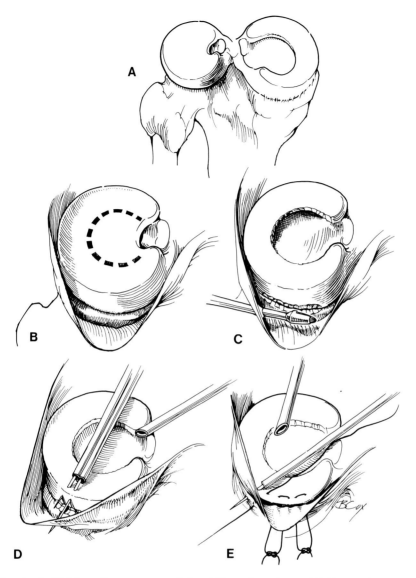

Fig. 114-34. Repair of a Wrisberg ligament type of discoid lateral meniscus. **(A)** The meniscotibial ligaments are absent along the posterior horn. **(B)** A central partial meniscectomy is performed. **(C)** The periphery of the meniscus, synovium, and capsule are abraded to stimulate a healing response. **(D,E)** Sutures are placed to secure the posterior horn to the synovial capsular junction by a technique used for repair of posterior peripheral meniscal tears.

tory studies have shown that the meniscus heals by fibrous scar and not by regeneration.[10,14]

With this information several authors proposed anew the concept that the meniscus could be preserved, and a new treatment option of repair of peripherally located meniscal tears devel-oped.[37,54,148,198,304] Meniscal repairs were reported in conjunction with collateral ligament repairs by Palmer[262] in 1938 and by Price and Allen[272] in 1978. With this information several surgeons performed open repairs of tears involving the most peripheral aspects of the meniscus. Wirth[318] in

1981 published a series of 10 cases. In 1981 DeHaven[83,85] reported meniscal repairs in the athlete; this was followed by Cassidy and Shaffer's report[54] of a series of 28 peripheral meniscal repairs. In 1983 Hamberg and Gillquist[140] reported on 50 meniscal repairs, 64 percent of which were evaluated by a repeat arthroscopy. They reported an 11 percent incidence of rupture at the initial repair site and a 9 percent incidence of rupture at a new site. Henning[150] was one of the first to popularize arthroscopic techniques for meniscal repairs. Subsequently several additional authors proposed various other arthroscopic meniscal repair techniques.[16,59,144,149,151,152,242,287,288,293,305,314] These techniques have expanded the indications for meniscal repair to include the outer 25 to 30 percent of the meniscus.

Many orthopaedists feel that the arthroscopic method is technically easier to perform than open repair, and early results of the arthroscopic technique appear encouraging. Because of these results and because of the high incidence of long-term degenerative changes in postmeniscectomy knees, repair of all peripheral tears should be performed whenever possible. The current indications for meniscus repair include: peripheral detachments through the coronary ligaments, longitudinal vertical cleavage tears located in the peripheral third of the meniscus, and some very selected radial or horizontal cleavage tears in the vascular zone. Repairs of other types of meniscal lesions, including complex, radial, and more central longitudinal (vertical or horizontal) tears are also being performed by Henning.[150–152] Longer follow-up with a large number of patients is needed in order to determine the efficacy of meniscus repairs for these types of lesions.

There are two basic techniques for arthroscopic repair of meniscus tears, the so-called inside-out and outside-in techniques. Several different cannula guide systems are available that facilitate inside-out techniques. Early reports are encouraging, but there have been no studies comparing results of various arthroscopic techniques. Early in this era arthroscopic repairs were done by placing needles from within the joint to the outside of the joint and tying the sutures over bolsters. This technique initially gave rise to an alarming incidence of major neurovascular injuries and of infections secondary to tying of the sutures outside the skin.[86,242] Because of these risks it has become universally recommended that a small posteromedial or posterolateral incision be made for retraction of neurovascular structures, for retrieval of needles, and for tying the sutures over the capsule.[59,144,150,151,242,293,314]

Longitudinal peripheral tears through the coronary ligaments can be repaired either by open arthrotomy techniques or by one of several arthroscopic techniques. Proponents of open repair feel that the advantages of the open techniques include the ability to place the sutures in the vertical, rather than horizontal, orientation in order to ensure anatomic positioning of the entire height of the meniscus rim to the capsular bed.[86] It also has been suggested that preparation of the repair site and abrasion of the meniscal synovial junction are more easily accomplished during an open arthrotomy procedure. Furthermore, the risk of neurovascular injuries from a needle passage would be lower with the open technique. Those who advocate arthroscopic techniques, however, have shown that with the limited posteromedial or posterolateral incision the risk of neurovascular injury is negligible and that the efficacy of the procedures appears to be equal.[144,150,151,287,288,293] The arthroscopic techniques offer several advantages over open techniques in that they make possible repair of longitudinal tears that are several millimeters central to the meniscal synovial junction. Tears in this location cannot be adequately reached by the open arthrotomy technique. Posterior horn tears of the lateral meniscus offer a difficult if not impossible exposure by the open technique whereas they are accessible by the arthroscopic techniques.

Many authors have shown successful meniscus repairs by open arthrotomy as well as arthroscopic techniques.[16,54,85,140,149,151,242,287,293,304,318] We compared the two procedures in a retrospective study of 71 meniscus repairs with a minimum 2-year follow-up,[144] of which 28 were accomplished by open arthrotomy and 53 by arthroscopic techniques. Our follow-up examination included a clinical examination of all patients as well as a repeat arthroscopy in 22 of them. There were no neurologic or vascular complications in either group. We defined a failure as either failure of the original tear to heal or appearance of a new tear, even if it was not located through the original repair site. The overall failure rate was 8.4 percent, with three failures in each group. The failure rate was 11 percent in the open repair group versus 6.7 percent in the arthroscopic repair group. This may not represent a significant difference, as the open group had a longer follow-up period and a greater percentage of anterior cruciate ligament instabilities.

In 1985 DeHaven[85] showed that the rate of repeat tears in cruciate-stable knees was 10 percent versus a 30 percent failure rate of meniscus repair in anterior cruciate–deficient knees. We found a 6.3 percent failure rate in the anterior cruciate–stable knee versus a 13 percent failure rate in the unstable knee.[144] Other authors have also documented that results of meniscus repair are better in stable knees.[287,288,293] Even though we feel that

cruciate stability presents a more favorable environment, it is certainly not mandatory for a successful meniscus repair. In individuals who do not desire anterior cruciate ligament reconstruction, we still strongly favor meniscus repair over the alternative treatment, which would be subtotal meniscectomy in most cases. Long-term studies are currently underway to determine if meniscus repair can prevent the previously recorded high incidence of degenerative changes found in postmeniscectomy knees. The role of anterior cruciate ligament stability may be critical in prevention of the arthritic changes.

Several arthroscopic techniques and cannula systems have been developed. Although we use the inside-out technique with the double-cannula system (Acufex Microsurgical, Norwood, MA) developed by Graf and Clancy,[59] this technique may not

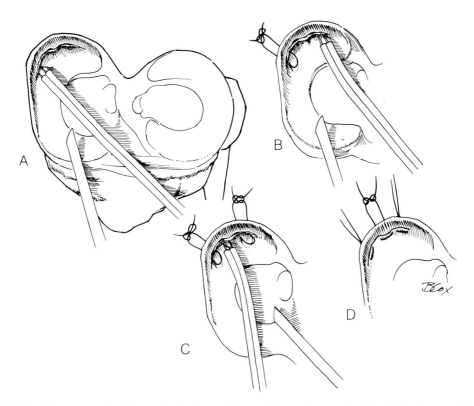

Fig. 114-35. Inside-out repair of the posterior horn of the medial meniscus using the double-lumen guides. **(A)** A straight cannula is shown placing the first suture into the meniscal body while viewing from the medial portal. **(B)** The cannula is positioned to place the most posterior suture. A limited posteromedial incision is made for retraction and direct retrieval of the needles. **(C)** The arthroscope and operating portals can be interchanged to facilitate placement of the sutures. **(D)** The meniscal tear is adequately stabilized by the sutures.

be superior to any of the other techniques to be described. Results published to date reveal most techniques to be equally successful.

Double-Cannula Technique

The double-cannula system for meniscus repair uses straight as well as curved cannulas.[59] These cannulas can be used from an ipsilateral or contralateral portal (Figs. 114-35 to 114-37). They are designed with varying shapes and curves, which can be used for tears in different locations — there is a straight cannula, a cannula curved to the right or left, and a straight cannula curved upward or downward at the tip. Sutures can be placed on either the superior surface or the inferior surface of the meniscus. The vast majority of sutures are placed on the superior surface of the torn body of the meniscus because it is more accessible and simply easier to visualize.

Preparation of the meniscal repair bed has been stated by many authors to be crucial to the success of the procedure.[86,150,288,293] Some have advocated rasping, abrading, or even burring the meniscal-synovial junction with hand or motorized instruments to produce a bleeding surface. Experimental studies by Arnoczky et al.[11] have shown that injecting a fibrin clot into the tear may aid in healing of the meniscal tear lesions. Further work is needed to document the necessity of adding this fibrin clot. In our retrospective review we found that in many patients the bed was not prepared with hand or motorized instruments, but none of our failures were associated with lack of bed preparation.[144] Until more data are available, however, meniscal bed preparation should be performed prior to suture placement.

After completion of a diagnostic examination and confirmation that a reparable meniscal lesion exists, the location and extent of the tear are re-

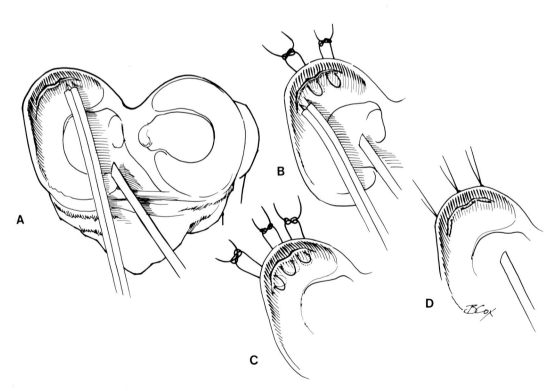

Fig. 114-36. Medial meniscus repair using the double-lumen cannula from the ipsilateral portal. **(A)** The posterior suture. **(B)** Placement of additional sutures. **(C)** After placement of the sutures. **(D)** The sutures are tied over the synovial capsular layers.

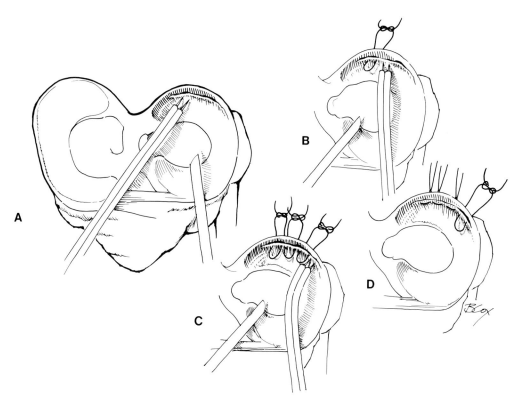

Fig. 114-37. Lateral meniscus repair using the double-lumen guide. **(A)** While viewing from the lateral portal, the straight guide is positioned and the needles are advanced and retrieved through the limited posterolateral exposure. **(B,C)** Additional sutures are placed through the contralateral or ipsilateral portals. **(D)** The sutures stabilize the meniscal tear.

corded and the number of sutures necessary for repair is estimated. Any displaced portion of the meniscus is reduced into position by use of a probe.

The meniscal bed is then prepared by debridement of the torn margins and abrasion of the adjacent synovial tissues. In acute tears with hemorrhage at the site of the peripheral tear, extensive debridement and preparation are probably unnecessary. In chronic tears, however, it is important to abrade and debride the edges to stimulate the vascular access channels.

The majority of tears of the medial meniscus are in the posterior horn or near the junction of the middle and posterior thirds of the meniscus. To accomplish the repair, the knee is flexed approximately 80 degrees, and the posteromedial joint line is palpated. A 1-inch vertical incision is made over the posteromedial joint line, and the posteromedial capsule is identified with sharp and blunt

dissection. During placement of the sutures a retractor is placed posteriorly to protect the neurovascular structures. With the arthroscope in the anterolateral or anteromedial portal, a curved cannula is placed through the opposite portal and is positioned on the superior surface of the meniscus at the level of the tear (Figs. 114-35, 114-36). Two 10-inch needles with a 2-0 polydiaxone suture (PDS) (Ethicon, Somerville, NJ) are placed through the cannula at the appropriate spot on the meniscal body. The needles are then pushed through the body of the meniscus approximately 2 cm. Care is taken to locate the needles in the posteromedial incision as they exit through the capsule. The cannula is removed, and the knee is then flexed to 90 degrees. Under direct visualization and palpation the needles are grasped with a needle holder and pulled through the posteromedial incision. The procedure is repeated for placement of as many sutures as necessary. The sutures should be spaced approximately 4 to 5 mm apart. No studies have proved that either the number or placement of the sutures is critical for a successful result as long as enough sutures are placed to produce a stable meniscus.

In the past many different suture materials, including both absorbable and permanent sutures, have been used by various authors. Repeat arthroscopy and clinical studies by several authors, confirmed by our study, have not shown any significant difference in results based on the type of suture used for the repair. Our preferred suture is 2-0 PDS, which is absorbed in 3 months. Repeat arthroscopy studies by Rosenberg et al.[287] have not shown any injurious effects on the articular cartilage from the sutures.

In tears of the most posterior aspect of the medial meniscus, it is safer to place the arthroscope in the inferomedial portal and the cannula through the inferolateral portal for placement of the most posterior sutures. It may be difficult to position the cannula over the tibial spine. With persistence and tenacity it is usually possible to insert either a straight or a curved cannula behind the tibial spine and have it spear the meniscus and exit at the appropriate position. Once all the sutures are placed, tension is applied on the sutures and the meniscal tear is probed to ensure that the tear is adequately stabilized. The sutures are then tied over the capsule, and the skin is closed in the usual fashion.

Postoperatively the leg is immobilized in a Bledsoe brace locked in approximately 30 degrees of flexion. The position of immobilization should be determined at the time of surgery by observing whether there is any separation of the repaired tear with the knee in various angles of flexion prior to tying the sutures.

The patient is kept on two-crutch ambulation for 4 weeks, non-weight bearing. Electrical stimulation and straight leg exercises are used to prevent muscle atrophy. At week 4 the Bledsoe brace is set to allow a 60 degree arc of motion, usually from approximately 10 to 70 degrees. Partial weight bearing using crutches is initiated and strengthening of the quadriceps is continued. Whirlpool is begun for range of motion. Gentle active flexion and extension exercises are permitted in the brace. At week 6 full weight bearing, as well as full active

and passive range of motion out of the brace, is permitted. The patient is advanced to a full program of progressive resistance exercises as tolerated. Guidelines for return to athletic activities include a full painless range of motion, ambulation without a limp, and satisfactory restoration of both quadriceps and hamstring strength as demonstrated by strength testing. When these criteria have been met, the patient is started on a graduated running program. Although there is no set time constraint, return to athletic activities is, in general, not recommended for 3 to 4 months.

In patients who have undergone combined anterior cruciate ligament reconstruction and meniscal repair, the postoperative rehabilitation is the same as for anterior cruciate ligament reconstruction alone. We feel that the complications of flexion contracture and anterior knee pain, previously noted to be associated with extensive immobilization following anterior cruciate ligament reconstruction, are more likely to occur if the patient does not work on early motion.[99,253,255] The risk of failure of meniscus healing appears small even with early motion.

For repair of a lateral meniscus tear, the arthroscope is placed in the inferolateral portal and the leg is placed in the figure-four position. The meniscal tear is probed and inspected. If a reparable lesion is confirmed, the bed of the tear is prepared as previously described. The posterolateral corner of the joint line is then palpated, and a longitudinal 2 to 3-cm incision is made at the interval between the posterior border of the iliotibial band and the biceps femoris tendon. Dissection is continued in this interval, and the posterolateral capsule is identified. With the leg flexed, the common peroneal nerve will lie posterior to the biceps tendon. A curved cannula is placed through the anteromedial portal and against the body of the meniscus. Two needles with 2-0 PDS are inserted into the cannula, the meniscal body, meniscal rim, and capsule. Retractors are placed in the previously made skin incision, and the needles are retrieved. It is essential to make sure that the needles exit above the anterior aspect of the biceps tendon to avoid injury to the common peroneal nerve. Additional sutures are then placed on either the superior or inferior surface of the lateral meniscus as necessary to stabilize the tear. Most lateral meniscal tears can be repaired by using the cannula through the antero-medial portal, but occasionally we have found it necessary to switch portals and insert the cannula through the anterolateral portal. Tension is placed on the sutures, and the meniscal tear is probed. If it is found to be stable, the sutures are tied over the posterior capsule. The skin is closed in the usual fashion, and postoperative rehabilitation is identical to that described for medial meniscus repairs.

Technique of Inside-Out Suturing Using the Single-Cannula System

Hendler,[149] Stone et al.,[304,305] and Henning et al.[150,151,293] have advocated use of straight, rigid, single-barreled cannulated guides through which the needles are passed. Because of some difficulty in placement of a straight rigid cannula in certain locations, Rosenberg[288] performed meniscal repair using curved, malleable 2.7-mm cannulas because of the greater maneuverability of these cannulas. A single cannula provides the freedom to vary the stitch size, and fewer sutures may be required than with the double-cannula technique. In addition, both horizontal and vertical mattress sutures can be placed from either the superior or inferior surface. The cannula is routinely placed from the contralateral portal while viewing from the ipsilateral portal. A posteromedial or posterolateral limited exposure as previously described is recommended to allow retraction and protection of neurovascular structures and for direct retrieval of needles. With the cannula in position, the needle is placed into the cannula and through the body of the meniscus, the peripheral rim, and the capsule, and the suture is pulled through the posterior incision. The cannula is repositioned, and the second needle is then placed and sutures passed in a similar fashion and tied.

Recently, because of some difficulty in suturing certain tears with use of the flexible cannula, Rosenberg has developed the zone-specific cannula system (Concept Inc., South Clearwater, FL). These cannulas are rigid single-lumen guides with preformed curves designated for suturing distinct anatomic locations, including anterior, middle, or posterior thirds of the meniscus (Fig. 114-38). The cannulas also have right and left curves. These cannulas were developed in order to facilitate more

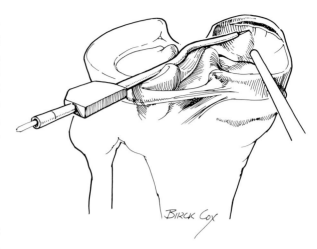

Fig. 114-38. The zone-specific cannulas are rigid single-lumen cannulas with preformed angles for placement of sutures in specific anatomic zones. This diagram shows the guide behind the intercondylar eminence for placing sutures in the posterior horn.

accurate needle passage. The curves of the posterior cannula are designed to pass over and behind the tibial eminence for suturing posterior tears. Further investigation will be needed to determine if these cannulas are superior to other available cannula systems.

Outside-In Technique for Meniscus Repair

Because of some of the early reported complications with transarticular or inside-out techniques prior to the adoption of limited posterior exposures, several orthopaedists have developed techniques for meniscus repair that involve placement of the needles or sutures from the outside position into the joint. Morgan and Casscells[242] and Warren,[314] in separate reports, describe a technique in which a small skin incision is made posteriorly along the posteromedial joint line for medial meniscus tears and posterolaterally for lateral meniscus tears. With the knee flexed 90 degrees, a posterolateral incision for lateral meniscus repairs is made over the posterolateral joint line anterior to the biceps tendon. After preparation of the meniscus bed and under arthroscopic visualization through the contralateral portal, an 18-gauge spinal needle is placed through the posterior incision from outside the joint and passed through the meniscus tear and body of the meniscus. Absorbable 2-0 PDS suture is placed through the spinal needle and is grasped from the anterior ipsilateral portal, and the suture is brought outside the joint to the knee (Fig. 114-39). A knot is tied in the end of the suture, which is then pulled back into the joint after removing the spinal needle. The knot on the end of the suture will bump against the meniscal body and pull the meniscus into its anatomic position. Several additional similar sutures are then placed, the number depending on the size of the tear. The ends of the sutures are then tied over the capsule posteriorly, and the meniscal lesion is re-probed to confirm stability. Postoperative rehabilitation is the same as that described for the double-cannula system.

Another technique for outside-in suturing uses the Meniscus Mender II System (Instrument Maker Inc., Okemos, MI). With this system a curved needle is inserted through a small posterior incision and penetrates the posterior horn tear (Fig. 114-40). A small wire loop passes through the needle and passes the suture into the joint. The suture

is then grasped with a miniature ligature holder. The second curved needle is passed several millimeters away from the first needle, and the tip of the suture is then passed through the wire loop, which is placed through the second needle. The wire loop is then withdrawn, pulling the suture into the posterior incision. The suture is tied taut, and the tear is reduced. Additional sutures are then placed sequentially as necessary depending on the length of the tear. Following suturing of the meniscus, the tear is probed to confirm stability. Closure of the wound is routine, and the postoperative rehabilitation previously described is followed.

SYNOVIAL LESIONS

The synovial lining of the knee joint has five basic pleats. Three of these pleats are considered distinct plicae, whereas two are considered minor folds.

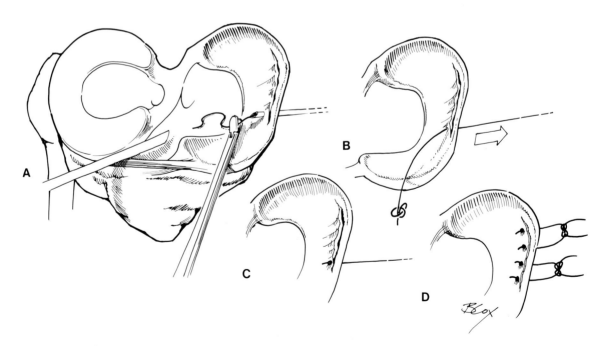

Fig. 114-39. The outside-in type of repair. **(A)** A spinal needle is inserted through the tear, and a suture is directed into the joint. The suture is grasped and is pulled through the ipsilateral portal. **(B)** A knot is tied on the end of the suture, and it is then pulled back into the knee. **(C)** When tension is placed on the suture, the knot will approximate the body of the meniscus to the peripheral rim of the meniscus. **(D)** Diagram of the sutures in position.

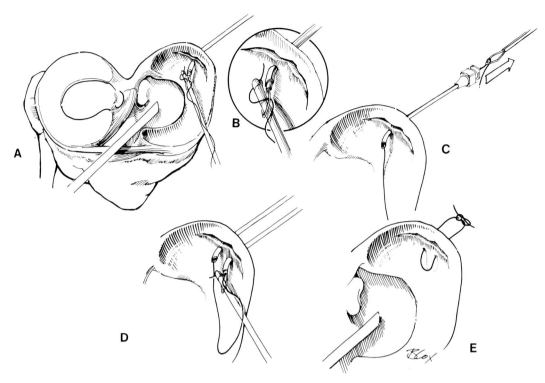

Fig. 114-40. The outside-in technique developed by Lanny Johnson. **(A)** A curved needle is placed through the meniscus, a wire loop is passed through the needle, and the suture is placed through the wire loop with use of a tiny ligature holder. **(B)** Close-up view showing threading of the suture. **(C)** The suture is pulled through the meniscus by withdrawing the wire loop. **(D)** The steps are repeated with the other end of the suture. **(E)** The suture is then tied, and additional sutures are placed as necessary. (Redrawn from Meniscus Mender II, Instrument Maker, Inc., Okemos, MI)

The five are the plica synovialis suprapatellaris, plica synovialis infrapatellaris, plica synovialis mediopatellaris, lateral synovial fold, and parapatellar fold.[264,265]

In order to assess whether or not a synovial lesion is pathologic, knowledge of the normal synovial structure is needed.[93,145,146] Lesions may be idiopathic problems of the synovium itself (i.e., localized pathologic plicae in the specific anatomic regions of the knee) or may be secondary to specific metabolic or systemic diseases presenting themselves with diffuse synovial manifestations. These diseases include arthrofibrosis, hemophilia, rheumatoid arthritis, pigmented villonodular synovitis, synovial osteochondromatosis, crystalline arthropathies, seronegative arthropathies, and osteoarthritis.

The role of arthroscopy in the past was purely diagnostic. However, arthroscopic surgical procedures can often be therapeutic in treatment of the entities listed.

Localized Synovial Lesions — Plica Resections

With trauma, the above-mentioned normal synovial folds can often become pathologic. These so-called fibrous adhesions very commonly follow minor insults to the joint, such as direct blows or subluxation of the patella, or more significant injuries, including anterior cruciate ligament tears or acute hemarthroses associated with the dislocating patella, as well as peripheral meniscus tears. A symptomatic, pathologic plica may present with a sensation of snapping, popping, and even tenderness to palpation on physical examination.[159,163,176,182,183,252,271,270] The exact location of the physical findings and symptoms are often quite consistent with the anatomic site of the previous normal synovial fold (Fig. 114-41).

A pathologic plica may be associated with visible articular cartilage changes (e.g., softening and fibrillation in the area directly in contact with the plica). There may be a diffuse synovitis, the manifestation of the release of cellular breakdown products and degradative enzymes, which in time incite a nonspecific inflammatory response.

Statistically, the most symptomatic plicae are those that are fenestrated (Fig. 114-42). Bordering the open areas, the plica is often quite thick and fibrous and can be excised by using the morselization and shaver-suction technique. The surgeon should be cautious in resecting normal synovial folds, as they might incite an inflammatory response and scar formation, producing an iatrogenic lesion. The surgical technique of synovial plica excision varies with the anatomic location of the lesion. The suprapatellar plica is best visualized and resected from an anterolateral portal, either the superior or inferior site. The resection is partial in that it should be limited to the fold itself and not include the synovium or the joint capsule. Usually with the fenestrated lesions, excision of the free margin is all that is necessary for relief of symptoms. Synovectomy usually requires a combination of basket, knife, and motorized instruments to complete the resection. One should intermittently decompress the joint to bring synovial tissue into closer proximity to the instruments. The surgeon's free hand must be used to palpate the knee and thereby displace tissue into juxtaposition with the instruments.

The medial pathologic plica is best viewed from the inferolateral portal. The plica can be resected either from an inferomedial portal or via a direct anterior portal though the patellar tendon. The exact location of the plica can be determined by insertion of an 18-gauge spinal needle under direct vision. An incision can then be placed directly anterior to the plica and a motorized instrument inserted. If the surgeon is already in an inferomedial portal for probing or other arthroscopic surgery, the motorized instrument can be placed in the joint via this portal, and with appropriate rotation of the trimmer, the resection can be completed. The medial pathologic plica often attaches in the region of the retropatellar fat pad and is therefore in continuity with the ligamentum mucosum. As a result resection of the femoral attachment of the ligamentum is often required to release the medial plica distally. A plica is pathologic only if associated with articular changes on the surface of the medial femoral condyle in direct contact with the plica.

The ligamentum mucosum is often resected during arthroscopy just to assist visualization. In cases of degenerative arthritis, the plica may be hypertrophic and associated with diffuse synovitis. In this specific instance it is possible to gain symptomatic relief following arthroscopic debridement.

Parapatellar synovitis, localized nodular synovitis, and small fibrotic bands are often found dur-

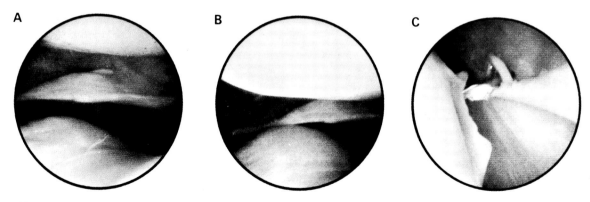

Fig. 114-41. Plica synovialis suprapatellaris. **(A)** Arthroscopic view revealing transverse course of pathologic plica. **(B)** Arthroscopic view with less distention of joint. **(C)** Needle localization of lesion as seen by arthroscopic position of 18-gauge spinal needle. (From Johnson,[186] with permission.)

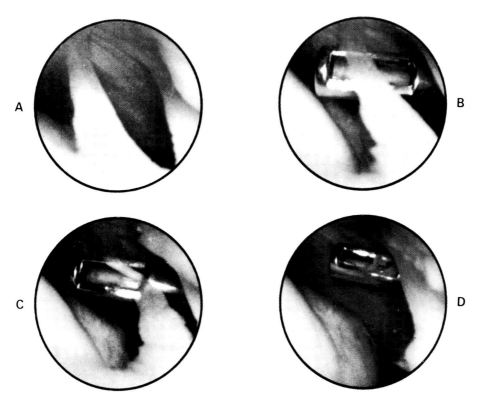

Fig. 114-42. Synovial plica lesions—medial fenestrated synovial plica. **(A)** Arthroscopic panoramic view of fenestrated lesion. **(B)** Intra-articular shaver. **(C,D)** Technique of resection technique of the free margin of the fenestrated lesion. Resection of the free margin is all that is needed to alleviate symptoms. (From Johnson,[186] with permission.)

ing arthroscopic surgery. The exact significance of these lesions is often unclear, but they usually indicate abnormal tracking or past trauma. These can be resected by the usual arthroscopic techniques.

Diffuse Synovial Lesions Requiring Generalized Synovectomy

Synovial lesions associated with rheumatoid arthritis, hemophilia, synovial osteochondromatosis, and pigmented villonodular synovitis require a more generalized synovectomy[153,154,197,263] (Figs. 114-43, 114-44). The procedure is tedious and time consuming. Familiarity with access through multiple portals is not only helpful but mandatory in order to effectively perform a synovectomy in each compartment. Instrumentation with variable-speed adaptations[8] is a must, in addition to the rou-

tine surgical setup. Interchangeable heads of sizes varying from 3.5 to 5.5 mm should be available: the 3.5-mm size is best suited for work about the menisci; the 4.5-mm head is best suited for soft tissue work in the intercondylar notch and the posteromedial and posterolateral compartments; and the 5.5-mm head is most effective in the anterior aspect of the knee and the suprapatellar pouch. A "whisker"-type synovial shaver for tiny areas and a full-radius resector for more aggressive cutting of thickened, dense tissue in wider areas can be extremely helpful (Fig. 114-45). A cannula system in each portal allows easy interchange of instruments and helps to speed up the procedure.

Johnson describes generalized synovectomy as being divided into six phases.[186] Phase 1 involves synovial resection of the suprapatellar pouch, the medial gutter, the anteromedial aspect of the knee, the parapatellar area, and the ligamentum muco-

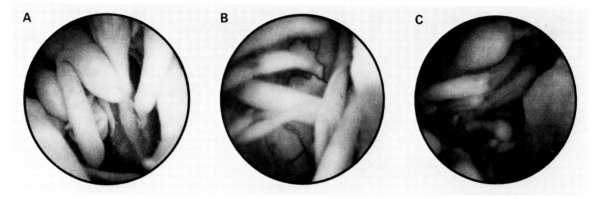

Fig. 114-43. Rheumatoid synovitis. **(A)** Dumbbell-like villous projections of the synovium. **(B,C)** The generalized nature of this synovitis is shown by these views, taken at different areas within the joint. (From Johnson,[186] with permission.)

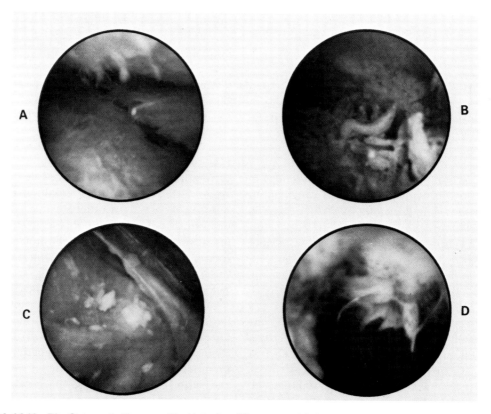

Fig. 114-44 (A–D). Osteoarthritic synovitis. Note the diffuse synovitis in the medial compartment secondary to degenerative disease and the distinct difference between the appearance of this condition and that of the rheumatoid synovium. Also note the degenerative free margin of the medial meniscus in Fig. A. (From Johnson,[186] with permission.)

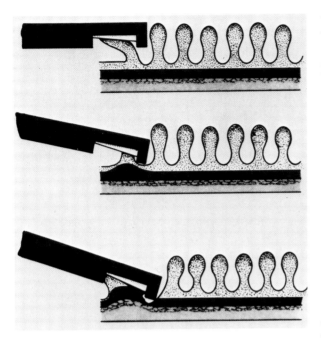

Fig. 114-45. Synovial resection technique: graphic depiction of intra-articular shaver resecting the synovium and adjacent structures to different depth. Level of resection depends on force applied to the instrument. Depth of the resection should be determined by the pathologic diagnosis of the lesion, (i.e., deeper for PVNS). The capsular structure should be spared unless the lesion is indeed invasive. (From Johnson,[186] with permission.)

sum. This is accomplished via an inferolateral portal for visualization and an inferomedial portal for instrumentation. The knee is kept at full extension and well distended.

In phase 2 synovectomy is carried out in the medial gutter and medial compartment. The instruments are placed in the same portals utilized in phase 1, but the knee is flexed, a valgus force is applied and the medial compartment is visualized in identical fashion to diagnostic arthroscopy. The small (3.5-mm) nonaggressive motorized instrument is used to resect tissue both beneath and above the meniscal surfaces.

Phase 3 is initiated by switching the arthroscope and instruments to the inferomedial and inferolateral portals, respectively. This allows additional inspection of the suprapatellar pouch from a different angle and aids in performing a synovectomy of the lateral gutter. Care must be taken with resec-

tion of the synovium in this area so as not to injure the popliteus tendon.

Phase 4 requires arthroscope placement in the posterolateral compartment and establishment of an accessory posterolateral portal in the manner previously described. With maximum distention of the knee joint, the posterolateral compartment may be palpated. A small incision is made in the skin and with blunt dissection is carried down to the capsule through the subcutaneous tissue. The lateral head of the gastrocnemius muscle is retracted along with the neurovascular structures in the popliteal fossa. A small incision is made in the capsule under direct visualization, and the shaver is inserted through this portal. Debridement and synovectomy of the posterolateral compartment are then carried out. If necessary, the portals for the arthroscope and the shaver can be exchanged.

Phase 5 can be accomplished blindly with the obturator in the sheath or under direct visualization by passing the telescope along the lateral aspect of the medial femoral condyle. A posteromedial portal is made in the same fashion described above for the posterolateral portal. Synovectomy of this compartment is performed not only along the surface of the synovial capsular attachments but along the posterior horn of the meniscus and the posterior cruciate ligament. Exchanging the portals for the arthroscope and shaver allows additional synovial resection.

Finally, phase 6 involves debridement of the Baker cyst, when present, via a double portal technique in the posteromedial compartment. The two posteromedial portals should be made under direct visualization and the Baker cyst inflated via a cannula placed through the intercondylar notch. Resection in this posterior region should be carried out only with the small (3.5-mm) whisker head.

The operator should be familiar with the maneuvers of the intra-articular motorized instrumentation to permit safe and accurate resection. These start with placement of the cutting tube against the synovial lining with its cutting window in direct apposition to the synovium to be resected. By simultaneously activating the shaver and suction, the synovial lining will be drawn into the resecting window. A "wiping" maneuver covers more surface area at a more rapid pace. More aggressive resection can be accomplished by applying external pressure to the knee to stabilize the synovial/capsular layer. The head of the motorized instrument is firmly applied to the lining of the knee joint and swept across its surface. Pressure aids in achieving the deeper resection that is often needed for more aggressive lesions (i.e., pigmented villonodular synovitis) (Figs. 114-45 to 114-47).

With the joint maximally distended, external pressure by the surgeon's opposite hand may be necessary to direct the tissue into the cutting instrument (Fig. 114-47). This technique can also be used to manipulate the tissue in front of a stationary motorized blade. The fluid pressure on the joint can be intermittently relieved so that the tissue relaxation permits the synovium to be more effectively drawn into the cutting window. These small but significant "tricks of the trade" enhance the efficiency of resection in each portal used and minimize instrument repositioning.

Tourniquet control is often necessary to allow adequate visualization. Generalized resection requires patience — more than 2 hours of tourniquet time may be necessary. Perfusion of the limb for approximately 15 minutes upon release of the tourniquet will permit the surgeon to finish the procedure following venous exsanguination. Generalized synovectomy does not necessarily mean complete synovectomy. Microscopic disease and inaccessible gross lesions may be left behind. Early work with a radioactive isotope such as dysprosium 165 is being evaluated, not only as a primary thera-

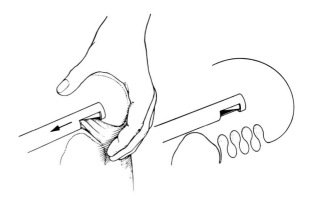

Fig. 114-47. Schematic depicting the importance of the surgeon's free hand in applying pressure against the soft tissue covering the knee to assist in synovial resection. (From Johnson,[186] with permission.)

peutic intervention but also for use following arthroscopic debulking synovectomies.

Postoperative Management

All portals are left open so that intra-articular fluid can drain, and a sterile bulky dressing is applied for general compression. Active and passive motion is instituted immediately, and the patient is permitted partial weight bearing as tolerated. Routine postarthroscopy wound care and rehabilitation instructions are followed.

Arthrofibrosis

Fibrous adhesions can develop following any insult to the knee joint (surgical procedures, plaster cast immobilization, etc.). The adhesions can be quite numerous and span any particular area of the joint. Such fibrous adhesions of the synovial lining of the knee joint result in limitation of the potential volume of the knee, thereby inhibiting knee motion, and may bind down the patella and patellar tendon. The posterior surface of the quadriceps mechanism proximally may be adherent to the anterior femoral cortex. Extensive fibrosis of this degree is commonly associated with open arthrotomies, particularly in ligament repairs and reconstructions (Fig. 114-48).

Arthroscopic release of arthrofibrosis is difficult but possible.[303] Following insertion of the instru-

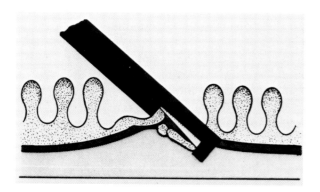

Fig. 114-46. Schematic showing: technique of "pawing." This allows the instrument to be moved back and forth over the synovial tissue in a motion resembling that of a dog scratching for fleas. (From Johnson,[186] with permission.)

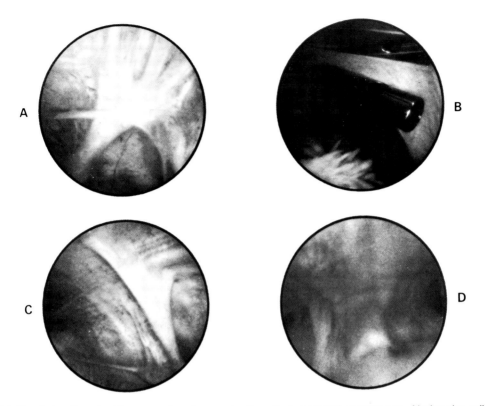

Fig. 114-48. Arthrofibrosis. The synovium has a significantly lamellated appearance. Notice the adhesions between the patella and femur in the patellofemoral groove in Fig. D. (From Johnson,[186] with permission.)

ments into the knee via the standard portals, the articular surface is inspected. This may be extremely difficult because of encasement fibrosis that markedly decreases the potential volume of the knee. Adhesions can be lysed and a joint space created by blunt dissection using the arthroscope sheath and blunt obturator. Blunt dissection is carried across the anterior surface of the femur and down the medial and lateral gutters. Additional dissection and resection can be carried out under direct visualization with basket forceps or scissors placed via the anteromedial portal. A superior suprapatellar release can be carried out by cutting from medial to lateral with a retrograde knife, almost in a subperiosteal fashion across the anterior surface of the femur. This can be accomplished via a superolateral or superomedial portal and requires maximum distention.

The same knife blade can be used via the inferomedial portal to perform the medial release, starting proximally and proceeding distally parallel to the patellar tendon. Changing the angle of attack from medial to lateral will allow performance of the lateral release, which in effect creates an inverted U about the quadriceps mechanism of the knee. At this point manipulation of the knee is carried out. Sterile conditions should be maintained. If further release is required, inspection of the potential volume of the knee at this point can lead the operator to the appropriate region. The retropatellar fat pad should be visualized and any adhesions of its posterior surface to the intercondylar notch resected. Care must be taken during release of these adhesions to avoid injury to the cruciate ligaments (Fig. 114-49).

Following careful documentation of motion obtained in the operating room, a pressure dressing is applied and the knee is immediately placed in a continuous passive motion machine. Generous use of ice and administration of narcotic analgesics are required to control pain. Active-assisted and passive range-of-motion exercises should be carried

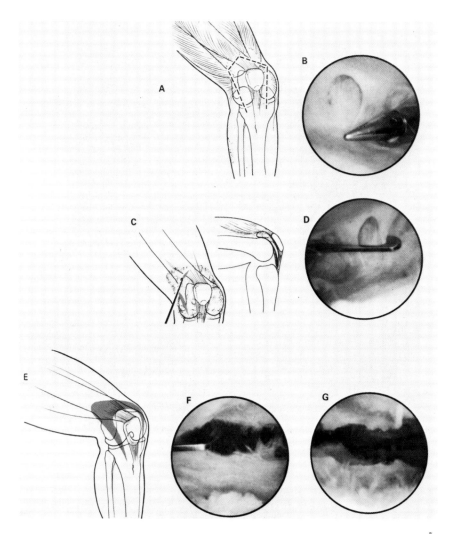

Fig. 114-49. Schematic and arthroscopic depiction of diffuse arthrofibrosis. **(A)** The inverted U reveals the areas requiring arthroscopic release to improve range of motion. Notice the area being concentrated around the patella and patellar tendon. **(B)** Fibrosis of the quadriceps mechanism to the anterior femur in the suprapatellar pouch. **(C, D)** Lateral gutter adhesions. **(E, F)** Medial gutter adhesions. **(G)** Creation of medial gutter at the end of the procedure. (From Johnson,[186] with permission.)

out under the guidance of a physical therapist. The patient should not be discharged from the hospital until the measured motion obtained in the operating room is achieved. If this cannot be achieved in 1 week, a repeat manipulation or debridement may be necessary. The patient is allowed to participate in progressive resistant exercises and other conditioning activities as tolerated.

Surgical Management of Synovial Lesions Amenable to Medical Treatment

Crystalline Arthropathies

Management of the crystalline arthropathies (i.e., gout and pseudogout) is mainly medical. Arthroscopy can be useful in those situations in which

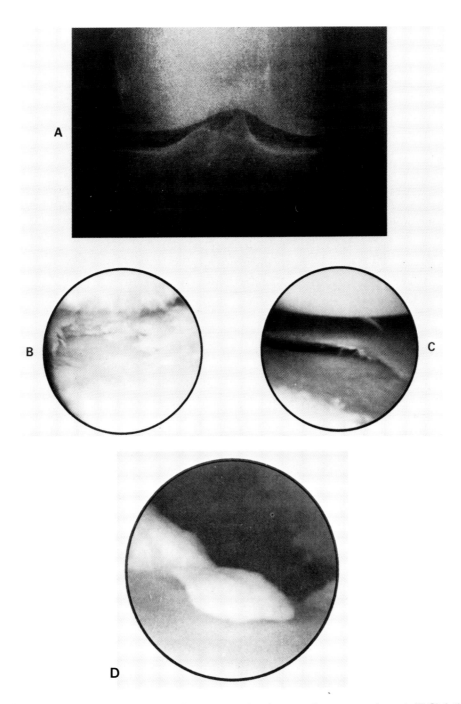

Fig. 114-50. **(A)** Radiographic appearance of chondrocalcinosis secondary to pseudogout. **(B,C)** Arthroscopic appearance of tibial plateau and meniscus with crystalline deposits. **(D)** Fibrinoid loose body often seen with Reiter's syndrome. (From Johnson,[186] with permission.)

sepsis must be ruled out.[258] An uncontrolled exacerbation can be relieved significantly with arthroscopic lavage and debridement, which can be performed under local anesthesia if desired. Large deposits of crystalline material may require the use of a synovial resector to remove the bulk of the lesion (Fig. 114-50A).

Seronegative Arthropathies

Reiter's syndrome and psoriatic arthritis rarely have indications for arthroscopic procedures. These conditions, however, can often be confused with a septic process. Joints affected in patients with Reiter's syndrome often show no articular changes and no synovial villus formation. These joints do, however, contain fibrinoid exudate, which flows freely in the joint (Fig. 114-50D). Lavage and debridement of this material may relieve the patient's symptoms significantly. The synovial hypertrophy process in psoriatic arthritis has a marked lacy, villous appearance. Within this villous synovial network the vascularity is quite developed and often is equated with a "rabbit ear"

appearance. Partial synovectomy and joint lavage may have a useful but limited role in psoriatic arthritis.

Degenerative Arthritis

The appearance of synovial inflammation accompanying degenerative arthritis is chronic. Even with the tourniquet deflated, the synovium is somewhat blanched and not very reactive (Fig. 114-44). Mechanical symptoms can be present, however, if a large nodule of the synovium exists. This specific lesion can be dealt with quite easily by localized synovectomy, together with caring for the underlying meniscal or articular disease.

If diffuse articular involvement is noted in the joint, acute inflammatory arthritis may be present along with the degenerative arthritis. The synovial inflammatory response associated with this acute inflammatory picture is quite proliferative and hemorrhagic. This particular entity may require a more generalized synovectomy, as described previously. Symptomatic relief of pain by debridement and lavage is extremely variable with respect

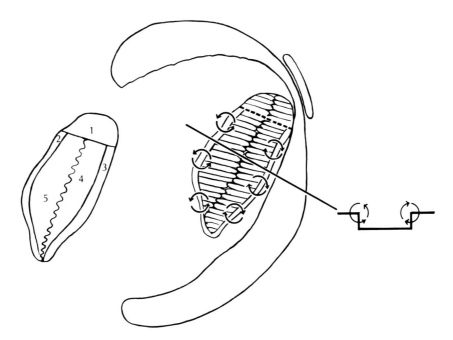

Fig. 114-51. Schematic depicting pattern of abrasion arthroplasty for tibial plateau articular lesion. Note the initiation of abrasion at the posterior margin of the plateau. Contouring of the intact cartilage margin with exposed bone allows a gradual drop-off. The central area of the lesion is finally abraded to the appropriate depth determined from the margins of the lesion. (From Johnson,[186] with permission.)

to both the magnitude and duration of symptom relief.

Arthroscopic Management of Osteoarthritis

Articular cartilage lesions in the degenerative knee vary from fibrillation and fragmentation to eburnated, exposed bone. Arthroscopy can be used not only to debride the fibrillated and fragmented areas but also to abrade or drill the eburnated areas.[113,170] This stimulates vascular ingrowth from the subchondral region, bringing primitive mesenchymal cells, which are capable of forming fibrocartilage, into the lesion. The work of Robert Salter[289,290] in Toronto and Lanny Johnson[186] in Michigan has substantiated this phenomenon.

Surgical Technique

Diagnostic arthroscopy is performed by using the standard portals and approach. Lesions of the medial femoral condyle are visualized best with a 30-degree telescope in the inferolateral portal and vice versa. The knee can be flexed and extended as needed to increase visualization of the articular surface. A curette and a basket forceps (placed through the inferomedial portal) are used to remove loose articular margins. A cannula placed through the portal is used to suction all loose fragments from the knee. Following the technique described by Johnson,[186] a motorized burr is used to penetrate the avascular subchondral plate to produce a bleeding bony surface. Small Kirschner (K-) wires or small drills can be used to make multiple perforations through the subchondral plate to a depth of approximately 5 mm. The articular margins of the medial condyle are inspected for any osteophytes that can be removed by the motorized burr. The burr must be held firmly so as not to create iatrogenic defects in the articular surface of either femur or tibia (Figs. 114-51 to 114-55).

High tibial osteotomy should be considered if significant angulatory deformities of the lower extremity exist. If this procedure is performed in one stage, the tibial osteotomy site must be adequately stabilized so that immediate postoperative motion can be instituted safely. If the surgeon is not familiar with internal or external fixation techniques for high tibial osteotomies that will permit immediate motion, the procedure should be performed in two stages. If the surgeon decides to perform the abrasion arthroplasty as the first stage, care must be taken not to perform the high tibial osteotomy too soon, as this might interfere with maintenance of motion and contribute to a higher incidence of infection.

Following an abrasion arthroplasty, patients should remain non-weight bearing for 4 to 6 weeks to take as much load as possible from the healing fibrocartilaginous tissue. Active and passive range-of-motion exercises, however, should be encour-

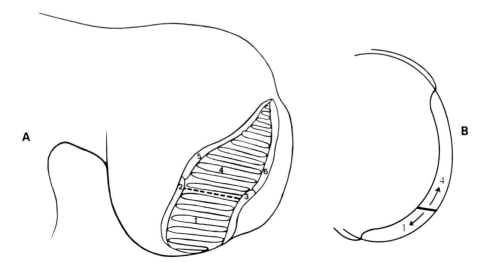

Fig. 114-52. Schematic of abrasion arthroplasty for a lesion of the femur. (See Fig. 114-51 caption.)

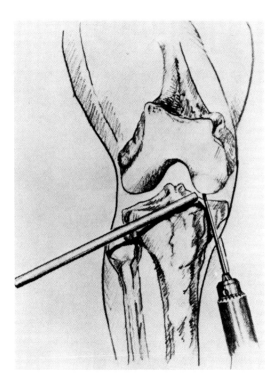

Fig. 114-53. Schematic revealing triangulation technique for drilling of medial femoral condyle eburnated lesion. (From Casscells,[51] with permission.)

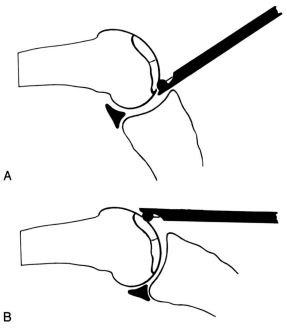

A

B

Fig. 114-54. Schematic depiction of the need for flexion and extension of the knee to increase visibility of femoral articular lesions. (From Johnson,[186] with permission.)

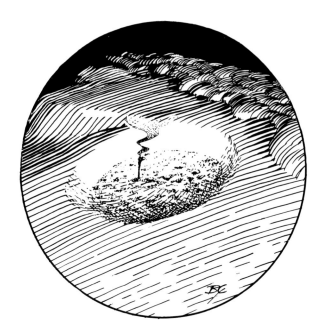

Fig. 114-55. Schematic depiction of depth of lesion with punctate bleeding.

aged at all times. The duration of symptomatic relief following abrasion arthroplasty is variable. Many patients report several years of significant relief, but some may have no relief at all (Fig. 114-56).

OSTEOCHONDRITIS DISSECANS

Osteochondritis dissecans remains an enigma. The pathophysiology remains unclear, and multiple theories about the etiology have been suggested. Two commonly mentioned theories implicate trauma and/or ischemia as the causes.

Classification of these lesions is based on radiographic location, size, and arthroscopic appearance. Special studies, including tomograms, bone scans, and bone age films, can help to categorize specific lesions (Fig. 114-57).

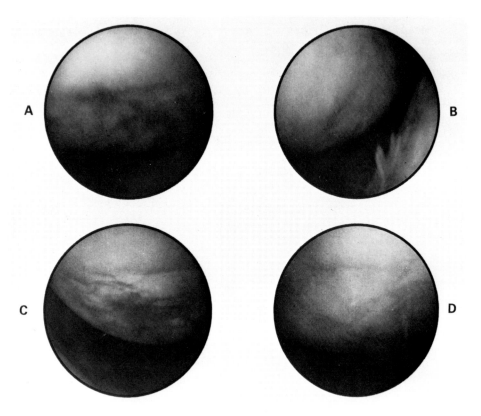

Fig. 114-56. Arthroscopic appearance following abrasion arthroplasty. (From Johnson,[186] with permission.)

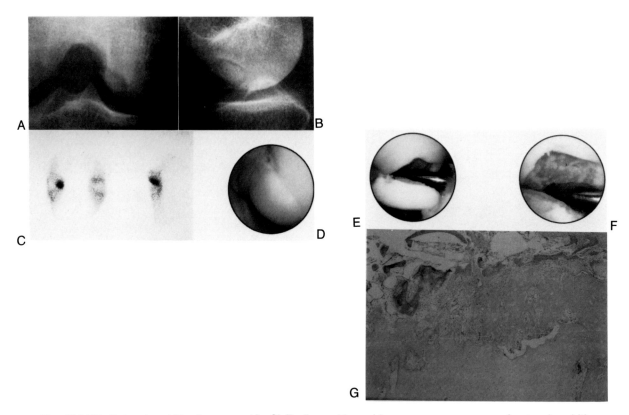

Fig. 114-57. Osteochondritis dissecans. **(A–C)** Radiographic and bone scan appearance of osteochondritis dissecans of the medial femoral condyle. **(D)** Arthroscopic appearance of the lesion, which is noted to be nondisplaced. **(E,F)** Arthroscopic displacement of osteochondritis dessecans fragment. **(G)** Microscopic appearance of osteochondral fragment. (From Johnson,[186] with permission.)

Arthroscopy is useful in characterizing the lesions into one of the several types described by Guhl.[136,138] Possible findings and important factors that must be assessed include articular surface continuity; articular surface continuity associated with softening and minimal motion of the articular fragment; partial detachment of the articular fragment; a free osteochondral fragment; and multiple free osteochondral fragments.

Lesions measuring less than 1 cm and lesions in patients less than 12 years of age are generally treated nonoperatively by immobilization. The period of immobilization is determined by signs of healing noted on subsequent radiographs and can vary from 1 to 4 months. Small lesions in older children are usually treated by excision of the lesion and debridement or drilling of the lesion bed.

Treatment of the osteochondritic lesion with an intact articular surface is especially difficult.[29,39,80,98,134] The patient usually presents with knee pain, and serial radiographs demonstrate a lesion, which may be revealed by arthroscopy and direct visual examination to be quite stable. There may be no breach in continuity of the articular cartilage or any visible degenerative changes. Several authors, including Johnson, suggest no surgical intervention, whereas others have suggested drilling of the lesion or retrograde bone grafting under arthroscopic and/or fluoroscopic control. The proper treatment remains controversial.[136,137,138,186,199,211,214]

For lesions in which the articular surface is in continuity but is soft or mobile, drill holes approximately 1.5 cm deep should be placed across the lesion. Retrograde bone grafting should be considered for large lesions (Figs. 114-58 to 114-60).

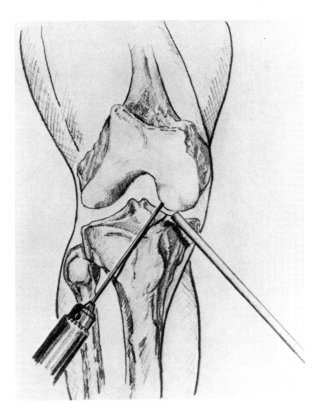

Fig. 114-58. Anterograde drilling of medial femoral condylar lesion. (From Casscells,[51] with permission.)

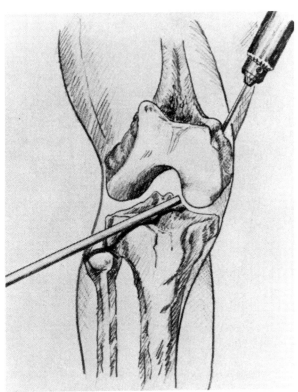

Fig. 114-59. Retrograde wire removal for retrograde bone reaming and grafting technique under arthroscopic control. (From Casscells,[51] with permission.)

A partially detached osteochondritic lesion is a surgical challenge. These lesions most commonly arise from the lateral aspect of the medial femoral condyle near the intercondylar notch and usually have a vascular pedicle from the synovial tissue originating in the intercondylar notch. The bone on the osteochondral flap and the base of the condylar lesion is usually covered with fibrous tissue, which must be removed prior to attempting to replace this bone fragment (Fig. 114-61). The fragment is reduced and held in place with a smooth K-wire. Pin breakage or migration is a potential complication of cannulated compression screws, but they offer the most secure fixation. For large fragments, two screws are required to control rotation. If the fragment is small and will not accommodate two screws, single screw fixation is the best alternative (see Fig. 114-62).

Free osteochondritic lesions have been extensively studied by Guhl.[136,138] Viability of the osteochondral fragment is assumed to be sustained by the synovial fluid. Both the condylar bed and the osseous surface of the free fragment need to be cleansed of fibrous tissue. Reduction of the fragment into its condylar bed is accomplished by probing and positioning with an arthroscopic grasping forceps. Occasionally, a bone graft is required in the base of the lesion to prevent an incongruous reduction of the free osteochondral fragment. The fragment is then temporarily secured with smooth K-wire pins, followed by permanent fixation with cannulated screws. The overall prognosis for these lesions, however, remains guarded.

For those patients who have multiple osteochondritic lesions, excision seems to be the treatment of

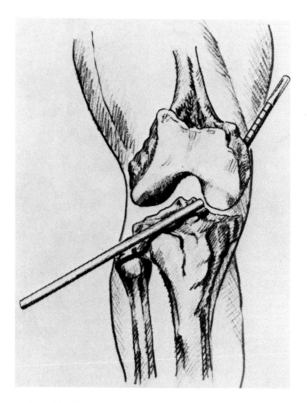

Fig. 114-60. The reamer is being driven to the subchondral region under direct arthroscopic visual control. Radiographic verification of exact depth of the reamer is necessary. Care must be taken to prevent articular cartilage injury. (From Casscells,[51] with permission.)

choice. The loose bodies should be removed from the joint, the base of the leisions debrided of soft tissue, and abrasion performed to produce a bleeding bony bed.

The use of free osteochondral allografts, as described by Gross (personal communication), is currently under investigation by several authors. Early results of this work are promising for posttraumatic and osteoarthritic conditions. Avascular lesions, however, have been largely associated with a poor outcome.

The majority of osteochondritic lesions occur on the medial femoral condyle, but lesions can also be found on the lateral femoral condyle, the femoral sulcus, and the patella. Treatment for each of these lesions should be individualized. Most of the lesions tend to be small and would therefore be best treated by excision and drilling of the defect.

Surgical Technique

A complete diagnostic examination is performed to detach any associated pathology and to search for possible loose bodies. The lesion is viewed from the inferolateral portal, and the base of the lesion and the flap of articular cartilage are debrided with a motorized shaver system. Care must be taken not to detach the vascular pedicle (if one exists) from the synovium of the intercondylar notch. If the fragment is only minimally detached, access to its osseous base can be achieved via surgical release of the margin of the lesion with an arthroscopic blade. The disection is carried along the superomedial and inferomedial margins, leaving the fragment to hinge on its base from the intercondylar notch. The arthroscope is placed in the inferomedial portal, and the fragment is reduced with a probe or grasping forceps inserted from the inferolateral portal. A smooth Kirschner wire is percutaneously drilled into the reduced lesion to secure the fragment to the femoral condyle. A cannulated screw is then inserted over the guide pin, and the screw head is countersunk so that it does not protrude beyond the surface of the articular cartilage. If the fragment is large, a second pin is placed percutaneously and a second screw inserted. The fragment is probed to confirm adequate reduction and stability of the lesion. Upon release of the tourniquet, some scant bleeding about the surface of the lesion should be noted. Potential complications include nonunion, fixation failure, fracture of the fragment, creation of iatrogenic surface lesions, and infection. Johnson has reported a reduction in the overall complication rate since adoption of the cannulated screw technique.[186]

Postoperatively the patient is kept non-weight bearing on crutches for 8 weeks. Weight bearing could cause injury to the tibial surface from the screw heads. As has been shown through Salter's work with rabbits and continuous passive motion, these patients should also undergo intensive therapy to maintain full range of motion of the joint.[289,290] The screws are removed at approximately 8 weeks postfixation. Participation in vigorous sports should be prohibited for approximately 6 months. Lesions managed by observation or simple drilling may be advanced to earlier weight bearing if serial radiographs display healing.

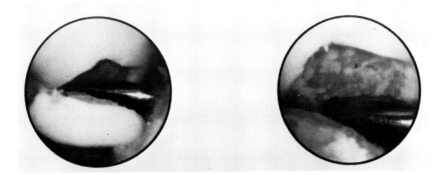

Fig. 114-61. Pedunculated lesion of the medial femoral condyle. Care must be taken to remove the fibrous tissue on both the pedunculated lesion and the base of the femoral condyle. (From Johnson,[186] with permission.)

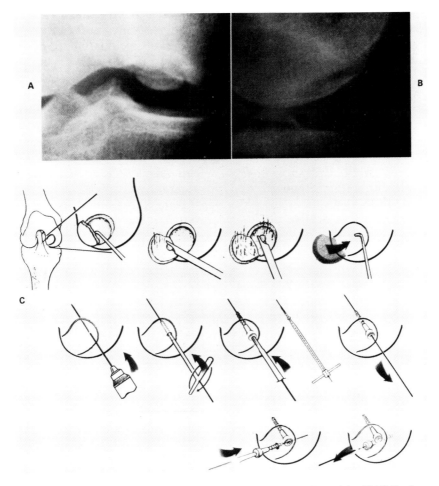

Fig. 114-62. Surgical technique for pedunculated lesion of medial femoral condyle. **(A,B)** Radiographic appearance. **(C)** Surgical release, debridement of soft tissue, and fixation with cannulated screws. (From Johnson,[186] with permission.)

ARTHROSCOPIC RECONSTRUCTION OF THE ANTERIOR CRUCIATE LIGAMENT

Treatment for anterior cruciate ligament instability has changed dramatically over the past decade.[3,32,90,105,126,181,187,209] Much work since the late 1960s has resulted in an acute sensitivity to and awareness of the importance of the anterior cruciate ligament in the function and longevity of the knee joint and in an appreciation of the frequency of anterior cruciate ligament injury in the acutely injured knee.[56,82,105,121,259] As older techniques for reconstruction have been refined and newer techniques have been developed, more surgeons are advocating operative treatment for the cruciate-deficient knee, not only to improve stability but also to prevent the subsequent meniscal tears and degenerative arthritis that are often seen in the unstable knee secondary to anterior cruciate ligament   tears.[12,52,60,58,57,104,107,112,116,160,189,190,193,205,223,267]

The diagnosis, pathogenesis, and classification of anterior cruciate insufficiency is well recognized.[4,38,49,62,74,87,103,106,118,119,156,161,206,219,251,258,297,308,321] The prime indication for reconstruction of this ligament is disability (i.e., the inability to perform activities of great importance to the patient, such as those of work and daily living). Anterior cruciate reconstruction is especially recommended in any young athletic individual who desires to continue participation in high-risk sporting activities. It is also indicated in other individuals who demonstrate a chronic instability that is refractory to nonoperative treatment and produces a disability for work or normal daily activities. A thorough discussion of this topic is included in Chapter   113.[3,32,90,105,126,162,166,181,187,209,246,292,326] The technique of arthroscopically assisted anterior cruciate ligament reconstruction will be presented in this section.[58,284]

Technique For Arthroscope Aided Anterior Cruciate Ligament Reconstruction

The arthroscopic technique offers several advantages over open techniques: smaller skin incisions, no capsular incisions, no disruption of the vastus medialis tendon, less postoperative pain, a lower incidence of infections, shorter hospitalization, and precise placement of the graft.[17,111,284] This technique allows early range of motion, more rapid rehabilitation, and a decreased potential for postoperative fibrosis or loss of range of motion.[18,41,99,218,245,253,268,296] The illumination and magnification provided by the arthroscope ensure a more precise and secure graft placement.

The procedure is performed under general or regional anesthesia with positioning, prepping, and draping similar to those for other arthroscopic procedures of the knee. Examination under anesthesia is performed first to document and assess the severity of the instability. The diagnostic arthroscopy[49,74,87] and treatment of meniscal pathology may be performed without use of the tourniquet. The arthroscopic portals and knee joint are infiltrated with approximately 30 ml of 0.5 percent Xylocaine with epinephrine diluted 1 : 200,000; 1 mg of epinephrine is added to each liter of irrigating solution. Systematic examination of the knee, resection or repair of meniscal injury, or treatment of other intra-articular injury may be performed prior to inflation of the tourniquet.

The reconstruction technique used is similar to that described by Clancy[57,58,60] and Rosenberg.[284] To harvest the graft, a 4- to 6-cm skin incision is made along the medial border of the patellar tendon, beginning at the level of the inferior third of the patella and extending distally to the middle of the tibial tubercle. Subcutaneous tissue and prepatellar fascia are incised, and the patellar tendon is identified. The fascia overlying the patellar tendon is incised and retracted medially and laterally so that the entire width of the patellar tendon is visualized. Proximally the prepatellar fascia is incised to the superior pole of the patella. The width of the patellar tendon just distal to the inferior pole of the patella is measured (the usual width ranges from 3.0 to 3.5 cm). The knee is flexed 30 degrees so that some tension is applied to the patellar tendon. A 1.0- to 1.2-cm strip of the central third of the patellar tendon is fashioned with a scalpel (Fig. 114-63A,B), and triangular bone block of identical width is harvested from the patella by use of an oscillating saw and a ½-inch curved osteotome. The bone block should not be levered with the osteotome for fear of fracturing it. Similarly, a tri-

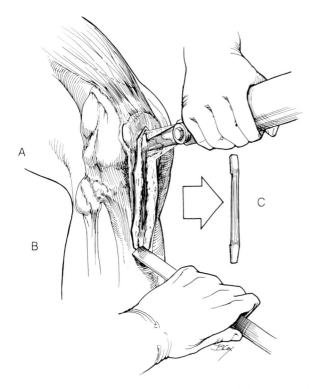

Fig. 114-63. **(A,B)** The patellar tendon graft is harvested by incising the central third of the patellar tendon. Triangular bone blocks are removed from the patella and tibial tubercle by using an oscillating saw and osteotomes. **(C)** The composite graft consists of a 12-cm long, 10-mm wide strip of patellar tendon with triangular bone blocks attached at each end.

angular bone block is harvested from the tibial tubercle. The length of the two bone blocks should be sufficient to produce a composite graft approximately 12 cm in length (Fig. 114-63C). The graft is further prepared by first sizing the diameter with a cylindrical sizer to ensure that the graft will pass through a 10-mm tunnel. The ends of each bone block are then smoothed and rounded into a bullet shape with a motorized Hall burr in order to facilitate passage of the bone plugs through the femoral and tibial tunnels. Three small drill holes are then placed in a longitudinal orientation through each bone plug, and a #2 Ti-cron suture (Davis and Geck, American Cyanamid Co., Danbury, CT) is placed through each drill hole. These sutures will be used for passing the graft through the tunnels and can be tied over a staple or screw if this type of fixation is chosen.

While the graft is being prepared by an assistant, the surgeon reinserts the arthroscope through the inferolateral portal, and the remnants of the cruciate are debrided. Any remaining soft tissues are then scraped from the medial wall of the lateral femoral condyle with a motorized shaver and curets. All soft tissues in the intercondylar notch must be removed to the posterior drop-off point at the junction of the notch roof and the wall of the lateral femoral condyle. The drop-off point is the site at which the roof of the intercondylar notch meets the posterior femoral condyle articular margin. It is identified with a probe. A notchplasty is performed to enlarge the space within the intercondylar notch in order to prevent impingement of the graft (Fig. 114-64), preferably by using curettes and a motorized arthroplasty burr. In most cases removal of 2 to 3 mm of bone and articular cartilage from the lateral wall and roof of the intercondylar notch is necessary to prevent graft impingement (Fig. 114-64). In patients with chronic anterior cruciate ligament insufficiency, osteophyte formation may necessitate removal of even more bone and overlying cartilage. After the notchplasty has been performed, the drop-off point is again identified. There is often a ridge on the medial wall of the lateral femoral condyle approximately two-thirds of the way towards the posterior drop-off point, which must not be confused with the true posterior margin of the intercondylar notch. A mistake in identification of the drop-off point could lead to anterior placement of the femoral tunnel. Once the drop-off point is precisely located, a pilot hole is placed by use of a small curet or motorized burr approximately 1 to 2 mm anterior to the drop-off point at the junction of the roof of the intercondylar notch and the medial wall of the lateral femoral condyle.

Prior to placing a guide pin, 4- to 6-cm skin incision is made over the distal lateral aspect of the femur just proximal to the lateral femoral epicondyle. The iliotibial band is identified, incised in its central portion, and retracted. The vastus lateralis is elevated from the linea aspera area and retracted anteriorly. The lateral aspect of the femoral shaft and metaphysis is exposed subperiosteally. A guide pin is placed through the lateral femoral condyle by one of two techniques, either freehand from inside the notch to outside at the lateral metaphysis or by using the anterior cruciate ligament rear entry

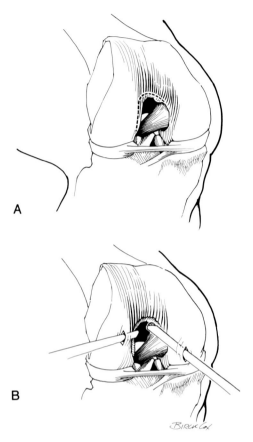

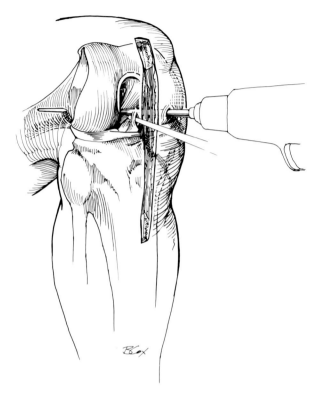

Fig. 114-65. Freehand technique for placement of the femoral tunnel guide pin. With the leg flexed about 110 degrees, the guide pin is placed in the starting hole just anterior to the drop-off point in the intercondylar notch. The guide pin is then drilled to exit on the lateral aspect of the femur.

Fig. 114-64. (A) Notchplasty. The dotted line represents the amount of articular cartilage and bone that should be removed to ensure that the graft will not impinge in the intercondylar notch. **(B)** The notchplasty is performed by using a motorized shaver, curettes, and a motorized arthroplasty burr inserted through the inferomedial portal while viewing from the inferolateral portal.

guide (Acufex Microsurgical, Norwood, MA). The freehand technique is performed by flexing the knee to approximately 100 degrees and placing the guide pin under arthroscopic guidance through the retinaculum adjacent to the patellar tendon just above the medial tibial plateau (Fig. 114-65). It is directed through the intercondylar notch into the pilot hole previously fashioned. The guide pin is directed toward the lateral femoral metaphysis to exit midway between the anterior and posterior cortices and approximately 1 cm above the start of the condylar flare. A 10-mm cannulated reamer is placed over the guide pin, and an osseous tunnel is drilled from lateral to medial (Fig. 114-66). The

guide pin and reamer are removed, and a #6 curette is passed down the tunnel to ensure that no ridges or bony spicules remain within the bony tunnel. Both the inner and outer edges of the tunnel are then chamfered so that no rough edges remain.

If one is unsuccessful in placing the guide pin after one or two attempts by the freehand technique, a rear entry or other suitable drill guide should be used. Many drill guides are available. We prefer the Acufex rear entry guide developed by Rosenberg[284] (Fig. 114-67). With this instrument a long, C-curved passer is placed through the inferolateral portal while viewing with the arthroscope from the inferomedial portal. The C-shaped passer is placed under the lateral femoral condyle in an "over-the-top" fashion, and the hooked portion of the guide is then attached to an eyelet on the passer

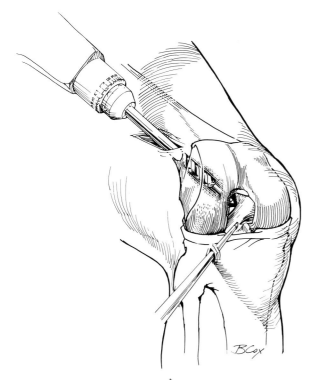

Fig. 114-66. The femoral tunnel is fashioned by using a 10-mm cannulated reamer over the guide pin.

and pulled back to the intercondylar notch. The passer is removed, the hook is placed in the starting hole just anterior to the drop-off point, the guide pin is drilled through the condyle, and the guide is removed. The femoral tunnel is created by using a cannulated reamer (Fig. 114-66). The edges of the femoral osseous tunnel are rounded, and the tunnel is filled with a polyethylene plug to prevent extravasation of fluid from the joint.

The proximal portion of the tibial metaphysis is identified subperiosteally near the insertion of the pes anserinus tendons. The tibial drill guide (Acufex Microsurgical) is inserted through the inferomedial portal while viewing from the inferolateral portal (Fig. 114-68). The guide pin should exit 1 to 2 mm anterior and medial to the original anatomic center of the anterior cruciate ligament insertion. This allows anatomic placement of the tendon graft in the tibial tunnel,[58] which is made by using the cannulated reamer over the guide pin. The edges of the tibial tunnel are chamfered so that there are no

sharp bony edges. Isometry of the tunnels is then checked by placing a suture (tied over a button) from the femoral tunnel through the intercondylar notch and through the tibial tunnel. A strain gauge (Acufex Microsurgical) is attached to the suture, and the knee is placed through a full range of motion. Isometric positioning of the graft is confirmed by an excursion of less than 3 mm on the strain gauge. If an excursion greater than 3 mm is encountered, the graft may need to be repositioned so that it lies posterior in the tunnel at the time of fixation. A plastic tube for passing the graft (DePuy Inc., Warsaw, IN) is tied to the suture and pulled through the tunnels. The sutures in the shorter of the two bone blocks of the graft are pulled through the plastic graft passer and used to slide the graft into position. The tendinous portion of the graft should be oriented posteriorly through both the femoral and tibial tunnels in order to ensure that the tendinous portion will be positioned as close as possible to the anatomic center of the original anterior cruciate ligament attachment. With the graft in position, the plastic graft passer is removed. We have found it easier to pass the graft through the femoral tunnel first and then pull it into the tibial tunnel (Fig. 114-69). While tension is then placed on both ends of the graft, Lachman's and pivot shift tests are performed to confirm stability.

Fixation of the graft can be accomplished by several different methods, including interference screw fixation, tying the sutures over a screw and washer, and tying the sutures over a staple. We believe that interference screw fixation is superior to the other methods. A 9-mm-diameter Kurosaka screw (DePuy), placed in the tibial tunnel, rigidly impacts the bone block into the tibial bone (Fig. 114-70). With the knee flexed 30 degrees and the tibia displaced posteriorly, maximum tension is placed on the graft by hand, and a Kurosaka screw of similar size is inserted to secure the femoral bone block to the femur (Fig. 114-71). Repeat examination should confirm stability of the knee and a full range of motion. Arthroscopic visualization is used to show that the graft is under good tension and to ensure that it does not impinge on the roof of the intercondylar notch when the leg is fully extended. If impingement occurs, additional notchplasty must be performed on the intercondylar notch. An extra-articular procedure can then be performed,

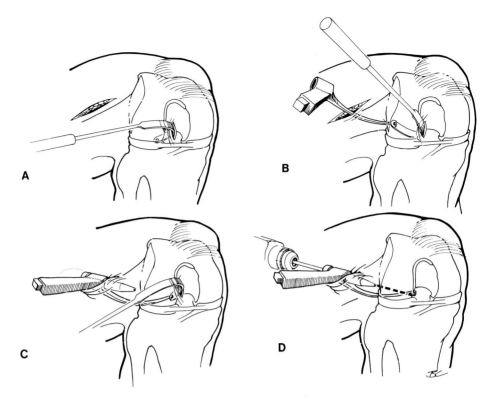

Fig. 114-67. Placement of femoral tunnel guide pin using the Acufex rear entry guide. **(A)** The C-shaped passer is placed in an over-the-top fashion. **(B)** The hooked portion of the guide is attached. **(C)** The hooked portion is pulled into the notch. **(D)** The guide is positioned just anterior to the drop-off point in the starting hole, and the guide pin is inserted.

if desired. The tourniquet is deflated, and the wounds are then closed in the usual manner. A soft tissue dressing is applied, and the patient is placed in a Bledsoe brace, which allows 30 to 60 degrees of knee flexion initially.

Rehabilitation Following Patellar Tendon Reconstruction of the Anterior Cruciate Ligament

On the first postoperative day the patient is allowed toe-touch weight bearing with two crutches, performs active range of motion from 30 to 60 degrees in the brace, and under a physical therapist's guidance is allowed passive range of motion in the range that is comfortable out of the brace. Leg lifts with the leg bent at 45 degrees are performed, and isometric contractions and neuromuscular stimulation of both quadriceps and hamstring muscles are permitted. Passive patellar mobilization is begun in the first postoperative week. In week 2 the brace is adjusted for a 15- to 60-degree range, and active range-of-motion exercises are continued in the brace. During physical therapy, passive extension to 0 degree and active 45- to 90-degree range-of-motion exercises are permitted. Standing hamstring curls with light weights are initiated. In week 3 the Bledsoe brace is opened between 15 and 90 degrees, and the patient is allowed out of the brace for bathing. Partial weight bearing is begun using two crutches, active flexion to 90 degrees and active extension to 45 degrees are permitted, and bent knee leg lifts and daily passive patellar mobilization are continued. Passive range of motion to full extension is emphasized. Patellar mobilization and active motion from 45 to 90 degrees are permitted.

During week 4 the brace is set at 10 to 120 degrees and may be removed for sleeping, and 50

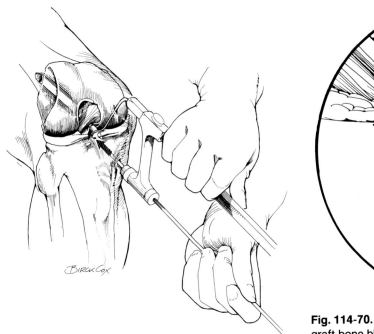

Fig. 114-68. The guide pin for the tibial tunnel is inserted under arthroscopic guidance with use of the Acufex tibial guide.

Fig. 114-70. Close-up of the Kurosaka screw securing the graft bone block to the femoral or tibial bony tunnel.

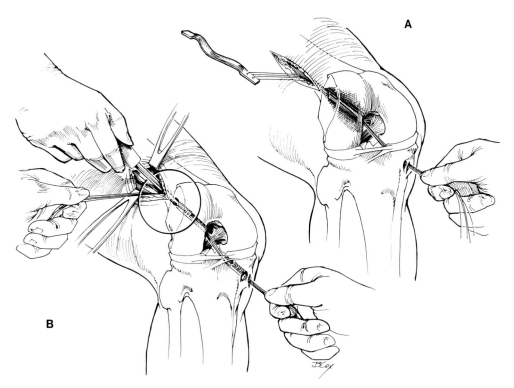

Fig. 114-69 (A). The patellar tendon graft is passed. The tendinous portion of the graft should be oriented in the posterior aspect of the bony tunnels. **(B)** The graft is secured under tension by using interference screws.

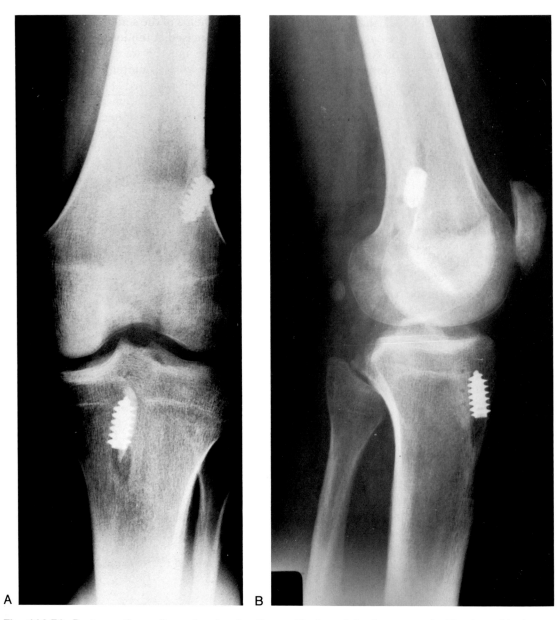

Fig. 114-71. Postoperative radiographs showing the positioning of the bony tunnels. The bone blocks are secured with 9-mm Kurosaka screws. **(A)** Anteroposterior view. **(B)** Lateral view.

percent weight bearing using two crutches is permitted. Concentric hamstring loading exercises as well as lightweight quadriceps extensions are initiated but are prohibited in the last 45 degrees of active extension. Use of an exercise bicycle is begun, and if full passive extension is not obtained

by the end of the fourth or fifth week, a Dynasplint is prescribed.

In week 6 the brace is discontinued for indoor activities. Bent leg raises are begun with progressively increasing weights. Partial weight bearing is permitted using one crutch, and swimming and bicycling are added. Full weight bearing is permitted in week 8, and isokinetic progressive resistance exercises are initiated. Quadriceps strengthening is permitted through a full range of motion, and the Bledsoe brace is discontinued. A functional derotation brace is measured and ordered.

Strength testing is performed on week 12. Slow, short jogging activities are permitted if strength of quadriceps and hamstrings has reached 85 percent that of the contralateral leg and provided there is a full range of motion with no pain or limp on ambulation. Strength testing is repeated at 4 months to determine the timing for graduated running activities. Return to athletic activities is individualized but generally is permitted between the sixth and tenth month based on the patient's overall progress. Even though use of a derotation brace is recommended for high-demand sporting activities, many of the patients choose to play without a brace and have done so without any problems.

Technique for Arthroscope-Aided Cruciate Reconstruction Using Semitendinosus and Gracilis Tendons

Reconstruction of the anterior cruciate ligament using hamstring tendons has been reported by many authors.[55,132,212,213,273] Arthroscopic reconstruction of this ligament using combined semitendinosus and gracilis tendon grafts begins with the procedure identical to that previously described for patellar tendon reconstruction. Diagnostic examination and treatment of intra-articular pathology, as well as notchplasty, preparation of the intercondylar notch, and identification of the femoral starting hole, are identical to those used in the patellar tendon reconstruction. The guide pin is inserted into the lateral condyle in a similar fashion.

From this point on there are several modifications. The femoral tunnel required for passage of the tendons need be only 9 mm in diameter. Harvesting of the tendon graft is performed by using a vertical incision approximately 4 cm in length near the insertion of the pes anserinus tendons. The fascia over the tendons is incised, and the semitendinosus and gracilis tendons are identified. Small fascial attachments of the semitendinosus and gracilis need to be incised. A tendon stripper is placed over each tendon and the tendon is stripped so as to release it at its musculotendinous junction. Both tendons are left attached at their distal insertion.

The tibial tunnel is then made using the tibial drill guide in a manner identical to that described for the patellar tendon reconstruction. The tibial tunnel enters the medial tibial metaphysis several millimeters superior to the insertion of the pes anserinus tendons. The semitendinosus and gracilis tendons are then passed underneath the remaining sartorius tendon, and a Bunnell-type suture is placed through the ends of the tendon, suturing them together with a #5 Ti-cron suture (Davis and Geck). Isometry is tested by the technique previously described, and the edges of the bony tunnels are beveled. A ligature passer is placed from lateral to medial through the femoral tunnel, through the intercondylar notch, and through the tibial tunnel. The suture from the tendon graft is then pulled through the bony tunnels with the tendons following. Firm tension is placed on the tendons, and Lachman and pivot shift tests are performed to confirm correction of the instability. The lateral aspect of the femoral shaft is then roughened with an osteotome. The tendons and suture are secured to the femur by one of several methods of fixation, including stapling the tendons to the femoral shaft, tying the sutures over a staple, and tying the sutures around a cortical screw placed in the distal femur. The knee is placed through a range of motion to ensure that full range of motion can be obtained. Stability testing is repeated.

Extra-articular tenodesis using the iliotibial band may be performed to augment the graft. Many extra-articular procedures have been reported.[5,43,95,96,109,110,115,167,200,215,307] Extra-articular tenodesis is usually not added when patellar tendon reconstruction is performed because of the excellent stability provided immediately. We feel that the tenodesis is indicated as a supplement to the primary procedure when the semitendinosus and gracilis grafts are used because fixation may not be as stable as the fixation of bone blocks with screws. Following tenodesis a lateral retinacular release is performed in order to decrease the lateral patellar-femoral pressures that could occur after closure of the iliotibial band defect.

Technique for Semitendinosus-Gracilis Reconstruction by the Over-the-Top Method

The procedure for the combined semitendinosus and gracilis reconstruction in an over-the-top fashion is similar to the previously described procedure except that no femoral tunnel is created.[230] The tendons are harvested in a similar manner, the tibial tunnel is prepared as described in the previous section, and a notchplasty is performed. No pilot hole or drill guide is used in the lateral femoral condyle. The C-shaped passer of the rear entry guide system (Acufex Microsurgical) is placed through the anterolateral portal while viewing through the anteromedial portal and is directed laterally between the posterior cruciate ligament and the lateral femoral condyle. A suture is placed through the hole of the C-shaped passer, and one end of the suture is held. The C-shaped passer is pulled into the intercondylar notch, dragging the suture with it into the knee and out the anterolateral portal. The suture is untied and is retrieved inside the knee by grasping it with a clamp passed through the tibial tunnel. The suture previously placed in the semitendinosus and gracilis graft is then tied to this suture. The sutures are pulled through the tibial tunnel, through the intercondylar notch, and over the posterior aspect of the lateral femoral condyle in an over-the-top fashion. After roughening of the distal lateral aspect of the femur, the tendons are attached to the bone by either a staple or a screw technique. Repeat testing and range of motion are also performed, as well as an extra-articular augmentation. A lateral retinacular release is performed in conjunction with an iliotibial band tenodesis in order to decrease the lateral patellar-femoral pressures that could occur after repair of the iliotibial band defect.

Postoperative rehabilitation for the semitendinosus-gracilis reconstruction differs from the previous rehabilitation scheme because we are reluctant to allow as much early aggressive physical therapy until some soft tissue healing of the graft has occurred. Thus, at the time of the operation the patient is placed in a Bledsoe brace locked at 30 degrees of flexion. After 2 weeks a 30- to 60-degree short arc is allowed in the brace. At 4 weeks the range of motion is increased to 30 to 90 degrees, and at 6 weeks range of motion is increased to 10 to 120 degrees in the brace. The patient is kept non-weight-bearing for 6 weeks on crutches, and gradual partial weight bearing is initiated at 6 weeks. At 8 weeks postsurgery range of motion is 0 to 120 degrees in the brace and progression to full weight bearing is allowed. Full active and passive range of motion and isokinetic exercises are begun 6 weeks postoperatively.

Authors' Preferred Method

Numerous procedures for repair or reconstruction of the anterior cruciate ligament with satisfactory results have been described in the literature.[17,34,35,63,207,220,221,313] The authors' preferred method of treatment for both acute and chronic anterior cruciate ligament insufficiency is an arthroscopically assisted anterior cruciate reconstruction using the central third patellar tendon. This places the strongest possible autogenous graft in an anatomic location.[33,135,157,235,254,286] Rigid bone-to-bone fixation with an interference screw allows more rapid mobilization and rehabilitation. Several investigators are now currently studying allograft reconstruction as well as prosthetic ligament reconstruction of the anterior cruciate ligament.[6,25,28,36,65,71,178,179,196,309,310,319,320] At this time there are not enough data to indicate conclusively that either of these methods is superior to autogenous reconstructions.

ARTHROSCOPY IN FRACTURES ABOUT THE KNEE

Arthroscopy has been shown to be useful in management of selected fractures about the knee.[44,45,46,180,231,277] Arthroscopic techniques can be used to evaluate as well as to aid in reduction and fixation of anterior intercondylar eminence fractures of the tibia and some tibial plateau fractures.

Tibial Eminence Fractures

Meyers and McKeever[236,237] have devised a useful classification system for intercondylar eminence fractures. A type I fracture has minimal or no displacement, and a type II fracture has one-half or one-third of the eminence slightly elevated. These fractures can be adequately treated with closed manipulation and casting in near full extension. The treatment of type III fractures with complete separation has been controversial, and various modes of reduction and fixation have been proposed.[19,61,81,231,237,280,281,323] Most open procedures are associated with considerable morbidity and generally with a slow return to normal activity.

McLennan[231] in 1982 reported on 35 patients with type III fractures treated by arthroscopic reduction followed by either cast immobilization or percutaneous pin fixation; the treatment was shown to be effective, and morbidity and hospitalization were significantly reduced. An advantage of the arthroscopic treatment is that it allows thorough inspection of the joint in order to rule out any other soft tissue injuries, including meniscal tears or articular cartilage lesions. The procedure is performed by using a standard arthroscope inserted in the inferomedial or inferolateral portal. The joint is irrigated, the fracture site is identified and visualized, and any small osteochondral fragments are removed. A probe is introduced and used to reduce the fracture. The knee is extended while the fracture interface is visualized to ensure maintenance of reduction. A radiograph is taken. If the fragment remains reduced with less than 2 mm of displacement, the leg is immobilized in a cylinder cast in full extension for 5 to 6 weeks. Following removal of the cast, an exercise program to regain strength and motion is initiated.

If the reduction is not maintained in extension, percutaneous pinning is performed. The pins can be introduced by either of two methods. The first method as described by McLennan[231] involves crosswise insertion of two or three smooth K-wires 0.5 cm proximal to the tibial tuberosity on each side of the patellar tendon. Proper placement of the pins is confirmed by image intensification and by arthroscopic inspection. An alternative method of pinning is under arthroscopic guidance. With the knee flexed at approximately 70 degrees, the pins are inserted through separate skin incisions adjacent to the medial and lateral edges of the inferior pole of the patella and directed into the tibial eminence. Proper pin position is confirmed both by image intensification and by arthroscopy. The pins are cut below the surface of the skin, and the knee is immobilized in a cast at 20 degrees of flexion. The pins are removed under local anesthesia 6 weeks later, and active range of motion exercises are initiated. Postoperatively 5 of the 35 patients in McLennan's series[231] showed a positive Lachman test, and 6, all of whom had had an associated repair of the meniscus or a collateral ligament at the time of treatment of the tibial eminence fracture, showed a mild flexion contracture.

In conclusion, operative arthroscopy provides an effective alternative to arthrotomy in the diagnosis and treatment of tibial eminence fractures, as well as in the treatment of the associated injuries of the menisci.

Tibial Plateau Fractures

There is a long history of controversy over the appropriate techniques for management of tibial plateau fractures.[155] Accurate classification and identification of the fracture are essential for proper treatment. Routine radiographs and tomograms are helpful in the identification of fracture patterns but often do not adequately show the severity of the fracture.[97,240,244] In addition, several other injuries can be associated with tibial plateau fractures, including meniscal tears and collateral and cruciate ligament tears, as well as articular surface damage.[222,241,295] Diagnosis of these associated injuries may be difficult in the presence of a tibial plateau fracture. Arthroscopy is a tool that can aid in the diagnosis of associated injuries as well as in identification of fracture configurations.[46,180,277]

To date this technique has been used sparingly. Caspari[44-46] has reported 30 cases of tibial plateau fracture treated by arthroscopic reduction and internal fixation. The extremity is sterilely prepped and draped in the routine fashion, and the contralateral iliac crest is prepared and draped to harvest a bone graft. A large-bore inflow cannula is inserted, and the joint is thoroughly lavaged of any blood and debris. Small bone and articular fragments are removed. A systematic examination is performed to rule out any additional associated intra-articular lesions, especially to the menisci and cruciate ligaments. Both posterior compartments should be visualized to detect the presence of any small fragments of cartilage and bone. The tibial plateau is then inspected, and the amount of displacement and/or depression of fragments is determined. After thorough inspection a decision regarding management should be made. Treatment options include closed reduction, closed reduction and percutaneous fixation, open reduction, or a combination of these techniques.[7,27,29,94,155,180,241,276,279,312] Fracture types that have been amenable to arthroscopic reduction and fixation include a longitudinal split, which may be reduced under arthroscopic visualization and fixed with lag screws or one or more Webb bolts.[44-46]

Depressed fractures are somewhat more difficult and require an anterior limited incision.[44-46] A 1-inch transverse incision is made anteriorly below the flare of the tibia, and the anterior cortex of the tibia is exposed subperiosteally and predrilled to permit removal of a cortical window with a ½-inch osteotome. The depressed fragments are then elevated while observing the articular cartilage arthroscopically. When a satisfactory reduction is obtained, the fragments are stabilized with either Webb bolts, cannulated screws, or standard cancellous lag screws. If there was significant depression (more than 5 mm), an iliac crest bone graft is harvested, inserted through the cortical window in the anterior cortex, and impacted into position. In all cases intraoperative radiographs and/or image intensification should be used to confirm radiographic reduction of the fracture in addition to the arthroscopic reduction of the articular surface. Fractures with a combined longitudinal split and central depression can also be treated by this technique.[44-46] As they become more complex, however, one needs to consider a more standard open technique and buttress plating. Severely comminuted fractures are not amenable to arthroscopic treatment and are best treated by open reduction and internal fixation.

Although the arthroscopic management of these fractures seems to offer several advantages, arthroscopy should only be view as an adjunct tool for possible assistance in their treatment. The arthroscopic technique is demanding and requires considerable experience. The surgeon should not hesitate to open these fractures or treat them in a more conventional manner whenever there is a question about adequacy of reduction and/or fixation.

PATELLOFEMORAL DISORDERS

Arthroscopy can be useful in the diagnosis and treatment of many patellofemoral disorders, the list of which includes anterior knee pain, patella alta or baja, excessive lateral pressure syndrome, malaligned/subluxating patella, osteochondral fracture, osteoarthrosis, patella tendonitis, fat pad fibrosis and tumor, osteochondromatosis, and reflex sympathetic dystrophy.

Anterior knee pain can be an enigma, and arthroscopy may be invaluable in determining whether or not a surgically correctable lesion exists.[88,208,274] If no such disorder or condition exists, the patient and the family can be counseled and reassured. Arthroscopy makes possible direct observation and documentation of patella malalignment and positioning superiorly or inferiorly. The tracking of the patella and its docking into the sulcus can be visualized from the superolateral portal. If late docking past 30 degrees of flexion occurs while the knee is put through a range of motion, consideration should be given to a lateral retinacular release, provided that physical examination and radiographic findings are compatible with a diagnosis of significant subluxation of the patella.[22,64,147,232,238] The retinaculum is incised adjacent to the patella from the vastus lateralis to the inferior pole. The patella should be mobilized enough to rotate 90 degrees along the longitudinal axis and figuratively sit on its articular margin.

Distal or proximal realignment should be considered in the surgical management of malalignment-subluxation syndrome. (A more detailed discussion can be found in Chapter 115.) Fibrosis of the fat pad can be treated by excision of the fat pad and knee joint manipulation. Results from treatment of fibrosis can be quite disappointing in that range of motion may be permanently limited. Osteochondromatosis may also be treated by excision with arthroscopic instrumentation. It would be prudent, however, to perform a standard arthrotomy to excise a fat pad extensively involved with large osteochondromatous lesions.

Acute osteochondral lesions from a patellar subluxation or dislocation injury should be treated by irrigation and debridement. The healing of articular cartilage is very poor following trauma or in the presence of noxious substances.[40] An obvious defect in the retinaculum should be repaired by open surgical techniques if warranted. A closed technique has been described by Lanny Johnson.[186] Osteoarthritis can be treated by irrigation and debridement, and often one must consider changing the dynamics of the patellofemoral articulation by proximal or distal realignment or by tibial tubercle advancement.

Arthroscopy is a valuable detective tool for use in attempting to unravel the mystery and the differential diagnosis of patellofemoral disorders. It has an equally important role in the successful treatment of many of these disorders.

THE SEPTIC KNEE

Septic arthritis is a disease most commonly found in young children, the debilitated, or elderly patients. In addition, one must also consider a sexually related septic arthritis (e.g., gonococcal arthritis) in the young, healthy patient.

The possible routes of entry for bacteria into the knee include hematogenous spread, direct inoculation from a puncture wound, and postsurgical infection. In children one must consider the direct extension of osteomyelitis into those joints whose capsule originates or inserts proximal or distal to the metaphyseal flare. This anatomic variation permits spontaneous decompression of the osteomyelitis directly into the joint. The joints that can be plagued by this particular problem include the hip, knee, ankle, and shoulder joints.

The most common organisms involved in septic arthritis are *Staphylococcus aureus* and *Streptococcus* spp. The bacteriology of septic arthritis varies with the age of the patient. Other common organisms include *Hemophilus influenzae* in the 6- to 24-month-old child and *Neisseria gonorrhoeae* in any age group.

Diagnosis

The diagnosis of a septic knee joint is made by exclusion. Clinically the patient may present with a painful, tensely swollen knee, which is very sensitive to any flexion or extension. However, presentations are not always so dramatic, especially in the debilitated patient.

A patient with gonococcal arthritis may be a young, healthy individual with an arthralgia, migratory in nature, who may also present with a rash or dermatitis or transient tenosynovitis. Occasionally presentation will be with severe monoarticular arthralgia and a tensely swollen joint.

The nongonococcal forms of septic knee joints usually present with a warm, tense, swollen joint, which is quite painful. Patients are usually very young children or more elderly debilitated persons. Included in this group of patients are those with rheumatoid arthritis or other collagen-vascular diseases and cancer patients who are also taking steroids or other immunosuppressive therapeutic agents. These individuals may also present with other sites of infection leading to septic knee via hematogenous spread.

Systemic symptoms in the form of fever, anorexia, and irritability may be present but often are not. The peripheral white blood count may or may not be elevated. As a result, aspiration of the suspected septic knee joint is mandatory to establish the diagnosis.

The joint should be aspirated without delay in all patients even remotely suspected of having a septic process. Aspiration is performed by a sterile technique, and the fluid should be tested for complete cell count with differential count, Gram stain, glucose (compared with simultaneous blood glucose), mucin clot, crystals, and cultures. Enough fluid should be sent for aerobic, anaerobic, fungal, and tuberculosis cultures. Recent work has also indicated that lactic acid levels are often elevated in a joint that is involved with a septic process.

The usual joint fluid findings in a septic knee include a white blood cell count greater than 35,000 to 40,000; often the white cell count is greater than 75,000. The differential may show over 90 percent polymorphonuclear forms, and the glucose is at least 40 mg percent less than that of a simultaneous blood sample. The Gram stain may be helpful but in approximately 40 percent of cases does not show any organisms. Simultaneous blood cultures should be drawn to detect any bacteremia, which could indicate a systemic infection such as subacute bacterial endocarditis.

Treatment

Treatment of septic arthritis is dependent on the type of organism responsible for the sepsis and the stage in which the disease presents. Treatment varies from repeated aspiration and antibiotics to arthroscopy and finally to formal arthrotomy. Indications for nonoperative treatment of a septic joint are limited but include gonococcal septic arthritis, joints involved early in a septic process with very thin joint fluid, and patients responding extremely well to aspiration and immediate antibiotic therapy. All other septic joints should be treated operatively. Any patient who fails to respond rapidly (within 6 to 12 hours) to aspiration and antibiotics should have arthroscopic debridement or formal arthrotomy without delay.

Prognostic factors in treating septic joints include the time interval between the onset of the infection and treatment and the age of the patient. Other factors include concomitant systemic diseases (including rheumatoid arthritis), malignancies, present medication, and the overall health of the patient. Any delay in treatment causes loss of proteoglycans, followed by secondary collagen loss and articular cartilage damage. If adequate therapy is delayed longer than 48 hours, over two-thirds of the glycosaminoglycan content and up to one-third

of the collagen content of the articular cartilage may be lost. Because of frequent delays in diagnosis, infants usually have a poorer prognosis than older children and adults. Infants and children are more likely to have an adjacent osteomyelitis with a secondary decompressive septic arthritis. Antibiotic therapy is instituted once proper cultures and diagnostic studies of the synovial fluid have been obtained.

Arthroscopic Technique for Drainage of a Septic Knee

The primary goal in the drainage of a septic knee joint is to remove the infectious material while maintaining adequate volume in the knee joint so that adhesion formation does not obliterate the potential space of the knee.[117,122] This requires that all adhesions created by the inflammatory process be lysed so that the potential space can be preserved. The arthroscope sheath is usually inserted in the inferior lateral portal. The blunt obturator is left in the sheath, and the arthroscope sheath is passed about the knee joint. The sheath is swept from the suprapatellar pouch to the lateral gutter, back across the patellofemoral groove, and down to the medial gutter. This provides the gentle maneuver necessary to break down the multiple adhesions already formed. The joint should then be thoroughly irrigated with lactated Ringer's solution in order to wash out as much debris as possible. The joint should be inspected to ensure that all potential spaces in it have been decompressed. Simultaneous inspection of the cartilage at this point will reveal the extent of the articular injury. Articular cartilage color and firmness to palpation should be noted. Loose or sequestrated fragments of bone or cartilage may be present and should be removed. During the procedure cultures of any material evacuated from the joint should be sent to the laboratory.

The arthroscope is then removed, but the sheath is left in the joint. A ⅛-inch plastic drainage tube can be inserted into the joint through the arthroscope sheath; the sheath is then removed, leaving the drainage tube within the joint.

The joint is then again distended with fluid, and a second stab wound is made in the suprapatellar region. The arthroscope sheath is then introduced in the joint and a second ⅛-inch plastic drainage tube is inserted. The cannula is withdrawn, leaving the plastic drainage tube in situ.

At this point the joint has been decompressed of the purulent material and a debridement performed. The joint has been inspected again and drained adequately with two ⅛-inch plastic tubes. The tubes are used to irrigate and distend the joint to provide ongoing mechanical debridement and lysis of early adhesions. Small amounts of a mucolytic agent or heparin can be added to the drainage solution to prevent clogging of the drainage tubes. In the past antibiotics were added to the irrigating solution, but studies have indicated that adequate intra-articular levels of antibiotic are reached with intravenous therapy alone.

With one tube used for instillation and the second for evacuation of fluid, the distention/irrigation process can then be initiated. Slow infusion of the physiologic saline solution is carried out over a 3-hour period. As the joint becomes distended, mechanical lysis of adhesions occurs. Recesses of the joint are also irrigated and cleansed. At this point the inflow is discontinued, the outflow tube opened to low continuous suction, and the knee drained for approximately 90 minutes. This allows evacuation of most of the instilled fluid. The cycle is repeated over a 24- to 48-hour interval. Intravenous antibiotics are administered simultaneously, with appropriate adjustments in therapy made according to the microbiologic analysis.

The distention-irrigation process is usually discontinued after 48 hours. Secondary infection can occur if the tubes are left for a prolonged period of time. Postoperatively the patient is gradually mobilized but is kept on protected weight bearing for approximately 6 weeks. This permits the potentially weakened articular cartilage to recover, thereby decreasing its susceptibility to compressive and shear stresses.

Results with arthroscopic debridement have been quite favorable.[172,299] Jackson has indicated that results in those patients treated with the distention-irrigation arthroscopic technique were better than in those treated by formal arthrotomy.[172] The former group showed an excellent range of motion and no sign of recurrence at the time of follow-up. It appears that prevention of

adhesions and loculation of infected fluid in the recesses of the knee joint are the major advantages of this technique. As therapeutic levels of antibiotics in the knee joint are reached with systemic administration, direct irrigation of the joint with antibiotic fluid is not indicated.

Debridement of the joint by arthroscopic techniques must be used judiciously. The occurrence of bleeding with aggressive synovectomies during these procedures could contribute to excessive adhesion formation. A fine line must be drawn between excessive and inadequate debridement. If the surgeon can restore the potential volume of the knee joint, a patient treated by this distention-irrigation technique should do well without aggressive synovectomy. For patients whose treatment has been long delayed, however, formal arthrotomy and debridement may be the most judicious procedure.

Suspicion of a knee joint infection is a diagnostic and perhaps a surgical emergency. The diagnostic workup must be aggressive and prompt. Arthroscopy can be extremely helpful in establishing the diagnosis and in carrying out a formal treatment plan.

ARTHROSCOPIC MANAGEMENT OF LOOSE BODIES IN THE KNEE JOINT

There are several entities associated with loose bodies present within the knee joint. Factors involved in the production of these lesions include metabolic disorders, synovial disorders, growth disturbances, meniscal lesions, and traumatic disorders.[1,2] Foreign bodies also have been implicated in formation of intra-articular loose bodies of the knee joint.

Traumatic intra-articular loose bodies may vary in their consistency. They may be purely cartilaginous or osteocartilaginous depending upon the depth of injury. Mechanical symptoms from these traumatic loose bodies can arise either from bodies that float freely around the joint, causing impingement at multiple locations, or from those that are still flapped or pedunculated, causing symptoms primarily in one location. Statistically, the femoral condyle and the patella are the major sources of these cartilaginous or osteocartilaginous loose bodies.

Synovial lesions, including synovial osteochon-dromatosis, are a common source of multiple "rice bodies." This diffuse metaplastic formation of osteocartilaginous lesions results in a characteristic radiographic appearance of the joint (Figs. 114-72, 114-73). Crystalline arthropathies such as gout or pseudogout may produce changes in the micro-

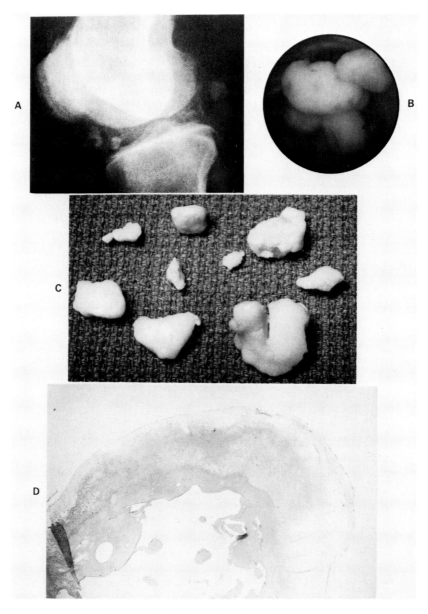

Fig. 114-72. Synovial osteochondromatosis. **(A)** Lateral radiographic appearance of knee diffusely involved with synovial osteochondromatosis. **(B)** Intra-articular view via arthroscopic technique of large multiloculated lesion. **(C)** Gross appearance. (From Johnson,[186] with permission.)

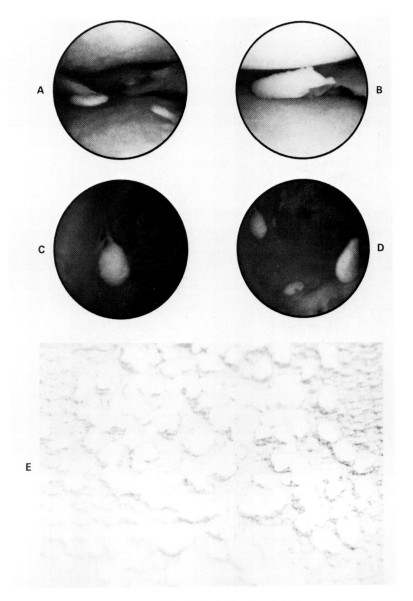

Fig. 114-73. **(A–D)** Arthroscopic appearance of multiple rice bodies. **(E)** Thousands of rice bodies can often be removed via an arthroscopic cannula connected to constant low-grade suction. (From Johnson,[186] with permission.)

structure of the articular cartilage such that chondral fragmentation occurs quite readily. Foreign bodies within the joint can be introduced either by iatrogenic sources (e.g., broken arthroscopic instruments) or by penetrating injuries such as gunshot wounds or lacerations. With penetration injuries the loose body is often so large that formal arthrotomy is indicated for removal.

Clinical Presentation

Patients presenting with loose bodies often give a history of unpredictable instability or locking. They are plagued with recurrent episodes of "giving way," which can occur at any time. This is quite unlike the history of patients with ligamentous instability, who can often identify the exact activity that will cause them to have a giving-way episode. Some patients will even experience a migratory prominence across the joint, depending on where the loose body has presented itself. At times, an area of palpable tenderness can be identified if the lesion has originated from a femoral condyle or the peripheral margin of the articular surface of the patella.

Preoperative evaluation of these patients should include not only a thorough history and physical examination but also standard radiographs, including AP, lateral, tunnel, and sunrise views to identify any possible lesions. Oblique views are occasionally necessary to localize a particular lesion. The actual size and number of loose bodies is often underestimated by routine radiography.[72,77,158,226]

Surgical Treatment

The surgical management of osteocartilaginous loose bodies originating from osteochondritis dissecans has been discussed in a previous section.

Excision of cartilaginous or osteocartilaginous loose bodies can tax the resourcefulness of the surgeon. The multiple recesses of the knee joint often preclude easy visualization and expeditious removal. A thorough diagnostic arthroscopy must be performed to identify the exact location of the loose body. If the lesion is quite small, as in the multiple rice bodies of synovial osteochondroma-

tosis, insertion of a large-bore cannula attached to low continuous suction can often remove numerous small fragments. Many loose bodies, however, are too large to be removed so easily. It is often helpful to stabilize a loose body to prevent it from floating freely by inserting a spinal needle through the skin and capsular tissue directly into the loose body itself (Figs. 114-74, 114-75). Another method to try to gain control of the loose body is to insert a suction cannula into the compartment containing the body, thereby pulling the body up to the cannula. Following either of these methods, a grasping forceps is inserted to capture the loose body (Fig. 114-76). The loose body is retracted and gently placed against the synovial lining of the knee joint so that it can be palpated through the skin. A generous incision over the loose body should be made so that the lesion can be removed without difficulty.

At times the loose body is not easily accessible, and inspection and probing using accessory portals may be required. The loose bodies can either be directly removed from or dislodged from the posterior compartment via the accessory portals. Use of the 70-degree arthroscope is helpful for visualizing the posterior compartments. The time required for loose body removal can be prolonged in many cases, but with patience and persistence most loose bodies can be found and removed.

Arthroscopic surgeons in the United States most often use a fluid medium for their surgical proce-

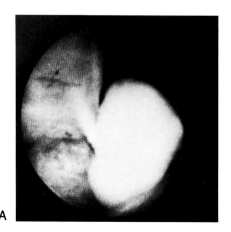
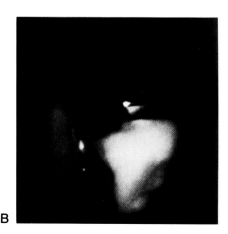

A   B

Fig. 114-74. Loose bodies. **(A)** Arthroscopic appearance of loose body in the suprapatellar pouch. **(B)** The loose body localized with an intra-articular needle. (From Casscells,[51] with permission.)

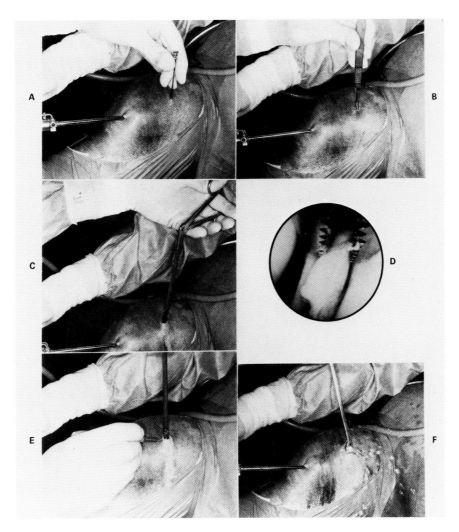

Fig. 114-75. Stage photographs of needle localization of a loose body. **(A)** Percutaneous puncture for localization. **(B)** Incision directly over loose body. **(C,D)** Grasping of the loose body. **(E,F)** Enlarging portal to allow removal of the loose body. (From Johnson,[186] with permission.)

dures, but it should be mentioned that gas distention of the knee joint is often quite beneficial with respect to removing intra-articular loose bodies. Gas distention not only allows increased visualization over a wider area, but it allows the loose body to remain immobile inside the joint.[101]

Arthroscopic removal of loose bodies is potentially one of the more frustrating surgical procedures for the novice as well as for the experienced arthroscopic surgeon. Surgeons should carefully plan their surgical approaches and familiarize themselves with the multiple portals that may be necessary. They should allow a reasonable time for the procedure, which may be short but could be prolonged.

SUMMARY

Many significant advances have been made in arthroscopic surgery of the knee in the past decade. Arthroscopic techniques have increased dra-

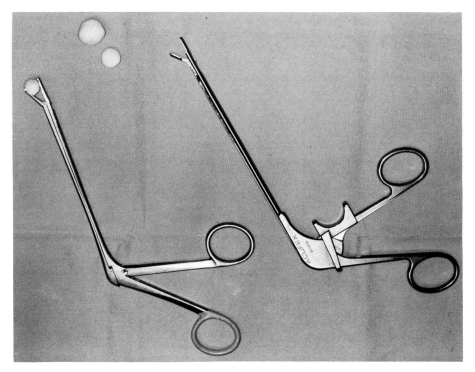

Fig. 114-76. Photograph depicting various graspers aiding the removal of intra-articular loose bodies.

matically in both number and complexity. Many procedures that previously required arthrotomies are now easily treated by arthroscopic techniques. Arthroscopy has proved to be an invaluable tool for the diagnosis and treatment of lesions of the synovium, the articular cartilage and the meniscus. The applications of arthroscopic techniques for treatment of ligamentous injuries and fractures have recently gained popularity. As present techniques are refined and newer techniques are developed, arthroscopy will undoubtedly play an even greater role in the treatment of injuries and diseases about the knee.

REFERENCES

1. Aicroth P: Osteochondritis dissecans of the knee: a clinical study. J Bone Joint Surg 53B:440, 1971
2. Aicroth P: Osteochondral fractures and their relationship to osteochondritis dissecans of the knee. J Bone Joint Surg 53B:448, 1971
3. Andrews JR: Management of acute anterolateral rotatory instability of the knee. Strategies Orthop Surg 1(3):Jan. 1981
4. Andrews JR, Axe MJ: The classification of knee ligament instability. Orthop Clin North Am 16:69, 1985
5. Andrews JR, Sanders R: A "mini-reconstruction" technique in treating anterolateral rotatory instability (ALRI). Clin Orthop 172:93, 1983
6. Andrish JT, Woods LD: Dacron augmentation in anterior cruciate ligament reconstruction in dogs. Clin Orthop 183:298, 1984
7. Apley AG: Fractures of the lateral tibial condyle treated by skeletal traction and early mobilization. A review of sixty cases with special reference to long-term results. J Bone Joint Surg 38B:699, 1956
8. Aritomi H, Yamamoto M: A method of arthroscopic surgery: clinical evaluation of synovectomy with the electric resectoscope and removal of loose bodies in the knee joint. Orthop Clin North Am 10:565, 1979
9. Arms SW, Pope MH, Johnson RJ, et al: The biomechanics of anterior cruciate ligament rehabilitation and reconstruction. Am J Sports Med 12:8, 1984
10. Arnoczky SP: The blood supply of the meniscus

and its role in healing and repair. In American Academy of Orthopaedic Surgeons Symposium on Sports Medicine: The Knee. CV Mosby, St. Louis, 1985

11. Arnoczky SP, McDevitt CA, Warren RF, et al: Meniscus repair using an exogenous fibrin clot—an experimental study in dogs. Orthop Trans 10:327, 1986

12. Arnoczky SP, Tarvin GB, Marshall JL: Anterior cruciate ligament replacement using patellar tendon: an evaluation of graft revascularization in the dog. J Bone Joint Surg 64A:217, 1982

13. Arnoczky SP, Warren RF: Microvasculature of the human meniscus. Am J Sports Med 10:90, 1982

14. Arnoczky SP, Warren RF: The microvasculature of the meniscus and its response to injury. An experimental study in the dog. Am J Sports Med 11:131, 1983

15. Arnoczky SP, Warren RF, Kaplan N: Meniscal remodeling following partial meniscectomy: an experimental study in the dog. Arthroscopy 1:247, 1985

16. Barber FA, Stone RG: Meniscal repair—an arthroscopic technique. J Bone Joint Surg 67B:39, 1985

17. Barlett EC: Arthroscopic repair and augmentation of the anterior cruciate ligament in cadaver knees. Clin Orthop 172:107, 1983

18. Baugher WH, Warren RF, Marshall JL, Joseph A: Quadriceps atrophy in the anterior cruciate insufficient knee. Am J Sports Med 12:192, 1984

19. Baxter MP, Wiley JJ: Fractures of the tibial spine in children. J Bone Joint Surg 70B:228, 1988

20. Bergstrom R, Hamberg P, Lysholm J, Gillquist J: Comparison of open and endoscopic meniscectomy. Clin Orthop 184:133, 1984

21. Berson BL, Hermann G: Torn discoid menisci of the knee in adults. J Bone Joint Surg 61A:303, 1979

22. Betz RR, Lonergan R, Patterson R, et al: The percutaneous lateral retinacular release. Orthopedics 5:57, 1982

23. Bircher E: Die Arthroendoskopie. Zentralbl Chir 48:1460, 1921

24. Bircher E: Beitrag zur Pathologie und Diagnose der Meniscusverletzungen (Arthroendoskopie). Beitr Klin Chir 127:239, 1922

25. Blazina ME: Prosthetic ligaments—indications. In Schultiz KP, Krahl H, Stein WH (eds): Late Reconstructions of Injured Ligaments of the Knee. Springer-Verlag, Berlin-Heidelberg-New York, 1978

26. Bots RAA, Slooff TJJH: Arthroscopy in the Evaluation of Operative Treatment in Osteochondritis Dissecans. Orthop Clin North Am 10:685, 1979

27. Bowes DN, Hohl M: Tibial condylar fractures. Evaluation of treatment and outcome. Clin Orthop 171:104, 1982

28. Bright R, Green W: Freeze-dried fascia lata allografts: a review of 47 cases. J Pediatr Orthop 1:13, 1981

29. Brown GA, Sprague BL: Cast brace treatment of plateau and bicondylar fractures of the proximal tibia. Clin Orthop 119:184, 1976

30. Burman MS: Arthroscopy or the direct visualization of joints: an experimental cadaver study. J Bone Joint Surg 8:669, 1931

31. Burman MS, Finkelstein H, Mayer L: Arthroscopy of the knee joint. J Bone Joint Surg 16:255, 1934

32. Burnett AM, Fowler PJ: Reconstruction of the anterior cruciate ligament. Historical overview. Orthop Clin North Am 16:143, 1985

33. Butler DL, Noyes FR, Grood ES, et al: Mechanical properties of transplants for the anterior cruciate ligament. Orthop Trans 3:180, 1979

34. Cabaud HE, Feagin JA: Experimental studies of acute anterior cruciate ligament injury and repair. Am J Sports Med 7:18, 1979

35. Cabaud HE, Feagin JA, Rodkey WG: Acute anterior cruciate ligament injury and augmented repair: experimental studies. Am J Sports Med 8:395, 1980

36. Cabaud HE, Feagin JA, Rodkey WG: Acute anterior cruciate ligament injury and repair reinforced with a biodegradable intraarticular ligament: experimental studies. Am J Sports Med 10:259, 1982

37. Cabaud HE, Rodkey WG, Fitzwater JE: Medial meniscus repairs. An experimental and morphologic study. Am J Sports Med 9:129, 1981

38. Cabaud HE, Slocum DB: The diagnosis of chronic anterolateral rotatory instability of the knee. Am J Sports Med 5:99, 1977

39. Cameron M, Piliar R, Macnab I: Fixation of loose bodies in joints. Clin Orthop 100:309, 1974

40. Campbell CJ: The healing of cartilage defects. Clin Orthop 64:45, 1969

41. Campbell DE, Glenn W: Foot-pounds of torque of the normal knee and the rehabilitated post-meniscectomy knee. Phys Ther 59:418, 1979

42. Carson RW: Arthroscopic meniscectomy. Orthop Clin North Am 10:619, 1979

43. Carson WG Jr: Extra-articular reconstruction of the anterior cruciate ligament: lateral procedures. Orthop Clin North Am 16:191, 1985

44. Caspari RB: Arthroscopy and the management of fractures of the tibial plateau. In O'Connor's Textbook of Arthroscopic Surgery. JB Lippincott, Philadelphia, 1984

45. Caspari RB: The techniques for arthroscopic man-

agement of tibial plateau fractures. In McGinty JB (ed): Arthroscopic Surgery Update. Aspen Systems Corp., Rockville, MD, 1985

46. Caspari RB, Hutton PMJ, Whipple TL, Meyers JF: The role of arthroscopy in the management of tibial plateau fractures. Arthroscopy 1(2):76, 1985

47. Casscells SW: Arthroscopy of the knee joint, a review of 150 cases. J Bone Joint Surg 53A:287, 1971

48. Casscells SW: The torn or degenerated meniscus and its relationship to degeneration of the weight bearing areas of the femur and tibia. Clin Orthop 132:196, 1978

49. Casscells SW: The place of arthroscopy in the diagnosis and treatment of internal derangement of the knee: an analysis of 1000 cases. Clin Orthop 151:135, 1980

50. Casscells SW: The technique of arthroscopy. Orthopedics 6:1498, 1983

51. Casscells SW: Arthroscopy: diagnostic and surgical practice. Lea & Febiger, Philadelphia, 1984

52. Casscells SW: The torn meniscus, the torn anterior cruciate ligament, and their relationship to degenerative joint disease. Arthroscopy 1(1):28, 1985

53. Casscells SW: The place of 35 mm still photography in arthroscopic surgery. Arthroscopy, 1:116, 1985

54. Cassidy RE, Shaffer AJ: Repair of peripheral meniscus tears—a preliminary report. Am J Sports Med 9:209, 1981

55. Cho KO: Reconstruction of the anterior cruciate ligament by semitendinous tenodesis. J Bone Joint Surg 57A:608, 1975

56. Clancy WG Jr: The role of arthrography and arthroscopy in the acutely injured knee. Med Times 109:20, 1981

57. Clancy WG Jr: Anterior cruciate ligament functional instability: a static intra-articular and dynamic extra-articular procedure. Clin Orthop 172:102, 1983

58. Clancy WG Jr: Intra-articular reconstruction of the anterior cruciate ligament. Orthop Clin North Am 16:181, 1985

59. Clancy WG Jr, Graf BK: Arthroscopic meniscal repair. Orthopedics 6:1125, 1983

60. Clancy WG Jr, Nelson DA, Reider B, Narechania RG: Anterior cruciate ligament reconstruction using one-third of the patella ligament augmented by extra-articular tendon transfers. J Bone Joint Surg 64A:353, 1982

61. Clanton TO, DeLee JC, Sanders B, Neidre A: Knee ligament injuries in children. J Bone Joint Surg 61A:1195, 1979

62. Collins HR: Reconstruction of the athlete's injured knee. Anatomy, diagnosis, treatment. Orthop Clin North Am 2:207, 1971

63. Collins HR, Hughston JC, DeHaven KE, et al: The meniscus as a cruciate ligament substitute. Am J Sports Med 2:11, 1974

64. Corta H: Zur Therapie der habituellen patellaren Luxation. Arch Orthop Unfallchir 51:256, 1959

65. Cotton FJ, Merrison GM: Artificial ligaments at the knee: technique. N Engl J Med 210:1331, 1934

66. Coventry MB: Osteotomy about the knee for degenerative and rheumatoid arthritis. J Bone Joint Surg 55A:23, 1978

67. Coventry MB: Upper tibial osteotomy for gonarthrosis: the evolution of the operation in the last 18 years and long term results. Orthop Clin North Am 10:191, 1979

68. Cox JS: The degenerative effects of medial meniscus tears in dogs' knees. Clin Orthop 125:236, 1977

69. Cox JS, Nye CE, Schaefer WW, Woodstein IJ: The degenerative effects of partial and total resection of the medial meniscus in dogs' knees. Clin Orthop 109:178, 1975

70. Curran WP Jr, Woodward EP: Arthroscopy: its role in diagnosis and treatment of athletic knee injuries. Am J Sports Med 8:415, 1980

71. Curtis R, DeLee J, Drez D: Reconstruction of the anterior cruciate ligament with freeze-dried fascia lata allografts in dogs: a preliminary report. Am J Sports Med 13:408, 1985

72. Dandy DJ: Arthroscopic surgery of the knee. Br J Hosp Med 17:360, 1982

73. Dandy DJ: The bucket handle meniscal tear: a technique detaching the posterior segment first. Orthop Clin North Am 13:369, 1982

74. Dandy DJ, Flanagan JP, Steenmeyer V: Arthroscopy and the management of the ruptured anterior cruciate ligament. Clin Orthop 167:43, 1982

75. Dandy DJ, Jackson RW: The impact of arthroscopy on the management of disorders of the knee. J Bone Joint Surg 57B:346, 1975

76. Dandy DJ, Jackson RW: The diagnosis of problems after meniscectomy. J Bone Joint Surg 57B:349, 1975

77. Dandy DJ, O'Carroll PF: The removal of loose bodies from the knee under arthroscopic control. J Bone Joint Surg 64B:473, 1982

78. Daniel D, Daniels E, Aronson D: The diagnosis of meniscus pathology. Clin Orthop 163:218, 1982

79. Day B, MacKenzie WG, Shim SS, Leung G: The vascular and nerve supply of the human meniscus. Arthroscopy 1(1):58, 1985

80. DeBacker A, Casteleyn PP, Opdecam P: Osteochondritis dissecans of the knee: Present state. The role of arthroscopy and arthroscopic surgery. Acta Orthop Belg 49:468, 1983

81. DeHaven KE: Acute injury to the knee. In American Academy of Orthopaedic Surgeons, Symposium on Arthroscopy and Arthrography of the Knee. CV Mosby, St. Louis, 1978

82. DeHaven KE: Diagnosis of acute knee injuries with hemarthrosis. Am J Sports Med 8:9, 1980

83. DeHaven KE: Peripheral meniscal repair: an alternative to meniscectomy. J Bone Joint Surg 63B:463, 1981

84. DeHaven KE: Principles of triangulation for arthroscopic surgery. Orthop Clin North Am 13:329, 1982

85. DeHaven KE: Meniscus repair in the athlete. Clin Orthop 198:31, 1985

86. DeHaven KE: Meniscus repair — open vs. arthroscopic. Arthroscopy 1:173, 1985

87. DeHaven KE, Collins HR: Diagnosis of internal derangements of the knee: the role of arthroscopy. J Bone Joint Surg 57A:802, 1975

88. DeHaven KE, Dolan WA, Mayer PJ: Chondromalacia patella in athletes — clinical presentation and conservative management. Am J Sports Med 7:1, 1979

89. DeLee JC: Complications of arthroscopy and arthroscopic surgery: results of a national survey. Arthroscopy 1:214, 1985

90. DelPizzo W, Norwood LA, Kevlan RK, et al: Analysis of 100 patients with anterolateral rotatory instability of the knee. Clin Orthop 122:178, 1977

91. Dickason JM, DelPizzo W, Blazina ME, et al: A series of ten discoid medial menisci. Clin Orthop 168:75, 1982

92. Dickhaut SC, DeLee JC: The discoid lateral-meniscus syndrome. J Bone Joint Surg 64A:1068, 1982

93. Dorfmann H, Orengo P, Amerenco G: Pathology of the synovial folds of the knee: value of arthroscopy. Rev Rhum Mal Osteoartic 49:67, 1982

94. Drennan DB, Locher FG, Maylahn DJ: Fractures of the tibial plateau. Treatment by closed reduction and spica cast. J Bone Joint Surg 61A:989, 1979

95. Ellison AE: Distal iliotibial-band transfer for anterolateral rotatory instability of the knee. J Bone Joint Surg 61A:330, 1979

96. Ellison AE: The pathogenesis and treatment of anterolateral rotatory instability. Clin Orthop 147:51, 1980

97. Elstrom J, Pankovich AM, Sassoon H, Rodriguez J: The use of tomography in the assessment of fractures of the tibial plateau. J Bone Joint Surg 58A:551, 1976

98. Elsworth C: Locked knee and osteochondritis dissecans. JR Soc Med 76:1030, 1983

99. Enneking WF, Horowitz M: The intraarticular effects of immobilization on the human knee. J Bone Joint Surg 54A:973, 1972

100. Eriksson E, Sebik A: A comparison between the transpatellar tendon and the lateral approach to the knee joint during arthroscopy: a cadaver study. Am J Sports Med 8:103, 1980

101. Eriksson E, Sebik A: Arthroscopy and arthroscopic surgery in a gas versus a fluid medium. Orthop Clin North Am 13:293, 1982

102. Fairbank TJ: Knee joint changes after meniscectomy. J Bone Joint Surg 30B:664, 1948

103. Feagin JA Jr: The syndrome of the torn anterior cruciate ligament. Orthop Clin North Am 10:31, 1979

104. Feagin JA Jr, Cabaud E, Curl WW: The anterior cruciate ligament: radiographic and clinical signs of successful and unsuccessful repairs. Clin Orthop 164:54, 1982

105. Feagin JA Jr, Curl WW: Isolated tears of the anterior cruciate ligament: 5-year follow-up study. Am J Sports Med 4:95, 1976

106. Fetto JF, Marshall JL: Injury to the anterior cruciate ligament producing the pivot-shift sign: an experimental study on cadaver specimens. J Bone Joint Surg 61A:710, 1979

107. Fetto JF, Marshall JL: The natural history and diagnosis of anterior cruciate ligament insufficiency. Clin Orthop 147:29, 1980

108. Finkelstein H, Mayer L: The arthroscope. A new method of examining joints. J Bone Joint Surg 13:583, 1931

109. Fleming RE Jr, Blatz DJ, McCarroll JR: Lateral reconstruction for anterolateral rotatory instability of the knee. Am J Sports Med 11:303, 1983

110. Fox JM, Blazina ME, Del Pizzo W, et al: Extra-articular stabilization of the knee joint for anterior instability. Clin Orthop 147:56, 1980

111. Fox JM, Sherman OH, Markhoff K: Arthroscopic anterior cruciate ligament repair. Preliminary results and instrumented testing for anterior stability. Arthroscopy 1:175, 1985

112. Fried JA, Bergfeld JA, Weiker G, Andrish JT: Anterior cruciate reconstruction using the Jones-Ellison procedure. J Bone Joint Surg 67A:1029, 1985

113. Friedman MJ, Bevasi CC, Fox JM, et al: Preliminary results with abrasion arthroplasty in the osteoarthritic knee. Clin Orthop 182:200, 1984

114. Fujikawa K, Iseki F, Mikura Y: Partial Resection of the Discoid Meniscus in the Child's Knee. J Bone and Joint Surg 63B:391, 1981

115. Fujisawa Y, Masuhara K, Shiomi S: The effect of high tibial osteotomy on osteoarthritis of the knee: an arthroscopic study of 54 knee joints. Orthop Clin North Am 10:585, 1979

116. Funk FJ: Osteoarthritis of the knee following ligamentous injury. Clin Orthop 172:154, 1983

117. Gainor BJ: Instillation of continuous tube irrigation in the septic knee at arthroscopy: a technique. Clin Orthop 183:96, 1984

118. Galway R: Pivot-shift syndrome. J Bone Joint Surg 54B:558, 1972

119. Galway R, Beaupre A, McIntosh DL: Pivot-shift: a clinical sign of symptomatic anterior cruciate insufficiency. J Bone Joint Surg 54B:763, 1972

120. Gillquist J, Hagberg G: A new modification of the technique of arthroscopy of the knee joint. Acta Chir Scand 142:123, 1976

121. Gillquist J, Hagberg G, Oretorp N: Arthroscopy in acute injuries of the knee joint. Acta Orthop Scand 48:190, 1977

122. Gillquist J, Hagberg G, Oretorp N: Therapeutic arthroscopy of the knee. Injury 10:128, 1978

123. Gillquist J, Hagberg G, Oretorp N: Arthroscopic examination of the posteromedial compartment of the knee joint. Int Orthop 3:13, 1979

124. Gillquist J, Hagberg G, Oretorp N: Arthroscopic visualization of the posteromedial compartment of the knee joint. Orthop Clin North Am 10:545, 1979

125. Gillquist J, Karpf PM: Arthroscopic knee surgery. Fortschr Med 21, 100:51, 1982

126. Gillquist L, Liljedahl SO, Lindvall H: Reconstruction for old rupture of the anterior cruciate ligament. Injury 2:271, 1971

127. Gillquist J, Oretorp N: Different techniques for diagnostic arthroscopy: a randomized comparative study. Acta Orthop Scand 52:353, 1981

128. Gillquist J, Oretorp N: Arthroscopic partial meniscectomy: technique and long-term results. Clin Orthop 167:29, 1982

129. Gillquist J, Oretorp N: The technique of endoscopic total meniscectomy. Orthop Clin North Am 13:363, 1982

130. Glinz W: Diagnostic arthroscopy and arthroscopic surgery: experiences with 500 knee arthroscopies. Helv Chir Acta 46:25, 1979

131. Glinz W, Segantini P, Kägi P: Arthroscopy in acute trauma of the knee joint. Endoscopy 12:269, 1980

132. Gomes JLE, Marczyk LRS: Anterior cruciate ligament reconstruction with a loop or double thickness of semitendinosus tendon. Am J Sports Med 12:199, 1984

133. Grana WA, Connor S, Hollingsworth S: Partial arthroscopic meniscectomy: a preliminary report. Clin Orthop 164:78, 1982

134. Green WT, Banks HH: Osteochondritis dissecans in children. J Bone Joint Surg 35A:26, 1953

135. Grood ES, Noyes FR: Cruciate ligament prosthesis: strength, creep, and fatigue properties. J Bone Joint Surg 58A:1083, 1976

136. Guhl JF: Arthroscopic treatment of osteochondritis dissecans: preliminary report. Orthop Clin North Am 10:671, 1979

137. Guhl JF: Operative arthroscopy. Am J Sports Med 7:328, 1979

138. Guhl JF: Arthroscopic treatment of osteochondritis dissecans. Clin Orthop 167:65, 1982

139. Guhl JF: Excision of flap tears. Orthop Clin North Am 13:387, 1982

140. Hamberg P, Gillquist J, Lysholm J: Suture of new and old peripheral meniscus tears. J Bone Joint Surg 65A:193, 1983

141. Hamberg P, Gillquist J, Lysholm J: A comparison between arthroscopic meniscectomy and modified open meniscectomy: a prospective randomized study with emphasis on postoperative rehabilitation. J Bone Joint Surg 66B:189, 1984

142. Hamberg P, Gillquist J, Lysholm J, Oberg B: The effect of diagnostic and operative arthroscopy and open meniscectomy on muscle strength in the thigh. Am J Sports Med 11:289, 1983

143. Hanks GA, Joyner DM, Kalenak A: Anterolateral rotatory instability of the knee—an analysis of the Ellison procedure. Am J Sports Med 9:225, 1981

144. Hanks GA, Kalenak A, Handal JA, Gause T: Repair of peripheral meniscus tears. Presented at the Pennsylvania-New York–New Jersey Orthopaedic Society Meeting, Aruba, Netherlands Antilles, April 1988

145. Harrewyn JM, Aignan M, Renoux M, et al: Synovial folds of the knee (plicae synoviales): treatment under arthroscopy. Rev Rhum Mal Osteoartic 49:3, 1982

146. Harty M, Joyce JJ III: Synovial folds in the knee joint. Orthop Rev 10:31, 1977

147. Harwin SF, Stern RE: Subcutaneous lateral retinacular release for chondromalacia patellae: a preliminary report. Clin Orthop 156:207, 1981

148. Heatley FW: The meniscus—can it be repaired? An experimental investigation in rabbits. J Bone Joint Surg 62B:397, 1980

149. Hendler RC: Arthroscopic meniscal repair. Clin Orthop 180:163, 1984

150. Henning CE: Arthroscopic repair of meniscus tears. Orthopedics 6:1130, 1983
151. Henning CE, Clark CE, Lynch MA, et al: Arthroscopic meniscus repair with a posterior incision. In American Academy of Orthopaedic Surgeons, Instructional Course Lectures. Vol. 37. CV Mosby, St. Louis, 1988
152. Henning CE, Lynch MA, Clark JR: Vascularity for healing of meniscus repairs. Arthroscopy 3:13, 1987
153. Highgenboten CL: Arthroscopy synovectomy. Orthop Clin North Am 13:399, 1982
154. Highgenboten CL: Arthroscopic synovectomy. Arthroscopy 1:190, 1985
155. Hohl M: Treatment methods in tibial condylar fractures. South Med J 68:985, 1975
156. Holden DL, Jackson DW: Treatment selection in acute anterior cruciate ligament tears. Orthop Clin North Am 16:99, 1985
157. Hoogland T, Hillen B: Intra-articular reconstruction of the anterior cruciate ligament: an experimental study of length changes in different ligament reconstructions. Clin Orthop 185:197, 1984
158. Hotchkiss RN, Tew WP, Hungerford DS: Cartilaginous debris in the injured human knee: correlation with arthroscopic findings. Clin Orthop 168:133, 1982
159. Hughston JC, Whatley GS, Dodelin RA, Stone MM: The role of the suprapatellar plica in internal derangement of the knee. Am J Orthop 5:24, 1963
160. Hughston JC: Complications of anterior cruciate ligament surgery. Orthop Clin North Am 16:237, 1985
161. Hughston JC, Andrews JR, Cross MJ, Moschi A: Classification of knee ligament instabilities. Part I. The medial compartment and cruciate ligaments. J Bone Joint Surg 58A:159, 1976
162. Hughston JC, Barrett GR: Acute anteromedial rotatory instability. Long-term results of surgical repair. J Bone Joint Surg 65A:145, 1983
163. Hughston JC, Stone M, Andrews JR: The suprapatellar plica: its role in internal derangement of the knee. J Bone Joint Surg 55A:1318, 1973
164. Iino S: Normal arthroscopic findings of the knee joint in adults. J Jpn Orthop Assoc 14:467, 1939
165. Ikeuchi H: Arthroscopic treatment of the discoid lateral meniscus. Clin Orthop 167:19, 1982
166. Insall J, Joseph DM, Aglietti P, Campbell RD Jr: Bone-block iliotibial-band transfer for anterior cruciate insufficiency. J Bone Joint Surg 63A:560, 1981
167. Ireland J, Trickey EL: MacIntosh tenodesis for anterolateral instability of the knee. J Bone Joint Surg 62B:340, 1980
168. Jackson JP: Degenerative changes in the knee after meniscectomy. Br Med J 2:525, 1968
169. Jackson RW: Arthroscopy of the knee. In Ahstrom JP (ed): Current Practice in Orthopaedic Surgery. Vol. 5. CV Mosby, St. Louis, 1973
170. Jackson RW: The role of arthroscopy in the management of the arthritic knee. Clin Orthop 101:28, 1974
171. Jackson RW: Current concepts review: arthroscopic surgery. J Bone Joint Surg 65A:416, 1983
172. Jackson RW: The septic knee, arthroscopic treatment. Arthroscopy 1:194, 1985
173. Jackson RW, Abe I: The role of arthroscopy in the management of disorders of the knee: an analysis of 200 consecutive cases. J Bone Joint Surg 54B:310, 1972
174. Jackson RW, Dandy DJ: Arthroscopy of the knee. Grune & Stratton, Orlando, FL, 1976
175. Jackson RW, DeHaven KE: Arthroscopy of the knee. Clin Orthop 107:87, 1975
176. Jackson RW, Marshall DJ, Fujisawa Y: The pathological medial shelf. Orthop Clin North Am 13:307, 1982
177. Jackson RW, Strizak AM: Present status of videoarthroscopy. Contemp Orthop 2:521, 1980
178. Jenkins DHR: The repair of cruciate ligaments with flexible carbon fibre. J Bone Joint Surg 60B:520, 1978
179. Jenkins DHR, McKibbin B: The role of flexible carbon-fibre implants as tendon and ligament substitutes in clinical practice: a preliminary report. J Bone Joint Surg 62B:497, 1980
180. Jennings JE: Arthroscopic management of tibial plateau fractures. Arthroscopy 1:160, 1985
181. Jensen JE, Slocum DB, Larson RL, et al: Reconstruction procedures for anterior cruciate ligament insufficiency: a computer analysis of clinical results. Am J Sports Med 11:240, 1983
182. Johnson LL: Diagnostic arthroscopy of the knee joint. In Excerpta Medica, Elsevier, New York, 1974
183. Johnson LL: Diagnostic arthroscopy of the knee. In Ingwersen OS (ed): The Knee Joint: Proceedings of the International Congress, Rotterdam, September, 1973, Excerpta Medica, Amsterdam, 1974
184. Johnson LL: Comprehensive Arthroscopic Examination of the Knee. CV Mosby, St. Louis, 1977
185. Johnson LL: Diagnostic and Surgical Arthroscopy: The Knee and Other Joints. 2nd Ed. CV Mosby, St. Louis, 1981

186. Johnson LL: Arthroscopic Surgery: Principles and Practice. 3rd Ed. CV Mosby, St. Louis, 1986

187. Johnson RJ, Eriksson E, Haggmark T, Pope MH: Five-to-ten-year follow-up evaluation after reconstruction of the anterior cruciate ligament. Clin Orthop 183:122, 1984

188. Johnson RJ, Kettelkamp DB, Clark W, Leverton P: Factors affecting late results after meniscectomy. J Bone Joint Surg 56A:719, 1974

189. Jones KG: Reconstruction of the anterior cruciate ligament using the central one-third of the patellar ligament. J Bone Joint Surg 52A:1302, 1970

190. Jones KG: Use of the central one-third of the patellar ligament to compensate for anterior cruciate ligament deficiency. Clin Orthop 147:37, 1980

191. Joyce J III: History of arthroscopy. In Arthroscopy. Upjohn, 1977

192. Kalenak A: Saphenous nerve entrapment as a cause of anterior knee pain. Presented at University of Wisconsin Sports Medicine Symp, Madison, 16 May 1986

193. Kannus P, Jarvinen M: Conservatively treated tears of the anterior cruciate ligament. Long term results. J Bone Joint Surg 69A:1007, 1987

194. Kaplan EB: Discoid lateral meniscus of the knee joint. J Bone Joint Surg 39A:77, 1957

195. Keene JS, Dyreby JR Jr: High tibial osteotomy in the treatment of osteoarthritis of the knee: the role of preoperative arthroscopy. J Bone Joint Surg 65A:36, 1983

196. Kennedy J, Willis RB: Synthetic cruciate ligaments: preliminary report. J Bone Joint Surg 58B:142, 1976

197. Kim HC, Klein K, Hirsch S, et al: Arthroscopic synovectomy in the treatment of hemophilic synovitis. Scand J Haematol suppl., 40:271, 1984

198. King D: The healing of semilunar cartilages. J Bone Joint Surg 18:333, 1936

199. Koshino T, Okamoto R, Takamura K, Tsuchiya K: Arthroscopy in spontaneous osteonecrosis of the knee. Orthop Clin North Am 10:609, 1979

200. Krackow KA, Brooks RL: Optimization of knee ligament position for lateral extraarticular reconstruction. Am J Sports Med 11:293, 1983

201. Krause WR, Pope MH, Johnson RJ, Wilder DG: Mechanical changes in the knee after meniscectomy. J Bone Joint Surg 58A:559, 1976

202. Kreuscher PH: Semilunar cartilage disease. A plea for early recognition by means of the arthroscope and early treatment of this condition. IMJ 47:290, 1925

203. Kroiss F: Die Verletzungen der Kniegelenkszwis-chenknorpel und ihrer Verbindungen. Beitr Klin Chir 66:598, 1910

204. Kurosaka M, Yoshiya S, Ohno O, Hirohata K: Lateral discoid meniscectomy. A 20 year follow-up. Presented at American Academy of Orthopaedic Surgery Meeting, San Francisco, January 1987

205. Lambert KL: Vascularized patellar tendon graft with rigid internal fixation for anterior cruciate ligament insufficiency. Clin Orthop 172:85, 1983

206. Larson RL: Combined instabilities of the knee. Clin Orthop 147:68, 1980

207. Larson RL: Augmentation of acute rupture of the anterior cruciate ligament. Orthop Clin North Am 16:135, 1985

208. Larson RL, Cabaud HE, Slocum DB, et al: The patellar compression syndrome. Clin Orthop 134:158, 1978

209. Laurin CA, Beauchamp P: The real challenge of cruciate ligament substitution. J Bone Joint Surg 59B:511, 1977

210. Lindenbaum BL: Complications of knee joint arthroscopy. Clin Orthop 160:158, 1981

211. Lindholm S, Pylkkanen P: Internal fixation of the fragments of osteochondritis dissecans of the knee by means of a bone pin. Acta Chir Scand 140:626, 1974

212. Lipscomb AB, Johnston RK, Snyder RB, Brothers JC: Secondary reconstruction of anterior cruciate ligament in athletes by using the semitendinosus tendon: preliminary report of 78 cases. Am J Sports Med 7:81, 1979

213. Lipscomb AB, Johnston RK, Snyder RB, et al: Evaluation of hamstring strength following use of semitendinosus and gracilis tendons to reconstruct the anterior cruciate ligament. Am J Sports Med 10:340, 1982

214. Lipscomb PR Jr, Lipscomb PR Sr, Bryan RS: Osteochondritis dissecans of the knee with loose fragments: treatment by replacement and fixation with readily removed pins. J Bone Joint Surg 60A:235, 1978

215. Losee RE, Johnson TR, Southwick WO: Anterior subluxation of the lateral tibial plateau. J Bone Joint Surg 60A:1015, 1978

216. Lysholm J, Gillquist J: Arthroscopic examination of the posterior cruciate ligament. J Bone Joint Surg 63A:363, 1981

217. Mariani PP, Gillquist J: The blind spots in arthroscopic approaches. Int. Orthop 5:257, 1982

218. Markey KL: Rehabilitation of the Anterior Cruciate Ligament Deficient Knee. Clin Sports Med 1:513, 1985

219. Marshall JL, Girgis FG, Zelko RR: The biceps fe-

moris tendon and its functional significance. J Bone Joint Surg 54A:1444, 1972

220. Marshall JL, Warren RF, Wickiewicz TL: Primary surgical treatment of anterior cruciate ligament lesions. Am J Sports Med 10:103, 1982

221. Marshall JL, Warren RF, Wickiewicz TL, Reider B: The anterior cruciate ligament: a technique of repair and reconstruction. Clin Orthop 143:97, 1979

222. Martin AF: The pathomechanics of the knee joint, the medial collateral ligament and lateral tibial plateau fractures. J Bone Joint Surg 42A:13, 1960

223. McDaniel WJ Jr, Dameron TB Jr: Untreated ruptures of the anterior cruciate ligament: a follow-up study. J Bone Joint Surg 62A:696, 1980

224. McGinty JB: Closed circuit television in arthroscopy. Int Rev Rheumatol 45, 1976 (Special edition devoted to arthroscopy)

225. McGinty JB: Arthroscopy of the knee: Update and review. Orthop Dig 7(11/12):17, 1979

226. McGinty JB: Arthroscopic removal of loose bodies. Orthop Clin North Am 13:313, 1982

227. McGinty JB, Freedman PA: Arthroscopy of the knee. Clin Orthop 121:173, 1976

228. McGinty JB, Guess LF, Marvin RA: Partial or total meniscectomy. J Bone Joint Surg 59A:763, 1977

229. McGinty JB, McCarthy JC: Endoscopic lateral retinacular release. Clin Orthop 158:120, 1981

230. McIntosh DL, Tregonning RJA: A follow-up study and evaluation of "over the top" repair of acute tears of the anterior cruciate ligament. J Bone Joint Surg 59B:511, 1977

231. McLennan JG: The role of arthroscopic surgery in the treatment of fractures of the intercondylar eminence of the tibia. J Bone Joint Surg 64B:477, 1982

232. Merchant AC, Mercer RL: Lateral release of the patella: a preliminary report. Clin Orthop 103:40, 1974

233. Metcalf RW: Operative arthroscopy of the knee. In American Academy of Orthopaedic Surgeons, Instructional Course Lectures. Vol. 30. CV Mosby, St. Louis, 1981

234. Metcalf RW: p. 131. In Casscells SW: Arthroscopy: Diagnostic and Surgical Practices. Lea & Febiger, Philadelphia, 1984

235. Meyers JF, Grana WA, Lesker PA: Reconstruction of the anterior cruciate ligament in the dog: comparison of results obtained with three different porous synthetic materials. Am J Sports Med 7:85, 1979

236. Meyers MH, McKeever FM: Fractures of the Intercondylar Eminence of the Tibia. J Bone Joint Surg 41A:209, 1959

237. Meyers MH, McKeever FM: Fractures of the intercondylar eminence of the tibia. J Bone Joint Surg 52A:1671, 1970

238. Micheli LJ, Stanitski CL: Lateral patellar retinacular release. Am J Sports Med 9:330, 1981

239. Miller GK, Maylahn DJ, Drennan DB: The treatment of idiopathic osteonecrosis of the medial femoral condyle with arthroscopic debridement. Arthroscopy 2:21, 1986

240. Moore TM, Harvey JP Jr: Roentgenographic measurement of tibial plateau depression due to fracture. J Bone Joint Surg 56A:155, 1974

241. Moore TM, Meyers MH, Harvey JP Jr: Collateral ligament laxity of the knee: long term comparison between plateau fractures and normal. J Bone Joint Surg 58A:594, 1976

242. Morgan CD, Casscells SW: Arthroscopic meniscus repair: a safe approach to the posterior horns. Arthroscopy 2(1):3, 1986

243. Nathan PA, Cole SC: Discoid meniscus. Clin Orthop 64:107, 1969

244. Newburg AH, Greenstein R: Radiographic evaluation of tibial plateau fractures. Radiology 126:319, 1978

245. Nicholas JA: Bracing the anterior cruciate ligament deficient knee using the Lenox Hill derotation brace. Clin Orthop 172:137, 1983

246. Nicholas JA, Minkoff J: Iliotibial band transfer through the intercondylar notch for combined anterior instability. Am J Sports Med 6:341, 1978

247. Nole R, Munson NM, Fulkerson JP: Bupivacaine and saline effects on articular cartilage. Arthroscopy 1:123, 1985

248. Northmore-Ball MD, Dandy DJ: Long-term results of arthroscopic partial meniscectomy. Clin Orthop 167:34, 1982

249. Northmore-Ball MD, Dandy DJ, Jackson RW: Arthroscopic, open partial, and total meniscectomy: a comparative study. J Bone Joint Surg 65B:400, 1983

250. Norwood RA, Andrews JR, Meisterling RC, Clancy GL: Acute anterolateral rotatory instability of the knee. J Bone Joint Surg 61A:704, 1979

251. Norwood LA, Cross MJ: The intercondylar shelf and the anterior cruciate ligament. Am J Sports Med 5:171, 1977

252. Notlage WM, Sprague NF, Auerbach BJ, et al: The Medial Patellar Plica Syndrome. Am J Sports Med 11:211, 1983

253. Noyes FR: Functional properties of knee ligaments and alterations induced by immobilization. Clin Orthop 123:210, 1977

254. Noyes FR, Butler DL, Grood ES, et al: Biomechan-

ical analysis of human ligament grafts used in knee-ligament repairs and reconstructions. J Bone Joint Surg 66A:344, 1984

255. Noyes FR, Butler DL, Paulos LE, Grood ES: Intra-articular cruciate reconstruction. I: Perspectives on graft strength, vascularization, and immediate motion after replacement. Clin Orthop 172:71, 1983

256. Noyes FR, Matthews DS, Mooar PA, Grood ES: The symptomatic anterior cruciate–deficient knee. II: The results of rehabilitation, activity modification, and counseling on functional disability. J Bone Joint Surg 65A:163, 1983

257. Noyes FR, Mooar PA, Matthews DS, Butler DL: The symptomatic anterior cruciate-deficient knee. I: The long-term functional disability in athletically active individuals. J Bone Joint Surg 65A:154, 1983

258. O'Connor RL: The role of arthroscopy in the management of crystal synovitis. J Bone Joint Surg 56A:206, 1974

259. O'Connor RL: Arthroscopy in the diagnosis and treatment of acute ligament injuries of the knee. J Bone Joint Surg 56A:333, 1974

260. O'Connor RL: Arthroscopy. JB Lippincott, Philadelphia, 1977

261. O'Connor RL, Shahriaree H: Meniscal lesions and their treatment. In O'Connor's Textbook of Arthroscopic Surgery. JB Lippincott, Philadelphia, 1984

262. Palmer I: On the injuries to the ligaments of the knee joint. A clinical study. Acta Chir Scand Suppl 53, 1938

263. Paradus LH: Synovectomy for rheumatoid arthritis of the knee. J Bone Joint Surg 57A:95, 1975

264. Patel D: Arthroscopy of the plicae-synovial folds and their significance. Am J Sports Med 6:217, 1978

265. Patel D: Proximal approaches to arthroscopic surgery of the knee. Am J Sports Med 9:296, 1981

266. Patel D: Superior lateral-medial approach to arthroscopic meniscectomy. Orthop Clin North Am 13:299, 1982

267. Paulos LE, Butler DL, Noyes FR, Grood ES: Intra-articular cruciate reconstruction. II: Replacement with vascularized patellar tendon. Clin Orthop 172:78, 1983

268. Paulos LE, Noyes FR, Grood ES, Butler DL: Knee rehabilitation after anterior cruciate ligament reconstruction and repair. Am J Sports Med 9:140, 1981

269. Pettrone FA: Meniscectomy: arthrotomy versus arthroscopy. Am J Sports Med 10:355, 1982

270. Pipkin G: Lesions of the suprapatellar plica. J Bone Joint Surg 32A:363, 1950

271. Pipkin G: Knee injuries: the role of the suprapatellar plica and suprapatellar bursa in simulating internal derangements. Clin Orthop 74:161, 1971

272. Price CT, Allen WC: Ligament repair in the knee with preservation of the meniscus. J Bone Joint Surg 60A:61, 1978

273. Puddu G: Method for reconstruction of the anterior cruciate ligament using the semitendinous tendon. Am J Sports Med 8:402, 1980

274. Radin E: A rational approach to the treatment of patellofemoral pain. Clin Orthop 144:107, 1979

275. Radin EL, De LaMotte F, Maquet P: Role of the menisci in the distribution of stress in the knee. Clin Orthop 185:290, 1984

276. Rasmussen PS: Tibial condylar fractures: impairment of knee joint stability as an indication for surgical treatment. J Bone Joint Surg 55A:1331, 1973

277. Reiner MJ: The arthroscope in tibial plateau fractures: its use in evaluation of soft tissue and bony injury. JAOA 81:704, 1982

278. Resnick D, Goergen TG, Kay JJ, et al: Discoid medial meniscus. Radiology 121:575, 1976

279. Roberts JM: Fractures of the condyles of the tibia. An anatomical and clinical end result study of 100 cases. J Bone Joint Surg 50A:1501, 1968

280. Roberts JM, Lovell WW: Fractures of the intercondylar eminence of the tibia. J Bone Joint Surg 52A:827, 1970

281. Rockwood CA Jr, Green DP: Fractures. Vol. 2. 2nd Ed. JB Lippincott, Philadelphia, 1984, p. 1475

282. Rockwood CA Jr, Green DP: Fractures. Vol. 3. 2nd Ed. JB Lippincott, Philadelphia, 1984, p. 940

283. Rosenberg TD, Metcalf RW, Gurley WG: Arthroscopic meniscectomy. In Bassett FH (ed): American Academy of Orthopaedic Surgeons, Instructional Course Lectures. Vol. 37. CV Mosby, St. Louis, 1988

284. Rosenberg TD, Paulos LE, Abbott PJ: Arthroscopic cruciate repair and reconstruction: an overview and descriptions of technique. In Feagin JA (ed): The Crucial Ligaments. Churchill Livingstone, New York, 1988

285. Rosenberg TD, Paulos LE, Parker RD, et al: Discoid lateral meniscus: case report of arthroscopic attachment of a symptomatic Wrisberg-ligament type. Arthroscopy 3:227, 1987

286. Rosenberg TD, Rasmussen GL: The function of the anterior cruciate ligament during anterior drawer and Lachman's testing: an in vivo analysis in normal knees. Am J Sports Med 12:318, 1984

287. Rosenberg TD, Scott SM, Coward DB, et al: Arthroscopic meniscal repair evaluated with repeat arthroscopy. Arthroscopy 2:14, 1986

288. Rosenberg TD, Scott SM, Paulos LE: Arthroscopic surgery: repair of peripheral detachment of the meniscus. Contemp Orthop 10:43, 1985

289. Salter RB, Field P: The effects of continuous compression: an experimental investigation. J Bone Joint Surg 42A:31, 1960

290. Salter RB, Simmonds DF, Malcolm BW, et al: The biological effect of continuous passive motion on the healing of full thickness defects in articular cartilage: an experimental investigation in the rabbit. J Bone Joint Surg 62A:1232, 1980

291. Schonholtz GJ: The use of closed circuit television in arthroscopy. Orthopedics 7:342, 1984

292. Scott WN, Ferriter P, Marino M: Intra-articular transfer of the iliotibial tract: two- to seven-year follow-up results. J Bone Joint Surg 67A:532, 1985

293. Scott GA, Jolly BE, Henning CE: Combined posterior incision and arthroscopic intra-articular repair of the meniscus. J Bone Joint Surg 68A:847, 1986

294. Shahriaree H: O'Connor's Textbook of Arthroscopic Surgery. JB Lippincott, Philadelphia, 1984

295. Shelton ML, Neer CS II, Grantham SA: Occult knee ligament ruptures associated with fractures. J Trauma 11:853, 1971

296. Sherman WM, Plyley MJ, Pearson DR, et al: Isokinetic rehabilitation after meniscectomy. A comparison of two methods of training. Physician Sportsmed 11:121, 1983

297. Slocum DB, James SL, Larson RL, Singer KM: Clinical test for anterolateral rotatory instability of the knee. Clin Orthop 118:63, 1976

298. Smillie IS: The congenital discoid meniscus. J Bone and Joint Surg 30B:671, 1948

299. Smith M: Arthroscopic treatment of the septic knee. Arthroscopy 2:30, 1986

300. Sprague NF III: Arthroscopic debridement for degenerative knee joint disease. Clin Orthop 160:118, 1981

301. Sprague NF, III: The bucket handle meniscal tear: a technique using two incisions. Orthop Clin North Am 13:337, 1982

302. Sprague NF III: Operative arthroscopy. Clin Orthop 167:4, 1982

303. Sprague NF III, O'Connor RL, Fox JM: Arthroscopic treatment of postoperative knee fibroarthrosis. Clin Orthop 166:165, 1982

304. Stone RG: Peripheral detachment of the menisci of

the knee: a preliminary report. Orthop Clin North Am 10:643, 1979

305. Stone RG, Miller GA: A technique of arthroscopic suture of torn menisci. Arthroscopy 1:226, 1985

306. Takagi K: Practical experiences using Takagi's Arthroscope. J. Jpn Orthop Assoc 8:132, 1933

307. Teitge RA, Indelicato PA, Kerlan RK, et al: Iliotibial band transfer for anterolateral rotatory instability of the knee: Summary of 54 cases. Am J Sports Med 8:223, 1980

308. Torg JS, Conrad W, Kalen V: Clinical diagnosis of anterior cruciate ligament instability in the athlete. Am J Sports Med 4:84, 1976

309. Townley CO, Fumich RM, Shall LM: The free synovial graft as a shield for collagen ingrowth in cruciate ligament repair. Clin Orthop 197:266, 1985

310. Tremblay GR, Laurin CA, Drovin G: The challenge of prosthetic cruciate ligament replacement. Clin Orthop 147:88, 1980

311. Veth RPH: Clinical significance of knee joint changes after meniscectomy. Clin Orthop 198:56, 1985

312. Waddell JP, Johnson DWC, Neidre A: Fractures of the tibial plateau: a review of ninety-five patients and comparison of treatment methods. J Trauma 21:376, 1981

313. Warren RF: Primary repair of the anterior cruciate ligament. Clin Orthop 172:65, 1983

314. Warren RF: Arthroscopic meniscal repair. Arthroscopy 1:170, 1985

315. Watanabe M: Arthroscopy of the knee joint. In Helfet AJ (ed): Disorders of the Knee. JB Lippincott, Philadelphia, 1974

316. Watanabe M, Takeda S, Ikeuchi H: Atlas of Arthroscopy. Igaku, Shoin, Ltd., Tokyo, 1957

317. Whipple TL, Bassett FH: Arthroscopic examination of the knee. Polypuncture technique with percutaneous intra-articular manipulation. J Bone Joint Surg 60A:4:444, 1978

318. Wirth CR: Meniscus repair. Clin Orthop 157:153, 1981

319. Woods GW: Synthetics in anterior cruciate ligament reconstruction: a review. Orthop Clin North Am 16:227, 1985

320. Woods GW, Homsy CA, Prewitt JM III, Tullos HS: ProPlast leader for use in cruciate ligament reconstruction. Am J Sports Med 7:314, 1979

321. Woods GW, Stanley RF, Tullos HS: Lateral capsular sign: x-ray clue to a significant knee instability. Am J Sports Med 7:27, 1979

322. Young RB: The external semilunar cartilage as a complete disc. In Cleland J, Mackay JY, Young RB

(eds): Memoirs and Memoranda in Anatomy. Williams & Norgate, London, 1889

323. Zaricznyj B: Avulsion fracture of the tibial eminence: treatment by open reduction and pinning. J Bone Joint Surg 59A:1,111, 1977

324. Zarins B: Arthroscopic surgery — Basic techniques and instruments. Contemp Orthop 6(3)1983

325. Zarins B: Knee arthroscopy: basic technique. Contemp Orthop 6:25, 1983

326. Zarins B, Rowe CR: Combined anterior cruciate ligament reconstruction using semitendinosus tendon and iliotibial tract. J Bone Joint Surg 68A:160, 1986

The Patellofemoral Joint

115

Andrew A. McBeath

A normal patellofemoral joint is necessary for optimal knee function. The surge of participation in athletic activities has charged physicians with obtaining better results in treating afflictions of the patellofemoral joint. The diagnosis and treatment of patellofemoral disease, however, can be extremely difficult. More than one abnormality may exist; the abnormalities may or may not be related. Despite considerable knowledge of this joint, conflicting conclusions and unsubstantiated opinions still appear in the literature.

This chapter summarizes the relevant literature, points out—if not resolves—conflicts, and focuses on those areas in need of investigation. First, a review of the function and the clinical evaluation of the patellofemoral joint is presented, followed by a discussion of major problems, including acute patellar dislocation, malalignment of the patella, chondromalacia, and osteoarthrosis of the patellofemoral joint, and fracture of the patella.

FUNCTION OF THE PATELLOFEMORAL JOINT

Functions of the Patella

Most recent reports[7,67,104,106] relating to the function of the patella indicate that the structure of the patella is highly important; preservation is desirable if at all possible. The greatest advantage of an intact patella is that it lengthens the moment arm[7,31,67,99,104] of the quadriceps muscle, thereby diminishing the muscle force necessary for knee extension. This effort is most apparent between 15 and 60 degrees of flexion, the range used for most activities of daily living.[68] In cadaver studies, Kaufer[67] showed that 15 to 30 percent more force on the quadriceps tendon was needed to obtain knee extension after patellectomy as compared with an intact knee. O'Donoghue et al.[92] and Sutton et al.[107] measured the functional strength of the

3433

quadriceps in patients after patellectomy and found 30 to 50 percent loss of functional strength compared with the unoperated side. Lack of the patella has been calculated to increase the tibiofemoral joint tangential force by 250 percent.[31] The patella serves as a protective mechanism for the anterior aspect of the knee. The low friction coefficient of the hyaline cartilage enhances the efficiency of the extensor mechanism. If the patellofemoral relationship is normal, extensor mechanism stability is enhanced. A patella also allows a knee to appear normal.

Area and Force of Contact

As the knee flexes, the areas of the patellofemoral contact change, and the amount of contact force increases.[7,97] As the knee flexes, the area of contact on the femoral condyle moves from proximal to distal, whereas on the patella it moves from distal to proximal. For the first 90 degrees of knee flexion, the total area of contact increases, but the increase in total force with increasing flexion is greater than the increase in area, so that the force/unit area increases as flexion increases.[39] Table 115-1 shows the total patellofemoral compression force for various degrees of knee flexion; the reason that patellofemoral pain increases in stair climbing becomes evident in that the total calculated force is 2.5 times body weight.[87,97,104] This force has been calculated to reach 5 times body weight if a subject's femora approach the horizontal position when the subject is standing on both feet.[31]

If the patellofemoral joint is painful, isometric quadriceps setting exercises should be performed with the knee in full extension; in this position, the contact force is negligible.

Tensile Stress on the Extensor Mechanism

Tensile stress on the extensor mechanism has been investigated in a variety of ways,[31,97,104] and different absolute values have been reported. However, all studies show that with increasing flexion these values increase markedly, as noted in Table 115-2.[86,87,97,104] These values also increase with activities other than level walking. Denham and Bishop[31] reported calculated and experimental values for tensile forces in the extensor mechanism showing that the tensile force in the patellar ligament for normal activities was frequently less than that in the quadriceps tendon.

Role of the Quadriceps

Lieb and Perry[72] did much to clarify the function of the quadriceps muscle and its separate components. In their cadaveric experiments, these workers investigated the effectiveness of each portion of the muscle in achieving knee extension. The vastus medialis was considered as two functional units, the vastus medialis longus (VML) and the vastus medialis obliquus (VMO).

The vastus intermedius was found to be the single most effective knee extensor muscle. Almost twice the quadriceps force was needed to achieve

Table 115-1. Patellofemoral Compression Force (× Body Weight)

Activity	Knee Flexion Angle (Degrees)				
	5	15	30	45	60
Isometric contraction (Smidt)[104]	0.8	1.6	2.2	2.5	2.6
Static loading (Perry et al.[97])	0	0.2	0.6	1.2	2.1
Walking (Morrison[86,87])	—	0.6	—	—	—
Ramp, up	—	—	0.9	—	—
Ramp, down	—	1.9	—	—	—
Stairs, up	—	—	—	2.5	—
Stairs, down	—	—	—	—	2.5

(From Kettelkamp,[68] with permission.)

Table 115-2. Quadriceps Tension (× Body Weight)

Activity	Knee Flexion Angle (Degrees)				
	5	15	30	45	60
Static loading (Perry et al.[97])	0.3	0.7	2.1	2.6	3.8
Isometric contraction (Perry et al.[97])	1.82	3.37	3.97	—	6.08
Isometric contraction (Smidt[104])	1.73	2.2	2.7	3.0	3.2
Walking (Morrison[86,87])	—	0.9	—	—	—
Ramp, up	—	—	1.1	—	—
Ramp, down	—	2.7	—	—	—
Stairs, up	—	—	—	2.8	—
Stairs, down	—	—	—	—	2.4

(From Kettelkamp[68] with permission.)

the last 15 degrees of extension against gravity as was needed to achieve extension from 90 to 15 degrees. Contrary to the belief of some investigators, the VMO provided no extension force; it was concluded that the main function of the VMO is to stabilize the patella medially, preventing lateral subluxation caused by the vastus lateralis. The prominence of the VMO is thought to be related to the obliqueness of its fibers, its low insertion, and the thin fascia overlaying it. Atrophy of the VMO, so readily visible, is considered a reflection of generalized quadriceps atrophy, not a selective process.

Perry et al.[97] demonstrated the undesirable effect of knee flexion contractures on the quadriceps force necessary for knee stability. These investigators showed that a quadriceps force equal to 20 percent of average quadriceps strength was needed to stabilize a weight-bearing knee with a 15-degree flexion contracture. This force must increase to 50 percent of average quadriceps strength, if the contracture is 30 degrees.

CLINICAL EVALUATION

An excellent detailed treatise on physical and radiographic evaluation of the patellofemoral joint was recently written by Carson et al.[19]

History

A history is the first step in identifying specific patellofemoral problems and differentiating patellofemoral problems from other problems within the knee. The mechanism of injury is frequently significant, as are factors accentuating and relieving a complaint.

Physical Examination

A physical examination is the second step in reaching a diagnosis, and it must extend from hips to feet. Before attention is focused on the knee, the patient should be observed while he or she is walk-ing. The alignment in the frontal plane and the rotational attitude of the lower extremities are noted. The direction in which the patella points can be an aid in diagnosing increased femoral neck anteversion. The direction in which the feet point while the patient is walking and the status of the arch are noted. With the patient standing, the amount of varus and valgus is observed. With the patient on the examining table, estimates of femoral neck anteversion and tibial rotation can be made. It is pertinent to assess the tightness or laxity of a patient's ligaments. The quadriceps is inspected or measured for detection of atrophy and is palpated to assess tone. The tightness of the rectus femoris is determined. Only the aspects of the knee examination most pertinent to the patellofemoral joint are mentioned here.

At full extension, alignment of the extensor mechanism is assessed by measuring the Q angle. This angle is formed by the intersection of a line drawn from the anterior superior iliac spine to the center of the patella and a line drawn from the center of the patella to the tibial tubercle (Fig. 115-1). This angle is usually 15 degrees or less. An angle greater than 20 degrees is considered definitely abnormal and is frequently associated with patellofemoral pathology. Also noted is the direction in which the patellae point when the patient sits with knees flexed 90 degrees; the patellae should point straight ahead and not deviate laterally, as they often do in malalignment. The path taken by the patella while the knee is put through a range of active and passive motion is noted. The stability of the patella at full extension is determined by pushing the patella both medially and laterally. Lateral displacement of the patella in the fully extended or slightly flexed position as the chief complaint, or a contraction of the quadriceps, constitutes a positive apprehension test, as is common in malalignment syndromes. When the patella is pushed medially and laterally, any asymmetric travel is noted. The degree of flexion at which the patella becomes engaged is noted, that is, when it can no longer be easily pushed laterally. The patella should engage at about 30 degrees of knee flexion.

Both the medial and lateral facets of the patella are palpated for tenderness, which is frequently found with chondromalacia. The pain of this prob-

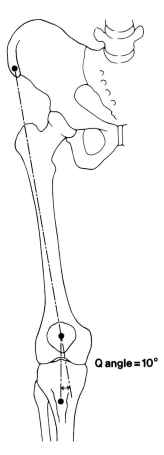

Fig. 115-1. Determination of Q angle.

lem can often be reproduced by asking the patient to perform an isometric contraction of the quadriceps while the examiner pushes the patella distally and posteriorly with the thumb and index finger. This maneuver is repeated with the patient's knee flexed approximately 20 degrees as well; this test can produce pain in an asymptomatic knee. The soft tissues around the patella are also palpated for tenderness or a defect. Any crepitation or effusion is noted.

Radiographic Evaluation

A routine radiographic evaluation includes anteroposterior, lateral, tunnel, and tangential views. Of these, the lateral and the tangential views are the most pertinent for assessment of the patellofemoral joint. Ficat and Hungerford[39] present an

inclusive summary of a radiographic study of the patellofemoral joint.

The AP view is useful in delineating patellar fractures and certain anatomic variants. Patellar position in relationship to the joint line or elevation is best determined from the lateral view. For many years, the criteria of Blumensaat[14] were accepted; he described a line that is an anterior extension of the inferior border of the intercondylar fossa. To be normal, the inferior pole of the patella should touch this line with the knee flexed 30 degrees. The need for exactly 30 degrees of knee flexion makes the technique somewhat impractical; the technique is now considered inaccurate.

Insall and Salvati[60] and later Jacobsen and Bertheussen[61] found that most patellae were positioned well above this line. Insall and Salvati proposed a more practical method that related the greatest diagonal patellar length (LP) to the patellar tendon length (TL) (Fig. 115-2). The knee may be positioned between 20 and 70 degrees of flexion. The average ratio was found to be 1.0, with 1.2 as the upper limit of normal. Jacobsen and Bertheussen

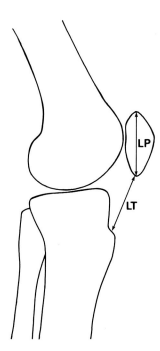

Fig. 115-2. Method for determining patellar position on lateral radiograph. (From Insall,[60] with permission.)

confirmed these results but considered 1.3 the upper limit of normal.

A wide variety of techniques have been proposed for obtaining a tangential view of the patellofemoral joint. The variables with these techniques include degree of knee flexion, patient position, radiograph tube position, and cassette position. Although the technique described by Hughston[52] is popular, the technique described more recently by Laurin et al.[70,71] (Fig. 115-3) apparently offers several advantages over the Hughston technique and the methods of others. The Laurin et al. technique permits the radiograph to be taken with the knee in 20 degrees of flexion, the position of the greatest patellar instability, and the cassette to be perpendicular to the beam. The supine position eliminates any distortion that might be caused by the weight of the limb applying pressure to the patella when the patient is in the prone position. Even with the beam directed cephalad, the eyes are not exposed to the x-ray beam. A wide variety of indices exist for assessing the patellofemoral relationship in the tangential view,[39] but the method described by Laurin et al.[71] apparently is both accurate and simple (Fig. 115-4). Two lines are drawn, one along the lateral patellar facet and the other across the femoral condyles; the angle

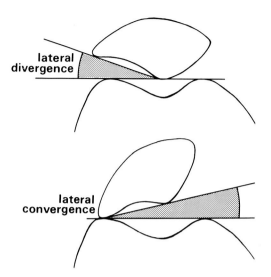

Fig. 115-4. Laurin technique for assessing the patello-femoral relationship on tangential view. (From Laurin,[71] with permission.)

formed by these lines is then noted. If the lines diverge laterally, the relationship is normal; if they are parallel or convergent laterally, subluxation must be strongly suspected. Laurin et al.[71] offered additional indices for evaluating the patellofemoral joint on the tangential view.

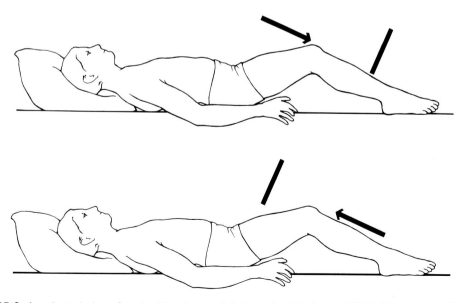

Fig. 115-3. Laurin technique for obtaining tangential view of patellofemoral joint. (From Laurin,[71] with permission.)

One study[85] indicates greater radiographic patellofemoral incongruence associated with chondromalacia and patellar instability when the symptomatic knee was compared with an asymptomatic knee rather than with an arbitrary value.

Computed tomography (CT) may well be more effective in detecting malalignment problems than any of the conventional tangential views.[79,102] This most probably is a result of the knee being in full extension when CT is performed because malalignment tends to normalize as the knee flexes.

Arthrography

Ficat and Hungerford[39] consider arthrography an important aid in evaluating patellofemoral joint surfaces. I have not had sufficiently satisfactory experience with tangential arthrography for the technique to be helpful.

Arthroscopy

Arthroscopy is a valuable technique in evaluating the patellofemoral joint surfaces and patellar tracking. Manipulation of the patella permits examination of all joint surfaces.

ACUTE DISLOCATION OF THE PATELLA

Acute dislocation of the patella is a painful condition. Most dislocations are lateral; most result from indirect trauma, but they may result from direct trauma. External rotation of the tibia in relationship to the femur is the most frequent mechanism of indirect violence causing lateral dislocation. Lateral patellar dislocation can occur at any age, but several authorities[15,46,50] document the mid-teens as the most common age for an initial dislocation. Usually the dislocation is or has been reduced by the time a patient is seen by an orthopaedist, but the diagnosis can usually be established.

The acute pathology may involve both soft tissue and bone. Medial structures, unless very lax, must tear to some degree to permit complete patellar dislocation. Most often, this is a tear of the medial retinaculum. Recently, disruption of the oblique portion of the vastus medialis has been described[6,8] as an avulsion of the VMO and of the adductor magnus from the adductor tubercle, with proximal migration of both. Osteochondral fractures from either the patella or the lateral condyle of the femur frequently occur (Fig. 115-5). Careful in-

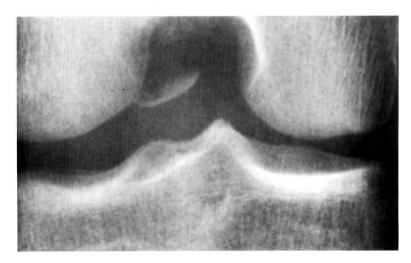

Fig. 115-5. Obvious osteochondral fracture fragment after lateral dislocation of the patella.

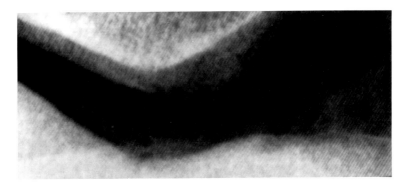

Fig. 115-6. Subtle defect on undersurface of patella indicating osteochondral fracture after acute dislocation of the patella.

spection of high-quality radiographs is necessary to detect these fractures if the fragment contains little bone (Fig. 115-6).

In addition to acute pathology, most knees sustaining a patellar dislocation have preexisting pathology. Preexisting conditions that may predispose the patella to dislocation are multiple and include patella alta, hypoplastic lateral femoral condyle, hypermobile patella, generalized ligamentous laxity, increased Q angle, external tibial torsion, increased femoral neck anteversion, and genetic predisposition.[8,17,46,52,59,84] Although knee valgus is frequently listed as a predisposing factor, the literature does not support this.[50,91]

Treatment

If no fractures are found, the options for therapy range from closed reduction of a dislocation (if it is still present) followed by immobilization to surgical procedures designed to correct preexisting pathology and to repair acutely torn structures.

Most primary dislocations without associated fractures are treated closed. Aspiration of the he-

marthrosis may enhance patient comfort. The knee is then immobilized with a plaster cast or a knee immobilizer for 2 to 4 weeks. In a series reported by McManus et al.[81] (Table 115-3), knees were immobilized 6 weeks; 5 of 26 knees so treated redislocated. In a series reported by Cofield and Bryan,[24] the immobilization period was variable but averaged 3.5 weeks. Of 48 knees, 21 redislocated. Hawkins et al.[47] related 3 of 20 redislocations to preexisting abnormalities rather than to immobilization time. In this series, 11 knees were immobilized an average of 3 weeks, and 9 knees were not immobilized. During immobilization, the patient should perform isometric quadriceps drills.

If closed treatment is chosen, the patient must be warned that symptoms, including redislocation, may be present when immobilization is removed. In a series of 48 patellar dislocations reported by Cofield and Bryan,[24] 21 patients had at least one redislocation, and 13 underwent corrective surgery. Of the 35 remaining patients not having surgery, 11 had recurrent dislocation, 22 had no or mild symptoms, and 3 had severe symptoms. Of 26 cases reported by McManus et al.,[81] 5 patients were subsequently operated on because of redislo-

Table 115-3. Follow-up Evaluation of Treated Knees

Investigators	Total	Redislocation	Late Surgery	Not Operated	Recurrent Dislocation	Significant Symptoms	Mild or No Symptoms
Cofield and Bryan[24]	48	21	13	35	11	3	22
McManus et al.[81]	26	5	5	21	0	11	10
Hawkins et al.[47]	20	3	NS	NS	0	10	10

NS, not stated.

cation, 11 felt insecure or apprehensive but had no pain or redislocation, and 10 were asymptomatic.

If the results of closed treatment are as dismal as reported, why not operate on all primary dislocations? Boring and O'Donoghue[15] and DePalma[33] advocate primary repair usually with some type of realignment procedure. If all primary dislocations were treated surgically, a significant number of knees would be operated unnecessarily. The largest end-result study is that of Boring and O'Donoghue. They reported an 8.2-year average follow-up of 17 knees treated with primary surgery. No redislocations occurred, but 12 knees were reported as painful and 7 were subject to effusions. Rorabeck and Bobechko[100] reported 10 cases with primary repair and realignment and no dislocation. Neither length of follow-up nor prevalence of symptoms was reported. Although redislocation can be markedly diminished with primary surgery, the incidence of residual symptoms is still significant.[47] If the results of surgery for recurrent dislocation[27,44,46] can be extrapolated, it is seen that surgery for these knees, frequently the Hauser procedure, does not eliminate symptoms or prevent arthritis. Unless long-term follow-up of currently used procedures shows improved functional results and less late arthritis than the results now available, routine surgery for a primary dislocation has no basis.

Indications for Surgery

Although routine surgical repair of an acute dislocation is not advocated, indications for surgery do exist. An osteochondral fracture other than on the medial side of the patella is an indication for primary surgery. The medial fragments are generally extraarticular and do not require removal.[39,100] Gross avulsion of soft tissue from the medial and superior aspects of the patella after a complete dislocation should be repaired. When this type of gross avulsion occurs, the articular surface of the patella is readily palpated with only the skin intervening. A relative indication for primary repair occurs when an individual has a knee with a grossly evident predisposing condition for redislocation and when the individual has a firm reason for minimizing the possibility of a redislocation.

Surgical Procedures for Dislocation

Specific realignment procedures are considered in the section on recurrent dislocations and subluxations. Most osteochondral fragments are removed, but if they are large and contain a sufficient amount of bone, an attempt should be made to replace them. All torn structures must be repaired. Special attention is paid to the oblique portion of the vastus medialis muscle. If this is avulsed from its origin and retracted proximally, it is brought distally and sutured in place. If a realignment procedure is undertaken, it should emphasize proximal realignment.[27] In children, tibial tubercle transfer should be avoided to prevent growth disturbances in the proximal tibia.[74]

Postoperative Care

Care after surgery obviously is determined by the specific procedure performed. If it is an arthroscopy or a simple arthrotomy for excising a small osteochondral fragment, immobilization is unnecessary. Partial weight bearing is prescribed for 2 weeks while motion is being regained. During this time, isometric quadriceps-strengthening exercises are performed. About 2 weeks postoperatively, an isokinetic or isotonic program appropriate for the patient is begun. If osteochondral fragments are replaced, the knee must be immobilized, and weight bearing must be restricted until the fragment heals; 8 weeks is usually adequate. Major repairs or realignment are discussed in the postoperative program in the following section.

MALALIGNMENT PROBLEMS OF THE PATELLA: RECURRENT SUBLUXATION AND DISLOCATION

Recurrent subluxation and dislocation of the patella are considered together because they have similar symptoms, underlying pathology, and treatments. Hughston[52] has done much to define the more minor forms of patellar malalignment as a cause of knee impairment; he has pointed out that the problem involves males as often as it does females.

"Giving way" and "catching" are frequent symptoms of patellar malalignment. Thus, the problem is frequently confused with meniscus pathology. Often the symptoms and signs of chondromalacia are present.

The underlying associated anatomical variations are the same as those listed for acute dislocation of the patella. In addition to those variations, an abnormal attachment of the iliotibial tract is reported as a rare cause of recurrent dislocation.[63]

Nonoperative Treatment

The initial treatment for malalignment problems should be nonoperative because (1) the nonoperative approach is frequently effective, and (2) the long-term results of operative treatment are far from ideal.[27,46,74] Hughston[52] emphasizes quadriceps strengthening with the knee in extension before surgery is considered. He believes this step is especially important in children because the patellofemoral joint may be capable of favorable remodeling during the last year or two of bone growth. Heywood[50] reported that 16 knees, 15 percent of his series of dislocating patellae, became symptom free after quadriceps development; his patients noted the onset of symptoms about the time of skeletal maturity. Henry and Crosland[48] reported that 76 percent of 145 patients with subluxing patellae improved after performing a vigorous and extensive exercise program and using a knee support. Straight-leg raising in the supine position, hip abduction in the lateral decubitus position, and hip flexion while sitting were performed by the patients. Thirty repetitions three times per day with weight added as tolerated was prescribed. The exercises were performed for a 6-week period and thereafter as needed. The knee support was a horseshoe-shaped piece of felt held in place by an elastic bandage. Of the improved patients, 76 percent found the exercise helpful, and 64 percent thought the support helpful. Those helped noted improvement by 6 weeks.

Operative Treatment

The indication for operative treatment of patellar malalignment is basically failure of nonoperative treatment for a knee with resultant functional impairment or limitation of a desired life-style. Because patellar realignment may actually hasten degenerative arthritis, the offer of surgery, much less the encouragement of surgery, must be made with great caution and after careful consideration.[27,46,74]

Necessary Overview Before Surgery

Before any specific surgical procedure can be selected, four principles must be considered and remembered.

Exploration of the Joint

Intraarticular pathology exists sufficiently often to merit routine exploration of the knee joint. In the past, this meant an arthrotomy, but now this requirement can sometimes be resolved by arthroscopy and arthrography. Crosby and Insall[27] reported significant associated pathology requiring surgery in 35 of 40 knees: chondromalacia of the patella in 20, chondromalacia of the lateral femoral condyle in 5, loose bodies in 7, and torn menisci in 3. In a series of 133 procedures, Hughston[53] found 17 tears of the medial meniscus, 18 tears of the lateral meniscus, 44 osteochondral fractures, and 81 knees with chondromalacia of the patella or the femoral condyles that required debridement.

Avoidance of Tibial Tubercle Surgery in Children

Fielding et al.[40] reported only one growth disturbance after 24 procedures on the tibial tubercle in children, but other investigators report growth disturbances as a problem. Macnab[74] reported that five of six children who had tibial tubercle surgery developed complications. Crosby and Insall[27] reported five cases of genu recurvatum in the knees of 27 children after this type of procedure. Because a sufficient number of alternatives exist and because of exposure to the risk of a growth disturbance secondary to tibial tubercle surgery, the procedure is not justified in children.

Avoidance of Overcorrection

The often-used Hauser procedure has now produced such a number of poor results[27,46,74] that it probably should be discarded, although DeCesare[29] reported good results with this procedure. At least three possible reasons exist for this common long-term failure; two relate to overcorrection. One reason is that the tibial tubercle may be transferred too far distally. Another reason is that it may be transferred too far medially, to the point of producing a medial dislocation (Fig. 115-7). Huberti and Hayes[51] showed in an experimental study that by increasing or decreasing the Q angle 10 degrees, peak patellofemoral contact pressures were markedly increased. Chrisman et al.[23] reported three medial dislocations in a series of 47 Hauser procedures. Crosby and Insall[27] considered the transfer medially was more detrimental than the transfer distally.

A third reason for failure could be increased joint forces after the medial transfer because the moment arm of the quadriceps is shortened. This shortening occurs because medial displacement of the tibial tubercle by the Hauser technique creates an associated posterior displacement caused by the contour of the tibia[39] (see Fig. 115-12C). After completion of the repair, the patella must move freely and smoothly as the knee is flexed to 90 degrees; it must not be bound down. Hughston[53] even advocates occasional proximal advancement of the tibial tubercle if the extensor mechanism is too tight.

Emphasizing Soft Tissue Procedures

Soft tissue procedures have less tendency to overcorrect the malalignment problem. Two series have been reported that compare the Hauser procedure with soft tissue procedures: both indicate the superiority of soft tissue procedures. Crosby and Insall[27] reported 75 percent acceptable results with soft tissue procedures and 59 percent with the Hauser procedure. Chrisman et al.[23] compared results of the Roux-Goldthwait procedure with lateral retinacular release and medial retinacular plication with the results of the Hauser procedure and found 93 percent and 72 percent acceptable re-

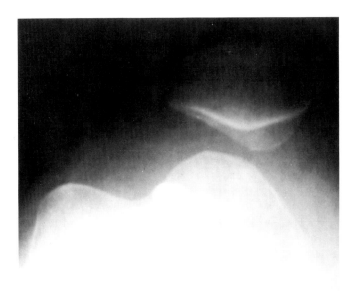

Fig. 115-7. Medial dislocation of patella following overcorrection with the Hauser procedure.

sults, respectively. Both studies reported less arthritis after the soft tissue procedures. Chrisman et al. experienced fewer complications with the soft tissue procedure: 15 percent versus 45 percent. Even though the series reported by Fondren et al.[41] does not offer a direct comparison, it lends credence to this concept. These workers report 91 percent good and excellent results in 47 knees followed an average of 5.8 years after a soft tissue procedure similar to that of Chrisman et al. These investigators switched to this procedure after experiencing frequent complications with the Hauser operation. In contrast to those reports, Madigan et al.[75] reported only 58 percent acceptable results after vastus medialis advancement; they associated the poor results with excessive valgus and preoperative synovitis. Perhaps more significantly, they performed a lateral release only occasionally and released the origin of the oblique portion of the vastus medialis. This release would tend to negate the patellar stabilizing function of this muscle.

Modifications of the Elmslie tibial tubercle transfer are now greatly used. Cox[25] reported that 88 percent of these patients had good or excellent results, but when the follow-up time was increased, the percentage of good and excellent results decreased to 66 percent.[26] Hughston[53] and Hughston and Walsh[54] reported good results using this type of osteotomy as an adjunct to a proximal realignment. The long-term results of the Elmslie-type procedure, however, need further documentation. If these results should prove favorable, the concept of emphasizing soft tissue procedures will need future modification to include this type of bony surgery that provides "gentle correction."

Specific Procedures

Many procedures have been described to correct patellar malalignment. The procedures are categorized as follows: (1) proximal realignment, (2) transfer of the patellar tendon insertion, (3) tenodesis, (4) osteotomy of the distal femur, and (5) patellectomy. Most often, a repair will combine elements from more than one category. Proximal realignment may be done separately, but performance of an isolated distal procedure without proximal realignment[54] remains questionable.

Proximal Realignment

Lateral Release   The release may be used occasionally as an isolated procedure for treating malalignment and lateral retinacular tightness associated with anterior knee pain. Two reports[21,49] endorse only a lateral release for the correction of lateral maltracking of the patella. Its inclusion is essential to any repair of lateral malalignment; therefore, it is the most frequently used component of any realignment operation. The release includes the lateral retinaculum and the inferior insertion of the vastus lateralis; thus, the release must extend 5 to 7 cm superior to the patella and down to the patellar ligament inferiorly. The synovium is not incised intentionally, but if so, it need not be repaired. Technique (as an isolated procedure) is shown in Figure 115-8.

Open Release   The release may be performed as an entirely open procedure through a lateral parapatellar incision.

Subcutaneous Release   After a small stab wound is placed lateral to the patella, minimal subcutaneous

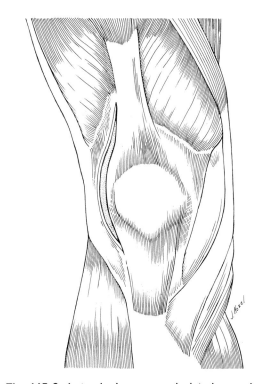

Fig. 115-8. Lateral release as an isolated procedure.

dissection is performed. The lateral retinaculum is then cut in both directions with a meniscotome. The stab wound is often an inferior lateral wound used for arthroscopy.

Arthroscopic Release Some operative arthroscopists perform the procedure from within the joint using scissors.

Postoperative Care The knee is immobilized for 1 or 2 days in a bulky dressing; quadriceps-setting exercises are instituted immediately. Active range of motion is begun when the bulky dressing is removed. Muscle strengthening is prescribed according to a patient's needs.

Vastus Medialis Advancement This advancement is either a simple distal advancement (Fig. 115-9A) or a distal and lateral advancement (Fig. 115-9B) onto the anterior surface of the patella.

Technique An anterior midline skin incision is made 5 cm proximal to the patella, extending distally along the side of the tibial tubercle. Incision of the fascia and capsule (Fig. 115-9) extends proxi-

mally into the quadriceps tendon, leaving a few fibers of tendon on the vastus medialis to facilitate suturing. The incision extends distally along the medial aspect of the patellar ligament. This incision allows for a two-layer closure with interrupted figure-of-8 Vicryl sutures from the proximal end of the wound to about the midportion of the patella. If the straight distal advancement is done, a small "dog ear" remains distally on the medial side of the capsule. Advancement is 1 cm or less for the routine case. Advancement must not be so great as to rotate the patella. A lateral release is done. The tourniquet is released temporarily before the repair is completed, and hemostasis is achieved. Suction drainage is used.

Postoperative Care See under Preferred Method for Realignment.

Proximal Tube Realignment This procedure, described by Insall et al.,[57] is a modification of an earlier method.[58] It is advocated for knees with patellar dislocation or subluxation and for knees with painful chondromalacia with an increased Q

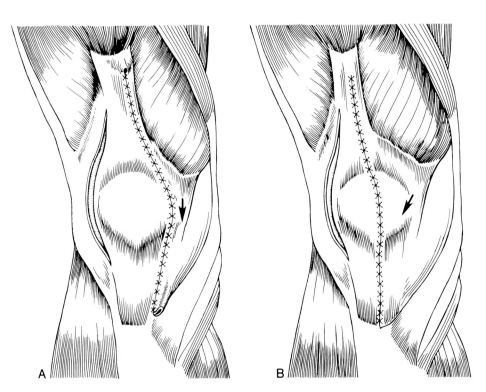

Fig. 115-9. Vastus medialis advancement. **(A)** Distal advancement. **(B)** Distal and lateral advancement.

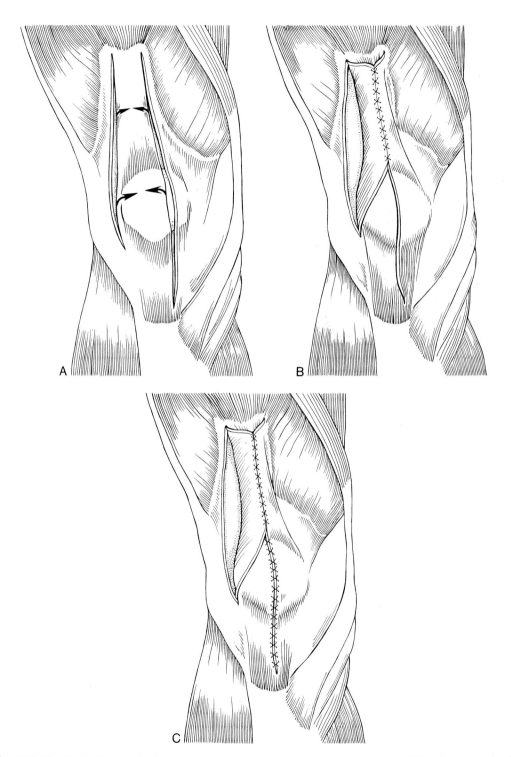

Fig. 115-10. (A–C) Proximal tube realignment by the method of Insall. (From Insall,[57] with permission.)

angle or patella alta. My experience with this procedure has been limited. It attains a gentle realignment and creates a suture line without tension. Postoperative strength requires evaluation because of the extensive lateral release.

Technique An 18-cm mid-line skin incision is used to expose the extensor mechanism (Fig. 115-10). The medial and the lateral aspects of the patella are exposed by subcutaneous dissection. The medial deep incision begins 10 cm proximal to the patella in the quadriceps tendon, about 5 mm from the vastus medialis, extending across the medial border of the patella and ending distally in the medial aspect of the patellar ligament. The quadriceps expansion is dissected sharply from the patella so that the longitudinal fibers remain intact. The lateral incision begins distally in the lateral retinaculum and extends proximally 10 cm, remaining 1.2 cm from the quadriceps tendon. The tourniquet is released and hemostasis is achieved. The vastus medialis is advanced and sutured to the stump of the vastus lateralis. The joining of these two structures ceases near the superior pole of the patella, just before the lateral patella starts to lift. The distal medial structures are sutured as they lie.

Postoperative Care The knee is immobilized in a Robert Jones dressing for 2 days. A knee immobilizer is suitable for the first 2 weeks, during which weight-bearing as tolerated is permitted. Flexion and extension exercises are begun at 2 weeks. Everyday activities are allowed at 6 weeks, but sports are not allowed for 6 months.

Other Procedures Simple imbrication of the medial capsule has been reported but has little rationale and is rarely used. The Campbell procedure uses a proximally based strip of medial capsule to wrap around the quadriceps tendon.[4] The strip is sewn back on the medial side to act as a tether; this is totally passive and could well stretch. The procedure has not received wide acceptance.

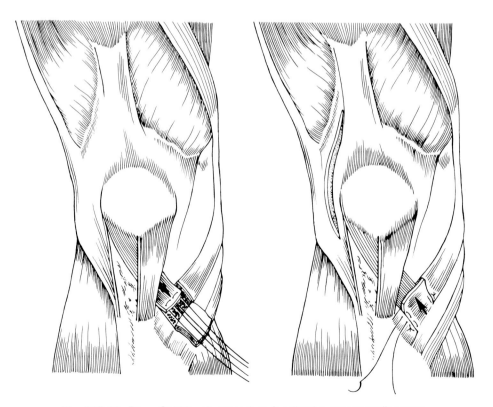

Fig. 115-11. Roux-Goldthwait procedure for distal extensor realignment.

Transfer of Patellar Tendon Insertion

Roux-Goldthwait Procedure After a medial parapatellar or midline skin incision, the lateral one-half of the patellar tendon is released from the tibial tubercle and is divided longitudinally (Fig. 115-11). The lateral one-half is then brought medially beneath the remaining medial one-half. A distally based osteoperiosteal flap is created over the medial tibia. The freed lateral one-half is then pulled into place with two #1 Vicryl sutures. The tendon and the flap can then be secured with a staple or a few additional sutures. Equal tension must be applied to each segment to the split insertion; a lateral release is done.

Postoperative Care See under Preferred Method for Realignment.

Elmslie Type (Modified by Trillot and Goutallier and Debeyre[39]) This type of tibial tubercle transfer permits limited medial transfer and very little associated distal transfer. It minimizes retropulsion of the tubercle, with resultant shortening of the quadriceps moment arm (Fig. 115-12).

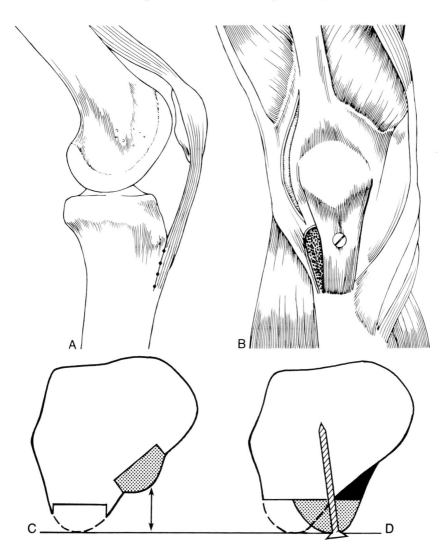

Fig. 115-12. (A,B) Basic technique for Elmslie-type tibial tubercle transfer. **(C)** Retropulsion of tubercle caused by Hauser procedure. **(D)** Avoidance of retropulsion with Elmslie technique. (From Ficat,[39] with permission.)

Technique In this technique (Fig. 115-12), a medial or lateral parapatellar incision is suitable. With an osteotome, an incomplete osteotomy of the tibial tubercle is made in the frontal plane that frees the tubercle proximally but leaves it attached distally by an osteoperiosteal flap. Brown et al.[18] advocate creating the osteotomy in an oblique fashion from posterolateral to anterior medial, to achieve some anterior displacement of the tibial tubercle. The tubercle is then swung 5 to 10 mm medially and fixed with a cancellous bone screw. A bit of bone placed medially behind the transferred tubercle augments the repair. If the intact distal bone is thick, a few drill holes will permit sufficient mobility for the transverse. A lateral release is done.

Postoperative Care See under Preferred Method for Realignment.

Tenodesis

Two recently described methods of tenodesis attach the distally based tendon of the semitendinosis to the patella or to the medial or lateral half of the patellar tendon.[5,69] Attachment to the patellar tendon appears to offer nothing that cannot be accomplished with the Roux-Goldthwait procedure. Baker et al.[5] reported 81 percent good or excellent results in 53 knees after an average of 5 years. Similar results were found by Hall et al.,[45] if patients with ligamentous laxity were not considered. The concept allows distal realignment without violating the tibial tubercle in growing children. I have used the tenodesis to the patella only twice, both times after other procedures failed. Both operations were successful.

In the technique for Galeazzi-Baker transfer (Fig. 115-13), either a long medial parapatellar incision or two shorter incisions are used. If two incisions are used, the anterior incision is shorter and a posterior incision over the muscle-tendon junction of the semitendinosis is made. The semitendinosis is cut at the muscle-tendon junction. The proximal end is sutured into the semimembranosis. After the patella is dissected free, an oblique hole is made in the direction of the transfer. The tendinous portion of the semitendinosis, with its insertion still intact, is brought anteriorly, passed through the drill hole medially to laterally, and then brought across the

front of the patella and sutured to itself. A routine closure and lateral release are performed.

Postoperative Care See Preferred Method for Realignment.

Osteotomy of the Femur

Although valgus alignment is often mentioned as a cause of chronic malalignment and osteotomy mentioned as a treatment, the procedure has never achieved wide acceptance. Heywood[50] reported seven supracondylar osteotomies of the femur for recurrent dislocation of the patella, with five failures.

Patellectomy

Patellectomy is a last resort. Only if the patella is grossly destroyed is patellectomy performed. Plastic procedures with realignment are preferred, although the remodeling may leave only cancellous bone. A patellectomy can always be performed.

If patellectomy is elected in the presence of gross malalignment, the extensor mechanism must be realigned such that it will not subluxate. The method of patellectomy that advances the vastus medialis, described by West and Soto-Hall,[113] will accomplish this objective.

West and Soto-Hall Technique The skin incision of choice is selected (Fig. 115-14). The originators advocated a U-shaped incision. The quadriceps expansion is incised in a U fashion with the inferior portion over the junction of the middle and distal third of the patella. The vastus medialis is released with a vertical medial parapatellar incision. The patella is removed by sharp dissection. The lateral flap is brought distally and medially 1.5 to 2.0 cm and sutured with #1 Vicryl figure-of-eight sutures, leaving a gap laterally that is not closed. The vastus medialis is then shifted distally and laterally and sutured into place. A routine closure is done.

Other Techniques See under Chondromalacia.

Postoperative Care The knee is immobilized for 3 weeks, and isometric quadriceps exercises are begun immediately. For 3 to 6 weeks, immobilization is discontinued to permit active range-of-motion exercises several times a day. At 6 weeks, iso-

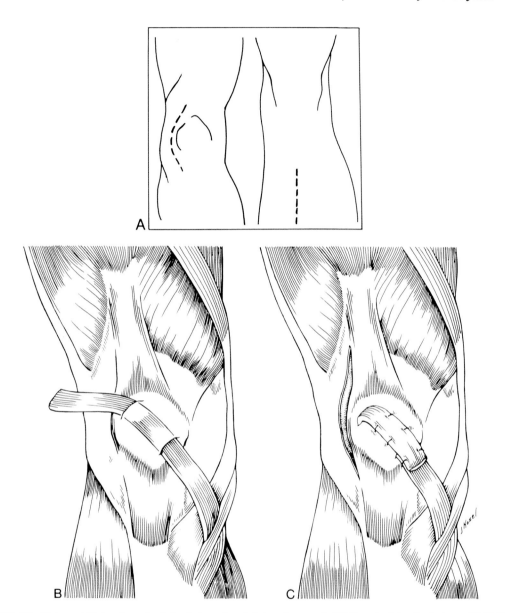

Fig. 115-13. Galeazzi-Baker tenodesis technique for distal realignment. **(A)** Two-incision technique. **(B,C)** Technique of tenodesis. (From Baker,[5] with permission.)

tonic or isokinetic exercises appropriate for the patient are prescribed.

Author's Preferred Method for Realignment

A nearly midline skin incision is used, although other surgeons advocate lateral or medial incisions. The joint is opened medially and explored. For many adults and for all children, a lateral release and a vastus medialis advancement is combined with a Roux-Goldthwait procedure. The advancement is either distally or distally and laterally on top of the patella, or both (Fig. 115-9). If the malalignment is more severe, advancement distally and laterally is the choice. If the Q angle exceeds 20 degrees, the Elmslie-type tibial tubercle transfer is

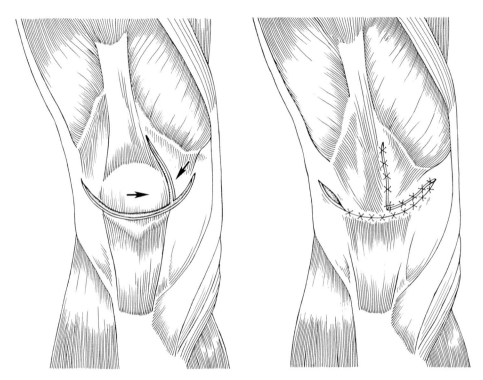

Fig. 115-14. West and Soto-Hall method of patellectomy. (From West,[113] with permission.)

performed with the use of a screw for fixation. The tourniquet is released before the repair is completed so that bleeders can be clamped; it is then reinflated. After repair is completed, the knee must easily flex passively to 90 degrees while the repair remains intact. The patella must track smoothly. Treatment of articular cartilage damage is discussed in the section on chondromalacia. The repair is accomplished with #1 Vicryl. A running subcuticular suture is used to close the skin.

Postoperative Care Two large suction catheters are used for the first 24 to 36 hours. The leg is initially immobilized in a Robert Jones type of dressing, a roll of cotton covered by a plaster stirrup extending from the groin around to the foot to the greater trochanter. Two days after surgery, a long-leg cast or a cylinder plaster cast or a knee immobilizer is applied. The knee is rarely immobilized for as long as 6 weeks. Most patients are placed in a removable knee immobilizer; 2 to 4 weeks after surgery, they are started on a gentle active range-of-motion program that does not exceed 40 degrees.

Active quadriceps setting is begun as soon as possible after surgery. Preoperative instruction in quadriceps setting facilitates the postoperative program. Six weeks after surgery, the patient is started on a vigorous active range-of-motion program. When 90-degree flexion is obtained, either an isokinetic or an isotonic program of muscle strengthening is begun for the quadriceps, hamstring, and hip abductors.

Complications

Peroneal Nerve Palsy This problem has been reported as a complication of extensor realignment[23,25,43,53] and is believed to be secondary to hemarthrosis. Prevention is the best treatment. Preventive measures include careful hemostasis, release of the tourniquet before closure, use of suction drainage, and a Robert Jones dressing (less constricting than a rigid cast) immediately after surgery.

Lack of Flexion This distressing problem can follow distal transfer of the tibial tubercle; it should occur less often as use of the Hauser procedure declines. Shorter immobilization times should decrease this problem. No matter what type of repair is used, it must allow 90-degree flexion at the time of surgery. If the knee fails to flex to 90 degrees with the repair intact, the repair is too tight. A gentle manipulation with the patient under anesthesia may be necessary to resolve this problem.

Patellofemoral Pain This problem can plague a patient after an ideal repair. Again, the repair must not be too tight or the correction too severe. A lateral release must be performed in almost all cases. Aspirin may be helpful. If this type of pain is present, isometric rather than isotonic or isokinetic exercises are emphasized for rehabilitation. The Maquet procedure may prove helpful. Occasionally, if plastic procedures have failed, patellectomy is necessary.

Medial Dislocation This obviously results from overcorrection (see Fig. 115-7), and the treatment is a transfer of the tibial tubercle to a more lateral position. We have found that optimal alignment is more easily obtained with the patient awake and able to move the knee actively.[108]

Recurrent Dislocation If the problem is sufficiently symptomatic to warrant further surgery, greater correction must be judiciously titrated into the knee to achieve stability.

Degenerative Arthritis Present knowledge[23,27] indicates that a predilection to arthritis is decreased by avoiding overcorrection. Elimination of the Hauser procedure should diminish this complication. Crosby and Insall[27] found less arthritis after proximal realignment than after the Hauser procedure. Chrisman et al.[23] found the Roux-Goldthwait procedure to produce less arthritis than the Hauser procedure.

Growth Disturbances in the Proximal Tibia Although careful transfer of the tibial tubercle in a growing child can produce few complications,[68] it should be avoided. A sufficient number of soft tissue procedures exist, so the risk of growth disturbance need not be taken.

Necrosis of Transferred Patellar Ligament This necrosis is best prevented by careful tissue handling and avoidance of strangulation when the ligament is anchored. If the results for tibial transfer with minimal bone continue to be successful, the Roux-Goldthwait procedure can be eliminated in adults, as advocated by Hughston and Walsh,[54] who transfer the tibial tubercle if the Q angle exceeds 10 degrees.

Rupture of the Quadriceps This problem can only be the result of an overzealous lateral release.[12]

Compartment Syndrome This syndrome problem has been reported[110] after the Hauser procedure mainly in the anterior compartment but in other compartments as well. It is thought to occur because of bleeding from vessels terminating on the lateral aspect of the tibial tubercle. Prevention involves the hemostasis and suction drainage, as well as treatment, recognition, and fasciotomy.

Lateral Tibial Rotation This problem is often mentioned[27] as a consequence of distal bony alignment; its occurrence indicates the importance of proximal realignment.

CHONDROMALACIA

No affliction of the patellofemoral joint is accompanied by as much speculation, confusion, and uncertainty as the patellofemoral pain syndrome often attributed to chondromalacia. Careful clinical evaluation and arthroscopy have been responsible for delineating a few soft tissue problems such as a painful plica and inflammation of the quadriceps insertion and patellar ligament insertion on the patella as a cause of anterior knee pain. The biggest impediment to progress on this subject has been, and still is, the tendency to attribute most cases of anterior knee pain to "chondromalacia," which is strictly an anatomic diagnosis. The literature offers little help because it presents a plethora of short-term results of patients treated with heterogeneous preoperative diagnosis, often with multiple procedures. Frequently the results are contradictory. Although the syndrome of anterior knee pain is easily recognized clinically, the cause(s), primary pathology, and treatment of the problem are not agreed on. Most surgeons concur that this clinically described condition can be associated with degeneration of the articular cartilage of the patella. But there the agreement ends. Because of this lack of agreement, this section must remain noncommittal.

Unresolved Questions

Does chondromalacia, that is, softening of the articular cartilage of the patella, cause the typical symptoms of anterior knee pain? Hughston et al.[55] recorded anterior knee pain in 48 percent of 97 patients without chondromalacia and in 45 percent of 249 patients with chondromalacia. Is chondromalacia an early form of degenerative arthritis? Is it a separate condition? Both Outerbridge and Dunlop[96] and Chrisman and Snook[22] believe that it is early degenerative arthritis because the pathologic and biochemical changes in the two are similar. Goodfellow et al.[44] believe that two distinct entities are present based on the location of the degeneration. In a long-term follow-up study, Karlson[65] reported that most patients in whom chondromalacia was diagnosed clinically and treated nonoperatively did not develop arthritis; this would indicate two separate entities.

In which layer of the cartilage does the degeneration begin? Most descriptions focus on the surface degeneration and its progression. But Goodfellow et al.[44] consider surface degeneration to be age related and not true chondromalacia. They describe chondromalacia as starting with basal degeneration and involving the superficial layer secondarily. What area of the patella is most apt to be involved? Many say it is the medial facet. Insall et al.[58] found that most lesions were centered about the midpoint of the central ridge, with extension having equal frequency onto the medial and lateral facets. What is the source of the pain? The cartilage has no nerves. Is it from underlying bone? From an inflamed synovium? All are provocative questions that remain to be answered.

Associated or Causative Conditions

The associated or causative conditions are categorized as those relating to (1) the primary carti-

lage injury, and (2) the patellar bone (Table 115-4) with secondary cartilage injury.

A blow to the anterior aspect of the knee is a commonly accepted cause of chondromalacia, as is an insult from an acute patella dislocation. The most common chronic cause of cartilage injury is malalignment. An increased Q angle is a more readily accepted finding than is patella alta,[58] but this has been refuted.[78] One study found the prevalence of abnormalities of joint laxity, Q angle, genu valgum, and femoral neck anteversion no greater in a group of teenagers with anterior knee pain than in an asymptomatic control group.[36] Excessive lateral compression syndrome, caused by a thickened lateral retinaculum, was well described by Ficat and Hungerford.[39] Perineural fibrosis and demyelination of lateral retinacular nerves has been associated with anterior knee pain.[42] The frequent association of chondromalacia and a torn meniscus is well known,[105] as is patellofemoral pain following a knee arthrotomy. Outerbridge[94] proposed a prominent medial supracondylar ridge on the femur as a patellar irritant, but this proposed pathogenesis has received little support. Wiberg[114] thought his type III patella might be a cause, but this possibility has been refuted by Outerbridge.[95]

Associated changes in patellar bone that might be causative have been reported. For example, Darracott and Vernon-Roberts[28] reported local-

Table 115-4. Conditions Causing or Associated with Chondromalacia

Direct injury to cartilage
Acute injury
Anterior blow
Acute patellar dislocation
Chronic irritation
Malalignment
Recurrent dislocation or subluxation
Increased Q angle
Patella alta
Excessive lateral pressure syndrome
Meniscus tear
Postarthrotomy
Prominent medial supracondylar ridge
Wiberg type III patella
Bone-related
Osteoporosis or osteopenia
Increased bone density
Differences in bone density
Overuse for a particular individual

ized or generalized osteopenia of patellar trabecula as the primary cause of patellofemoral pain. Stougard[106] found increased bone density of the lateral patellar facet. Abernethy et al.[1] proposed differences in patellar bone stiffness that lead to differential cartilage deformation as a cause of cartilage degeneration. Venous congestion in the patella visualized by venography has been found in patients with chondromalacia and degenerative arthritis.[109] Simple overuse must also be considered as a cause for this perplexing problem.

Treatment

Nonoperative Treatment

In most cases, the symptoms attributed to chondromalacia can be improved with nonoperative treatment. Spontaneous healing of surface cartilage damage has been reported and could be a cause of decreased symptoms. The essentials of treatment include (1) rest or avoidance of painful activities until symptoms decrease, (2) performance of isometric quadriceps exercises, and (3) administration of nonsteroidal anti-inflamatory medication three or four times per day for 2 to 3 weeks. The exercise program should be continued for two or three times per week if symptoms are controlled, and should be intensified if symptoms increase. Aspirin taken before engagement in provoking activities is frequently effective.

Other modalities that may help include a flexible arch support, if flexible pes planus exists, as well as a knee support. Bicycling in low gears (with the seat properly adjusted for height) and gentle cross-country skiing can frequently diminish symptoms. If the rectus femoris is tight, stretching of this may be beneficial.

In a formal program, DeHaven et al.[30] treated 100 athletes who had clinically diagnosed chondromalacia using the principles mentioned. The program also included isotonic hamstring exercises and running. Significant improvement was reported in 82 percent of athletes.

Counseling of patients on this problem proves worthwhile; patients should be guided, if possible, into nonaggravating activities. Prolonged sitting with the painful knee in a flexed position must be avoided.

Operative Treatment

Nonoperative treatment must have been exhausted, and symptoms must be severe in order for operative treatment to be considered. Several procedures have been proposed; none has been universally accepted. Arthroscopy is contributing to an upsurge of patellofemoral surgery for symptoms attributed to chondromalacia. I sincerely hope that as this surgery is performed the pathology, the procedure performed, and the results will be documented and comprehensively reported.

Table 115-5 outlines the procedures available to relieve the symptoms of chondromalacia. Reported results are difficult to evaluate and compare because alignment is not mentioned in several reports comparing plastic procedures with patellectomy, and because multiple procedures are often performed simultaneously, making it difficult to evaluate the effectiveness of any single procedure. One 5-year follow-up study reports surgery to be beneficial for early disease in posttraumatic chondromalacia and chondromalacia associated with malalignment.[93]

Realignment Procedures

If clinical or radiographic evidence of malalignment is present, a potential cause for the cartilage damage exists. Patellar realignment is a relatively new concept in the treatment of chondromalacia. Earlier thinking was generally focused on either plastic procedures or patellectomy. Before realignment becomes the obvious solution for a large num-

Table 115-5. Surgical Procedures for Symptoms of Chondromalacia

Realignment
Lateral release
Proximal realignment
Distal realignment
Plastic procedures
Shaving
Open
Closed
Excision down to bone
Diminution of reactive force
Osteotomy of patella
Patellectomy

ber of patients with the symptoms of chondromalacia, the symptoms remaining after correction of malalignment (discussed under Malalignment Problems of the Patella) would well be reviewed.

Lateral Retinacular Release

This procedure, with or without plastic procedures, is frequently performed; it is indicated for a knee with malalignment. The ideal knee apparently is the knee with greater tightness of the lateral retinaculum than of the medial retinaculum. This is ascertained by passive movement of the patella both medially and laterally, with the knee fully extended and the quadriceps relaxed. Extreme lateral patellar movement as the knee achieves full active extension is an indication for lateral release. A patella that rides laterally on the Laurin view is another indication. The procedure is contraindicated in the normal knee and the knee with a hypermobile patella.

Results   See under Malalignment. Ficat and Hungerford[39] reported 76 percent good or excellent results in 174 cases of excessive lateral pressure syndrome followed for at least 6 months. Although these investigators differentiate this syndrome from chondromalacia, apparently it is more of a category of chondromalacia than a separate entity. Merchant and Mercer[83] reported excellent results in five knees showing radiographic evidence of malalignment after lateral release, but in only three of six knees that had no radiographic evidence of malalignment or patella alta had good or satisfactory results.

Technique   See under Malalignment.

Postoperative Care   Isometric quadriceps exercises are initiated as soon as possible after surgery. Partial weight bearing is maintained until any effusion resolves. If the patient desires high performance from the knee, isometric exercises in several positions of flexion are instituted about 1 week after surgery; otherwise, isometrics are performed only in full extension. If plastic procedures were extensive on the patella and exposed bone, an attempt is made to restrict a patient to partial weight bearing for 4 to 6 weeks, but this is rarely accomplished. During this period, pendulum exercises are prescribed in addition to the isometric exercises.

Proximal and Distal Realignment

If malalignment is severe, more than a lateral release must be considered. The orthopaedist is again faced with a choice — performing this procedure either proximally or distally. Devas and Golski[34] reported improvement in 17 of 20 knees treated by distal and medial transfer of the tibial tubercle. Insall et al.[58] reported 79 percent good results in 87 knees treated with either proximal or distal realignment in addition to plastic procedure on the patella. These workers stated that the results of proximal realignment were most satisfactory but that these patients were experiencing subjective dislocation, whereas those having a distal procedure had true dislocation. Patella alta and an increased Q angle were frequent findings. The proximal realignment presented in the preceding section, described by Insall et al.,[57] is a modification of the procedure just discussed.[58] Insall et al.[57] suggested that only blister lesions or gross erosions require plastic procedures. The modified procedure yielded 94 percent good or excellent results.

Plastic Procedures

Simple shaving of the pathologic cartilage has been a frequently performed procedure, with good results reported.[22,65,115,116] However, recent documented reports that isolated shaving produces lasting good results, except in posttraumatic chondromalacia, are lacking. Johnson[64] reported very good results of transcutaneous cartilage excision under arthroscopic control. If radiographic or clinical evidence of malalignment existed, he performed a lateral release as well (Johnson LL, personal communication). Goodfellow et al.[44] reported good results after local excision of the involved cartilage and drilling of the subchondral bone. In contrast to these reports, Bentley[9–11] reported on two occasions that patellectomy is the best procedure for chondromalacia. The first report[9] compares shaving with patellectomy but does not mention realignment. In the second[10] he compares patellectomy with shaving, excision and drilling, and realignment, but only one knee had both realignment and shaving. O'Donoghue[91] reported good results after facetectomy of the patella. Outerbridge[95] advocated excision of a sharp ridge at the superior aspect of the cartilage-bone junction on the medial femoral condyle.

Technique of Cartilage Shaving Cartilage shaving is performed if only the superficial layers are involved and the deep layers are firm to palpation. This procedure is simply a tangential shaving of the frayed superficial layers of cartilage and is most often done arthroscopically with a cartilage shaver. Postoperative management is not influenced by superficial shaving but is dictated by the major procedure performed.

Technique of Cartilage Excision and Bone Drilling This technique (Fig. 115-15) is performed if the pathology is well localized and involves the entire thickness of the cartilage. The defect is circumscribed with a scalpel blade held perpendicular to the surface. The involved cartilage is then removed with a curette (Fig. 115-15). The exposed subchondral bone is drilled with multiple holes. Although a drill bit generates debris that must be removed, it is preferable to a Kirschner (K-) wire because it produces better bleeding. Postoperatively the knee is held in a bulky dressing for 2 to 4 days. Isometric quadriceps exercises are begun immediately. Active range-of-motion and pendulum swing exercises are begun 4 to 5 days after surgery. An attempt is made to restrict full weight bearing for 4 to 5 weeks to enhance and protect the desired repair.

Diminution of Patellar Femoral Joint Force

Maquet[77] proposed the addition of anterior transposition of the tibial tubercle to the surgical armamentarium for the treatment of chondromalacia. The anterior transfer reduces the contact stresses by increasing the moment arm for the quadriceps mechanism and opening the angle of the quadriceps pull on the tibia. Recent laboratory studies have shown marked reduction in the contact surface areas with increased peak forces in the superior lateral aspect of the patella with 2.5-cm advancement.[38,90] Whether this procedure accom-

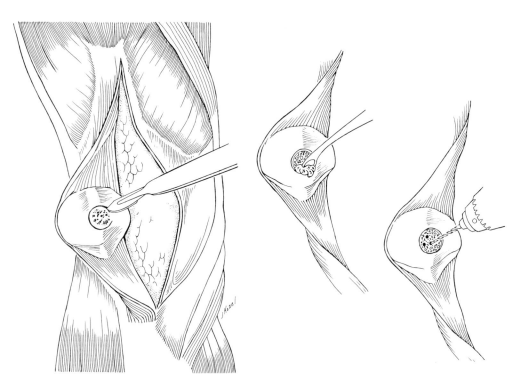

Fig. 115-15. Technique for focal full-thickness excision of diseased cartilage with bone drilling.

plishes the desired clinical result remains to be confirmed. To date, preliminary reports indicate mixed results.[37,77,99,101]

Operative Technique   Maquet[77] describes an anteromedial incision extending 10 to 13 cm inferior to the lower pole of the patella, 0.5 to 1 cm posterior to the tibial crest. Lateral, midline, and transverse incisions have also been advocated. Several drill holes are made in the frontal plane 0.7 cm posterior to the tibial crest (Fig. 115-16). The proximal end of the tubercle is then separated with either a saw or an osteotome, taking care to leave the distal end attached. A saw may be used without making drill holes. Two corticocancellous iliac grafts are then placed in the interval to maintain the forward displacement. Additional small grafts are placed in the interval. Even though Maquet states that a 2-cm advancement is necessary, biomechanical studies[38,90] show that more than 1.2 cm of elevation is of little practical value. Screw fixation is usually not necessary, but it may be used if considered necessary in a particular case. Maquet advo-

cates immediate mobilization, but I use a knee immobilizer for protection with intermittent range-of-motion exercises. A medial shift of the tubercle may be performed to achieve a distal realignment.

Osteotomy

A longitudinal osteotomy[88] has been proposed to increase contact of the medial patellar facet in Wiberg patella types III and IV and the "hunter's hat" form. A lateral release is done. Results reported so far are only preliminary.

Patellectomy

Patellectomy must be the last procedure considered for the treatment of chondromalacia. This view is taken despite favorable results reported by Bentley,[9] West,[112] and Jakobsen et al.[62] Bentley reported patellectomy the single most successful procedure, advocating the procedure for all but mild chondromalacia and in female patients under

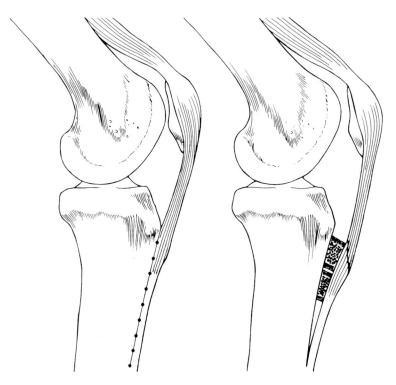

Fig. 115-16. Maquet procedure for tibial tubercle advancement. (From Maquet,[77] with permission.)

20 years of age. Despite these impressive results, I have not talked with any patient who has had a patellectomy and who desires an active life-style who is satisfied with the operated knee. The biomechanical studies referred to[107] provide adequate reason for this dissatisfaction.

Technique A transverse skin incision is often advocated, but a median parapatellar or midline incision is used because it is less restricting if future surgery is needed. Three basic techniques are available for patellectomy: (1) vertical incision (Fig. 115-17A), (2) transverse incision (Fig. 115-17B), and (3) excision with quadricepsplasty, as described by West and Soto-Hall[111] (see under Malalignment). In the first two techniques, the patella is removed by sharp dissection, taking care to preserve all soft tissues; the latter are then reapproximated with figure-of-8 sutures of #1 Vicryl. On the basis of cadaver studies, Kaufer[67] found a slight mechanical advantage to the transverse incision. If malalignment exists, excision with quadricepsplasty is the method of choice.

Postoperative Care The knee is immobilized for 3 to 4 weeks; isometric quadriceps exercises are started immediately. Gentle active range-of-motion exercises are begun when immobilization is ended; resistance exercises are started 7 to 8 weeks after surgery.

Complications

Subluxation of quadriceps mechanism after patellectomy: This usually results from failure to recognize malalignment initially and to perform the proper procedure. The technique of West and Soto-Hall[113] most often corrects malalignment at the time of patellectomy.

Disruption of repair after patellectomy: This is usually caused by infection, inadequate repair, or too vigorous mobilization. Three weeks should be the minimum period of immobilization; #1 Vicryl is used. All motion for the first 2 months must be active.

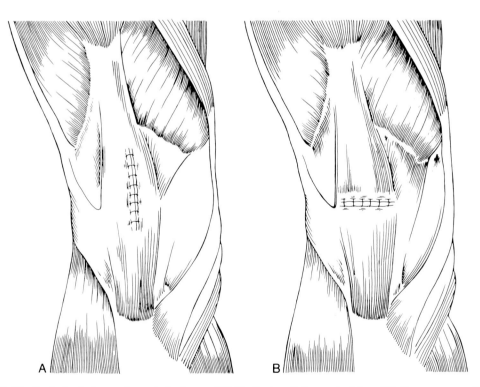

Fig. 115-17. Basic techniques for patellectomy. **(A)** Vertical soft tissue incision. **(B)** Transverse soft tissue incision.

Limited range of motion after patellectomy: This tends to occur after prolonged immobilization and may require gentle manipulation under anesthesia for correction.

Calcification at the site of patellectomy repair: This is probably of no consequence.

Weakness after patellectomy: This requires intense exercise to compensate for mechanical disadvantage. If this is insufficient for a patient's needs, anterior transposition of the tibial tubercle may be considered. This may be accomplished by the methods of Kaufer[67] or of Maquet.[77]

Pain after plastic or realignment procedures: If severe, this problem leaves only the Maquet operation or patellectomy for consideration.

Skin necrosis after a Maquet operation: This complication indicates excessive tension on the skin at the time of closure; limiting tubercle elevation to 1.0 cm will decrease the problem. Sufficient undermining of the skin flaps must be done to achieve wound closure with acceptable tension.

Pain when kneeling after a Maquet procedure: This may well be an inherent disadvantage to the procedure.

Lowering of the patella after a Maquet procedure: This problem has been reported in 8 of 72 patients. No etiology or solution is offered.[66]

Author's Preferred Method for Treatment

If nonoperative treatment fails, the knee is arthroscoped. If any indication of lateral tightness exists, a lateral release is performed. If articular damage exists, the damaged area is excised. If the damage is superficial and firm cartilage exists below the fibrillated area, only the superficial layers are removed. If the damage extends to bone, the entire lesion is excised to bone, and the subchondral bone is drilled in many areas. If malalignment exists, it is usually corrected by soft tissue procedures (as advocated under Malalignment) or by the soft tissue procedure advocated by Insall et al.[57] My experience with tibial tubercle advancement has been equivocal, but I will continue to use it before considering patellectomy.

OSTEOARTHRITIS OF THE PATELLOFEMORAL JOINT

Osteoarthritis confined to the patellofemoral joint fortunately is relatively rare, but when it does occur it presents a perplexing problem. Whether chondromalacia and osteoarthritis are on a continuum or not, the principles for treating both conditions are similar. If surgical treatment is necessary for osteoarthrosis, more extensive procedures are generally required than for chondromalacia.

The diagnosis of osteoarthrosis of the patellofemoral joint is straightforward with the aid of clinical evaluation and radiographic examination. Evaluation must include assessment of the alignment of the extensor mechanism as well as the disease of the articulating surface.

Nonoperative Treatment

The nonoperative treatment of osteoarthrosis of the patellofemoral joint is similar to that for chondromalacia of the patella. Generally the exercise program is less vigorous because these patients are usually not young and expect less from the knee. In addition to the emphasis on quadriceps drill and aspirin administration, performance of pendulum exercises is helpful.

Operative Treatment

Indications

Failure of nonoperative treatment is the main indication for surgical intervention.

Contraindications

Contraindications include the following:

Extensive disease in other compartments: This would eliminate knees with extensive flexion contractures and varus or valgus deformities.

Restricted motion: At least 90 degrees of flexion should be present if patellofemoral surgery is to be considered.

A nonmotivated or a debilitated patient: Any surgical procedure for patellofemoral arthritis requires much active rehabilitation for an adequate result. If a patient is not capable of adhering to such a program, a poor result is predicted.

Available Procedures for Osteoarthrosis

Realignment Procedures

Malalignment must be corrected as part of any surgical procedure, including patellectomy. These techniques are presented under Malalignment.

Maquet-Type Procedure

Radin[98] has reported 90 percent good results in patients with patellofemoral arthritis treated with a modified Maquet procedure. The tibial tubercle advancement was 2.0 to 2.5 cm.

Arthroplasties

Arthroplasties include the Cave-Rowe type.[20]

Cave-Rowe Type This procedure removes approximately the posterior three-fourths of the patella. The raw surface is then covered by the reflected fat pad. This salvage procedure is just short of a patellectomy; its inclusion may be primarily for historic completeness.

Technique A median parapatellar or midline incision is made sufficiently long to expose the infrapatellar fat pad and to allow the patella to be rotated laterally 180 degrees (Fig. 115-18). Care is taken to bluntly dissect approximately 15 percent of the quadriceps tendon medially with the vastus medialis, permitting firm anchorage for the closing sutures. The soft tissues are sharply dissected from the superior, lateral, and medial aspects of the patella. The posterior three-fourths of the patella are then removed with a saw. Care must be taken to prevent bone dust from entering the joint and to remove any that enters it. A superiorly based flap of the synovium of sufficient size to cover the exposed surface is created, consisting of the synovium over the intrapatellar fat pad and 2 to 3 mm of the un-

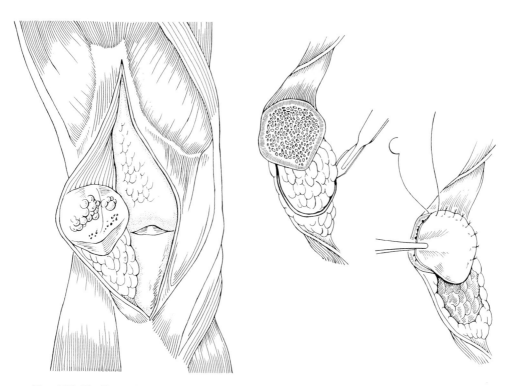

Fig. 115-18. Cave-Rowe patellar arthroplasty. (Modified from Cave,[20] with permission.)

derlying fat pad. This flap is reflected superiorly with the synovial surface against the patella and sutured in place with 2.0 interrupted Vicryl sutures. A routine closure is performed. Suction tubes are used. A bulky compression dressing is applied with the knee in full extension.

Isometric quadriceps exercises are instituted as soon as possible after surgery and are continued during the succeeding 4 weeks. On the third or fourth postoperative day, active range of motion is begun. The patient is kept on partial weight bearing for 5 to 6 weeks. At 4 weeks postsurgery, isokinetic or isotonic exercises for the quadriceps and hamstrings are begun.

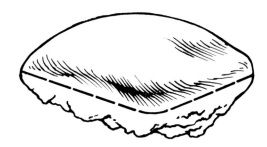

Fig. 115-19. Tangential view of patella, illustrating the amount of bone removed for subchondral exposure-type arthroplasty.

Subchondral Exposure

In this procedure, osteophytes are trimmed from the patella and the femoral condyles. The soft tissues are dissected sharply from around the patella. The subchondral bone and any remaining cartilage are cut from the posterior surface of the patella (Fig. 115-19). The normal angulation between the facets is maintained such that the articulating surface is still V shaped; this is done to attain maximum contact and stability. If the femoral condyles are eburnated, multiple drill holes are made on the surfaces, as advocated by Pridie and reported by Insall.[56] With the exceptions mentioned, the exposure, closure, and postoperative care are the same as for the Cave-Rowe procedure.

Hemiarthroplasty

The McKeever prosthesis[80] is a device fixed with a screw to the posterior aspect of the patella. Metallic prostheses fixed to the patella with methylmethacrylate have also been proposed.[3,117] For additional information and because these devices have not received wide acceptance, the reader is referred to the original articles.[3,80,117]

Total Patellofemoral Prosthesis

Resurfacing of the anterior surface of the distal femur with metal and the patella with polyethylene has been performed.[13,73] Both components are fixed with methyl methacrylate.

Patellectomy

Patellectomy is probably the most used procedure for patellofemoral arthrosis; the literature on this procedure[2,35] reports greater numbers of operations than for other procedures. The technique for patellectomy is described under Chondromalacia.

Author's Preferred Treatment

The subchondral arthroplasty without foreign material often with tibial tubercle advancement is preferred. If realignment is necessary, this is usually achieved with vastus medialis advancement and lateral release.

Complications and Results

None of these procedures except patellectomy has been sufficiently used to document numerically significant complications and results. The most common problem would most likely be lack of motion. Mobilization must be undertaken as soon as physically possible for any given procedure. Manipulation under anesthesia should also be considered. All investigators cited report encouraging results for the procedure presented. No one procedure has produced sufficiently dramatic results to justify its selection with enthusiasm. Even moderate improvement is considered a good result. It is hoped that future developments in implant arthroplasty surgery will produce better results for this problem.

FRACTURES OF THE PATELLA

Background

Fractures of the patella are predominantly intra-articular fractures of a sesamoid bone. The goals of treatment are restoration of the extensor mechanism and perfect restoration of the articulating surface. In contrast to most other intraarticular fractures, the selection of treatment must take into consideration tensile stress on the bone, as well as compressive stress. The literature contains numerous reports of varying quality pertaining to fractures of the patella, but the report by Boström[16] is probably the single most significant.

Fractures of the patella involve people of all ages, but the mean age generally falls within the fifth decade. Males are approximately twice as susceptible to these fractures as females. These frac-tures constitute approximately 1 percent of skeletal injuries.[16]

Mechanisms of Injury

Indirect force is an accepted mechanism of fracture, as is the more obvious application of direct force.[32,82] Fractures caused by indirect force are thought to occur if the quadriceps muscle forcibly contracts and the knee is partially flexed; this results if a person tries to recover equilibrium after a stumble or a fall. These types of fractures are usually transverse. The vulnerable position of the patella exposes it to direct violence, such as dashboard impact.

Classification

To determine therapy, patellar fractures must be classified in three models (Fig. 115-20): (1) open or closed fracture (integrity of the skin); (2) amount of

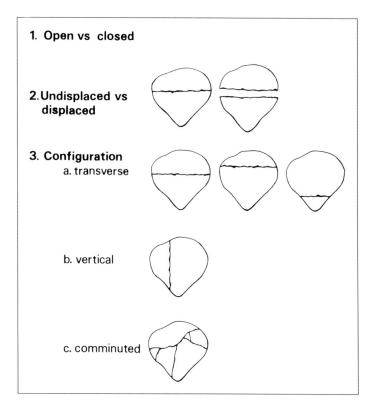

Fig. 115-20. Classification of patellar fractures.

displacement; and (3) configuration of fracture. The most common configuration of patellar fractures is the transverse.[16] This type can be subdivided into transverse fractures across the midportion of the patella and fractures of the upper and lower poles. Vertical and stellate, or comminuted, are the other two main patterns of fracture.

Diagnosis

The diagnosis of patellar fractures should present little difficulty. The presence of active knee extension must not dissuade the practitioner from making this diagnosis, as extension is possible if the retinaculum is intact. A defect in the bone or crepitation may be present with palpation. In most cases, anterior and posterior radiographs are sufficient for the diagnosis and determination of therapy. Before closed treatment is elected, however, a tangential view is necessary for detection of vertical fractures and determination of displacement. Knowledge of such anomalies as bipartite patella is necessary when one is interpreting radiographs.

Treatment

The treatment options vary from closed treatment to total patellectomy. At the middle of the spectrum are open reduction and partial patellectomy.

Nonoperative Treatment

Nonoperative treatment is indicated if the extensor retinaculum is intact and if displacement of fragments is minimal. The extensor retinaculum is intact if the patient can actively extend the knee. On the basis of a large follow-up study, Boström[16] accepts up to a 3- to 4-mm diastasis and up to a 2- to 3-mm stepoff between the fragments as the upper limits for nonoperative treatment. Most probably, these should be shaded for extremes in age and degree of desired physical activity. I would accept less displacement, especially stepoff, in a 20-year-old high-performance athlete and more displacement in an 80-year-old nursing home patient.

Nonoperative treatment consists of knee immobilization in full extension, in a plaster dressing for

4 weeks, with care to avoid hyperextension. For some conscientious patients, a knee immobilizer is a sufficient dressing. Aspiration of hematomata under aseptic conditions may be desirable. Crutch use with partial weight bearing is generally prescribed. Isometric quadriceps drill is performed during the period of immobilization.

Operative Treatment

Operative treatment is indicated for all open fractures and for those closed and displaced fractures that do not meet the criteria for closed treatment. For open fractures, the basic principles of wound care are followed. The timing of internal fixation must depend on a surgeon's appraisal of the wound. In many cases, definitive treatment can be carried out at initial surgery.

Open Reduction and Internal Fixation

Most displaced fractures are amenable to open reduction and internal fixation. The most effective suture material is 18-gauge wire. The wire may need to be removed after the fracture has healed, but little if any justification exists for using less adequate suture materials, which often fail. Repair of the medial and lateral retinaculum, if torn, must be performed after internal fixation has been achieved. Several methods of fixation exist that include various forms of wiring and screw fixation; four are presented below.

A recent biomechanical study[111] on the efficiency of various forms of fixation for transverse fractures showed that fixation with wire in direct contact with the bone was superior to forms without direct contact. When the specimens were stressed during range of motion, the tension-band method modified with longitudinal K-wires and the Magnuson techniques allowed negligible motion between the fragments, but under similar circumstances the conventional tension-band method and the circumferential wire method permitted much interfragment motion.

Transverse incisions are suggested by many authorities for operative treatment of patellar fractures. Although this type of incision is most often adequate for the initial procedure, its subsequent versatility is limited. Therefore, a median parapatellar incision is advocated.

Circumferential Wiring This is commonly used for both transverse fractures and for fractures with minimal comminution. The technique involves weaving the wire in the soft tissue around the patella and tightening the wire while the fracture is held in a reduced position (Fig. 115-21). The wire must be applied as close to the patella as possible to avoid slippage and loss of position. The wire is tightened with a wire tightener and is twisted. A common fault is to position the wire too far anteriorly such that the articular surface hinges open (Fig. 115-22).

Magnuson Technique This technique[76] is basically a horizontal mattress suture passing within the patella. It is used with transverse fractures (Fig. 115-23). Two drill holes are made from the superior pole of the patella on each side of the quadriceps tendon that exit on the fracture surface just posterior to the midfrontal plane. Two holes are then made in the distal fragment, exiting on each side of the patellar ligament. The wire is passed as shown in Figure 115-23. Care must be taken that the holes on the fracture surface of the two frag-

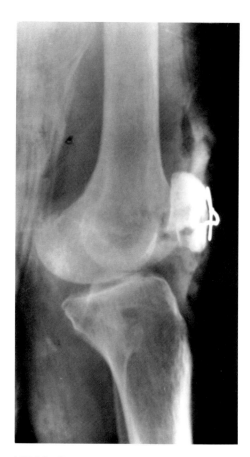

Fig. 115-22. Radiograph showing circumferential wire placed too far anteriorly, so that reduction was not maintained. This fracture went on to complete disruption.

ments correspond, or the reduction will be imperfect. The fragments are held reduced while the wire is tightened and twisted.

Standard Tension-Band Technique This technique[89] uses two longitudinal wires across the anterior aspect of the patella (Fig. 115-24). The first wire is passed as shown deep to both the insertion of the quadriceps tendon and the patellar ligament. The second wire is more superficial and passes at both poles through Sharpey's fibers. A slight overcorrection is sought that corrects with knee flexion. The originators of the technique consider immobilization unnecessary.

Modified Tension-Band Technique This technique (Fig. 115-25) was proposed for comminuted fractures,[89] but it works well for transverse frac-

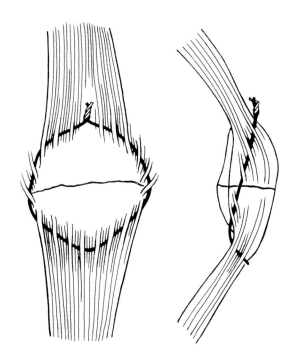

Fig. 115-21. Circumferential wiring for transverse patellar fracture.

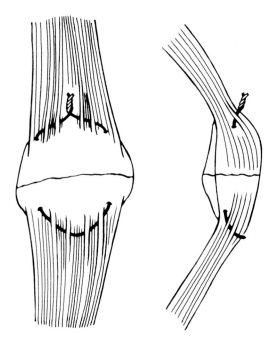

Fig. 115-23. Magnuson technique for fixation of transverse fracture of patella. (From Magnuson,[76] with permission.)

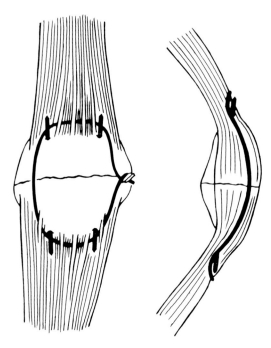

Fig. 115-25. Modified tension-band technique for fractures of the patella. (From Müller,[89] with permission.)

tures. Two vertical K-wires are drilled through the reduced fragments. A circumferential wire is passed around the K-wires where they exit from bone and is tightened. Figure 115-26 shows a variation of this technique.

Partial Patellectomy

Partial patellectomy is chosen if one pole can be saved and not the other. Most authorities[4,105] advocate excision of the lower pole, but Scapinelli[103] advocates excision of the upper pole. Scapinelli's recommendation was made because much of the patellar blood supply enters through the inferior pole, and avascular necrosis has been seen in the remaining superior pole. The decision as to which pole to excise is often superfluous; if a true choice exists, the whole patella usually can be saved. Partial patellectomy should be selected in preference to total patellectomy if at all possible because partial patellectomy offers better function.[16]

Technique A horizontal mattress technique similar to that of the Magnuson procedure is effective. The significant procedure is to reapproximate the

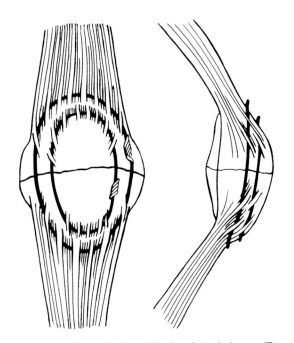

Fig. 115-24. Standard tension-band technique. (From Müller,[89] with permission.)

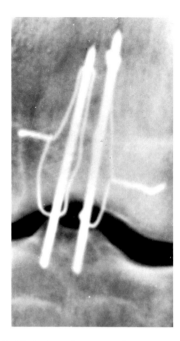

Fig. 115-26. Variation of the modified tension-band technique utilizing individual circumferential wires over each K-wire.

remaining soft tissue to the center of the fracture surface so that the patella does not tilt (Fig. 115-27). Some displaced vertical fractures are best treated by fragment excision. Most small marginal vertical fractures will heal; if they do not, the fragment should be excised.

Total Patellectomy

Total patellectomy is the procedure of choice only if no other patellar-saving procedure is feasible. If patellectomy is elected, the fragments are excised, and the soft tissues, including the retinaculum, are reapproximated. Small fragments of the two poles may be retained and reapproximated in an extraarticular manner. The retained fragments provide firm anchorage.

Author's Preferred Method for Treatment

My indications for open treatment are those stated. The modified tension-band wiring is the preferred method of fixation. The circumferential wire technique is used in some comminuted frac-

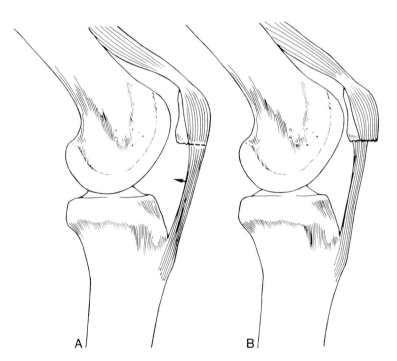

Fig. 115-27. Proper and improper techniques for partial patellectomy. **(A)** Patellar ligament sutured too far anteriorly, resulting in a tilted patella. **(B)** Proper position of patellar ligament.

tures that can be pulled together effectively by this technique.

Postoperative Care

Postoperative care is similar for all procedures except the unmodified tension-band technique. A soft cotton dressing with plaster splints is used for 2 to 3 days; this is followed by a plaster cylinder that is removed 4 weeks after surgery. Although the modified tension-band and Magnuson techniques provide rigid fixation,the originators of tension-band wiring advocate immediate motion, and the benefits of early motion are noted. I still use a cast or a knee immobilizer. If immobilization is not used, the patient is forced into a race between fixation failure and fracture healing. After motion is attained, a muscle-strengthening program appropriate for the patient is begun.

Complications

Breakdown of the repair is rare if metal fixation is used in a proper way and if immobilization is used. If there is disruption of a fracture, the only choice is to repeat the repair. Restriction of motion is avoided by limiting the period of immobilization after surgery and by prompt initiation of a rehabilitation program. If limited flexion is not improved by very gentle manipulation under anesthesia, I would probably perform an open lysis of the adhesions before resorting to a vigorous manipulation.

Avascular necrosis is thought rare, but Scapinelli[103] reported a 25 percent incidence in 165 transverse fractures; most necrosis occurred in the upper pole. Fortunately the problem did not influence the prognosis, and no special treatment was needed.

Osteoarthrosis may well result from the initial trauma. The one variable controlled by the physician is the achievement of the best reduction possible.

Prognosis

On the basis of a follow-up study of 320 patients, Boström[16] drew several conclusions regarding prognosis after patellar fractures. Excellent and good results were seen in 92 percent of the total series, 99 percent in those treated closed, and 79 percent in those requiring operative treatment. Patients with open fractures and concomitant injury were more likely to obtain a poor result. The results of partial patellectomy were equal to those of osteosynthesis and inferior to those achieved with patellectomy.

REFERENCES

1. Abernethy PJ, Townsend PR, Rose RM, et al: Is chondromalacia patellate a separate clinical entity? J Bone Joint Surg 60B:205, 1978
2. Ackroyd CE, Polyzoides AJ: Patellectomy for osteoarthritis. A study of eighty-one patients followed from two to twenty-two years. J Bone Joint Surg 60B:353, 1978
3. Aglietti P, Insall JN, Walker PS, et al: A new patella prosthesis. Clin Orthop 107:175, 1975
4. Stewart M: In Crenshaw AH (ed): Campbell's Operative Orthopaedics, 5th Ed. CV Mosby, St. Louis, 1971 Dislocations. p. 450.
5. Baker RH, Carroll N, Dewar FP, et al: The semitendinosus tenodesis for recurrent dislocation of the patella. J Bone Joint Surg 54B:103, 1972
6. Ballard A: Patellar dislocations. Presented at the Annual Meeting of the American Orthopaedics Society for Sports Medicine, New Orleans, July 1975
7. Bandi W: Chondromalacia patellae und femoropatellare Arthrose. Helv Chir Acta 1 (suppl):3, 1972
8. Bassett FH III: Surgery of the patellofemoral joint. p. 40. In American Academy of Orthopaedic Surgeons Instructional Course Lectures. Vol. 25. CV Mosby, St. Louis, 1976
9. Bentley G: The surgical treatment of chondromalacia patellae. J Bone Joint Surg 60B:74, 1978
10. Bentley G: Chondromalacia patellae. J Bone Joint Surg 52A:221, 1979
11. Bentley G: Articular cartilage changes in chondromalacia patella. J Bone Joint Surg 67B:769, 1985
12. Blasier RB, Ciullo JV: Rupture of the quadriceps tendon after arthroscopic lateral release. Arthrosc Rel Surg 2:262, 1986
13. Blazina ME, Fox JM, Del Pizzo W, et al: Patellofemoral replacement. Clin Orthop 144:98, 1979
14. Blumensaat C: Die Lageabweichungen und Verrenkungen der Kniescheibe. Ergeb Chir Orthop 31:149, 1938

15. Boring TH, O'Donoghue DH: Acute patellar dislocation: Results of immediate surgical repair. Clin Orthop 136:182, 1978

16. Boström A: Fractures of the patella. Acta Orthop Scand 143 (suppl):1, 1972

17. Bowker JH, Thompson EB: Surgical treatment of recurrent dislocation of the patella. J Bone Joint Surg 46A:1451, 1964

18. Brown DE, Alexander AH, Lichtman DM: The Elmslie-Trillat procedure: evaluation in patellar dislocation and subluxation. Am J Sports Med 12:104, 1984

19. Carson WG Jr, James SL, Larson RL, et al: Patellofemoral disorders: physical and radiographic evaluation. I and II. Clin Orthop 185:165, 1984

20. Cave EF, Rowe CR: The patella. Its importance in derangement of the knee. J Bone Joint Surg 32A:542, 1950

21. Chen SC, Ramanathan EBS: The treatment of patellar instability by lateral release. J Bone Joint Surg 66B:344, 1984

22. Chrisman OD, Snook GA: The role of patelloplasty and patellectomy in the arthritic knee. Clin Orthop 101:40, 1974

23. Chrisman OD, Snook GA, Wilson TC: A long-term prospective study of the Hauser and Roux-Goldthwait procedures for recurrent patellar dislocation. Clin Orthop 144:27, 1979

24. Cofield RH, Bryan RS: Acute dislocation of the patella: Results of conservative treatment. J Trauma 17:526, 1977

25. Cox JS: An evaluation of the Elmslie-Trillat procedure for management of patellar dislocations and subluxations: a preliminary report. Am J Sports Med 4:72, 1976

26. Cox JS: Evaluation of the Roux-Elmslie-Trillat procedure for knee extensor realignment. Am J Sports Med 10:303, 1982

27. Crosby EB, Insall J: Recurrent dislocation of the patella: relation of treatment to osteoarthritis. J Bone Joint Surg 58A:9, 1976

28. Darracott J, Vernon-Roberts B: The bony changes in chondromalacia patellae. Rheum Phys Med 11:175, 1971

29. DeCesare WF: Late results of Hauser procedure for recurrent dislocation of the patella. Clin Orthop 140:137, 1979

30. DeHaven KE, Dolan WA, Mayer PJ: Chondromalacia patella in athletes. Am J Sports Med 7:5, 1979

31. Denham RA, Bishop RED: Mechanics of the knee and problems in reconstructive surgery. J Bone Joint Surg 60B:345, 1978

32. DePalma AF: Diseases of the Knee. JB Lippincott, Philadelphia, 1954

33. DePalma AF: The Management of Fractures and Dislocations. An Atlas, p. 1463. WB Saunders, Philadelphia, 1970

34. Devas M, Golski A: Treatment of chondromalacia patellae by transposition of the tibial tubercle. Br Med J 1:589, 1973

35. Dinham JM, French PR: Results of patellectomy for osteoarthritis. Postgrad Med J 48:590, 1972

36. Fairbank JCT, Pynsent PB, Poorvliet JA, Phillips H: Mechanical factors in the incidence of knee pain in adolescents and young adults. J Bone Joint Surg 66B:685, 1984

37. Ferguson AB Jr: Elevation of the insertion of the patellar ligament for patellofemoral pain. J Bone Joint Surg 64A:766, 1982

38. Ferguson AB, Brown TD, Fu FH, et al: Relief of patellofemoral contact stress by anterior displacement of the tibial tubercle. J Bone Joint Surg 61A:159, 1979

39. Ficat RP, Hungerford DS: Disorders of the Patellofemoral Joint. Williams & Wilkins, Baltimore, 1977

40. Fielding JW, Liebler WA, Tambakis A: The effect of a tibial-tubercle transplant in children on the growth of the upper tibial epiphysis. J Bone Joint Surg 42A:1426, 1960

41. Fondren FB, Goldner JL, Bassett FH III: Recurrent dislocation of the patella treated by the modified Roux-Goldthwait procedure. J Bone Joint Surg 67A:993, 1985

42. Fulkerson JP, Tennant R, Jaivin JS, Grunnet M: Histologic evidence of retinacular nerve injury associated with patellofemoral malalignment. Clin Orthop 197:196, 1985

43. Garland DE, Hughston JC: Peroneal nerve paralysis: a complication of extensor reconstruction of the knee. Clin Orthop 140:169, 1979

44. Goodfellow J, Hungerford DS, Woods C: 1. Patello-femoral joint mechanics and pathology. 2. Chondromalacia patellae. J Bone Joint Surg 58B:291, 1976

45. Hall JE, Micheli LJ, McManama GB Jr: Semitendinosus tenodesis for recurrent subluxation or dislocation of the patella. Clin Orthop 144:31, 1979

46. Hampson WGJ, Hill P: Late results of transfer of the tibial tubercle for recurrent dislocation of the patella. J Bone Joint Surg 57B:209, 1975

47. Hawkins RJ, Bell RH, Anisette G: Acute patellar dislocations: The natural history. Am J Sports Med 14:117, 1986

48. Henry JH, Crosland JW: Conservative treatment

of patellofemoral subluxation. Am J Sports Med 7:12, 1979

49. Henry JH, Goletz TH, Williamson B: Lateral retinacular release in patellofemoral subluxation: indications, results, and comparison to open patellofemoral reconstruction. Am J Sports Med 14:121, 1986

50. Heywood AWB: Recurrent dislocation of the patella: a study of its pathology and treatment in 106 knees. J Bone Joint Surg 43B:508, 1961

51. Huberti HH, Hayes WC: Patellofemoral contact pressures: the influence of Q-angle and tendofemoral contact. J Bone Joint Surg 66A:715, 1984

52. Hughston JC: Subluxation of the patella. J Bone Joint Surg 50A:1003, 1968

53. Hughston JC: Reconstruction of the extensor mechanism for subluxating patella. J Sports Med 1:6, 1972

54. Hughston JC, Walsh WM: Proximal and distal reconstruction of the extensor mechanism for patellar subluxation. Clin Orthop 144:36, 1979

55. Hughston JC, Walsh WM, Puddu G: Patellar Subluxation and Dislocation. WB Saunders, Philadelphia, 1984

56. Insall JN: Intra-articular surgery for degenerative arthritis of the knee. A report of the work of the late KH Pridie. J Bone Joint Surg 49B:211, 1967

57. Insall JN, Bullough PG, Burstein AH: Proximal "tube" realignment of the patella for chondromalacia patellae. Clin Orthop 144:63, 1979

58. Insall J, Falvo KA, Wise DW: Chondromalacia patellae: a prospective study. J Bone Joint Surg 58A:1, 1976

59. Insall J, Goldberg V, Salvati E: Recurrent dislocation and the high-riding patella. Clin Orthop 88:67, 1972

60. Insall J, Salvati E: Patella position in the normal knee joint. Radiology 101:101, 1971

61. Jacobsen K, Bertheussen K: The vertical location of the patella. Acta Orthop Scand 45:436, 1974

62. Jakobsen J, Christensen KS, Rasmussen OS: Patellectomy—a 20-year follow-up. Acta Orthop Scand 56:430, 1985

63. Jeffreys TE: Recurrent dislocation of the patella due to abnormal attachment of the ilio-tibial tract. J Bone Joint Surg 45B:740, 1963

64. Johnson LL: The treatment of chondromalacia of the patella by a transcutaneous arthroscopic method using the intra-articular shaver: a new surgical device. Orthop Trans 3:289, 1979

65. Karlson S: Chondromalacia patella. Acta Chir Scand 83:349, 1939

66. Karlsson J, Bunketrop O, Lansinger O, et al: Lowering of the patella secondary to anterior advancement of the tibial tubercle for the patellofemoral pain syndrome. Arch Orthop Trauma Surg 105:40, 1986

67. Kaufer H: Mechanical function of the patella. J Bone Joint Surg 53A:1551, 1971

68. Kettelkamp DB, DeRosa GP: Surgery of the patellofemoral joint. p. 25. In American Academy of Orthopaedic Surgeons Instructional Course Lectures. Vol. 25. 1976

69. Kummel BM, Crutchlow WP: Stabilization of the subluxating patella by semitendinosus transfer to the lateral third of the infrapatellar tendon. Am J Sports Med 5:194, 1977

70. Laurin CA, Dussault R, Levesque HP: The tangential x-ray investigation of the patellofemoral joint: x-ray technique, diagnostic criteria and their interpretation. Clin Orthop 144:16, 1979

71. Laurin CA, Levesque HP, Dussault R, et al: The abnormal lateral patellofemoral angle: a diagnostic roentgenographic sign of recurrent patellar subluxation. J Bone Joint Surg 60A:55, 1978

72. Lieb FJ, Perry J: Quadriceps function. J Bone Joint Surg 50A:1535, 1968

73. Lubinus HH: Patella guide bearing total replacement. Orthopedics 2:120, 1979

74. Macnab I: Recurrent dislocation of the patella. J Bone Joint Surg 34A:957, 1952

75. Madigan R, Wissinger HA, Donaldson WF: Preliminary experience with a method of quadricepsplasty in recurrent subluxation of the patella. J Bone Joint Surg 57A:600, 1975

76. Magnuson PB: Fractures. 3rd Ed. JB Lippincott, Philadelphia, 1939

77. Maquet PBJ: Biomechanics of the Knee, With Application to the Pathogenesis and the Surgical Treatment of Osteoarthritis. p. 204. Springer-Verlag, Berlin, 1976

78. Marks KE, Bentley G: Patella alta and chondromalacia. J Bone Joint Surg 60B:71, 1978

79. Martinez S, Korobkin M, Fondren FB, et al: Diagnosis of patellofemoral malalignment by computer tomography. Computer Assist Tomog 7:1050, 1983

80. McKeever DC: Patellar prosthesis. J Bone Joint Surg 37A:1074, 1955

81. McManus F, Rang M, Heslin DJ: Acute dislocation of the patella in children: the natural history. Clin Orthop 139:88, 1979

82. McMaster PE: Fractures of the patella. Clin Orthop 4:24, 1954

83. Merchant AC, Mercer RL: Lateral release of the patella. Clin Orthop 103:40, 1974

84. Miller GF: Familial recurrent dislocation of the patella. J Bone Joint Surg 60B:203, 1978

85. Møller BN, Krebs B, Jurik AG: Patellofemoral incongruence in chondromalacia and instability of the patella. Acta Orthop Scand 57:232, 1986

86. Morrison JB: Function of the knee joint in various activities. Biomed Eng 4:573, 1969

87. Morrison JB: The mechanics of the knee joint in relation to normal walking. Biomechanics 3:51, 1970

88. Morscher E: Osteotomy of the patella in chondromalacia: preliminary report. Arch Orthop Traumatol Surg 92:139, 1978

89. Müller ME, Allgöwer M, Willenegger H: Manual of Internal Fixation. Springer-Verlag, New York, 1979

90. Nakamura N, Ellis M, Seedhom BB: Advancement of the tibial tuberosity: a biomechanical study. J Bone Joint Surg 67B:255, 1985

91. O'Donoghue DH: Facetectomy of the patella. In Proceedings of the International Knee Society, April 26, 1979

92. O'Donoghue DH, Tompkins F, Hays MB: Strength of quadriceps function after patellectomy. West J Surg Obstet Gynecol 60:159, 1952

93. Ogilvie-Harris DJ, Jackson RW: The arthroscopic treatment of chondromalacia patellae. J Bone Joint Surg 66B:660, 1984

94. Outerbridge RE: The aetiology of chondromalacia patellae. J Bone Joint Surg 43B:752, 1961

95. Outerbridge RE: Further studies on the aetiology of chondromalacia patellae. J Bone Joint Surg 46B:179, 1964

96. Outerbridge RE, Dunlop JAY: The problem of chondromalacia patellae. Clin Orthop 110:177, 1975

97. Perry J, Antonelli D, Ford W: Analysis of knee-joint forces during flexed-knee stance. J Bone Joint Surg 57A:961, 1975

98. Radin EL: The Maquet procedure — anterior displacement of the tibial tubercle. Clin Orthop 213:241, 1986

99. Radin E, Leach R: Anterior displacement of tibial tubercle for patello-femoral arthrosis. Orthop Trans 3:291, 1979

100. Rorabeck CH, Bobechko WP: Acute dislocation of the patella with osteochondral fracture. J Bone Joint Surg 58B:237, 1976

101. Rozbruch JD, Campbell RD, Insall J: Tibial tubercle elevation (Maquet operation): a clinical study of thirty-one cases. Orthop Trans 3:291, 1979

102. Sasaki T, Yagi T: Subluxation of the patella: investigation by computerized tomography. Intern Orthop (SICOT) 10:115, 1986

103. Scapinelli R: Blood supply of the human patella. Its relation to ischaemic necrosis after fracture. J Bone Joint Surg 49B:563, 1967

104. Smidt GL: Biomechanical analysis of knee flexion and extension. J Biomech 6:79, 1973

105. Smillie IS: Injuries of the Knee Joint. 5th Ed. Churchill Livingstone, Edinburgh, 1978

106. Stougard J: Chondromalacia of the patella. Incidence, macroscopical and radiographical findings at autopsy. Acta Orthop Scand 46:809, 1975

107. Sutton FS, Thompson C, Lipke J, et al: The effect of patellectomy on knee function. J Bone Joint Surg 58A:537, 1976

108. Templeman D, McBeath AA: Iatrogenic patellar malalignment following the Roux-Goldthwait procedure, corrected by dynamic intraoperative realignment. J Bone Joint Surg 68A:1096, 1986

109. Waisbrod H, Treiman N: Intra-osseous venography in patellofemoral disorders. J Bone Joint Surg 62B:454, 1980

110. Wall JJ: Compartment syndrome as a complication of the Hauser procedure. J Bone Joint Surg 61A:185, 1979

111. Weber MJ, Janecki CJ, McLeod P, et al: Efficacy of various forms of fixation of transverse fractures of the patella. J Bone Joint Surg 62A:215, 1980

112. West FE: End results of patellectomy. J Bone Joint Surg 44A:1080, 1962

113. West FE, Soto-Hall R: Recurrent dislocation of the patella in the adult. End results of patellectomy with quadricepsplasty. J Bone Joint Surg 40A:386, 1958

114. Wiberg G: Roentgenographic and anatomic studies on the femoropatella joint. With special reference to chondromalacia patellae. Acta Orthop Scand 12:319, 1941

115. Wiles P, Andrews PS, Bremner RA: Chondromalacia of the patella. A study of the later results of excision of the articular cartilage. J Bone Joint Surg 42B:65, 1960

116. Wilppula E, Vahvanen V: Chondromalacia of the patella. Acta Orthop Scand 42:531, 1971

117. Worrell RV: Prosthetic resurfacing of the patella. Clin Orthop 144:91, 1979

Articular Fractures of the Proximal Tibia

116

Mason Hohl
Tillman M. Moore

The diagnosis and management of articular fractures of the proximal tibia continue to improve. Careful analysis of a large series reporting on fractures has provided a better scientific basis for treatment, with the result that an even greater percentage of injured knees than previously have achieved near-normal appearance, function, and stability.[4,5,7,9,14,15,17,18,22,25,35,37,41,53,55,56,59,69,71] The principles of accurate articular restoration and early resumption of knee movement are reaffirmed as basic to obtaining a good result.

We approach this broad subject with a classification of fracture types designed to aid in the selection of the most appropriate and effective treatment in a given situation. This chapter emphasizes the key elements of diagnosis, treatment, and aftercare of the various fracture types, with our preferences clearly delineated.

DIAGNOSTIC TECHNIQUES

Decision making regarding the treatment of a particular knee fracture is aided if the surgeon knows the patient, the mechanism of injury, the clinical stability of the knee, and its radiographic appearance. The mechanism causing the plateau fracture together with the radiographic appearance often predicts the likelihood of associated ligamentous injury.

Clinical evaluation of the injured knee by stress testing has proved particularly useful in deciding whether surgical treatment would be helpful. The reason for knee instability may be loss of articular level from fracture, ligament injury, or both. Rasmussen[56] suggested that a fractured knee with less than 10 degrees of instability in extension be considered stable and with 10 degrees or more of instability be considered unstable; the stable knee achieves a generally acceptable result by nonsurgical means, and the unstable knee is improved by surgical treatment. This concept has been used by many surgeons and has proved of considerable value. We use clinical stress testing under analgesia or anesthesia with the knee in extension and also in 20 to 30 degrees of flexion to detect instability and to aid in formulating therapeutic decisions. Stress films are usually necessary to document the exact cause of the instability, but in any event surgical treatment is usually beneficial to unstable knees.[13,15,30,36,59,71]

Radiographic examination using anteroposterior (AP) and lateral projections usually reveals the fracture but often leaves considerable doubt as to depth of depression or amount of displacement and fracture configuration. In order to make the best treatment decisions and especially in the event that surgery is contemplated, the surgeon should document the fracture completely and clearly. For this reason, other radiographs, such as obliques, plateau views, tomograms, and computed tomograms (CT), are ordered selectively. The oblique views help to determine the AP location of fracture, while the plateau view and tomograms delineate articular depression with greater accuracy.[19,50] The plateau view taken as an anteroposterior 10 to 15-degree caudal projection is especially helpful in compression-type fractures.[48] CT scans clearly indicate the displacement of articular fragments.[16,54]

The diagnosis of associated ligament injury is suggested in routine radiographic views by widening of the cartilage space on the side opposite the fracture or the finding of avulsion fractures from the femoral or tibial condyles, fibular head, or intercondylar region.[1,44,73] This presumptive evidence should be substantiated by stress testing in valgus and varus and as necessary in the anteroposterior plane.[20] Also, in those fractures with clinical instability, the reason for the instability should be documented by radiography (Fig. 116-1). In patients for whom surgery is going to be performed this study can be deferred to the operating room and done after induction of anesthesia. It should be noted that the forces exerted during stress testing are small compared with those that initially produce the fracture, so that although the fracture may

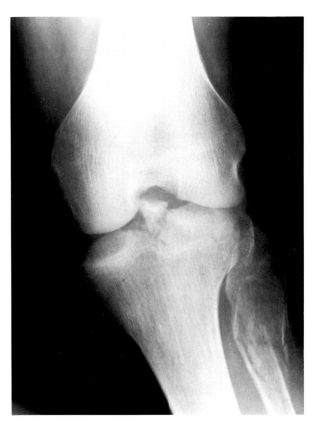

Fig. 116-1. This 48-year-old man was struck by an automobile. Note entire condyle fracture with separate intercondylar fragment and medial widening in this stress film.

displace during stress testing it will spring back to its original position subsequently without permanent harm to the knee.

Arthroscopic examination is being used increasingly to evaluate the menisci, cruciate ligaments and fracture configuration.[10,33,52,57] An added advantage may be the elimination of debris from the joint.

FRACTURE SEQUELAE

To know the problems and treatment complications of proximal tibial articular fractures is to be forewarned and forearmed against them. Understanding the reasons that these sequelae develop provides a background from which to make optimal treatment and postoperative decisions so as to ensure the best possible result for the patient. The sequelae discussed here are the most frequent and include limited movement, instability, angular deformity, and traumatic arthritis. Nonunion is rare, but malunion is quite frequent.[29,65]

The fractured knee evokes a tremendous fibrous and bony healing reaction. The more extensive the injury or invasive the treatment, the greater the reaction that is provoked. Such an injured knee, when immobilized, stiffens progressively as fibrous pannus grows from fractured areas to adjacent synovia, eventually forming cords of dense adhesive scar.[31,40] These dense adhesions lyse only slowly and incompletely during the months following termination of immobilization, often leaving an unacceptable degree of permanent stiffness. Experimental work on primates demonstrated conclusively that early movement prevents the formation and maturing of these adhesions.[31]

Clinical studies indicate that although motion begun in the first week after injury or surgery is probably best, motion in 3 to 4 weeks can still lead to the recovery of full movement.[22] When traction treatment is used, knee movement through a 90 degree range should be provided for with an exerciser device.[2,32,42,59] The advantage of a cast-brace or open reduction after secure internal fixation is the ability to move the knee early.

Continuous passive motion machines are being used by many to provide early knee movement in the recovery room and for a few days thereafter.[61,62] The advantages include greater patient comfort, and early recovery of up to 90 degrees of knee motion. The disadvantages include the possibility of skin incisional problems. It is only applicable after rigid internal fixation.

We advocate and practice early mobilization of proximal tibial articular fractures that are uncomplicated by associated injuries. We also advocate aggressive treatment of ipsilateral femoral or tibial fractures to permit early knee movement.

A knee lacking full extension by 5 to 10 degrees is impaired because of the inevitable limp, walking inefficiency, and tiring produced. Unfortunately, this is an all-too-common sequel to proximal tibial articular fractures, and it is preventable in many instances. The avoidable cause is treatment of the fracture in flexion, with either a flexed-knee cast or traction in flexion, permitting intra-articular adhesions to bind down the fat pad and menisci. Prevention by treatment with a straight-knee cast or with the resting fraction position in extension is far easier than the repetitive therapy usually prescribed after a contracture has developed.

Residual instability of the knee occurs because of articular depression, ligament laxity, or both. It is generally accepted that the unstable knee tends to develop traumatic degenerative changes at an accelerated rate. Instability may be predicted by the initial clinical stress testing, with appropriate surgical means employed to restore and maintain normal articular level and to repair ligament injuries. Late surgical treatment of instability is unsatisfactory and incomplete; thus, it is doubly important to diagnose and restore stability early.[15]

Angular deformity into valgus or varus occurs to some extent after many tibial plateau fractures because of failure to achieve and maintain the correct articular level of one or both condyles.[25] The loss of 4 to 5 mm of articular height creates an angular deformity that may not be significant, but generally an 8 to 10-mm displacement will lead to a very recognizable deformity. Although it is true that the knee tolerates valgus deformity better than varus, valgus is still a problem best avoided rather than treated late by osteotomy.

Traumatic arthritis is the degenerative reaction of an injured knee to articular surface incongruity, joint instability, or angular deformity, especially into varus. Avoidance or minimization of causative factors should, in most patients, lessen the need for subsequent measures to treat arthritis. Traumatic arthritis has been variously estimated to occur in 10 to 50 percent of injured knees.[25,46] The wide range of these figures is testimony to the lack of definition of the problem and failure to measure the changes against the opposite knee as a control.

Pain and loss of strength are not frequent sequelae at long-term follow-up; when present, they are usually seen in those patients with traumatic arthritic changes or varus knees. From this group of patients will often come those few subsequently requiring osteotomy or arthroplasty of the knee.

CLASSIFICATION

Articular fractures of the proximal tibia are classified to aid the clinician in thinking about the therapeutic problems peculiar to a particular fracture configuration. Most published classifications recognize compression, wedge, and bicondylar types, and a few authorities have included other types on the basis of their own observations of a change in behavior or different fracture line. Some have attempted to subclassify into types that are stable — thus minor and posing no treatment problem — or unstable — thus major and requiring sophisticated knowledge and judgment.

We have used the Hohl classification for many years, recognizing that some observed fractures did not fit the six categories either by anatomic configuration or behavior (Fig. 116-2). It was fur-

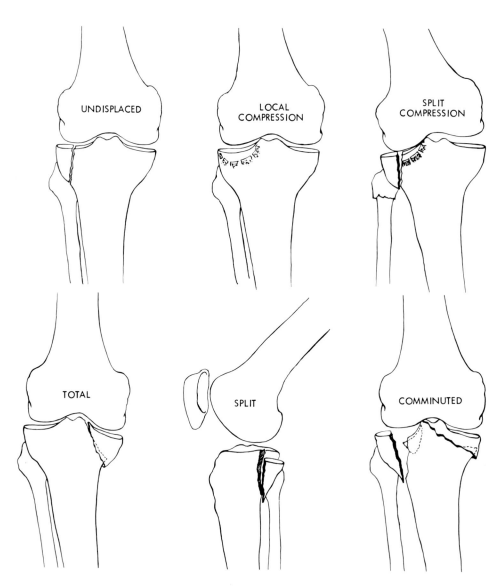

Fig. 116-2. Classification of tibial condylar fractures. (From Hohl,[24] with permission.)

ther observed by one of us (T.M.M.) that many of these unclassified fractures had a high incidence of soft tissue injury, poorer results, and represented 11 percent of upper tibial fractures.[47] A classification of proximal tibial articular fractures was thus developed, including fracture dislocations of the knee (Fig. 116-3).

The split fracture of the plateau fracture classification, by virtue of its nature, was moved into the fracture dislocation group. With this change, the plateau fractures represent those reproducible in the experimental laboratory as compression fractures of the articular surface, total condyle depression, or bicondylar fractures.[34] The fracture dislocations are those produced by much greater violence, and they have a 60 percent incidence of ligament injury and a much enhanced risk of an inferior result if not recognized for what they are.[47] Plateau fractures, however, are not exempt from coexisting ligament injury, and such should be considered when one is performing stress tests and selecting definitive treatment.[20]

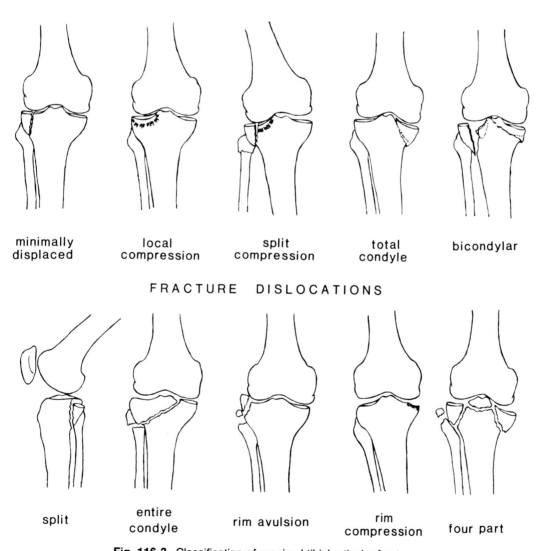

TIBIAL PLATEAU FRACTURES

minimally displaced   local compression   split compression   total condyle   bicondylar

FRACTURE DISLOCATIONS

split   entire condyle   rim avulsion   rim compression   four part

Fig. 116-3. Classification of proximal tibial articular fractures.

SOFT TISSUE INJURIES

Coexisting injuries to vessels, nerves, ligaments, or menisci are observed with sufficient frequency that the possibility of soft-tissue injury must be considered in evaluation of a fracture of the proximal tibia. It goes without saying that neurovascular injury must be tested for immediately and subsequent to the initial definitive treatment in all fractures, but certainly the incidence of such injuries is known to be higher in the fracture-dislocation group.[47] The surgeon also must remain aware of the rare possibility of compartment syndrome developing after fracture or following open reduction.

Ligamentous injury was discussed in the section on diagnosis. The incidence of injury to collateral ligaments has been variously estimated at between 10 and 50 percent of all proximal tibial articular fractures, the percentage depending somewhat upon the criteria and diligence used in diagnosis.[13,15,20,30,36,71] Moore doubts the significance of ligament injury in the plateau fracture group because in a followed series instability seemed to be accounted for by residual articular depression.[49] Moore believes that the fracture-dislocation group must be carefully assessed for ligament injury, which could significantly affect the end result. In the age group of most patients sustaining articular fractures of the proximal tibia, ligament injuries occur to a considerable extent through the ligament insertion to bone rather than through the substance of the ligament. The rapid and often complete healing that occurs with immobilization treatment of avulsive ligament injuries tends to support Moore's impression of the significance of many of these injuries. Most agree, however, that when combined bone and ligament injuries occur, surgical repair of both will lead to the most stable knee and the most predictable result.

Meniscal injuries occur in 10 to 20 percent of fractures and are less frequent than previously reported.[46] Some of these represent peripheral tears, which tend to heal with closed methods of treatment or after surgical resuture because of the intense healing pannus that accompanies the fracture. The current use of arthroscopic examination of the knee may identify and correct meniscal injuries more effectively. We advise that menisci—unless torn transversely or damaged irreparably—be preserved and resutured with little future expectation of the need for late meniscal surgery.[72]

CLOSED TREATMENT METHODS

A wide variety of treatment methods have been available over the years, with the latest development being the cast brace. Each method has advantages and disadvantages that must be considered in the selection of treatment for a particular fracture.[26,27,29]

The long-leg cast has probably been used in the treatment of more plateau fractures than all other methods combined. Unfortunately, the ease and convenience of its use are more than balanced by the restriction of movement, lack of extension, and angular deformity seen so frequently at follow-up. Prolonged immobilization favors the toughening of intra-articular adhesions to the point that months of exercise may not result in an acceptable range of motion or full extension. Apley has called this plaster disease. When using a cast, the knee is placed in extension to guide the pannus in such a way that extension is not prevented. The duration of immobilization should be 6 weeks or less, if a good final range is to be achieved, optimally less than 3 weeks. The usual long-leg cast does not efficiently control valgus or varus, especially as atrophy of thigh muscles proceeds. Fractures that have the propensity to lose position will almost inevitably do so in a cast regardless of bowleg or knock-knee stress placed on the cast.[26,29]

The cast brace, and before that the hinged cast, is the logical further development from the cast. With this device, guided movement is permitted, minimizing loss of strength and adhesion formation. It is not surprising that the cast-brace technique is being used increasingly as a primary treatment of some fractures and after traction or open reduction in others.[8,11,14,45,66] A significant advantage would appear to be that valgus or varus stress may be applied at the time hinges are affixed to effectively unweight one condyle. Caution must be observed in using the cast-brace for primary treatment; Sarmiento et al. report many unfavorable results after fracture-brace or cast-brace treatment.[63]

Traction has been and remains a dependable and effective means of maintaining reasonable alignment while permitting both movement of the knee and fracture healing. A variety of techniques for utilizing traction are in current use, but certainly Apley's system is one of the simplest and best.[2] The general principle of keeping the knee extended at rest is important, but of equal importance is insisting upon first passive and later active movement through 90 degrees in traction. The major drawback of traction is that it does not effect complete reduction in most fractures, and in some, involving both condyles or the medial condyle, it tends to decrease or eliminate the normal knee valgus. Badgley and O'Connor used traction with an alignment brace to prevent this problem,[3] and such a system is currently in use by one of us (T.M.M.).

Manipulative-reduction techniques include anesthesia, traction, and manipulation of fragments followed by some means of holding them in the final position. Today these techniques are seldom used because of the uncertainties of reduction and difficulties of maintaining position and alignment. It is useful when conditions do not permit open reduction. However, in certain fractures such treatment is compatible with a good result. Our preferred technique was learned from Ilfeld and utilized distal tibial or os calcis pin traction with 27 kg (60 pounds) on a fracture table.[32] After knee aspiration, a compression bandage is applied and radiographs are taken. Normal condylar level is restored by pushing or pounding major fragments into position; when this has been demonstrated by radiography, the fragments are compressed and impacted by a Bohler clamp or "giant nutcracker." This also should be checked by radiography. If it is satisfactory, the patient should be transferred into bed with 9 kg (20 pounds) of traction in a knee exerciser.[24] Knee motion should be started as discomfort decreases, and as the fracture solidifies traction weights should be appropriately lessened. After 5 to 6 weeks, traction can be discontinued in favor of a cast-brace or bivalved cast, used until healing is complete.

OPEN REDUCTION

Open reduction is currently used in about 45 percent of proximal tibial articular fractures; thus a thorough understanding of approaches, methods of reduction, fixation, grafting, and postoperative management is necessary. Arthroscopic techniques are being perfected to accomplish reduction and fixation.

Most fractures that require open reduction involve the lateral condyle, but a similar approach is used on the medial side. A skin incision starting just proximal to the joint line and cephalad to the fibular head passes to the patellar tendon and distally 4 to 5 cm (Fig. 116-4). With the patient's knee flexed, some iliotibial band fibers are reflected from Gerdy's tubercle, and the capsular incision is made along the proximal tibia through the meniscotibial ligament distal to the meniscus (Fig. 116-5). With some varus stress the entire meniscus is easily inspected from below. The meniscus should not be removed unless it is torn transversely or is otherwise irreparably damaged. The tibial articular surface is easily seen except for the posterior margin, which if necessary can be exposed by extending the capsular incision further posteriorly

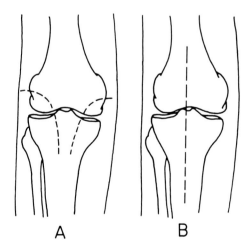

Fig. 116-4. Useful skin incisions to treat proximal tibial articular fractures. **(A)** Curvilinear skin incisions, either medial or lateral. **(B)** Midline incision for simultaneous approach to both the medial and lateral compartments of the knee.

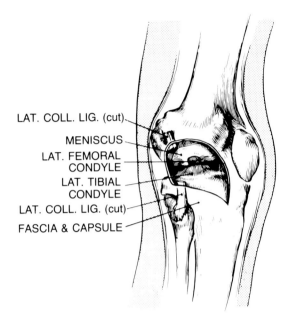

LAT. COLL. LIG. (cut)

MENISCUS

LAT. FEMORAL CONDYLE

LAT. TIBIAL CONDYLE

LAT. COLL. LIG. (cut)

FASCIA & CAPSULE

Fig. 116-5. Inframeniscal capsular approach. Lateral collateral ligament usually need not be cut. (From Hohl,[29] with permission.)

and dividing the lateral collateral ligament. Cortical bone grafts may be obtained from the lateral surface of the upper tibia by extending this skin incision down the tibial shaft.

Some bicondylar fractures require simultaneous exposure of both medial and lateral condyles. This is best accomplished by a long midline incision similar to the approach for knee replacement. The joint is entered through a parapatellar capsular incision or through separate lateral and medial capsular approaches in the inframeniscal intervals.[26,51] With comminuted proximal tibial fractures it is best to avoid osteotomy of the tibial tubercle. Should wider exposure be needed consider division of the patellar tendon in a linear fashion and proximal reflection of the patella. Careful resuture and protection is needed after this procedure. Y-shaped incisions should be used cautiously due to the incidence of skin slough, which has been noted.

Ligament injuries are repaired through conventional approaches after completion of the bony reconstruction. Structures such as the patellar tendon, fibular collateral ligament, meniscotibial ligament, and capsule should be carefully repaired as closure is effected.

POSTOPERATIVE MANAGEMENT

The best reduction and fixation of a tibial plateau fracture is no guarantee of a good result; such a result also depends upon the successful early resumption of knee motion.

Open reduction can convert a difficult and unstable fracture to an undisplaced fracture, with treatment by early motion in the manner of Rombold,[60] if rigid internal fixation is obtained. Some internal-fixation systems employ contoured buttress plates and cancellous screws and thus supply sufficient internal stability to allow the patient to begin movement after a few days in a splint or immediately in a continuous passive motion machine. Standard available internal fixation materials consisting of plates, bolts, and screws can also permit the same postoperative regimen. Compression-type fractures with elevation and grafting may use a cast brace to unweight the elevated condyle until revascularization and healing take place. Traction should be employed when open internal fixation is not completely stable, with transfer to a cast brace as stability improves.

Unreliable patients are best managed a few weeks in an extended-knee long-leg cast regardless of the stability of the fracture or its fixation. When both bony and ligamentous repair have been necessary, it is probably best to support the repairs in a cast with the optimum flexion position for ligament healing. After 4 to 6 weeks a cast brace may be used for additional support with provision for the resumption of knee movement.

Light weight bearing in a cast brace may be permitted early in an occasional fracture, but this usually is deferred for 8 to 10 weeks. Full weight bearing must await bony healing and revascularization, usually 2 to 4 months after the fracture.

TIBIAL PLATEAU FRACTURES

Minimally Displaced Fractures

Nearly one-fourth of proximal articular fractures present with depression or displacements of less than 4 mm. When these fractures are clinically stable the knees — almost regardless of treatment — are expected to do well.[31] A few days of Buck's traction with early knee movement and a knee splint removable for exercise should encourage the optimal result (Fig. 116-6).

Should the fracture involve the medial condyle or be unstable by clinical or radiographic stress testing, much more concern and thought must go into a treatment plan. The reason for clinical instability must be recognized and treated, whether it be bony instability or ligament rupture. In some fractures, especially those resembling total or entire condylar depression on the medial side, a cast-brace stressed into the knock-knee position may be tried.[12] However, it is important to obtain radiographs frequently and to change treatment promptly if the fracture begins to lose position.

Usually after 8 weeks, fracture union is secure, and further protection is not needed.

Minimally displaced fractures carry a favorable prognosis in 90 percent of cases. Most of the unsatisfactory results have either limited motion, instability, traumatic arthritis, or, rarely, angular deformity from fractures that displaced further under treatment.

Compression Fractures

Almost one-half of proximal tibial articular fractures are compression or impression fractures. Axial loading forces combined with valgus stress drive the femoral condyle into the lateral tibial plateau, creating either a local or a split compression fracture configuration (Fig. 116-3). Because the

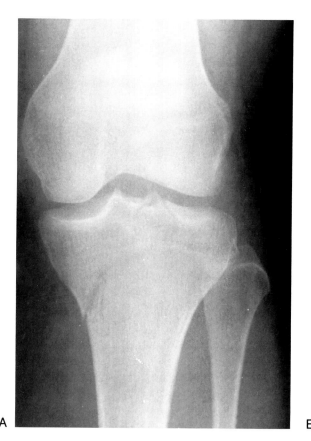

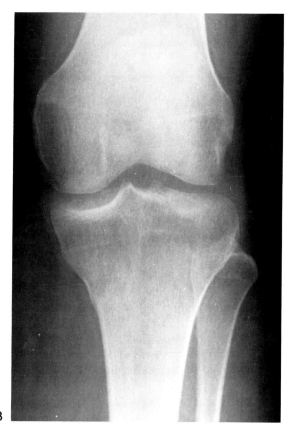

A

B

Fig. 116-6. This 21-year-old woman had an undisplaced fracture extending from the intercondylar area to the medial upper tibia, treated in plaster. **(A)** Note good fracture position. **(B)** Four months later, the fracture is well healed. (From Hohl,[29] with permission.)

approach, treatment, and prognosis of the two types are different, they are discussed separately.

Local Compression Fractures

The shape of the femoral condyle is imprinted into the tibial condyle by the creation of several fractures, often with a mosaiclike appearance of the articular surface (Fig. 116-7). The AP location of maximum depression depends on the flexion angle of the knee at the time of fracture. With the knee fractured in full extension the depressed area will be anterior and usually less than 6 to 7 mm deep. With greater degrees of flexion, the area will be further toward the middle or posterior aspects of the lateral condyle and can be 10 to 30 mm deep. The AP location and depth of depression should be ascertained by appropriate radiographic studies, such as tomography or the plateau view. Clinical stress testing helps in determining how unstable the knee will ultimately be in various flexion angles, if surgical correction is not done.

No treatment other than surgical reconstruction of articular level will restore alignment and stability if these are lacking initially; however, a variety of closed methods will restore movement and strength in spite of significant articular damage. Cast treatment until the early pain is gone, followed by active non-weight-bearing exercise, will restore movement almost as well as a period of early traction. Cast bracing as a primary treatment is not indicated.

The decision for or against surgical elevation is made on the basis of the patient's future requirements, clinical stress testing, and the radiograph. In general, fractures in the anterior to middle portion of the condyle with depression of 8 mm or more benefit by articular restoration; those exhibiting instability with less than 8-mm depression will also do better with surgery.[25,46]

Open reduction is accomplished by exposing the articular surface, making a window in the lateral tibial flare, and pushing the depressed fragments with a generous amount of attached cancellous bone to normal articular level with an impactor, elevator or broad osteotome. A radiograph in surgery is the only certain way of assuring complete reduction. The large cavity that remains under the elevated plateau fragments must be filled with some type of bone graft. Cancellous packing has been used successfully by many surgeons with bone harvested from the ilium or femoral condyle; packing must be very firm for this method to succeed. Cortical grafting has the advantage of slow absorption and rigidity giving a positive support of the elevated fragments. One of us (M.H.) prefers the use of tibial cortex removed from the proximal lateral tibia exposed by extending the skin incision distally. Actually, either iliac or tibial cortex can be used. The sheet of bone is driven through a separate contoured opening in the lateral tibial flare in direct contact with the cancellous bone of the previously elevated fragments. The graft is driven medially into intact cancellous bone in the area of the intercondylar notch. Immediately after surgery a splint or cast is applied, followed in a few days by a cast brace stressed into varus as the hinges are affixed. The cast brace is used for about 8 weeks. Arthroscopic-assisted reduction of mild to moderately depressed local compression fractures is being utilized more frequently because of the decreased operative morbidity and early indications of a high number of satisfactory results. Our technique is as follows. First, iliac bone graft is obtained and the wound closed. Then, a small (5- or 7-cm) incision is made, exposing the lateral tibial flare, and a window created. This wound is temporarily packed with a sponge. An arthroscope is inserted and the knee irrigated and debrided to permit complete visualization of the lateral compartment. The meniscus is typically seen to lie in proper relationship to the femoral condyle but the compressed articular fragments lie in a depressed position. Using curved impactors through the tibial flare window the depressed fragments are gently elevated to meet the meniscus. A check radiograph indicates restoration of articular height. When reduction is satisfactory, the bone grafts are packed tightly under the elevated fragments. Antibodies are used routinely. A cast brace stressed into varus for 8 weeks protects the reductions.

Rarely, the lateral articular surface is so comminuted and devoid of blood supply that consideration should be given to replacing the surface with an iliac cortical graft.[21,38,67,68] Such a graft fixed in place can substitute satisfactorily for articular surface and can result in a normally aligned and functioning knee in many instances. Such grafting also

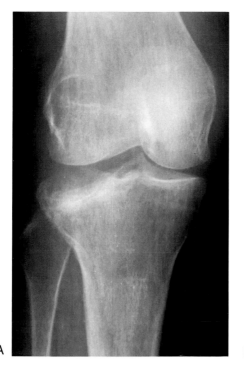

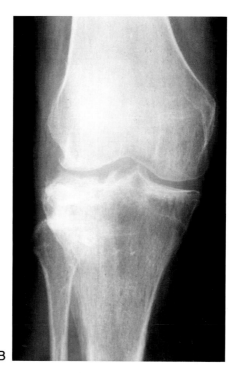

A   B

Fig. 116-7. This 62-year-old woman fell from a stepladder, sustaining a local compression fracture treated by open reduction and iliac cortical and cancellous grafting. **(A)** Original radiograph, demonstrating the articular depression. **(B)** Six months after open reduction. **(C)** Six years after injury, with adequate knee function and stability.

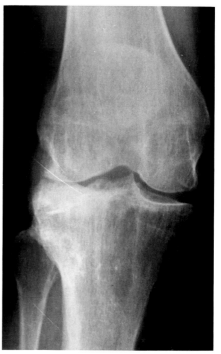

C

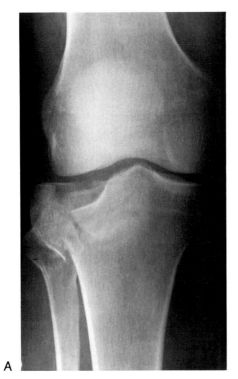

A

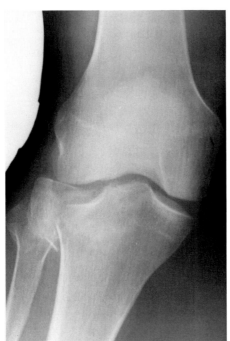

B

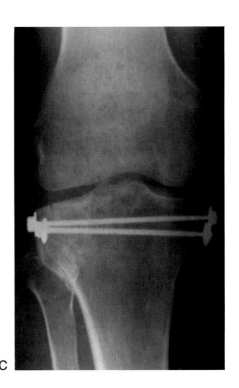

C

Fig. 116-8. This 37-year-old man was injured in a motorcycle accident. **(A)** Split-compression fracture shown. **(B)** Stress film at surgery demonstrates minimal medial opening. **(C)** Five months after open reduction without bone grafting. *(Figure continues.)*

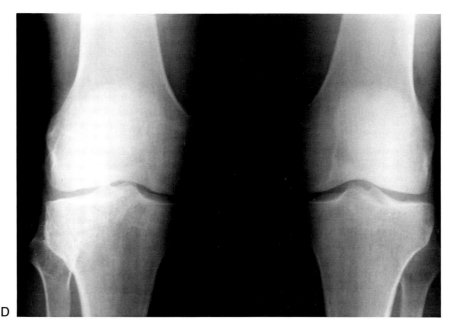

D

Fig. 116-8 *(Continued).* **(D)** Both knees are shown, 5 years after fracture. Clinical result is excellent, and the patient has fully resumed sports activities.

provides a scaffold, should future knee replacement be required.

Late articular defects have been restored by the use of allografts of articular cartilage and bone. This technique restores alignment as well as a smooth articular surface. Results from centers performing these procedures would suggest late allografting as a reasonable consideration.[23,39]

Most operated local compression fractures at follow-up have good motion and strength. The amount of instability and angular deformity depends upon the degree of restoration of normal articular level. When the surface has been well restored and protected and early motion instituted, a near-normal knee can be anticipated in the short term, with a low incidence of significant posttraumatic changes developing over the years.

Split Compression Fractures

These fractures are characterized by the presence of a wedge-shaped articular fragment split off the lateral tibial plateau, with the more central surface depressed. Because of this fragment, treatment considerations are quite different from those of the local compression type of fracture. If the fragment can be made to heal at normal articular level, thus giving support to the femoral condyle, angular deformity will not result. The objective of treatment — whether it be closed or open — is the support of the femoral condyle by this fragment. There are occasional cruciate and medial collateral ligament injuries that occur with this fracture; one must examine for these early in the course of treatment by stress testing and radiography, and repair should be carried out if they are identified.

Closed treatment, such as traction, manipulative reduction, or a cast-brace, may succeed in producing a good result if the split fragment can be made to heal in its normal position, regardless of the more central depressed area. If the femoral condyle is not supported and the upper tibia is thus widened, reduction must be accomplished. The traction-compression method followed by treatment in traction can succeed, but most surgeons prefer the assurance given by a well-performed internal fixation.[5,7,28,46,56,58,64,70] The split compression fracture type has the highest incidence of successful surgical management.

With the standard inframeniscal approach the

split fracture gap is encountered. With retraction or a spreader used to open this interval, the depressed fragments can be well seen and can be brought to articular level by use of an elevator. The split fragment is then opposed to the upper tibia and fixed firmly, either by plate and screws or by compression bolts, depending on cortical stability along the shaft. An intraoperative radiograph is then taken to make certain of the accuracy of reduction. The defect beneath the elevated articular fragments may be grafted by local bone, but this is not required, since the split fragment will effectively prevent the femoral condyle from redepressing these fragments while they revascularize and strengthen. Postoperatively a cast brace works effectively for restoration of motion and strength if internal fixation is not optimally strong and secure (Fig. 116-8).

One of us (M.H.) performs open reduction in two-thirds of these fractures, providing as a rule sufficient internal fixation that external support, a cast, or a cast brace is not required after surgery except for the unreliable patient.

The prognosis is quite good following treatment of these fractures if the femoral condyle is supported by the opposing tibial condyle.[25] Restoration of motion is possible early, and alignment is controlled by the fixation of the split fragment.

Total Depression

Instead of a portion of the articular surface, the entire condyle may be depressed (Fig. 116-9). The fracture line is more oblique than vertical and enters the articular surface in the fractured compartment. This type constitutes about 6 percent of plateau fractures, primarily those involving the lateral plateau. The fracture tends to impact, and it is difficult to reduce in traction. If the lateral condyle is significantly depressed, the fibular head or neck is often fractured.

Occasionally, the spine of the intercondylar eminence in the involved compartment may be depressed, and this should not be overlooked at the time of diagnosis or management. Total depression fractures frequently have some degree of cortical comminution in the metaphysis, which may lead to further condylar depression as the fracture heals. If

this problem is not corrected promptly, an unacceptable varus or valgus malalignment may result.[29] Meniscal and ligament injuries are uncommon, but they must be looked for with appropriate stress films and inspection of the meniscus at surgical reduction.

Buck's traction can be used initially for lateral condylar depression of less than 5 mm, but Buck's traction will routinely produce loss of normal valgus when used for medial condylar fractures.[46,63] A long-leg cast, even when "stressed" into varus or valgus, will not reliably prevent progressive malalignment in fractures of either plateau. Because of the impaction, manipulation is not usually successful, and maintenance of the reduction becomes a challenge should reduction be obtained. An occasional fracture will reduce in a modified Badgley traction apparatus,[46] and movement in traction is encouraged until healing provides stability.[3]

We prefer open reduction and rigid fixation for most total depression fractures, especially those involving the medial condyle.

The inframeniscal approach permits inspection of the meniscus and anatomic reduction of the joint surface under direct vision. The condyle can be adequately stabilized with two or three cancellous lag screws only if the distal cortex is not comminuted and reduction is accurate. If the elevated condyle cannot be adequately supported because of the comminuted distal cortex, a buttress plate will provide much better fixation than screws alone. Autogenous bone grafts from local sources or the iliac crest provide additional support in the area of the defect and are used in most cases. Radiographs should always be made prior to closure to confirm restoration of the plateau to its anatomic position. During the postoperative period we use a continuous passive motion machine, after which the patient can be protected in a cast brace for about 6 weeks. Full weight-bearing is not allowed for at least 12 weeks.

Because there is only one fracture line involving the joint surface, articular reduction at surgery is relatively easy. If the fractured condyle is minimally displaced initially or has been adequately reduced and stabilized at surgery, a well-functioning knee with good alignment should be obtained in most cases.

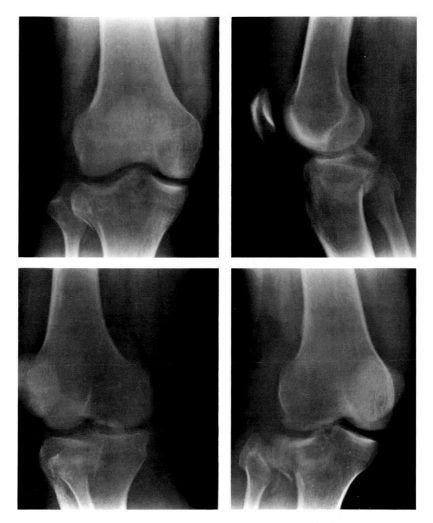

Fig. 116-9. Total depression lateral plateau fracture in anteroposterior, lateral, and oblique projections. There is increased valgus on the AP view and associated fractures of the posterior spine and fibular head. The knee was aligned by elevation, bone graft, and plating. All ligaments were intact on stress films.

Bicondylar Fractures

About 15 percent of plateau fractures involve both the medial and lateral condyles, producing a bicondylar or comminuted fracture. The fracture patterns in this type are more variable than in those previously described. The typical patterns are some form of inverted T, Y, or V, each of which presents unique problems. Ligament injury is rarely encountered, but meniscal damage is more frequent than in other types. At times, the whole proximal third of the tibia is shattered. In such

cases, the tibial tuberosity can penetrate the thin overlying skin owing to pull of the quadriceps. Manipulation or operative reduction must be considered in such cases to prevent skin slough over sharp bone spicules or the tibial tubercle.

The inverted T and Y patterns are often associated with a subcondylar transverse fracture of the proximal tibia, which may contraindicate early knee motion or, if knee motion is allowed, may contribute to delayed union or nonunion of the transverse fracture. Also, the condyles are occasionally dissociated by differential rotation about the transverse axis or angulated at the proximal tibia, producing osseous recurvatum or flexion. The 10 to 15-degree posterior slope of the plateaus[48] must be restored by the means of management selected. If the fibula is intact, as it is in up to one-half of cases, it will exert a deforming varus force.[63]

The inverted V type tends to allow the intercondylar eminence to impinge on the femoral notch if the condyles settle, resulting in painful limited movement. Closed management can be employed successfully only if the fracture is totally stable, which is unusual. Buck's traction is contraindicated if the medial condyle is unstable, since tibial traction will cause loss of normal valgus. Also, a long-leg cast or fracture brace usually results in a varus knee. A modification of the Badgley traction apparatus is our preferred method of closed management.

Most of these fractures are maintained or reduced by this device, but about one-third require surgery for optimum reduction, stabilization, and early knee motion. We prefer a midline or long median parapatellar approach which can provide

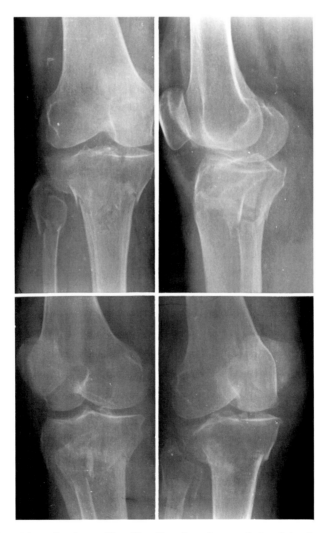

Fig. 116-10. Bicondylar plateau fracture with a T pattern in anteroposterior, lateral, and oblique projections. Acceptable reduction and alignment were achieved by traction in a plaster knee exercizer using a distal tibial pin.

access to both fractured condyles (see Fig. 116-4). Subperiosteal dissection and inframeniscal exposure provide direct vision.

Reduction is accomplished by systematically fitting the fragments and fixing them with Kirschner wires. T or Y fracture patterns are usually fixed with a single T plate on the lateral side unless there is comminution at the base of the medial condyle. V fracture patterns optionally can be fixed with three or four long cancellous screws, but if there is distal comminution of one of the condyles, a T plate is placed on the side with the comminution. Plating of both condyles is done infrequently because, in our experience, this has caused difficulty with wound closure and healing in these massive injuries (Fig. 116-10).

Postoperative management after rigid fixation is a continuous passive motion machine for a few days, depending on the healing of the wound. Thereafter, encouragement of active motion and protection from weight bearing is used. Unreliable patients are best managed in a cast brace. If reduced to near-anatomic position by traction or surgery this type of fracture can result in minimum long-term knee disability, but most fractures have some residual problem. A valgus malalignment is better tolerated than varus in the long term.

FRACTURE DISLOCATIONS

Most fractures of the proximal tibial articular surfaces are easily recognized on radiography as one of the types of plateau fractures just described. They occur in the sagittal plane, involve part or all of the tibial support for the opposing femoral condyle, and rarely are complicated by significant occult ligament injuries, avulsions of the anterior spine, or proximal fibular structures. Avulsion fractures of the anterior spine and the fibular styloid, involving tibial attachment of the posterior cruciate, and the "lateral capsular sign" [44,73] are associated with varying degrees of knee joint instability. Some investigators have included a few articular surface fractures associated with otherwise classic knee dislocations, but there is no con-

sistent pattern in this rare and unusual group. In addition to these recognized fractures, another significant group recently has been described in some detail.[47]

This group is termed *fracture dislocation,* an injury commonly recognized in other joints but one that has not previously been described about the knee. These injuries cause knee instability because of ligament laxity combined with major intra-articular fractures, and they have a relatively high neurovascular injury rate compared with plateau fractures. Fracture dislocations of the knee occur in the coronal plane or involve the rims of the joint surfaces, which distinguishes them from standard plateau fractures, with which they have previously been included. Many of the fracture dislocation knees are grossly unstable on initial clinical examination, as compared with plateau fractures. Injuries to cruciate and collateral ligaments usually occur by avulsion of ligament insertions, which is apparent on radiography, but some ligaments also rupture in their substance. Intrasubstance ligament ruptures constitute occult injury unless they are suspected and diagnosed by stress examination and radiography. Fracture dislocations are not as common as plateau fractures, occurring in an approximate ratio of 1 : 7 in one series,[47] but they are much more frequent than classic knee dislocations or eminence fractures. The average age of patients with fracture dislocations is less than that of patients with plateau fractures but greater than that of patients with knee dislocations.

There are two reasons to test knee instability under anesthesia in fracture dislocations. First, recognition of the fracture dislocation pattern on radiography does not always indicate significant instability; the soft tissue lesions may be partial instead of complete. About one-third of fractures will be stable enough to offer the surgeon an option of closed management.[46] Second, if the fracture dislocation is found to be unstable, the location of occult ligament ruptures is best diagnosed by comparative stress films of both knees, assessing both valgus-varus and anteroposterior instability. Knee stability is restored in fracture dislocations mainly by attention to soft tissue injuries. We believe that operative repair of disrupted ligaments provides optimum long-term functional results.

As might be expected, there is a close association

between ligament injury and neurovascular injury in fracture dislocations. Knee stability, particularly in the lateral structures, protects the peroneal nerve from stretch injury. Thus, this nerve is not frequently injured in plateau fractures. AP instability of the knee predisposes the popliteal artery to injury. This type of instability occurs in fracture dislocations but rarely in plateau fractures.

Table 116-1 shows that the incidence of neurovascular injury increases progressively in each fracture type, reaching about 50 percent in type 5 fracture dislocation. Overall, fracture dislocations can be expected to have a 15 percent associated incidence of neurovascular injury, which approaches that seen in traditional knee dislocations.[43] Recognition of these patterns of fracture and appreciation of their serious implications will alert the surgeon to suspect associated instability and neurovascular complications and the difficult management problems that they present.

Meniscus injuries occur in 20 percent of cases, slightly more frequently than in plateau fractures,[47] they consist mostly of major tears in the meniscal substance. Opportunities for repair of simple peripheral detachments are rare in this group, but such repair should be done when possible.

The surgical approaches used for stabilization and repair of fracture dislocations are the same as those used for plateau fractures. Modifications of these incisions can be anticipated following vascular repair or to allow for exploration of the peroneal nerve. In addition, if fasciotomies have been done for prophylaxis or treatment of compartment syndrome, or if there has been a delay in arterial repair,[43] modifications of the incisions may be required. We prefer medial and lateral demofascio-

tomies for simplicity and safety, using delayed skin closure or immediate split-thickness skin grafts.

In the long run, fracture dislocations are more disabling than plateau fractures but are not as disabling as classic knee dislocations, which is due in part to the devastating effects of associated neurovascular injuries in the knee dislocation and fracture dislocation groups. Patients who have sustained neurovascular injury as a complication of their fracture dislocation will require a prolonged and intensive rehabilitation program and will have more eventual knee disability. Also, stability is easier to maintain or restore in plateau fractures because the essential lesion is osseous. In fracture dislocation, isolated avulsed ligament insertions heal quickly and permit earlier rehabilitation of the limb. The intrasubstance ligament ruptures associated with classic knee dislocations are known to heal more slowly. That dislocations and fracture dislocations occur in a younger age group than do plateau fractures is also a factor because the older patient is less active and usually requires less from an injured knee. Finally, clinical observations suggest that plateau fractures generally result from less energetic trauma than dislocations and fracture dislocations, and thus the final results should be more favorable in plateau fracture, all other factors being equal.

Segregation of fracture dislocations from other fractures of the proximal tibial articular surfaces began with the split type of fracture.[24] This fracture was recognized as differing from the others in Hohl's classification because of instability and difficulty in management. Our radiographic classification (Fig. 116-3) closely relates to the clinical instability that characterizes this group (Table 116-1). It also relates closely to the incidence of occult

Table 116-1. Incidence of Neurovascular Injury

Type of Fracture Dislocation	Split (Type 1) (%)	Entire Condyle (Type 2) (%)	Rim Avulsion (Type 3) (%)	Rim Compression (Type 4) (%)	Four-Part (Type 5) (%)
Frequency	37	25	16	12	10
Clinically unstable	58	60	90	90	93
Occult ligament injury	0[a]	22	63	66	—[b]
Neurovascular injury	2	12	30	12	50

[a] Capsule massively torn if unstable.
[b] All ligaments attached to loose fragments.

ligament injury and the frequency of neurovascular injury in each of the five types, as shown.

Type I, or split fracture dislocation, has been considered to be a plateau fracture in the past, constituting about 5 percent of plateau fractures in classifications used by each of us and published first in 1956.[31] While it can produce knee instability associated with a fracture through the central articular surface, the other attributes of this injury separate it from plateau fractures.

Type 2, or entire condyle, and type 5, or four-part fracture dislocations, resemble plateau fracture types II and V but are distinguished from them by the presence of fracture of the eminence, usually as a separate fragment. This finding on radiography indicates inherent cruciate instability and suggests that the collateral ligaments may also have sustained ruptures in their substance.

Type 3, or rim avulsion fractures, occur almost exclusively on the lateral side, where avulsion of the iliotibial tract is indicated,[1,44] or of the lateral capsular insertions,[73] and there is often disruption of the lateral collateral complex with one or both cruciates. Collateral instability therefore occurs on the side of the knee where the radiograph shows the avulsion.

Type 4, or rim compression fractures, indicate disruption of the collateral complex across the knee from the fracture and, in addition, possibly one or both of the cruciates. Collateral instability therefore occurs on the opposite side of the knee from the fracture.

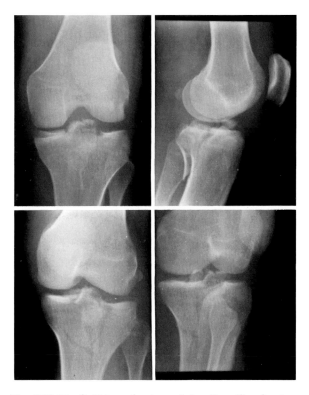

Fig. 116-11. Split-type fracture dislocation. The fracture involves the medial condyle and is displaced distally. This is appreciated in the AP view, where two levels of joint surface are seen. Ligamentous instability was associated with avulsion fractures in the median eminence.

Split Fracture Dislocations

The major fracture in this type is most frequently posterior and occurs only on the medial side, displaces only distally, and is usually uncomminuted. The fracture line is in the coronal plane, forming an angle of about 45 degrees with the medial compartment joint surface on the lateral radiographic view. If the fragment is displaced, the medial femoral condyle subluxes posteriorly with the fracture fragment on knee flexion, but the fragment and subluxation tend to reduce with full extension.

On the AP view, if the fragment is displaced, the medial tibial articular surface is seen at two levels (Fig. 116-11). At times the fracture extends into the lateral compartment, which can suggest a variant of a bicondylar plateau fracture unless oblique views are carefully interpreted. Avulsion fractures of the fibular styloid, the anterior spine, or Gerdy's tuberosity are fairly frequent. Peroneal nerve injuries are uncommon, and vascular injury has not been observed.

About one-half of the split-type fracture dislocations are stable on stress films and can be managed nonoperatively by a cylinder cast, a long-leg cast, or balanced suspension in extension. We believe that the inherent instability of the fracture dislocations makes their initial management in cast brace or functional cast brace unwise. If a long-leg cast is used, it must be positioned in extension and therefore may lead to some long-term limitation of flexion. A variant of this type of fracture dislocation includes fracture dislocation of the entire medial condyle, which can lead to varus malalignment of the limb if closed management is elected. This variant and the unstable fractures are best managed by operative reduction and fixation.

We prefer to place the stable split fracture dislocations in a modified Badgley apparatus in distal tibial pin traction[47] to allow for carefully monitored early motion for 3 weeks, after which a protective functional cast brace can be used for an additional 4 to 6 weeks. Graded weight bearing is then allowed. Unstable split injuries are approached with a medial plateau incision and reduced by extending the knee; the fragment is stabilized with two or three cancellous screws. Associated ligament injuries and a large capsular tear, which is always present, are repaired before closure. After ligament injuries are repaired, the knee is protected in a long-leg cast for a minimum of 6 weeks.

Even if the knee is initially stable or is stabilized by surgery, some patients can expect a near-normal knee; most will have some degree of instability and loss of flexion range. Eventual function will depend largely on the patient's motivational level during rehabilitation and the surgeons' persistence in de-manding an intensive and prolonged knee reconditioning program.

Entire Condyle Fracture Dislocations

This injury is distinguished from a type **IV** plateau fracture by the location of the intraarticular fracture. It extends beneath the intercondylar eminence and into the opposite compartment (Fig. 116-12). Either condyle can be fractured, and at times the intercondylar eminence is a separate fragment. When the knee is unstable, the femur subluxes out of the opposite compartment, accompanying the displaced tibial condyle (Fig. 116-12). The opposite collateral complex is disrupted in about half the cases; the fibular head or neck is frequently fractured or the proximal tibiofibular joint is dislocated. Neurovascular and meniscal injuries are more common than in the split type.

Occult ligament injuries may be suspected by recognition of this pattern on radiography but require stress testing under anesthesia for confirmation. They occur in about one-fifth of cases and are

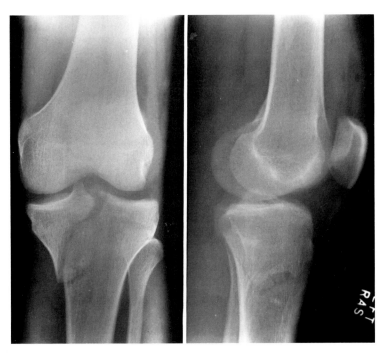

Fig. 116-12. An entire medial condyle fracture dislocation showing a mild medial subluxation of the femur from the lateral compartment and an undisplaced avulsion of the fibular styloid.

associated with neurovascular damage in about 12 percent of cases of this type of fracture dislocation.

If stable, entire condyle fracture dislocations can be managed by long-leg cast with frequent radiographic monitoring of position in balanced suspension, or by a fracture or cast-brace until the fracture becomes stable and then with protection until weight bearing is allowed (at about 8 weeks). If they are unstable, we prefer a routine plateau operative approach for reduction and fixation of the condyle with two or three cancellous lag screws and fixation of the intercondylar eminence. Collateral ligament repair is done by standard techniques.

The medial approach may require modification if a vascular repair has been required. If the knee is initially stable or if a reasonably anatomic reduction and ligament repair is done, management will result in a moderately functional knee.

Rim Avulsion Fracture Dislocations

This type of fracture dislocation occurs almost exclusively on the lateral side of the knee, and it is characterized by an avulsion of the lateral capsular attachment, Gerdy's tubercle, or a portion of the plateau (Fig. 116-13). The fibular styloid or head also is occasionally avulsed. Occult anterior or posterior cruciate ligament disruption occurs in about one-third of cases. In the uncommon case with medial rim avulsion, there is usually a split compression lateral plateau fracture, but the medial collateral complex rarely shows significant laxity on stress testing. Almost all lateral rim avulsions are unstable, and neurovascular injury occurs in about 30 percent of cases. Meniscal injury is uncommon.

If the fracture dislocation of this type is stable, a long-leg cast will protect the partially damaged ligaments until healing occurs. When operative repair is necessary, we prefer a lateral plateau approach to permit repair by suture or a cancellous screw or two in the plateau fragment. We prefer to reattach the avulsed fibular styloid or head by sutures passed through drill holes in the fibular head. Cruciate injury is repaired by a method of the surgeon's choice. A long-leg cast is then applied for 6 weeks. Rim avulsion fracture dislocations often result in a moderately impaired knee, even when adequate repair has been done.

Rim Compression Fracture Dislocations

This type of fracture dislocation is characterized by an anterior, middle, or posterior rim compression fracture of either plateau. Middle rim injuries

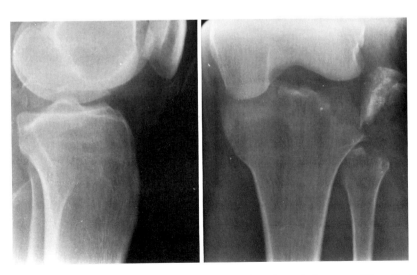

Fig. 116-13. A rim avulsion fracture dislocation involving most of the lateral plateau and the attached head of the fibula. The posterior cruciate is avulsed from the tibia, and the anterior cruciate was totally disrupted in its substance.

are apparent on AP view, but anterior and posterior rim compressions can be overlooked unless adequate films, including oblique projections, are carefully interpreted. Almost all these injuries are unstable because the collateral complex in the opposite compartment must be disrupted to allow the femoral condyle to impinge on the rim of the plateau (Fig. 116-14). Occasionally, a "medial capsular sign" is seen, indicating medial complex laxity. Anterior or posterior cruciate disruption by avulsion or rupture occurs in three-fourths of cases. Neurovascular injury is not as common in rim compression fracture dislocations as in the rim avulsion type (see Table 116-1). Meniscal injuries may occur on the side with the compressed rim.

If the fracture is stable on stress examination (which is unusual), a long-leg cast will protect the damaged ligaments, until healing occurs. If operative repair is necessary, we prefer the midline plateau incision, which will also adequately expose the opposite compartment for collateral ligament re-pair. Exposure of the crushed rim is necessary to remove intraarticular cartilage and bone fragments and to inspect the meniscus and repair it if it is damaged. If the impacted rim fragment is stable, it can be ignored; if it is loose, it should be stabilized or removed. A long-leg cast is used to protect the ligament repair for 6 weeks, after which the patient begins graduated weight bearing.

If adequate ligament repairs are done, a minimally lax knee should result; it should be moderately functional, but high patient motivation is necessary for optimum rehabilitation.

Four-Part Fracture Dislocations

This type of fracture dislocation is the most unstable of this group and is fortunately also the least common, representing only about 1 percent of all proximal tibial articular fractures. It is distinguished from the bicondylar plateau fracture only

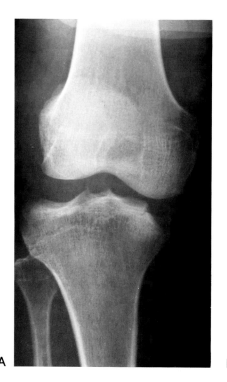 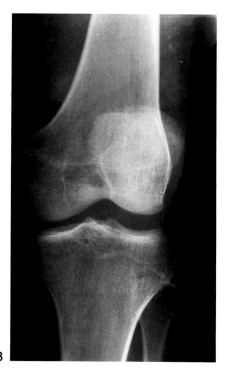

A   B

Fig. 116-14. Rim compression fracture dislocation **(A)** compared with the normal knee on varus stress films **(B)**. The lateral collateral complex and the anterior cruciate were completely disrupted, and the posterior cruciate was 80 percent disrupted. There was an axontemesis of the peroneal nerve.

by the presence of a fracture of the whole intercondylar eminence, which disrupts one or both cruciates. This separate fragment is the "fourth part" (Fig. 116-15). Because the capsule and collateral complexes are attached to loose condyles, there are no intact stabilizing elements. Often, these injuries also disrupt the fibular attachment of the biceps and collateral ligament, leaving only skin and muscle to stabilize the knee. About one-half of the cases of four-part fracture dislocations have nerve or vascular injury, and more than one-third have combined peroneal nerve and popliteal artery injuries. Meniscus injuries have not been noted in this type, but the meniscus should be examined in all fracture

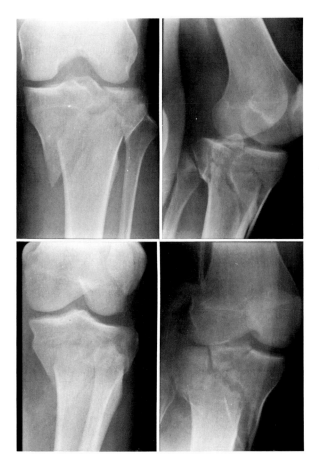

Fig. 116-15. Four-part fracture dislocation, showing the entire eminence as a separate fragment on the lower right. There was a peroneal nerve deficit and a thrombosis of the popliteal artery. Residual arteriographic contrast medium is also seen on the lower right.

dislocations if surgery is performed. In the rare case demonstrating initial stability, a long-leg cast for several weeks should maintain fragment position and permit healing.

We use the bicondylar plateau approach for operative repair, modified as necessary if vascular repair has been done. Maintaining reduction of the eminence is difficult; at times, it can be stabilized by sandwiching it between the condyles, which are compressed together with lag screws. A suture through drill holes in the anterior rim of the tibia or a malleolar screw will also provide stability and maintain reduction. We prefer to stabilize the condyles to the tibial shaft with a T plate, placing it electively on the lateral side unless the medial is comminuted at the distal cortex. Postoperatively, the patient with vascular injury is placed in a bivalved long-leg cast until circulation is ensured, after which a long-leg cast is applied and maintained for a minimum of 4 weeks. A functional brace or cast brace is then used for an additional 4 weeks of protection.

Probably because of the neurovascular injuries and the high energy level of the inciting trauma, patients with four-part fracture dislocations will have significant residual impairment of knee function. If the eminence is not reduced, drawer instability can be disabling, particularly when combined with failure to regain quadriceps circumference and strength.

Complications

Ipsilateral lower lateral limb injuries and polysystem trauma are occasionally associated with plateau fractures and occur in up to 20 percent of fracture dislocations. The implications of foot and ankle, tibial, femoral, hip, and pelvis injuries on management of an unstable knee fracture must be considered carefully. A femur fracture — particularly when distal — will seriously interfere with knee rehabilitation unless the femur is stabilized. We prefer closed intramedullary rodding of the femur when possible, and this should be done before the knee repair.

If loss of reduction occurs during closed management or postoperatively, it must be carefully evaluated; in general, it should be approached aggressively if optimum results are sought. Reoperation carries an increased risk of infection and thromboembolism, interferes with rehabilitation, and is difficult because of the bone and soft tissue atrophy of disuse. These risks, the age of the patient, the surgeon's experience, and the degree of loss of reduction must all be considered. In carefully selected cases, we have done delayed elevation of plateau fractures after rehabilitation is no longer productive. This type of surgery is most difficult, and it probably should not be attempted, unless the surgeon is prepared to perform a cartilage allograft.

Open plateau and fracture dislocations of the knee are likely to be unstable because of the massive trauma. A decision regarding whether to do an immediate or a delayed repair depends upon the number and degree of associated injuries, the time elapsed from injury, the amount of local soft tissue damage, and the surgeon's skill and experience. Debridement and skin coverage under antibiotic protection followed by delayed reconstruction in a week or so, is safer in general but will make the eventual knee repair more difficult. We elect to do definitive initial repair only if all conditions are optimal.

When an arterial injury has occurred in a fracture dislocation, reestablishment of blood flow must take priority over stabilization of the knee and absolutely must precede the orthopaedic procedure. A postoperative arteriogram should be done following the knee repair and prior to closure to assure patency of the arterial repair. We prefer to immobilize the limb in a bivalved long-leg plaster cast or a heavy gutter long-leg splint to avoid possible constriction and to allow observation of pulses and compartment integrity.

Peroneal nerve injuries should be explored at the time of surgery with intent to effect repair if possible and to establish the prognosis of return of peroneal nerve function. In our experience, stretch injury is a common finding in fracture dislocations.

The complications of treatment of fracture dislocations, classic knee dislocations, and plateau fractures are similar. Wound infection and thromboembolism are the most serious early problems; short-term broad-spectrum antibiotic coverage of all operative cases and aggressive mobilization of the patient's limb will help minimize their inci-

dence. If thrombophlebitis or thromboembolism occurs, immediate anticoagulation is indicated and should be continued until the patient is fully ambulatory. Knee and limb motion should be restricted until therapeutic anticoagulation is attained; motion may then cautiously be started again. Infection must be treated promptly by removal of skin sutures and institution of adequate drainage. If there is any suspicion of pyarthrosis, the knee should be immediately aspirated for Gram stain and culture. A pyarthrosis is serious, frequently producing long-term loss of function and degenerative arthritis. We prefer to institute specific antibiotics and perform repetitive arthrocenteses, provided that this management regimen controls the infection.

Peroneal nerve deficits, knee instability, and degenerative arthritis are the most frequent of the serious long-term problems encountered. Foot drop is best managed by early application of an orthosis, to permit ambulation to be resumed in as nearly a normal fashion as possible. More than one-half the fracture dislocations will have some degree of knee instability because of combined ligament laxity and muscle atrophy. A prolonged, intensive, and carefully supervised graded exercise program is mandatory if optimum results are to be obtained. Quadriceps, hamstrings, and gastrocnemius muscle strength must be regained as quickly as possible, with use of a progressive-resistance exercise program. This should start within 4 weeks for plateau fractures, stable fracture dislocations, and those unstable knees in which laxity of soft tissue constraints has been caused by avulsion fractures. If intraligamentous disruptions have occurred, resistive exercises should be delayed until 6 to 8 weeks. It is expected that a minimum of 6 months will be required for these exercises, and the patient may need to return to such a program intermittently for an indefinite period of time.

The cause, natural course, prevention, and treatment of degenerative arthritis of the knee are poorly understood. Fracture dislocations have only recently been recognized; thus the incidence here cannot be discussed with any confidence. Early observations suggest that arthritis will occur more frequently in fracture dislocations than in plateau fractures.

Nonunion is rare in proximal tibial articular fractures and has responded to bone grafting with internal fixation as required. Malalignment of the limb, not correctable by delayed elevation of articular surfaces, can be improved by proximal tibial osteostomy if the problem is moderate in degree; if it is severe, a total knee implant should be considered.

REFERENCES

1. Abdalla FH, Tehranzadeh J, Horton JA: Avulsion of the lateral tibial condyle in skiing. Am J Sports Med 10:368, 1982
2. Apley AG: Fractures of the tibial plateau. Orthop Clin North Am 10:61, 1979
3. Badgley CE, O'Connor SJ: Conservative treatment of fractures of the tibial plateau. Arch Surg 64:506, 1952
4. Bakalim G, Wilppula E: Fractures of the tibial condyles. Acta Orthop Scand 44:311, 1973
5. Blokker CP, Rorabeck CH, Bourne RB: Tibial plateau fractures. An analysis of the results of treatment in 60 patients. Clin Orthop 182:193, 1984
6. Bomler J, Arnoldi CC: Resurfacing of depression fractures of the lateral tibial condyle. Acta Orthop Scand 52:231, 1981
7. Bowes DN, Hohl M: Tibial condylar fractures. Evaluation of treatment and outcome. Clin Orthop 171:104, 1982
8. Brown GA, Sprague BL: Cast brace treatment of plateau and bicondylar fractures of the proximal tibia. Clin Orthop 119:184, 1976
9. Burri C, Bartzke G, Coldewey J, Muggler E: Fractures of the tibial plateau. Clin Orthop 138:84, 1979
10. Caspari RB, Hutton PMJ, Whipple TL, Meyers JF: The role of arthroscopy in the management of tibial plateau fractures. J Arthrosc 1:76, 1985
11. Daniel D, Rice T: Valgus-varus stability in a hinged cast used for controlled mobilization of the knee. J Bone Joint Surg 61A:135, 1979
12. DeCoster T, Nepola J, El-Khoury G: Cast brace treatment of proximal tibial fractures: a ten year followup. Clin Orthop 231:196, 1988
13. Dejour H, Chanbat P, Caton J, Melere G: Les fractures des plateaux tibiaux avec lesion ligamentaire. Rev Chir Orthop 67:593, 1981
14. Delamarter R, Hohl M: The cast brace and tibial plateau fractures. Clin Orthop in press, 1989
15. Delamarter R, Hohl M, Hopp E Jr: Ligament injuries in tibial plateau fractures. Orthop Trans 9:571, 1985 (abst)
16. Dias J, Stirling A, Finlay D, Gregg P: Computerised axial tomography for tibial plateau fractures. J Bone Joint Surg 69B:84, 1987
17. Dovey H, Heerfordt J: Tibial condyle fractures. A follow-up of 200 cases. Acta Chir Scand 137:521, 1971
18. Drennan DB, Locher FG, Maylahn DJ: Fractures of the tibial plateau. J Bone Joint Surg 61A:989, 1979
19. Elstrom J, Pankovich AM, Sasson H, et al: The use of tomography in the assessment of tibial plateau fractures. J Bone Joint Surg 58A:551, 1976
20. Forster E, Mole L, Coblentz J: Etude des lesions ligamentous dans les fractures du plateau tibial. Ned Tijdschr Geneeskd 105:2173, 1961
21. Freehafer A, Goldman S, Chapman K: Stubbins' arthroplasty for fractures of the tibial condyle. Clin Orthop 90:140, 1973
22. Gausewitz S, Hohl M: The significance of early motion in the treatment of tibial plateau fractures. Clin Orthop 202:135, 1986
23. Gross A, McKee N, Pritzker K, Langer F: Reconstruction of skeletal deficits at the knee. A comprehensive osteochondral transplant. Clin Orthop 174:96, 1983
24. Hohl M: Tibial condylar fractures. J Bone Joint Surg 49A:1455, 1967
25. Hohl M: Tibial condylar fractures: Long-term follow-up. Texas Med 70:46, 1974
26. Hohl M: Fractures and dislocations of the knee. p. 1157. In Rockwood CA, Green DP (eds): Fractures, Vol. 2. JB Lippincott, Philadelphia, 1975
27. Hohl M: Treatment methods in tibial condylar fractures. South Med J 68:985, 1975
28. Hohl M: Management of tibial condylar fractures. p. 95. In Symposium on Reconstructive Surgery of the Knee. CV Mosby, St. Louis, 1978
29. Hohl M: Complications of fractures of the knee. p. 486. In Epps CH (ed): Complications in Orthopedic Surgery, Vol. 1. 2nd Ed. JB Lippincott, Philadelphia, 1986
30. Hohl M, Hopp E: Ligament injuries in tibial condylar fractures. J Bone Joint Surg 58A:279, 1976 (abst)
31. Hohl M, Luck JV: Fractures of the tibial condyles. A clinical and experimental study. J Bone Joint Surg 38A:1001, 1956
32. Ilfeld FW, Hohl M: Closed reduction treatment of tibial condylar fractures. J Bone Joint Surg 42A:534, 1960 (abst)
33. Jennings J: Arthroscopic management of tibial plateau fractures. J Arthrosc 1:160, 1985

34. Kennedy JC, Bailey WH: Experimental tibial-plateau fractures. J Bone Joint Surg 50A:1522, 1968

35. Kennedy WR: Fractures of the tibial condyles. A preliminary report on supplementary fixation with methyl methacrylate. Clin Orthop 134:153, 1978

36. Loechlin P, Nael J, Bonnet J, et al: Ligament injuries associated with fractures of the tibial plateau. Acta Orthop Belg 49:751, 1983

37. Lansinger O, Bergman B, Korner L, Andersson G: Tibial condylar fractures. A twenty year followup. J Bone Joint Surg 68A:13, 1986

38. Lee H: Osteoplastic reconstruction in severe fractures of the tibial condyles. Am J Surg 94:940, 1957

39. Locht R, Gross A, Langer F: Late osteochondral allograft resurfacing for tibial plateau fractures. J Bone Joint Surg 66:328, 1984

40. Luck JV: Response of joints to trauma. Presented at the Annual Meeting of The American Academy of Orthopaedic Surgeons, New York, 1950

41. Lucht V, Pelgaard S: Fractures of the tibial condyles. Acta Orthop Scand 42:366, 1971

42. Marwah V, Gadegone W, Magarkar D: The treatment of fractures of the tibial plateau by skeletal traction and early mobilisation. Intern Orthop 9:217, 1985

43. Meyers MH, Moore TM, Harvey JP: Traumatic dislocation of the knee joint. J Bone Joint Surg 57A:430, 1975

44. Milch H: Cortical avulsion fracture of the lateral tibial condyle. J Bone Joint Surg 18:159, 1936

45. Mooney V: Cast bracing. Clin Orthop 102:159, 1974

46. Moore TM: Management of tibial plateau fractures. p. 56. In Moore TM (ed): Symposium on Trauma to the Leg and Its Sequelae. CV Mosby, St. Louis, 1981

47. Moore TM: A classification of fracture-dislocation of the knee. Clin Orthop 156:128, 1981

48. Moore TM, Harvey JP Jr: Roentgenographic measurement of tibial plateau depression due to fracture. J Bone Joint Surg 56A:155, 1974

49. Moore TM, Meyers MH, Harvey JP: Collateral ligamentous laxity of the knee — Long term comparison between fractures and normal. J Bone Joint Surg 58A:594, 1976

50. Newberg AH, Greenstein R: Radiographic evaluation of tibial plateau fractures. Diagn Radiol 126:319, 1978

51. Perry CR, Evans LG, Rice S, et al: A new surgical approach to fractures of the lateral tibial plateau. J Bone Joint Surg 66A:1236, 1984

52. Pino A: The role of arthroscopy in the diagnosis and treatment of fractures about the knee. Orthop Trans 10:633, 1986 (abst)

53. Porter BB: Crush fractures of the lateral tibial table. J Bone Joint Surg 52B:676, 1970

54. Rafii M, Firooznia H, Golimbu C, Bonamo J: Computed tomography of tibial plateau fractures. AJR 142:1181, 1984

55. Rasmussen PS: Lateral condylar fracture of the tibia. Acta Orthop Scand 42:429, 1971

56. Rasmussen PS: Tibial condylar fractures. J Bone Joint Surg 55A:1331, 1973

57. Reiner S, Rinott M, Kaufman B: Trans-arthroscopic monitoring of reduction and percutaneous internal fixation of minimally displaced intraarticular fractures about the knee. Orthop Trans 10:98, 1986 (abst)

58. Rinonapoli E, Aglietti P: Comparison of treatment by open and closed reduction of comparable cases of articular fractures of the proximal tibia. Ital J Orthop Traumatol 3:99, 1977

59. Roberts JM: Fractures of the condyles of the tibia. J Bone Joint Surg 50A:1505, 1968

60. Rombold S: Depressed fractures of the tibial plateau. J Bone Joint Surg 42A:783, 1960

61. Salter R, Hamilton H, Wedge J, et al: Clinical application of basic research on continuous passive motion for disorders and injuries of synovial joints. J Orthop Res 1:325, 1984

62. Salter RB, Simmonds DF, Malcolm BW, et al: The biological effect of continuous passive motion on the healing of full-thickness defects in articular cartilage. J Bone Joint Surg 62A:1232, 1980

63. Sarmiento A, Kinman PB, Latta LL: Fractures of the proximal tibia and tibial condyles. Clin Orthop 145:136, 1979

64. Schatzker J, McBrown R, Bruce D: The tibial plateau fracture. The Toronto experience. Clin Orthop 138:94, 1979

65. Schatzker J, Schulak DJ: Pseudarthrosis of a tibial plateau fracture. Clin Orthop 145:146, 1979

66. Scotland T, Wardlow D: The use of cast-bracing as treatment for fractures of the tibial plateau. J Bone Joint Surg 63B:575, 1981

67. Segal D, Franchi A, Campanile J: Iliac autograft for reconstruction of severely depressed fracture of the lateral tibial plateau. J Bone Joint Surg 67A:1270, 1985

68. Sisk T: Autogenous patella transplantation for severe tibial plateau fractures. Jefferson Orthop 9:23, 1980

69. Tscherne H, Lobenhoffer P, Russe O: Proximale intraartikulaere Tibiafrakturen. Unfallheilkunde 87:277, 1984

70. Waddell JP, Johnston DWC, Neidre A: Fractures of the tibial plateau: A review of ninety-five patients

and comparison of treatment methods. J Trauma 21:376, 1981

71. Wilppula E, Bakalim G: Ligamentous tear concomitant with tibial condylar fracture. Acta Orthop Scand 43:292, 1972

72. Wirth CR: Meniscus repair. Clin Orthop 157:153, 1981

73. Woods GW, Stanley RF, Tullos HS: Lateral capsular sign: X-ray clue to a significant knee instability. Am J Sports Med 7:27, 1979

Musculotendinous Problems About the Knee

117

John P. Albright

THIGH CONTUSIONS AND MYOSITIS OSSIFICANS

Crush injury to the distal and central portion of the thigh sufficient to damage the quadriceps muscle fibers is the most common of the musculotendinous problems discussed in this chapter. Regardless of severity, these contusions can be differentiated from strains not only because of the direct nature of the injury producing the force and the frequent association with femoral fractures but because of the potential for the development of myositis ossificans.

The time-related response to soft tissue damage resulting from a direct blow is usually characteristic. At first, the contused area remains soft and painful during voluntary contraction of the surrounding muscle. Initially, even the most severe injury can appear quite benign. For a few minutes after the immediate pain of injury subsides, the range of motion remains full. Often the only reliable sign of significant tissue damage is the demonstration of weakness through inability to perform a one- or two-legged squat. The initially softened area then becomes tense from hemorrhage and edema. As the tension develops, the clinical picture also changes. Within a few hours of the injury, the discomfort intensifies and the tolerable range of motion may diminish.

Feagin and Jackson[18] demonstrated the great clinical value of a functional classification of the severity of injury through the picture that evolves within the first day or two. It is at this point (24 to 48 hours), that the hemorrhage and edema usually stabilize and that the clinical manifestations truly reflect the severity of the tissue damage and relate to the prognosis for the injury.

Mild quadriceps contusions are those which, at their worst, display only pain in the face of a full range of motion and relatively normal muscle strength. Moderate contusions are distinguished by a grossly enlarged, tense and tender thigh that exhibits extreme pain with attempts to passively flex the knee beyond 90 degrees. In the severe contusion, the thigh becomes greatly swollen, tender, and painful to the point that the patient may even be incapable of voluntarily initiating contraction of the muscle. In this instance, passive flexion is not tolerated beyond 45 degrees and any attempt to stretch or actively contract the muscle mass initiates excruciating pain and spasm. Clinically, those patients at very high risk of the development of myositis ossificans are those with severe contusions.

Myositis ossificans is a well-recognized post-traumatic form of local heterotopic formation of bone and cartilage occurring in an area of necrosis of voluntary muscle tissue. There is experimental evidence that prolonged recovery and the development of myositis ossificans are most likely when the tissue damage is severe enough to also disrupt the periosteum of the femur.[33,76]

Pathologically, the process is very similar to callus formation. Fibroplastic cells from the endomysium and mesenchymal cells from the injured fascia give rise to osteoid and chondroid tissue as early as 4 to 5 days after injury. This process is first noted at the outer margins of the necrotic area and progresses inward toward the center. The reactive bone is gradually replaced in the same order by mature lamellar bone. The histologic hallmark in this condition is the centripetal pattern of ossification and maturation.

In the muscle belly, complete resorption may be completed within a few years. Clinically, those patients at very high risk of the development of myositis ossificans are those with severe contusions. However, location near the musculotendinous junction, repeated crush injuries, and untimely surgery increase the likelihood of permanent impairment from mechanically disruptive masses of nonresorbable bone.

Indications

Surgical interventions in cases of myositis are rarely indicated; with proper nonoperative management there is little chance that any significant functional impairment will ever result. Local excision of the ectopic ossification is indicated only when the patient is symptomatic with pain, restriction of motion, or vulnerability to repeated trauma because of the size and location of the mass.

The radiographic features of myositis ossificans are helpful in assessing the maturity of the process.[52] Barring repeated trauma, myositis is usually visible radiographically within 3 to 4 weeks after injury. By 6 to 8 weeks, a lacy pattern of new bone is sharply circumscribed by cortex around the periphery, similar to the phenomena observed histologically. By 4 to 6 months, the lesion usually has ceased to expand in size and so the bone appears to be lamellar in nature. However, complete maturation of the nucleus may not occur for another 6 to 12 months, when this resorption of the bony mass usually begins.

Lysis of adhesions or quadricepsplasty may be indicated when fibrosis in the quadriceps muscle is severe enough to create an unacceptable loss of flexion. This likelihood is increased when the muscle injury is accompanied by associated comminuted or distally located femoral fracture.

Contraindications

No surgery should be attempted for 6 to 12 months after the last trauma; or at least sufficient time to give the myositis process a chance to reach complete maturity. Furthermore, because they will prolong the disability of the initial injury and worsen the eventual prognosis, the following should be avoided: (1) aggressive early attempts to regain motion; (2) a premature or an early return to physical activity; and (3) use of irritating therapeutic modalities (e.g., ultrasound, diathermy). Prolonged immobilization can also lead to restriction of motion from cicatrix formation between tissue planes. Manipulation to speed the return of motion in a worrisome knee will only retard the progress. Surgical excision or biopsy of an immature mass of heterotropic bone is contraindicated because it will invariably lead to an exacerbation of the myositis process. Furthermore, the biggest diagnostic mistakes have come when the lesion has been biopsied. The cellular variation in early myositis ossificans can look identical to those seen with sarcomatous changes.[74]

Clinically, differentiation between sarcomatous change and myositis ossificans traumatica is also occasionally a problem. However, the history of appropriate trauma with decreasing pain and a consolidating mature periphery of myositis with the accompaniment of a normal alkaline phosphatase level should obviate the confusion.

Treatment Alternatives

Hematoma aspirations and steroid injections[55] as well as femoral nerve blocks have helped lessen total disability time. However, in light of their potential adverse effects, the evidence for their effectiveness is not convincing enough to recommend their usage.

Author's Preferred Treatment

A proper initial treatment plan should include rest, ice, a compressive dressing, and elevation (RICE), immobilization, and a strong anti-inflammatory agent until after the acute inflammatory reaction to the injury subsides. Hospitalization is recommended when a lack of patient compliance is anticipated.

While the specifics of the best treatment method have not been clearly defined, some studies provide interesting observations for a frame of reference that favors obtaining motion as soon as possible.[33-35] For example, in the contused rat gastrocnemius, mobilization produced more of an initial inflammatory reaction and, eventually, more scar tissue. However, the speed of repair and the final tensile strength of the wound were greater in the group that was moved during the repair process.

Rehabilitation of the quadriceps unit is begun when the initial symptoms of pain and tenderness subside and a full range of motion is achieved. It is critical that the early phases of the strengthening program proceed very slowly on a "to tolerance" basis. Whether or not myositis ossificans develops, this protective program should be followed using the same functional guidelines regardless of the time since injury.[42]

Operative Technique

Excision of a troublesome mass can be very successful if careful operative technique and rehabilitative control are maintained. Exposure should be made with sharp dissection centered directly over the entire mass, without vigorous retraction. The incision should be carried down sharply through the skin, subcutaneous tissue, muscle fibers, and capsule directly onto the mass. Hemostasis should be obtained at each step of the way, especially through the muscle splitting phase. Once contact with the mass is made, sharp dissection should be carried around its borders. To avoid unnecessary trauma to the surrounding soft tissues, great care must be taken to follow the outline of the mass toward its attachment to the bone. It is pertinent to remember that three forms of myositis ossificans masses occur. The two most likely to require excision have a stalk or a broad-based pedestal connection to the adjacent femur. Therefore, the delineation between the femoral cortex and the mass is very plain. The mass should be divided from the femur by a sharp osteotome.

Once the mass is removed, all shreds of devitalized tissue should be carefully dissected away without invading the healthy muscle mass itself. Maximum hemostasis should be achieved to avoid any hemorrhagic condition similar to that which occurred at the time of the original injury. Closure is then accomplished with absorbable sutures beginning in the periosteal layer nearest the femur. The muscle edges should be closed as closely as possible over closed suction tubing or Penrose drain, but no sutures should constrict the muscle tissue itself. An absorbable synthetic suture is placed subcuticularly to avoid the need for suture removal after discharge.

Postoperative Care

A Jones pressure dressing is applied in the operating room with cotton batting and a posterior splint. The patient is placed in balanced suspension to obviate the need for contraction of the quadriceps and yet allow an early, gentle, passive range-of-motion exercise. The drain is removed at 24 to 48 hours, or whenever drainage has ceased. In 5 to 7 days a snug-fitting cylinder cast brace with drop locks is applied with elastic plaster in order to allow the patient to ambulate non-weight bearing on crutches and continue a gentle range-of-motion program progressing on a "to tolerance" basis.

At the end of 3 to 4 weeks, the cast brace is removed and the wound is inspected. If continuity of the contracted muscle mass is secure and there is no undue reaction or tenderness, a knee exercise program is begun with nongravity active range-of-motion exercises. A long knee immobilizer or crutches can be used for protection during ambulation.

This rehabilitation process is extremely slow. Three to 4 months may be needed for achieving complete flexion of the knee, and 8 to 12 months may be required before contact sports or other vigorous physical activities can be permitted even with protective equipment.

Results

The results of early aggressive nonoperative management are extremely encouraging. Feagin and Jackson[18] reported that in over 250 quadriceps contusions all but one patient resumed unrestricted full activity. Their treatment heavily emphasized hospitalization and early bedrest followed by a very slow rehabilitation program without massage or stretching to achieve motion.

The duration of disability is related to the severity of the injury. Mild contusions regain full strength and motion within 1 week. Moderate contusions require 3 to 8 weeks before all symptoms are resolved. Eight to 10 weeks may elapse before an individual with a severe contusion has recovered enough to return to normal flexion, strength, and activity level.

The predictive value of the 24- to 48-hour clinical assessment is reinforced by the correlations reported by Feagin and Jackson.[18] Athletes with greater than 90 degrees of flexion 48 hours after injury had a mean disability of 6½ days while those with less than 90 degrees had a mean disability of 66 days.

Even though radiographic evidence for the development of myositis ossificans nearly doubles the disability time; the adequacy of eventual resorption of the mass is unrelated to the time of return to full function.

Complications

Most significant surgical complications that occur are postoperative scar tissue adhesions and contractures related to prolonged immobilization of the extremity. If possible, a period of complete immobilization should be avoided but not at the expense of tissue breakdown. Unfortunately, a delayed manipulation to speed the return of motion may not be effective and may even cause more stiffness.

STRAIN SYNDROMES

The spectrum of injuries to the actively contracted quadriceps musculotendinous unit ranges from dramatic but rare ruptures to the much more commonplace minor chronic strain syndromes. They have in common the fact that they are all a result of mechanical overloading with forces that are relatively greater than the extensor mechanism is capable of withstanding. The location and severity of any of these pathologic entities are related to intrinsic, as well as extrinsic, causative factors.

Important extrinsic factors include the magnitude, direction, and site of application of the applied loads, as well as the relationship of both the state of contraction of the muscle and the position of the knee at impact. A strategic factor in the development of chronic problems is a sudden increase in the demand for power or endurance during a work session.[1] They are more likely to occur when the participant has not prepared for the demand by gradually achieving a proper level of fitness prior to exposure (e.g., early season team workouts, weekend recreational athletes).[64]

Influential intrinsic factors include the generalized effects of advancing age, inactivity, and systemic disease.[15] Furthermore, sites of local pathology (i.e., secondary to previous trauma or steroid injections) can predispose any site to subsequent injury.[11,15,38,47,53,75]

Also associated with the occurrence of these musculotendinous injuries is the preinjury status of the knee joint. Knee joint pain, instability, articular surface pathology resulting in increased friction, and restricted motion are all factors that may indirectly affect the vulnerability of the limb to injury.[60]

Distinct from direct contusions and lacerations, muscle strains are injuries usually caused by stretching an actively contracting unit. Such injuries are consistently found to be major causes of time loss from a variety of competitive sports as well as recreational activities. The most common lower-extremity sites are the quadriceps and hamstring units. For almost all degrees of severity, the most common site of pathology is at the myotendinous junctions. While this fact is of limited clinical value in localizing the site of a tear, it does serve to remind us that the muscle fibers generally run obliquely and that tendons of origin and insertion extend throughout most of the length of muscle. For the sake of clarity, the discussion of this group of injuries is divided into categories of severity and anatomic location.

Delayed Muscle Soreness

First introduced by Hough at the beginning of the twentieth century,[31] delayed muscle soreness is a universally experienced syndrome in which pain or discomfort appears 24 to 72 hours after exercise. While commonly conceptualized as appearing only after particularly spirited ventures, it is the untrained muscle tissues of the weekend athletes that are the most susceptible. The soreness is associated with rhabdomyolysis, myoglobinuria, serum elevation of intramuscular enzymes, and localized muscle fiber necrosis on biopsy.[21,29,39] Of the various enzymes that are measurable, creatine kinase is the most frequently used for evidence of muscle damage. This enzyme is elevated for at least 24 hours after marathon races.[3] With the tissue damage and the soreness, there is a measurable muscle weakness, with normal strength usually returning from within a few days to weeks.[5,16,40]

This mildest form of muscle strain is more likely to result from muscle-lengthening (eccentric) rather than from isometric or muscle-shortening (concentric) exercises.[4] For the most part, this mild-level injury creates the best prognostic situation for the regeneration process in that the extracellular matrix, the blood, and the nerve supply are all left intact, and the damage is confined to the muscle fiber. If there has been significant connective tissue breakdown, urinary level of hydroxyproline will also be elevated.

Most modern-day athletes who indulge in weight training believe that maximum strength and power require tearing down existing muscle tissue. Therefore, soreness for a brief period after lifting sessions is expected and invited as a sign of advancement. Whether the soreness is a necessary part of the process is not yet clear. Actually, muscle fiber degeneration occurs routinely after both weight-lifting sessions and endurance events and is often accompanied by muscle soreness. It is speculated that the regenerated fibers are those that can stand the new level of demand. Nevertheless, the extent of our basic knowledge about this phenomenon is at least consistent with the weight coach recommendation that while maintenance lifting can be repeated daily, attempts to make major strides toward increasing strength should be limited to three sessions per week.

A few general approaches to training are commonly employed in these sessions to maximize strength gains. First, and most popular with the general public because of the exposure from the Olympic games, is the attempt to perform a single concentric contraction lift of a poundage that is at or just beyond the lifter's previous maximum. The second approach involves taking the targeted muscle group to exhaustion by concentically lifting a submaximal weight for a limited number of repititions. Eccentric muscle contractions are featured in a third general weight-lifting technique commonly referred to as burnouts, in which the force applied to the contracting muscle in eccentric exercises exceeds the muscle force, causing the muscle to lengthen rather than shorten. While gaining in popularity, this technique requires either a partner or very expensive equipment. The last approach of emphasizing eccentric exercise may hold the most promise for prevention of injury to muscles and joints during sports.

Partial Strains

While ruptures are the newsworthy soft tissue injuries, it is the partial tears of hamstring and quadriceps muscle groups that are so common in both competitive and recreational sports that they are a major reason for time lost from competition and from the workplace.[2,23,58] In animal studies, Nikolaou and associates[51] showed that in this mild form of injury, sites of torn fibers and limited hemorrhage are followed by a cellular-based inflammatory response. This process takes up to 4 days in the rabbit and is manifested by edema, acute inflammatory cells, granulation tissue vascularity, and fibrous tissue deposition. By 1 week, the scar tissue appeared sufficient and muscular strength had returned to normal. Present imaging technology will enable more clinical knowledge to be gained in the near future. In a study of hamstring injuries, Garrett et al.[22] demonstrated that intramuscular hematomas appear as areas of high electron density, while low electron density indicates an inflammatory process with edema formation. This ability to observe pathology in vivo without interrupting the natural process of injury and repair means that a major barrier to performing clinical research has been removed.

While clinical management of the mild and moderate injuries still consists mainly of rest and symptomatic treatment, some advancements have been made. For instance, it is now clear that one of the biggest residual problems of this type of injury is a very subtle loss of length of the musculotendinous unit. The amount of flexion in the position of immobilization is critical to avoiding a permanently weakened and contracted muscle in the injured patient. As for contusions, maintaining early and full motion generally offers the best treatment plan. However, if the extremity must be immobilized, it is well to remember that muscles immobilized in extension are larger and more resistant to tear and can generate more force than those contained in a flexed position.

Strain Syndromes

Prevention of strains is possible mainly through proper warm up technique. Safran et al.[64] recently lent scientific support to the common practice of warming up prior to any strenuous physical activity to reduce the likelihood of injury. These authors' results indicate that greater force and increased length are needed to tear isometrically preconditioned muscle.

ACUTE STRAINS

Ruptures of the extensor apparatus present some of the least common, but most dramatic, injuries to occur about the knee. They are dramatic because they occur following a single violent episode and result in the immediate loss of control of knee extension. Depending on the nature of the extrinsic and intrinsic causative factors, ruptures occur in a variety of locations along the quadriceps unit ranging from its separate origins on the pelvis and proximal thigh to the common tendinous insertion on the tibia tubercle.

The injuries that result from blunt trauma or laceration of the extensor mechanism are most likely to result in partial rather than complete disruption. However, ruptures in muscle substance at midthigh or through the body of the patella do occur by this mechanism if the direct blow occurs at the time of maximum quadriceps muscle contraction.[7]

Actually, fractures to the body of the patella represent the most common type of extensor unit rupture about the knee. Clap[13] found that patellar fractures accounted for 62 of 70 injuries that resulted in a complete loss of ability to actively extend the knee. These injuries are discussed elsewhere in this chapter.

The remaining ruptures have in common the fact that they occur to the flexed knee during attempts to prevent a fall. Further knee flexion results as the maximally contracted quadriceps unit is overpowered by the violent resultant force. This force is created from the weight of the body, the applied extrinsic force, the tremendous lever action on the acutely flexed knee and the floor reaction force at the foot.

Exactly where the rupture will occur and just how violent the episode must be to cause a complete tear appears to depend on the health of the tendon. In 1933, McMaster[44] based some still pertinent conclusions about the causes and locations of tendon and muscle ruptures on his clinical and experimental studies. He observed that a very great strain was required to rupture a normal musculotendinous unit, while very slight forces would rupture through a diseased segment. Furthermore, he discovered that in the normal unit the location of rupture was not through the tendon but at its junction with bone or muscle, the substance of the muscle, or its own bony origin.

Clinical experience has supported McMaster's ideas to the point that when a rupture has occurred or in the substance any tendon in the absence of an appropriate history, the surgeon must be aware that predisposing factors existed that may also affect the repair process postoperatively. In such pathologic ruptures modifications of the standard methods of treatment may need to be employed to assure an acceptable result.

As the severest form of strain syndrome, quadriceps unit ruptures are clinically important because of (1) the knee and whole body functional impairment associated with loss of extensor power; (2) the frequency of delays in diagnosis and treatment; and (3) relationship between the delay in treatment and quality of result.

The prognosis is poor for the patient who receives no treatment after a total disruption of extensor power. From the instant of injury, there is a total functional instability of the bent knee. Standing with the knee locked in full extension is usually possible. However, locomotion is difficult on flat ground and impossible on stairs or even on a slight decline.

Although the time limit varies according to the site or rupture, repairs that are done early yield consistently good to excellent results, whereas those performed after degeneration, retraction, and fibrosis of the tissue ends has taken place may not do as well.

Costly delays in treatment of these ruptures are frequent because of failure of either the patients or the physicians to recognize the significance of the injury. In review of 72 extensor ruptures about the knee, Rao and Siwek[61] found that in 28 patients (39 percent), the diagnosis was missed on the initial exam. Thirteen (18 percent) of these were not appreciated before more than 2 weeks after the injury.

Ramsey and Mueller[60] found that 7 of his 17 patients were not treated until 14 days to 1 year after their injury because the severity of the condition was not appreciated on the initial physical examination. These presenting signs and symptoms of these ruptures generally depend on the extent of time delay from injury as well as the mechanism

of the accident, the extent and location of associated tissue damage, the degree of separation of the fragments, the presence of other injuries, and the preinjury ambulatory status of the individual.

In patients with pathologic ruptures seen on a delayed basis the tendency for underdiagnosis stems from the lack of impressive pain, negative radiographic findings, and the absence of an appropriately violent history. These patients eventually seek attention mainly because of continued buckling of their knee and not because of pain. Prior to injury, these patients often are less ambulatory, older, and have obvious predisposing factors such as: inactivity, arthritis, systemic lupus erythematosus, renal failure, age-related degeneration, or a previous history of local trauma or injections. Even in fresh injuries seen shortly after violent trauma, hemarthrosis and subcutaneous hematoma may mislead the examiner away from the associated soft tissue defect.

Regardless of the presentation, diagnosis of a rupture should not be difficult in a patient with a history of anterior thigh or knee pain. The examiner must merely remember to look for the ability to extend the knee voluntarily or to even maintain the knee isometrically in a reasonable degree of extension against the force of gravity. Regardless of presence of a hematoma, complete ruptures are always associated with the presence of a palpable soft tissue defect at rest that widens with the upward migration of the proximal fragment during voluntary muscle contraction (Fig. 117-1).

Ruptures of the extensor mechanism can be classified by their anatomic location as well as the tissue type through which the rupture occurs. In the proximal thigh, the most common injury occurs to the origin of the rectus femoris muscle and results in an avulsion fracture from the ilium. In the midthigh, the ruptures occur through the muscle substance of the rectus femoris. In the distal thigh, several types of ruptures have been reported. Isolated ruptures of the vastus medialis and rectus femoris can occur at the musculotendinous junction. Complete extensor unit ruptures can occur in the supra- and infrapatellar region of the quadriceps tendon. Since the population at risk, mechanism of injury, examination findings, details of pathologic anatomy indications and results of treatment vary

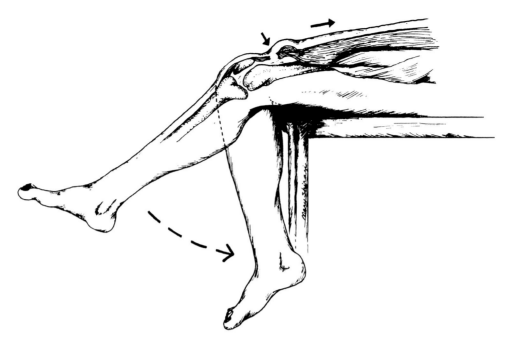

Fig. 117-1. Quadriceps tendon rupture. A soft tissue defect is palpable at rest that widens during attempts at knee extension. When the defect is complete, the patient is unable to maintain the extension against the force of gravity.

with the location of the rupture, each common site will be discussed separately.

Rectus Femoris Origin Avulsions

Disruption of the rectus femoris from one or both of its origins on the pelvis usually occurs either in the adolescent nearing skeletal maturity or in the very elderly. Often there has been a chronic prior history of symptoms and perhaps even of steroid injections.

Diagnosis

Typically, patients with these injuries present with sudden, severe anterior hip pain while running. The pain appears at pushoff on a maximally extended hip and moderately flexed knee. Localized to the anterior inferior iliac spine, this pain is exacerbated at examination by active flexion of the knee against resistance and by passive knee flexion with the hip fully extended. A defect may not be easily palpable in the area of maximum tenderness because of the location of its origin. Radiographs

are helpful in that an avulsion fragment is often present.

Indications

Surgical repair is rarely indicated because of the excellent functional result that can be expected without it. This muscle represents only one of the four units of the knee extensor mechanism and it is at best only a poor hip flexor. A relative surgical indication, provided there is radiographic evidence of an avulsion fragment, is a strong desire on the part of a competitive athlete. When indicated, surgical reattachment should then be performed before shortening of the muscle makes it technically difficult.

Another indication for surgical treatment of this injury is actually limited to late surgical excision of a large ossified segment in the tendon or muscle origin because of persistent pain. Peterson[56] reports the necessity for excision of a calcific mass in the origin of the rectus femoris that became painful with active flexion in a football player. Local excision in this instance will often allow a return to painless function.

Contraindications

Delay in diagnosis, absence of a bone fragment, a history of steroid injections, or a debilitated status or advanced age of the patient makes the technical aspects of a tendon-to-tendon repair difficult enough to provide a relative contraindication to surgical reattachment.

Treatment

Symptomatic nonoperative treatment includes rest, ice, and anti-inflammatory agents followed by a gradual rehabilitation program once the acute symptoms have subsided. The use of pain as a guide to rehabilitation progress is essential to optimizing the return to full activity without complication. Surgical repair of the avulsed fragment, although rarely worth considering, can usually be accomplished by direct suture to the original site of at-tachment through two parallel drill holes at the anterior iliac spine in the bone (Fig. 117-2).

If there has been too great a time delay and the contracture of the muscle will not allow for rehabilitation to be reattached to the origin, resuturing to a more distal point on the pelvis or proximal femur will provide satisfactory results. Usually, the tendon end has not migrated more than 3 or 4 cm distally because it is tethered by the attachment of the reflected head to just above the acetabulum.

Postoperative Care

Bedrest with the hips slightly flexed and knee straight provides sufficient comfort in the early postoperative period. Touch weight bearing with crutches is begun after a few days and maintained for the first 3 weeks. This is followed by a gradual return to full weight bearing and isometric muscle

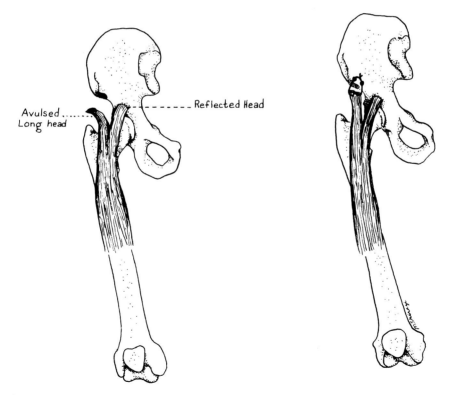

Fig. 117-2. Avulsion rectus femoris origin. Note the intact long head attachment to just above the acetabulum. Reattachment of the long head can usually be accomplished by direct suture through drill holes in the cortex and over the bone fragment in the detached tendon. Distal migration of the avulsed fragment is usually restricted by the intact reflected head.

contraction. An active muscle-strengthening program that includes hip flexion against resistance should not be started for at least 6 weeks or until there is no tenderness at the repair site.

Results

Function of the leg after an untreated proximal rupture is usually excellent with no apparent weakness or pain. Early and delayed operative reattachments have also been generally reported to be successful. No studies have been done to document any measurable loss of strength or athletic performance resulting from nonoperative management.

Complications

Rerupture is a problem after surgery because of the difficulty of protecting the hip in an advantageous position. Persistent pain can be seen occasionally after either nonoperative or operative treatment and is usually activity related. In one patient, the pain was the result of an entrapped motor nerve to the rectus femoris secondary to intermuscular adhesions. Neurolysis improved but did not relieve the symptoms.

Quadriceps Muscle Substance Ruptures

Occurrence

Quadriceps unit ruptures through the muscle tissue itself occur mostly in the isolated midthigh belly of the rectus femoris and distal portion of the vastus medialis. Ruptures of the rectus femoris usually occur from the combination of direct trauma to the forced stretch of the maximally contracted muscle.

Diagnosis

A muscle tear should be suspected when, in the absence of fracture or dislocation, the maximum pain and tenderness are located in the middle one-third of the anterior aspect of the thigh. The diagnosis may be difficult because the muscle is just one of four that extends the knee. As O'Donoghue[54] points out, the typical patient is at first treated for the more commonplace thigh contusion because they appear able to demonstrate some knee extension and have anterior thigh pain, swelling, and tenderness as a result of the direct blow. The depression is palpable at rest but is usually masked by hematoma. Also, the tell-tale bulge seen with contraction of the muscle may not be appreciated initially because of the voluntary or reflex inhibition of muscle contraction secondary to pain. Ruptures of the vastus medialis occur after patellar dislocations and are discussed elsewhere in this chapter.

Indications

Treatment plans should be aimed at establishing end-to-end continuity of the muscle unit through a strong, pliable fibrous band of scar that permits freedom and independent motion of the muscle belly with relationship to the adjacent tissue plane. Since surgical intervention can increase scarring, the critical question that must be carefully assessed initially is: Can operative approximation provide better results than those expected from nonoperative treatment? The expected results will vary according to the age of the patient; the type, location, and status of the tissue injured; the time delay since injury, and the results of alternative nonoperative treatment.

Although advocated by Smillie,[68] late surgical repair of quadriceps muscle ruptures have often failed. Therefore, the surgeon's decision to operate on a complete disruption of the midmuscle or musculotendinous portions of the quadriceps should be made during the first days post trauma. However, even early surgical treatment for complete tears is indicated only when the degree of expected loss of function that will result from nonoperative treatment is unacceptable to the patient's lifestyle.

In making the proper management decisions, several principles can be used as guidelines:

1. Muscle tissue does not regenerate, but contractile strength can return to near normal regardless of cosmetic appearances if some continuity can be maintained through scar tissue.
2. Healing of ruptured muscle tissue requires initial immobilization to establish continuity of the scar. This is followed by early motion to develop

a strong, pliable, fibrous band that is free of any adhesions to other tissue planes. Stearns[70] documented experimentally, that early movement of the injured tissue is required in order to obtain an orderly fibrillary network in the scar tissue.

3. Muscle tissue itself is extremely difficult to suture, and even the most diligent attempts can result not only in failure but more necrosis and scar tissue as a result of the surgery.
4. Ruptures occurring after a direct blow, such as a contusion, myositis ossificans, or laceration contain wide areas of edematous and friable tissue. A decision to repair these surgically may result in the dilemma of excising necrotic tissue, which shortens the mass of the healthy muscle and creates a larger and irreparable defect that must fill in with even more scar tissue.

It is my experience that if ever indicated, surgical repair of complete tears of the substance of the rectus femoris muscle should only be attempted if done soon after injury. Furthermore, it should be attempted only in the equivalent of young athletes and manual laborers; where even relatively minor losses of power or speed will have major functional consequences. The best results will be obtained within the first few days when the muscle appears to be at normal resting length and displays the proximal bulge only when contracted. The main goal of surgery is to reestablish an end-to-end continuity of the muscle unit that is strong enough to allow an effort to gain motion to begin within a 3-week period.

Late excision of the detached muscle ends may be indicated in the rare instance where localized significant pain and tenderness become disabling after only moderate physical therapy modalities. Surgery is not indicated in the instances where cramping can be relieved by a passive stretching program. Rather than a recent tear, this cramping is more indicative of a muscle-scar-muscle repair unit that has healed in continuity.

Contraindications

When muscle tissue is involved, delaying treatment of more than 3 to 5 days is a relative contraindication to attempting surgical reapproximation of rupture ends. In such instances, retraction of the muscle edges as well as necrosis and friability of tissues may already have occurred to make reinjury likely.

Treatment

Nonoperative treatment should consist of a few weeks of immobilization emphasizing only gentle isometric contraction of the muscle. Nongravity, active flexion exercises are then cautiously begun as tolerated. Straight leg lifting and progressive resistance muscle strengthening are not begun until 90 degrees of flexion is achieved without pain.

Operative Technique

In my hands, repair of quadriceps muscle ruptures is only attempted within the first few days after injury. A 20-cm-long midline anterior thigh incision is centered over the rupture (Fig. 117-3A). The hematoma is aspirated and the entire muscle belly sheathed and surrounding tissues are inspected closely for damage and salvage ability. The necrotic ends of the muscle tissue are debrided.

The main surgical goal is to establish continuity of the muscle unit through a scar that allows freedom of motion with relationship to the adjacent compartment. Therefore, after debridement of the necrotic muscle fibers, with the tourniquet deflated an assessment is made of the gap that must be bridged. If the gap is as much as 3 to 6 cm, either an iliotibial band or Dacron tape reinforcement will be required for approximation. Suturing muscle fibers directly together is fruitless, and successful repair depends on the availability of tough fibrous tissue for reapproximation. The best tissue is usually located at the base of the wound in the sheath of the vastus intermedius and in the more superficial but thick and expansive tendon of the rectus femoris. Heavy chromic catgut horizontal mattress sutures are first inserted but not tied in the deepest layers. If reapproximation proves difficult, a 12-cm-long and 1.5-cm-wide iliotibial band graft should be obtained from the lateral aspect of distal and midthigh (Fig. 117-3B). The graft is then sectioned into two 6-cm pieces; dependent on the width of the gap to be closed and be placed 3 cm on either side of the tear sutured to one side and tightened by the assistant prior to tying the deep vastus intermedius sheath sutures (Fig. 117-3B). Postop-

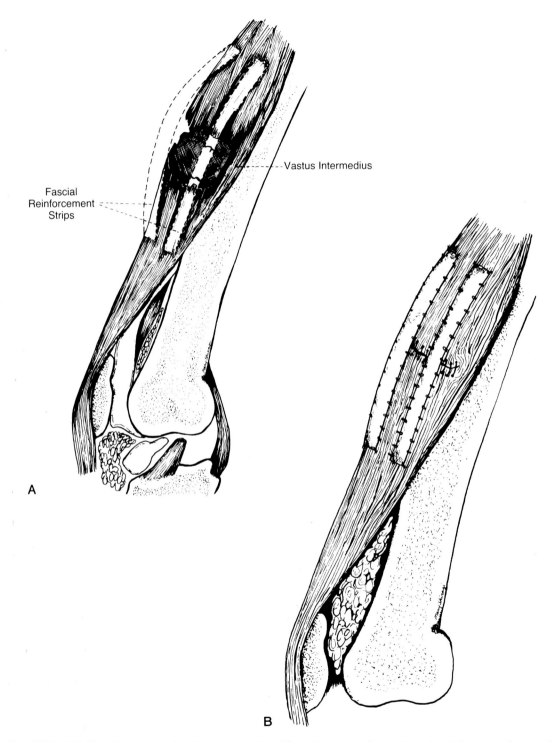

Fig. 117-3. (A) Quadriceps muscle substance rupture. Hematoma must be aspirated and the necrotic muscle fibers in frayed fascial sheath must be debrided. Do not resect any viable tissue and do not place sutures in the muscle belly. The best tissue for sutures is usually the vastus intermedius fascia at the base of the wound. **(B)** Fascial graft strips should be used to close the entire rupture site.

erative care is basically the same for the quadriceps tendon rupture.

Results

Successful maintenance of the reapproximation of tissue is technically difficult even when the repair is done early. Because of the high risk of pain, limited motion, and recurrence, there is a question of whether early attempts at repair in this area should ever be made postoperatively. Late excision of painful scar or muscle tissue relieves pain.

In my experience, a few fresh ruptures of the extensor mechanism in relatively healthy patients whose muscle ruptures were repaired early have given excellent results. On the contrary, late repair or repair in patients with preexisting soft tissue pathology greatly diminishes the chance of regaining satisfactory postoperative function. In general, more satisfactory results are obtained when there has been an avulsion from the bony attachment of the extensor unit and when an exact reapproximation has been achievable and early strengthening and range-of-motion exercises have been instituted.

Complications

As pointed out by Nagel and Jameson,[48] the potential for developing some type of complication after any kind of surgery on a musculotendinous unit is high enough to temper even the most enthusiastic surgeons. However, the repair of a complete disruption of the extensor mechanism of the thigh is particularly fraught with hazards because of (1) the basic nature of the tissue in this mass of muscle fibers with relatively little fascial covering; (2) the high incidence of preexisting pathology at the injury site; and (3) the magnitude of the strength demands that are placed on this structure during activities of daily living. Specifically, the most common complications include residual extensor weakness, delayed wound healing, pain and ankylosis of the knee joint, and patellofemoral joint pain.

Weakness from failure to reestablish continuity may result from quadriceps unit ruptures which are unrecognized and therefore go untreated or at least inadequately protected. Weakness is also a common occurrence even after surgical intervention has been attempted because of the lack of sufficient amounts of firm tissue for reattachment; the size of the gap to be made up; or the lack of sufficient postoperative immobilization. Significant thigh atrophy has been found after quadriceps and patellar tendon repairs, despite a return to a functionally normal strength for the patient's daily needs.[67]

Delayed healing can be expected to occur commonly and will lead to rerupture if caution is not exercised at surgery and during the early postoperative periods. This is particularly true for pathologic ruptures at the site of steroid injections, after long-term systemic steroid therapy, or in the presence of severe systemic disease affecting the wound healing process. Inspection of the viability and the friability of the tissues and biopsy analysis of the margins of the rupture can help firmly establish the likelihood of this complication in the surgeon's mind. Since early motion is generally desirable during the postoperative period, a primary goal of surgical intervention is to establish adequate integrity and inherent stability of the repair to allow motion to begin without risk of rerupture.

Significant postoperative limitation of motion with or without pain is enough of a concern in those patients that a considerable effort must be directed toward these technical details of the operative procedures, which may help in prevention of this complication.

Preexisting pathology of the patellofemoral joint is common and should be assessed intraoperatively. The need for immediate or delayed reconstructive knee surgery should not be overlooked as this may have been the primary problem which lead to the eventual disruption of the extensor unit. If simultaneous total knee replacement and reapproximation of the extensor unit is being considered, it is helpful to remember that a patellar button will increase the tension on the extensor unit and that a prosthesis with a femoral flange alone can significantly reduce the patellofemoral pain.

Significant postoperative patellofemoral pain can develop even in a previously normal joint. Patellofemoral problems can easily result if the patellar tendon or the quadriceps tendon is excessively shortened. This situation creates undue compression and incongruity between the joint surfaces and may produce rapid articular erosion. Testing for the ability to fully flex the knee to 90 degrees at the operating table prior to skin closure will help avoid this major complication.

Quadriceps Tendon Ruptures

Occurrence

According to an extensive review by Siwek and Rao,[67] in 117 cases published from 1880 to 1978 in which the age of patient was given, there were 69 quadriceps tendon ruptures with an average age of 48.2 years. Sixty-five (88 percent) of these ruptures occurred in patients who were 40 years old or older. While 38 (80 percent) of those patients with ruptures below the patella were younger than 40 years.

Several investigators have reported that tissue biopsies from fresh rupture sites of the quadriceps tendon showed local degenerative changes already present, including decreased collagen content, fibrotic degeneration and infiltration.[65,76] Thus, it is not surprising that these dramatic injuries can result from a moderately stressful incident such as a mere attempt to avoid crashing to the ground after stumbling over an embankment. Bilateral quadriceps tendon ruptures are indeed indicative of the severe preexisting basic system disease process.[78] When the injury occurs bilaterally, the initial diagnosis may be very difficult to make because often there is no swelling or any other sign, symptoms or history of trauma.

In the great majority of cases, tear of the quadriceps tendon occurs when the knee is in a semi-flexed position. The tear first occurs in the central portion of the tendon usually at the superior border of the patella.[10] However, it may also occur as much as 4 to 5 cm more proximal. The ruptures may be limited to the tendon or rectus femoris or may expand to include the aponeurotic expansions of the vasti as well. When the rupture extends into deeper planes, the synovial lining becomes involved and a large hemarthrosis is evident.[15]

Diagnosis

The signs of symptoms of this condition depend entirely on the time and manner of occurrence of the injury as it relates to the degree of separation and the fragments and the extent of the rent that has occurred. The cardinal symptom is the inability to voluntarily extend the knee (see Fig. 117-1). The patient has only a modest amount of suprapatellar pain and tenderness. In the complete disruption, one immediately notices a profuse hemarthrosis with an especially prominent bulge when the hematoma has been distributed subcutaneously through the rupture site. One can palpate the anterior aspect of the femoral condyles and the supracondylar area and the patella is easily movable and lying at a slightly lower than normal level.

Except for an occasional avulsion fragment and the usual presence of some degree of degenerative arthritis of the knee, no pathology will be evident radiographically.[60] Bilateral knee films may reveal a significant difference in the distance from the patella to its tibial insertion.

During the attempt to actively extend the leg, the thigh contour becomes obviously abnormal at the site of the defect as it is accentuated by the bulge of the retracting proximal quadriceps edge. Unfortunately, when seen shortly after injury, this telltale bulge often remains much less than obvious with the leg at rest because the adjacent defect is initially filled with hematoma. Furthermore, an early pain-related voluntary reflex inhibition can often make the bulge difficult to detect at all. My experience with patients with complete ruptures involving medial and lateral vastus attachments has been an impressive lack of extensor function to the degree that they have occasionally been suspected of a peripheral neuropathy. By contrast, those less extensive ruptures with nearly complete extension are thought to have a mild ligament sprain, bruise, or locked knee from interarticular pathology. Incomplete extension and hemarthrosis have even lead to arthroscopy, with immediate diffusion of irrigation fluid into the thigh. In very difficult diagnostic situations, a computed tomography (CT) scan has proved very helpful at identifying the nature and exact location and extent of the injury.

Clinically, it is extremely important for the examiner to carefully look for any continuity of fibers by checking for the rigidity of the proximal muscle mass, the medial lateral extent of the bulge, and the looseness of the patella to passive motion both up and down and side to side during a voluntary quadriceps contraction.

Indications

The diagnosis of rupture of the complete extensor mechanism at the tendon-bone junction is a definite indication for surgical repair regardless of the time elapsed since surgery because of the poor results of the nonsurgical management and the degree of functional impairment incurred without the extensor mechanism.

The most difficult management decision is encountered where there is a delay in orthopaedic referral. A patient noted initially to have no extensor strength is usually experiencing a partial return of active extension against gravity within a few weeks. As the strength slowly improves, the indications for surgery become less clear. However, this improvement usually has a definite limit that is far short of providing support while walking down an incline. In this instance, critical to choosing the best course of treatment is the assessment of the possibility of the reestablishment or any continuity. If surgery is to be delayed for even a short time, a definite quadriceps contraction force must be palpated to be directly transmitted through the defect to the patella. If there is some return, a definitive time frame should be established to assess any further progress. Whenever it becomes apparent that strengths will remain inadequate for stooping, climbing stairs, and so forth, surgery deserves careful consideration.[20]

Contraindications

When surgical repair is delayed to the point of retraction of the proximal flap in a patient with a marginal medical or functional status, a relative contraindication exists for surgery. The surgeon is faced with a choice of either allowing the patient to be up in braces or remain wheelchair bound or to risk loss of knee flexion at the expense of reestablishing control of extension.

Author's Preferred Treatment
(Early Repair)

Within the first 48 hours of injury, there usually is enough pliability of the tissues to reestablish continuity directly through end-to-end repair. However, since, as already discussed, one of the primary goals of surgery is to provide enough strength in the repair to allow early motion, some reinforcement over the single end-to-end suture line is usually deemed necessary.

Operative Technique

A midline anterior longitudinal skin incision is begun approximately 15 cm above the proximal pole of the patella and extended distally toward the joint line. After aspiration of the hematoma, the breadth of the entire quadriceps mechanism should be inspected for tissue damage and salvageability.

The most superficial layer of the tendon is usually torn distally, at or near the superior pole of the patella. The middle and deep layers of the quadriceps tendon are each torn more proximally in the

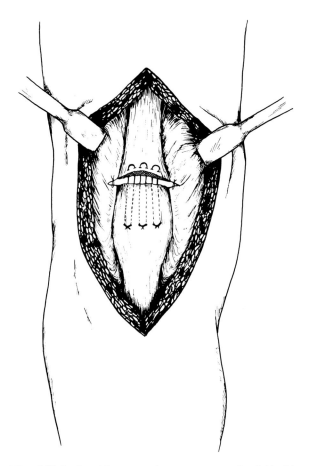

Fig. 117-4. Quadriceps tendon rupture repair. Critical in the repair is reattachment of the rectus tendon fibers through drill holes to a prepared bed on the patella.

soft tissues. The suprapatellar pouch must also be inspected thoroughly, as it is usually also disrupted.

The necrotic and frayed edges of fascia and muscle should be carefully debrided and the synovium should be closed. Despite the fact that it may be difficult to identify precise anatomic planes, attempts should be made with heavy absorbable horizontal mattress sutures to reapproximate the edges of the tendon as accurately as possible. This should start deep with the intermedius and proceed outwards through the middle layer of the two vasti to the most anterior major tendon for the rectus femoris. During the initial resuturing, ten-

sion may be kept off the suture line by deflating the tourniquet and placing a towel clip proximally in the rectus tendon and pulling the quadriceps mechanism distally. The tough fibers of the rectus femoris tendon should be sutured directly through drill holes to a prepared bed on the patella (Fig. 117-4).

When reinforcement of the suture line is needed to allow early motion, a Scuderi[65] flap is usually fashioned and turned down over the suture line (Fig. 117-5A). This triangular flap should be carefully dissected to create a uniform thickness of 3 mm. The apex should be centered 8 cm above the site of rupture and extend distal to the medial and

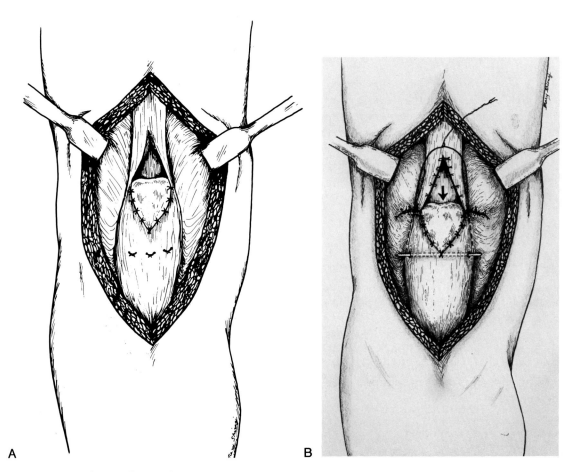

A   B

Fig. 117-5. (A) Scuderi flap reinforcement. This triangular flap is based 2 cm above the site of the rupture. It is 5 cm wide at its base and approximately 6 to 8 cm long. The flap should be approximately 3 mm thick. **(B)** If approximation of the rupture edges proves difficult, a Bennett type quadriceps tendon lengthening is performed by completing the Scuderi flap incision down through the full thickness of the tendon. A retention suture with a pull-out wire is fastened to a Steinmann pin in the patella.

lateral margins of the thick rectus femoris tendon to form a base approximately 2 cm above the site of the rupture. This usually results in a flap that is at least 5 cm wide at its base. Then heavy resorbable sutures are used to tack down the flap to the tough prepatellar tissue.

Late Repair

Shortening of the quadriceps muscle becomes a progressively more pertinent problem with increasing time delay from surgery. If the surgery has been merely delayed to the point that the gap can be closed but there is a problem with tension at the suture line from proximal retraction of the tissue, iliotibial band or Dacron tape reinforcement should be used as a retention extending from the base of the Scuderi flap into drill holes across the proximal patella.

When the gap of the resting quadriceps muscle reaches 5 cm or more, it is unlikely that direct reapposition of the tendon ends will be possible. In this instance, after the flap is fashioned, the inverted V incision is completed down through the full thickness of the extensor mechanism to allow the edges of the rupture site to be closed in a manner similar to that described by Scuderi and credited to Codvilla.[65] The repair is protected with a patellar pin distally and proximally based pull-out wires (Fig. 117-5B). When this same poorly correctable situation occurs in elderly or debilitated patients with marginal preinjury knee extensor strength, anterior transfer of the biceps and semitendinosis tendons is indicated[32,65,78] (Fig. 117-6).

At the conclusion of the operative procedure, adequacy of the repair should be tested by lifting the thigh to 90 degrees of flexion allowing the knee to gradually flex passively. Barring preinjury limitations of motion, 90 degrees of flexion should be achievable in the operating room from the weight of the leg without undue stress at the suture line. If there is doubt about the surgical repair to withstand an early range-of-motion program, a McLaughlin[43] tibial bolt and pull-out wire threaded through the proximal tendon is used. This reinforcement can remain for protection of the repair as much as 6 weeks until full extension and active flexion to 90 degrees has been achieved.

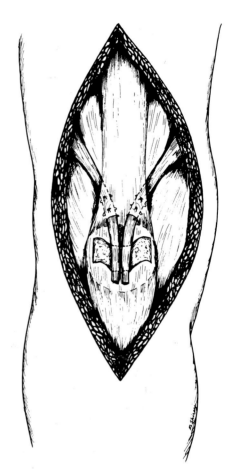

Fig. 117-6. Anterior hamstring transfer. The semitendinosis and biceps femoris tendon are subcutaneously transferred anteriorly and attached to the extensor mechanism in two places. Each is first tunneled through the proximal tendon fragment and then attached to its periosteal flap on the anterior aspect of the patella.

Postoperative Management

A compressive dressing is reinforced with either a posterior plaster splint or a large knee immobilizer. After 3 days, the wound is inspected and a snug cylinder cast with drop lock joint is applied with the knee in full extension. Quadriceps setting and straight-leg raising are encouraged from the outset. Partial weight bearing with crutches is allowed as tolerated. Gentle, passive range of motion is begun after the first week under the supervision of the therapist.

If the age of the patient and the condition of the patellofemoral joint cause major concern with limitation of motion, patient is kept in the hospital and left initially in a knee immobilizer so that they may begin inpatient physical therapy with range of motion beginning on the third to seventh day. Prior to discharge, at least 40 degrees of motion should be achieved and a drop-lock cylinder cast should be applied.

At 3 weeks the cast and skin sutures are removed and quadriceps control is assessed. A long knee immobilizer is applied and the patient is sent to therapy for supervised active and gentle active assistance range of motion exercises as well as a gradually progressive quadriceps- and hamstring-strengthening protocol.

Results

Fresh ruptures of the extensor mechanism in relatively healthy patient's repaired early give excellent results. Siwek and Rao[67] found that all 30 of their patients had excellent results with direct suture and cylinder cast support. On the contrary, late repair or repair in patients with preexisting pathology in the soft tissues themselves greatly diminishes the chance of regaining satisfactory function postoperatively. Siwek and Rao[67] found that only 3 of 6 results were optimum due to lack of 90 degrees of flexion and significant quadriceps atrophy. One of the 6 patients required a Codvilla quadricepsplasty. In general, the most satisfactory results are obtained when there has been an avulsion from the bony attachment of the unit and reapproximation has been easily achievable.

Complications

As noted by Siwek and Rao,[67] stiffness of the knee joint is the most common complication. However, surgery in this area is fraught with all of the complications pointed out by Nagel and Jameson[48] (see under Quadriceps Muscle Substance Ruptures).

Patellar Tendon Ruptures

Occurrence

Rupture of the patellar tendon is extremely rare, occurring with an incidence about equal to that of the quadriceps tendon. Mostly occurring in people under 40, they are usually located at either end of the patellar tendon rather than its middle. The relatively more common ruptures are at the inferior patellar pole. They are associated with steroid injections or previous history of patellar tendinitis.[53,72]

Disruption of the distal patellar tendon insertion on the tibial tubercle is very rare in mature adults and has not been reported except after steroid injection, previous laceration or contusions, or Osgood-Schlatter's disease.[68] I have also seen this injury occur twice after patellar tendon transfer was done to correct malalignment at the time of total knee replacement. In adolescents, the disruption of this distal tibial insertion of the tendon has been reported to occur as a displaced avulsion fracture of the tibial tubercle.[55] Bilateral rupture has also been reported in patients with systemic lupus erythematosus and rheumatoid arthritis.[61,62,71]

Diagnosis

The diagnosis of patellar tendon rupture is not difficult to make. On clinical examination, the patient is unable to extend the knee at all despite visible and palpable contraction of the quadriceps muscle and concomitant proximal migration of the patella. A defect can be palpated in the patellar tendon and an avulsion fragment is frequently visible on radiography. When present, this fragment can aid in identification of the extent of the proximal migration of the tendon. With the knee in full extension and the quadriceps mechanism at rest, the patella may not have an unusually high-riding appearance to the examiner but, as the knee is passively flexed or actively extended, this defect becomes very obvious.

Indications

Surgical repair is indicated whenever sufficient damage has occurred that leg extension against resistance is not mechanically possible and patellar migration is demonstrable. If the patellar tendon is damaged but there is no proximal migration of the patella, nonoperative treatment should be considered initially. This is possible because the retinacular attachments of the medialis and lateralis as well as the superficial attachments of the rectus femoris tendon can allow some extension of the knee when the tear is completely through the patellar tendon itself. However, even incomplete tears of the patella tendon should be considered for repair when the patella has demonstrated any tendency to migrate proximally.

Contraindications

Relative surgical contraindications include: a history of recurrent injury, fixed proximal migration of patella, preexisting severe systemic vascular or neuromuscular disease, treatment with long-term steroids, and generally debilitated elderly patients with other medical problems that in themselves restrict their mobility.

Treatment Alternatives

Most of the variations in the surgical approach emanate from the concern with the late repair and are attempts to provide a means of easing tension from the repair site. McLaughlin[43] suggested a wire loop around the superior pole of the patella which is fixed to a bolt in the tibial tuberosity. Chandler[12] described the use of the circular wire through transverse drill holes in the patella and the

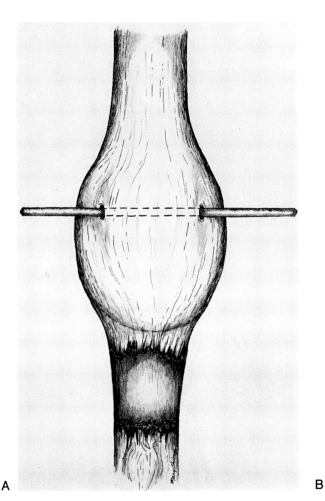
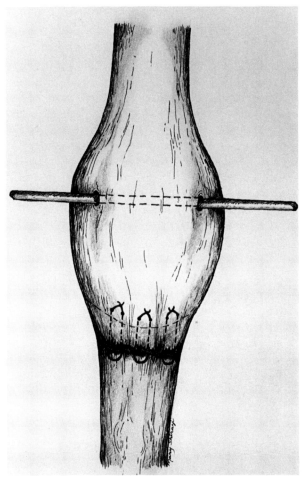

A

B

Fig. 117-7. (A) Proximal patellar migration. Delayed repair of patellar tendon occasionally requires distal traction preoperatively. The pin site should be in the proximal one-half to reserve the inferior region for fixation of patellar tendon or reinforcement. **(B)** Delayed primary repair of patellar tendon rupture was accomplished by intraoperative distal pin traction.

tibial tuberosity. Siwek and Rao[67] described the use of the pins and wires method beginning with preoperative traction by means of a Steinmann pin placed through the patella. A second pin is placed in the tibia at the time of surgery, and the two parallel pins are connected by #7 wires meant to hold the patella in its anatomic position. They also used a fascia lata graft reinforcement of the suture line incorporated in both ends of the ruptures in a figure-of-eight fashion. Kelikian et al.[37] used the semitendinous tendon to bridge the tendonous gap. Ecker[17] added the gracilis to the semitendinous for reinforcement, by the distal patellar skeletal traction intraoperatively only and reinforced the repair with wire fixation.

In light of the fact that restriction of motion is a problem in this instance Blair and Pontarelli[8] suggest the most novel answer with an ambulatory dynamic patellar tendon traction using a cast brace assembly to correct early proximal migration of the patella prior to any infrapatellar reconstruction. They describe applying distal traction with rubber bands attached proximally to transpatellar threaded Steinmann pin and distally to wire loops projecting from the tibial portion of the cast brace. The patient is allowed to ambulate full weight bearing with a hinged cast locked in extension.

Author's Preferred Treatment

Immediate repair of ruptures of the patellar tendon is accomplished using end-to-end sutures, avoiding strangulation of the patellar tendon blood supply by not including too much tissue with each suture. Reinforcement of the suture line is usually unnecessary in early cases with the rupture at the tendon-to-bone attachment.

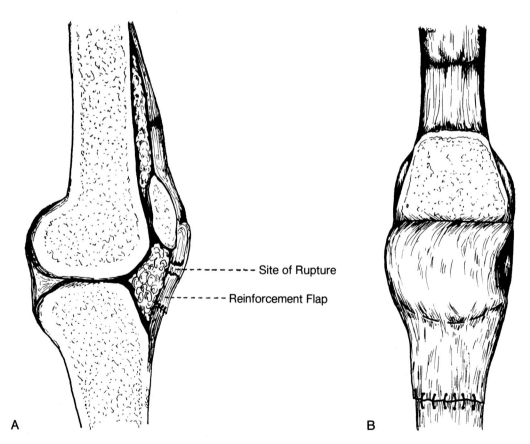

Site of Rupture

Reinforcement Flap

A

B

Fig. 117-8. Patellar tendon rupture reinforcement. This flap is similar to the one described for reinforcement of the quadriceps tendon rupture except that the donor site extends across the anterior surface of the patella. Ruler measurement should be used to estimate the proximal extent of the donor flap prior to dissection.

Repairs of the patellar tendon that are performed 2 weeks or more after injury can cause problems in repair or reconstruction especially if enough time has elapsed for fixed proximal migration of the patella.

In delayed repairs, the need for a preoperative traction has not been considered necessary and has been avoided whenever possible because of a fear of infection. Intraoperatively, a Steinmann pin is placed in the superior portion of the patella, and distal traction is applied (Fig. 117-7). If reapproximation of the patellar tendon edges is possible on the delayed basis, an adaptation of the Scuderi turn-down flap has also been used to reinforce the patellar tendon when its mass is insufficient (Fig. 117-8). If there is need for bridging the tendinous gap, drill holes are placed transversely through the inferior pole of the patella and the tibial tubercle. The semitendinosus is then looped through these holes and sewn back down onto itself at the tibial tubercle (Fig. 117-9). The Steinmann pin is then removed, and a Dacron graft can be placed through this proximal patellar tunnel. A second more distal drill hole is placed in the tibial tubercle for distal attachment of this graft. Both the biologic and Dacron material have the advantage over wire or Steinmann pins in the early motion can be begun without fear of it breaking or becoming infected. Also, a second procedure is not needed for removal of pins or wires. When approved in this country, the use of carbon filament sutures is attractive because of their initial tensile strength, the stimulation of fibrous tissue reaction, and their biodegradability.

The main reason for the concern with reinforcement is that limitation of knee motion is a major problem after patellar tendon repairs. Those patients with the best results are those who have been able to move their knee throughout a range of motion relatively early in the postoperative period.

Postoperative Care

Postoperative care is the same as for the quadriceps tendon ruptures.

Results

In the 26 patients reported by Siwek and Rao,[67] 20 had excellent results of immediate repair. Four

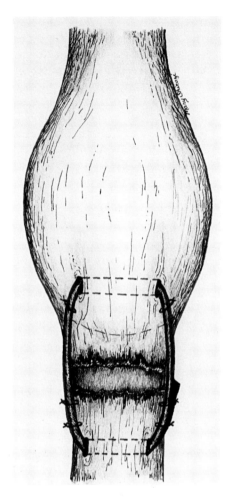

Fig. 117-9. Fixed proximal patellar migration. Dacron or fascial graft should be passed securely through drill holes in patella and tibia.

patients experienced less than 90 degrees of motion and 2 patients reruptured 8 weeks after surgery. In the 7 patients with delayed patellar tendon repair, two were "excellent," and three were "good" postoperatively.

Complications

Infection, rerupture, and painful ankylosis of the knee are the three primary complications of surgical repair in this area. Necrosis of the patella and its tendon is also possible if attempts to overcome a fixed proximal migration of the patella result in overzealous circumferential surgical dissection. When the tautness of the repair makes extension contracture a concern, the best choice would appear to await the results of an early motion program. Other procedures can be performed on a delayed basis, if necessary (see discussion of stiff knee).

CHRONIC STRAINS

Jumper's Knee

In this chronic strain syndrome the chief complaint is pain of insidious origin located at the extensor tendon attachment to the inferior or superior pole of the patella. It is associated with the cumulative effects of repetitive strains during periods of sustained vigorous physical activity but has also been noted to occur after arthroscopy performed through a transpatellar tendon portal.

The initial symptoms are suggestive of a mild to moderate acute strain, with very localized pain lasting a few hours to a few days. If insufficient time is allowed for recovery, the symptoms recur after resumption of the same physical activity. Sports that involve a great deal of running and jumping are the most aggravating. Stiffness may be experienced after just sitting, squatting, or climbing stairs, but the symptoms are not disabling.

If the offending activity is still continued, the problem may become more severe and be accompanied by the more diffuse pain of generalized synovitis across the anterior aspect of the knee. The severity of the symptoms can progress to the point of being disabling not only for competition but even for simple activities of daily living. The acute symptoms will usually subside spontaneously if the frequency and intensity of the physical demands are lessened or ceased.

Although several investigators have considered this entity to be a rare problem that invariably requires surgical management, my primary care-level experience is quite different. In athletes, the symptoms frequently develop as a secondary part of an impressive picture of chondromalacia patella and synovitis. Whether of primary or secondary origin, only a few people with acute symptoms ever progress to the chronic persistent syndrome that leads to orthopaedic consultation.

The pathology is difficult to identify surgically without invading the substance of the tendon. In the middle and deep layers of that portion of the tendon under clinical suspicion, a region can be identified by its loss of continuity to the attachment of the tendon fibers to the patella. This area contains varying degrees of tissue degeneration as well as a fibrous tissue response in the absence of a remarkable inflammatory cell infiltrate.[6] Microscopically, the torn edge of the surgical specimen exhibits demarcated areas of normal and abnormal tendon fibers and necrotic debris surrounded by granulation tissue at the zone of bony attachment. The necrotic areas may also contain spotty calcifications.

Except for the usual absence of radiographic changes, this adult syndrome appears to be clinically related to osteochondritis of the lower pole of the patella described in adolescents by Sinding-Larson in 1921 and by Johansson in 1922.[45] In this adolescent's syndrome, ossicles are usually present in the specimen. These ossicles consist of a central core of trabecular bone with a peripheral zone of cartilage surrounded by normal appearing tendons. At the patellar tendon-bone junction, varying degrees of the injury and repair process are present. This may include evidence of callus formation, which is indicative of avulsion fracture.

Diagnosis

As mentioned above, symptoms of jumper's knee may exist alone or be part of a confusing complex which includes symptoms of coexisting entities such as chrondromalacia patella, pes bursitis, and generalized synovitis. Regardless of other manifestations in patients with jumper's knee, the pain and tenderness are uniquely located adjacent to the inferior pole of the patella and can be readily identified as originating from within rather than deep to this extensor mechanism. In the early stages, the diagnosis is made by the location of the point of maximum tenderness at the center of the tendon-bone junction and the reproduction of the symptoms during attempts at manually resisted extension regardless of the position of the knee. Tenderness can also be elicited in any degree of knee flexion. However, greater sensitivity is present in full extension and with increasing tautness of the extensor mechanisms. When the knee is flexed, greater applied pressure is required to elicit the tenderness. Localized transient fullness just inferior to the patellar pole is occasionally detectable acutely in the area of maximal tenderness. This is sometimes followed by a subtle defect when compared to the contralateral knee.

Other than osteopenia, no diagnostic radiographic changes are usually seen.[63] In my experience, one 18-year-old woman displayed an avulsion fracture just off the inferior patellar pole (Fig. 117-10). In longstanding cases, a local calcification in the patellar tendon has been reported.[6]

The differential diagnosis in these early stages

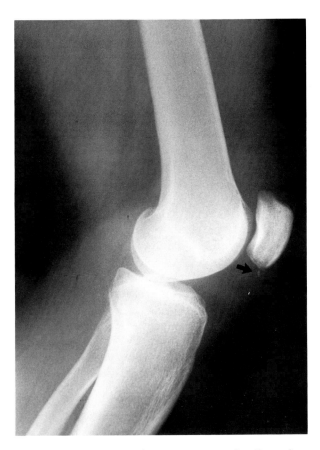

Fig. 117-10. An avulsion fracture may occasionally confirm the diagnosis of jumper's knee. However, most often no radiographic changes are present. An elongated and rarefied patellar pole may eventually develop.

should include prepatellar bursitis, chondromalacia of the patella, Hoffa's disease,[15] anterior meniscal tear, synovitis with tender alar folds, and/or painful plica syndrome.

In chronic prepatellar bursitis, the location of the point of maximum tenderness usually overlaps the inferior or superior pole of the patella into the patellar capsule. However, in contrast to the symptoms in jumper's knee, the thickened rim of the prepatellar bursa can usually be easily palpated to extend well beyond the medial and lateral limits of the patellar tendon.

In patients with jumper's knee, compression of the patella itself does not reproduce the symptoms as it does in chondromalacia patella.

Passive extension of the knee to its full extent does not cause the impingement pain in jumper's knee as it will in Hoffa's disease[15] or in the presence of an anterior meniscal tear. Furthermore, in the presence of pathology deep to the patellar tendon, tensing the quadriceps muscle tends to push the examiner's finger away from the tender spot.

Indications

Because this entity is often persistent but self-limiting, the choice of treatment should be appropriate to the nature and duration of the symptoms and the goals of the patient. This must be followed by a carefully controlled rehabilitation and conditioning program. The best chance for cure is immediately after the initial injury with an aggressive immobilization program. In the chronic state, pain and tenderness will improve with immobilization but tend to quickly return if there is a premature resumption of the offending physical activity. The patient always has the luxury of avoiding the symptoms by avoiding the situation that causes it originally.

Surgery is indicated in a small well-defined group of patients with chronic symptoms resistant to nonoperative treatment. In most of these surgical candidates, the pathologic process has developed to a point beyond the body's capacity for repair. Surgical excision may be preferred by these individuals because it offers the only chance left for a cure and the restrictions required for adaptation to the physical impairment are not tolerable. A few patients requiring surgery are athletes whose goals are to return to action with a reasonably functional level of performance.

In both instances, the best results are seen when the surgeon is convinced that elimination of this specific problem will significantly alter the patient's clinical picture. Enhancing the surgeon's confidence are (1) the consistent presence of localized tenderness and a palpable defect in the patellar attachment of the tendon; (2) radiographic evidence for local changes at the patellar pole; (3) a persistent extensor lag due to a pain related disuse atrophy despite the maximum efforts of a reliable patient; or (4) disinterested party verification that the significant functional impairment is obvious in the patient's daily environment and that the alleged symptoms are not providing significant secondary gain.

Contraindications

Operative treatment is contraindicated in the absence of a specific diagnosis or when the patient maintains unrealistic postoperatively goals. The diagnosis should definitely be established preoperatively, and the symptoms should have become intolerably limiting to make a surgical venture worthwhile. One of the greatest potential problems with active athletes is experienced when the patient has unreasonable expectations that an operation can bring about an immediate cure. The decision to operate on such patients without their first gaining an understanding of the nature of the problem will prove unsatisfactory to both patient and surgeon. Injections of cortisone should not be used in the treatment of this injury because of their lack of long-term relief and the potential for subsequent rupture.[27] Furthermore, lidocaine (Xylocaine) injections for temporary relief during competition are also potentially dangerous and unnecessary. If the symptoms are so severe that the anti-inflammatory medications, ice, and transcutaneous electrical nerve stimulation are not effective at pain relief, such patients may be in danger of causing further damage to the tendon if they return to full activity.

Treatment Alternatives

Successful early nonoperative treatment of the mild to moderate acute injuries mainly requires immediate and adequate immobilization. In addition to the use of routine anti-inflammatory agents, topical application of hydrocortisone may aid in decreasing the inflammatory symptoms. This is accomplished by the phonoporesis process using ultrasound as an energy source to transport the 5 to 10 percent hydrocortisone lotion transcutaneously to the problem area. This must be accomplished over a 10- to 14-day period to avoid counterproductive irritation from the energy source.

Since most patients with jumper's knee whom I have seen also have symptoms of acute soft tissue inflammation and perhaps even chondromalacia patella, a trial of transcutaneous electrical nerve stimulation (TENS) can be most helpful in improving the physician's diagnostic and prognostic capabilities by temporarily relieving the pain of the surrounding inflamed tissue. In doing so, the examination is much more reliable as the patient is less apprehensive; the actual contribution of the tendon injury to the total pain picture can be unveiled and the short-term success of nonoperative management can be predicted. In a study of 50 patients with anterior knee pain from a variety of causes, a high percentage of transient pain relief (i.e., 50 to 100 percent improvement) from the brief TENS trial correlated well with the success of short-term nonoperative management when local and systemic anti-inflammatory improvement agents were included along with appropriate rest or immobilization.

Immobilization may be accomplished most effectively with a cylinder cast or, to provide complete freedom from pain for 2 to 12 weeks, by a reinforced canvas knee immobilizer. Once pain free and nontender, most individuals can return to full activity status without recurrence. However, critical to a successful return is whether enough time is allowed for gradual progressive rehabilitation and conditioning programs, which restore the strength and mass of the extensor mechanism. The activity level is regulated by the absence of symptoms at each step.

Often, isometrics and straight-leg lifting without weights are the only exercises tolerated at the outset. Pain often diminishes as strength improves and the extensor lag disappears. A progressive resistance program is then indicated to the point that a one-legged squat can be performed to 90 degree flexion without pain. Use of a patellar tendon strap is sometimes of value in relieving pain. The best placement site and the prognosis for the success of this strap can be determined by manual testing in the clinic setting. The patients first performs a one-legged squat to the point of pain. Pressure is then exerted through the examiner's thumb onto the middle or distal tendon while the squat test is repeated. Use of the strap is indicated if some relief of pain is noted with this maneuver.

Three surgical options are mentioned in the literature but none of them has yet had adequate followup to assess their relative indications. Smilie,[69] with the idea of improving blood supply to the tendon attachment, suggests placement of multiple drill holes in the affected pole of the patella through a short lateral incision. Bassett et al.[6] prefer a vertical incision in the tendon for local excision of the degenerative portion and resuturing of the remaining healthy tendon.

The third option, described by Blazina et al.,[9] involves detachment of the entire patellar or quadriceps tendon with resection of the diseased segment, excision of the involved patellar pole and surgical reattachment of the tendon to the nonarticular patellar surface. This is accompanied by rein-

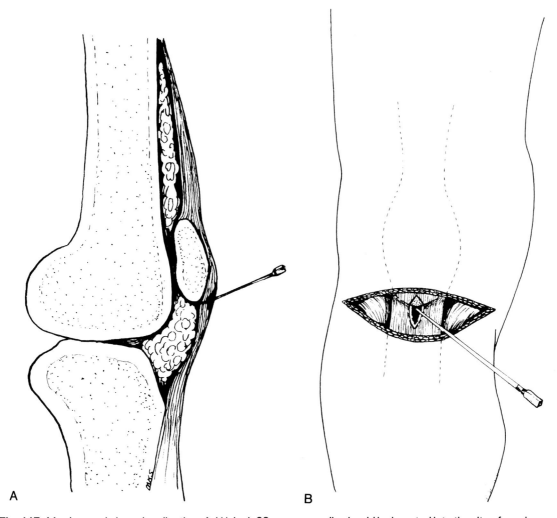

A   B

Fig. 117-11. Jumper's knee localization. A 1½-inch 22-gauge needle should be inserted into the site of maximum tenderness with the patient awake. Confirmation can be obtained by relief with 1 to 2 ml Xylocaine. Later localization may be eased either by injecting 1 or 2 drops of methylene blue or by leaving the needle in place for the surgical approach.

forcement of the repair with the medial patellar retinaculum.

Author's Preferred Treatment

Local resection of the diseased portion of the tendon in a manner similar to that described by Bassett[6] is preferred. The fact that this technique does not sacrifice the adjacent healthy portion tendon attachment makes the recovery period short compared with the more radical procedure. We have never yet found complete tendon resection necessary but believe it would be indicated for instances of extensive injury spanning the entire width of the tendon or for failure of a less invasive procedure.

Operative Technique

Identification of the precise location of the lesion is essential to the success of this procedure. This can either be done using local anesthesia and the cooperativeness of the patient or by general anesthesia and the cooperativeness of the anesthesiologist. In the later instance, the knee should be prepared and draped and flexed 90 degrees, prior to the initiation of anesthesia. In the instance where the diffuse clinical symptoms prevent the surgeon from becoming confident of pinpointing lesion, the area of maximum tenderness should be localized and marked for later operative identification with a 22-gauge spinal needle (Fig. 117-11A). The needle, with its stylette, is inserted into the most tender area of pathology with or without further verification by injection of 2 to 3 ml of 1 percent Xylocaine solution. To mark the correct area either a drop or two of methylene blue solution is instilled or the needle is firmly embedded into the correct area prior to anesthesization of the patient.

Surgery is begun with the knee still flexed at 90 degrees to tighten the patellar tendon. A transverse skin incision is made along the lines of Langer just distal to the bony prominence of the patellar pole, near the entry point of the needle (Fig. 117-11B). After visualizing the entire width of the tendon-bone attachment, a longitudinal incision into the tendon is centered over the needle puncture site with the dissection carried down to the needle tip. Once the pathologic tissue and its

borders are identified, a local resection is carried out extending to the tendon-bone junction (Fig. 117-12). The cortical surface of the patella is then curretted and then drilled with a small dental burr.

With the knee in full extension, absorbable synthetic sutures are used to approximate the split healthy tendon edges starting at the point most distant from the patellar attachment. Occasionally, the defect is large enough that the final sutures, located nearest the patella, are mattressed at a 45-degree angle starting through the drill holes placed in the nonarticular portion of the bone in the normal plane of attachment. At the time of closure, the prepatellar bursa is excised only if it has become enlarged and indurated and symptomatic. The skin

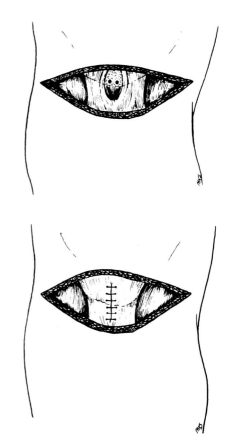

Fig. 117-12. Jumper's knee excision. After the pathologic area has been excised, the adjacent patellar surface is denuded and drill holes are placed in it to anchor the mattress sutures.

is then closed with a subcuticular stitch of absorbable synthetic material.

Postoperative Management

A cylinder cast is applied in the operating room and left on for 3 to 4 weeks or longer depending on anticipated patient compliance. Straight-leg raises are encouraged during this period of plaster immobilization. After cast removal, a knee immobilizer is initially worn at all times except for the twice-daily exercise periods.

Supervised exercise begins with straight-leg raising program and an active no gravity range of motion. When the active range of motion has become full, hamstring-strengthening exercises are begun. This is followed later by a gradually progressive resistance quadriceps-strengthening program. This sequence allows an extended time for strengthening of the suture line and delays the tendency of the athlete to return to action too soon. When strength reaches 90 percent of normal without recurrence of symptoms, the more vigorous conditioning programs are initiated. As preoperatively, the speed of the return to a preactivity level is regulated by the absence of symptoms within each step of the rehabilitation-conditioning protocol.

Results

The results of treatment are usually satisfactory to the surgeon and the patient but depend on the goals of the treatment to begin with. Although in our experience, return to a higher level of competition is feasible without surgical intervention. The attitude, industry, and patience of the patient are extremely critical to the prognosis during the 2- to 6-month rehabilitation period that may be required.

Complications

Avascular necrosis of otherwise healthy tendon is possible if the blood supply is compromised by a too-vigorous attempt to develop an exceptionally strong retention type suture line. Subsequent recurrence of the symptoms or even complete rupture is possible postoperatively if there is a premature resumption of the offending activity.

THE STIFF KNEE

Extension Contracture

As pointed out by Nicoll,[50] in contrast to the consequences in the ankle, spine, wrist, and other joints, stiffness of the knee can severely disable some patients to the point that their occupational and leisure pursuits are drastically affected. Historically, aggressive attempts to regain knee motion have gained unpopularity because of high complication rates and disappointing results. Limited knee motion can emanate from either intra- or extra-articular problems. Modern experience has shown that when stiffness is due to soft tissue adhesions rather than a bony block, consideration of the responsible structures and of alternative treatment methods can be worthwhile. As pointed out by Smillie[51]: "the primary source of stiffness (although usually due to multiple causes) is most often localized to one of the following: (1) the synovial cavity; (2) the capsule and peri articular tissue; (3) the quadriceps extensor unit; (4) the fascia lata; and (5) skin and subcutaneous tissue."

Fractures of the femur or upper tibia which require prolonged immobilization occasionally cause stiffness because of extraarticular adhesions of the extensor mechanism.[10,24,46,56,59,67] These adhesions usually occur in one of four ways: (1) fibrosis of the vastus intermedius with tethering of the rectus femoris to the femur (Fig. 117-13); (2) shortening and adhesion of the medial and/or lateral vastus expansions over the distal femur; (3) adhesions of the patella to the femoral condyles; and (4) shortening of the rectus femoris itself.

Often leading to intra-articular adhesions of the knee are distal femoral fractures supracondylar skeletal traction pins, infections, soft tissue injuries to the knee joint itself as well as prolonged periods of immobilization for any reason. Sites that are most frequently involved include adhesions between (1) the patella and the femur; (2) opposing synovial layers in the suprapatellar pouch; (3) meniscal adhesions to the capsule and tibia; and (4) the infrapatellar fat pad adhesions to the patellar tendon, the meniscus, or tibia.

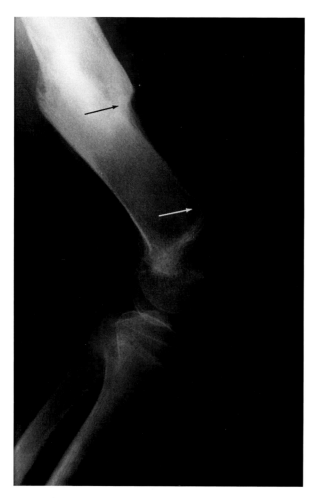

Fig. 117-13. Adhesion sites after femoral fracture. Range of motion was 20 to 70 degrees with a 20-degree extensor lag.

Diagnosis

Loss of flexion from extra-articular scarring of the extensor mechanism alone will result in an abrupt stop to passive and active knee flexion without loss of rotation. There also will be an associated extension lag initially with passive motion measurably greater than that achievable actively. Eventually, if this situation persists and the passive motion is not used daily, a flexion contracture will also develop.

Intra-articular adhesions are usually detectable by the limited rotation that is associated with lack of flexion and extension. Patellar adhesions are usually detectable by its decreased mediolateral excursions to passive motion in the relaxed, extended knee. Also, the patient can usually provide valuable aide to the examiner by localizing the specific maximally tender site that restricts patellofemoral and tibiaofemoral motion.

Indications

When selected properly, salvage treatment of the stiff knee can be very successful. However, patient selection should be confined to those persons in whom the expected handicap is severe enough to otherwise force a major change in their way of life. For example, whereas a 70-degree range of motion may prove tolerable to most people leading rather sedentary life, a stop at 110 degrees may provide insurmountable impairment to someone involved in an occupation demanding flexibility (e.g., telephone lineman, coal miner, tile worker, cab driver).

Determining the best management plans depends on knowledge about the source, duration, and degree of the limitation as well as the age and goals and motivation of the patient. Surgical release and closed manipulation of the stiff knee under anesthesia should be considered only as a last resort. Closed manipulation should be used when, despite maximally supervised rehabilitation efforts, progress in regaining motion has been halted. Manipulations are most favorable when done to release relatively avascular adhesions localized inside the capsular borders of the joint, in the absence of significant inflammation. In contrast to warnings by Smillie[69] and Helfet,[26] early postoperative manipulation has recently been reported to be successful after synovectomy or total knee replacement when done for a sluggish return of motion. The author has little experience with this indication since excellent results are achievable with supervised range of motion exercises on an active and active-assisted basis in the hospital setting. From a scientific standpoint, proof of the contribution of manipulation to the success of an early rehabilitation program will require a well-controlled, prospective study with randomized selection of patients.

If a supervised, active-assistance range-of-motion program has failed, admission of the patient to the hospital is indicated. Here a rigorous physical therapy program can be administered twice a day as described below. Also indicated is a search for reasons for the failure. This includes observations about motivation, pain tolerance, and an assessment of the possible negative factors in the environment, which may have been counterproductive. If this program does not show promise within the first few days, closed manipulation or surgical intervention is considered.

Surgical intervention should be considered in those patients (1) where all nonoperative attempts have failed; (2) where closed manipulation is contraindicated because of disuse osteoporosis or where the tensile strength of the adhesions is sufficient to create a high risk of fracture or unwanted soft tissue trauma from manipulation; (3) who are young and well motivated to realize postoperatively the surgically gained new motion; and develop the necessary muscle strength to maintain it; (4) in whom the primary limitation of motion is located in the extensor mechanism; (5) in whom only a moderate amount (20 to 70 degrees) of improvement in the motion range is necessary for good function; and (6) for whom sufficient time has elapsed to allow the adhesions to become mature.

Contraindications

It is generally held that recent, vascular, adhesions should not be manipulated nor otherwise forcibly stretched by the therapist. Such treatment can delay or permanently inhibit the recovery of motion by producing inflammation and edema and fresh, more extensive adhesions. The past history of recent or extensive infection also provides a relative contraindication to surgery because the tissue in the adhesions is more avascular and more likely to harbor an infection. The presence of bony deformity from prolonged knee stiffness is also a contraindication to releasing soft tissue adhesions. The intra-articular presence of a bony obstruction makes any method of increasing range of motion doomed to failure but may provide an indication for osteotomy to place the available motion in the functional range.

As already mentioned, a contraindication to closed manipulation but an indication for surgical release is disuse osteoporosis sufficient to increase the risk of femoral fracture.

Treatment Alternatives

Active range-of-motion exercises are the mainstay of any program to regain motion early after injury or surgical procedure. Because an unsupervised home program has failed, the initial hospital program consists of supervised (1) isometric and isokinetic muscle strengthening; (2) active assistive range of motion; and (3) mobilization exercises in physical therapy to increase the maximum range of motion. "Mobilization therapy" of the extensor mechanism consists of manipulating the patella in a medial and lateral direction to loosen the adhesions between the patella and femur. Similarly, internal and external rotation exercises of the tibia on the femur are emphasized to loosen the adhesions of intra-articular structures at the joint line. Control of the discomfort during therapy sessions may be offered with heat, transcutaneous electrical nerve stimulation, or anti-inflammatory agents. An active program is also established for the patient to continue throughout the day. It is aimed at improving the "functional range" of motion that the patient feels comfortable with and can rapidly accomplish without assistance.

The progress of the patient is closely monitored by the therapist on a daily report card that the patient takes back to his room to show to the physician. Muscle strengths of the extensor and flexor mechanisms are listed on the card because increases in motion cannot be expected to be maintained without sufficient muscular control. The patient's progress can be accurately assessed by monitoring the maximum limits of the patient's motion and the extensor lag, as well as the effort-free range of motion. Short-term modifications in the treatment plan are based on the progress. If the activity is not producing signs of excessive joint irritation, the knee can be continued on the activity program. If inflammation or pain is evidenced and the maximum range of motion is increasing without a concomitant increase in the functional range, appropriate anti-inflammatory medications are administered and the exercise therapy is continued. If the functional range of motion improves but the maximum that can be obtained passively does not, manipulation or surgical release are considered.

Closed Manipulation

This procedure is best performed under a short acting general anesthetic to provide a brief, but complete, state of total muscle relaxation. Since disastrous iatrogenic bony or ligament injury is possible, a carefully controlled technique of manipulation must be developed so the surgeon feels confident he will sense whenever minor changes in resistance occur.

Prior to anesthetizing the patient, the following are determined: (1) the sites of maximum pain and tenderness; (2) the degree of maximum active versus passive sagittal plane motion; (3) the degree of tibiofemoral rotation; (4) the amount of patellar mobility; (5) the abruptness of increased resistance at the motion end point and the magnitude of the force required to reach it; and (6) the functional range of motion that is achieved rapidly and comfortably by the patient.

With the patient fully anesthetized, the range of motion is reassessed by slowly flexing the thigh to at least 110 degrees or more and noting the maximum amount of flexion the knee will assume from gravity alone.

The manipulation is performed with the knee in the position illustrated in Figure 117-14 with the distal tibia held under the surgeon's axilla. Flexion is slowly accomplished by gradually increasing the downward force of the physician's body weight onto the flexed hip and knee. This allows a slow, well-controlled increase in resistance as well as allowing both hands to be free to palpate the pre-marked adhesions sites.

When the timing has been right, one or several "pops" should be palpable or even audible as the tough, avascular adhesions are lysed. Increasing flexion to the point of tethering of the major adhesions sites is accompanied by an increasing resistance. At this point, it is important to avoid bouncing or otherwise abruptly increasing the flexion force. Rather, internal and external rotation are first stressed before resuming the attempt to gain flexion. If, 30 to 60 seconds after resuming the same attempt to gain more flexion, a gradually decreasing resistance is not detected, the force is increased by 2 to 5 pounds and maintained for another 30 to 60 second period. This process is repeated until either a satisfactory range has been achieved or until a plateau is reached at a magnitude of resistance that prohibits further manipulation. The full range of motion is then repeated with

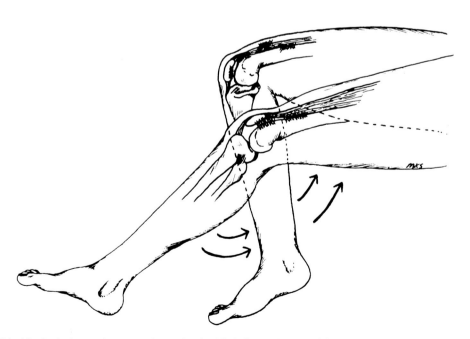

Fig. 117-14. Manipulation under general anesthesia. Hip is flexed beyond 90 degrees and the flexion force at the knee is generated through a downward force applied at the distal tibia.

only a small amount of force being applied toward both flexion extension and rotation. A recheck of the gravity assisted flexion is then made.

The same general process is now repeated for increasing extension. For this procedure, towels or folded sheets are placed under the Achilles tendon and distal calf. The surgeon transmits a slowly increasing force by shifting his body weight through extended arms to hands placed just above and below the joint line. This maneuver is not heavily pursued if there is a significant flexion contracture of 10 to 25 with tibial subluxation.

The gravity affected limit to extension is also checked pre- and postmanipulation. At the completion of the procedure, the amount of hemorrhage is noted and 15 to 20 cc of 0.5 percent Marcaine is injected. As soon as he is awake, the patient is sent for a radiograph, followed by reinstitution of physical therapy.

Complications

In my experience two fractures of the femur have been produced in patients with multiple trauma who developed osteoporosis from prolonged immobilization and a history of joint infection prior to manipulation. Postmanipulation hemorrhage and the subsequent inflammatory reaction can lead to decreased range of motion and further adhesions if patients are not selected carefully. Therefore, if an initial manipulation attempt decreases or even fails to increase the range of motion, the procedure is not repeated. Repeated attempts at manipulation have been associated with muscle and ligamentous damage manifested by ossifications detectable on radiograph.

Results

Very few patients with stiff knees even require hospitalization. Of those hospitalized, very few require manipulation under anesthesia. Of those selected for manipulation, the results are promising when physical therapy can be immediately resumed and the patient is well motivated.

Surgical Management

Lengthening of the quadriceps tendon as described by Bennett[7] is the best-known procedure for increasing an otherwise permanent loss of knee

flexion. It is based on the idea that the restriction of motion is most frequently attributable to pathology in the extraarticular extensor mechanism and that the development of stiffness within the joint capsule is entirely a secondary affair that will take care of itself. The procedure begins with exposure of the extraarticular adhesions and freeing of them by blunt dissection. A distally based quadriceps tendon flap is then constructed: two parallel incisions of the tendon extending distally from the infrapatellar area and narrowing gradually to end at a point 4½ inches proximally in the rectus femoris tendon (Fig. 117-15). The incision must be deep enough to include the tendinous section of the vastus intermedius. The flap is then freed from underlying structures and the knee is flexed to at least 90 degrees, where the tendon is reattached to the vasti with some heavy synthetic resorbable sutures in a mattress stitch fashion. This procedure is not recommended unless the inevitable loss of control of active extension is appropriate for the goals of the patient.

Patellectomy alone has not proved successful when the degenerative changes noted have appeared secondarily to the soft tissue contractures. Although some increased motion can result, these results are not nearly as good as when a soft tissue release as described below is added.

Total knee replacement to improve motion of the stiff knee is performed when significantly bony impingement is present or when the soft tissue contractures have existed long enough that severe degenerative changes exist between the femur and tibia. Arthroscopic release of plica and interarticular adhesions combined with lateral retinacular release may be very successful if patient localizes the site of the restricted motion appropriately. However, occasionally, when the capsular adhesions are too extensive, arthroscopic release can be combined with a two-incision limited surgical release, as described by Smillie.[69] In this procedure, digital and scissor separation of the intraarticular adhesions is performed through two 4-cm-long parapatellar incisions.

Author's Preferred Treatment

Modification of the original Thompson[73] quadricepsplasty technique has been shown to be very effective[27,36,49,50] at increasing motion without

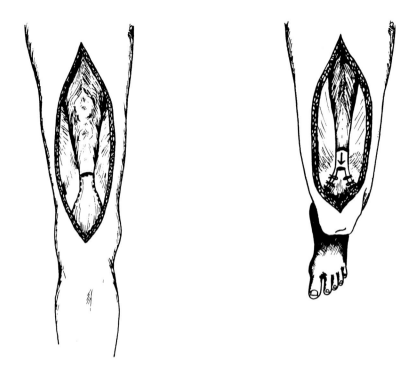

Fig. 117-15. Bennett quadriceps tendon lengthening. An inverted V incision is made through the depth of the entire quad mechanism. The knee is manipulated into flexion and the flap is resutured to the edges of the vasti.

compromising the power of the extensor mechanism. Its success does require vigorous postoperative therapy and thus a well-motivated patient. It also requires that the rectus femoris can be freed from all adhesions while its integrity is retained, complete with its patellar and tibial attachments.

Operative Technique

A vertical median parapatellar skin incision is begun 4 inches above the superior pole of the patella and extended distally to the joint line. The junctions of the vastus medialis and lateralis with the rectus femoris are visualized by subcutaneous dissection. Here, as before the operation, the knee is flexed to identify the sites of adhesions by flexing and rotating the knee and moving the patella medially, laterally, proximally and distally.

The exact sequence of the incisions varies according to the locations of the adhesions. However, until proved otherwise, the lateral parapatellar incision is first extended proximally and distally as for a lateral release. This incision flares laterally at the joint line to end approximately 1 to 2 cm wide of the patellar tendon. It also proceeds up the junction between the vastus lateralis and rectus femoris the full length of the skin incision (Fig. 117-16A). This can be extended more proximally if there has been scarring to a femoral fracture or soft tissue injury of the thigh. However, isolation of the rectus above the middle one-third of the femur may endanger its nerve and blood supply.

After this and each step of the surgical release, flexion of the knee is attempted to identify sites of adhesion. In particular, the suprapatellar pouch is inspected for contracture and evidence of tethering of the extensor mechanism to the femur. This is usually accompanied by adhesions between the rectus femoris and the vastus intermedius. If present, the intermedius is excised (Fig. 117-16B). Next a search is conducted along the femoral condyles for adhesions between the retinacular attachments of the vastus and the femur. If there is restriction to medial displacement of the patella, a mirror image medial release is extended from just proximal to the joint line to 2 inches above the patella through the junction of the vastus medialis and rectus femoris.

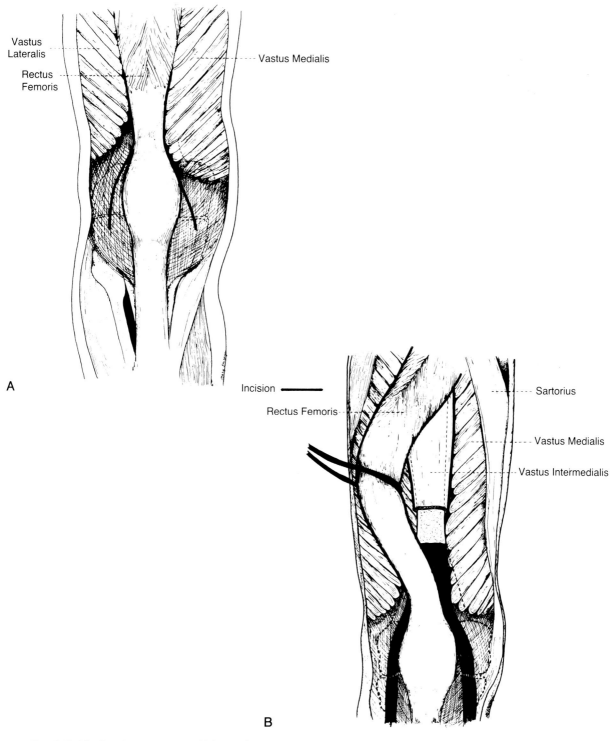

Fig. 117-16. Quadricepsplasty. **(A)** Lateral and medial parapatellar capsular incisions are flared about 0.5 cm near the joint line. These release incisions are then carried proximally to isolate the rectus femoris. **(B)** The intermedius tendon is excised and any remaining adhesions are released.

If, at this point, the knee does not flex to 120 degrees with minimal force, intra-articular adhesions are looked for at the tibiofemoral joint line itself. Hypertrophy and scarring of the fat pad is associated with loss of flexion as well as extension.[26,30] Normally it is a mobile structure which appears to adapt itself to the contours of the anterior part of the knee joint and provide a cushion as it flexes and extends. Following prolonged immobilization or injury this vascular fat pad can become very fibrotic and adherent to the tibia or to the anterior horn of one or both of the menisci. Fibrosis of the alar folds that span from the medial and lateral margins of the joint to the femoral notch may tether the fat pad to the joint capsule or to plical extensions. Surgical excision of the scar and careful mobilization of its attachments to the tibia are favored over complete removal of the fat pad because of its importance in providing vascularity to the patella and the cruciates.

When there is adherence of the anterior rims of the semilunar cartilages to the fat pad or to the tibia, tibiofemoral rotation is noticeably limited. Adherence to the tibia is usually a result of fibrosis of the coronary ligament. The body of the meniscus itself can also become fibrotic and lose its pliability. Toward the same end, the anterior horn has also been noted to separate from its anterior tibial attachment, retract, and thicken to the point of becoming a mechanical block. If the meniscus is thickened and retracted or is fibrotic and nonpliable, it should be excised. Careful surgical release of remaining meniscal adhesions should be followed by manipulation. If manipulation fails to this point, complete meniscectomy may be necessary.

Other intracapsular adhesions are usually demonstrable in the femoral recess just above the medial joint line between the femur and the capsule. It may also be dissected or sharply snapped by closed manipulation. Finally, if further limitation of flexion is encountered, more proximal scarring in the extensor mechanism should be looked for and a more proximal release of all attachments to the rectus femoris should be accomplished.

Postoperative Management

At completion of the procedure, hemostasis is achieved and subcutaneous and skin layers are closed loosely over a Penrose drain for the first 24 to 48 hours. A compression dressing is applied using cotton batting and oversize knee immobilizer for the first 72 hours.

The knee is immobilized and the wound compressed for the first days until recurrent bleeding is not a problem. Then, the active and active assistive physical therapy program, as prescribed preoperatively, is resumed.

Complications

Care must be taken to avoid any injury to rectus femoris extensor mechanism itself. In the suprapatellar pouch, care must be taken to not excise the fat pad that lies underneath the synovium. When both medial and lateral incisions have been made during the quadricepsplasty, care must be taken to avoid totally devascularizing the patellar tendon when the fat pad is released.

Flexion Contracture

Knees that are stiff in a flexed, rather than extended, position are not only more common but more disabling to the point of even preventing ambulation. Seen most often in adults with degenerative or rheumatoid arthritis, Smillie[69] feels that most functionally significant contractures occur chiefly as a result of mismanagement of acute inflammatory processes. In any acute disease state, there is a tendency to reduce the pain of the swollen knee by allowing it to assume the most comfortable position at about 30 degrees flexion. Especially in patients with moderate or advanced chronic arthritis, loss of the ability to completely extend the knee creates an increase in the forces required of the extensor muscle to maintain the erect position.

Fixed flexion deformity of greater than 20 to 25 degrees will often be complicated by posterior subluxation and external rotation of the tibia due to (1) the pull of the hamstring muscle; (2) tethering of the iliotibial band; (3) shortening of the anterior cruciate ligament; and (4) contracture of the posterior capsule. Forced attempts at straightening the knee cause hinging rather than the normal gliding motion. The resulting anterior impingement can cause irreversable articular surface changes.[80]

Indications

The ease of treatment of an established flexion contracture is related to the severity and duration of the deformity. The consequences of allowing a residual flexion contracture depends on its severity the health of the joint, the prior ambulatory status, and age, as well as the future activity goals of the patient. Mild deformities of less than 10 degrees can usually be managed by the patients themselves with a program to be designed for home or for physical therapy unit. This includes an "active" range-of-motion program combined with manual attempts at stretching. If the manual program is insufficient, a "passive" program can be instituted in which a light (5- to 10-pound) weight is hung from a sling placed directly over the knee. The weight, in turn, is suspended in midair by placement of the heel on a chair or stool. Accompanied by quadriceps-strengthening exercises, this procedure should be continued for 30 to 60 minutes at a time, several times each day. A straight knee immobilizer or plaster shell is worn at night.

Moderate deformities of recent origin with no more than 25 to 30 degrees of flexion can benefit from the additional use of a felt-padded plaster posterior shell designed by Smilie so that successive layers of felt can be removed from the plaster as further extension is gained.

Contraindications

Care must be taken to fully establish the competency of the vascular system in the lower extremity. Marginal occlusive arterial disease may require popliteal bypass prior to any attempt to eliminate a severe flexion contracture in a debilitated patient. It is my experience that for the rheumatoid patient prior to total knee replacement, the ordeal is of such magnitude that careful reconsideration should be given at each step of the danger of losing the limb. Too rapid or vigorous attempt at straightening the contracted knee can easily result in loss of peroneal nerve function. Hinging action of the posteriorly subluxed tibia will also serve to increase this stretching phenomenon on the nerve and artery in the popliteal space. Such signs and symptoms of neurovascular compromise are definite contraindications to pursuing that particular line of treatment further.

Supracondylar osteotomy may be performed to alter the existing range of motion to a more functional arc. This is the salvage procedure of choice when the flexion deformity is the result of uncorrectable intra-articular pathology.

Treatment Alternatives

For moderately severe longstanding contractures the constant forces of serial cylinder casts or of Russell's traction applied to the skin can be very effective if properly done. With contractures of 25 degrees or more in which there is posterior subluxation of the tibia, proper procedure must avoid a hinging action. The proximal tibia must be pulled forward and the femur depressed posteriorly to recreate the gliding motion.

Manipulation under anesthesia is not generally as effective as it may be for extension contractures. It may be best used for relatively new flexion contractures of mild severity.

For severe longstanding flexion contractures, proximal tibial skeletal traction can be employed (Fig. 117-17). If the patient's general medical condition tolerates it, this can be a very effective method of correcting a deformity. The Pearson attachment is attached directly to the tibial pin and provides merely a balanced suspension for the anterior pull of the skeletal traction. If the skeletal traction fails to correct a long-term 20- to 35-degree flexion contracture with posterior tibial subluxation, the anterior cruciate ligament can also be cut in selected patients. Since this maneuver can result in permanent problems with instiability, it should be reserved for situations in which the long-range goals do not include demanding levels of ambulation.

Although often useful in neuromuscular disease in children, the indications for surgical release of the posterior soft tissue structures in the adult are very rare. These indications would include the presence of a severe flexion contracture, resistant to the above nonoperative methods of correlation in a patient who is potentially ambulatory or in whom mere nursing care is a problem because of the flexed knees.

Author's Preferred Treatment (Posterior Release)

A lateral vertical incision is made beginning just proximal to the fibular head distally and extended up to the femoral attachment of the fibular collat-

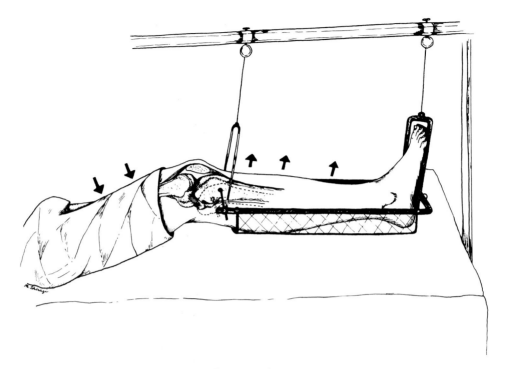

Fig. 117-17. During extension, skeletal traction for severe flexion contracture with posterior subluxation. Proximal pin skeletal traction can avoid hinging effect.

eral ligament and then another 2 inches proximally along the interval between the extensor and flexor mass of the thigh. After identifying the peroneal nerve, the biceps tendon is isolated and severed at its attachment to the fibular head. If tension is apparent as the knee is forcibly extended, the iliotibial band is then excised obliquely to allow suturing in a more relaxed position if needed at closure.

At this point the medial hamstrings are exposed through a vertical skin incision that begins just anterior to the tibial collateral ligament below the joint line and extends proximally to the femoral attachment of the collateral ligament and further proximally 3 inches along the interval just anterior to the sartorius. Again, as flexion is forced passively, the presence of tension on the semitendinosus, sartorius, and gracilis warrants their surgical release as far distally as possible. The semimembranosis is finally lengthened in a Z-plasty manner starting distally at the posterior border of the medial collateral ligament.

If extension is not yet acceptable, the contribution of the neurovascular structures of the popliteal space is made at this time. If the neurovascular bundle is not under great tension, the posteromedial capsule, the fibular collateral ligament, the popliteus and arcuate ligament are all released as needed. The posterior and anterior cruciates may also require release before full extension can be easily obtained. Posterior cruciate can be reached through a small anterior lateral parapatellar incision by putting traction on the ligament with a button hook and cutting it with a Smillie meniscitome. During each of the above steps, the surgeon should continually apply a gentle extension force sufficient to identify that structure under the greatest tension. The neurovascular bundle in the popliteal space should be checked repeatedly, and, if tension develops, the procedure should be terminated in favor of postoperative serial casting.

Postoperative Management

For severe deformities requiring operative intervention, patients placed in a compressive dressing over hemovac drains for the first 24 hours with an immobilizer in a balanced suspension system with Buck's traction applied with 3 to 5 pounds of weight allowing the knee to be flexed as it was prior to surgery and slowly straightening the knee over the next 10 to 14 days so that the function of the nerve must be observed. When the knee has been straightened to at least 15 to 20 degrees, a mini hip spica cast with dial drop-lock hinges can be applied from the iliac crest to the toes. Resting extension is increased until 0 is reached and sessions of range-of-motion exercises are employed on a daily basis. At 5 weeks the cast is replaced with a long leg brace again with droplock joints at the knee to allow walking in full extension but flexion while sitting.

Results

At least on a short-term basis, most flexion contractures can be significantly improved. However, the chances of success of the procedure is highly dependent on several factors which must all be considered (i.e., the functional expectations of the procedure, the magnitude of the required surgical insult, the potential for complications, and the likelihood of recurrent deformity).

As in other joints, the chances of recurrence of a knee-flexion contracture depend on its etiology originally (e.g., muscle imbalance, pain, lack of motivation). Permanent success will be limited or nonexistent if these factors remain dominant after the surgery.

Complications

Neurovascular complications are of special concern after release of contractures in the knee. These include peripheral compromise of the popliteal and peroneal nerve segments. Peroneal nerve palsies have been noted after release of contractures of as little as 25 to 35 degrees.

Severe flexion contractures have even required femoral-popliteal artery bypass surgery prior to and traction or serial casting after release has been accomplished.

The development of residual ligamentous instability and/or greater impairment from anklyosis also present as calculated risks.

REFERENCES

1. Anzel S, Cobey K, Weiner A, et al: Disruption of muscles and tendons: an analysis of 1,014 cases. Surgery 45:406, 1959
2. Apple DV, O'Toole J, Annis C: Professional basketball injuries. Phys Sports Med 10:81, 1982
3. Apple FS, Rogers MA, Casal DC, et al: Creatine kinase-MB isoenzyme adaptations in stressed human skeletal muscle of marathon runners. J Appl Physiol 58:149, 1985
4. Armstrong RB: Muscle damage and endurance events. Sports Med 3:370, 1986
5. Armstrong RB, Ogilivie RW, Schwane JA: Eccentric exercise-induced injury to rat skeletal muscle. J Appl Physiol 54:80, 1983
6. Bassett F, Soucacos P, Carr W: Jumper's knee: patellar tendinitis and patellar tendon rupture. In AAOS Symposium on the Athlete's Knee. CV Mosby, St. Louis, 1978
7. Bennett G: Lengthening of the quadriceps tendons. J Bone Joint Surg 4: 1922
8. Blair W, & Pontarelli W: Ambulatory dynamic patellar traction. Clin Orthop 169:145–147, 1982
9. Blazina M, et al: Jumper's knee. Orthop Clin North Am 4:665, 1973
10. Böhler L: The Treatment of Fractures. Vol 5. Grune & Stratton, New York, 1958
11. Brewer B: Mechanism of injury to the musculotendinous unit. In American Academy of Orthopaedic Surgeons. Instructional Course Lectures. Vol 17. CV Mosby, St. Louis, 1960
12. Chancler F: Patellar advancement operation; A revised technique. J Int Surg 3:433, 1940
13. Clap L: Les ruptures de pappareil extensaur de la pambe. Tbise de Paris, 1921
14. Convery FR, et al: Flexion deformities of the knee in rheumatoid arthritis. Clin Orthop 74:90:3, Jan 1971
15. Conway F: Ruptures of the quadriceps tendon. Am J Surg 50:3, 1940
16. Davies CTM, White MJ: Muscle weakness following eccentric work in man. Pfluegers Arch 392:168, 1981
17. Ecker ML: Late reconstruction of the patellar tendon. J Bone Joint Surg 61A:884, 1979
18. Feagin J, & Jackson D: Quadriceps contusion in young athletes. J Bone Joint Surg 55A:95, 1973
19. Fichat RP, Hungerford DS: Disorders of the Patello-Femoral Joint. Williams & Wilkins, Baltimore, 1977
20. Francis K: The surgical treatment of tears of the

quadriceps tendon. Bull NY Orthop Hosp 1:18, 1957

21. Friden J, Sjostrom M, Ekblom B: Myofibrillar damage following intense eccentric exercise in man. Int J Sports Med 4:170, 1983

22. Garrett WE Jr, Rich FR, Nikolaou PK, et al: Computed tomography of hamstring muscle strains. Am J Sports Med. In press

23. Garrick JG, Requa RK: Epidemiology of women's gymnastics injuries. Am J Sports Med 8:261, 1980

24. Gunn D: Contracture of the quadriceps muscle. J Bone Joint Surg 46B:492, 1964

25. Harand BA, et al: Severe hyperextension following correction of flexion contracture of the knee. A report of two cases. J Bone Joint Surg 56A:1722, 1974

26. Helfet: Disorders of the Knee. JB Lippincott, Philadelphia, 1974

27. Herndon C: Tendon transplantation at the knee and Foot. p. 145. In American Academy of Orthopaedic Surgeons. Instructional Course Lectures. Vol 18. CV Mosby, St. Louis, 1981

28. Hesketh K: Experiences with the thompson quadricepsplasty. J Bone Joint Surg 45B:491, 1963

29. Hikida RS, Staron RS, Hagerman RC, et al: Muscle fiber necrosis associated with human marathon runners. J Neurol Sci 59:185, 1983

30. Hoffa A: The influence of the adipose tissue with regard to the pathology of the knee joint. JAMA 43:795, 1904

31. Hough T: Ergographic studies in muscular soreness. Am J Physiol 7:76, 1982

32. Jakubowki S, et al: The treatment of flexion contracture of the knee joint with posterior capsulotomy in rheumatoid arthritis. Acta Scand 45:235–240, 1974

33. Jarvinen M: Healing of a crush injury in rat striated muscle. 2. A histological study of the effect of early mobilization and immobilization on the repair process. Acta Pathol Microbiol Scand 83:269, 1975

34. Jarvinen M: Healing of a crush injury in rat striated muscle. 3. A microangiographical study of the effect of early mobilization on capillary ingrowth. Acta Pathol Microbiol Scand 84:85, 1976

35. Jarvinen M: Healing of a crush injury in rat striated muscle. Acta Pathol Microbiol Scand 142:47, 1976

36. Judet R: Mobilization of the stiff knee. J Bone Joint Surg 41B:853, 1959

37. Kelikian H, Riashi E, Gleason J: Restoration of quadriceps function in neglected tear of the patellar tendon. Surg Gynecol Obstet 104:200, 1957

38. Kennedy J, Willis R: The effects of local steroid injections on tendons: a biomechanical and microscopic correlative study. Am J Sports Med 4:11, 1976

39. Knochel JP: Rhabdomyolysis and myoglobinuria. Annu Rev Med 33:435, 1982

40. Komi PV, Burskirk ER: Effect of eccentric and concentric muscle condition on tension and electrical activity of human muscle. Ergonomics 15:417, 1972

41. Levi J, Coleman C: Fracture of the tibial tubercle. Am J Sports Med 4(6):254, 1976

42. Lipscomb G, Thomas D, Johnson R: Treatment of myositis ossificans trauma in athletes. Am J Sports Med 4(3):111–120, May-June 1976

43. McLaughlin H: Treatment of midthigh muscle ruptures. Am J Surg 74:758, 1947

44. McMaster P: Tendon and muscle ruptures. ACIA Orthop Scand 46:700, 1975

45. Medlar R, Lyne E: Sinding-Larsen-Johansson disease. J Bone Joint Surg 60A:1113, 1978

46. Mira A, Carlisle K, Greer R: A critical analysis of quadriceps function after femoral shaft fracture in adults. J Bone Joint Surg 62A:61–67, 1980

47. Morgan J, McCarty D: Tendon ruptures in patients with systemic lupus erythematosus treated with cortical steroids. Arthrit Rheumat 17:1033–1035, 1974

48. Nagel D, Jameson R: Complications of surgery on muscles, fascia, tendon sheaths, ligaments and bursae. In Epps C Jr, (ed): Complications in Orthopaedic Surgery. JB Lippincott, Philadelphia, 1978

49. Nes C: Quadricepsplasty. J Bone Joint Surg 44B:954, 1962

50. Nicoll E: Total quadricepsplasty. J Bone Joint Surg 45B:483, 1963

51. Nikolaou PK, MacDonald BL, Glisson RR, et al: Biomechanical and histological evaluation of muscle after controlled strain injury. Am J Sports Med 15:9, 1987

52. Norman A, Dorkman H: Juxtacortical circumscribed myositis ossifican: evolution and radiographic features. Radiology 96:301–306, 1970

53. Noyes F, Grude F, Neusbaum N, et al: The effect of intraarticular corticosteroids on ligament properties. Clin Orthop 123:1977

54. O'Donoghue D: Injuries of the thigh. In Treatment of Injuries to Athletes. WB Saunders, Philadelphia, 1970

55. Ogden J, Tross R, Murphy M: Fractures of the tibial tuberosity in adolescents. J Bone Joint Surg 62A:205, 1980

56. Peterson T: Injuries to the anterior thigh region. In AAOS Symposium on the Athletes Knee. CV Mosby, St. Louis, 1978

57. Piero A, Ferandis R, Garcia L, et al: Simultaneous and spontaneous bilateral rupture of the patellar tendon.

58. Pritchett JW: High cost of high school football injuries. Am J Sports Med 8:197, 1980
59. Rakolta G, Omer G: Combat sustained femoral injuries. Surg Gynecol Obstet 128:813, 1969
60. Ramsey R, Mueller G: Quadriceps tendon rupture: a diagnostic trap. Clin Orthop 70:161, 1970
61. Rao J, Siwek K: Bilateral spontaneous rupture of the patellar tendons. Orthop Rev 7:51, 1978
62. Rascher T, Marcolin L, James P: Bilateral sequential rupture of the postellar tendon in systemic lupus erythematosus. J Bone Joint Surg 56A:821, 1974
63. Roels J, Martens M, Mulier J, et al. Patellar tendinitis (jumper's knee). Am J Sports Med 6(6):362, 1978
64. Safran M, Garrett W, Seaber R, et al: The role of warmup in muscular injury prevention. Am J Sports Med 16:123, 1988
65. Scuderi C: Ruptures of the quadriceps tendon. Am J Surg 95:626, April 1958
66. Schwartzmann J, Crego C: Hamstring tendon transplantation for the relief of quadriceps femoris paralysis in residual polio myeolitis. J Bone Joint Surg 30A:541, 1948
67. Siwek C, Rao J: Ruptures of the extensor mechanism of the knee joint. J Bone Joint Surg 63A:932, 1981
68. Smillie IS: Injuries of the Knee Joint. 4th ed. Churchill Livingstone, Edinburgh, 1933
69. Smillie IS: Diseases of the Knee Joint. Churchill Livingstone, Edinburgh, 1974
70. Stearns M: Studies of the development of connective tissues in transparent chambers in the rabbit ear. Am J Anat 67:55, 1940
71. Stegeck J, Popelka S: Bilateral rupture of the patellar ligaments in systemic lupus erythematosus. Lancet 2:714, 1969
72. Tarsney F: Catastrophic jumper's knee: a case report. Am J Sports Med 9(1):60, 1981
73. Thompson T: Quadricepsplasty to improve knee function. J Bone Joint Surg 26:366–379, 1944
74. Thorndike A: Myositis ossificans traumatica. J Bone Joint Surg 22:315–323, April 1940
75. Unvesferth L, Olix M: The effect of local steroid injections on tendons. J Sports Med 1:31, 1973
76. Walker J: Rupture of the quadriceps extensor muscle and its tendon above and below the patella. Am J Sci 3:638, 1896
77. Wener J, Schein A: Simultaneous bilateral ruptures of patellar tendon and quadriceps expansion in systemic lupus erythematosus. J Bone Joint Surg 56A:823, 1974
78. Wiesemann G: Tendon transfers for peripheral nerve injuries of the lower extremity. In symposium on peripheral nerve injuries. Orthop Clin North Am 12(2):459, 1981
79. Williams P: Quadriceps contracture. J Bone Joint Surg 50B:278, 1968
80. Wilson P: Posterior capsulotomy in certain flexion contractures of the knee. J Bone Joint Surg 11:40, 1929

Synovial and Bursal Lesions About the Knee

118

Robert P. Mack
Mack L. Clayton

SYNOVIAL LESIONS

The function of normal synovium is to secrete fluid for purposes of lubrication and nutrition of the articular cartilage of the knee joint. Normal synovium has a single synovial cell layer with an irregular villous surface resulting in a large surface area. Most intra-articular problems within the knee joint are associated with irritation of this synovial lining, resulting in excessive fluid secretion and thickening of the synovium, i.e., synovitis. The clinical picture of synovitis is pain, effusion, increased local warmth, and stiffness of the knee. Presented with this picture, the clinician must make a proper diagnosis before instituting treatment. Aspiration of the knee with observation and study of the fluid is usually the first step (Fig. 118-1). Grossly bloody fluid is usually the result of trauma.

Yellow thickened synovial fluid with an elevated white blood cell (WBC) count is indicative of synovitis. Depending on the color, WBC count, and turbidity, the clinician must consider the following: arthritis (rheumatoid and osteoarthritic) septic arthritis, meniscal derangement, medial plica syndrome, pigmented villanodular synovitis, osteochondromatosis, and synovial hemangioma.

Rheumatoid Arthritis

The knee joint is the most commonly involved joint in patients with rheumatoid arthritis (RA). The synovium is the target organ; it results in the early symptoms of pain and stiffness associated with effusion and thickening of the synovium. The synovial membrane becomes hypertrophied with diffuse infiltration of plasma cells and secretes an abnormal fluid characterized by a WBC count of 5,000 to 50,000 as well as poor mucin and increased protein. Unabated synovitis will produce cartilage destruction either by direct invasion by pannus or by chemical destruction of cartilage by lysozymal enzyme action combined with frictional use (rheumatoid synovial fluid is a poor lubricant compared with normal fluid).

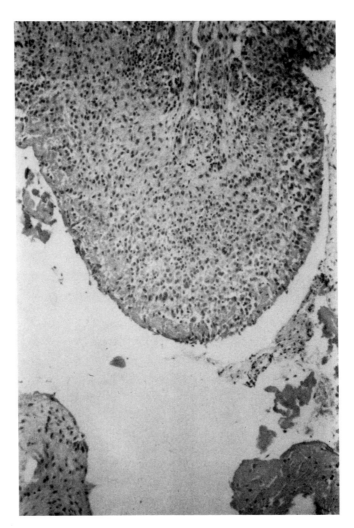

Fig. 118-1. Synovitis. Nonspecific synovitis. Specimen from an arthroscopic synovectomy showing a hyperplastic synovial layer supporting edematous connective tissue incorporating numerous lymphocytes, plasma cells, and scattered neutrophils. (×100)

Indications for Surgery

General medical treatment of RA is aimed at suppression of the synovitis. Failure of medical control of the synovitis after 5 months of conservative treatment[22] with resulting chronic effusion and a thickened synovium is the prime indication for surgical synovectomy. It is essential that the surgical candidate have no or minimal loss of joint space as confirmed by weight bearing and stress films of the knee. Further criteria for surgical intervention are good range of motion of the knee with less than a 20-degree flexion contracture and no significant valgus deformity. Ideally, the patient should be capable of walking on crutches, partial weight bearing, and participating in a vigorous physical therapy program consisting of early range of motion and quadriceps progressive resistive exercises.

Operative Technique

Surgical excision (synovectomy) has been performed since 1888. Enthusiasm for the procedure has waxed and waned over the years. The procedure should be considered palliative, as the synovium regenerates and usually again becomes destructive.[27] How quickly this occurs depends on the completeness of the synovectomy and the activity of the rheumatoid arthritis in the individual patient. Most patients enjoy relief of pain, improved function, and decreased effusion of the knee. How long this clinical improvement lasts is unpredictable but usually lasts[14,15] longer than 2 years.

No technique[19] for synovectomy allows for total removal. The more complete the synovectomy the better the results.[28] The difficult area to reach is the posterior compartments of the knee joint. When this procedure was done open, a double skin and capsular technique was recommended. However, today this procedure is best done arthroscopically.

As many as six arthroscopic portals may be indicated; superior medial and lateral, mid-medial and lateral, and anteromedial and lateral (Fig. 118-2). Posteromedial and posterolateral portals also can be quite helpful. A high-speed reversible 4.5-mm synovial power resector is an essential tool. The resector should be a wide opening side cutter (Fig. 118-2). A high-flow technique makes this technique easier.

The arthroscopic synovectomy is best done systematically with wide sweeping semicircular movements pivoting around each portal. Synovial resection should be started in the suprapatellar pouch (medial and lateral), using the midanterior, parapatellar portals (medial and lateral); the synovium is resected anteriorly to the joint line and including the fat pad as necessary. Using the anteromedial and lateral portals, the synovium can be resected from the medial and lateral gutters, the medial and lateral capsule, and under the medial and lateral meniscus (small end cutter, 2.8 mm). The arthroscope may be pushed through the notch into the posterior compartments, then with posteromedial and lateral portals the synovial resector can be introduced and a posterior synovectomy may be performed.

Postoperative Management

Because of the extensive surface area involved, considerable bleeding may be encountered postoperatively. A large Hemovac drain and a compression dressing may help prevent a postoperative

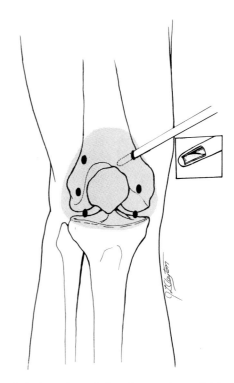

Fig. 118-2. Location of the six portals useful in arthroscopic synovectomy. **(Inset)** Synovial resector—essential power tool for arthroscopic synovectomy.

hematoma. Early range of motion is facilitated by the continuous passive motion machine, usually started on the first postoperative day. Ambulation with crutches or walker is started on day 2 with partial weight bearing. Active range of motion and quadriceps isometric exercises are started on day 2. Following arthroscopic synovectomy, the patient generally regains preoperative motion rapidly, and manipulation is seldom required. Full weight bearing is delayed until the patient demonstrates satisfactory range of motion and good quadriceps strength.

Results

The results of synovectomy in rheumatoid arthritis of the knee[8,9] show good pain relief with suppression of clinical activity. Radiologic deterioration of an inflamed knee joint is delayed for approximately 3 years in RA patients who do not respond to conservative treatment within a period of 5 months.[22] Probable or definite recurrences approach 50 percent after several years, although function is still improved; the longer the follow-up, the more recurrences in a given series.

The results and incidence of recurrence are time dependent and proportional to the general activity of the disease as well as to the extent of joint damage present at the time of operation. By doing the synovectomy arthroscopically as opposed to open, the long-range expectations of the procedure have not changed. Arthroscopic synovectomy has decreased the postoperative morbidity and recovery time and shortened the hospital stay considerably.[30]

Rheumatoid arthritis is a generalized disease. If the disease remains active, the new synovium can become rheumatoid.[26] Although destruction of the knee joint may be the ultimate outcome, the combination of good medical control and a properly timed synovectomy may delay this inevitability.

Pigmented Villanodular Synovitis

Pigmented villanodular synovitis is an uncommon synovial disease characterized by proliferation of the synovial tissue into numerous nodular villous masses.[16,33] Ninety percent of cases are found at the knee joint. This condition presents as a painful knee with recurrent effusions. The effusions are usually bloody. This disease can mimic rheumatoid arthritis, and the synovium can invade bone in the unusual case. The diagnosis can be suspected with recurrent bloody effusions but is not confirmed until the time of arthroscopy and synovial biopsies.[13]

Pathologic study reveals grossly thickened synovium; changes are consistent with old hemorrhage, usually a brownish discoloration. Microscopic examination shows a considerable amount of hemosiderin pigment in the irregular villous area. The synovial lining cells can fuse into the cells of adjacent villi to form narrow clefts. There is proliferation of synovial lining cells until they are several cells thick. Multinucleated giant cells tend to be present in the nodular area.

Treatment

The treatment of choice is arthroscopic synovectomy. The technique is identical to that described for RA. The more complete the synovectomy, the better the result. Recurrence rate should be low as this is a localized disease. However, with recurrence, repeat arthroscopic synovectomy is indicated. Aftercare and concern for regaining motion in the knee joint are the same as described for RA.

Osteochondromatosis

Osteochondromatosis is an unusual disease, seen in several joints but most common in the knee.[12,23] The patient presents with an internal derangement of the knee joint, with persistent effusion, pain, and catching in the knee joint. Radiographs are often negative, although loose bodies may be seen. Diagnostic arthroscopy is indicated because of persistent symptoms of internal derangement. The joint has the appearance of a glass paperweight filled with snowflakes. Literally, hundreds of small, white, loose bodies are seen. Most of these will be cartilaginous, although osteocartilaginous bodies may be seen; these loose bodies originate from the synovial membrane.

Treatment

The treatment of choice is synovectomy. This can be attempted arthroscopically using a widebore shaver. However, this may be an impossible task because of frequent clogging of the equipment with the tiny loose bodies. The surgeon may revert to open classic synovectomy in this case. Medial and lateral parapatellar incisions are usually best. The joint is cleared of loose bodies by open irrigation. The synovium is then dissected from the capsule throughout the entire knee joint. Aftercare and rehabilitation are as previously described.

Synovial Hemangiomas

Synovial hemangiomas have been described in various joints of the body, but by far the most frequent site has been the knee joint.[24] It may present clinically as an internal derangement but usually has an insidious beginning. Hemangioma seems to involve males and females approximately equally: 75 percent of patients will have symptoms before the age of 16. No cases of bilateral involvement have been reported. Skin overlying the synovial hemangioma is often described as normal, but there have been vascular involvements of superficial skin described as bluish, as telangiectasia, or as hemangioma in about one-half of cases. Radiographs may show no abnormalities or some soft tissue thickening. Arthrocentesis often yields blood-tinged fluid. Arthrography is not particularly helpful; arthroscopy is very helpful.

There are essentially two types of synovial hemangiomas: (1) localized sessile, and (2) the infiltrated diffuse. There are also histologic types, such as capillary or cavernous. The best results are noted following synovectomy, radiotherapy, or partial synovectomy. The more localized type of tumor is more amenable to total excision and offers a better prognosis. Where a total excision cannot be performed, recurrence is very common. The present status of radiotherapy is in question, and it should not be used in a benign condition. Total synovectomy is indicated only in a case of the infiltrative type.

In summary, the lesion most frequently affects the child or adolescent; it is slightly more common and is found symptomatically earlier in girls. Most patients have recurrent symptoms of pain, swelling, and frequently loss of knee motion. Boggy synovitis is palpable. Leg-length discrepancies are variable, and vascular changes in the skin may be observed. It is a diagnosis to be considered with unexplained repeated hemarthroses. Routine radiographs may show soft tissue thickening or may show joint phleboliths. Arthroscopy is helpful for diagnosis. Treatment of choice is total excision of the mass by synovectomy. Occasional recurrences have been noted after surgery. Radiotherapy is not recommended for a benign condition.

LESIONS OF THE PATELLAR FAT PAD

The fat pad lies posterior to the patellar tendon and is anchored between the tibial spines by the retinaculum. It is covered by synovial membrane. There have been many descriptions of hypertrophy of the fat pad, pinching, and so on; it is hard to determine the true pathology. A ganglion cyst is the most common lesion.[25] Calcification may fol-

low injury; it may be painful and require excision. Any disease that involves the synovium will involve a portion of the fat pad, and it may be necessary to include its excision if the general treatment requires an operation.

EXTRA-ARTICULAR LESIONS

Prepatellar Bursitis

Prepatellar bursitis presents as a painful swelling over the anterior aspect of the knee joint. Septic bursitis must be distinguished from a nonspecific inflammatory bursitis. Aspiration of the prepatellar bursa will usually distinguish between septic and nonseptic bursitis. Often there is a history of a recent puncture wound associated with septic prepatellar bursitis. If purulent exudate is found, immediate incision and drainage are indicated. Because the lymphatic drainage of the prepatellar bursa leads directly to the knee joint, this becomes important in order to avoid secondary contamination and possible infection of the knee joint.

A small, 1- to 2-inch, incision is made over the most fluctuant area. Through this incision, the bursa is irrigated and debrided as necessary. A small drain is then left in place to establish drainage. IV antibiotics are started as soon as the diagnosis is made. The knee is splinted and protected from weight bearing. The drain is advanced at 24 hours and is usually removed at 48 hours. Antibiotics are continued until the infection is eradicated.

Frequent observation of the knee joint is important in order to make certain that the infection has not invaded the knee. Rehabilitation is started as soon as the infection is clinically subsiding. This begins with straight-leg raise quadriceps rehabilitation and progressing to active range-of-motion exercises.

The history may be one of insidious onset associated with repeated trauma, such as in a carpet layer, wrestler, or football lineman. If the aspirate is normal-appearing synovial fluid, one may be dealing with an inflammatory prepatellar bursitis. In this situation, cortisone injection into the bursa

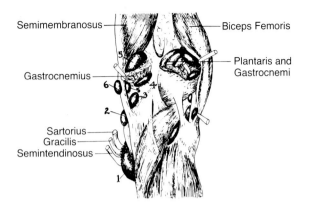

Fig. 118-3. Semimembranosus bursa in relationship to popliteal cyst. Bursa around the knee. Numbers 4 and 5 are the ones most commonly involved with a popliteal cyst. (From Wilson[32] with permission.)

as well as splinting and a compression dressing will often solve the problem. Occasionally, prepatellar bursitis will become chronic with a very large thickened bursa. If this conservative treatment fails, surgical excision is indicated.[27]

Operative Technique

A vertical midline 2-inch incision directly over the patella is generally used. The thickened bursa is dissected from the overlying subcutaneous tissue and the underlying patellar periosteum and is removed in its entirety. A Hemovac and compression dressing are used to prevent hematoma. Splinting is important postoperatively. The patient is started on active straight-leg raises immediately. Range of motion exercises are delayed until the incision is healed and there is no sign of prepatellar effusion.

Popliteal Cysts

Cysts in the popliteal space are the most common extra-articular synovial lesions; they were first described in 1840. Baker[1] in 1877 described eight popliteal cysts that he concluded were herniations from the posterior aspect of the knee secondary to osteoarthritis of the joint.

In 1938 Wilson and Francis[32] (Fig. 118-3) described six primary bursae in the popliteal space and medial aspect of the knee:

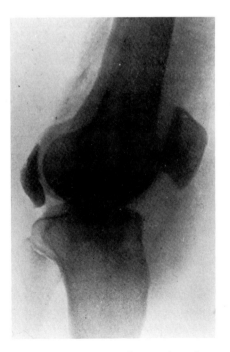
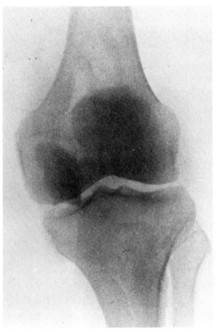

Fig. 118-4. Injection of gastrocnemius-semimembranosus bursa with radiopaque material. (From Wilson,[32] with permission.)

1. A bursa between the tendons of insertion of the pes anserinus and the superficial medial collateral ligament
2. A bursa between the medial collateral ligament and the semimembranosus insertion
3. A bursa between the semimembranosus and the medial condyle of the tibia
4. A bursa between the medial gastrocnemius head and posteromedial capsule of the knee
5. A bursa between the medial gastrocnemius head and the semimembranosus
6. A bursa between the semimembranosus and the semitendinosus

(Any type of synovial lesion may occasionally involve these bursae. The gastrocnemius-semimembranosus bursa (Nos. 4 and 5) is adjacent to the posterior capsule of the knee joint; in more than one-half of cases, this is the usual point of communication between the knee joint and the bursa. The bursa is seen by radiography when it is injected with paraffin and lipodol in cadaver studies (Fig. 118-4).

Dahlin and co-workers[3] studied the histology of 81 popliteal cysts excised: 46 were of bursal origin, 26 were considered posterior herniations, and 11 could not be classified. The pathology was divided

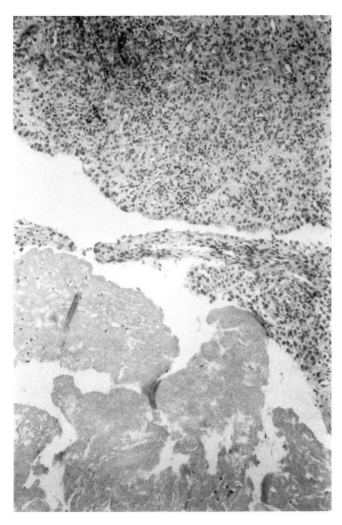

Fig. 118-5. Microscopic slide showing fibrous tissue wall of a popliteal cyst lined with hypertrophic synovial tissue. (×100)

between fibrous cysts with a fibroblastic lining and synovial cysts with a thick lining of synovial cells (Fig. 118-5). There was correlation between the point of origin and the type of cyst.

A popliteal cyst is a distended synovial gastrocnemius-semimembranosus bursa at the back of the knee. It can arise in the bursa, or it can be secondary; that is, it communicates with the knee joint and is related to a synovitis within the knee joint.[18]

The history is usually one of painless swelling in the posterior aspect of the knee; mild aching and stiffness may be noted. In the Case Western Reserve University Hospital series, only 8 of 39 patients had symptoms.[21] A tense cystic mass is palpable just below the flexion crease on the medial aspect of the popliteal fossa and is more prominent with the knee in hyperextension.[20] Homan's sign may be positive.

The differential diagnosis considers the following features:

1. Thrombophlebitis
2. Benign tumors (lipoma, xanthoma)
3. Malignant tumors (fibrosarcoma, rhabdomyosarcoma)
4. Vascular tumors (aneurysm, arteriovenous fistula, hemangioma)
5. Pyogenic abscess

Diagnosis

The cyst does not show on routine radiographs. An arthrogram is helpful.[11] Double-contrast arthrography is useful in examination for intraarticular lesions. The patient is told to exercise the knee joint to facilitate passage of air and/or dye into the popliteal cyst (Fig. 118-6).

Ultrasound B scanning is a useful noninvasive tool for outlining popliteal cysts, irrespective of their communication with the knee joint.

Treatment

Childress[4-7] presented the thesis that posterior horn tears of medial meniscus are frequently associated with popliteal cysts; he advocated meniscectomy without excision of the cyst. Bryan et al.[2] reported that in one-half of their cases (young adults), the cysts were associated with meniscal tears; they removed the meniscus and cyst in one operation.

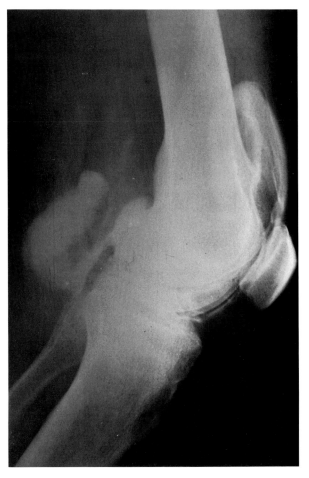

Fig. 118-6. Note the large popliteal cyst as seen after injection of dye and air into the knee joint and patient exercising of the joint by walking and active motion.

Popliteal cysts in children differ in that they rarely communicate with the joint and in that they usually regress spontaneoulsy.[10,19,21] The overall incidence drops off significantly after the age of 10. At this time, we recommend that popliteal cysts in children be observed and not excised.

It is important clinically to differentiate thrombophlebitis from a popliteal cyst. Not infrequently, patients have been given anticoagulants for mistaken phlebitis and have hemorrhaged into a popliteal cyst.

Venography is often necessary in a doubtful case. Extremely large popliteal cysts can occur and dissect down the leg, even to the ankle joint. These are associated with intra-articular disease, resulting in an effusion that expands into the popliteal cyst secondary to the increased intra-articular pressure, continuing to expand by dissecting along anatomic lines of least resistance. The same synovial process in the joint is present in the cyst.

Figure 118-7 illustrates the case of 55-year-old man with RA who had a popliteal cyst extending almost to the ankle. He had a mild pain in his knee and calf and noted swelling of the calf over a 6-month period. The knee had mild synovial thickening, free motion, and good stability. The mass was excised, and more than 300 ml of fluid was found in a thickened synovial sac that microscopically was consistent with RA.[29] (Today arthroscopic synovectomy of the knee should probably be performed at the same procedure if there is active synovitis.)

What is the mechanism of production of popliteal cysts of such gigantic proportions? It is believed that the communication between the joint capsule and the gastrocnemius-semimembranosus bursa is a one-way valve. When pressure increases within the joint, fluid is pumped into the bursa, owing to knee motion. When the pressure in the knee drops, the fluid cannot return because of the valve.

This theory is supported by the fact that radiopaque injections directly into the cyst never move into the joint, although on an arthrogram the dye can be forced into the cyst. Also, once a rheumatoid process begins in the cyst, it can be a self-perpetuating synovitis.

Indications for Surgery

In the patient who presents with symptoms of internal derangement of the knee and an asymptomatic (or mildly symptomatic) popliteal cyst, arthrography is indicated. If the cyst communicates with the joint, arthroscopy only is indicated. A lesion is found in the medial or lateral meniscus is treated appropriately arthroscopically, and the popliteal cyst is left alone. The cyst will usually regress spontaneously with the treatment of the intra-articular pathology.

In RA with a chronic synovitis of the knee and a symptomatic popliteal cyst, a combined procedure is usually indicated. This consists of arthroscopic synovectomy of the knee and then turning the patient prone and performing an excision of the popliteal cyst. In those patients who have had an arthroscopic meniscectomy and in whom the popliteal cyst persists and is painful, excision of the popliteal cyst is indicated.

Operative Technique

A thigh tourniquet is used. The patient is turned to the prone position. A bayonet-type incision is used: a 2- to 3-inch verticle arm laterally on the thigh, a 3- to 4-inch transverse portion at the flexion crease, and then a vertical medial portion over the medial head of the gastrocnemius muscle. The dissection is carried through the popliteal fascia,

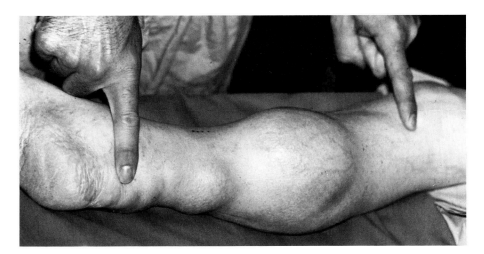

Fig. 118-7. Note large swelling of calf due to popliteal cyst in rheumatoid arthritis. The total extension of the process is between the two palpating fingers, from the knee to the ankle.

care being taken to protect the popliteal artery, nerve, and vein. The cyst is usually protruding posterolaterally to the tendon of the semimembranosus. The cyst is dissected carefully from the surrounding tissues. The stalk of the cyst is traced down to its communication to the knee joint and is excised at its junction with the posterior capsule. The capsule is oversewn to close the opening into the knee joint.

Postoperatively, the patient is immobilized in a removable knee splint and started on early range of motion. Isometrics and partial weight bearing are started on day 2. The rehabilitation program becomes aggressive after soft tissue healing is satisfactory, usually at 10 to 14 days postoperatively.

Summary

A popliteal cyst is an enlarged gastrocenemius-semimembranosus bursa of varying synovial etiology. Primary popliteal cysts probably do occur; they result from hyperplasia of normal synovial cells in the bursa. In adults most popliteal cysts are secondary to a pathologic process within the knee joint that produces a joint effusion. All patients with cysts must be checked for intra-articular pathology. It is very important to differentiate between a popliteal cyst and thrombophlebitis. In adults with popliteal cysts that communicate with the knee joint and that are secondary to a torn medial meniscus, only meniscectomy is indicated.

Other bursae around the knee can be involved in the same way by the same type of pathology; for example, cystic degeneration of the medial meniscus has been noted to dissect along the semimembranosus with a swelling along the surface, rather than in the typical popliteal cyst area.

Ganglion (synovial) cysts in the neighborhood of the knee can arise within the joint and protrude outward, such as a cyst of a lateral meniscus. Another type may arise from the tibiofibular joint.[31] The problem depends on the direction in which these cysts expand along the anatomic planes. Anterior expansion usually produces simply a swelling, while posterior expansion may involve the peroneal nerve and its tunnel at the neck of the fibular area. Some ganglia are actually intraneural and may or may not have any connection to a joint or bursa. The cyst should be excised, but intraneural dissec-

tion should be kept to a minimum to minimize nerve damage.[31]

REFERENCES

1. Baker WM: On the formation of synovial cysts in the leg in connection with disease of the knee joint. St. Bartholomew Hosp Rep 13:245, 1877
2. Bryan RS, DiMichelle JD, Ford GL: Popliteal cysts. Clin Orthop 50:203, 1967
3. Burleson RJ, Bickel WH, Dahlin DC: Popliteal cyst. J Bone Joint Surg 38A:1265, 1956
4. Childress HM: Popliteal cysts associated with undiagnosed posterior lesions of the medial meniscus. J Bone Joint Surg 36A:1233, 1954
5. Childress HM: Posterior medial meniscus lesions and popliteal cysts. J Bone Joint Surg 47A:1272, 1965
6. Childress HM: Popliteal cysts and posterior lesions of the medial meniscus. Clin Orthop 18:136, 1960
7. Childress HM: Popliteal cysts associated with undiagnosed posterior lesions of the medial meniscus. J Bone Joint Surg 52A:1487, 1970
8. Cleland LG, Treganza R, Dobson P, Arthroscopic synovectomy a prospective study. J. Rhematol 13:907, 1986
9. Cohen S, Jones R: An evaluation of the efficacy of arthroscopic synovectomy of the knee in RA: 12–24 month result. J Rheumatol 14:452, 1987
10. Dinham JM: Popliteal cysts in children. J Bone Joint Surg 57B:69, 1975
11. Doppman JL: Baker's cyst and the normal gastrocnemio-semimembranosus bursa. AJR 94:646, 1965
12. Dunn AW, Whisler JH: Synovial chondromatosis of the knee with associated extracapsular chondroma. J Bone Joint Surg 44A:1747, 1973
13. Ganel A, Horoszowski H, Militeanu J, et al: Arthrographic diagnosis of pigmented villonodular synovitis. Orthop Rev 9:92, 1980
14. Geens S: Synovectomy and debridement of the knee in rheumatoid arthritis. I. Historical review. J Bone Joint Surg 51A:17, 1969
15. Geens S, Clayton ML, Leidholt JD, et al: Synovectomy and debridement of the knee in rheumatoid arthritis. II. Clinical and roentgenographic study of thirty-one cases. J Bone Joint Surg 51A:626, 1969
16. Granowitz SP, D'Antonio J, Mankin HL: The patho-

genesis and long-term end results of pigmented villonodular synovitis. Clin Orthop 114:335, 1976

17. Gristina AG, Wilson PD: Popliteal cysts in adults and children. Arch Surg 88:357, 1964
18. Haggart GE: Posterior hernia of the knee joint. J Bone Joint Surg 20:363, 1938
19. Higgenboten CL: Arthroscopic synovectomy. Orthop Clin North Am 13:399, 1982
20. Hoffman BK: Cystic lesions of the popliteal space. Surg Gynecol Obstet 116:551, 1963
21. Mack RP: Popliteal cysts. p. 195. In Funk FJ (ed.): American Academy of Orthopaedic Surgeons Symposium of the Athlete's Knee. Surgical Repair and Reconstruction. CV Mosby, St. Louis, 1980
22. Meijers HA, Valkenberg, Cats A: A synovectomy trial and the history of early knee synovitis in RA, Rheumatol Int 3:161, 1983
23. Milgram JW, Addison RG: Synovial osteochondromatosis of the knee. Chondromatous recurrence with possible chondrosarcomatous degeneration. J Bone Joint Surg 58A:264, 1976
24. Moon NF: Synovial hemangioma of the knee joint. A review of previously reported cases and inclusion of two new cases. Clin Orthop 90:183, 1973
25. Muckle DS, Monahan P: Intra-articular ganglion of the knee. Report of two cases. J Bone Joint Surg 54B:520, 1972
26. Patakis MJ, Mills DM, Bartholomew BA, et al: A visual, histological and enzymatic study of regeneration rheumatoid synovium in the synovectomized knee. J Bone Joint Surg 55A:287, 1973
27. Quayle JB, Robinson MP: An operation for chronic prepatellar bursitis. J Bone Joint Surg 58B:504, 1976
28. Ranawat CS, Ecker ML, Straub LR: Synovectomy and debridement of the knee in rheumatoid arthritis (A study of 60 knees). Arthritis Rheum 15:571, 1972
29. Schmidt MD, Workman JB, Barth WF: Dissection or rupture of a popliteal cyst. Arch Intern Med 134:694, 1974
30. Shibata T, Shiraoka LK, Takubo N: Comparison between arthroscopic and open synovectomy for the knee in RA. Arch Orthop Trauma Surg 105:257, 1986
31. Stener B: Unusual ganglion cysts in the neighborhood of the knee joint. A report of six cases — three with involvement of the peroneal nerve. Acta Orthop Scand 40:392, 1969
32. Wilson PD, Francis JD: A clinical and anatomical study of the semimembranosus bursa in relation to popliteal cysts. J Bone Joint Surg 20:963, 1938
33. Wu KK, Ross PM, Guise ER: Pigmented villonodular synovitis: a clinical analysis of twenty-four cases treated at Henry Ford Hospital. Orthopedics 3:751, 1980

Tibial Osteotomy

119

Donald B. Kettelkamp

Osteotomy of the tibia for varus or valgus deformity at the knee is based on the principle of restoring limb alignment to relieve excessive force on one tibial plateau. Tibial osteotomy distal to the tubercle for degenerative arthritis was reported by Wardle[47] to have been performed in Liverpool since the time of Sir Robert Jones. Jackson and Waugh reported the results of a dome-type osteotomy just below the tibial tubercle in 1961.[20] Larson, in 1960, taught me a technique for a dome osteotomy above the tubercle.

The foundation for and the popularity of proximal tibial osteotomy in this country emanated from a publication by Coventry in 1965. Coventry's criteria for the osteotomy are as applicable today as in 1965 and merit a direct quote[6]:

> The osteotomy should (1) fully correct and, in fact, slightly reverse the varus or valgus deformity, (2) be near the site of the deformity, (3) involve bone that will heal rapidly—the bone should be primarily cancellous, (4) allow early motion of the knee and early bearing of weight, (5) provide convenience for exploration of the knee at the time of

osteotomy, if such is indicated, and (6) present no undue technical difficulties or potential hazards.

Many subsequent investigators[2,4,6-12,15,16,19,21,27, 30,31,36,40,41,43-48] have substantiated the applicability of these criteria for tibial osteotomy, although the specific surgical technique may vary. The efficacy of proximal tibial osteotomy for the relief of pain and improvement of function in unicompartmental degenerative arthritis is without question.

The pathomechanics of unicompartmental degenerative arthritis have been defined by Maquet[33] and Chao.[5] The primary problem is loss of articular cartilage and subsequent loss of subchondral bone secondary to excessive stress. The etiology of the excessive stress is usually unknown; however, the specific effects of meniscectomy, plateau fracture, osteonecrosis[28] and residual angular deformity after tibial or femoral diaphyseal fractures are well documented. Once angular deformity and cartilage loss occur, the severity of the deformity and of the arthritis tends to increase with time. This course is not always unremitting over a 5- to 11-year interval, as pointed out by Miller et al.[34] Their study mitigates against prophylactic osteotomy.

INDICATIONS

The ideal indication for proximal tibial osteotomy is a patient under 60 years of age[18] who has unicompartmental degenerative genu varum, stable knee ligaments, no flexion deformity, and more than 100 degrees of flexion range. The lateral joint space and patellofemoral compartments should be normal.[4,9] The angular deformity would require 10 to 12 degrees of correction. Relative and specific contraindications will be given because proximal tibial osteotomy is frequently indicated in less than this ideal situation. As a general rule, the younger the patient, the greater his or her weight, and the more strenuous the occupational requirements, the more likely I would be to recommend osteotomy in less than ideal circumstances.[4]

Relative contraindications include age over 70 years, severe patellofemoral arthritis, and lax collateral ligaments. Patients over 70 years of age may do well with osteotomy; however, their activity level and general health must be weighed against the longer convalescence associated with osteotomy as compared to implant replacement.[3,18] Severe patellofemoral arthritis will be symptomatic with flexed knee activities after closing-wedge osteotomy. The barrel-vault osteotomy of Maquet provides some decompression of the patellofemoral joint. The results of combining a closing-wedge proximal tibial osteotomy with a tibial tubercle elevation (sometimes called the Maquet procedure) have been reported by several investigators[9,17,38]; however, the complication rate is greater than with either procedure alone or with the Maquet barrel-vault osteotomy. Patellar subluxation or dislocation must be corrected.

Ligamentous laxity of greater than a mild degree may contraindicate osteotomy. In general, laxity is better tolerated when it is on the concave side of the corrected limb (e.g., lateral side after correction of a varus deformity into valgus). Specific contraindications include valgus deformity of greater than 10 degrees,[40] flexion deformity greater than 20 degrees, excessive bone loss from the tibial plateau or femoral condyle,[26] and rheumatoid arthritis.

The correction of valgus deformity by proximal tibial osteotomy produces obliquity of the tibial surface at least equal to the correction. If more than 10 to 15 degrees of correction is required, the osteotomy should be in the distal femur.[40]

Up to 20 degrees of flexion deformity can be corrected with a closing-wedge proximal tibial osteotomy; however, this does not improve the decreased weight-bearing area associated with knee flexion. If more than a 20-degree deformity exists, or if a barrel vault osteotomy is to be done,[33] the deformity must be corrected before osteotomy.

Many authorities have suggested that more than 15 degrees of varus is a contraindication. Correction of a greater deformity by closing-wedge osteotomy leaves very little contact for healing, and more than 20 degrees correction by curved osteotomy with fibular osteotomy increases the risk to the foot and ankle dorsiflexors.[39] In my experience, this degree of deformity is usually associated with bone loss from the medial tibial plateau. If the bone loss exceeds about 1 cm, weight bearing on both plateaus after osteotomy may not occur—the teeter effect.[26] This gives an unstable knee and a poor result. Occasionally, a similar situation occurs when one is considering tibial osteotomy for the residuals of a lateral plateau fracture. If the depression is enough to prohibit some weight bearing on both plateaus after osteotomy, another procedure should be chosen. Tibial osteotomy for angular deformity in rheumatoid arthritis has not produced good results in any reported series, and rheumatoid arthritis should be considered a contraindication for this procedure.

EVALUATION

The primary motivations behind surgical treatment of unicompartmental arthritis are alleviation of the patient's pain and improvement of activity level. Throughout the discussion of indications, it is assumed that the patient's symptoms and disability are of sufficient magnitude to warrant surgical intervention. The first question is: Are the symptoms sufficiently severe? In my experience the patient who wishes to have surgery usually has pain with all weight bearing, can walk fewer than three blocks because of pain, and has great difficulty negotiating stairs. Occasionally, a working person will be less limited yet still request surgical treatment. The second question is: Are the patient's goals or needs compatible with the expected results? This question has various answers and may require that the surgeon and patient spend considerable time in discussion.

A thorough medical evaluation is necessary, including coagulation studies. Our presurgery coagulation evaluation includes partial thromboplastin time, prothrombin time, bleeding time, platelet count, fibrinogen, and platelet agglutination. Abnormalities should be corrected before surgery. Obesity should be reduced preoperatively, if possible, to improve the effectiveness of plaster immobilization, decrease the risk of pin-tract infections if compression techniques are used, and decrease the risk of phlebitis.

Distal arterial blood supply must be intact. We have not considered varicosities or a previous history of phlebitis as specific contraindications to osteotomy; however, both increase the risk.

The entire lower extremity must be evaluated for range of motion and alignment. Ipsilateral hip disease with restricted motion and deformity should be corrected before tibial osteotomy to enable the surgeon to calculate the tibial correction. Angular deformity of the femur or tibia secondary to previous fracture may require correction as a preliminary procedure. Such correction may obviate the necessity for tibial osteotomy.

The knee must be evaluated for significant instability of the posterior capsule, posterior cruciate, medial collateral ligament, and anterolateral rotatory instability, any of which may contraindicate tibial osteotomy. Apparent laxity of the collateral ligaments may occur because of joint opening secondary to cartilage and bone loss. With apparent laxity there is a firm end point, and the tibiofemoral alignment cannot be corrected past normal.

Stress radiographs will assess ligament stability and demonstrate the presence of a joint space on the unaffected plateau. The patient should be observed walking. Prodromos et al.[37] noted a greater failure rate in patients with a higher adduction moment-lateral thrust. While this is not a contraindi-

cation to osteotomy both the surgeon and the patient should recognize the increased risk of a less than satisfactory result.

Radiographic examination includes the following views: anteroposterior (AP) weight-bearing, lateral, tunnel, and Merchant. An AP weight-bearing film that extends from the hip to the ankle is obtained to measure the mechanical angle for calculation of correction. A stress film will evaluate the joint space on the unaffected side and ligament stability. Lateral shift of the tibia seen on the weight-bearing films and not corrected on the stress film is associated with a greater incidence of unsatisfactory results and should be considered by both the surgeon and patient in making their decisions. Arthroscopy has not been of value for preosteotomy evaluation of the articular surfaces.[9,23]

CALCULATION OF CORRECTION

The mechanical angle, the angle formed by a line from the center of the femoral head to the center of the knee with a line from the center of the ankle to the center of the knee, is measured from the long AP film. I prefer Maquet's desired correction, which is the normal (0-degree) mechanical angle plus 2 to 4 degrees for a varus deformity and minus 1 to 3 degrees for a valgus deformity.[31-33]

This correction approximates 8 to 10 degrees anatomic valgus for a varus deformity and 3 to 4 degrees anatomic valgus for a valgus deformity.[33] These ranges are similar to those of other authors.[2,6,7,15,19,27,30,36,45] The correction is drawn on tracing paper and the anatomic angle measured (for use in the operating room) from the corrected tracing.

OPERATIVE TECHNIQUE

There are two fundamental techniques for proximal tibial osteotomy: the barrel-vault, as described by Maquet,[31,33] and the closing-wedge.

Maquet Barrel-Vault Tibial Osteotomy

This procedure is done without a tourniquet. The initial incision is over the fibula at the middle third (Fig. 119-1). Skin and subcutaneous tissue are incised, and the plane is found between the muscles on the lateral border of the fibula. The muscles are subperiosteally elevated to permit resection of 1 cm of fibula. Great care must be exercised to avoid traumatizing the veins along the medial border of the fibula. If injured, considerable bleeding will ensue; it must be controlled, an often difficult and time-consuming task; 1 cm of fibula is removed with a rongeur. The wound may be packed open until termination of the procedure.

An incision is then made over the patellar tendon and the tibial tubercle. Maquet[31,33] describes a 4-cm incision; however, a somewhat longer incision facilitates exposure. The incision is carried through skin and subcutaneous tissue. Care must be taken to avoid incising the patellar tendon. Skin is then retracted medially and laterally. An incision is made parallel and adjacent to the medial and lateral margins of the patellar tendon. Veins are usually present and must be clamped and cauterized. The medial surface of the proximal tibia is exposed subperiosteally to the posterior medial corner. At this level, the lateral border of the tibia at the distal portion of the wound is almost vertical and is exposed subperiosteally. This subperiosteal dissection should not be extended too far distally, where the anterior tibial artery could be traumatized or compromised. The curved marking jig is then placed under the patellar tendon immediately above or against the upper part of the tubercle. It may be necessary to elevate 0.5 to 1 cm of patellar tendon from the tubercle to permit greater distal

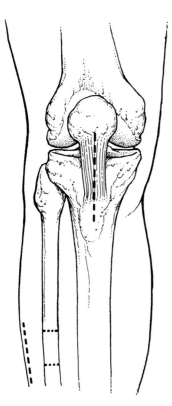

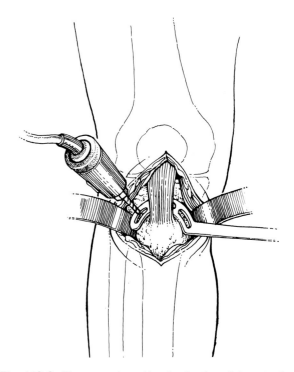

Fig. 119-1. The skin incisions for the Maquet barrel-vault osteotomy consist of a lateral incision over the lower middle third of the fibula for fibular osteotomy and an incision over the proximal tibia that extends from the lower pole of the patella to just below the tibial tubercle.

Fig. 119-2. The curved marking jig is placed deep to the patellar tendon. Under image intensification the jig is properly located. Holes in the anterior cortex of the tibia are then drilled using a powered K-wire placed through the slots in the curved marking jig. The posterior cortex does not need to be perforated.

placement of the curved marker. With valgus rotation of the distal fragment after osteotomy, it is desirable to leave somewhat more proximal tibia on the medial side. Position is checked with an image intensifier. With a power drill containing a Kirschner (K-) wire, the anterior surface of the tibia is marked through the slot in the curved jig with a series of holes (Fig. 119-2). The wire only needs to pass through the anterior cortex. Passage of the wire through the posterior cortex runs the risk of perforating the popliteal and/or posterior tibial vessels. Using image intensification for control and a power drill, a 4- to 5-mm smooth Steinmann pin is inserted through the proximal tibia. A short vertical incision is made on the lateral side of the proximal tibia before placement of the pin. The pin

should be proximal to the apex of the curve for the osteotomy and may be started just below the subchondral cortex on the lateral side and angled medially and distally. As the pin approaches the skin on the medial side, the skin is again incised longitudinally and the pin passage completed. The angle guide is then passed over the pin on the lateral side (Fig. 119-3). Frequently, the hole in the angle guide is larger than the pin size. Wobble, and therefore potential error, can be avoided by inserting the cannulated soft tissue drill protectors from an AO set in the angle guide. The distal pin is then placed through the anterior compartment muscles from the lateral side. As the pin is inserted through the muscles, an assistant has a hand on the patient's toes. If the toes twitch with pin passage, the pin should be removed and replaced. The distal pin is held in a hand chuck and inserted through the tibia with a twisting to-and-fro motion. This is time consuming and difficult but much less risky than using

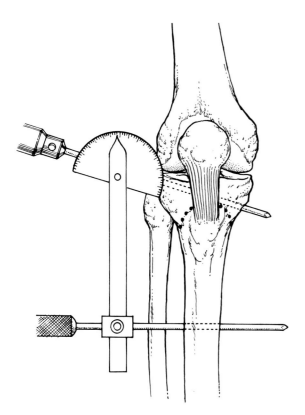

Fig. 119-3. Using the angle guide and the image intensifier, the surgeon places a Steinmann pin through the proximal tibial fragment. The angle guide is then set for the desired angle of correction. The distal pin is placed using a hand chuck. An assistant should grasp the patient's toes during placement of the distal pin; if the toes twitch, the pin site should be changed.

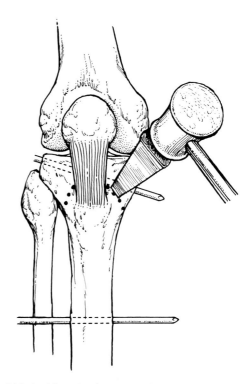

Fig. 119-4. After pin placement, the osteotomy is cut from anterior to posterior using the thin marked otolaryngology osteotomes. Care must be taken to avoid penetration past the posterior cortex.

a power drill for this pin insertion. After the pins have been placed, a large goniometer set at the desired angle is placed inside the pins. The image is then used to ascertain that the pins are, in fact, parallel to each arm of the goniometer, thereby making the correct angle. Attention is now turned to the osteotomy.

The osteotomy is cut from anterior to posterior (Fig. 119-4). The osteotome should be thin and straight. I have found the marked osteotomes used by the otolaryngologist most satisfactory. Great care must be exercised to avoid penetrating beyond the posterior cortex. Once the osteotomy has been completed, the knee is flexed and the surgeon angulates the distal tibia forward at the osteotomy site (Fig. 119-5). The distal tibia should be displaced 1 cm anterior to its former position and moved in a valgus direction such that the pins are parallel. Two Synthes clamps, previously set, are placed over the pins and tightened (Fig. 119-6). If the skin is under tension because of the pin placement, the incisions for the pins should be lengthened. Stability can be checked under direct vision.

Hemovac drains are placed in both the fibular and tibial wounds. Fascia is not closed. Subcutaneous tissue is approximated with interrupted sutures and the skin is closed with interrupted sutures. A gauze dressing is applied and either a splint or a knee mobilizer used for initial support of the extremity. The Hemovac drains are usually removed at 48 hours or when drainage is minimal. Active straight-leg raising without external support and active knee flexion can usually be started 4 to 7 days after surgery depending on the patient's comfort.

The clamps should be tightened at 2 weeks and may need to be tightened again during the subsequent 6 weeks. Pins are customarily left in place for 8 weeks.

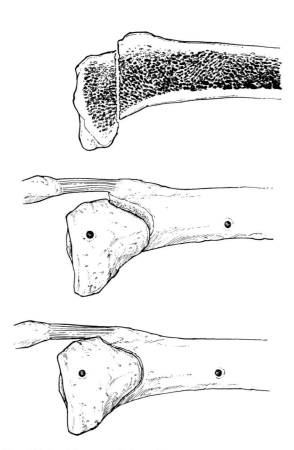

Fig. 119-5. After completion of the osteotomy, the knee is flexed and the distal tibial fragment angled forward at the osteotomy site, permitting 1-cm anterior displacement of the distal tibia.

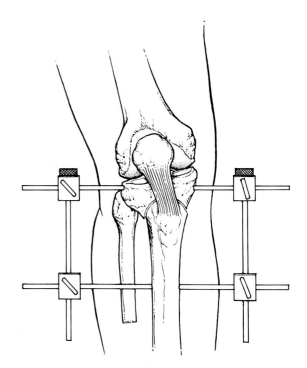

Fig. 119-6. After anterior displacement, correction is accomplished by the application of two Synthes clamps, which are tightened such that the pins are parallel. Position is again checked using an image intensifier or radiograph.

Technical Points

The most severe complications of this procedure have been anterior compartment syndrome and/or peroneal nerve palsy. Perforation of the popliteal artery has also occurred. Consequently, there are several points during the procedure at which great attention must be paid to detail:

1. The distal pin must be placed with a hand chuck. The site must be moved if twitching of the toes occurs as the pin passes through the muscle.
2. It is safer to mark only the anterior cortex of the tibia rather than penetrating the posterior cortex with the pin.
3. It is imperative that the surgeon have the "feel" of the osteotome as the posterior tibial cortex is infracted to avoid penetrating the posterior structures.
4. It is important to obtain hemostasis at the site of fibular osteotomy before closure.
5. It is important to use Hemovac drains in both incisions.
6. The periosteum and fascia should not be closed at either incision.
7. Correction can be changed a few degrees during the first 7 to 10 postoperative days by tightening or loosening the appropriate compression clamp.

Closing-Wedge Osteotomy

There are a number of technical variations in performing a closing-wedge proximal tibial osteotomy. Two techniques, Coventry's[6] and the one I prefer,[24] are given in detail; some of the other variations are then discussed.

Coventry Closing-Wedge Osteotomy

In Coventry's technique,[6-9] after sterile preparation of the leg and inflation of the tourniquet, the knee is flexed 90 degrees. The incision begins anterior to the fibular head, extending up across the joint line to the iliotibial band, which is split longitudinally (Fig. 119-7). The distal part of the incision in the iliotibial band is parallel and anterior to the fibular collateral ligament. The tendon of the biceps femoris muscle and the fibular collateral lig-

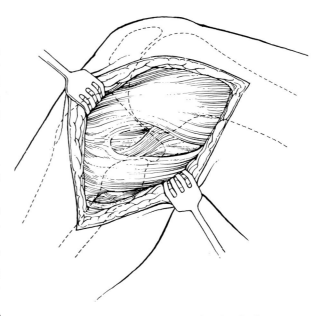

Fig. 119-7. The iliotibial band is split longitudinally, exposing the fibular collateral ligament. The incision in the iliotibial band is parallel and anterior to the fibular collateral ligament. The fibular collateral ligament, proximal fibula, and biceps tendon are identified.

ament are then identified and removed by dissection from the head of the fibula as a Y-conjoined tendon (Fig. 119-8). The fibular head is then excised with an osteotome proximal to the peroneal nerve. The peroneal nerve is not dissected free and isolated but is protected by a finger placed on it to avoid injury. The lateral lip of the lateral tibial plateau is then identified manually or with a small incision through the capsule, care being taken not to interfere with the joint space or lateral meniscus. Soft tissues are elevated from the front of the tibia as far as the patellar tendon and posteriorly for the full width of the posterior surface of the proximal tibia. Two-wires are inserted at the appropriate angle. The proximal pin is 2 cm distal to the articular surface, and the distal pin is directed at the proper angle for the desired wedge. Placement of the pins is facilitated by image intensification control, which is simpler than control by radiographs. Roughly, the base of a wedge of 1 mm equals 1 degree of correction up to 10 degrees of correction. Beyond 10 degrees of correction less added wedge is needed for the additional correction required. The wedge is removed with flat osteo-

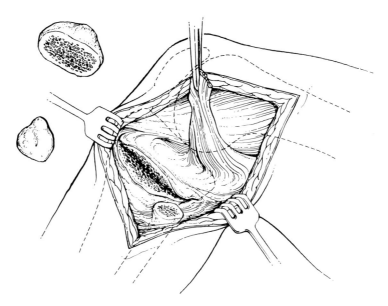

Fig. 119-8. The conjoined tendon and fibular collateral ligament are removed from the head of the fibula, and the proximal fibula is excised with an osteotome. Subperiosteal dissection exposes the tibia lateral to the patellar tendon and posteriorly across the back of the tibia. The osteotomy angle is then marked with K-wires and checked with an image intensifier, and a wedge is removed using osteotomes.

tomes. The medial tibial cortex is perforated with a narrow osteotome to provide easy infraction with wedge closure. The K-wires are removed, the knee extended, and the wedge closed and held with a step staple (Fig. 119-9). The tourniquet is then released and blood vessels coagulated. The 45-degree flexion position is used throughout closure. The biceps femoris tendon and fibular collateral ligament are reattached by suture through a drill hole to the neck of the fibula and reinforced by sutures through the iliotibial band and the anterior crural fascia. The incision in the fascia lata is approximated with horizontal mattress sutures. Hemovac drainage is inserted posteriorly before complete closure of the wound. A modified Robert Jones dressing is applied for the first 8 days after surgery, followed by a cylinder cast. Weight bearing with crutches is then allowed.

Author's Preferred Technique: Closing-Wedge Proximal Tibial Osteotomy

In the closing-wedge proximal tibial osteotomy, the technique I prefer,[24] the leg is prepped and draped in the usual manner and a tourniquet is used. The incision begins 1 to 1.5 cm medial to the medial border of the patellar tendon at the level of the proximal edge of the tibial tubercle. The incision continues transversely following the lateral ridge of the lateral plateau at the level of origin of the anterior tibial muscle to just anterior to the anterior portion of the head of the fibula and then curves distally for another 1 to 1.5 cm. The incision is continued through skin and subcutaneous tissue. On each side of the patellar tendon the veins are clamped and cauterized. A vertical incision is made in the periosteum on the medial side of the patellar tendon and the medial periosteum elevated with a Cobb elevator to the posteriormedial corner of the tibia.

The fat pad is freed deep to the patellar tendon so that it can be moved proximally. This usually does not require any specific dissection but merely passage of a retractor deep to the tendon. The patellar tendon is then released from the tubercle for a distance of about 1 cm. On the lateral side, the incision is continued to bone in line with the skin incision to the level of the proximal tibiofibular joint where the fascia overlying the muscles is split longitudinally just anterior to the head of the fibula.

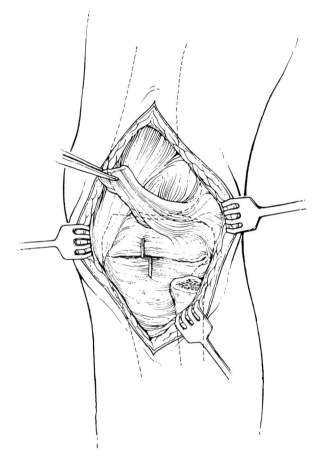

Fig. 119-9. The wedge is closed and held with one or more stepped staples. The fibular collateral ligament and biceps tendon are resutured to the neck of the fibula.

This allows exposure to the anterior surface of the head of the fibula. The periosteum on the proximal tibia lateral to the patellar tendon is elevated with sharp dissection. Similarly, sharp dissection is used to begin the periosteal elevation of the anterior tibial muscle from the tibia. Once this has been carried inferiorly to Gerdy's tubercle, continued elevation can usually be done with a periosteal elevator. Caution is taken to avoid deep elevation of the periosteum posteriorly, although it usually needs to be elevated more distally nearer the crest of the tibia. The muscle is reflected from the anterior part of the proximal tibiofibular joint. With the anterior surface of the head of the fibula thus exposed, the anterior cortex is removed with an osteotome. The contents of the head of the fibula are

removed with a curette, including the interior surface of the corical bone, such that the fibular head will collapse with closure of the osteotomy. Retractors are placed medially, under the patellar tendon, laterally exposing the proximal tibia and osteotomy site. A wedge of the proper angle is then marked. This can be drawn out on a piece of sterilized tin foil and placed over the tibia. Approximately 1 mm of bone resection at the base equals 1 degree to about 10 degrees.

An alternate method of measuring the desired wedge is that described by Slocum et al.[41] The wedge is drawn preoperatively and the width of the base is measured at 4, 5, 6, and 7 cm from the apex (Fig. 119-10). The initial transverse saw cut is made 2 cm below the articular surface and a ruler inserted in the cut. The width of the base of the wedge is then measured with a second ruler and marked[41] (Fig. 119-11). Once the anterior cuts are marked, the anterior portion of the tibia is removed with a saw. This is carried posteriorly stopping short of the posterior cortex. This wedge of bone is then removed with a narrow osteotome. Any remaining cancellous bone anterior to the posterior cortex of the tibia is removed with currettes. The posterior cortex to past the midline from lateral to medial is removed with a narrow jawed Lexel rongeur. The posterior jaw of the rongeur is used as a periosteal elevator, and all cuts are made bringing the rongeur anteriorly (Fig. 119-12). The posterior medial cortex of the tibia is infracted with a narrow osteotome. With the retractors placed as described, the proximal tibial plateau can be observed during wedge closure. If closure does not occur easily, the fibular head should be inspected again to be certain that sufficient bone has been curretted to permit collapse, and one should again check the medial cortex to make sure it is ade-

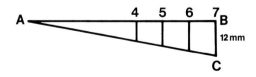

Fig. 119-10. The correct-angle wedge is drawn. The amount of bone to resect at 4, 5, 6, and 7 cm is measured directly from the tracing. (After technique of Slocum et al.) (Redrawn from Slocum,[41] with permission.)

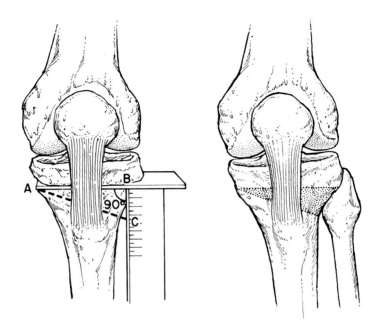

Fig. 119-11. After the transverse cut has been made across the tibia, a ruler is placed in the cut. The measurement for the base of the wedge then depends on the width of the tibia from medial to lateral side. The amount based on the drawing described in Figure 119-10 is then marked, and the wedge is removed. (From Slocum,[41] with permission.)

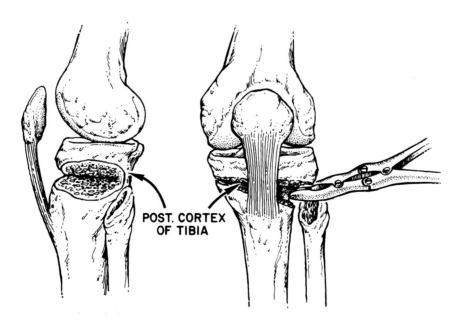

Fig. 119-12. The posterior cortex of the tibia is cut past the midline using a narrow jawed Lexel rongeur with the posterior blade serving as a periosteal elevator. All cuts are made by pulling the rongeur anteriorly.

quately infracted. Should the tibial plateau fracture, attention must be directed to the fibular head and the medial cortex to be certain those areas are loose. The normal relationship of the medial and lateral tibial plateaus must be restored and fixed with a pin or screw before again attempting to close the wedge. After the wedge has been closed, it is held in position with stepped, Stone, or standard staples. Usually some of the resected wedge is used as a bone graft placed along the lateral side of the osteotomy. Hemostasis is obtained after removal of the tourniquet and before complete wound closure. A Hemovac drain is placed on the lateral side in the area of elevation of the anterior tibial muscle. The anterior tibial muscle is reattached to the periosteum proximally with interrupted sutures. Subcutaneous tissues are approximated with interrupted sutures and skin closed with vertical mattress sutures. A long leg cast is applied with the knee in slight flexion. The cast can be applied most easily by applying the foot and calf portion of the cast, letting this dry, and then maintaining valgus stress on the leg as the upper portion of the cast is applied. This same procedure should be used for subsequent cast change.

Alternate Techniques

MacIntosh and Welsh[30] and Ha'eri and Wiley[14] advocated arthrotomy at the time of osteotomy. Early mobilization of the knee is provided by fixation with compression clamps with the MacIntosh technique; Ha'eri and Wiley use a blade plate. Andrews has been using internal fixation with an AO semitubular four-hole plate and cancellous screw (Andrews JR: personal communication). In this technique, the plate is driven into the plateau from the lateral side leaving one screw hole out. The protruding end of the plate is bent 45 degrees distally and a cancellous screw is inserted through the plate into the distal tibia. Compression and fixation are provided by tightening the screw. A buttress plate and screws have also been used for immediate fixation of the osteotomy. These techniques permit early knee motion.

The fibula may be managed in varying ways. Coventry excised the fibular head,[6] I prefer currettage and collapse[24]; MacIntosh[30] uses more distal osteotomy, as does Maquet[31] and Evarts et al.[11] re-

sected the medial portion of the fibular head and displaced the remaining fibular head posteriorly. All methods provide for shortening of the fibula. Osteotomy of the fibula has more associated morbidity and complications than does partial excision or collapsing the fibular head.[22,48] If fibular osteotomy is used there is no agreement as to the safest site,[9,22,33,39,48] however, 5 cm[9] and 10 to 20 cm[24] distal to the fibular head may be the areas of greatest risk for peroneal nerve palsy.

POSTOPERATIVE MANAGEMENT

The postoperative management of proximal tibial osteotomy varies only in relation to the method of fixation. Antibiotics are started intravenously in the operating room before surgery and are continued until the removal the Hemovac drains. Further use depends on the patient's course and the surgeon's preference.

Phlebitis prophylaxis consists of aspirin twice daily beginning after surgery. We have had no experience with Dextran. Coumadin, in our clinical experience, has been associated with slow bone healing and loss of correction. Although Stinchfield et al.[42] suggest such a relationship, Harris (personal communication) did not have a similar clinical impression in hip fracture healing. As a result, we would advise carefully noting bone healing in patients receiving Coumadin prophylaxis.

Postoperative immobilization varies with the surgical technique and is given in the operative technique. Usually cast immobilization is continued for 6 to 8 weeks with weight bearing as tolerated with crutches. Compression clamps are continued for 8 weeks with weight bearing as tolerated. Quadriceps sets, straight-leg raising, and dorsiflexion and plantar-flexion exercises are started with both methods as soon as tolerated by the patient. Knee flexion exercises can usually be started 7 to 10 days after surgery if compression techniques are used and after cast removal if staple fixation is used. Progressive resistance exercises are not begun until union of the osteotomy is without question. Crutches are continued until there is solid union, full return of motion, and good muscle control. This usually takes 4 to 6 months after surgery. If symptoms persist after bony union with optimum correction, the patient's gait should be carefully analyzed for walking pattern and the knee carefully examined for specific evidence of internal mechanical derangement. The knee will often seem to have to retrack, and this may take 1 year or more. Under these circumstances, the decision for secondary surgery should only be for a specific diagnosis, until after 1-year follow-up. Symptoms associated with loss of correction and nonunion may be treated by reoperation at any time as the situation dictates.

COMPLICATIONS

The most frequent complication of tibial osteotomy is undercorrection or loss of correction.[27] Undercorrection usually represents inaccurate measurement of the deformity or inaccurate estimation of the correction. The fact that there is no certain method of controlling rotation for the radiograph makes small degrees of error inescapable. Obesity and technical imprecision further add to the problem. The barrel-vault osteotomy offers some advantages over the closing-wedge in this regard since some alteration in correction can be done during the first postoperative week by selectively tightening clamps.

Loss of correction can occur because of insecure fixation, bone settling, and slower-than-average healing. Correction loss can be minimized by closely observing and protecting the extremity until union is stable. Medications such as heparin, coumadin, diphenylhydantoin (Dilantin), and steroids may retard bone union.

Undercorrection and loss of correction can be remedied more easily by repeat osteotomy than can overcorrection. Delayed union and nonunion can be treated by bone graft or repeat osteotomy when associated with loss of correction.

Phelbitis and pulmonary embolism are potential complications of any major lower-extremity surgery. Maquet believes that doing the osteotomy without tourniquet may prevent phlebitis.[33] Early mobilization of the foot, ankle, and knee may be desirable with any technique used. Because heparin and coumadin may delay bone healing, we use salicylates for prophylaxis of phlebitis.

Peroneal nerve palsy appears to be related to the type of osteotomy and the amount of correction. Most reported peroneal nerve palsies occurred in cases which used pins and compression clamp fixation.[25] Osteotomy of the fibula has also been associated with peroneal nerve palsy, particularly when 15 to 20 degrees of correction were required.[25,39] Shargorodsky[39] found that correction of 15 to 20 degrees, when associated with fibular osteotomy, produced tension in the branches of the peroneal nerve. He found the incidence of palsy was greatest with osteotomy of the fibular neck followed by osteotomy in the middle and distal thirds. The trauma associated with pin placement through the anterior compartment may contribute to this complication.

Maquet reported paresthesias of the foot, 4.8 percent, and paresis of the foot dorsiflexors in 1.7 percent with the barrel-vault osteotomy, which uses pins and fibular osteotomy.[32] Sundaram and co-authors used a similar technique and had three patients with weakened dorsiflexors and four with paresthesias out of 105 osteotomies.[43] Bleeding into the anterior compartment from the tibial osteotomy, the fibular osteotomy, or the pin placement may also be a causative factor. Gibson et al.[13] measured anterior compartment pressures in 20 patients after closing-wedge osteotomy and found lower pressures in those who had their wounds drained postoperatively. Three of their twenty patients including both groups had weakness of toe dorsiflexors. The wider dissection necessary for use of plate fixation may also lead to anterior artery compromise.[9,48] For the past few years, I have routinely done prophylactic anterior fasciotomies with the barrel-vault osteotomy. Whatever the mechanism, the greater reported frequency of peroneal palsy and anterior compartment problems with those techniques which use pin and clamp fixation and fibular osteotomy must enter into the choice of operative method.

Infection has been an infrequent complication.[25] Pin-tract infections have about 10 percent incidence with the pin-compression techniques.[25] Arterial injury is also an infrequent complication.[25,48] Arterial injury can occur with any surgical method, and care must be taken to avoid damage to the popliteal and anterior tibial vessels.

RESULTS

Proximal tibial osteotomy for degenerative genu varum produces good and acceptable results in a high percentage of patients. Most authorities agree that the single most important factor in a determining the result is adequate correction, generally conceded to be 10 degrees of anatomic valgus.[4,5,7–9,16,19,27,29,30,33,36,44,46] As would be expected, the results do deteriorate with time. Long follow-up studies demonstrate this effect. Insall et al.[19] reported 97 percent excellent or good results at 2 years, 85 percent at 5 years, and 63 percent subsequently. Aglietti et al.[1] found 64 percent good and excellent results after 10 years. These figures are similar to those reported by Coventry,[9] with pain relief in 67.5 percent at 4 years and 61.8 percent at 10 years. Maquet[35] reports a slightly higher percentage of good and fair results with the barrel-vault technique. This may be due in part to slightly more accurate correction and decompression of the patellofemoral joint.

CORRECTION OF VALGUS DEFORMITY

The pathomechanics and evaluation of degenerative genu valgum are the same as for varus deformity. The desired correction is a 0- to 5-degree valgus anatomic tibiofemoral angle. On the basis of the mechanical angle, the correction is the mechanical angle less 1 to 3 degrees. If the medial collateral ligament is lax the correction should be based on the angle with the medial joint space closed. Tracings of the corrected position are recommended.

OPERATIVE TECHNIQUE

Valgus Deformity of 10 to 15 Degrees

For valgus deformity of 10 to 15 degrees, correction may be in the proximal tibia using either the closing-wedge or barrel-vault technique. Fibular osteotomy is not required for a correction of less than 15 degrees.

Closing-Wedge Osteotomy

The technique is the same as for varus deformity except that the fibula requires no surgery. The superficial portion of the medial collateral ligament is sectioned distally and reflected proximally or retracted posteriorly. The popliteus muscle and posterior periosteum are reflected from the tibia and a medially based wedge removed. The apex of the wedge should be at the level of the proximal tibiofibular joint. The closed osteotomy is fixed with one or more staples, and the medial collateral ligament is imbricated if it was sectioned. Postoperative care is the same as for closing-wedge for varus deformity.

Barrel-Vault Osteotomy

The barrel-vault osteotomy for valgus deformity, developed by Maquet,[33] is the same as for varus deformity except that the fibula need not be osteotomized for less than 15 degrees correction and the angles of the pins are reversed.

Valgus Deformity of More Than 10 to 15 Degrees

Correction of valgus deformity of more than 10 to 15 degrees should be done at the distal femur to avoid excessive obliquity of the articular surface of the tibia. Calculation of the desired correction is the same as for correction in the proximal tibia in the preceding section. Tracings should be made with the osteotomy in the distal femur just proximal to the adductor tubercle.

Distal Femoral Osteotomy

AO Group Technique

According to the AO group, the medial femoral condyle and medial distal femoral shaft are exposed through a longitudinal incision. The varus osteotomy guide is applied to the medial cortex (Fig. 119-13), the angle of correction is measured and a K-wire is inserted into the femoral condyles to serve as a guide for the seating chisel and the blade of the right-angle plate. An image intensifier will help during the insertion. Perform the osteotomy with the seating chisel in place, and then apply the right angle plate with either the 15- or 20-mm offset. The amount of offset and length of the blade are determined preoperatively from the tracings. The osteotomy is reduced and the tension device inserted. The first cancellous screw is then inserted, the tension device is tightened, and the os-teotomy compressed. The plate is fixed to the shaft and the tension device removed. After surgery, the hip and knee are placed at 90 degrees. The knee should be mobilized the day after surgery, and the patient should be allowed out of bed in 4 to 5 days.

Andrews Technique

The Andrews technique permits a lateral release of the patella, which is frequently needed in a knee with valgus deformity. A lateral iliotibial band splitting incision is used to approach the femur. A K-wire is placed through the joint to demonstrate the relationship of the femoral condyles. The AO seating chisel is inserted into the femoral condyles at the desired angle as determined from tracings to result in correction to the desired angle, using a 95-degree blade plate. The femur is marked for rotational orientation, and the osteotomy is per-

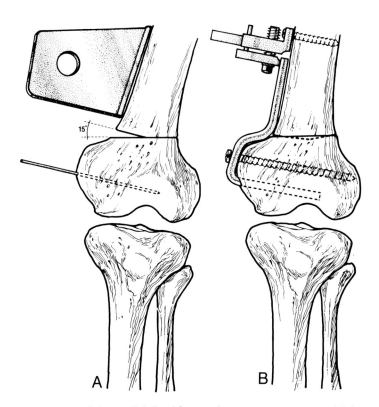

Fig. 119-13. (A) After exposure of the medial distal femur, the varus osteotomy guide is applied to the medial cortex. The angle of correction is measured, and a Kirschner wire is inserted into the femoral condyle to serve as a guide for the seating chisel. **(B)** After placement of the seating chisel, the osteotomy is completed and the offset blade plate inserted and fixed. (From Müller,[35] with permission.)

formed 3 cm above the seating chisel. If the osteotomy slants slightly from distal lateral to proximal medial, removal of a medial wedge is usually not necessary. The medial side is impacted, the blade plate inserted. The AO system of compression is used. Intraoperative radiographs confirm the alignment. A knee immobilizer is applied postoperatively. Quadriceps exercises are started the day of surgery. Range of motion and partial weight bearing are not permitted until there is radiographic evidence of healing. Usually this occurs about 6 to 8 weeks after surgery, and crutches are continued for an additional month or longer depending on the patient's progress.

Maquet Technique

In the Maquet technique, tracings of the correction are made from the radiograph (as for proximal tibial osteotomy) with the site of correction in the distal femur. Correction equals the mechanical angle minus 1 to 3 degrees. This correction usually leaves the knee in a few degrees of anatomic angle valgus.

The medial metaphyseal portion of the distal femur is exposed through a longitudinal incision between the vastus medialis and the medial hamstrings. Two parallel Steinmann pins are drilled through the femur distal to the site of osteotomy. Care should be taken to avoid entering the knee joint. The distance between the pins will vary depending on the type of compression clamps used. Avoiding the joint is easier if the pins are close together; the Synthes clamps permit closer placement than do double Charnley clamps. The protractor guide used for the barrel-vault osteotomy has two pin guides for the distal limb of the protractor which facilitates parallel placement. Two proximal pins are then placed in the diaphysis with the protractor guide at the desired angle to correspond to the drawings. A transverse osteotomy is performed in the metaphyseal area just proximal to the distal pins (Fig. 119-14). The lateral cortex is completely cut and impacted with osteotomy closure. The proximal bone is bevelled so that it can compress into the distal fragment. The clamps are applied and then tightened until the pins are parallel. The position is checked by radiography, a He-

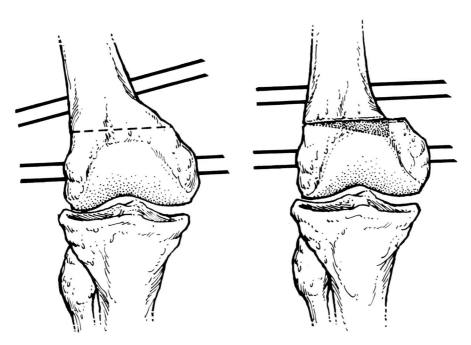

Fig. 119-14. Pin placement and osteotomy configuration for distal femoral osteotomy using the Maquet technique. The proximal medial fragment is compressed into the distal fragment on the medial side. (From Maquet,[33] with permission.)

movac drain is inserted, and the wound is closed and dressed. We use a knee immobilizer or posterior splint until the leg is comfortable enough for knee motion, ambulation, and partial weight bearing with crutches. The pins are removed when there is radiographic evidence of sufficient union, usually after 8 weeks. The extremity should be protected until union is complete. Because the osteotomy is in cancellous bone the proximal fragment may impact into the distal after clamp and pin removal if unprotected weight bearing occurs prematurely.

Technical Points

With all the techniques of distal femoral osteotomy, the surgeon must be cognizant of the femoral artery and vein and should avoid traumatizing them. Depending on approach, either the superior medial or superior lateral geniculate vessels will need to be ligated. The dissection about the distal femur should be on bone and extrasynovial to avoid the risk of intraarticular scarring and loss of joint motion.

COMPLICATIONS

Bone union at the distal femur takes longer than at the proximal tibia, and therefore, the limb must be protected for a longer time.

RESULTS

Proximal tibial osteotomy for degenerative genu valgus deformity produces approximately 70 percent good results. Distal femoral osteotomy produced somewhat better results as reported by Maquet[33] and Andrews. Distal femoral osteotomy offers the advantage of avoiding obliquity of the tibial plateau.

REFERENCES

1. Aglietti P, Rinonapoli E, Stringa G, Taviani A: Tibial osteotomy for the varus osteoarthritic knee. Clin Orthop 176:239, 1983
2. Bauer GCH, Insall J, Koshino T: Tibial osteotomy in gonarthrosis (osteoarthritis of the knee). J Bone Joint Surg 51A:1545, 1969
3. Broughton NS, Newman JH, Bailey RA: Unicompartmental replacement and high tibial osteotomy for osteoarthritis of the knee. A comparative study after 5-10 years follow-up. J Bone Joint Surg 68B:447, 1986
4. Brueckmann FR, Kettelkamp DB: Proximal tibial osteotomy. Orthop Clin North Am 13:3 1982
5. Chao EYS: Biomechanics of high tibial osteotomy. p. 143. In American Academy of Orthopaedic Surgeons Symposium on. Reconstructive Surgery of the Knee. CV Mosby, St. Louis, 1978
6. Coventry MB: Osteotomy of the upper portion of the tibia for degenerative arthritis of the knee. A preliminary report. J Bone Joint Surg 47A:984, 1965
7. Coventry MB: Osteotomy about the knee for degenerative and rheumatoid arthritis. J Bone Joint Surg 55A:23, 1973
8. Coventry MB: Upper tibial osteotomy for gonarthrosis. The evolution of the operation in the last 18 years and long term results. Orthop Clin North Am 10:191, 1979
9. Coventry MB: Current concepts review. Upper tibial osteotomy for osteoarthritis. J Bone Joint Surg 67A:1136, 1985
10. Devas MB: High tibial osteotomy for arthritis of the knee. J Bone Joint Surg 54B:95, 1969
11. Evarts CM, DeHaven K, Nelson CL: Proximal tibial osteotomy for degenerative arthritis of the knee. Orthop Clin North Am 2:231, 1971
12. Fujisawa Y, Nasuhara K, Shiomi S: The effect of high tibial osteotomy on osteoarthritis of the knee. An arthroscopic study of 54 knee joints. Orthop Clin North Am 10:585, 1979
13. Gibson MJ, Barnes MR, Allen NJ, Chan RNW: Weakness of foot dorsiflexion and changes in compartment pressures after tibial osteotomy. J Bone Joint Surg 68B:784, 1986
14. Ha'eri GB, Wiley AM: High tibial osteotomy combined with joint debridement: a long term study of results. Clin Orthop 151:153, 1980
15. Harding ML: A fresh appraisal of the tibial osteot-

omy for osteoarthritis of the knee. Clin Orthop 114:223, 1976

16. Harris WR, Kostuik JP: High tibial osteotomy for osteoarthritis of the knee. J Bone Joint Surg 52A:330, 1970

17. Hofmann AA, Wyatt RWB, Jones RE: Combined Coventry-Maquet procedure for two compartment degenerative arthritis. Clin Orthop 190:186, 1984

18. Insall JN, Joseph DM, Msika C: High tibial osteotomy for varus gonarthrosis. A long term followup study. J Bone Joint Surg 66A:1040, 1984

19. Insall J, Shoiji H, Mayer V: High tibial osteotomy. A five year evaluation. J Bone Joint Surg 56A:1397, 1974

20. Jackson JP, Waugh W: Tibial osteotomy for osteoarthritis of the knee. J Bone Joint Surg 43B:746, 1961.

21. Jackson JP, Waugh W, Green JP: High tibial osteotomy for osteoarthritis of the knee. J Bone Joint Surg 54B:89, 1969

22. Jokio PJ, Ragni P, Lindholm TS: Management of the fibula in high tibial osteotomy for arthritis of the knee. Union times and complications. Ital J Orthop Trauma 12:41, 1986.

23. Keene JS, Dyreby JR Jr: High tibial osteotomy in the treatment of osteoarthritis of the knee. The role of preoperative arthroscopy. J Bone Joint Surg 65A:36, 1983

24. Kettelkamp DB: Proximal tibial osteotomy. Clin Orthop 103:46, 1974

25. Kettelkamp DB: A review of proximal tibial osteotomy for degenerative arthritis. J Cont Ed Orthop 7:11, 1979

26. Kettelkamp DB, Leach RE, Nasca R: Pitfalls of proximal tibial osteotomy. Clin Orthop 106:232, 1975

27. Kettelkamp DB, Wegner DR, Chao EYS, et al: Results of proximal tibial osteotomy. The effects of tibiofemoral angle, stance-phase flexion-extension, and the medial plateau force. J Bone Joint Surg 58A:952, 1976

28. Koshino T: The treatment of spontaneous osteonecrosis of the knee by high tibial osteotomy with and without bone-grafting or drilling of the lesion. J Bone Joint Surg 64A:47, 1982

29. Koshino T, Tsuchiya K: The effect of high tibial osteotomy on osteoarthritis of the knee. Clinical and histological observations. Int Orthop 3:37, 1979

30. MacIntosh DL, Welsh P: Joint debridement-A completion to high tibial osteotomy in the treatment of degenerative arthritis. J Bone Joint Surg 59A:1094, 1977

31. Maquet P: Valgus osteotomy for osteoarthritis of the knee. Clin Orthop 120:143, 1976

32. Maquet P: The treatment of choice in osteoarthritis of the knee. Clin Orthop 192:108, 1985

33. Maquet PGJ: Biomechanics of the Knee. Springer-Verlag, New York, 1976

34. Miller R, Kettelkamp DB, Laubenthal KN, et al: Quantitive correlations in degenerative arthritis of the knee. J Bone Joint Surg 55A:956, 1973

35. Müller ME, Allgöwer M, Schneider R, et al: Manual of Internal Fixation. 2nd Ed. Springer-Verlag, Berlin, 1979, p. 376

36. Myrnerts R: Optimal correction in high tibial osteotomy for varus deformities. Acta Orthop Scand 51:689, 1980

37. Prodromos CC, Andriacchi TP, Galante JO: A relationship between gait and clinical changes following high tibial osteotomy. J Bone Joint Surg 67A:1188, 1985

38. Putnam MD, Mears DC, Fu FH: Combined Maquet and proximal tibial valgus osteotomy. Clin Orthop 197:217, 1985

39. Shargorodsky FS: Traumatic neuritis of the peroneal nerve complicating the surgical correction of tibia vara. Orthop Traumatol Protez 5:32, 1969

40. Shoji H, Insall J: High tibial osteotomy for osteoarthritis of the knee with valgus deformity. J Bone Joint Surg 55A:963, 1973

41. Slocum DB, Larson RL, James SL, et al: High tibial osteotomy, Clin Orthop 104:239, 1974

42. Stinchfield FE, Sankaran B, Samilson R: The effect of anticoagulant therapy on bone repair. J Bone Joint Surg 38A:270, 1956

43. Sundaram NA, Hallett JP, Sullivan MF: Dome osteotomy of the tibia for osteoarthritis of the knee. J Bone Joint Surg 68B:782, 1986

44. Tjornstrand BAE, Egund N, Hagstedt BD: High tibial osteotomy. A 7 year clinical and radiographic follow-up. Clin Orthop 160:124, 1981

45. Torgerson WR Jr, Kettelkamp DB, Igorz RA Jr, et al: Tibial osteotomy for the treatment of degenerative arthritis of the knee. Clin Orthop 101:46, 1974

46. Vainionpa AS, Laike E, Kirves P, Tiusanen P: Tibial osteotomy for osteoarthritis of the knee. J Bone Joint Surg 63A:938, 1981

47. Wardle EN: Osteotomy of the tibia and fibula. Surg Gynecol Obstet 115:61, 1962

48. Waugh W: Tibial osteotomy in the management of osteoarthritis of the knee. Clin Orthop 210:55, 1986

Cementing Techniques in Total Knee Arthroplasty

120

Jo Miller
Kwan-Ho Chan

Acrylic cement was first used in total knee arthroplasty almost 20 years ago and continues to be the most popular method for the fixation of implants. Throughout this history, loosening has been recognized as the problem that dominates knee reconstruction. During the early 70s, the first resurfacing devices appeared, all designed to be used with cement. The earliest of these devices was Gunston's Polycentric knee,[43,44] followed by the Geometric[23] and the Freeman-Swanson.[35,36] Some were moderately constrained by the congruous femoral and tibial articular surfaces and were subject to loosening. The initial results of the Gunston-type polycentric knee arthroplasty were impressive, with greater than 80 percent good results at 2 years; with longer follow-up, however, there was a significant increase in failure, secondary to loosening of the tibial track and subluxation of the knee.[12,24,44,73] Similar results were recorded with the Geometric and the Freeman-Swanson, with a relatively high incidence of loosening of the tibial component but infrequent loosening of the femoral component.[24,35,36]

Typically, radiolucent lines between cement and bone appeared within months of implantation, becoming more prominent with the passage of time. Eventually, gradual or sudden sinkage of the implant into the upper tibia occurred with bone destruction, loss of leg alignment, and progressive deformity. In the same era, other problems caused concern. Infection, malalignment, polyethylene failure, knee instability, and limited range of motion, when considered together with loosening, were of a magnitude such that knee arthroplasty seemed unreasonably risky.

With the advent of progressively less constrained designs and improved surgical techniques and instrumentation, some of these problems diminished significantly. The second-generation unhinged knee prostheses, as exemplified by the Total Condylar and Townley, represented a clear advance in design, as reflected in the reduced tendency to loosen. Insall and Ranawat[58,59,87,101] and others[3] reported excellent long-term survival with the total condylar design, which continues to be used today, essentially unmodified from its original form.[87] These and other more modern designs and the recognition of the importance of limb alignment and ligament balancing have resulted in long-term performance of total knee arthroplasty at least on a par with that of total hip replacement.

In spite of these encouraging results, loosening, with its implication of bone damage and technically difficult revisions, continues to be the problem of greatest concern to the knee implant surgeon. The appearance, during the early 1980s, of cementless fixation[52,53] reflected the dissatisfaction felt by the orthopaedic community with traditional cementing techniques. Cementless fixation has not been problem free, however. This, together with improving techniques and results with cement, has sustained interest in acrylic cement for the fixation of knee implants.

To summarize, the modern-day orthopaedic surgeon has access to a variety of unconstrained condylar-type prostheses and also to excellent instrumentation, facilitating leg alignment, soft tissue balancing, and accurate bone resection. The quality of fixation thus becomes the single most important factor in the long-term survival of the reconstructed knee. It is the purpose of this chapter to discuss the problems related to fixation of knee implants with acrylic cement and to describe modern cement techniques that enhance the quality of fixation.

on the concept that once ingrowth has taken place it will remain indefinitely, a point that still requires confirmation. Cementless techniques impose greater technical demands on the surgeon and require a relatively long period of protected weight bearing. Failure of ingrowth,[22,46,47] which is not rare, results in micromovement, possible gross loosening, and, under some circumstances, damage to the porous surfaces with loose beads.[92] The implications of increased ion release from porous surfaces into adjacent tissues and the general body environment are not yet fully understood.[9,109] Leg pain, possibly originating from failed fixation, is commonplace and well documented in the hip[31] and is also recognized in the knee but is still a poorly defined entity.

Cemented fixation is indicated in the elderly or in patients for whom prolonged crutchwalking might represent a problem. Cementless implants should be used preferentially in patients who are young or in those patients in their 60s or 70s who have a higher-than-average activity level.

Mixed or so-called hybrid fixation has been used by many surgeons. The femoral and perhaps the patellar components are implanted without cement and are rarely a problem, but the tibial component, which is most likely to loosen, is fixed with cement.

INDICATIONS FOR USE OF ACRYLIC CEMENT

Currently the orthopaedic community uses both cement and biologic fixation in knee arthroplasty. There are obvious advantages and disadvantages to both cement and cementless methods, which determine the indications for use. Cement gives immediate and secure fixation, compensates for small surgical errors and bone irregularities, uses a less complex prosthesis, and permits early full weight bearing. It has the disadvantages of uncertain endurance and damage to bone, which is inevitable when a cemented interface loosens.

Cementless devices with porous surfaces achieve biologic fixation by ingrowth. This type of system has implications of long endurance, based

FACTORS THAT INFLUENCE FIXATION ENDURANCE

Much of the blame for failure of cemented implants can be attributed to the perception that cement acts as a glue that will function successfully even in the face of indifferent surgical technique. To the contrary, acrylic cement neither adheres to the osseous tissue nor forms a chemical bond with the skeleton to which it is applied. Fixation depends entirely on physical interlock between irregularities in bone surfaces and corresponding conformities formed by the cement in its prepolymerized state. The quality of this interface, created by the surgeon, is a major factor in the endurance of the implanted prosthesis.

Implant loosening can be attributed to a disparity between the strength of the fixation system and the mechanical demands imposed upon it. These demands include overall load, load distribution, impact load, and load repetition. Loads that exceed the capacity of the fixation system will lead to a gradual or acute failure that may be initiated in the prosthesis, cement, or bone or at either of the interfaces; it may involve several sites as disruption progresses. A number of different factors that contribute to implant loosening can be identified.

Prosthesis Design

Several aspects of prosthesis design influence the endurance of fixation. Some are related to the magnitude of load imposed on the fixation system and others to the quality of fixation.

Constraint

Constraint refers to the extent to which forces other than axial load are transferred from one component of the knee implant to the other. For exam-

ple, in a very unconstrained design, the femoral component articulates with a flat or almost flat tibial component. Rotary and shear loads are resisted to a very limited degree by the contours of the implant itself and are not transmitted to the fixation system but are absorbed by ligaments and capsule, as occurs in the normal knee (Fig. 120-1A). By contrast, more congruent implant designs transmit a greater portion of shear, rotary, and angular load from one component to the other,[40,41] placing high loads on the fixation (Fig. 120-1B). These constrained implants, and even more so, the hinged or linked designs, are notorious for their high rate of radiolucency and loosening.[66]

The need for constrained or stabilized implants has decreased with improved understanding of leg alignment and ligament balancing. Their use is now rare in primary total knee arthroplasty, based on a survey of prominent knee surgeons.

Metal-Backed Tibial Components

Metal-backed tibial components have come into general use during the past 10 years. The change was based on the perception that polyethylene de-

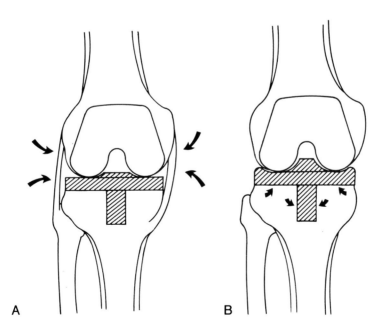

A   B

Fig. 120-1. (A) In minimal constrained design, the rotary and shear loads are resisted to a very limited degree by the contours of the implant itself and are not transmitted to the fixation system but are absorbed by ligaments and capsule as occurs in the normal knee. **(B)** More congruent implant designs transmit a greater portion of shear, rotary, and angular load from one component to the other, placing high loads on the fixation.

vices are subject to gross deformation under some loading conditions.[30,104] The flexible plastic, when cyclically loaded, imposes bending deformation (Fig. 120-2) of the underlying cement, bone, and interface shear, resulting in cement fracture, the development of a radiolucent line, and perhaps cancellous failure with subsidence of the implant.[30] Metal backing, either in the form of a tray or integrated with the plastic itself, stiffens the tibial component, resulting in a more even distribution of load and lower stresses in the underlying cement and bone.[8,74,82,104]

The metal backing provides an additional advantage for enhanced fixation. A textured or porous surface can be applied and improves the cement-prosthesis interface.

Stem Versus No Stem

The use of a stem versus no stem on the tibial component is an issue that has been debated for many years. The original resurfacing devices such as the Geometric and Polycentric designs were essentially stemless and had high failure rates.[12,24,23,44] The Total Condylar and the Townley designs introduced a substantial stem to resist angular and shear displacements of the prosthesis relative to the tibia and to increase the area of cement-bone interface and had a lower incidence of gross failure.[58,59,100] They often showed a typical radiologic pattern of a well-fixed stem but large radiolucencies under the plateaus[58] of the implant

(Fig. 120-3), probably as a result of micromovement of the flexible polyethylene wings or stress shielding. Finite element analysis studies seem to show that the stems reduce the level of load on the upper surface of the tibia[8] and, by implication, are advantageous.

In more recent years, tibial components in which the stems have been replaced by two to four short positioning pegs have become popular and perform well. In contrast to earlier stemless devices, the more modern designs are provided with porous metal backing and are designed to be used with advanced cement techniques. The large majority have shown good early evidence that they will not loosen,[21,79] as did their predecessors.

Sinkage has occurred in a small number of stemless tibial components for a number of reasons, related to prosthetic design, surgical technique, and

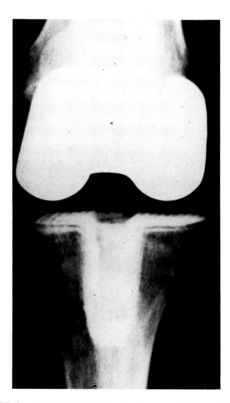

Fig. 120-3. A well-fixed stem can be associated with radiolucencies under the plateaus of the implant as a result of micromovement of the flexible polyethylene wings or from stress shielding when the stem takes a large proportion of the load.

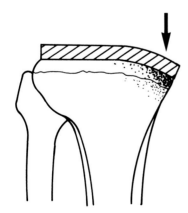

Fig. 120-2. Deformation of the flexible plastic tibial component can cause fracture of the underlying cement and cancellous bone.

patient selection. Osteoporosis or osteopenia as seen in rheumatoid arthritis is probably the single most important contributing factor.

Should stemmed devices be used routinely? The excellent survival of the total condylar device[58,59,87,101] tends to support the concept. However, nonstemmed devices are more conservative and less intrusive and, in the non osteoporotic patient, appear to have equally good prospects.

Prosthesis Alignment

Malalignment of the implant, as an independent error, appears to be a less serious concern than malalignment of the leg. In the well-aligned limb, minor valgus or varus orientation of the prosthesis is well tolerated. Indeed, Hungerford and Kenna[52] advocate placing the tibial component in 3 degrees of varus and the femoral component in a corresponding valgus position. Rand and Bryan[86] pointed out that in an attempt to align the tibial component in slight varus, many of their cases resulted in varus malalignment of the entire limb. Excessive malalignment produces a shear effect with a corresponding increase in load on the fixation system; it may contribute to loosening, especially of the tibial component. In a review of total knee replacement in varus knees, Laskin[71] found that there is a modest increase in tibial component bone-cement radiolucent lines when the reconstructed knee is in varus with well-aligned components or when the tibial component is in varus in a well-aligned limb. However, there is a significant

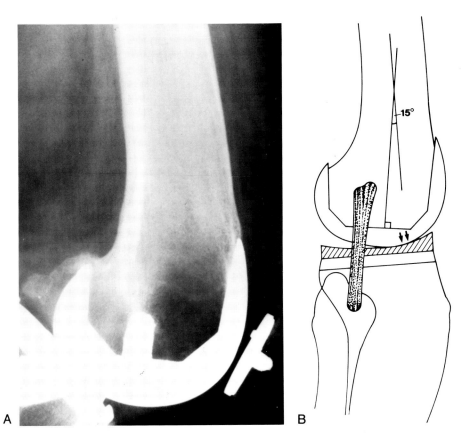

Fig. 120-4. (A, B) An excessively flexed femoral component is the commonest malalignment error in the flexion-extension plane, resulting in relative hyperextension of the components when the limb is fully extended. This can result in anterior impingement and excessive load transmitted anteriorly to the tibial component.

increase in radiolucent lines when both the limbs and the tibial components are in varus.

Rotary malalignment of one or both components may result in abnormal loading of components or impingement at some point in the range of movement. The most common malalignment error in the flexion-extension plane is a flexed position of the femoral component (Fig. 120-4). This, in effect, places the two components into a hyperextension relationship and, in certain designs, results in anterior impingement that may contribute to anterior sinkage of the tibial implant (Fig. 120-5). Posterior tilt of the tibial component is recommended in many knee systems and is well tolerated, but excessive tilt sacrifices strong bone and may overload the prosthesis posteriorly with sinkage (Fig. 120-6).

Leg Alignment

Malalignment of the leg into varus or less frequently into valgus is the most common error in knee implant surgery and has a high correlation with implant failure.[7,10,56,77,73] Ideally, the mechanical axis of the leg, running from hip to ankle, should pass through the center of the knee (Fig. 120-7A). Malalignment moves the mechanical axis away from the center of the knee (Fig. 120-7B), with consequent overloading of one compartment, leading to collapse of bone or failure of cement.

Recent gait studies[84] have demonstrated that even in the well-aligned limb, there is a varus thrust with every step. This is in keeping with previous studies[48,62,81] showing the total compressive load to

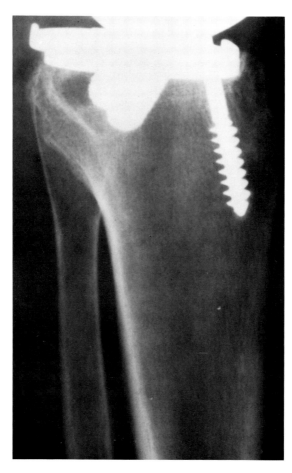

Fig. 120-5. Anterior sinkage of tibial component, which may be secondary to an excessively flexed femoral component. (Courtesy of Anthony K. Hedley, MD.)

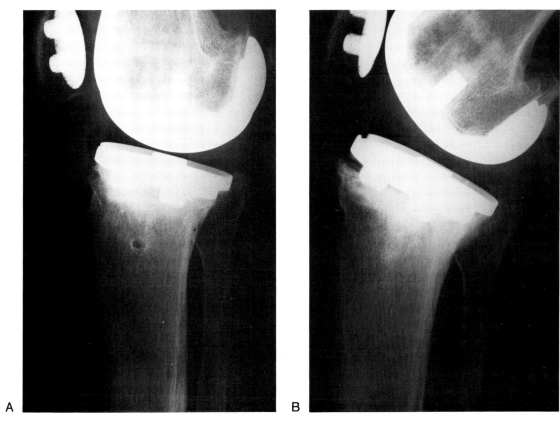

Fig. 120-6. Posterior sinkage of tibial component secondary to excessive posterior tilting of the tibial component. **(A)** Immediately postoperatively. **(B)** Two years postoperatively.

be greater in the medial than in the lateral compartment. These findings suggest that the reconstructed knee can perhaps tolerate a small error in valgus, as measured from the mechanical axis but at all costs should not incorporate an error into varus.

Recurvatum of the knee is uncommon and can be attributed to excess resection of bone or to the use of components, usually the tibial, which are thinner than required. The resulting laxity of collateral and of posterior soft tissues produces hyperextension of the knee. Theoretically, anterior impingement might occur, leading to fixation failure, but loosening due to hyperextension has not been reported in the literature.

Persistent flexion contracture following knee replacement is exceedingly common. Contractures, even in excess of 10 degrees, are compatible with excellent function. Patient complaints about an inability to extend the knee fully are rare. The loads imposed on the articular surface of the knee during weight bearing have been calculated and increase proportionately as the knee moves from extension into increasing degrees of flexion.[81] In spite of these data, there is no evidence to suggest that postoperative flexion contracture can be incriminated in implant loosening.

Patient Selection

Three elements in the area of patient selection, popularly quoted in regard to implant loosening, are obesity, age, and activity level. Obesity is frequently cited as a contributing factor in the loosening of hip replacements.[16,97] In knee arthroplasty, heavier weight of the patient has been implicated as a factor in loosening.[29,99] However, according to a survey of prominent knee surgeons, obesity, as an

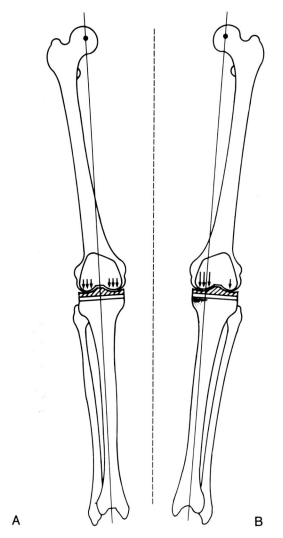

Fig. 120-7. (A) The mechanical axis of the leg is a line in the frontal plane running from the center of the hip to the center of ankle and normally passes through the center of the knee. **(B)** Malalignment moves the mechanical axis away from the center of the knee with consequent overloading of the compartment that the mechanical axis is closer to.

isolated factor, does not appear to raise the incidence of loosening in reconstructions that are otherwise well done.

Youth and activity levels are related variables. The higher failure rate of hip arthroplasty in the younger and more active patient is well documented.[16] Common sense dictates that the same phenomenon will occur in the reconstructed knee, but this has not been recorded in a published series,

perhaps because knee arthroplasty is not commonly performed in the young active patient with monarticular arthritis. A recent review by Ewald and Christle[32] suggested that in the case of a group of patients under the age of 45, most of whom had inflammatory arthritis, cemented total knee arthroplasty in these patients is comparable to that of the older patients.

Bone Stock Influence

An understanding of tibial fixation requires a knowledge of the distribution of cancellous bone in the proximal tibial metaphysis. Figure 120-8 shows contact radiographs of mid-coronal and transverse slabs of bone, each 5 mm thick, taken from a pair of tibias from a 56-year-old female donor. The cortex thins out rapidly in the metaphyseal area and consists of a condensation of cancellous bone rather than true compact bone. The trabeculae are generally oriented vertically and have the greatest density under the weight-bearing areas of the tibial plateaus, with sparsity of trabeculae in the center. The best quality of cancellous bone with higher density and strength is in the anterior part of the medial plateau and the posterior part of the lateral plateau.[54,63] At the level at which the tibia is customarily resected for total knee arthroplasty, the medial surface is almost always larger than at the lateral surface (Fig. 120-8).

The strength of the bone to which a prosthetic component is applied is critical to the survival of the reconstructed knee. Resection of subchondral bone removes the structure that ties together the upper ends of the trabecular array. The structural integrity is restored by the application of cement; if it interlocks with the trabeculae, it reestablishes an equivalent to the subchondral plate. The appearance of a new plane of corticated bone immediately adjacent to cement (Fig. 120-9) is a reparative process provoked by micromovement that indicates that the cement-bone interlock has not been established.

Osteopenia

Early in the history of knee resurfacing, it was determined that progressive radiolucencies and loosening were more common in the osteoarthritic knee than in the rheumatoid knee.[60] It was gener-

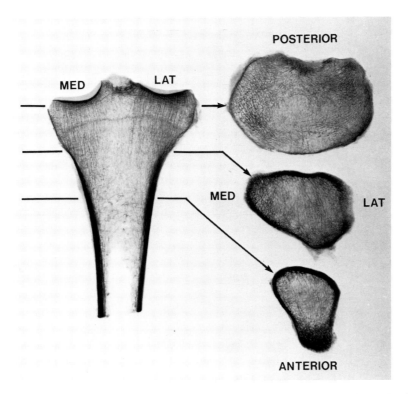

Fig. 120-8. Contact radiographs of 5-mm-thick midcoronal and transverse slabs of proximal tibias from a 56-year-old female donor. Note the sparsity of cancellous bone at the center, the thin "metaphyseal shell" in the most proximal 2 cm and, in the most proximal transverse cut, the medial plateau is larger than the lateral and the cancellous bone is most dense in the anterior medial and posterior lateral regions.

ally agreed that the rheumatoid knee presented less dense bone, providing an opportunity for cement interlock, and that the lower activity level of the patient with multiple joint involvement would place fewer demands on the reconstructed joint. In the current era, improved cementing techniques have reduced the incidence of radiolucencies in both rheumatoid and osteoarthritic knees. However, a small incidence of tibial component sinkage occurs in the well-fixed implant, probably as a result of failure of weak cancellous trabeculae associated with osteopenia. Clearly, the surgeon should be aware of the vulnerability of osteoporotic bone and should use whatever special measures are available to improve fixation and coverage.

Full Coverage of the Tibia

An important element in the reduction of loosening is a prosthesis that maintains full coverage of the tibia.[6] In the early era of resurfacing, all that was available was a single size of implant (or, at best, few sizes). It was commonplace to see, on postoperative radiographs, a tibial component that was much smaller in its mediolateral and anteroposterior (AP) dimensions than the tibia to which it was applied—a situation that necessarily imposes a less than optimum distribution of load with associated failure in some cases. It is clearly advantageous to distribute a given load over an area of cancellous bone that is as large as possible[7,33,69] by achieving full coverage of the upper tibia by the prosthesis. An understanding of the problem has now resulted in a much larger selection of implant sizes, and it is the general impression that this has contributed to a reduced incidence of loosening.

It is not essential to have an exact fit of prosthesis to the upper tibia. Perfect peripheral rim contact is not expected to increase the load-bearing capacity

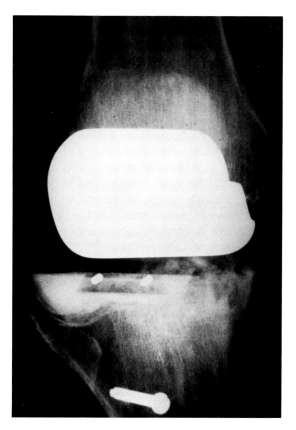

Fig. 120-9. Formation of corticated bone adjacent to cement is indicative of a reparative process provoked by movement.

of the proximal tibia significantly, as there is no true cortical shell.[20,55]

Level of Resection

The level of resection is clearly related to the strength of bone with which the implant will interface. A number of studies focusing on the strength of the cancellous bone of the proximal tibia[7,63,94] suggest that bone strength diminishes from the proximal to distal levels. However, this is disputed by other investigators.[54] What is clear is that in going from proximal to distal, good-quality cancellous bone remains peripheral, and full coverage should be used. Major defects should not be a basis for more radical resection. Rather, the surgeon is wise to resect conservatively and to deal with the defect in one of several acceptable ways, including bone grafting, special prostheses, or special cement techniques.

Cement Techniques

The lack of understanding of proper cement techniques has undoubtedly contributed to a higher incidence of radiolucent lines, cement fracture, and a combination of the two. Inevitably, the blame for poor results has been placed on the cement itself, which has been labeled the weak link or grout. More probably, inattention by the surgeon to the many details that constitute good cement technique and the attitude that fast surgery is crucial are the important factors in loosening.

There has been a steady increase in interest in the proper use of acrylic cement. The emphasis on improved technique has resulted in an improved record for knee implants fixed with cement. Increased awareness of the importance of bone preparation by lavage, the use of cement in a less doughy stage, and the application of pressure to improve intrusion[67,78] have dramatically reduced the incidence of radiolucent lines[79,105] and loosening.

Sepsis

The characteristic of an infected total knee is pain at rest as well as on weight bearing. In the presence of a complete and widening radiolucent line or patchy radiolucency around the prosthesis at the bone-cement interface, an ongoing infection must be considered.[57] Even in a well-fixed prosthesis, sepsis leads to implant loosening in almost every case. There are rare occasions when a septic knee has been successfully opened, debrided, and closed without implant removal and treated with high doses of antibiotics. However, in most cases, removal of the implant together with cement is essential to the control of the infection. Interestingly, the incidence of infection is less with the less constrained prosthesis.[42]

THE PATHOPHYSIOLOGY OF LOOSENING

The cemented knee implant is subject to failure in a variety of modes, related to the implant itself, the cement, and the underlying bone, and perhaps more importantly, to the interfaces between cement and bone and cement and implant. It is probable that all cases of loosening are initiated on a mechanical basis; other elements, such as thermal damage,[1,61,98] chemical necrosis of bone,[76] and immunologic effects,[17] are unproved. Once loosening has been initiated, a variety of nonmechanical mechanisms come into play. If the initiation of loosening can be understood on a mechanical basis, the same basis can be used to evolve measures for prevention. Four separate but somewhat interdependent mechanisms for loosening can be identified.

Gross Movement

There is a tendency for the implant, as a whole, to move with respect to the adjacent bone. The degree and direction of movement depend on the shape, design, and fit of the implant; the nature and magnitude of the applied load; and the quality of fixation. Gross movement has implications of lifting the prosthesis from the bone surface, of uneven transmission of load between the prosthesis and bone, and, most important, of micromovement at the interface. Gross movement of the tibial component may be on the basis of an uneven resection of the articular surface, such that the prosthesis, in effect, wobbles on the irregularity, and on the basis of eccentric loading of the prosthesis, with elastic deformation of the underlying cancellous bone.[102] If there is a poor interlock, micromotion can also occur at the interfaces as a result of differential deformation of the prosthesis, cement, and bone because of difference in elastic moduli.

Loosening of the tibial component is a relatively common problem in knee replacements. By contrast, the femoral component, because of its shape, is more stable and is far less likely to loosen.[65] The implant is applied to the distal femur, covering anterior, distal, and posterior surfaces, in effect achieving fixation on the basis of its gross configuration. This fixation resists compression, shear, and rotational displacement in several axes. By increasing the area of fixation and the mechanical moment of fixation, pegs and stems reduce gross movement.

Gross movement leads to implant failure through two other mechanisms. The first is micromovement at the interface between cement and bone, inducing progressive bone resorption,[78,80] and the second is the failure or collapse of cancellous surfaces

that support the prosthesis, resulting in subsidence, often with loss of limb alignment.

Micromovement

Small movements occurring at either the cement-prosthesis or the cement-bone interface are termed micromovement. This movement can be a local phenomenon involving segments of the interface as short as a few millimeters, or it may take place over the complete interface and be inseparable from gross movement. Its occurrence is highly dependent on the presence or absence of microfixation which, in the case of the cemented prosthesis, results from cement intrusion into bony interstices, and, in the cementless prosthesis, by ingrowth of bone into a porous surface. Both can be termed microinterlock. In the presence of poor interlock, micromovement can also occur as a result of differential deformation of prosthesis, cement, and bone because of differences in elastic moduli.

Load applied to the reconstructed joint must necessarily cross the cement-bone interface and appear as compressive, shear, and tensile stresses. Where cement is poorly intruded (Fig. 120-10A–C), micromovement between cement and bone is induced and bone is resorbed and replaced with a fibrous membrane. This phenomenon can be appreciated radiographically as a radiolucent line. Mechanically, it represents a loss of contact between cement and bone, a site that will be ineffective in resisting shear or tensile load. Microinterlock sites should be as close together as possible, optimally at intervals of 1 mm or less, as is achieved when cement is pressurized into cancellous bone surfaces (Fig. 120-10D). With such ideal fixation, forces that would otherwise have produced micromovement are absorbed as strain or deformation in adjacent layers of cancellous bone or cement[18]; these forces are well tolerated.

Macrointerlock, or cement interfacing with large irregularities or contours on the bone surface, is ineffectual in preventing micromovement. Micromovement can be a local phenomenon, limited to a small part of the interface with associated resorption of bone. It is not uncommon to see a small radiolucency at one site in a radiograph of a well-fixed knee implant, with no other evidence of radiographic change (Fig. 120-11).

To recapitulate, micromovement is a phenome-

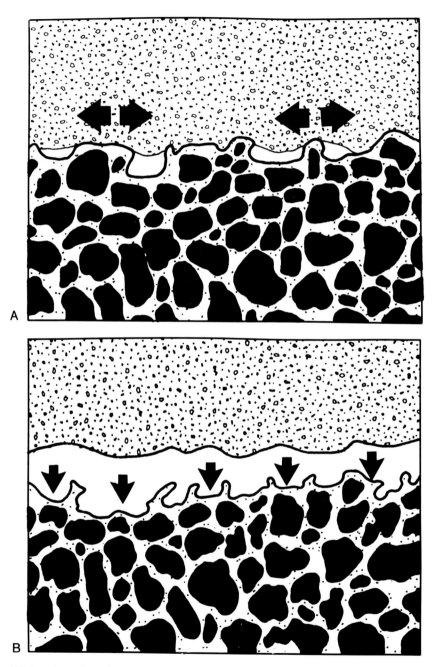

Fig. 120-10. (A) Poor intrusion of cement allows micromovement at the cement–bone interface. **(B)** Micromovement leads to bone resorption. *(Figure continues.)*

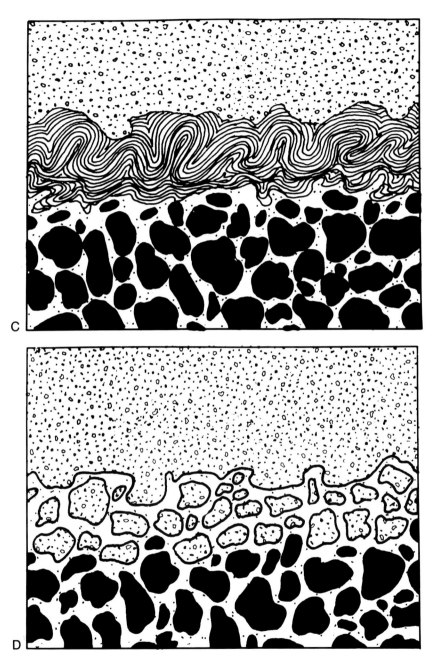

Fig. 120-10 *(Continued).* **(C)** The formation of a fibrous membrane. **(D)** Good cement intrusion produces microinterlock and prevents micromovement.

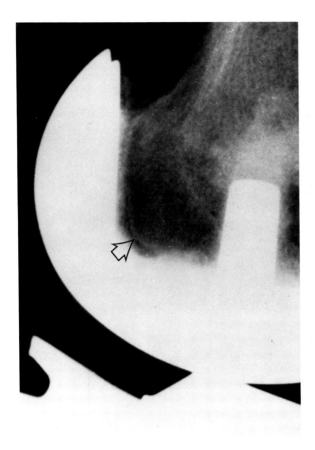

Fig. 120-11. Local area of radiolucency may be the result of local micromovement.

non that should be thought of in terms of very small increments of the cement-bone interface. Partial radiolucencies represent a local failure to achieve microinterlock, hence a defect in a small portion of the fixation system. The remainder of the interface, well fixed, carries the load transmitted between prosthesis and bone. When the functioning parts of the interface, those with microfixation, are small, or when excessive demands are placed on the joint, the areas with microfixation begin to fail and, as a result, the radiolucency will be seen to extend and even become complete.

Cancellous Failure

Loads applied to cancellous bone in excess of its mechanical capacity will lead to cancellous failure. Failure may take a variety of forms.

Subclinical subsidence: This subtle form of cancellous failure of knee implants detected by roentgen stereophotogrammetry[39,93] is gradual, perhaps associated with micromovement and bone resorption. Loss of alignment is not necessarily a feature and the reconstructed joint, in many cases, continues to function well.

Excessive loading: This form of cancellous failure appears to result from excessive loading. Two mechanisms may apply. The poorly aligned reconstruction, most often in varus (see Fig. 120-7B), concentrates load in one compartment of the knee to the point where the underlying trabecula fails, either gradually or suddenly, with subsidence of the prosthesis (Fig. 120-12). This mechanism is commonly superimposed on a failing interface where a radiolucent line of increasing width has been observed. Cancellous failure with subsidence may also occur in the well-aligned leg, often in the presence of a complete radiolucency. Momentary eccentric loading during normal gait[4] is accompanied by downward displacement of the loaded side of the prosthesis, as the underlying cancellous bone elastically deforms (see Fig. 120-14). The downward displacement is unopposed by the incompetent fixation on the unloaded side, and the prosthesis tends to lift off.[102] Deformation of cancellous trabeculae on the loaded side may lead to failure either acutely, as a result of a single overload, or because of fatigue failure as a result of repeated deformations.

Sudden failure in the well-fixed implant: This problem may occur as a result of osteopenia. Rheumatoid patients with knee implants well fixed by modern cement techniques and with no radiolucent lines may begin to experience pain, sometimes following a trivial traumatic event. Immediate radiographs show no change in the interface, but subsequent radiographs 2 months later demonstrate clear evidence of subsidence. The advent of subsidence, without preexisting evidence of loosening, suggests that fracture of osteoporotic cancellous bone adjacent to the cement is the probable mechanism.

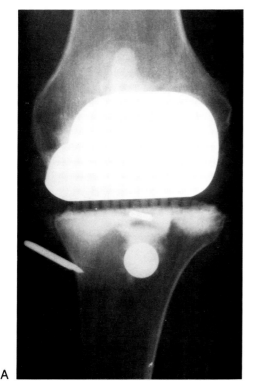
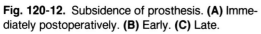
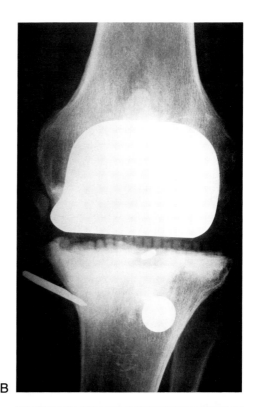

Fig. 120-12. Subsidence of prosthesis. **(A)** Immediately postoperatively. **(B)** Early. **(C)** Late.

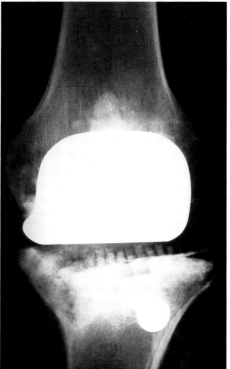

Biologic Mechanisms

Mechanical factors can be considered, in the absence of sepsis, to be the initiating factor in implant loosening but biologic mechanisms are responsible for the actual changes that constitute loosening, that is, bone resorption.

The fibrous membrane that develops as bone resorbs is highly variable in appearance and function.[49] Membranes found adjacent to implants that are not grossly loose and where no change has occurred, either clinically or radiologically for several years, consist of collagen fibers in organized patterns and relatively few cells. Giant cells are sparse or absent. Around an implant that is grossly loose or where the radiolucent line is progressively widening, the membrane is more active with a cellular appearance, including giant cells and histiocytes.

The destruction of bone appears to be enzymatic either on the basis of round cell activity[106,107] or by chemical compounds, prostaglandin E_2 (PGE_2), and collagenase, secreted by synovial-like cells in the fibrous membrane.[38]

Histiocytes are invariably present. Once thought to be characteristic of the fibrous membrane around acrylic cement,[34] they are now acknowledged to be around any type of implant material, even those that are most bioinert.[95] They are more frequent where there is a greater surface of foreign material, particularly loose cement, or in association with polyethylene wear debris.

Wear debris and particulate material is an almost constant finding in the examination of the fibrous membrane around implants. Acrylic fragments from broken or loose cement and polyethylene wear particles are most common and provoke a dramatic cellular response. Much of the literature on this subject is in reference to hip arthroplasty. Willert[107] postulated that large amounts of debris and the associated cellular mass overloads the lymphatic system, accumulates in the joint and in the interfaces, and provokes bone destruction on the basis of cellular enzymes. The catastrophic loosening experienced by Charnley[19] with Teflon acetabular implants is an example. Harris and associates[49] described massive osteolysis, undoubtedly a related phenomenon. The occurrence of an isolated area of osteolysis in an otherwise securely fixed total hip seems to implicate wear debris rather than cement particles as a precipitating factor. Massive osteolysis is rarely reported in total knee replacements.[45] Wear debris has on rare occasion been implicated in accelerating total knee prosthesis loosening.[26]

COMPOSITE STRUCTURE FIXATION

Fixation of a cemented implant, in which both the interfaces are secure, converts the three elements — bone, cement, and prosthesis — into a single unit (Fig. 120-13). This is composite structure fixation.[80] The achievement of this kind of fixation has two obvious benefits in the prevention of loosening.

The first relates to the cement bone interface. Microinterlock between cement and cancellous interstices produced by modern cement techniques significantly reduces the incidence of radiolucencies as compared with interfaces produced by traditional techniques.[79,80] The second benefit relates to the competence of both cement-bone and cement-prosthesis interfaces in resisting tensile loading. In contrast to the lift-off that occurs in the poorly fixed implant with eccentric loading, as illustrated in Fig. 120-14, secure fixation resists lift off on the unloaded side of the implant (Fig. 120-15). This produces a transfer to the tensile side of some of the deforming force, which otherwise is concentrated on the loaded side of the implant. The entire interface now functions in load transfer, resulting in a more even load distribution.

The achievement of microinterlock between cement and bone is accomplished by forcing cement into the carefully prepared and clean cancellous surface. A variety of techniques that produce cement penetration are outlined later in this chapter.

The interface between cement and prosthesis is optimized when cement either interlocks with a microporous surface such as sintered beads (Figs. 120-13, 120-15) or fiber metal, or, as an alternative, forms a strong adhesive bond to a prosthesis having an acrylic precoat. An interface formed by either method is characterized by successful transmission of load in compression, shear, and tension.

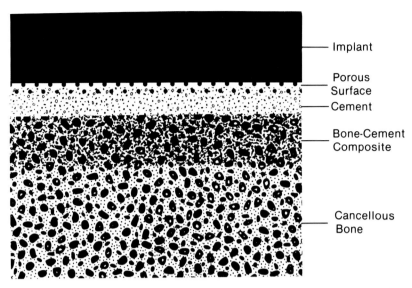

Fig. 120-13. Composite structure fixation. Mechanically secure interfaces between prosthesis and cement, and between cement and bone.

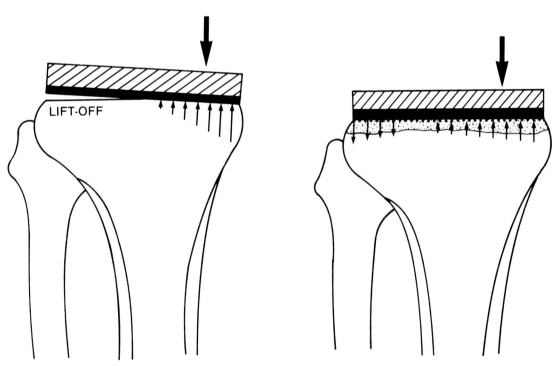

Fig. 120-14. Under eccentric loading, lift-off can occur on the opposite side if the interfaces are unable to resist tension.

Fig. 120-15. Secure composite structure fixation permits transmission of both compressive and tensile load, hence a more even load distribution.

The more even distribution of load thus achieved cannot be accomplished by traditional prostheses with macrocontours designed for cement anchoring.

ENHANCED USE OF BONE CEMENT

Since the introduction of acrylic cement in orthopaedic surgery, its major chemical constituents have remained almost unchanged. However, there have been some alterations in its composition and in the methods of handling the cement, enhancing its effectiveness in the fixation of orthopaedic implant.

Precoat

The surface of a prosthesis accumulates a layer of absorbed contaminants during the processing of the metal and the manufacturing and handling of the prosthesis. When methyl methacrylate is applied to this surface, a nonuniform and unreliable bonding is obtained. The shear strength of this interface is significantly degraded when exposed to saline for as short a period as 30 days.[2,85]

The bonding between cement and the prosthesis can be enhanced using a technique of industrial precoating of the implant surface with PMMA. The process requires meticulous cleaning of the surface of the implant, followed immediately by passivation to obtain a uniform oxide layer. A thin coating of acrylic is then applied to the surface; when cured, this coating bonds by adhesion to the oxide layer.[25] At surgery, the cement chemically unites with the precoat to produce an enhanced interface. The strength of this bond is two to three times greater than that achieved by the application of surgical cement directly to an unprecoated interface and does not degrade when tested in saline or in vivo for periods of up to 2 years.[15]

Porosity Reduction

It has been recognized that acrylic cement is relatively weak and is particularly prone to fail in tension. More recently, work by Harris and associates[14,27,37] showed (1) that testing cement by cyclic loading might be a more sensitive indicator of true cement performance than is static testing, and (2) that air bubbles trapped in cement can severely impair its fatigue life.

Cement, mixed by hand in the traditional way, contains numerous entrapped air bubbles. A number of factors contribute to a higher content of air bubbles, and this includes vigorous mixing and the use of high viscosity cement.

Several techniques have been proposed for the reduction of entrapped air. Centrifuging effectively reduces the porosity by removing larger bubbles with an associated improvement in mechanical characteristics. Testing in tension gives an increase in static strength of 20 to 30 percent[14,75] and a 500 percent improvement in fatigue life.[14] Mixing cement under partial vacuum has been reported to reduce porosity with similar improvement in tensile and fatigue properties.[108]

If air is to be removed from cement either by centrifuging or vacuum mixing, it is an essential requirement that the cement be in a low-viscosity state and that there be a sufficient working time. This requires that the surgeon either choose a low-viscosity cement or convert standard cement into a low-viscosity state and prolong the working time by chilling of the monomer before mixing.[27,108] Certain brands of cement have little or no low-viscosity phase and do not respond to chilling of the monomer. These cements are unsuitable for air removal by either centrifugation or vacuum mixing.

Alternative methods to fatigue testing have been used to evaluate cement. A study that differs in that it employs fracture toughness has cast some doubt on the concept that the removal of air enhances the mechanical characteristics of cement.[90] It is difficult to be certain which method of testing is most meaningful within the context of use of cement in surgery, but it seems rational that until this uncertainty is resolved, porosity reduction be used as a possibly advantageous step.

Choice of Cement

A variety of surgical cements are available for implant fixation. All are polymethylmethacrylate with, in some cements, the addition of a copolymer. All are supplied in the form of two components, a polymer powder and a monomer liquid, combined to form the working cement.

When monomer is added to powder, a process is initiated that passes through a series of stages. The powder wets out and then enters a low-viscosity stage, followed by a doughy stage (Fig. 120-16). The process continues with the cement becoming first rubbery and then hard.

All cements contain chemical materials that influence the polymerization process. These compounds, including an inhibitor, an accelerator, and a catalyst, can be adjusted during the manufacturing process to control a variety of characteristics of the cement. In addition, the physical character of the powder itself, with respect to particle size and surface characteristics, very much influences the rate of polymerization and the viscosity characteristics of the wet cement.

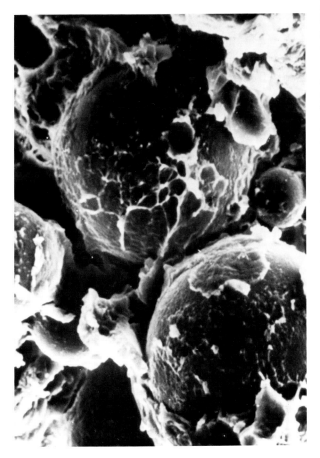

Fig. 120-16. Scanning electron micrograph of cement, showing the polymer beads and the liquid monomer in its early stage of polymerization (reaction stopped with liquid nitrogen). (Courtesy of Dr. Klaus Draenert.)

A particular cement may wet out slowly or quickly or may have relatively long low viscosity or doughy phases, and it may set rapidly or more slowly. Expressions such as dough time, which marks the first moment that cement can be handled, as well as working time and set time are largely self explanatory and are usually outlined in manufacturers' specifications, packaged with the product.

Handling characteristics is a general term to describe the physical qualities of the cement between mixing and setting, most specifically the rate of the process and the changes in viscosity. These qualities very strongly influenced the techniques that the surgeon must employ. The traditional doughy cements were formulated for manual use, that is, to be applied to bone or prosthesis during the dough phase by the gloved hand of the surgeon. This method is familiar to most orthopaedic surgeons and benefits from its simplicity, relatively long working time, and ease of cleanup.

In recent years, a number of manufacturers have developed low-viscosity cements, designed specifically for use with cement guns or delivery systems. These cements remain in a fairly constant low-viscosity state during a major portion of their working time and then quickly become doughy and set during the last 2 to 5 minutes. This provides a sufficient length of time for the surgeon to pressurize the cement, in the low-viscosity state, into cancellous bone. These products have the potential for superior intrusion into bone with attendant better fixation but carry the penalty of being technically more difficult to use.

The handling characteristics of all cements are very much affected by ambient temperature and humidity.[5,70] A cement designed to be hard 12 minutes after mixing when used at 70°F will require 2 or 3 extra minutes if used at 65°F and conversely, will harden at 8 or 9 minutes if used at 75°F. Similarly, water vapor accelerates the polymerization process. Humidity in the operating room might vary from 20 percent to 60 percent, depending on geographic location, season of year, and efficiency of air-conditioning equipment. Higher humidity can shorten set time by as much as 2 or 3 minutes.[70]

As an additional precaution, it should be noted that acrylic cement, still in the package, tends to equilibrate with the surrounding environment within a few hours. Therefore, cement brought from a non-air-conditioned storage room or otherwise exposed to temperature and humidity extremes will, if used within an hour or two, act very differently than cement stored in the operating theater itself.

Intrusion of cement into bone describes the process by which microinterlock and microfixation are achieved. The ability of cement to intrude is related to its viscosity, to the pressure application, and to the porosity characteristics and cleanliness of the bone to which it is applied.[67,72,104] Ideally, cement should be made to penetrate cancellous surfaces to a depth of 3 to 5 mm. Less penetration does not ensure microinterlock, and penetration beyond 5 mm is not only unnecessary but may result in the necrosis of the most deeply buried trabeculae, on either a thermal[61,98] or a nutritional basis.

Viscosity is measured in units of Newtons per second per square meter ($N/sec/m^2$) and is expressed as false apparent viscosity, as a reflection of the complexity of the subject and the indirect methods used for measurement. Viscosity of most doughy cements is in the range of 300 to 500 units during the working period while a low-viscosity cement measures in the region of 100 units. The techniques required to achieve intrusion of these very different cements are described later in this chapter.

The application of pressure to cement to induce intrusion has certain important prerequisites. Low-viscosity cement will require relatively low pressure to be effective, while doughy cements require high pressure.[68] It is important to understand that, to be optimally effective, the pressure must be applied in a sustained fashion. This requirement is based on the fact that cement flow, like that of all fluids, is rate dependent. The sustained pressurization allows the cement time to penetrate the very tiny interstices of cancellous bone. By contrast, pressurization produced by hammering produces a very high pressure but of short duration, and the flow of cement into bone may be less effective.

Addition of Antibiotics

Antibiotic cement was first advocated by Buchholz[13] for use in the revision of infected total hips. Gentamicin, added to the methacrylate powder, either by the surgeon or during manufacture, is slowly released into the tissue surrounding the implant at levels that appear to be effective[103] for a limited time at least.[50] Clinical studies in Sweden[64] suggest that antibiotic cement effectively reduces the incidences of infection in nonrevision hip implant surgery.

There are no published data related to the use of antibiotics in knee arthroplasty. Antibiotic cement is, at this time of writing, still not approved by regulatory agencies for manufacture or sale in the United States. It is, however, in wide use elsewhere in the world.

SURGICAL TECHNIQUE

Cementing must simultaneously achieve two interrelated objectives: (1) gross fixation of the implanted prosthesis to bone, and (2) creation, if possible, of a microscopic interlock between cement and bone, over the entire interface.

The achievement of gross fixation alone is relatively simple. Even the crudest of surgical techniques gives the immediate impression of effectiveness. The poor quality of a newly formed interface is usually not apparent either at surgery or on the basis of immediate postoperative radiologic evaluation. Only months later, the appearance of a radiolucency announces that the cement-bone interface is undergoing a degradation, which is the first stage of mechanical failure.

The successful production of a microinterlock between cement and bone is directly related to the technique employed by the surgeon. The use of special steps will result in effective interlock and an optimistic prospect for enduring fixation. The special measures required can be summarized simply by stating that acrylic cement must be induced to penetrate bone surfaces.

Exposure

Exposure of the bone surfaces to which the cemented implant is applied is essential to optimum fixation. An ample incision facilitates proper positioning of instruments, accurate and well-executed bone cuts, proper cleaning of the cancellous surfaces, and, most important, sufficient room to maneuver during the application of cement to bone, placement and impaction of the implant, and cleanup.

In tricompartmental replacement, where the anterior cruciate ligament is sacrificed, there should be little difficulty in creating satisfactory exposure. Lateral displacement and eversion of the patella give full access to its articular surface. The same maneuver fully exposes the anterior and distal portions of the distal femur. Access to the posterior surfaces of the distal femur is less easy and is directly dependent on the degree of knee flexion that can be achieved during surgery.

The upper tibia must be seen in its entirety. With the knee flexed to at least 90 degrees, a periosteal elevator or Hohmann retractor, inserted behind the tibia and levered against the femur, will bring the upper tibia forward in the manner of an anterior drawer test, and its entire surface will be visible. This maneuver is not always possible before the articular surface of the tibia has been resected, but thereafter it can be done in virtually every case. The only remaining element in the exposure is the displaced patellar tendon and fat pad, which tends to obscure the lateral edge of the tibia and adjacent cut surface. This can easily be solved by inserting a small Hohmann retractor downward along the lateral cortex of the upper tibia and levering those structures away. This maneuver is so effective that excessive resection of the fat pad is now rarely required. Care must be taken, however, not to over-retract the laterally placed Hohmann, as this may apply excessive force to the patellar tendon attachment.

In some situations, such as arthroplasty following previous high tibial osteotomy or revision arthroplasty, complete exposure of the upper tibia may be impossible or difficult without a dangerous degree of retraction. The difficulties are almost entirely related to apparent tightness of the extensor apparatus. Displacement and eversion of the patella may be impossible or may be accomplished only under tension so excessive as to threaten avulsion of the patellar tendon. Under such circumstances, the surgeon may be tempted to compromise, accepting incomplete exposure and jeopardizing the quality of fixation that can be achieved.

More complete exposure under these circumstances requires radical release of the extensor apparatus either distally or proximal to the patella. Detachment of the tibial tubercle, together with the patellar tendon, immediately resolves the problem of exposure but requires a meticulous and secure reattachment that is not always easy to achieve. The postoperative program for remobilizing the knee and reambulating must be modified to prevent disruption of the reattachment, which is difficult to deal with and may result in permanent disability.

Proximal mobilization consisting of a radical division of the quadriceps tendon in one of several patterns is currently being advocated and certainly improves exposure but has an associated increased morbidity. In spite of the obvious difficulties associated with these maneuvers, they must be employed in problem cases in which exposure of the upper tibia cannot otherwise be achieved.

Preparation of Bone

The resection of worn articular surfaces will be carried out in accordance with the prosthetic design and instrument system employed by the surgeon. Ideally, thin cuts will expose surfaces of relatively dense and strong cancellous bone. The presence of certain deformities will necessitate the excision of thicker cuts, thereby exposing less strong bone or, with a conservative resection, will leave areas of corticated bone to which cement must be applied. This problem is discussed later in this chapter. Thermal and mechanical damage to cancellous structures during resection with power equipment can be minimized by new and sharp saw blades and by the use of copious saline irrigation for cooling.

Cleaning of the cut surface is an essential step in the precementing preparation. Cancellous interstices, which are the potential sites for cement penetration, are obstructed with small fragments of bone produced by the action of the saw. Blood clot is not an important factor when surgery is conducted under tourniquet.

Method Cleaning is best achieved with a thin high-pressure stream of sterile saline. A power-driven pulsating water jet is commonly used (Fig. 120-17), but similar results can be achieved with

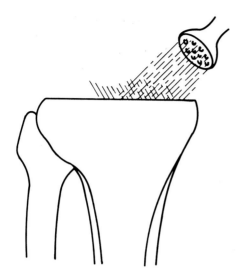

Fig. 120-17. Pulsating jet lavage for cleaning of cut cancellous surfaces.

simpler devices. Even a large-capacity syringe and an 18-gauge needle will be effective. Removal of saw debris and some intracancellous marrow changes the cut surface to a pale buff color, an indication of complete cleaning. Drying of the surface is easily accomplished with a sponge but is probably not essential, since small residuals of saline do not prevent penetration of cement.

Cement Technique

The traditional method of using acrylic cement employs so-called insertional pressurization, whereby the force imparted to the interface by the seating of the prosthesis induces cement to intrude into bone. Other methods of achieving cement penetration that are now in use force cement into bone before the prosthesis is positioned and are described as preinsertional pressurization

Insertional Pressurization

Insertional pressurization is the traditional cement technique. It is the method that requires the least effort and has the advantage of minimal spill and easy cleanup. It has the disadvantage of using cement with a relatively high viscosity and therefore poor intrusion characteristics. As the implant

is seated and impacted, excess cement tends to escape from the interface around the edges of the prosthesis. This results in a relatively low pressure, and therefore poor cement intrusion into bone near the edges, but better pressure and penetration toward the center of the interface. If a stemmed device is used, considerable pressure rise around the stem will occur with impaction, resulting in excellent intrusion. This technique is responsible for the commonly seen radiological picture of a stemmed tibial component with lucencies beneath the wings of the prosthesis but a perfect interface between cement and bone around the stem, obviously as a result of microinterlock.

Method   Cement, in the doughy phase, is formed into a patty of approximately the same shape and size as that of the implant, 5 to 10 mm thick, and is applied either to bone or to the prosthesis. The prosthesis is forced into place by manual pressure and by hammering, compressing the cement into a layer 1 to 2 mm thick. Excess cement squeezed out from beneath the prosthesis should be separated using a scalpel rather than by tearing, which may remove essential cement from beneath the edges of the prosthesis. Firm but not excessive pressure on the prosthesis should be maintained until the cement has hardened. This measure is particularly important when operating without a tourniquet, since oozing of blood from deep in the cancellous bone can actually displace the unpolymerized cement and lift the prosthesis.

An alternative method requires implanting both femoral and tibial components with the same mix of cement. The tibial component is inserted as described above; after rapid provisional removal of excess cement, the femoral component with its cement layer is positioned by manual pressure. Final compression is achieved by straightening the knee and holding in full extension until the cement hardens.

Preinsertional Pressurization

Digital Technique

This technique requires that the surgeon force the cement into the well-prepared cancellous surface using the gloved finger or thumb (Fig. 120-18A). The prerequisites for success are a scru-

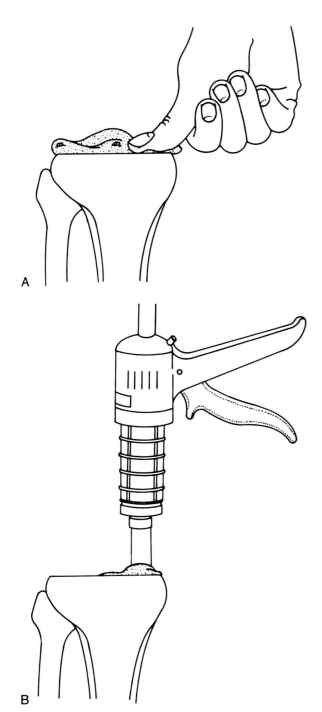

A

B

Fig. 120-18. Preinsertional pressurization. **(A)** Digital technique with doughy cement. **(B)** Cement gun with low-viscosity cement.

pulously well-prepared bone surface by pulsating lavage and cement that is just becoming doughy (after mixing for less than 3 minutes) and therefore has intrusion characteristics superior to cement in the advanced doughy state.[28]

Method The surgeon places a thin patty of cement on the cancellous surface and, with repeated finger or thumb thrusts, presses cement into bone at many sites over the entire cut surface. The procedure should be repeated, after wiping away any extruded fat or blood, by applying additional cement over the first layer, which is once again forced in with digital pressure. Cement is placed on the prosthesis, which is then impacted into place. The layers of cement bond together securely. Lamination with associated weakness is not a problem.

Cement Gun Using Low-Viscosity Cement

This second technique of preinsertional pressurization has been used since 1979[80] and has been shown to be effective. Low-viscosity cement with its improved intrusion characteristics cannot be applied manually, since it adheres to the gloved hand and therefore must be used with a cement delivery system that, in effect, injects the cement into the cancellous surface.

The surgeon may choose a proprietary low-viscosity cement or may elect to use one of several standard cements that has a brief period of low viscosity. This period can be prolonged by chilling the monomer, thereby slowing the polymerization process. Laboratory data suggest that chilling may diminish the strength of the polymerized cement unless either vacuum mixing or centrifuging is used to reduce porosity.[27,96]

Method Low-viscosity cement is prepared in a cement gun that has an attached nozzle suitable for use with cancellous bone surfaces. In the case of the tibia, cement is applied to the prosthesis before being pressurized into bone but, in the case of the femur and patella, cement is applied to the prosthesis after pressurizing bone.

The nozzle of the gun is placed and held firmly on the cancellous surface (Fig. 120-18B). The gun is activated, extruding 2 or 3 ml of liquid cement that penetrates the bone. Some cement inevitably escapes from around the edge of the nozzle onto the bone surface. The process is repeated to cover the entire surface. The cement reaches a depth of 3 to 6 mm. Penetration to greater depths is rare as the resistance to intrusion increases exponentially with the depth reached. For this reason, inadvertent repressurization of the same site will not result in excessive penetration. When the pressurization is complete, some excess may be removed from the bone surface to diminish the magnitude of spill. The prosthesis is then seated into position with hammering, if necessary.

Certain precautions are worth mentioning. The technique is complex, and timing is essential to success. The technique involves considerable spillage of low-viscosity cement and can be termed messy. The surgeon who is unfamiliar with the technique

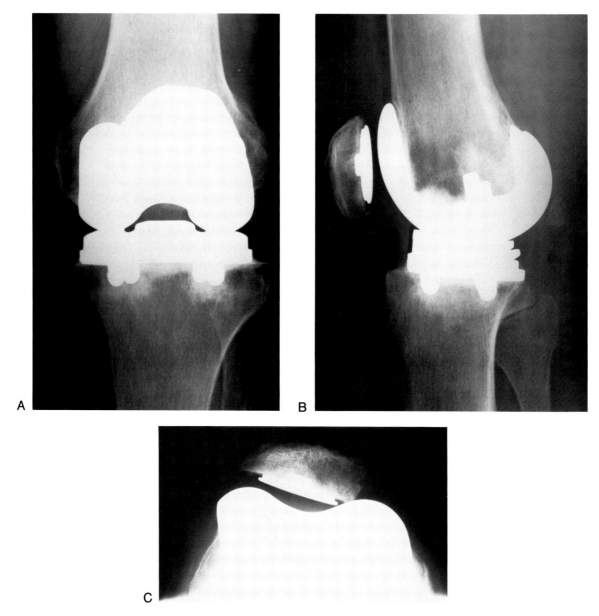

Fig. 120-19. (A–C) Views of a total knee 6 years postoperatively. Low-viscosity cement was pressurized into tibial and femoral surfaces.

is well advised to learn the method at a workshop or by scrubbing with a more experienced colleague. Rehearsal by the surgical team with a cadaver bone is useful.

The cement nozzle, to be effective, must be pressed firmly against the cancellous bone and aligned to achieve a seal with the bone. Placing the nozzle over a defect, irregularity, cut, or hole made in the cancellous surface will render the pressurization ineffective. In effect, pressurization can only be accomplished on a flat cancellous surface. Its use is not advised on curved surfaces or in the context of revision.

Some bone, particularly in the center of the upper tibia, is soft. Injudicious handling of the gun may result in penetration of the nozzle itself deep into the bone surface and should be avoided. Pressurization near the edge of the cut surface encounters dense bone with resulting poor penetration. Rheumatoid bone is less dense and requires careful pressure on the nozzle and modest activation of the gun.

The concept of creating holes into which a cement gun nozzle can be inserted is tempting but should be avoided, except in special situations. The dynamics of intrusion are very much altered by the nozzle-in-hole method and will result in cement penetration of bone to depths far beyond the ideal limits.

Cement spilled in the low-viscosity state is difficult to clean up and tends to fragment and stick to soft tissue. The surgeon should make no effort to remove excess cement until it has progressed to a doughy state and is then easily removed from soft tissue. Cement on the edges or surfaces of the prosthesis is most easily removed after it has polymerized.

The use of pressurized low-viscosity cement has virtually eliminated the existence of complete or progressive radiolucent lines in total knee arthroplasty.[79] Small lucencies at the edge of the tibia, where the bone is dense and pressurization is technically difficult, are not uncommon, but these become nonprogressive after 6 to 12 months. With respect to the femoral component, a lucency associated with the posterior cut surface of the bone, where poor access makes pressurization impossible, is very common and does not affect the overall fixation of the implant. The large majority of total knees done by this method look pristine after 6 to 7 years (Fig. 120-19).

SPECIAL PROBLEMS

Certain circumstances may exist in which the standard techniques are not capable of producing an optimum fixation interface. They require that the surgeon employ special techniques or measures. The extra time and effort expended in these situations is justified by the enhanced results and prognosis.

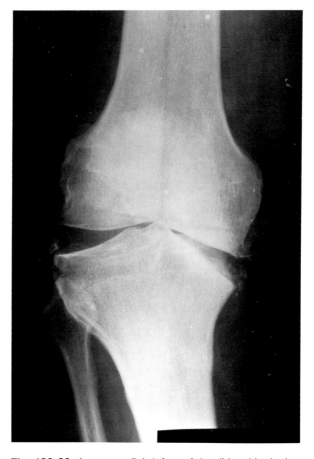

Fig. 120-20. Large medial defect of the tibia with sloping and sclerotic surface.

Deformed Articular Surface

It is common to encounter grossly deformed articular surfaces, which constitute a decisional and a technical problem to the surgeon. As an example, a marked varus knee shows, on radiographic evaluation and surgical exposure, a relatively normal lateral tibial plateau but a medial plateau that is depressed, sloping, and sclerotic (Fig. 120-20). A decision must be made about the level of resection. A conservative level with respect to the lateral plateau leaves a large defect on the medial side. A radical resection reduces or eliminates the medial defect but sacrifices valuable bone from the lateral plateau; this choice is a poor one. A compromise between the two extremes is usually the best choice, removing slightly more than the minimal amount from the lateral compartment and leaving a partial or a marginal defect on the medial side (Fig. 120-21).

Fixation of the implant to the resected tibia with a marginal defect requires a decision. The simple solution of filling the defect with cement is unsatisfactory. The acrylic, poorly fixed to the corticated surface of the defect, tends to fracture with deleterious effect on the overall support of the prosthesis.

Three workable options are available. A small autogenous bone graft held in place with screws reconstitutes the surface of the tibia and provides support for the prosthesis[86] (Fig. 120-22A). Often bone resected from the distal femoral condyle or tibial eminence constitutes an adequate amount for grafting. A stemmed implant reduces the load on the grafted area.[89] Care should be exercised to prevent cement from intruding between graft and adjacent bone. A period of protected weight bearing is advisable.

The second option involves the use of an augmented prosthesis. The defect is, in effect, filled with prosthetic material rather than cement or bone. The surgeon may elect to use a custom made prosthesis (Fig. 120-22B) or a system in which augmenting elements can be attached in a modular fashion[11] (Fig. 120-22C). The considerations with respect to this choice relate to cost, fit, and inventory.

The third option involves filling of the defect with acrylic cement used in such a way as to enhance its fixation to both bone and prosthesis. Bonding of the cement to the undersurface of the prosthesis that is either porous or precoated is advantageous. The cement-bone interface can be reinforced by the insertion of two or more surgical screws into the defect.[91] The heads of the screws are left protruding to the level of the adjacent cut surface of the tibia and act as reinforcing members for the cement filling the defect (Fig. 120-22D).

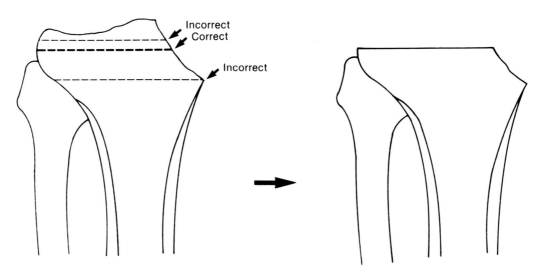

Fig. 120-21. A compromise between the two extremes of bone resection leaves a residual medial defect that is technically easy to deal with.

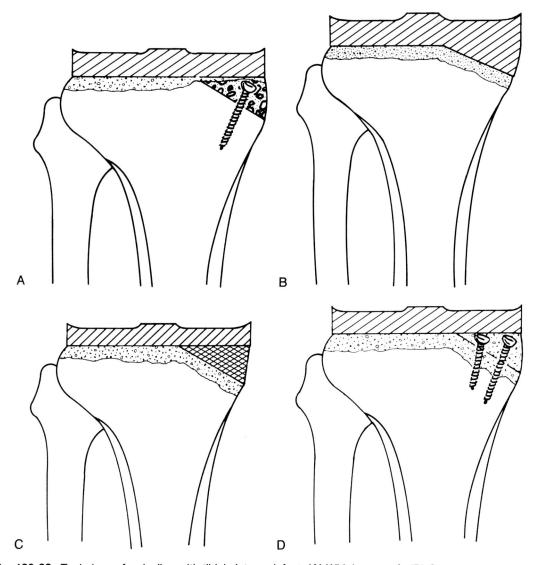

Fig. 120-22. Techniques for dealing with tibial plateau defect. **(A)** With bone graft. **(B)** Custom prosthesis. **(C)** Modular prosthetic inserts. **(D)** Cement reinforced with screws. *(Figure continues.)*

An alternative treatment for the cement-bone interface involves the penetration of the sclerotic subchondral bone on the base of the defect with several ¼-inch drill holes of a depth sufficient to enter cancellous bone. Using a cement delivery system and a suitable nozzle, small amounts of low-viscosity cement are pressurized into each hole (Fig. 120-22E). The nozzle is then exchanged for a cancellous nozzle and the undeformed part of the interface is pressurized as previously described and the prosthesis seated. Extra cement is introduced as necessary into the defect. This technique has been used for almost 10 years and has all the characteristics of composite structure fixation. The cement in the defect is well attached to the prosthesis and is microinterlocked with bone at several sites. These secure interfaces make the cement highly resistant to displacement or fracture.

Femoral defects are smaller and less common than tibial defects and are usually less difficult to

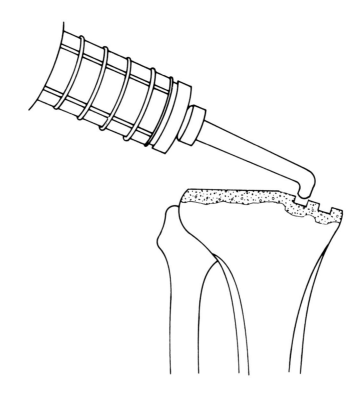

E

Fig. 120-22 *(Continued).* **(E)** Shallow drill holes through sclerotic bone to permit pressurization of cement.

resolve. Major defects are amenable to solutions similar to those outlined for the tibia.

Central Plateau Defects or Cortication

It is common, particularly in the rheumatoid knee, to find defects at the center of the medial or lateral tibial plateau occupied by encysted synovial material. Tiny defects can be cleared of soft tissue but otherwise ignored. Large and occasionally huge defects are found; these should not be filled with cement. Cancellous bone, usually obtained from the resected articular surfaces, is ideal and should be compacted into the defects. Cement laid on top of the grafted area or pressed into its superficial layers does not affect the eventual incorporation of the graft.

Corticated areas may persist at the center of the medial or lateral tibial plateau surfaces after resec-

tion or occasionally on the distal femoral surfaces result from the conservative removal of deformed articular structures, particularly where there has been some subchondral sclerosis. Typically, the prepared tibia will show good-quality cancellous bone over the entire surface, except for an irregular area at the center of the medial plateau, which is white, nonporous, and obviously sclerotic. This bone does not permit cement to interlock and will eventually evolve a radiolucent line as a result of micromovement-induced bone resorption. Precutting the tibia at a slightly deeper level has the advantage of simplicity but sacrifices valuable bone and should be discouraged.

The most commonly employed option is to treat the corticated area in a fashion similar to that outlined earlier. The sclerotic surface is drilled at many sites to a depth sufficient to enter cancellous bone. Using a delivery system, cement is carefully pressurized into the drill holes and then applied to the remainder of the cancellous surface by one of the methods outlined. This technique dramatically reduces the tendency for the corticated area to develop a major radiolucency.

Cementing in Revision Surgery

The damaged and irregular surfaces that present themselves to the surgeon at the time of revision surgery are not ideal for cement fixation. No single solution or set of rules is applicable to all situations. Obviously, if a very limited further resection of bone produces a flat, clean, virginlike surface amenable to the cement techniques outlined for primary surgery, this is the best approach. In situations in which more extensive damage to bone has occurred, further resection sacrifices valuable tissue and length and is contraindicated. A more logical approach may be to attempt to reconstitute damaged tissue with either allograft or preferably autogenous bone and to create a firm flat base suitable to accept a cemented prosthesis.

A careful surgical exposure is used to preserve all remaining bone and particularly cortical structures, no matter how thin or fragile. All traces of fibrous membrane and other soft tissue are meticulously removed along with all cement. Small pieces of cortical bone may be required to reestablish a metaphyseal cortical configuration, but in most cases, cancellous bone will suffice. Large intramedullary defects from previous stemmed devices should be cleared of cement and fibrous tissue and filled with graft.

There is merit in the idea of using a revision prosthesis with the stem inserted into the medullary canal surrounded with graft rather than cement and using doughy cement only on the grafted upper surface. A porous or precoated implant will be beneficial in terms of protecting the cement from fracture. Pressurization techniques are contraindicated when the cement is being applied to graft material rather than to viable and previously undisturbed cancellous bone. A prolonged period of protected weight bearing is indicated. Implants designed for use in revision surgery are indispensable. Augmentation of the prosthesis to compensate for asymmetric bone loss reduces the need for grafting or for resection.

SUMMARY

The most effective use of acrylic cement is directly related to the creation of secure interfaces between cement and prosthesis and cement and bone. Knowledge regarding fixation is now sufficiently advanced to enable the caring orthopaedic surgeon to create ideal fixation both predictably and reproducibly. The ability of surgeons to achieve these ends is proportional to their awareness of the issues and to their interest, patience, and skill in implementing their objectives. Better cement techniques will result in better fixation, which in turn will yield more enduring fixation. In the future, loosening of knee implants should be an uncommon occurrence.

REFERENCES

1. Ahmed AM, Nair R, Burke DL, et al: Transient and residual stresses and displacements in self-curing bone cement. II. Thermoelastic analysis of the stem fixation. J Biomech Eng 104:28, 1982
2. Ahmed AM, Raab S, Miller JE: Metal/cement interface strength in cemented stem fixation. J Orthop Res 2:105, 1984
3. Aglietti P, Rinonapoli E: Total condylar knee arthroplasty. A five-year follow-up study of 33 knees. Clin Orthop 186:104, 1984
4. Andriaccchi TP, Stanwyck TS, Galante JO: Knee biomechanics and total knee replacement. J Arthroplast 1:211, 1986
5. Anuta DA, Young KA, Gilbertonson LN: Influence of humidity on setting characteristics and fracture toughness values of poly(methyl methacrylate) bone cement. p. 2. In Transactions of the Seventh Annual Meeting of the Society for Biomaterials, 1981
6. Bargren JH, Blaha JD, Freeman MAR: Alignment in total knee arthroplasty. Correlated biomechanical and clinical observations. Clin Orthop 173:178, 1983
7. Bargren JH, Day WH, Freeman MAR, Swanson SAV: Mechanical tests on the tibial component of

non-hinged knee prosthesis. J Bone Joint Surg 60B:256, 1978

8. Bartel DL, Burstein AH, Santavicca EA, et al: Performance of the tibial component in total knee replacement. J Bone Joint Surg 64A:1026, 1982

9. Black J: Metallic ion release and its relationship to oncogenesis. p. 199. In Fitzgerald RH Jr (ed): The Hip. Proceedings of the Thirteenth Open Scientific Meeting of the Hip Society. CV Mosby, St. Louis, 1985

10. Boegard T, Brattstrom H, Lidgren L: Seventy-four Attenborough knee replacements for rheumatoid arthritis. A clinical and radiographic study. Acta Orthop Scand 55:166, 1984

11. Brooks PJ, Walker PS, Scott DS: Tibial component fixation in deficient tibial bone stock. Clin Orthop 184:302, 1984

12. Bryan RS, Peterson LFA: Polycentric total knee arthroplasty - A prognostic assessment. Clin Orthop 145:23, 1979

13. Buchholz HW, Engelbrecht H: Uber die dipotwirkung einiger antibiotica bei vermischung mit dem kunstharz palacos. Chirurgie 41:511, 1970

14. Burke DW, Gates EI, Harris WH: Centrifugation as a method of improving tensile and fatigue properties of acrylic bone cement. J Bone Joint Surg 66A:1265, 1984

15. Chan KH, Johnson JA, Miller J, et al: Effect of prolonged exposure of wet environment on bond strength of PMMA precoat. Manuscript in preparation, 1988

16. Chandler HP, Reineck FT, Wixson RL, et al: Total hip replacement in patients younger than thirty years old. J Bone Joint Surg 63A:1426, 1981

17. Charnley J: Sensitivity to acrylic resins. p. 79. In Acrylic Cement in Orthopaedic Surgery. 1st Ed. E & S Livingstone, Edinburgh, 1970

18. Charnley J: The theory of mechanical fastenings in bone surgery. p. 10. In Acrylic Cement in Orthopaedic Surgery. 1st Ed. E & S Livingstone, Edinburgh, 1970

19. Charnley J: In Robert Jones Lecture. Combined Meeting of the English Speaking Orthopaedic Associations, London, 1976

20. Cheal EJ, Hayes WC, Lee CH, et al: Stress analysis of a condylar knee tibial component. Influence of metaphyseal shell properties and cement injection depth. J Orthop Res 3/4:424, 1985

21. Cloutier J-M: Results of total knee arthroplasty with a non-constrained prosthesis. J Bone Joint Surg 65A:906, 1983

22. Collier JP, Mayor MB, Townley CO, et al: Histology of retrieved porous-coated knee prosthesis. Presented at the Fifty-third Annual Meeting of the American Academy of Orthopaedic Surgeons, New Orleans, 1986 (paper 14)

23. Coventry MD: Two-part total knee arthroplasty: evolution and present status. Clin Orthop 145:29, 1979

24. Cracchiolo A III, Benson M, Finerman GAM, et al: A prospective comparative clinical analysis of the first-generation knee replacement: polycentric vs geometric knee arthroplasty. Clin Orthop 145:37, 1979

25. Crowninshield RD, Hawkins M, Price H: Poly(methylmethacrylate) precoating of orthopaedic implants. p. 67. In Harris WH (ed): Advanced Concepts in Total Hip Replacement. Slack, Thorofare, NJ, 1985

26. Dannenmaier WC, Haynes DW, Nelson CL: Granulomatous reaction and cystic bony destruction associated with high wear rate in a total knee prosthesis. Clin Orthop 198:224, 1985

27. Davies JP, Burke DW, O'Connor DO, et al: Comparison of the fatigue characteristics of centrifuged and uncentrifuged Simplex P bone cement. J Orthop Res 5:366, 1987

28. Dorr LD, Boiardo RA: Mechanisms of failure of total knee arthroplasty. p. 9. In Scott WN (ed): Total Knee Revision Arthroplasty. Grune & Stratton, Orlando, FL, 1987

29. Dorr LD, Lindberg JP, Claude-Faugere M, Malluche HH: Factors influencing the intrusion of methylmethacrylate into human tibiae. Clin Orthop 183:147, 1984

30. Ducheyne P, Kagan A, Lacey JA: Failure of total knee arthroplasty due to loosening and deformation of tibial component. J Bone Joint Surg 60A:384, 1978

31. Engh CA, Bobyn JD, Glassman AH: Porous-coated hip replacement. The factors governing bone ingrowth, stress shielding and clinical results. J Bone Joint Surg 69B:45, 1987

32. Ewald FC, Christie MJ: Results of cemented total knee replacement in young patients. Orthop Trans 2(3):442, 1987

33. Figgie HE, Davy DT, Heiple KG, Hart RT: Load-bearing capacity of the tibial component of the total condylar knee prosthesis. An in-vitro study. Clin Orthop 183:288, 1984

34. Freeman MAR, Bradley GW, Revell PA: Observations upon the interface between bone and polymethylmethacrylate cement. J Bone Joint Surg 64B:489, 1982

35. Freeman MAR, Sammuelson KM, Levak B, et al: Knee arthroplasty at the London hospital 1975–1984. Clin Orthop 205:12, 1986

36. Freeman MAR, Todd RC, Barnert P, et al: ICLH—

arthroplasty of the knee 1968–1978. J Bone Joint Surg 60B:339, 1978

37. Gates EI, Carter DR, Harris WH: Comparative fatigue behavior of different bone cements. Clin Orthop 189:294, 1984

38. Goldring SR, Schiller AL, Roelke M, et al: The synovial-like membrane at the bone–cement interface in loose total hip replacements and its proposed role in bone lysis. J Bone Joint Surg 65A:575, 1983

39. Green DL, Bahnuik E, Liebelt RA, et al: Biplane radiographic measurements of reversible displacement (including clinical loosening) and migration of total joint replacements. J Bone Joint Surg 65A:1134, 1985

40. Greenwald AS, Black JD, Matejczyk MB: Stability characteristics of total knee designs. p. 238. In American Academy of Orthopaedic Surgeons' Instructional Course Lectures. Vol. 30. CV Mosby, St. Louis, 1981

41. Greenwald AS, Matejczyk MB, Postak PD: Stability characteristics of total knee replacements. Scientific Exhibit, Presented at the Meeting of the American Academy of Orthopaedic Surgeons, San Francisco, 1987

42. Grogan TJ, Dorey F, Rollins J, et al: Deep sepsis following total knee arthroplasty: Ten-year experience at the University of California at Los Angeles Medical Center. J Bone Joint Surg 68A:226, 1986

43. Gunston FH: Polycentric knee arthroplasty — prosthetic simulation of normal knee movement. J Bone Joint Surg 53B:272, 1971

44. Gunston FH, MacKenzie RI: Complications of polycentric knee replacement. Clin Orthop 120:11, 1976

45. Habermann ET: Revision arthroplasty for failed total knee replacement. p. 219. In Hungerford DS, Krackow KA, Kenna RV (eds): Total Knee Arthroplasty. A Comprehensive Approach. Williams & Wilkins, Baltimore, 1984

46. Haddad RJ, Cook SD, Thomas KA, et al: Histologic and microradiographic analysis of noncemented retrieved PCA knee components. Presented at the Fifty-third Annual Meeting of the American Academy of Orthopaedic Surgeons, New Orleans, 1986 (paper 15)

47. Haddad RJ, Cook SD, Thomas KA: Histologic analysis of retrieved noncemented porous-coated implants. Presented at the Fifty-fourth Annual Meeting of the American Academy of Orthopaedic Surgeons, San Francisco, 1987 (paper 224)

48. Harrington IJ: Static and dynamic loading patterns in knee joints with deformities. J Bone Joint Surg 65A:247, 1983

49. Harris WH, Schiller AL, Scholler J: Extensive localized bone resorption in the femur following total hip replacement. J Bone Joint Surg 58A:612, 1976

50. Hoff SF, Fitzgerald RH Jr, Kelly PJ: The depot administration of Penicillin G and Gentamicin in acrylic bone cement. J Bone Joint Surg 63A:798, 1981

51. Huiskes R: Some fundamental aspects of human joint replacement. Acta Orthop Scand 185(suppl):109, 1980

52. Hungerford DS, Kenna RV: Preliminary experience with a total knee prosthesis with porous coating used without cement. Clin Orthop 176:95, 1983

53. Hungerford DS, Krackow KA, Kenna RV: Two- to five-year experience with a cementless porous-coated total knee prosthesis. p. 215. In Rand JA, Dorr LD (eds): Total Arthroplasty of the Knee. Proceedings of the Knee Society 1985–1986. Aspen, Rockville, MD, 1986

54. Hvid I, Christensen P, Sondergaard J, et al: Compressive strength of tibial cancellous bone. Acta Orthop Scand 54:819, 1983

55. Hvid I, Jensen J, Nielsen S: Contribution of the cortex to epiphyseal strength. Acta Orthop Scand 56:256, 1985

56. Hvid I, Neilsen S: Total condylar knee arthroplasty. Prosthetic component position and radiolucent lines. Acta Orthop Scand 55:160, 1984

57. Insall J: Infection of total knee arthroplasty. p. 319. In Anderson LD (ed): The American Academy of Orthopaedic Surgeons Instructional Course Lectures. Vol. 35. CV Mosby, St. Louis, 1986

58. Insall JN, Hood RW, Flawn LB, et al: The total condylar knee prosthesis in gonarthrosis — a five to nine-year follow-up of the first one hundred consecutive replacements. J Bone Joint Surg 65A:619, 1983

59. Insall J, Kelly M: The total condylar prosthesis. Clin Orthop 205:43, 1986

60. Insall J, Ranawat CS, Aglietti P, et al: A comparison of four models of total knee replacement prosthesis. J Bone Joint Surg 58A:754, 1976

61. Jefferiss CD, Lee AJC, Ling RSM: Thermal aspects of self-curing polymethylmethacrylate. J Bone Joint Surg 57B:511, 1975

62. Johnson F, Leitl S, Waugh W: The distribution of load across the knee. J Bone Joint Surg 62B:346, 1980

63. Johnson JA, Krug WH, Nahon D, et al: An evaluation of the load bearing capability of the cancellous proximal tibia with special interest in the design of knee implants. p. 403. Presented at the Transac-

tions of the Twenty-ninth Annual Meeting of the Orthopaedic Research Society, Anaheim, CA, 1983

64. Josefsson G, Lindberg L, Wiklander B: Systemic antibiotics and gentamicin-containing bone cement in the prophylaxis of postoperative infections in total hip arthroplasty. Clin Orthop 159:194, 1980

65. King TV, Scott RD: Femoral component loosening in total knee arthroplasty. Clin Orthop 194:285, 1985

66. Knutson K, Lindstrand A, Lidgren L: Survival of knee arthroplasties. A nation-wide multicentre investigation of 8000 cases. J Bone Joint Surg 68B:795, 1986

67. Krause WR, Krug WH, Miller JE: Strength of cement–bone interface. Clin Orthop 163:290, 1982

68. Krause WR, Miller J, Ng P: The viscosity of acrylic bone cements. J Biomed Mater Res 16:219, 1982

69. Krug WH, Johnson JA, Sovaid DJ, et al: Anthropomorphic studies of the proximal tibia and their relationship to the design of knee implants. p. 402. Presented at the Transactions of the Twenty-ninth Annual Meeting of the Orthopaedic Research Society, Anaheim, CA, 1983

70. Krug WH, Kelebay LC, Miller JE, Krause WR: The effect of temperature and humidity on the handling and setting characteristics of acrylic bone cement. p. 249. Presented at the Transactions of the Twenty-eighth Annual Meeting of the Orthopaedic Research Society, New Orleans, 1982

71. Laskin RS: Varus knee deformities: a review of ten years' experience. p. 30. In Rand JA, Dorr LD (eds): Total Arthroplasty of the Knee. Proceedings of the Knee Society 1985–1986. Aspen, Rockville, MD, 1987

72. Lee AJC, Ling RSM: A device to improve the extrusion of bone cement into the bone of the acetabulum in the replacement of the hip joint. J Biomed Eng 9:522, 1974

73. Lewallen DG, Bryan RS, Peterson LFA: Polycentric total knee arthroplasty. A ten year follow-up study. J Bone Joint Surg 66A:1211, 1984

74. Lewis JL, Askew MJ, Jaycox DP: A comparative evaluation of tibial component designs of total knee prostheses. J Bone Joint Surg 64A:129, 1982

75. Lidgren L, Drar H, Moller J: Strength of polymethlmethacrylate increased by vacuum mixing. Acta Orthop Scand 55:536, 1984

76. Linder L: Reaction of bone to the acute chemical trauma of bone cement. J Bone Joint Surg 59A:82, 1977

77. Lotke PA, Ecker ML: Influence of positioning of prosthesis in total knee replacement. J Bone Joint Surg 59A:77, 1977

78. Miller J, Burke DL, Staciewicz JW, et al: The pathophysiology of loosening of femoral components in total hip arthroplasty. A clinical and experimental study of cement fracture and loosening of the cement–bone interface. p. 64. In The Hip. Proceedings of the Sixth Open Scientific Meeting of the Hip Society. CV Mosby, St. Louis, 1978

79. Miller J, Clayton M, Dunn H: Composite structure fixation in total knee arthroplasty: a preliminary report of a multicentre clinical trial. J Bone Joint Surg 66B:300, 1984

80. Miller JE, Kelebay, Bobyn D, et al: The development of a fibrous membrane (radiolucent line) between implants and bone—prevention by "microinterlock." p. 254. Presented at the Transactions of the Twenty-sixth Annual Meeting of the Orthopaedic Research Society, Atlanta, 1980

81. Morrison JB: The mechanics of the knee joint in relation to normal walking. J Biomech 3:51, 1970

82. Murase K, Crowninshield RD, Pedersen DR: An analysis of tibial component design in total knee arthroplasty. J Biomech 16:13, 1983

83. Noble PC, Swarts E: Penetration of acrylic bone cements into cancellous bone. Acta Orthop Scand 54:566, 1983

84. Prodromos CC, Andriacchi TP, Galante JO: A relationship between gait and clinical changes following high tibial osteotomy. J Bone Joint Surg 67A:1188, 1985

85. Raab S, Ahmed AM, Provan JW: Thin film PMMA precoating for improved implant bone–cement fixation. J Biomed Mater Res 16:679, 1982

86. Ranawat CS: How to compensate for bone loss. p. 95. In Ranawat CS (ed): Total-Condylar Knee Arthroplasty. Technique, Results and Complications. Springer-Verlag, New York, 1985

87. Ranawat CS, Rose HA: Clinical and radiographic results of total-condylar knee arthroplasty: a 3- to 8-year follow-up. p. 140. In Ranawat CS (ed): Total-Condylar Knee Arthroplasty. Technique, Results, and Complications. Springer-Verlag, New York, 1985

88. Rand JA, Bryan RS: Alignment in porous coated anatomic total knee arthroplasty. p. 111. In Dorr LD (ed): The Knee. Papers of the First Scientific Meeting of the Knee Society. University Park Press, Baltimore, 1985

89. Reilly D, Walker PS, Ben-Dov M, et al: Effects of tibial components on load transfer in the upper tibia. Clin Orthop 165:273, 1982

90. Rimnac CM, Wright TM, McGill DL: The effect of centrifugation on the fracture properties of acrylic bone cements. J Bone Joint Surg 68A:281, 1986

91. Ritter MA: Screw and cement fixation of large defects in total knee arthroplasty. J Arthroplasty 1(2):125, 1986

92. Rosenqvist R, Bylander B, Knutson K, et al: Loosening of the porous coating of bicompartmental prostheses in patients with rheumatoid arthritis. J Bone Joint Surg 68A:538, 1986

93. Ryd L: Micromotion in knee arthroplasty—a roentgen stereophotogrammetric analysis of tibial component fixation. Acta Orthop Scand 220 suppl):57, 1986

94. Sneppen O, Christensen P, Larsen H, et al: Mechanical testing of trabecular bone in knee replacement. Int Orthop 5:251, 1981

95. Spector M: Implant materials. Presented at Symposium on Total hip replacement—critical issues and prognostications, Hot Spring, VA April 30, 1987

96. Stubbs BE, Mathews LS, Sonstegard DA: Experimental fixation of fractures of the femur with methylmethacrylate. J Bone Joint Surg 57A:317, 1975

97. Sutherland CJ, Wilde AH, Borden LS, et al: A ten-year follow-up of one hundred consecutive Muller curved-stem total hip replacement arthroplasties. J Bone Joint Surg 64A:970, 1982

98. Swenson LW, Schurman DJ: Finite element temperature analysis of a total hip replacement and measurement of PMMA curing temperatures. J Biomed Mater Res 15:83, 1981

99. Thornhill TS, Dalziel RW, Sledge CB: Alternatives to arthrodesis for the failed total knee arthroplasty. Clin Orthop 170:131, 1982

100. Townley CO: The anatomic total knee resurfacing arthroplasty. Clin Orthop 192:82, 1985

101. Vince KC, Insall J, Kelly M, et al: Total condylar knee prosthesis: ten to twelve year follow-up and survivorship analysis. Orthop Trans 2(3):443, 1987

102. Vince KC, Johnson JA, Krygier JJ, et al: Tibial component tilting in total knee arthroplasty. p. 360. Presented at the Transactions of the Thirty-second Annual Meeting of the Orthopaedic Research Society, New Orleans, 1986

103. Wahlig H, Dingeldein E, Buchholz HW, et al: Pharmacokinetic study of gentamicin-loaded cement in total hip replacements. Comparative effects of varying dosage. J Bone Joint Surg 66B:175, 1984

104. Walker PS, Greene D, Reilly D, et al: Fixation of tibial components of knee prostheses. J Bone Joint Surg 63A:258, 1981

105. Walker PS, Soudry M, Ewald FC, et al: Control of cement penetration in total knee arthroplasty. Clin Orthop 185:155, 1984

106. Willert HG: Reactions of the articular capsule to wear products of artificial joint prostheses. J Biomed Mater Res 11:157, 1977

107. Willert HG, Ludwig J, Semlitsch M: Reaction of bone to methacrylate after hip arthroplasty. A long-term gross, light microscopic and scanning electron microscopic study. J Bone Joint Surg 56A:1368, 1974

108. Wixson RL, Lautenschlager EP, Novak MA: Vacuum mixing of acrylic bone cement. J Arthroplasty 2:141, 1987

109. Woodman JL, Jacobs JJ, Galante JO, et al: Metal ion release from titanium-based prosthetic segmental replacements of long bones in baboons: a long-term study. J Orthop Res 1(4):421, 1983

Arthroplasty of the Knee

121

Clement B. Sledge

The clinical results of replacement of the arthritic knee now equal or exceed the success of hip replacement in terms of frequency of pain relief, satisfactory function, and survival of the implant at 10 years.[15,32] These results have been achieved, not by any one person or center, but by the combined efforts of engineers and surgeons from many countries. It has been a slow evolution of concepts, techniques, and designs over the past 30 years with enormous strides occurring in the past 15 years.

To appreciate fully the current status and future directions of knee arthroplasty, it is necessary to review some landmarks in this evolution, the kinetics of the normal knee, and the pathology of the arthritic knee, as well as to discuss the controversies that remain and describe current techniques and results.

EVOLUTION OF KNEE ARTHROPLASTY

Resection arthroplasty of the knee was first reported in 1861 by Ferguson.[36] Frequent failures, secondary to either excessive instability or sponta-neous fusion, prevented widespread use of this procedure. To prevent the latter complication, a variety of interpositional materials was tried over the years with little success until Campbell, in 1940,[20] reported the use of a metallic mold over the distal femur to provide a new articular surface. A similar device, derived from experience with cup arthroplasty of the hip, was implanted by Smith-Petersen in 1953 and used sporadically until the end of the 1960s.[70] This implant, developed at the Massachusetts General Hospital, was called the MGH femoral arthroplasty. A similar concept, hemiarthroplasty of one of the articular surfaces, was applied to the tibial surface by McKeever in 1952[97] and by MacIntosh in 1958.[88] These latter two prostheses are still used with satisfactory results in some patients considered not to be candidates for total knee arthroplasty (Fig. 121-1). Long-term evaluation of these implants has shown stable, satisfactory results in most patients.[31,127] In view of the controversy surrounding the recent introduction of uncemented knee replacements, it is interesting to note that the MGH femoral stem hemiarthroplasty and the tibial hemiarthroplasty of MacIntosh and McKeever usually failed because of destruction of the unresurfaced articulating member, not through loosening or migration of the uncemented metallic components.

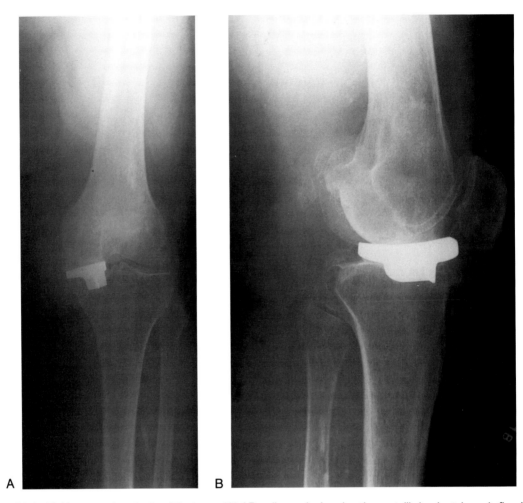

A   B

Fig. 121-1. McKeever arthroplasty of the knee. **(A)** AP radiograph showing the metallic implant, loosely fixed by a keel-like structure into the tibial plateau. **(B)** Lateral radiographic view.

Modern attempts to replace both surfaces of the arthritic knee can be traced to early hinged designs of Walldius,[169] first in acrylic and later in chrome cobalt. Although earlier sporadic efforts used hinge replacements for the knee, none achieved widespread use until the Walldius design.

The Walldius prosthesis, the somewhat similar Shiers,[136] and the later GUEPAR[27,96] were capable of providing 90 degrees (or more with the GUE-PAR) of painless motion in patients with severe deformities and restricted motion as they sacrificed all ligaments, enabling the deformities to be corrected. Because of their excessive constraint, however, failure of fixation was common (Fig. 121-2).

Accumulation of metallic debris from the metal-on-metal axle resulted in an inflammatory reaction with chronic effusion and frequent late infections.

One report analyzed 90 total knee arthroplasties using the Walldius prosthesis. There were four infections, one wound dehiscence, and four patellar tendon ruptures, for a failure rate of 9 percent. This high success rate was attributed to the avoidance of cement fixation. Radiolucent zones developed around most of these prostheses, but this finding was not usually associated with pain or clinical instability.[106,175]

Other series, most using cemented hinges, have reported high initial failure rates and even higher

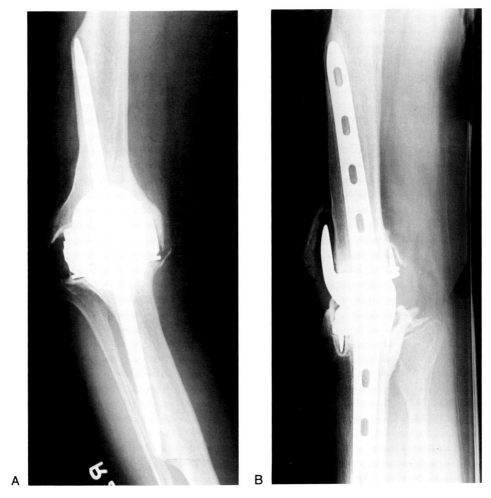

Fig. 121-2. Walldius hinge prosthesis in place for more than 15 years. **(A)** AP radiograph showing recurrent varus deformity with migration of the implant stems through the lateral cortex of the femur and tibia. The implant was uncemented. **(B)** Lateral radiograph showing migration of the stem into the anterior cortex of the femur. Fenestrations in the implant stem for bone ingrowth are well seen.

long-term failure rates.[56] We reported on 144 Walldius hinges in 1976.[144] These implants had been used between 1970 and 1975 and provided an average follow-up of 4 years. There were 6 revisions for aseptic loosening and 10 for sepsis, giving a failure rate of 11 percent at that early interval. Continued surveillance has demonstrated other later failures, and more are sure to come. Most centers have now abandoned the fixed-axis metal-bearing hinges entirely.

In England, the Stanmore hinge is still used at some centers with reports of satisfactory results by Lettin and co-workers.[81] Although early enthusiasm was expressed and good long-term results are still being reported, enthusiasm has lessened. A 1984 analysis of 103 sequential Stanmore knee replacements, with a maximal follow-up period of 9 years, 3 months, demonstrated that the prosthesis was successful in alleviating pain, stabilizing an unstable knee, and modestly increasing the arc of flexion. Walking capacity was increased and flexion contractures were reduced. There were seven cases of infection and four of fracture around the prosthesis. Two knees with both fracture and infection required amputation. Eight knees were revised for aseptic loosening for a combined failure rate of 19 percent, and a further 14 were found to have radiologic signs of loosening.[49]

The insertion of a polyethylene bushing to decrease metallic wear and provide some "sloppiness" of articulation produced the Spherocentric and the Kinematic Rotating Hinge. A recent report by the developers of the Spherocentric[94,95] listed a 10 percent loosening rate, 51 percent with lucent lines, 12 percent with patellar pain, and 9 percent with reoperation. Early results with the Kinematic Rotating Hinge were reported from the Mayo Clinic,[112] where 50 arthroplasties (15 primary arthroplasties and 38 revisions) produced 14 excellent results, 12 good results, 5 fair results, and 5 poor results, with 16 percent infection, 22 percent patellar instability, and 6 percent breakage of the implant.

Failure rates are higher with these highly constrained devices than with the unlinked designs.[138] There is now rarely an indication for such constrained devices, as most problems (90 to 99 percent), including revisions of hinge failure, can be salvaged by unlinked devices with thick components, to produce appropriate tension of the soft tissue envelope and provide the necessary lateral stability.[60,159,160]

The modern era of knee arthroplasty began with Frank Gunston in 1970.[51] Working in Charnley's unit, he developed the first unlinked knee replacement using polyethylene as one of the articulating surfaces. This prosthesis and the others that immediately followed, were successful in relieving pain and providing about 90 degrees of flexion. To achieve stability, they relied on conforming geometry, which limited flexion and imposed excessive constraint. These prostheses usually failed because of loss of fixation at the methacrylate-bone interface.[52,85]

To overcome the problems of inadequate motion and frequent loosening, Walker[166] pioneered the development of more anatomic condylar replacements, from which most current designs are derived (Fig. 121-3). Virtually all modern knee prostheses attempt to duplicate the normal knee in terms of motion and stability. The various methods used to achieve this goal can best be understood by an analysis of the kinetics of the normal knee.

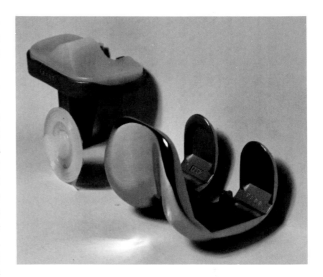

Fig. 121-3. Posterior cruciate-sparing total condylar prosthesis with a one-piece metal tray, cruciate recess in the back of the tibial component, and a polyethylene patellar button.

KINETICS OF THE NORMAL KNEE

Motion

The knee joint achieves both flexion and rotation by low femorotibial conformity, especially in the lateral compartment, and by reduction in the sagittal radius of the femoral condyles from front to back.[143] The ligaments and capsule are relatively inelastic and change their length very little during motion.[83] There is thus a preferred path of rotation, as flexion proceeds in synchrony with the resultant force and moment vectors of the muscles.[76] The relative conformity of the medial articulation and the nonconformity of the lateral compartment produce rotation about an axis centered toward the medial side of the joint.[76,162] The medial condyle remains relatively stationary, while the lateral condyle moves backward by about 17 mm as flexion proceeds from 0 to 120 degrees with the knee loaded.[76] This produces a total external rotation of the tibia of some 20 degrees (Fig. 121-4). This combination of external rotation and rollback of the lateral femoral condyle permits flexion approach-

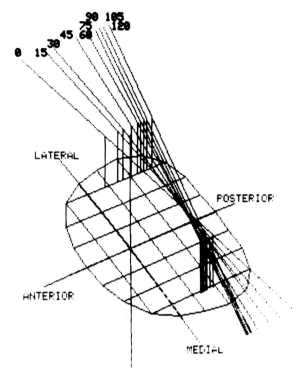

Fig. 121-4. Rotation of the femur on the tibia during flexion. The transverse angled lines represent the axis through the centers of the femoral condyles. The pivot point is close to the medial side with greater excursion of the femoral condyle on the lateral tibial plateau. (From Insall,[60] with permission.)

ing 140 degrees. Without this mechanism, impingement of the posterior rim of the tibia and the soft tissues behind the knee would limit flexion to between 90 and 105 degrees.

Stability

The unloaded knee joint displays considerable laxity, particularly in rotation and anteroposterior motion when no compressive load is acting.[55,92,170,171] This laxity decreases progressively as compressive load is applied but, even at loads of three times body weight, the laxity is still significant. In laboratory tests, the more the joint is forced to move in a restricted path in one plane, the less are the laxities in other planes.[92,108] It therefore appears that laxity performs the very important function of attenuating the forces on the joint

surfaces by permitting additional freedom of motion of the joint, transferring forces to the ligaments and muscles. Conversely, excessive constraint in one plane (such as a highly conforming patella-femoral joint) may limit motion in other planes. Clearly, there are strong reasons for designing replacement joint surfaces that provide laxity characteristics similar to those of the normal knee.

Stability in the normal joint depends on a complex interaction of the muscles, the ligaments, and the joint surfaces. In most situations, force analysis shows that the knee is not stabilized by muscle action alone, but that certain force imbalances are borne by the ligaments and joint surfaces (Fig. 121-5).

In the arthritic knee, the musculature is often weak, but the posterior cruciate ligament and the collateral ligaments are usually intact, although the latter may display a length imbalance. Assuming optimal alignment, it is axiomatic that the external forces and moments that are not stabilized by muscles are stabilized by the remaining ligaments and by the geometry of the prosthetic surfaces. The aims of joint replacement (other than replacement of the bearing surfaces) are to restore adequate stability and motion to the joint.

The mechanism of stability in a prosthetic joint is essentially an interaction between the geometry of the condylar surfaces and the remaining soft tissue structures. If conforming surfaces are chosen for stability, wear is reduced, but motion is sacrificed and stress is transferred to the interface. By contrast, if nonconforming geometry is chosen, motion is gained and interface stresses are lowered, but surgical technique is more exacting to ensure adequate stability and the problem of wear is acclerated.

Mediolateral Translation

The femorotibial force in this direction has been estimated to be from 0.2 × body weight,[102,103] to 2.5 times this force.[105] In any case, the force will be borne primarily by the intercondylar eminence.[92] The excessive translation that can result from the absence of such an eminence on a prosthesis has been demonstrated and was a common cause of

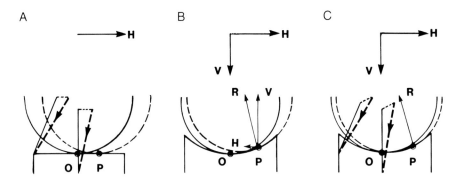

Fig. 121-5. Mechanisms of stability to a horizontal force. **(A)** Stability is first from the cruciate ligament, second from the collateral ligament. The joint surfaces provide no stability. **(B)** Stability is entirely from the partially conforming surfaces. **(C)** Stability is from the surfaces, the cruciate ligaments, and the vertical collateral ligaments. (From Insall,[60] with permission.)

failure of hemiarthroplasties and early bicompartmental prostheses.[33]

Anteroposterior Translation

Nissan[105] calculated forces in level walking of up to 200 newtons forward force on the femur relative to the tibia and 100 newtons in the other direction; these forces translate into 400 newtons and 200 newtons in the posterior and anterior cruciates, respectively. However, walking upstairs or up a ramp produces as much as 1,200 newtons and 500 newtons, respectively, in the posterior cruciate.[102] In stooping, the anterior shear force of the femur on the tibia was calculated at 1.3 body weight, giving about twice that force in the posterior cruciate.[26,135] The highest demands are placed on the posterior cruciate; in a prosthesis, these forces must be stabilized either by a retained posterior cruciate ligament, by the conformity of the bearing surfaces (including cruciate substituting pegs), or by both. For a conforming geometry, the surfaces carry all the forces, and stability is unaffected by the presence or absence of the cruciates[93] (Fig. 121-6). In a partially conforming geometry, it is difficult to arrange for a sharing of the force. If there is close conformity, most of the force will be carried by the condylar surfaces. As flexion proceeds, however, the smaller radius of the posterior femoral condyles comes into play concurrent with a rollback of the contact point. In this situation, the condyles will offer little stability. In tests of force

transmission in prosthetic components of different curvatures, with and without the posterior cruciate ligament, the shear force transmitted to the tibial interface was always substantially higher in the absence of the posterior cruciate.[150,151]

Further aspects that would affect the force distribution are stiffness of the cruciate ligament, tightness after prosthetic insertion, and variation in tightness, attributable to prosthetic geometry and position, through the range of flexion.[85] This association has been clearly shown in bench tests before and after insertion of knee prostheses of various geometries, with and without the cruciates. Conforming geometry with cruciate retention produces excessive forces in the ligaments and at the interfaces; nonconforming geometry requires additional stability from either an intercondylar peg or the posterior cruciate.[83,93] Such considerations explain the practical difficulty of retaining both cruciate ligaments. To achieve effective functioning of both throughout the range would require accuracy of design and placement to within an estimated 2 mm of the ideal.

Varus-Valgus Angulation

During normal activities, such as walking, a few degrees of varus-valgus motion occur. This is caused by the general flexibility of the menisci and cartilage surfaces, some sliding of the femoral condyles on the changing slope of the tibial surfaces and, in extreme cases, to lift off on one side.[92] As the

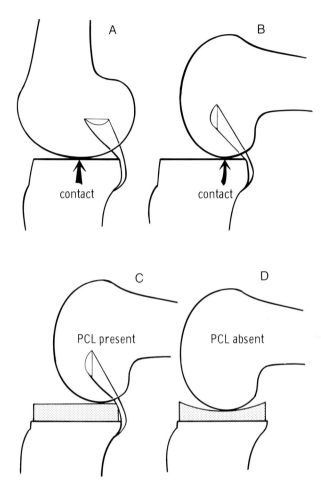

Fig. 121-6. The effect of posterior cruciate retention on prosthetic design. **(A,B)** Because of the rollback enforced by the posterior cruciate ligament (PCL) the prosthetic tibial surface must be flat to permit this movement. **(C)** When the PCL is absent, a dished tibial plateau is used for stability. (From Insall,[60] with permission.)

arthritic knee is usually deformed in the varus-valgus plane, resistance to tilting is an advantage. A prosthesis with a broad base of contact and preservation of one or both cruciate ligaments will assist the prime stabilizers, the collateral ligaments.

Rotation About the Tibial Axis

In vivo studies have recorded rotations in the range of 10 to 20 degrees occurring during normal activities. Recent work[76] has shown that this trans-verse rotation occurs by rolling backward of the lateral femoral condyle, with the medial condyle being stationary or even moving forward. This rotational laxity in full extension is small, constrained by tense collateral and cruciate ligaments, combined with conformity of the joint surfaces and the menisci. In flexion, however, there is considerable rotational laxity, primarily because of the loss of conformity of the joint surfaces and slackening of the ligaments. It appears that laxity of rotation, particularly in flexion, will allow the knee to accommodate readily to different activity patterns by adjusting its rotational path.[1,2] Prosthetic geometry that prevents or restricts laxity will not provide these characteristics and will transfer loads to the bone-cement interface.

THE POSTERIOR CRUCIATE LIGAMENT

It is evident that the posterior cruciate ligament (PCL) is involved both in passive attenuation of knee forces and in actively controlling knee motion. As the knee flexes, the eccentric position of the PCL femoral origin produces a tensile force in the ligament. Because of the nonconforming low-friction articulation, this tensile force is converted into a translatory force, shifting the tibia forward (or forcing the femur to roll back). This rollback produces two major effects: posterior clearance is increased, permitting greater flexion without impingement, and the moment arm of the quadriceps is increased by 20 to 30 percent (Fig. 121-7).

Total knee designs that resect the PCL must provide AP stability by having congruent geometry in flexion to avoid sagittal instability (Fig. 121-8). This geometry permits essentially uniaxial flexion with less flexion arc[1,2] and produces a quadriceps force that is demonstrably weaker[151] (Fig. 121-9). Posterior cruciate function may be built into the prosthesis by an appropriately shaped intercondylar tibial eminence articulating in flexion with the femoral component.[65] This design maximizes flexion and quadriceps power but transfers shear forces normally absorbed by the posterior cruciate

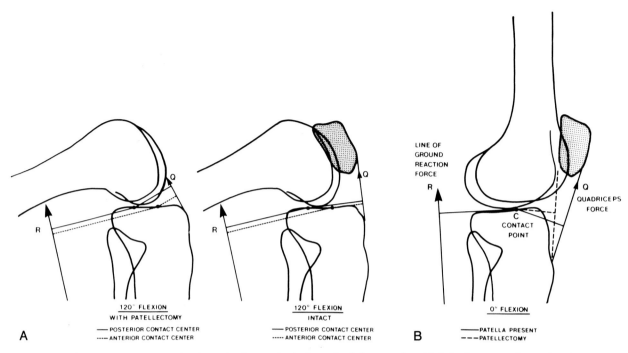

Fig. 121-7. Forces about the knee in the sagittal plane. In full extension **(right)**, the ground reaction force moment arm *(R-C)* is balanced by the quadriceps moment arm *(Q-C)*. In flexion **(left, center)**, as the contact point rolls posteriorly, the quadriceps moment arm increases by approximately 30 percent. This mechanism enhances the strength of the quadriceps, hence the ability of patients to ascend and descend stairs. (From Insall,[60] with permission.)

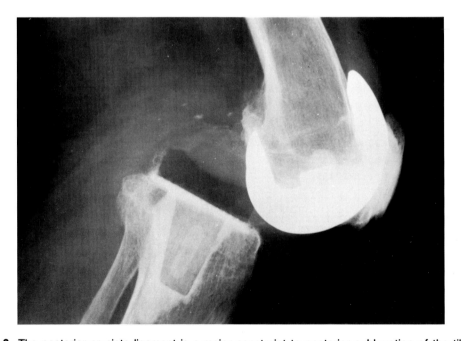

Fig. 121-8. The posterior cruciate ligament is a major constraint to posterior subluxation of the tibia. In its absence (especially if the patella is also absent), subluxation may occur in cruciate-excising knee replacements, unless secondary constraints such as the collateral ligaments and posterior contour of the tibial component provide sufficient stability. (From Insall,[60] with permission.)

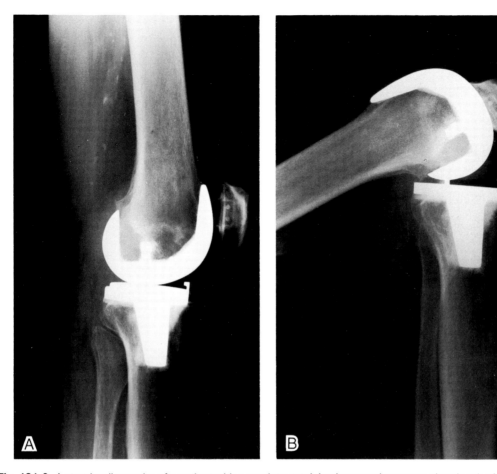

Fig. 121-9. Lateral radiographs of a patient with a cruciate-retaining knee replacement, showing the full range of motion with the contact point moving from an anterior position **(A)** to a posterior position **(B)**. The excursion in this instance was about 10 mm. (From Insall,[60] with permission.)

ligament to the bone-cement interface. High stresses are also transferred to the patella and fractures have been reported with increased frequency.[60]

The PCL is not often involved in osteoarthritis, but in juvenile rheumatoid arthritis with long-standing flexion deformity of severe degree, the ligament and the posterior capsule are often shortened and must be resected to correct the flexion deformity. In that situation, it is necessary to use a cruciate-substituting prosthesis. In osteoarthritis or adult-onset rheumatoid arthritis, however, deformity or absence of the ligament is exceedingly rare. Indeed, in more than 3,000 total knee arthroplasties done in our unit, the ligament has been absent or severely attenuated only three times and

contracted enough to produce a flexion deformity in three additional patients. Thus, in only six cases of 3,000 has a cruciate-substituting device been necessary in primary arthroplasties.

Criticism of the concept of cruciate retention includes some of the following disadvantages:

1. The anterior cruciate, posterior cruciate, and the bone separating their origins and their insertions consitute a rigid four-bar link, defining the envelope of motion of the knee in the sagittal plane. If both ligaments are retained, the arthroplasty surfaces must conform to that envelope (in both design and placement) within about 2 mm if "jamming" and excessive stress transfer are to be avoided. It is unrealistic to

expect enough implant sizes or sufficient surgical accuracy of placement to meet that requirement.

2. It is easier to resect the entire upper tibia, including the intercondylar spine, than to save the 1 cm posterior block that protects the posterior cruciate ligament tibial insertion.

3. The normal function of the PCL is to produce rollback of the femur on the tibia. If this is extreme (from an overly tight PCL), the tibial component will be alternately loaded in its central portion, then posteriorly, producing a seesaw effect (Fig. 121-10) with some threat to tibial fixation. (These stresses are offset by the intermedullary stem on the tibial component. Less secure tibial fixation might be suspect.)

4. The geometry of the tibial surface must be nearly flat posteriorly to permit rollback without impingement or excessive stress on the tibial fixation. This diminished congruity between femur and tibia results in greater stress concentration in the high-density polyethylene with the risk of increased wear[178] (Fig. 121-11).

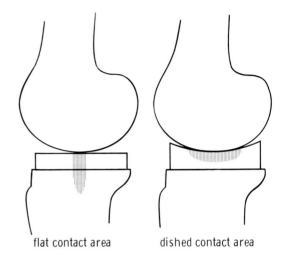

flat contact area   dished contact area

Fig. 121-11. The disadvantage of a flat tibial component (in addition to decreased saggital stability) is the high concentration of stress in the polyethylene tibial surface. (From Insall,[60] with permission.)

In 8- to 10-year follow-up studies it has been demonstrated that both cruciate retention and cruciate resection techniques give similar results in terms of revision for loosening.[63,143] There have been virtually no instances of revision for excessive plastic wear with either concept. The major difference in the two approaches has been in range of motion and function. Cruciate retention results in an average of 109 degrees of flexion,[142] while cruciate excision has given an average of about 100 degrees.[64,125] Function is also improved by cruciate retention. The greater flexion facilitates rising from the seated position[68] and going up and down stairs.[2]

Cruciate Substitution

There is now wide agreement that the functions of the PCL (stress sharing, AP stability, and rollback) are useful in the prosthetic knee. The debate continues, however, over whether to provide these functions by retaining the ligament or by substituting for the ligament in the design of the implant. Insall and Burstein[65] have taken the latter approach with the posterior stabilized knee (Fig. 121-12). Because of the shape of the tibial intercondylar extension, articulating with the femoral compo-

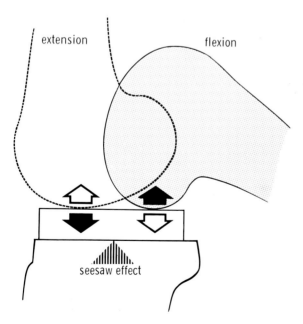

extension   flexion

seesaw effect

Fig. 121-10. If rollback is excessive and the tibial component is not stabilized by an intermedullary peg, a seesaw effect may be produced creating a rocking motion that may produce loosening. (From Insall,[60] with permission.)

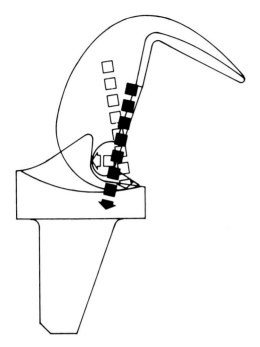

Fig. 121-12. One solution to the problem of allowing roll-back with its enhanced flexion arc while avoiding the see-saw effect is seen in the posterior stabilized condylar prosthesis. The contact point does move posteriorly with flexion, but the resultant force across the contact point is always directed through the fixation peg, minimizing rocking of the tibial component. (From Insall,[65] with permission.)

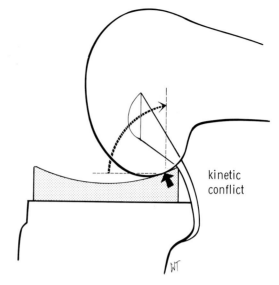

Fig. 121-13. It is important not to confuse the concepts of cruciate excision and cruciate retention. If the cruciate ligament is retained, the tibial component must be flat posteriorly to permit rollback. If a constrained tibial component is used and the cruciate ligament is retained, impingement and loss of flexion may result. (From Insall,[60] with permission.)

nent, rollback becomes obligatory. This increases potential flexion, increases quadriceps power, and permits better function. The price has been increased stress on the patella with more frequent patellar fractures.[60]

On balance, it seems preferable to retain the posterior cruciate ligament in knees undergoing primary replacement with moderate varus or valgus deformity and less than 30 degrees of permanent flexion deformity. In revisions, or in knees in which deformity is great and/or the PCL is a deforming structure, cruciate substitution is preferable. It must be emphasized that the surgical technique for the two approaches is different and the design of the prosthesis required for each is different; the PCL should not be retained when using a prosthesis in which there is a conforming geometry between femur and tibia in the sagittal plane (rolling pin-in-trough) (Fig. 121-13).

FIXATION OF IMPLANTS

Virtually none of the modern knee replacement designs has failed because of loss of fixation of the femoral component. An anatomic shape, capping the corticocancellous bone of the distal femur, has broad interface surfaces in both flexion and extension. With close contact between the condylar runners of the implant and the dense bone of the posterior femur, very little shear stress is transmitted to the bone-cement interface in flexion. In extension, the distal femur is well covered by the prosthesis and the cancellous bone is usually dense and supports stresses well.

Strength of Tibial Trabecular Bone

Failures of total knee replacements have largely been at the interface between the tibial component and the underlying tibial bone. The trabecular bone of the proximal tibia is highly variable in quantity and strength from place to place in the same knee, both the normal and arthritic.[59] There is a dramatic decrease in strength at increasing depth from the subchondral surface, suggesting that it is wise to minimize tibial resection to seat the component in the strongest available bone.[8] On the deformed side in an osteoarthritic knee, except in areas of cyst formation, the trabecular bone is much denser and stronger than normal; in rheumatoid arthritis, it is generally weaker and more porous and contains more cystic areas than does normal bone. The compressive strength of trabecular bone in the proximal tibia varies between 11 and 260 percent of normal, the higher values being for sclerotic bone in the lateral plateau of knees with valgus deformity[79,80]; the subchondral bone on the medial plateau, in rheumatoid bone, demonstrated about one-half the hardness of normal subchondral bone.

The limited data available suggest that some portions of the tibial trabecular bone, especially in rheumatoid arthritis (RA), are much weaker than normal. It might be considered that such bone would be inadequate for normal load-bearing, but presumably the limited usage and light weight of most patients with RA prevent excessive failure of the bone. After prosthetic replacement, it is expected that the activity level will increase significantly. Given the deficiencies in the properties of rheumatoid trabecular bone and areas of weakness in osteoarthritic bone, it is particularly important that the stresses on the implant-bone interface be minimized. Various types of tibial components have been compared in laboratory studies by subjecting them to a sequence of loads and moments and measuring the component-to-bone movements.[10,37,113,165,167,168] Modular components deflected the most, whereas the best performance overall was demonstrated by one-piece metal-backed components with one or two fixation pegs and with or without a posterior cruciate cut-out. Metal trays generally distributed the forces better and reduced the maximum compressive stresses on the underlying cancellous bone compared with the all-plastic components. Plastic pegs carry only a small percent of the compressive load, but metal pegs carry about 25 percent.[6,113]

The features of a metal tray, reduction in compressive stresses on cancellous bone attributable to better stress distribution and load carrying by the central peg, are seen as advantages in the weak bone, which may be relatively unstressed before arthroplasty but which will become more stressed as the patient resumes a more active life-style after joint replacement. In cruciate-substituting designs, the additional stability conveyed by a central peg or stem is desirable to offset the increased stress transmitted from the cruciate-substituting intercondylar eminence.

Fixation with Methyl Methacrylate

Regardless of the sophistication of design and retention of the PCL, stresses will be transmitted to the tibial implant-bone interface. If acrylic cement is used for fixation, interdigitation with strong cancellous bone is essential. The strongest available bone must be used by judicious resection of the upper tibia; deficient areas should be bone-grafted, and a tibial component providing maximal coverage of the resected plateau must be chosen. Interface strength will then depend on the amount of penetration of acrylic into the cancellous interstices. Figure 121-14A shows an example of trabecular bone in which the acrylic cement has barely penetrated the matrix. Many of the trabecular ends are not held at all by the cement, while only the tips of others are encased. When a shear force is applied, cement-bone micromotion will occur at the tips, while the high bending stresses in other trabeculae will lead to resorption or fracture; tensile forces will clearly lead to micromotion at the interface. In the example in Figure 121-14B, showing penetration of a few millimeters, the trabecular ends are firmly held, and the stiffness and resistance to compression, shear, and tension will be greatly enhanced.

Measurements of bond strength show the significance of penetration depth. Using trabecular bone from the knee, Krause et al.[75] obtained tensile strengths ranging from 2.5 to 8 mPa, with the higher values for more thorough bone cleaning and greater depth of penetration. Shear strength values also increased. However, the interface at the limit of penetration is much weaker, with strength of about one-third of these values.[53] As failures will

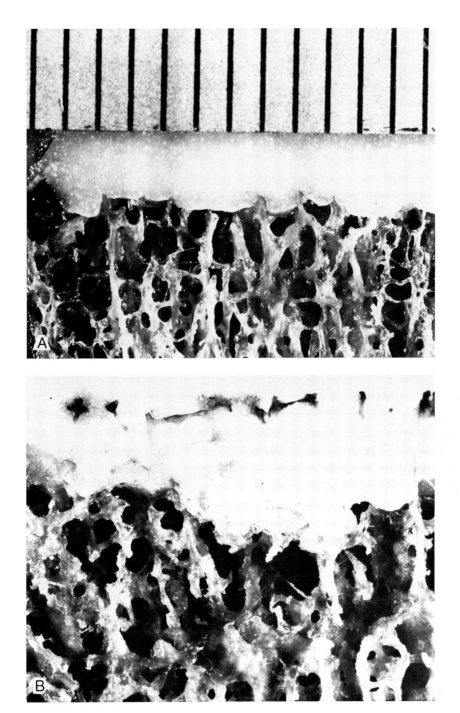

Fig. 121-14. (A) Trabecular bone and cement, showing poor penetration of cement after inadequate bone preparation and pressurization. **(B)** Improved penetration after surface cleaning and pressurization of the cement. (From Insall,[60] with permission.)

occur at the limit of penetration and the bone is weaker at these lower levels, the bone strength will be lower for excessive penetration. In addition, if failure does occur farther into the bone, much more bone has been lost for the revision. The viability of the bone encased in cement must also be questioned, as well as the weakening effect of the trabeculae on the cement mantle. Heat necrosis will almost certainly occur for penetration ≥5 mm.[57]

Taking all factors into consideration, it appears that the ideal penetration depth is 3 to 5 mm, which would effectively bond to many cross-struts of the trabecular bone as well as to the verticals. The aim of the surgical technique should be to choose the correct viscosity of cement and apply sufficient pressure to force it uniformly into the bone to this ideal depth.

Another aspect of tibial fixation that is often overlooked is the amount of coverage of the tibial surface by the component. Clinical failures in which an undersized component has gradually subsided into the bone are widely reported. Complete coverage has been shown to reduce the component-bone movement considerably under a variety of load conditions.[22,165]

On the basis of laboratory studies, confirmed by clinical experience, the tibial interface must be protected by appropriate prosthetic geometry, by adequate stiffness of the tibial component to equalize stresses, by minimal tibial resection to retain the strongest bone, and by utilization of the entire surface area available. In addition, cement techniques should be optimized (unless designs for uncemented use prove effective).

Fixation of the femoral component has been studied relatively little, probably because of a lower incidence of recognized loosening. However, principles similar to those discussed for the tibial side apply. A metallic component for better stress distribution and maximum area of coverage are two important aspects. The areas that generally give the highest incidence of interface failure are the patellar flange and the posterior condyles. It is important to note that these are areas of poor cement intrusion at surgery and have a high shear stress when loaded during walking. Fixation as a whole is preserved by the distal surface, as well as by the fixation pegs. The usefulness of a central

fixation stem has not been demonstrated but is often empirically chosen in rheumatoid patients in whom the quality of femoral cancellous bone is found to be particularly poor or during revision in which a large portion of the cancellous bone must be destroyed during the surgical procedure.

It has been difficult to obtain reliable laboratory data on implant fixation; bench tests may indicate the fate of cemented implants but give little indication of the role of biological fixation in uncemented implants. Studies on autopsy material, more closely resembling the in vivo situation, are too few to be

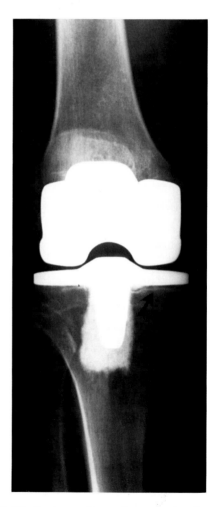

Fig. 121-15. Postoperative radiograph showing a broad lucent line under the medial side of the tibial component. There is no radiolucency at the bone-cement interface surrounding the intermedullary peg. The patient was entirely asymptomatic.

predictive. Radiographic analysis has shown a high (up to 60 percent) incidence of radiolucent lines in clinically successful implants (Fig. 121-15). Some portion of the tibial interface has shown such lucency in 35 percent of our cases with average 6-year follow-up but only 1 knee of 192 has required revision for tibial loosening. On the femoral side, 29 percent showed a lucent line in at least one zone, with no failures. Clearly, lucent lines are common, most are nonprogressive, and they do not predict failure unless extensive (more than 1.5 mm thick) or progressive.

Some indicator of insecure fixation, more sensitive than ordinary radiographs, is needed. In studies using roentgen stereophotogrammetric analysis (RSA) following implantation of small metal beads into the skeleton adjacent to the implant, the technique was found to have an accuracy 10 times better than conventional radiography. Two types of micromotion of the tibial component were identified: migration, or gradual motion over time, and deflection, or instant motion in response to external load. Eighty-nine clinically successful arthroplasties were studied from 2 to 5 years after surgery: 51 conventionally cemented all-polyethylene prostheses, 27 total and 24 unicompartmental, and 7 metal-backed tibial components were studied. Migration was found for all prostheses, with a mean maximum of 1.2 mm after 4 years. In all groups, the major part of the migration occurred during the first year, after which most components did not migrate further. Some prostheses, with greater migration during the first year, continued to migrate throughout the investigation. All prostheses showed reversible inducible displacement, the maximum deflection ranging from 0.2 to 1.0 mm. Ryd reported that "measurable migration and inducible displacement may be the rule rather than an exception in total knee arthroplasty. Accordingly, absolute rigid fixation may not be necessary for successful function of a TKA."[118,119]

Fixation by Bone Ingrowth

Reports thus far, analyzing bone ingrowth into uncemented tibial components, suggest that such ingrowth occurs rarely and to a limited extent of

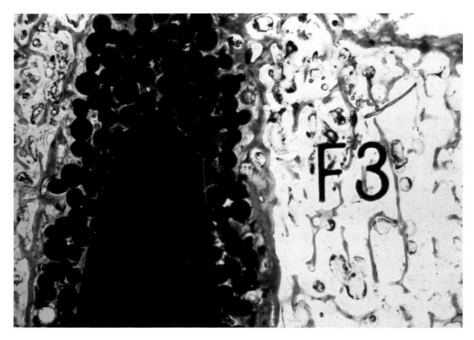

Fig. 121-16. Histologic section showing bone ingrowth into the beaded surface of the fixation peg of a femoral component removed at revision surgery. Such ingrowth is commonly seen on the femoral side, infrequently on the tibial side.

the available surface[110] (Fig. 121-16). This lack of predictable ingrowth into the tibial surface is probably related to unavoidable micromotion at the implant-bone interface.[118,119,154,163] Lack of rigid tibial fixation may not be associated with symptoms or early failure[58] but does result in less predictable clinical results[154] with a higher complication rate than cement fixation[111] and a higher reoperation rate.[15] Given the success rate of cemented knee arthroplasties with 6- and 10-year follow-up (our unpublished data; Insall[63]), further data on the long-term behavior of ingrowth prostheses should be awaited before wide acceptance of the concept.

Another approach to cementless fixation has been proposed by Freeman et al.[42,43] In this approach, polyethylene plugs with multiple horozontal fins are driven into the cancellous bone, providing immediate fixation.

THE PATELLOFEMORAL JOINT

Early surface-replacement designs (e.g., Polycentric, Geometric, Duocondylar,[34,164] ICLH[44]) ignored the patellofemoral joint and provided neither a resurfacing prosthesis for the patella nor a resurfacing of the patellar groove of the femur (Fig. 121-17). Pain, attributable to progression of the lesion in the patellofemoral joint, was common and became one of the most frequent causes for revision.[18,84,109,117,161] Because of this, designs such as the Duopatellar and Total Condylar quickly gained acceptance, as they provided an anterior femoral flange with automatic resurfacing of one side of the patellofemoral joint. The incidence of revision for patellofemoral pain diminished with those designs but did not disappear.[126,142]

The patella is routinely resurfaced in patients with RA. There is strong clinical and laboratory evidence that articular cartilage in the rheumatoid joint perpetuates the inflammatory response of the synovium.[24,141] With all cartilage excised, the inflamed synovium becomes quiescent. It is not necessary to perform a synovectomy at the time of knee replacement if all cartilage is removed. Furthermore, with the cartilage removed, the oper-

ated joint will not become involved in subsequent flares of rheumatoid activity. Conversely, a knee with the patellar cartilage retained may continue to be mildly inflamed and may participate in flares of inflammatory activity with the possibility of progressive destruction of the remaining patellar cartilage and the possiblity of resorption at the bone–cement interface.

In patients with osteoarthritis, controversy remains.[149] There are those who maintain that the quality of result after patellar resurfacing is improved to the point that it should be routine in all total knee arthroplasties[19,60,82,133] (Fig. 121-18). Others maintain a more selective approach, resurfacing those patellae that are badly arthritic or do not track well in the femoral groove, but leaving those with essentially normal articular cartilage on the patella (Fig. 121-19). This group maintains that the frequency of complications of patellar resurfacing outweighs the frequency of revision to correct an unresurfaced patella.[130] It would appear wise to err on the side of resurfacing most patellae. Patellar fracture or dislocation after such resurfacing is now less common than continued wear and pain produced by the articulation of imperfect articular cartilage with the metal femoral flange.

Patellectomy, as a solution to continued pain in the patellofemoral joint, must be discouraged. The patella is so important in its role of enhancement of power of extension that it should be preserved if at all possible. In patients who have undergone patellectomy prior to total knee arthroplasty, it must be borne in mind that the mechanics of the knee are altered and one of the major restraints to anterior dislocation of the femur has been removed.[7] In the presence of the patella, the patellar tendon is nearly parallel to the PCL; after patellectomy, the patellar tendon drops into the femoral groove during flexion and loses this parallel alignment. If the posterior cruciate ligament is excised in such a patient, there remains very little resistance to such dislocation. Therefore, in patients who have had patellectomy, it is mandatory to use either a posterior cruciate retaining or cruciate-substituting prosthesis that provides resistance to anterior translation of the femur on the tibia.

If the patella is to be replaced, the design of the component must be appropriate for the femoral component being used. To avoid excessive wear,

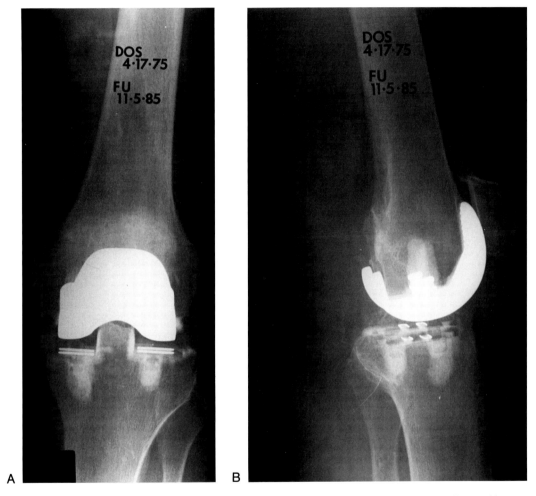

Fig. 121-17. **(A)** AP radiograph of a patient who underwent a Duopatellar total knee arthroplasty with separate plastic tibial components in 1975. This is a 10-year follow-up radiograph showing maintenance of optimal component position and the absence of significant radiolucent lines. **(B)** Lateral radiograph of the same patient. The patella was unresurfaced and remains asymptomatic.

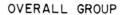

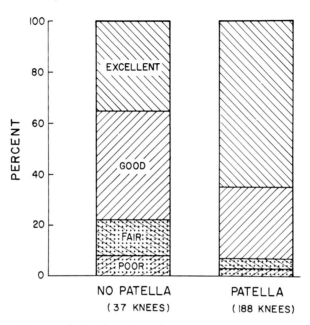

Fig. 121-18. Resurfacing of the patella in this series of patients produces some improvement in the overall clinical score. (From Insall,[60] with permission.)

congruence should be maximized; to avoid loosening, constraint, especially in rotation between patellar button and femur, should be minimized; to avoid fracture of the underlying patellar bone, resection should be minimal and fixation holes small. These requirements are best met by an all-plastic button that is a segment of a sphere and fixed to the patellar bone with small lugs. A metal tray, which has theoretical advantages, has been associated with some instances of acclerated wear between the edge of the metal tray and the matal flange of the femoral component, separated by only a very thin thickness of polyethylene (Walker PS, Ewald FC, personal communication) (Fig. 121-20).

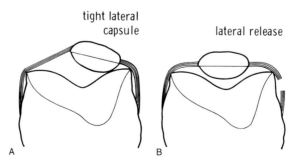

Fig. 121-19. A tight lateral capsule may produce either lateral tilting of the patella or frank lateral dislocation. Following adequate lateral release, tracking is improved. (From Insall,[60] with permission.)

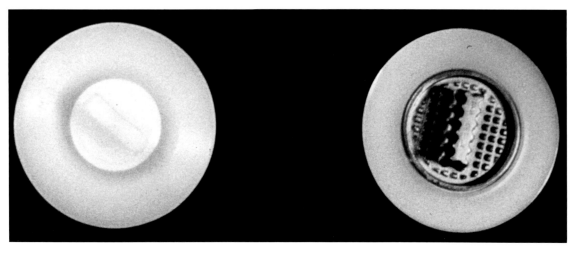

Fig. 121-20. Undersurface of two patellar prostheses. The one on the left is all plastic, and the one on the right has a metal tray and fixation lug.

ALIGNMENT

Alignment refers to the relationship of each prosthetic component to the relevant bone as well as the overall alignment of the limb. In the sagittal plane (lateral view), most techniques recommend placement of the implants at right angles to the long axis of the tibia and femur. Some techniques recommend a slight (5 to 10 degree) posterior slope of the tibial component to facilitate flexion by avoiding the possibility of excessive ligament tightness in flexion. Our studies indicate that the surgeon is very accurate in this plane; the femoral component averages 4 degrees of flexion, and the tibial component averages 1 degree of posterior slope. The range of error for both was very narrow, and no correlation was seen between the extremes of error and failure.

In the frontal or AP plane, however, alignment is thought to be critical; special devices should be used to ensure appropriate alignment during the surgical procedure.[4,35,40,41,54,61] Alignment can be described in reference to the weight-bearing axis from the center of the femoral head to the center of the ankle or to the relationship between the long axis of the femur and the long axis of the tibia (in

which case physiologic alignment is 7 to 9 degrees of valgus angulation). (Fig. 121-21). Ideally, the implants should be placed at right angles to the weight-bearing axis and would therefore be in 0 to 3 degrees of varus for the tibial component and 7 to 9 degrees of valgus for the femoral component (relative to the long axis of the femur). As it is easier to cut right angles than 3 degrees off the right angle and a varus error in the tibia is the most common error with significant implications, most techniques call for resection of the upper tibia at 90 degrees to its long axis.

The appropriate position of the femoral component can be chosen either by using an intramedullary alignment device to locate the long axis of the femur or by correctly positioning the entire limb so that the weight-bearing axis is straight with the femur resected parallel to the tibial resection (Fig. 121-22).

Valgus errors appear to be well tolerated, while varus errors are not.[40,62,86] One analysis of results with the ICLH prosthesis revealed that, in knees with overall alignment between 1 degree and 13 degrees of valgus, the success rate at 5 to 9 years follow-up was 89 percent. In patients with knees aligned between neutral and 8 degrees varus, the success rate was only 14 percent.[4,9] In another study, 49 of 56 failures were attributed to malalignment.[35]

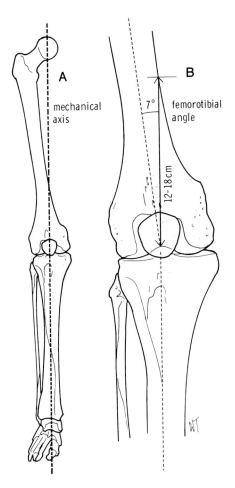

Fig. 121-21. (A) The mechanical axis of the knee is a line connecting the center of the femoral head with the center of the talus. Normally this line passes through the intercondylar notch of the tibia. (B) The anatomic axis is the midline of the femoral shaft and normally forms an angle of 7 to 9 degrees with the mechanical axis. (From Insall,[60] with permission.)

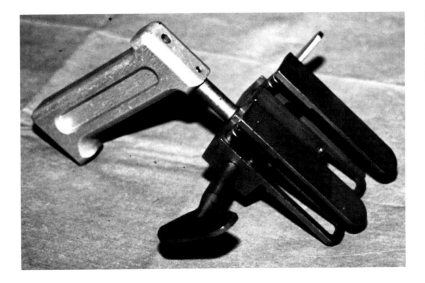

Fig. 121-22. A simple and effective device for adjusting ligament tension and assuring correct alignment of the resection cuts based on an intermedullary rod.

By contrast, Tew and Waugh[156] reported on 428 knee replacements followed for 1 to 9 years. They found that one-half of the failures occurred in knees correctly aligned at operation; stating that "malalignment, in itself, may not be the most important cause of failure, though it probably does compound failure from other causes."

Another aspect of alignment that appears to be important is the location of the implants relative to the normal joint line in the lateral view. Functional knee scores, range of motion, patellofemoral pain and mechanical symptoms, and the need for revision could all be statistically correlated with errors in location of the prosthetic joint line in a recent study.[38] Because of the wider gap created by cruciate excision, error in joint line placement is more likely with such prostheses, and an attempt must always be made to restore the normal location of the articulation. In revisions, this will often necessitate bone grafting to restore lost tibial or femoral height or use of a custom prosthesis with additional thickness of metal in areas of bone deficit.

INDICATIONS AND CONTRAINDICATIONS FOR KNEE ARTHROPLASTY

Indications for Knee Arthroplasty

Total knee arthroplasty has become so predictable in its outcome that it need no longer be used only as an alternative to arthrodesis. In a patient with severe pain and loss of function related to arthritis of the knee, total knee arthroplasty may be considered using the following guidelines:

In patients with rheumatoid arthritis there are virtually no alternatives for the painful knee with radiographic evidence of advanced destruction. Therefore, such patients may be considered for total knee arthroplasty regardless of their age. It is understood that such patients will rarely return to activity levels that will compromise the longevity of the implant and their functional improvement is so great that the benefits outweigh the risks for most patients.

In patients with osteoarthritis, several factors must be taken into account: age, weight, activity level, and the presence or absence of other limitations of function. In the young active patient with only one knee joint involved, every effort should be made to avoid total knee arthroplasty by medical management or tibial osteotomy for unicompartmental disease. It should be noted that a previous tibial osteotomy may make knee arthroplasty slightly more difficult, technically,[71] but the results are unaffected.[152]

Contraindications to Knee Arthroplasty

Most contraindications to knee arthroplasty are relative. Youthfulness of the patient is a relative contraindication and must be taken into consideration in the overall context of alternatives available (e.g., further conservative treatment, tibial osteotomy).

Excessive weight will almost certainly have a deleterious effect on the durability of the implant and/or its fixation, although precise data are not available, and function, in one study, was not affected by patient weight.[146] Every effort should be made to have patients achieve near-normal weight before surgery in order to lessen perioperative complications and prolong the life of the implant.

Isolated patellofemoral arthritis is not an indication for total knee replacement; this rare condition usually follows chondromalacia patellae of adolescence. In the fourth decade, some such patients develop isolated patellofemoral arthritis. This is occasionally severe enough to necessitate patellectomy. As patellectomy does not appear to prejudice the results of subsequent knee arthroplasty, it probably represents a better treatment for severe patellofemoral degeneration than does prosthetic replacement.

Neuropathic joints have shown high rates of failure in earlier series using constrained devices. More recent experience with unconstrained surface replacements suggests that adequate longevity of the implant can be expected in such patients if alignment is correct and proper ligament tension is reestablished.[148]

A solid bony arthrodesis of the knee is a contraindication to knee arthroplasty. The range of motion achieved after arthroplasty in such patients is not good.[104] It would be of questionable judgment to sacrifice a painless supportive arthrodesis for the uncertainty of arthroplasty with limited motion. Furthermore, the anticipated absence of collateral ligaments in this situation would probably necessitate the use of a constrained implant, with its attendant problems.

In patients with paralysis or gross weakness of the quadriceps muscle, a prosthetic knee will not function well, and the stresses transferred to the fixation interface by hyperextension will probably lead to early failure.

Acute pyogenic infection is an absolute contraindication to primary joint replacement. (The man-

agement of an infected prosthesis and one-stage revision of such prostheses are discussed in Ch. 167.) In patients with tuberculosis, thorough debridement after appropriate antituberculous medication appears to allow safe joint replacement as a primary procedure.

The destructive arthritis of the knee seen in some patients with hemophilia responds well to knee replacement.[77,90,145] The early fears that repeated bleeding might occur at the interface, leading to loss of fixation, have not been borne out by experience. Adequate replacement of factor VIII must be carried out, and precautions against transmission of acquired immune deficiency syndrome (AIDS) must be rigorous.

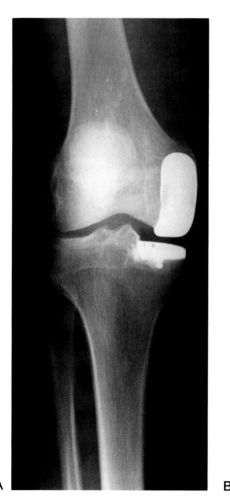
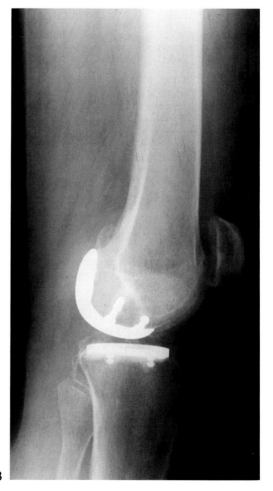

Fig. 121-23. AP and lateral radiographs illustrating the postoperative appearance of a patient who underwent unicompartmental arthroplasty on the medial side. Limb alignment and component alignment are ideal.

UNICOMPARTMENTAL KNEE REPLACEMENT

Unicompartmental replacement remains controversial. Some authorities have reported unacceptably high failure rates, due either to loosening of the prosthetic components[91,123] or to accelerated deterioration of the unreplaced compartment of the knee.[66] There are, however, numerous reports of excellent results, including some 5- to 10-year results.[3,67,128,137,158] A recent report compared two similar populations, one of which underwent high tibial osteotomy and the other unicompartmental replacement. At 5- to 10-year follow-up, the results of unicompartmental replacement were clearly superior.[13]

Our results have been comparable to the results of total knee arthroplasty with approximately 1 percent failure per year.[128] (Fig. 121-23). The advantages of unicompartmental replacement over tricompartmental replacement are that the range of motion following unicompartmental replacement is nearly normal and less bone stock is sacrificed so that either subsequent arthrodesis or revision to total knee arthroplasty can be carried out with sufficient bone stock.[5] Comparison with high tibial osteotomy suggests advantages in range of motion (which can be improved after unicompartmental replacement but not after tibial osteotomy), virtually complete elimination of pain versus partial relief for osteotomy and lack of a compensatory deformity (the 11 to 14 degrees of valgus following a tibial osteotomy). Disadvantages are related primarily to the use of prosthetic components with concerns about infection and loosening. Infection has been an infrequent complication of knee arthroplasty, in general, and failure rates of unicompartmental arthroplasty have been very similar to those for total knee arthroplasty. It has been argued that unicompartmental replacements would fail because the base of support for the prosthetic components is small, especially on the tibial side. The infrequency of that failure mode is probably attributable to the fact that the procedure is done in unicompartmental osteoarthritis (OA) where the subchondral bone of the femur and the tibia have undergone compensatory hypertrophy

with increased strength and stiffness. Early failures were attributable to the use of thin polyethylene without metal support, but most designs now incorporate a metal tray and thicker polyethylene tibial components. Retention of both cruciate ligaments allows nearly allows normal range of motion and function; both are also enhanced by retention of the patellofemoral joint.

BILATERAL KNEE ARTHROPLASTIES

Many patients (32 percent in our experience) will undergo bilateral knee replacements. In some cases, one knee is clearly much more symptomatic than the other, and replacement of the more symptomatic knee gives months to years of satisfactory function before the opposite knee requires surgery. Frequently, however, the patient's function will not be satisfactory until both knees are replaced. Should such patients undergo bilateral replacements on the same day, during the same hospitalization 7 to 10 days apart, or during separate admissions? Several studies have shown that simultaneous bilateral knee arthroplasties are associated with shorter hospitalization, quicker rehabilitation, and less financial burden to society (the complications of thrombophlebitis, pulmonary embolism, infection, and loosening are no higher following such simultaneous bilateral procedures).[12,98,101,147] In appropriate patients, therefore, simultaneous procedures have much to recommend them.

SURGICAL TECHNIQUES

Posterior Cruciate Retention: Author's Preferred Technique

Earlier use of curved median parapatellar incisions led to occasional necrosis of the skin edges, usually on the lateral flap at the superior pole of the patella, where the blood supply is most tenuous.

Because of the likelihood of deep infection in the face of such skin loss, most surgeons now favor straight vertical skin incisions over the patella with a curved parapatellar incision through the capsule (for a conflicting view, see Johnson et al.[69]) Wide exposure of the proximal tibia is useful in order to allow the tibia to be brought forward to visualize its upper surface. This is achieved by a sub-periosteal detachment of the soft tissues on the medial side (Fig. 121-24). Even if there is not a varus deformity, this dissection should include the deep insertion of the medial collateral ligament. If the anterior cruciate is intact, it should be resected. The upper tibia can then be exposed by inserting a dull instrument (e.g., a joker) through the intercondylar notch of the femur, parallel to the PCL, and

levering the tibia forward. The bone surrounding the PCL insertion is outlined using either a saw or osteotomes and a ½-inch osteotome inserted in front of the PCL to a depth of ½ inch to protect the ligament while the proximal tibia is resected. The posterior cruciate ligament inserts on the posterior aspect of the tibia behind and distal to the tibial intercondylar spines. It is therefore possible to resect the entire upper tibia without injuring the ligament, but it is usually desirable to leave a small square of posterior intercondylar eminence to ensure that the ligament is not damaged by the saw during tibial resection.

The tibial surface should be resected first to minimize the amount of bone removed from this vulnerable area (Fig. 121-25). This cut should be precisely parallel to the long axis of the tibia in both planes and just deep enough into the substance of the subchondral bone to provide an appropriate porous interface for interdigitation of cement. An amount of bone equal to the anticipated thickness of the prosthetic tibial component should be resected so that the location of the joint line can be maintained.[38] Massive resection to clear bone defects in the tibia should not be done; bone grafting should be used to fill such defects, minimizing the amount of tibia resected to stay in the strongest available bone and maximizing the surface area available by staying high on the cone-shaped proximal tibia. Small bone defects can be filled with polymethylmethacrylate, using screws into the base of the defect to maintain proper alignment of the component until the cement hardens. For defects greater than 8 to 10 mm, it is preferable to fill the defect with either bone or metal.[11,28,176] The first choice is autogenous bone from the resected femoral condyles if it is sufficient. If not, allograft bone (such as a femoral head) has been perfectly satisfactory. Both types of bone usually require screw fixation to the underlying tibia to avoid cement penetration into the bone-bone interface and provide secure initial fixation to facilitate healing.

Once the upper tibia has been resected, ligament balance can be assessed with the knee in extension and in flexion. The access provided by carrying out tibial resection before ligament release facilitates the latter, while failure to perform ligament release before femoral resection leads to excessive bone resection of the femur and the possibility of persist-

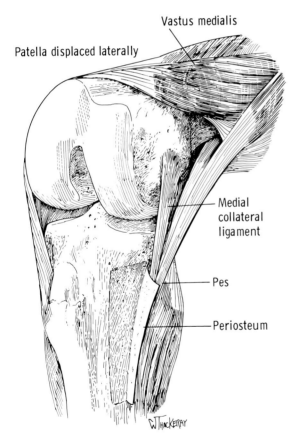

Vastus medialis

Patella displaced laterally

Medial collateral ligament

Pes

Periosteum

Fig. 121-24. Diagrammatic representation of the first stage of a medial release showing subperiosteal elevation of deep insertion of the medial collateral ligament and partial release of the superficial portion of the medial collateral ligament. (From Insall,[60] with permission.)

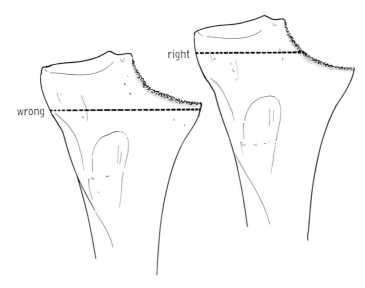

Fig. 121-25. Large defects on one or the other tibial plateau should not be entirely resected, rather the defects should be filled in by bone graft or a custom implant. (From Insall,[60] with permission.)

ent imbalance (Fig. 121-26 to 121-28). Tension in the collateral ligaments can be assessed by a number of different techniques, but the aim is to restore 7 to 9 degrees of valgus between the long axis of the femur and long axis of the tibia with both medial

and lateral collateral ligaments under equal tension and with the prosthetic components in proper static alignment. The techniques of carrying out this balance have been well described by Insall[60] and by Freeman and Insall.[41]

It is also important to restore ligamentous bal-

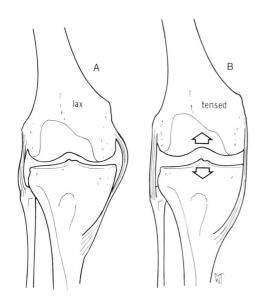

Fig. 121-26. Symmetric loss of bone and cartilage from both compartments in the knee, leading to uniform laxity of both collateral ligaments. Ligament release is not necessary to achieve appropriate alignment. (From Insall,[60] with permission.)

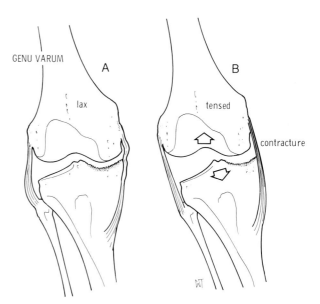

Fig. 121-27. With varus deformity, there is laxity of the lateral structures and contraction of medial structures. (From Insall,[60] with permission.)

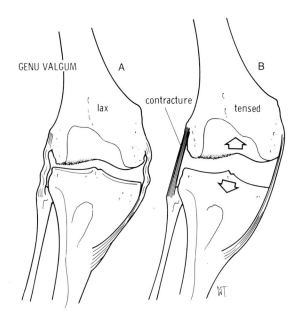

Fig. 121-28. With valgus deformity, the lateral structures are contracted and must be released to restore normal alignment. (From Insall,[60] with permission.)

ance with the knee flexed to 90 degrees to provide uniform distribution of stress to both collaterals and the PCL and to avoid rotational deformities in the femoral cut. As the posterior aspect of the femoral articular surface is rarely destroyed in OA, the gap between the posterior femoral condyle and the resected upper surface of the tibia should be uniform, both medially and laterally. (By contrast, with PCL removal, less bone should be removed from the lateral condyle to balance the ligaments in flexion.) If not, tight structures should be released until the tension in medial collateral and posterior cruciate ligaments is equal with the knee flexed to 90 degrees, upward distraction on the femur, and distal traction on the tibia (the lateral collateral will be slightly lax to permit excursion of the femoral component on the lateral tibial plateau during flexion). If this is accomplished, the knee will be stable in flexion and will not have rotary instability in spite of the flattened contours of the posterior aspect of the tibial component. Excessive tension in the posterior cruciate ligament, on the other hand, will lead to the possibility of rotary subluxation of the femoral component off the back of the tibial component in flexion.

Once the ligaments are balanced in both extension and flexion, the posterior femoral cut is made after the appropriate amount of resection is marked with the knee flexed and the ligaments under slight tension. The anterior femoral cut is made to accept the largest possible femoral component, seating the anterior flange snugly on the anterior femur but taking care to avoid notching the cortex.

In similar fashion, the distal femur is marked for resection with the knee extended, the collateral ligaments tensioned, and 6 to 9 degrees valgus alignment maintained. The aim is to produce precisely the same gap in extension as that produced in flexion so that stability throughout the arc of motion will be maintained with the prosthetic components in place (Fig. 121-29).

Particular attention should be paid to the fit between the posterior femur and the condylar portion of the femoral prosthesis. As it is difficult to apply cement to this interface, there must be a close fit between prosthesis and bone; otherwise, posterior forces in flexion will be resisted only by the cement between the distal femur and the prosthesis, which resists shear forces poorly.

Valgus Deformity

Lateral release is often necessary, especially in the rheumatoid knee, to correct valgus and external rotation deformities and to improve patellar tracking.[132] Because of the poor quality of the skin in many of these patients, we prefer to carry out all releases from within the joint, avoiding second incisions and large subcutaneous flaps. With the patella everted, the lateral synovium and capsule are incised vertically about 2 to 3 cm posterior to the lateral patellar border. This exposes the iliotibial band, which can be incised in the same vertical direction. The incision is carried distally to the tibia just behind Gerdy's tubercle, then curved anteriorly to detach the iliotibial band from the tubercle. Proximally the posterior margin of the vastus lateralis is defined and swept anteriorly off the lateral intermuscular septum. The superior lateral geniculate artery is carefully identified and preserved. With the artery retracted out of the way, the incision in the iliotibial band is carried proximally with scissors. If necessary, the vastus lateralis can be

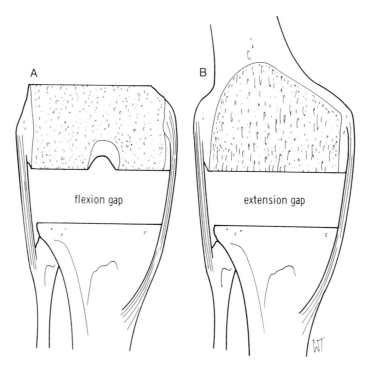

Fig. 121-29. As the combined thicknesses of the femoral and tibial components are equal in extension and flexion, the bony gap created by resection is also identical in flexion and extension with the ligaments under tension. (From Insall,[60] with permission.)

elevated from its distal femoral origin along the lateral intermuscular septum. The remaining intact portion of the iliotibial tract is the posterior band behind the vertical incision. If necessary, this remaining portion can be cut transversely proximal to the joint line. If the valgus deformity is still uncorrected, the popliteus muscle and lateral collateral ligament are detached from their femoral origin with a thin sliver of bone (Fig. 121-30). This step is rarely necessary if the iliotibial tract is sectioned as described above, but detachment of the popliteus tendon often facilitates correction of the external rotation deformity of the tibia.

The adequacy of the vertical component of the lateral release is tested by assessing patellar tracking. The patellar prosthesis should track in the groove of the femoral component easily and smoothly with no tendency to lateral dislocation. Tracking should be assessed before the capsule is closed, and the patella should remain in the groove during flexion without manual force.

Varus Deformity

In knees with varus deformity, the medial collateral ligament is lengthened in three stages. First, the deep fibers are excised from the tibial insertion; next, the arcuate capsular fibers immediately posterior to the tibial collateral ligament are detached from the medial and posterior rim of the tibia; and finally, if the deformity is not fully corrected, the superficial fibers of the medial collateral ligament are elevated from their tibial insertion under the pes anserinus using a curved $\frac{1}{2}$-inch osteotome as an elevator (Fig. 121-31). Correction must be tested repeatedly after each step in the release to avoid overcorrection and medial instability.

If patellar resurfacing is being carried out, the plane of resection is important. Enough patellar bone should remain to provide strength and avoid fracture; the plane should be parallel to the plane of femoral resection so that the patella sits well in the trochlear groove in flexion; and the prosthetic

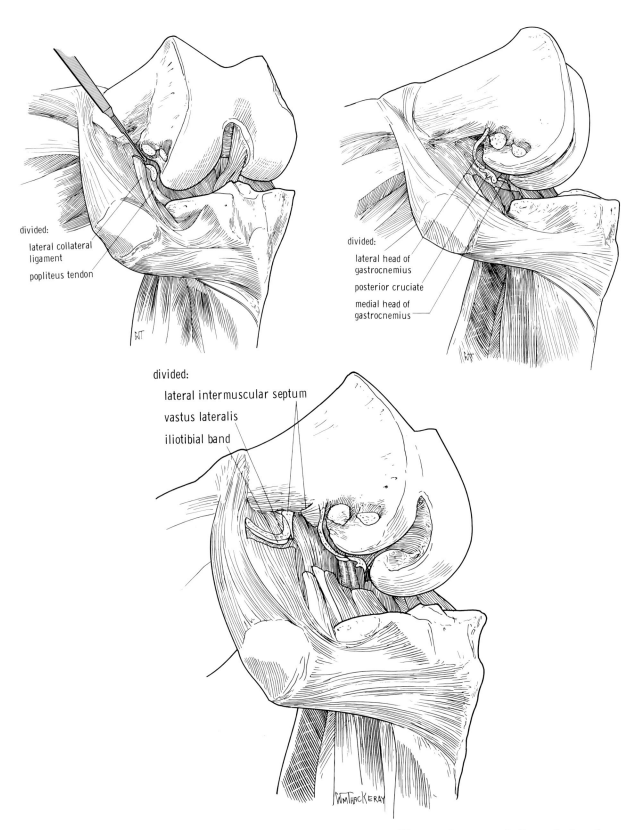

Fig. 121-30. Sequential stages in lateral release for valgus deformity. Alignment is assessed after each step of the release to ensure that only deforming tight structures are released. (From Insall,[60] with permission.)

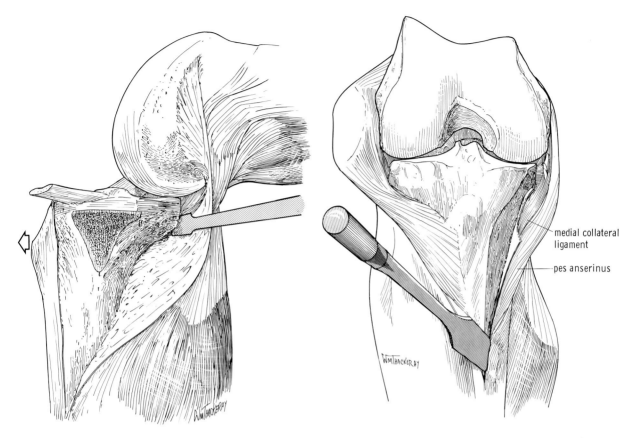

Fig. 121-31. With varus deformity, extensive medial release permits correction of the deformity and anterior subluxation of the tibia, to improve exposure. (From Insall,[60] with permission.)

patella should be placed as far as possible to the medial side of the resected patellar surface to reduce the angle between quadriceps and patellar tendon (the Q angle) and lessen the likelihood of lateral dislocation. Enough patellar bone should be resected so that the consined thinkness of bone and prosthesis restores normal patellar thickness (approximately 2 cm).

After completion of bone resection and ligament release, trial components are inserted to test alignment, proper tension of collateral and posterior cruciate ligaments, tracking of the patella, and the range of flexion and femoral rollback. The appropriate size of femoral component was chosen during creation of the flexion gap; the tibial component is chosen that most completely covers the exposed tibial cancellous bone. A slight overhang of the component is well tolerated and is preferable to undersizing of the component. If the compo-

nents are too tight in flexion, wedging may occur or the components may rock. If this happens, a thinner tibial component should be used, or an additional 1 or 2 mm of tibia should be resected. If the sequence of steps outlined above has been followed, this additional tibial resection will not produce excessive laxity in extension. Rather, the slight flexion deformity that usually accompanies excessive tightness in flexion will be corrected. The components should not rock during flexion and extension before cementing. If they do, persistent ligamentous imbalance should be corrected. The sole purpose of the technique described here is to minimize shear stress at the bone-cement interface. Ligament imbalance demonstrated by the rocking of the uncemented components will produce undesirable forces on the interface and on the weak trabecular bone. Patellar tracking is assessed with trial components in place. If there is a tendency for lateral subluxation, the position of the tibial component can be adjusted to more external rotation, producing relative internal rotation of the tibial tubercle, lessening the angle between quadriceps and patellar tendon and thus lessening the tendency of the patella to dislocate laterally. If the tendency for the patella to subluxate laterally persists, the adequacy of the lateral release (described above) should be assessed and corrected, if necessary.

Before the components are cemented in place, the tourniquet should be deflated to secure careful hemostasis. This is most easily done before the components fill the resection gap and obscure access to the posterior capsule, lateral gutter, and other bleeding sources. After the tourniquet is reinflated, the cancellous bone surfaces are cleaned with pulsating saline lavage, followed by aspiration of water and fat with suction.

To ensure adequate cement penetration, we prefer to insert both the femoral and tibial components simultaneously, so that the knee can be extended to achieve pressurization of cement. The use of pressure-sensitive film inserted between the components during this maneuver has demonstrated that nearly 1,000 newtons of force is generated on average — far greater than that possible with manual pressure alone.[168] It is not necessary to cement the femoral component at the same time as the tibial to achieve this effect. The femoral component can be inserted without cement, used to pressurize the tibial fixation, and then removed to facilitate removal of excess cement behind the tibial component after polymerization. The femur and patella can then be fixed simultaneously with a second mix of methyl methacrylate. After capsular closure, the knee should be flexed 105 to 110 degrees to ensure adequacy of the closure and proper patellar tracking and to demonstrate that postoperative physical therapy will not compromise the capsular closure.

The extremity is loosely wrapped in a bulky dressing and elastic bandage. Immobilization is provided by a commercial knee immobilizing splint. Prophylactic antibiotics, begun just before induction of anesthesia, are continued for 48 hours. Suction drainage tubes are removed at 24 hours, and at 48 hours the dressing is removed and gentle physical therapy begun. This consists of quadriceps

sets, assisted straight-leg raising, and side-lying active assisted flexion and extension. (Whether to use continuous passive motion machines to facilitate the return of motion is still controversial; most studies show that such units decrease hospital stay by accelerating the attainment of 90 degrees of flexion but do not effect the eventual range of motion.[25,177]) By day 4 or 5, independent straight-leg raising should be achieved. The patient is then allowed to sit on the edge of the bed with the operated knee flexed. Walking with two crutches is begun when the patient obtains 60 degrees of knee flexion and demonstrates muscular control of the extremity.[46] Seventy degrees of flexion should be reached by day 7 to 10, and bicycle exercises should be begun at that point. Ninety degrees of flexion should be achieved before discharge on day 10 to 14. If 90 degrees is not reached by that time, manipulation under anesthesia may be carried out (necessary in fewer than 10 percent of patients).[39] Patients are usually discharged from the hospital by day 10 to 14, walking independently on two crutches. Crutches are continued for 1 month while the patient carries out a formal program of exercises at home, including the use of a stationary bicycle. If these measures are effective in producing adequate motion and muscular strength at the 6-week follow-up, a single crutch can be used until all support is removed at 3 months.

Posterior Cruciate Substitution

Most of the steps for implantation of a cruciate-substituting knee prosthesis are identical to those for cruciate retention. The difference is in preparation of the flexion gap. With the PCL excised, a tensor should be inserted between the posterior femur and the resected tibial surface to ensure that the collateral ligaments will be snug in flexion; otherwise, instability might result. In addition, the extra width of the flexion gap allowed by cruciate resection dictates a thicker tibial component to fill the gap. It is helpful to create the flexion gap first and then carry out distal femoral resection to create an equal extension gap. If the extension gap is created first, it is likely to be too narrow.

In flexion, the PCL is nearly parallel to the lateral collateral ligament and becomes tense before the latter, enabling the lateral compartment of the normal knee to pivot around the PCL and permit rotation. When creating the flexion gap for a PCL-retaining prosthesis, the PCL limits the amount of gap created by distraction of the flexed knee, and nearly equal amounts of bone are resected from both posterior femoral condyles. With the PCL excised, the greater laxity of the lateral collateral permits asymmetric distraction of the flexed knee and must be offset by resecting less lateral condyle than medial to create a rectangular resection that will be filled by the prosthesis without creating lateral instability.

Unicompartmental Replacement

The first step in the procedure is to assess the quality of articular cartilage in the uninvolved or less involved compartment. If that cartilage is normal and the patient is young, debridement of osteophytes followed by tibial osteotomy should be considered.[89] If the patient is 60 or older and the level of demand not excessive, unicompartmental replacement will give excellent results and satisfactory longevity. If the less involved compartment shows softening and fibrillation, again age should be a major consideration. In the younger active patient, tibial osteotomy should perhaps still be considered, with unicompartmental replacement being favored in the middle-aged patient and tri-

compartmental replacement in the older patient. If there is obvious damage with areas of ulceration of articular cartilage, bi- or tricompartmental replacement should be carried out.

Having made the decision to carry out unicompartmental replacement, debridement of the tibial spine and intercondylar notch of the femoral condyle should be carried out, as there is often an abrasive ulcer between the tibial spine and the inner aspect of the femoral condyle that may be made worse by correction of the varus deformity. Osteophytes on the medial aspect of the femur and tibia should be removed to permit correction of deformity by relative elongation of the medial collateral ligament. If that is insufficient to permit correction of the varus deformity, medial release should be carried out as for total knee arthroplasty. Having corrected the soft tissue deformity, the involved compartment of the tibia is resected at right angles to the long axis of the tibia. Carrying out this step first facilitates access to the compartment and permits proper positioning of the femoral component. The femoral component is placed so that it will resurface all portions of the femur that will be in contact with the tibia from full extension to full flexion. The proximal portion of the femoral component should be countersunk into the bone to provide a smooth transition from bone to prosthesis for the patellar articulation. The size of the femoral component chosen should accurately replace the AP dimension of the femoral articular surface. The

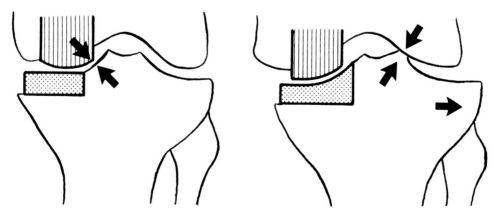

Fig. 121-32. If appropriate alignment between the femoral and tibial components of a unicompartmental replacement is not achieved, impingement may occur, either between the femoral component and the tibial spine or between the contralateral tibial spine and femoral condyle.

proper thickness of tibial component should be chosen to restore the tibial plateau to its normal height and provide proper tension in the collateral ligament and correct alignment of 4 to 7 degrees of valgus.

Attention must be paid to the relative location of the tibial and femoral components to avoid producing either subluxation of the knee or impingement between one component and an unresurfaced articulation (Fig. 121-32). Closure and aftercare are the same as for bi- or tricompartmental replacements, except that recovery is usually quicker and more flexion is achieved, both during the hospital stay and over the next several months.

RESULTS

Methods of Evaluation

It is difficult to compare results from various series or with different prostheses, as there is no agreement on how results should be evaluated. Many authorities use the Hospital for Special Surgery (HSS) knee score or a modification thereof. This scoring system, and other similar point systems, are insensitive. Thirty points out of 100 are awarded for relief of pain and an arthrodesis would, therefore, score 60 points. Function is poorly quantified with 22 points for walking distance, use of stairs, and transfers. Points are awarded for motion, regardless of the functional implication of the range; for example, the point score for a range from 45 degrees to 135 degrees is the same as for 0 degrees to 90 degrees in spite of the marked functional advantage of the latter range. In addition, it is not useful to lump the categories of pain relief, function, and range of motion to produce a global score. Each category should be kept separate so that accurate data on each type of outcome can be accumulated and used for reference and clinical decisions. For example, some patients with a need for maximal flexion (i.e., patients with polyarticular RA) would be happier with mild pain on walking but an ability to flex from 0 to 112 degrees rather than to have no walking pain but flex only to 80

degrees. Both situations would produce the identical score of 86.

Several attempts have been made to produce improved methods of evaluation. The British Orthopaedic Association developed one such scheme, which has objective data from the patients own evaluation as well as data on general function and disease in other joints.[157]

Several studies have used gait analysis to evaluate the outcome of knee replacements[1,2,14,78,107,139,172] and have shown near-normal gait in patients with successful arthroplasties. In the absence of a comprehensive universal method of analysis, comparison of results is semiquantitative at best.

COMPLICATIONS

In terms of frequency, complications involving the patella are most common. These problems include patellar dislocation,[100] stress fractures,[47,130] avascular necrosis,[174] progressive erosion of articular cartilage in unresurfaced patellae,[60] and loosening of the patellar prosthesis.[63] Altogether, these complications involving the patella occur in approximately 15 percent of knees that have undergone replacement of the patella. Patellar dislocation may be related to tight lateral structures (especially in the valgus knee), internal rotation of the tibial component (with resultant external rotation of the tibia and an excessive Q-angle), trauma, or incongruency of the unresurfaced patella articulating with the trochlear groove of the prosthetic femur. Periprosthetic fractures, especially involving the femur, are seen, usually in patients with severe osteoporosis or rheumatoid arthritis and bone loss.[17,99,140]

Deep venous thrombosis and pulmonary embolism are detected frequently if sought, but are infrequent sources of clinically evident problems. Nonetheless, the serious nature of these complications warrants routine prophylaxis, either with mechanical means (pulsatile stockings, CPM), antiinflammatory agents (antiplatelet activity), or warfarin.[87,153]

Occasionally one can find evidence of transient partial weakness and numbness in the distribution of the peroneal nerve. Rare instances of permanent peroneal nerve injury have been reported.[115] Although there are rare reports of vascular complications leading to amputation,[116] infection is the most serious complication of total knee replacement of significant frequency. Deep infection occurs in 0.5 to 2 percent of knee arthroplasties.[50,121] In our series of 266 consecutive arthroplasties, there were two infections during the immediate postoperative period and two infections (in one patient) at 2 years, for an overall incidence of 4 of 266 (1.5 percent).

The management of an infected knee arthroplasty is not the provenance of this chapter. It should be noted that aggressive treatment of early postoperative infections by intravenous antibiotics coupled with debridement and retention of the components may be successful (four out of four in our series). Procrastination to the point of bone involvement and sinus formation uniformly leads to the necessity for removal of the prosthesis and either exchange arthroplasty with prolonged intravenous antibiotics, or arthrodesis.

RESULTS REPORTED IN THE LITERATURE

At 10 years, 87.5 percent of patients with Total Condylar arthroplasties were functioning satisfactorily and 41 percent had radiolucent lines under the tibial component.[64] Average flexion arcs were the same 2 years after arthroplasty as were arcs before surgery in another series of patients with RA or OA.[125] Seventeen percent of patients had flexion deformities after surgery, compared with 61 percent before surgery.[155]

The Spherocentric, at average 8-year follow-up, had an infection rate of 5 percent and a reoperation rate of 15 percent,[94] the custom long-stem patellofemoral Spherocentric, at average 4-year follow-up, produced significant improvement in pain in 87 percent and an average range of motion of 88 degrees; 74 percent of patients were able to climb stairs independently. There was one infection in 86 operated knees.[72,95]

Townley[161] reports 2 percent loosening in 532 cemented arthroplasties followed 2 to 11 years with good or excellent results in 89 percent. Cloutier[23] reports 91 percent good to excellent results in 107 arthroplasties at 2 to 4.5 years follow-up. The Variable Axis design is reported to have no significant deterioration of results 2 to 9 years after implantation. Complications were patellar (6.9 percent), laxity (2.9 percent), aseptic loosening (1.2 percent), deep infection (2 percent), supracondylar fracture (1.2 percent), and peroneal nerve palsy (1.6 percent).[16,173] Similar results are reported for the Oxford Knee,[45] the Posterior Cruciate Condylar knee,[114] the Porous Coated Anatomic,[58] and the intramedullary adjustable prosthesis.[30]

A multicenter study of 8,000 cases from Sweden reported a probability of revision from infection by 6 years of 2 percent in OA and 3 percent in RA. Fusion was required in 2 percent of the cases followed 6 years, while 90 percent of the unicondylar replacements and 87 percent of the bi- or tricompartmental replacements were functioning satisfactorily. The most common mode of failure was loosening of the tibial component.[73,74]

RESULTS IN RHEUMATOID ARTHRITIS

It is a common misconception that patients with juvenile or adult-onset RA have a poorer outcome following joint replacement than do their counterparts with OA. Although it is true that the late infection rate is higher and that disease in other joints prejudices function following replacement of one joint, patients with inflammatory arthritis do quite well after joint replacement in general and following knee replacement, in particular.[142,143] There are occasional problems with atrophic skin in patients on long-standing steroids, skin contamination in psoriatic skin lesions in the operative field, and weak trabecular bone in the proximal tibia. A knowledge of these problems enables the surgeon to avoid most complications. It has been our experience that these patients achieve predictable pain relief and increased range of motion of the knee. Function of the knee is improved, although disease in adjacent joints will continue to compromise overall function. Patients with juvenile RA should be considered for synovectomy, soft tissue releases to resolve contractures and deformities, and other conservative measures, if possible. When the articular surfaces are destroyed, knee replacement can provide excellent results with the expectation that the implant will last for at least 10 years in these patients with limited activity.[21,120,122,129] When the implant fails for mechanical reasons (wear or loosening), revision can provide a second successful result.

RESULTS FROM THE AUTHOR'S INSTITUTION

Unicompartmental Knee Replacement

In the 2- to 6-year follow-up of the first 100 unicompartmental replacements carried out at our institution (Harvard Medical School, Brigham & Women's Hospital) 92 percent achieved satisfactory pain relief, the average knee flexion was 114 degrees, and 49 of the 100 knees had at least 120 degrees of flexion. Ninety percent required no walking aids after operation, 73 percent could walk unlimited distances without support, and 65 percent could go up and down stairs normally. Ten-year follow-up evaluation of the same group of patients has confirmed these results and has shown that the failure rate has remained consistent at about 1 percent per year.[5]

Bicompartmental Replacement

Between June 1978 and August 1981, 266 consecutive total knee replacements were carried out in 200 patients at the author's institution. A cruciate-preserving prosthesis was used (Fig. 121-33), and the surgery was carried out by any one of nine surgeons. This group of patients was recalled recently for evaluation from 5 to 8.6 years following surgery (average 6 years); 192 knees were available for review, of which 73 percent were in female patients and 25 percent in males. The diagnosis was RA in 50 percent, OA in 44 percent, juvenile RA in 4 percent, and psoriatic arthritis in 2 percent. The patella had been resurfaced in all patients with RA and in 48 of the 85 knees with OA. Patients were evaluated by a numerical score (Table 121-1). Overall, 90 percent achieved a good or excellent result and just over 5 percent had a poor result. Ninety-five of the patients with OA had a good or excellent result, compared with 83 percent in the RA population. Most of the poor results were found in the latter group.

Pain relief was virtually complete in 96 percent of patients with OA, and 84 percent of patients with RA (90 percent overall). The ability to go up and down stairs in reciprocal fashion without the use of supporting devices was restored in 68 percent of patients with OA and in 34 percent of patients with RA (50 percent overall); 97 percent of patients had no pain on level walking, and 83 percent of patients were able to walk at least four to six blocks. Eighty percent could climb stairs without aids, and 50 percent could climb stairs in reciprocal fashion. We were unable to ascertain any difference in stair-climbing ability in OA patients, regardless of whether patellar replacement had been carried out.

The average preoperative flexion was 104 degrees (102 degrees in OA, 106 degrees in RA). On average, postoperative flexion was 109 degrees (110 degrees in OA and 109 degrees in RA). Sixty-five percent of knees had more than 110 degrees of flexion, and the average increase in flexion was 5 degrees. There were no cases of AP instability, and only 3 percent of knees showed any medial or lateral instability on clinical testing.

Radiographic Analysis

Alignment

Ninety-four percent of rheumatoid knees were in preoperative valgus alignment and 6 percent in varus alignment. In patients with OA, 57 percent of knees were in varus and 3 percent in valgus. The

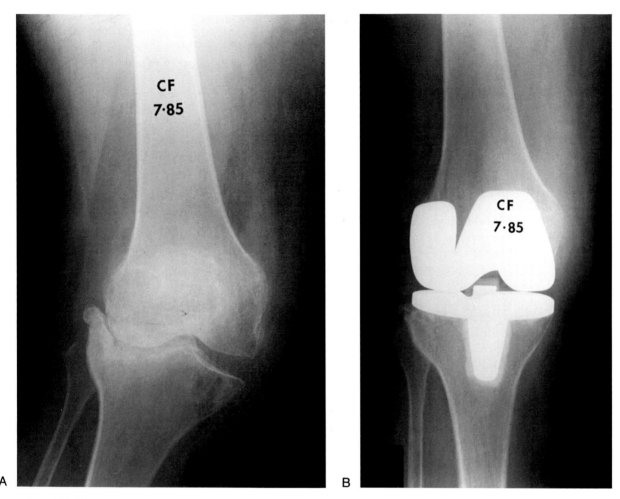

Fig. 121-33. **(A)** Preoperative radiograph showing severe valgus deformity in a patient with rheumatoid arthritis. Note the laxity at the medial collateral ligament and depression of the lateral tibial plateau. **(B)** Postoperative radiograph showing correction of the valgus deformity.

Table 121-1. Results of Knee Arthroplasty at 5- to 9-Year Follow-up

	% of Knees Achieving Result		
Clinical Result	All	OA	RA
Excellent	59	71	50
Good	29	24	33
Fair	6	4	8
Poor	6	1	9
No or minimal pain	90	96	84
Reciprocal stairs with or without handrail	50	68	34

Wright RJ, Walker PS, Ewald FC, personal communication.

average postoperative alignment was 5 degrees of valgus and did not differ in the two groups.

Radiolucent Lines

In the AP view of the tibial component, 39 percent of knees had a radiolucent line in at least one zone. These lines were usually under the lateral flange of the tibial component and only once involved the central peg. All lucencies were less than 1 mm in width and were nonprogressive. The incidence of these radiolucent lines was slightly less in RA knees than in OA knees (34 percent compared with 46 percent). No relationship could be demonstrated among alignment, component position, and the development of radiolucent lines.

Failures

Overall, six revisions have been carried out. In six of those knees, the patella was loose and in one case the tibial component was also loose, with a fractured tibial tray. The average time at revision was 4.7 years, with a range of 2 to 5.9 years. Only one of the patellar revisions was in a patient with OA giving a revision rate of 1.2 percent in the category. The other five revisions were in rheumatoid knees, for an overall revision rate of 5.2 percent. Twenty-one knees had postoperative surgical complications. Nine of these did not require reoperation. Four superficial wound infections were treated successfully with antibiotics. Two knees had hematomas, and one rheumatoid knee sustained a fractured patella that was treated conservatively. One patient had lateral subluxation of the patella that resolved spontaneously. One knee had a postoperative peroneal nerve palsy; this knee had been in 26 degrees of valgus preoperatively and was corrected to 6 degrees of valgus at surgery. All were resolved over 6 months.

Twelve of the 21 knees required reoperation. Four knees had a deep wound infection, two of which were early, and two knees (in one patient) became infected 2 years after operation following hematogenous seeding with *Staphylococcus aureus*. All four knees were treated with incision, drainage, and debridement with intravenous antibiotics. All four infections were controlled, and the knees are now doing well aside from limited flexion (three knees with 85 degrees and one knee with only 10 degrees of flexion). One rheumatoid knee sustained a patellar tendon rupture that was repaired. One patella dislocated laterally was treated by arthrotomy and quadriceps realignment. Six further cases required revision surgery for loose components.

From an analysis of these results, and those reported elsewhere,[29,124,131,134] it appears that total knee arthroplasty is very similar to total hip arthroplasty in terms of the predictability of good or excellent results, the infrequency of complications, and the ability to salvage most complications with an eventual satisfactory result.

ACKNOWLEDGMENTS

The collaboration of my colleagues in the Department of Orthopedic Surgery at the Brigham and Women's Hospital, Harvard Medical School, is acknowledged, especially Dr. F.C. Ewald, Dr. R.J. Wright, and Dr. P.S. Walker; Dr. Stuart Kozinn, Fellow in Reconstructive Surgery, was of invaluable assistance in the preparation of this chapter, as was Ms. Phyllis White, administrative assistant.

REFERENCES

1. Andriacchi TP, Andersson GBJ, Fermier RW, et al: A study of lower limb mechanics during stair-climbing. J Bone Joint Surg 62A:749, 1980
2. Andriacchi TP, Galante JO, Fermier RW: The influence of total knee-replacement design on walking and stair-climbing. J Bone Joint Surg 64A:1328, 1982
3. Bae DK, Guhl JF, Keane SP: Unicompartmental knee arthroplasty for single compartment disease. Clinical experience with an average four-year follow-up study. Clin Orthop 176:233, 1983
4. Bargren JH, Blaha JD, Freeman MAR: Alignment in total knee arthroplasty. Correlated biomechanical and clinical observations. Clin Orthop 173:178, 1983
5. Barrett WP, Scott RD: Revision of failed unicondylar arthroplasty. J Bone Joint Surg 69A:1328, 1987
6. Bartel DL, Burstein AH, Santavicca EA, et al: Performance of the tibial component in total knee replacement (conventional and revision designs). J Bone Joint Surg 64A:1026, 1982
7. Bayne O, Cameron HU: Total knee arthroplasty following patellectomy. Clin Orthop 186:112, 1984

8. Behrens JC, Walker PS, Shoji H: Variations in strength and structure of cancellous bone at the knee. J Biomech 7:201, 1974

9. Blaha JD, Insler HP, Freeman MAR, et al: The fixation of a proximal tibial polyethylene prosthesis without cement. J Bone Joint Surg 64B:326, 1982

10. Bourne RB, Finlay JB: The influence of tibial component intramedullary stems and implant-cortex contact on the strain distribution of the proximal tibia following total knee arthroplasty. An in vitro study. Clin Orthop 208:95, 1986

11. Brooks PJ, Walker PS, Scott RD: Tibial component fixation in deficient tibial bone stock. Clin Orthop 184:302, 1984

12. Brotherton SL, Roberson JR, DeAndrade JR, et al: Staged versus simultaneous bilateral total knee replacement. Orthop Trans 10:576, 1986

13. Broughton NS, Newman JH, Baily RA: Unicompartmental replacement and high tibial osteotomy for osteoarthritis of the knee. A comparative study after 5–10 years' follow-up. J Bone Joint Surg 68B:447, 1985

14. Brugioni DJ, Andriacchi TP, Rotti RA, et al: A relationship between gait, disease process, and radiographic appearance following total knee replacement. Orthop Trans 10:345, 1986

15. Bryan RS: Total knee arthoplasty revisited. Orthop Trans 10:171, 1986

16. Buchanan JR, Greer RB III, Bowman LS, et al: Clinical experience with variable axis total knee replacement. J Bone Joint Surg 64A:337, 1984

17. Cain PR, Rubash HE, Wissinger HA, McClain EJ: Periprosthetic femoral fractures following total knee arthroplasty. Clin Orthop 208:205, 1986

18. Callihan SM, Halley DK: Prospective analysis of Sheehan total knee arthroplasty. Clin Orthop 192:124, 1985

19. Cameron HU, Fedorkow DM: The patella in total knee arthroplasty. Clin Orthop 165:197, 1982

20. Campbell WC: Interposition of vitallium plates in arthroplasties of the knee. Preliminary report. Am J Surg 47:639, 1940

21. Carmichael E, Chaplin DM: Total knee arthroplasty in juvenile rheumatoid arthritis. A seven-year follow-up study. Clin Orthop 210:192, 1986

22. Cheal EJ, Hayes WC, Lee CH, et al: Stress analysis of a condylar knee tibial component: influence of metaphyseal shell properties and cement injection depth. J Orthop Res 3:424, 1985

23. Cloutier JM: Results of total knee arthroplasty with a non-constrained prosthesis. J Bone Joint Surg 65A:906, 1983

24. Cooke TD, Richer S, Hurd E, et al: Localization of antigen-antibody complexes in intra-articular collageneous tissues. Ann NY Acad Sci 256:10, 1975

25. Coutts RD, Rosenstein A, Stewart WT, et al: The effect of CPM and functional muscle stimulation on rehabilitation after total knee arthroplasty. Orthop Trans 10:171, 1986

26. Dalquist NJ, Mayo P, Seedholm BB: Forces during squatting and rising from a deep squat. Engin Med 11:69, 1982

27. Deburge A, GUEPAR: GUEPAR hinge prosthesis. Complications and results with two years follow-up. Clin Orthop 120:47, 1976

28. Dorr LD, Ranawat CS, Sculco TA, et al: Bone graft for tibial defects in total knee arthroplasty. Clin Orthop 205:153, 1986

29. Ecker ML, Lotke PA, Windsor RE, Cella JP: Long-term results after total condylar knee arthroplasty. Significance of radiolucent lines. Clin Orthop 216:151, 1987

30. Eftekhar NS: Total knee-replacement arthroplasty. Results with the intramedullary adjustable total knee prosthesis. J Bone Joint Surg 65A:293, 1983

31. Emerson RH, Potter T: The use of the McKeever metallic hemiarthroplasty for unicompartmental arthritis. J Bone Joint Surg 67A:208, 1985

32. Ewald FC, Jacobs MA, Miegel RE, et al: Kinematic total knee replacement. J Bone Joint Surg 66A:1032, 1984

33. Ewald FC, Scott RD, Thomas WH, Sledge CB: The importance of intercondylar stability in knee arthroplasty: comparison of McKeever, modular and duocondylar types. J Bone Joint Surg 57A:1033, 1975

34. Ewald FC, Thomas WH, Poss R, et al: Duopatellar total knee arthroplasty in rheumatoid arthritis. Orthop Trans 2:202, 1978

35. Farcy JP, McIlveen SJ: Modes of failure in total knee replacement. Orthop Trans 10:497, 1986

36. Ferguson W: Excision of the knee joint; recovery with a false joint and a useful limb. Med Times Gaz 1:601, 1861

37. Figgie HE III, Davy DT, Heiple KG, Hart RT: Load-bearing capacity of the tibial component of the total condylar knee prosthesis. An *in vitro* study. Clin Orthop 183:288, 1984

38. Figgie HE III, Goldberg VM, Heiple KG, et al: The influence of tibial-patellofemoral location on function of the knee in patients with the posterior stabilized condylar knee prosthesis. J Bone Joint Surg 68A:1035, 1986

39. Fox JL, Poss R: The role of manipulation following

total knee replacement. J Bone Joint Surg 63A:357, 1981

40. Freeman MAR: The surgical anatomy and pathology of the arthritic knee. p. 31. In Freeman MAR (ed): Arthritis of the Knee. Springer-Verlag, New York, 1980

41. Freeman MAR, Insall J: Tibio-femoral replacement using two un-linked components and cruciate resection. (The ICLH and total condylar prostheses.) p. 254. In Freeman MAR (ed): Arthritis of the Knee. Springer-Verlag, New York, 1980

42. Freeman MAR, McLeod HC, Levai JP: Cementless fixation of prosthetic components in total arthroplasty of the knee and hip. Clin Orthop 176:88, 1983

43. Freeman MAR, Samuelson KM, Bertin KC: Freeman-Samuelson total arthroplasty of the knee. Clin Orthop 192:46, 1985

44. Freeman MAR, Swanson SAV: Total prosthetic replacement of the knee. J Bone Joint Surg 54B:170, 1972

45. Goodfellow JW, O'Connor J: Clinical results of the Oxford knee. Surface arthroplasty of the tibiofemoral joint with a meniscal bearing prosthesis. Clin Orthop 205:21, 1986

46. Grace DL, Cracchiolo A III, Dorey FJ: The effect of early weight-bearing in total knee arthroplasty. Clin Orthop 207:178, 1986

47. Grace JN, Sim FH: Fracture of the patella following total knee arthroplasty. Orthop Trans 10:496, 1986

48. Green DL, Bahniuk E, Liebelt RA, et al: Biplane radiographic measurements of reversible displacement (including clinical loosening) and migration of total joint replacements. J Bone Joint Surg 65A:1134, 1983

49. Grimer RJ, Karpinski MR, Edwards AN: The long-term results of Stanmore total knee replacements. J Bone Joint Surg 66B:55, 1984

50. Grogan TJ, Dorey F, Rollins J, Amstutz HC: Deep sepsis following total knee arthroplasty. Ten-year experience at the University of California at Los Angeles Medical Center. J Bone Joint Surg 68A:226, 1986

51. Gunston FH: Polycentric knee arthroplasty. Prosthetic simulation of normal knee movement. J Bone Joint Surg 53B:272, 1971

52. Gunston FH, MacKenzie RI: Complications of polycentric knee arthroplasty. Clin Orthop 120:11, 1976

53. Halawa M, Lee AJ, Ling RS, et al: The shear strength of trabecular bone from the femur and some factors affecting the shear strength of the cement–bone interface. Arch Orthop Traum Surg 92:19, 1978

54. Hood RW, Vanni M, Insall JN: The correction of knee alignment in 225 consecutive total condylar knee replacements. Clin Orthop 160:94, 1981

55. Hsieh HH, Walker PS: Stabilizing mechanisms of the loaded and unloaded knee joint. J Bone Joint Surg 58A:87, 1976

56. Hui FC, Fitzgerald RH Jr: Hinged total knee arthroplasty. J Bone Joint Surg 62A:513, 1980

57. Huiskes R, Slooff TJ: Thermal injury of cancellous bone, following pressurized penetration of acrylic cement. Trans Orthop Res Soc 6:134, 1981

58. Hungerford DS, Krackow KA: Total joint arthroplasty of the knee. Clin Orthop 192:23, 1985

59. Hvid I, Hansen SL: Trabecular bone strength patterns at the proximal tibial epiphysis. J Orthop Res 3:464, 1985

60. Insall JN: Surgery of the Knee. Churchill Livingstone, New York, 1984

61. Insall JN: Reconstructive surgery and rehabilitation of the knee. p. 1870. In Kelley WN, Harris ED Jr, Ruddy S, Sledge CB (eds): Textbook of Rheumatology. Vol II. WB Saunders, Philadelphia, 1985

62. Insall JN, Binazzi R, Soudry M, Mestriner LA: Total knee arthroplasty. Clin Orthop 192:13, 1985

63. Insall JN, Hood RW, Flawn LB, Sullivan DJ: The total condylar knee prosthesis in gonarthrosis. A five to nine-year follow-up of the first one hundred consecutive replacements. J Bone Joint Surg 65A:619, 1983

64. Insall JN, Kelly M: The total condylar prosthesis. Clin Orthop 205:43, 1986

65. Insall JN, Lachiewicz PF, Burstein AH: The posterior stabilized condylar prosthesis. A modification of the total condylar design. Two to four year clinical experience. J Bone Joint Surg 64A:1317, 1982

66. Insall JN, Ranawat CS, Aglietti P, et al: A comparison of four models of total knee replacement prostheses. J Bone Joint Surg 58A:754, 1976

67. Jackson RW, Burdick W: Unicompartmental knee arthroplasty. Clin Orthop 190:182, 1984

68. Jergesen HE, Poss R, Sledge CB: Bilateral total hip and knee replacement in adults with rheumatoid arthritis: an evaluation of function. Clin Orthop 137:120, 1978

69. Johnson DP, Houghton TA, Radford P: Anterior midline or medial parapatellar incision for arthroplasty of the knee. A comparative study. J Bone Joint Surg 68B:812, 1986

70. Jones WN, Aufranc OE, Kermond WL: Mold arthroplasty of the knee. J Bone Joint Surg 49A:1022, 1967

71. Katz MM, Hungerford DS, Krackow KA, Lennox DW: Results of total knee arthroplasty after failed proximal tibial osteotomy for osteoarthritis. J Bone Joint Surg 69A:225, 1987

72. Kaufer H, Matthews LS: Spherocentric arthroplasty of the knee. J Bone Joint Surg 63A:545, 1981

73. Knutson K, Lindstrand A, Lidgren L: Survival of knee arthroplasties. A nation-wide multicentre investigation of 8000 cases. J Bone Joint Surg 68B:795, 1986

74. Knutson K, Tjornstrand B, Lidgren L: Survival of knee arthroplasties for rheumatoid arthritis. Acta Orthop Scand 56:422, 1985

75. Krause W, Krug W, Miller JE: Cement–bone interface — effect of cement technique and surface preparation. Trans Orthop Res Soc 5:76, 1980

76. Kurosawa H, Walker PS: A new method for describing the motion of the knee. Presented at the Sixth Annual Conference of the American Society of Biomechanics, Seattle, WA, 1982

77. Lachiewicz PF, Inglis AE, Insall JN, et al: Total knee arthroplasty in hemophilia. J Bone Joint Surg 67A:1361, 1985

78. Laughman RK, Stauffer RN, Ilstrup DM, Chao EY: Functional evaluation of total knee replacement. J Orthop Res 2:307, 1984

79. Lereim P, Goldie I: Relationship between morphologic features and hardness of the subchondral bone of the medial tibial condyle in the normal state and in osteoarthritis and rheumatoid arthritis. Arch Orthop Unfall-Chir 81:1, 1975

80. Lereim P, Goldie I, Dahlberg E: Hardness of the subchondral bone of the tibial condyles in the normal state and in osteoarthritis and rheumatoid arthritis. Acta Orthop Scand 45:614, 1974

81. Lettin AW, Kavanagh TG, Scales JT: The long-term results of Stanmore total knee replacements. J Bone Joint Surg 66B:349, 1984

82. Levai JP, McLeod HC, Freeman MAR: Why not resurface the patella? J Bone Joint Surg 65B:448, 1983

83. Lew WD, Lewis JL: The effect of knee-prosthesis geometry on cruciate ligament mechanics during flexion. J Bone Joint Surg 64A:734, 1982

84. Lewallen DG, Bryan RS, Peterson LF: Polycentric total knee arthroplasty. A ten-year follow-up study. J Bone Joint Surg 66A:1211, 1984

85. Lewis JL, Askew MJ, Jaycox DP: A comparative evaluation of tibial component designs of total knee prostheses. J Bone J Surg 64A:129, 1982

86. Lotke PA, Ecker ML: Influence of positioning of prosthesis in total knee replacement. J Bone Joint Surg 59A:77, 1977

87. Lotke PA, Wong RY, Ecker ML: Asymptomatic pulmonary embolism after total knee replacement. Orthop Trans 10:490, 1986

88. MacIntosh DL: Hemiarthroplasty of the knee using a space occupying prosthesis for painful varus and valgus deformities. J Bone Joint Surg 40A:1431, 1958

89. MacIntosh DL, Welsh RP: Joint debridement — a complement to high tibial osteotomy in the treatment of degenerative arthritis of the knee. J Bone Joint Surg 59A:1094, 1977

90. Magone JB, Dennis DA, Weis LD: Total knee arthroplasty in chronic hemophilic arthropathy. Orthop Trans 10:576, 1986

91. Mallory TH, Danyi J: Unicompartmental total knee arthroplasty. A five- to nine-year follow-up study of 42 procedures. Clin Orthop 175:135, 1983

92. Marklolf KL, Bargar WL, Shoemaker SC, et al: The role of joint load in knee stability. J Bone Joint Surg 63A:570, 1981

93. Markolf KL, Finerman GM, Amstutz HC: In vitro measurements of knee stability after bicondylar replacement. J Bone Joint Surg 61A:547, 1979

94. Matthews LS, Goldstein SA, Kolowich PA, Kaufer H: Spherocentric arthroplasty of the knee. A long-term and final follow-up evaluation. Clin Orthop 205:58, 1986

95. Matthews LS, Kaplan SI, Kaufer H: The role of long stemmed patellofemoral spherocentric arthroplasty in the treatment of patients with severe damage to the knee joint. Orthop Trans 10:170, 1987

96. Mazas FB, GUEPAR: Guepar total knee prosthesis. Clin Orthop 94:211, 1973

97. McKeever DC: Tibial plateau prosthesis. Clin Orthop 18:86, 1960

98. McLaughlin TP, Fisher RL: Bilateral total knee arthroplasties. Comparison of simultaneous (two-team), sequential, and staged knee replacements. Clin Orthop 199:220, 1985

99. Merkel KD, Johnson EW Jr: Supracondylar fracture of the femur after total knee arthroplasty. J Bone Joint Surg 68A:29, 1986

100. Merkow RL, Soudry M, Insall JN: Patellar dislocation following total knee replacement. J Bone Joint Surg 67A:1321, 1985

101. Morrey BF, Adams RA, Ilstrup DM, Bryan RS: Complications and mortality associated with bilateral or unilateral total knee arthroplasty. J Bone Joint Surg 69A:484, 1987

102. Morrison JB: Function of the knee joint in various activities. Biomed Eng 4:573, 1969

103. Morrison JB: The mechanics of the knee joint in relation to normal walking. J Biomech 3:51, 1970

104. Mullen JO: Range of motion following total knee arthroplasty in ankylosed joints. Clin Orthop 179:200, 1983

105. Nissan M: The use of a permutation approach in the solution of joint biomechanics of the knee. Engin Med 10:39, 1981

106. Oglesby JW, Wilson FC: The evolution of knee arthroplasty. Results with three generations of prostheses. Clin Orthop 186:96, 1984

107. Otis JC, Lane JM, Kroll MA: Energy cost during gait in osteosarcoma patients after resection and knee replacement and after above-the-knee amputation. J Bone Joint Surg 67:606, 1985

108. Piziali RL, Rastegar JC, Nagel D: The axis of varus-valgus rotation of the in-vitro human knee joint. Trans Orthop Res Soc 3:239, 1978

109. Ranawat CS: The patellofemoral joint in total condylar knee arthroplasty. Pros and cons based on five- to ten-year follow-up observations. Clin Orthop 205:93, 1986

110. Ranawat CS, Johanson NA, Rimnac CM, et al: Retrieval analysis of porous-coated components for total knee arthroplasty. A report of two cases. Clin Orthop 209:244, 1986

111. Rand JA, Bryan RS, Chao EYS: Porous coated anatomical total knee arthroplasty. Orthop Trans 10:169, 1986

112. Rand JA, Chao EYS, Stauffer RN: Kinematic rotating-hinge total knee arthroplasty. J Bone Joint Surg 69A:489, 1987

113. Reilly D, Walker PS, Ben-Dov M, et al: Effects of tibial components on load transfer in the upper tibia. Clin Orthop 165:273, 1982

114. Ritter MA, Gioe TJ, Stringer EA, Littrell D: The posterior cruciate condylar total knee prosthesis. A five-year follow-up study. Clin Orthop 184:264, 1984

115. Rose HA, Hood RW, Otis JC, et al: Peroneal-nerve palsy following total knee arthroplasty. A review of The Hospital for Special Surgery experience. J Bone Joint Surg 64A:347, 1982

116. Rush JH, Vidovich JD, Johnson MA: Arterial complications of total knee replacement. J Bone Joint Surg 69B:400, 1987

117. Rutledge R, Webster DA, Murray DG: Experience with the variable axis knee prosthesis. Clin Orthop 205:146, 1986

118. Ryd L: Micromotion in knee arthroplasty. A roentgen stereophotogrammetric analysis of tibial component fixation. Acta Orthop Scand 220(Suppl):1, 1986

119. Ryd L, Lindstrand A, Rosenquist R, Selvik G: Tibial component fixation in knee arthroplasty. Clin Orthop 213:141, 1986

120. Rydholm U, Boegard T, Lidgren L: Total knee replacement in juvenile chronic arthritis. Scand J Rheumatol 14:329, 1986

121. Salvati EA, Robinson RP, Zeno SM, et al: Infection rates after 3175 total hip and total knee replacements performed with and without a horizontal unidirectional filtered airflow system. J Bone Joint Surg 64A:525, 1982

122. Sarokhan AJ, Scott RD, Thomas WH, et al: Total knee arthroplasty in juvenile rheumatoid arthritis. J Bone Joint Surg 65A:1071, 1983

123. Schmidt RG, Lotke P, Rothman RH: Tibiofemoral resurfacing arthroplasty utilizing the Marmor modular prosthesis: a long term follow-up study. Orthop Trans 10:491, 1986

124. Schneider R, Soudry M: Radiographic and scintigraphic evaluation of total knee arthroplasty. Clin Orthop 205:108, 1986

125. Schurman DJ, Parker JN, Ornstein D: Total condylar knee replacement. A study of factors influencing range of motion as late as two years after arthroplasty. J Bone Joint Surg 67A:1006, 1985

126. Scott RD: Duopatellar total knee replacement: the Brigham experience. Orthop Clin North Am 13:89, 1982

127. Scott RD, Joyce MJ, Ewald FC, Thomas WH: Mckeever metallic hemiarthroplasty of the knee in unicompartmental degenerative arthritis: long-term clinical follow-up and current indications. J Bone Joint Surg 67A:203, 1985

128. Scott RD, Santore RF: Unicondylar unicompartmental replacement for osteoarthritis of the knee. J Bone Joint Surg 63A:536, 1981

129. Scott RD, Sarokhan AJ, Dalziel R: Total hip and total knee arthroplasty in juvenile rheumatoid arthritis. Clin Orthop 182:90, 1984

130. Scott RD, Turoff N, Ewald FC: Stress fracture of the patella following duopatellar total knee arthroplasty with patellar resurfacing. Clin Orthop 170:147, 1982

131. Scott RD, Volatile TB: Twelve years' experience with posterior cruciate-retaining total knee arthroplasty. Clin Orthop 205:100, 1986

132. Scott RD, Volatile TB, Gebhardt E: Total knee replacement in severe valgus deformity. Orthop Trans 10:490, 1986

133. Scott WN, Rozbruch JD, Otis JC, et al: Clinical and biomechanical evaluation of patella replacement

in total knee arthroplasty. Orthop Trans 2:203, 1978

134. Scott WN, Rubinstein M: Posterior stabilized knee arthroplasty. Six years' experience. Clin Orthop 205:138, 1986

135. Seireg A, Arvikar RJ: A mathematical model for the evaluation of forces in lower extremities of the musculoskeletal system. J Biomech 6:313, 1973

136. Shiers LGP: Arthroplasty of the knee. Preliminary report of a new method. J Bone Joint Surg 36B:553, 1954

137. Shurley TH, O'Donoghue DH, Smith WD, et al: Unicompartmental arthroplasty of the knee: a review of three-five year follow-up. Clin Orthop 164:236, 1982

138. Simison AJ, Noble J, Hardinge K: Complications of the Attenborough knee replacement. J Bone Joint Surg 68B:100, 1986

139. Simon SR, Trieshmann HW, Burdett RG, et al: Quantitative gait analysis after total knee arthroplasty for monarticular degenerative arthritis. J Bone Joint Surg 65A:605, 1983

140. Sisto DJ, Lachiewicz PF, Insall JN: Treatment of supracondylar fractures following prosthetic arthroplasty of the knee. Clin Orthop 196:265, 1985

141. Sledge CB, Ewald FC: Total knee arthroplasty experience at the Robert Breck Brigham Hospital. Clin Orthop 145:78, 1979

142. Sledge CB, Walker PS: Total knee arthroplasty in rheumatoid arthritis. Clin Orthop 182:127, 1984

143. Sledge CB, Walker PS: Total knee arthroplasty in rheumatoid arthritis. p. 697. In Insall JT (ed): Surgery of the Knee. JB Lippincott, Philadelphia, 1984

144. Sledge CB, Thomas WH, Arbuckle RH: Hinge arthroplasty of the knee. p. 344. In Evarts C McC (ed): American Academy of Orthopaedic Surgeons Symposium on Reconstructive Surgery of the Knee. CV Mosby, St. Louis, 1978

145. Small M, Steven MM, Freeman PA, et al: Total knee arthroplasty in haemophilic arthritis. J Bone Joint Surg 65B:163, 1983

146. Smith BE, Gradisar IA Jr, Martin JM, et al: The effect of obesity on the functional outcome of total knee arthroplasty. Orthop Trans 10:577, 1986

147. Soudry M, Binazzi R, Insall JN, et al: Successive bilateral total knee replacement. J Bone Joint Surg 67A:573, 1985

148. Soudry M, Binazzi R, Johanson NA, et al: Total knee arthroplasty in Charcot and Charcot-like joints. Clin Orthop. 208:199, 1986

149. Soudry M, Mestriner LA, Binazzi R, Insall JN:

Total knee arthroplasty without patellar resurfacing. Clin Orthop 205:166, 1986

150. Soudry M, Walker PS, Reilly DT, Sledge CB: Interface forces of tibial components: the effect of PCL sacrifice and conformity. Trans Orthop Res Soc 8:37, 1983

151. Soudry M, Walker PS, Reilly DT, et al: Effects of total knee replacement design on femoral-tibial contact conditions. J Arthroplasty 1:35, 1986

152. Staeheli JW, Cass JR, Morrey BF: Condylar total knee arthroplasty after failed proximal tibial osteotomy. J Bone Joint Surg 69A:28, 1987

153. Stulberg BN, Insall JN, Williams GW, Ghelman B: Deep-vein thrombosis following total knee replacement. An analysis of six hundred and thirty-eight arthroplasties. J Bone Joint Surg 66A:194, 1984

154. Stulberg SD: The biological response to uncemented total knee replacements. Orthop Trans 10:169, 1986

155. Tew M, Forster IW: Effect of knee replacement on flexion deformity. J Bone Joint Surg 69B:395, 1987

156. Tew M, Waugh W: Tibiofemoral alignment and the results of knee replacement. J Bone Joint Surg 67B:551, 1985

157. Tew M, Waugh W, Forster IW: Comparing the results of different types of knee replacement. A method proposed and applied. J Bone Joint Surg 67B:775, 1985

158. Thornhill TS: Unicompartmental knee arthroplasty. Clin Orthop 205:121, 1986

159. Thornhill TS, Dalziel RW, Sledge CB: Alternatives to arthrodesis for the failed total knee arthroplasty. Clin Orthop 170:131, 1982

160. Thornhill TS, Hood RW, Dalziel RE, et al: Knee revision in failed noninfected total knee arthroplasty — the Robert B Brigham and Hospital for Special Surgery Experience. Orthop Trans 6:368, 1982

161. Townley CO: The anatomic total knee resurfacing arthroplasty. Clin Orthop 192:82, 1985

162. Trent PS, Walker PS, Wolf B: Ligament length patterns, strength and rotational axes of the knee joint. Clin Orthop 117:263, 1976

163. Vince KG, Johnson JA, Krygier J, et al: Tibial component tilting in total knee arthroplasty. Orthop Trans 10:408, 1986

164. Volatile TB, Ewald FC: Ten year results of 171 duocondylar total knee replacements. Orthop Trans 10:491, 1986

165. Walker PS, Greene D, Reilly D, et al: Fixation of

the tibial components of knee prostheses. J Bone Joint Surg 63A:258, 1981

166. Walker PS, Hajek JV: The load-bearing area in the knee joint. J Biomech 5:581, 1972

167. Walker PS, Lawes P: The stability and fixation of knee prostheses. p. 195. In Hastings GW, Williams DF (eds): Mechanical Properties of Biomaterials. John Wiley & Sons, London, 1980

168. Walker PS, Thatcher J, Ewald FC: Variables affecting the fixation of tibial components. Engin Med 11:83, 1982

169. Walldius B: Arthroplasty of the knee joint using endoprosthesis. Acta Orthop Scand 24(suppl):19, 1957

170. Wang CJ, Walker PS: Rotatory laxity of the human knee joint. J Bone Joint Surg 56A:161, 1974

171. Wang CJ, Walker PS, Wolf B: The effects of flexion and rotation on the length patterns of the ligaments of the knee. J Biomech 6:587, 1973

172. Waters RL, Perry J, Conaty P, et al: The energy cost of walking with arthritis of the hip and knee. Clin Orthop 214:278, 1987

173. Webster DA, Murray DG: Complications of variable axis total knee arthroplasty. Clin Orthop 193:160, 1985

174. Wetzner SM, Bezreh JS, Scott RD, et al: Bone scanning in the assessment of patellar viability following knee replacement. Clin Orthop 199:215, 1985

175. Wilson FC, Fajgenbaum DM, Venters GC: Results of knee replacement with the Walldius and Geometric prostheses. A comparative study. J Bone Joint Surg 62A:497, 1980

176. Windsor RE, Insall JN, Sculco TP: Bone grafting of tibial defects in primary and revision total knee arthroplasty. Clin Orthop 205:132, 1986

177. Woods L, Wasilewski SA, Healy W: The value of continuous passive motion in total knee arthroplasty. Orthop Trans 10:576, 1986

178. Wright TM, Bartel DL: The problem of surface damage in polyethylene total knee components. Clin Orthop 205:67, 1986

Revision Total Knee Arthroplasty

122

James A. Rand

Failure of initial total knee arthroplasty designs leading to revision has been a problem. Failure rates have been progressive with time, and in some series failure by all mechanisms was an ongoing process as late as 10 years following arthroplasty.[30,47] The failure rate with the polycentric prosthesis at 10 years was 58 percent,[47] with the Stanmore prosthesis at 8 years was 58 percent,[30] and with the GUEPAR prosthesis at 5 years was 73 percent.[31] By contrast, the total condylar prosthesis at 10 years has been satisfactory in 87.5 percent of 40 knees.[40] Failure of total knee arthroplasty may be attributed to one or a combination of three basic reasons: (1) inadequate implant design, (2) improper patient selection, or (3) incorrect surgical technique. Occasionally, a fourth mechanism of abnormal tissue response such as heterotopic ossification or fat pad hypertrophy leads to failure but this mode of failure is infrequent.

FAILURE MECHANISM

Inadequate implant design was a contributing factor to failure in many early designs and continues to be a problem with some current implants. Inadequate implant design may contribute to failure by (1) excessive stress within the implant leading to breakage, (2) excessive stress at the bone-cement interface leading to loosening, or (3) a kinematic mismatch between the implant and soft tissues resulting in limited motion or abnormal mechanics. The polycentric and geometric tibial implant designs lead to areas of stress concentration in the metaphyseal bone of the tibia with subsequent loosening[58] (Fig. 122-1). Fixed hinge designs such as the GUEPAR (Fig. 122-2) did not permit the normal rotating motion of the knee resulting in loosening. The metal on metal-bearing surfaces resulted in metallic wear debris and syno-

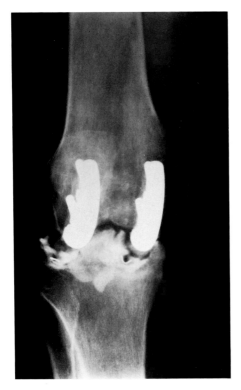

Fig. 122-1. Loose polycentric tibial component from subsidence.

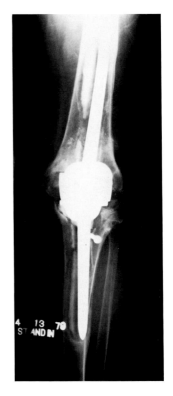

Fig. 122-2. Loose GUEPAR prosthesis.

vitis (Fig. 122-3). The shallow patellar groove of the fixed hinge devices allowed patellar subluxation and dislocation.[56] The geometric prosthesis was a kinematic mismatch between a constrained articular surface geometry with a single axis of rotation and retained cruciate ligaments.[46] For a geometric knee to flex beyond 60 degrees, there is a loss of joint congruity and a force of three to four times normal in the posterior cruciate ligament.[46] Some implants such as the older Herbert and newer kinematic rotating hinge have had areas of stress concentration in the design, which resulted in implant breakage (Fig. 122-4). In a review of 50 kinematic rotating hinge prostheses, there was a 10 percent incidence of implant breakage.[67] Implant breakage may also occur in condylar knee designs related to excessive stress by the patient, abnormal limb alignment and an unsupported tibial tray being stressed in cantilevered bending fatigue.[52,74] Newer porous-coated prostheses are potentially at an increased risk of breakage because the sintering process weakens the metal.[59]

With condylar implant designs, metal trays decrease motion between the implant and bone under load.[6,48,70,86] The use of a metal central stem reduces stress in the cancellous bone of the tibia from 16 to 39 percent compared with a plastic stem.[60,86] The length of the stem is important, with stress shielding occurring along the length of the stem.[9,85] Fixation peg designs are of even greater importance in porous ingrowth designs. For a cementless ingrowth prosthesis, failure will occur if there is inadequate initial fixation, which prevents bone ingrowth. Conversely, a long porous coated stem may permit ingrowth into the stem with stress shielding and failure of ingrowth on the articulating portion of the prosthesis.[8] One-piece tibial component designs give lower bone-cement interface stresses than do two-piece designs.[48] Implant design will affect stress levels on the bone-cement interface with a partially conforming implant that permits rotation, presenting less stress than a fully conforming implant.[10,77,87]

Improper patient selection may lead to implant

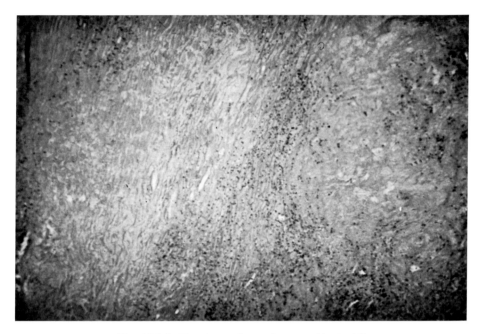

Fig. 122-3. Histology of metallic synovitis. (×16)

failure. The very young patient who resumes normal activities such as sports with impact loading or repetitive heavy lifting in an occupation will present increased stresses to the prosthesis and bone-cement interface. The obese patient will also place increased load on the implant and bone-cement interface with the potential for implant breakage or loosening.[83] Therefore, patients should be informed of activity limitations following total knee arthroplasty, and obese patients should

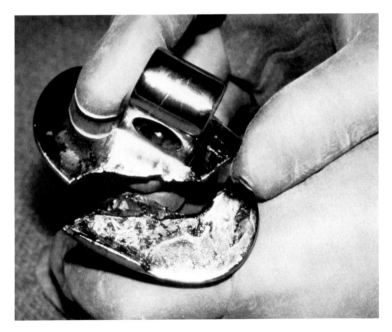

Fig. 122-4. Breakage of inner tibial bearing of kinematic rotating hinge.

be required to decrease their weight. The patient with severe osteoporosis will have inadequate structural support for the components that may lead to sinkage on the tibial or femoral side.[17] Femoral loosening related to severe osteoporosis occurred in 5 of 300 ICLH prostheses.[17]

Although failure may occur from inadequate implant design or improper patient selection, errors in surgical technique are a frequent problem leading to failure of a total knee arthroplasty. Errors in surgical technique result from failure to follow the principles of proper component orientation, soft tissue balancing throughout a range of motion,[55] and correct limb alignment.

The importance of correct limb alignment (tibial-femoral angle) and more recently a correct mechanical axis (a line passing from the center of the femoral head to the center of the ankle should pass through the center of the knee) has been emphasized[4,20,24,25,37,45,47,49,68,80] (Fig. 122-5). Errors in limb alignment result from errors in surgical technique. Errors occur with current instrumentation systems due to difficulty in defining anatomic landmarks at surgery. Performance errors by a surgeon in deviating as little as two or three degrees on a tibial or femoral cut may result in a significant deviation of limb alignment from ideal goals. Using an extramedullary alignment system, 48 percent of 29 knees were significantly malaligned.[62] The use of an intramedullary alignment device has improved the accuracy of alignment to within 2 degrees in 86 percent.[45] Failure to obtain correct alignment may also result from failure to obtain full-length radiographs preoperatively. Full-length radiographs are especially important in patients with bowing of the femoral or tibial shafts or posttraumatic deformity (Fig. 122-6). Deviation from a correct mechanical axis in either a varus or valgus direction will result in asymmetric loading and potential loosening. The exact amount of deviation of the mechanical axis from ideal that will adversely affect implant function is unknown, but any deviation is undesirable. Correct alignment and symmetric loading are essential in cementless prostheses due to limited fixation stems in soft cancellous bone.[2]

Malalignment of the limb predisposes to tibial component loosening. Varus limb alignment has correlated with stress fracture of the tibial plateau and loosening in the geometric knee.[68] In a study of

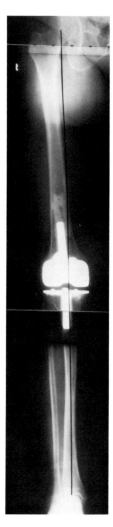

Fig. 122-5. Mechanical axis of the limb in porous-coated anatomic revision total knee arthroplasty.

209 polycentric knees, varus positioning or valgus positioning of greater than 8 degrees doubled the failure rate compared to neutral alignment.[47] For the ICLH prosthesis, there was a 91 percent failure rate with varus alignment, 100 percent failure with 0 degrees alignment, and 11 percent failure with valgus alignment in 32 knees.[4] In a study of 428 resurfacing arthroplasties, there was a 35 percent failure rate if less than 2 degrees of valgus, 24 percent failure rate if 3 to 12 degrees of valgus, and 55 percent failure rate if greater than 12 degrees of valgus.[80] In a review of 124 kinematic condylar knees, knees undercorrected to an average of 2

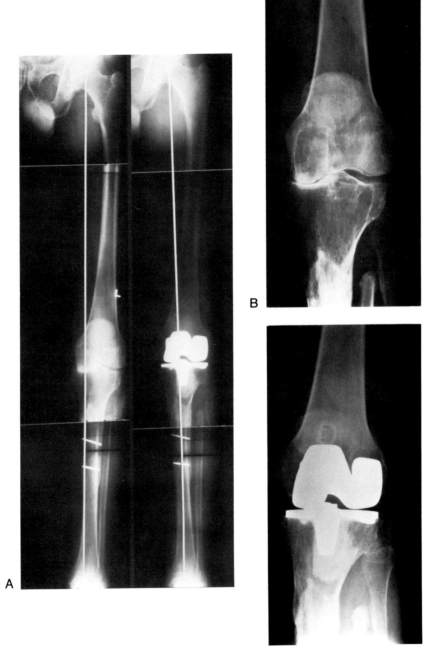

Fig. 122-6. **(A)** Full-length and short standing AP radiograph, **(B)** before, and **(C)** after total knee arthroplasty in a patient with a previous tibial fracture. A metal wedge has been used on the lateral aspect of the tibial component.

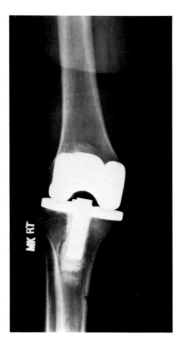

Fig. 122-7. Compensatory valgus femoral component placement for varus tibial component resulting in an overall correct limb alignment.

degrees of valgus had lucent lines significantly more frequently than did knees with 5 degrees of valgus.[24,25] In a review of 30 total condylar prostheses, alignment of 3 to 9 degrees of valgus resulted in significantly fewer radiolucent lines (35 percent) compared with varus (93 percent) or excessive valgus (67 percent).[20] Therefore, failure to obtain correct limb alignment with a correct mechanical axis is a frequent reason for failure.

Improper component orientation may occur in the presence of a correct mechanical axis of the limb. Varus placement of the tibial component in the coronal plane with a compensatory increase in valgus of the femoral component will provide a correct mechanical axis of the limb (Fig. 122-7). However, varus placement of the tibial component has been correlated with tibial component loosening.[19,20,24,25,68] Although some authorities have suggested a 2- to 3-degree varus inclination of the tibial component in the coronal plane relative to the mechanical axis of the limb, this objective is difficult to achieve.[34] In an attempt to achieve a 3-degree varus inclination of the tibial component,

4.6 degrees of varus occurred.[62] In a subsequent review of the cementless porous coated anatomic knee, varus orientation of the tibial component significantly correlated with lucent lines.[65] Varus orientation of five degrees of the tibial component significantly correlated with tibial radiolucent lines compared to one degree of varus in a series of 124 kinematic condylar prostheses.[24,25] Varus positioning of the tibial component of five degrees or more significantly correlates with tibial radiolucent lines in the total condylar prosthesis.[20] The angulation of the joint line probably increases shear forces on the tibial component contributing to loosening. An increased valgus placement of the femoral component to compensate for the varus tibia will compromise patellar tracking and may contribute to lateral patellar subluxation or dislocation.[21]

Sagittal plane component malalignment and malposition is also a problem. Anterior tilt of the tibial component will result in impingement between the posterior aspect of the tibial component and the femoral component in flexion. The wedging effect of contact between the components will be a loss of flexion. Furthermore, increased stress will be placed on the bone-cement and prosthesis-cement interfaces of the tibial component, potentially leading to loosening. Porous coated cementless implants are particularly at risk for tibial

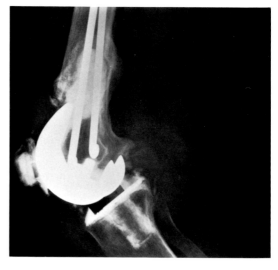

Fig. 122-8. Posterior rotation of the femoral component resulting in notching of the femur.

loosening due to limited tibial fixation. A posterior slope for the tibial component has been recommended to improve flexion.[20] Some implant designs have an inherent posterior slope to the articular surface. If either an excessive posterior slope is cut on the tibia or a posterior sloped prosthesis is placed on a posteriorly angled bone cut, sagittal plane instability may occur. An excessive posterior angle to the tibial cut may compromise the tibial attachment of the posterior cruciate ligament.

Posterior rotation of the femoral component in the sagittal plane may lead to notching of the femur in the supracondylar area, stress concentration and subsequent fracture (Fig. 122-8). Anterior rotation of the femoral component may result in patellar impingement between the trochlear surface of the femoral component and patella. Anterior rotation of the femoral component will lead to point loading of the tibial polyethylene and to potentially increased wear.

Incorrect placement of the femoral component in the anteroposterior plane may lead to failure. If the femoral component is anteriorly displaced or an undersized femoral component is used, there will be an excessive flexion space, leading to flexion instability[20,37] (Fig. 122-9). If an oversized femoral component is used, the extensor mechanism will be anteriorly displaced, limiting flexion. If the femoral component is posteriorly displaced, notching of the anterior femoral cortex will occur which may lead to a supracondylar fracture or the flexion space may be decreased leading to loss of motion. If excessive bone is resected from the posterior aspect of the femur and a correct size implant is used, the femoral component will be unsupported in flexion, leading to femoral loosening[43] (Fig. 122-10). Excessive posterior bone resection from the femur was the etiology of femoral loosening in 13 of 15 cases.[43]

Rotational malalignment of either the tibial or femoral component is a potentially severe problem. Internal rotation of the tibial component relative to the tibia will result in a lateral displacement of the tibial tubercle and extensor mechanism, leading to patellar instability. Internal rotation of the femoral component will impair the patella en-

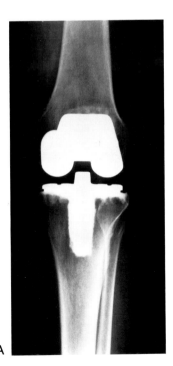
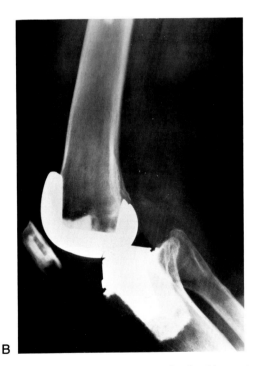

A   B

Fig. 122-9. **(A)** AP, and **(B)** lateral radiographs of Insall-Burstein prosthesis with undersized femoral component leading to flexion instability. *(Figure continues.)*

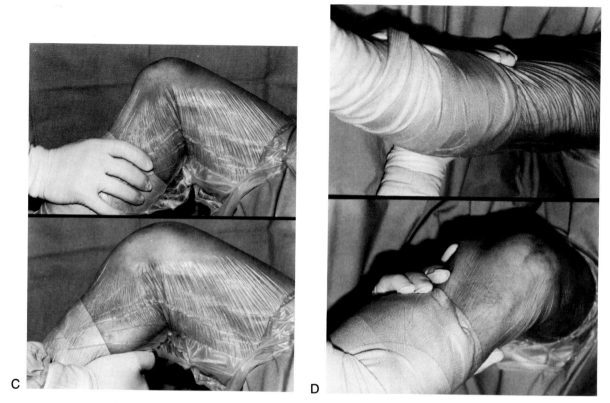

C   D

Fig. 122-9 *(Continued).* **(C)** Sagittal plane, and **(D)** coronal plane instability.

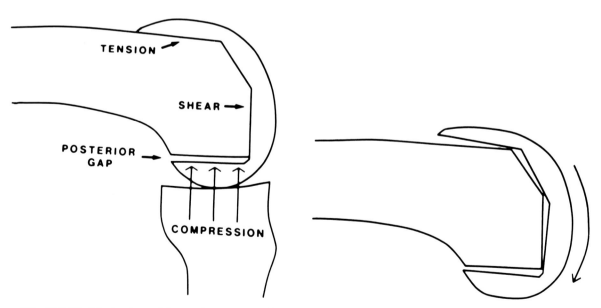

Fig. 122-10. Mechanism of femoral component loosening due to lack of support in flexion from excessive posterior bone resection from the femur. (From King,[43] with permission.)

tering the trochlear groove of the femur and patellar tracking. Excessive external rotation of the tibial component will result in posterior overhang of the tibial component on the lateral side with a decreased area for load transmission to the tibia and a potential for impingement with the femur on knee flexion. Mild external rotation of the femoral component appears to be well tolerated and has been advocated to aid in soft tissue balancing on the lateral side of the knee in flexion.[37]

Medial or lateral translocation of the components will alter load transmission across the joint.[32,57] Medial translocation of the tibial component beyond the medial cortex of the tibia can result in impingement between the medial collateral ligament and component with pain (Fig. 122-11).

The level of tibial bone resection is important. The mechanical strength of the tibial bone decreases from a proximal to distal level.[5,17,36,44,86] The bone of the proximal tibia is stronger medially and laterally than centrally[17] The strength of the femoral condyle is five times greater than the tibial

condyle.[17] Lucent lines adjacent to a total condylar prosthesis were significantly more frequent when 7 mm compared with 3 mm of proximal tibial bone was resected.[20] If excessive bone is removed from the proximal tibia and distal femur with the resultant space filled with a thick tibial component, the joint line will be displaced proximally. Proximal displacement of the joint line will alter ligament kinematics and may result in patellar impingement against the tibial component.[27] This problem of bone loss is common in revision surgery.

Tibial component sizing relative to the cut surface of the proximal tibia is important. If the tibial component does not cover the proximal tibia, strain distribution in the proximal tibia is lower than normal.[70] The adequacy of coverage of the tibial plateau by the prosthesis affects the quality of fixation and as large a prosthesis as possible should be used.[9,26] In vitro, a 21 to 89 percent improvement in single load to failure occurs with a prosthesis that conforms to the tibial surface compared to incomplete coverage.[9] Loss of tibial component-cortex contact in vitro results in a 30 to 60 percent decrease in proximal tibial strain values, which pre-

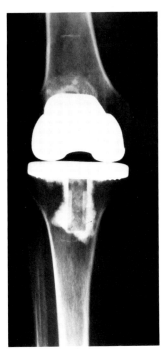

Fig. 122-11. Excessive implant size and medial translation of tibial component relative to tibia leading to painful impingement on medial collateral ligament.

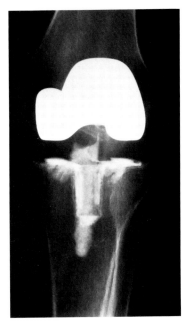

Fig. 122-12. Subsidence of a tibial component of a total condylar prosthesis after 5 years due to inadequate coverage of the proximal tibia in an osteoporotic patient.

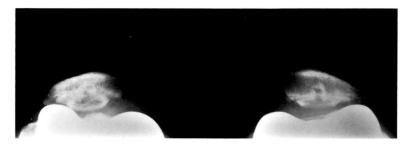

Fig. 122-13. Tilted patella (right knee) on Merchant view due to asymmetric bone cut.

disposes the cancellous bone of the proximal tibia to increased loading with possible component subsidence or loosening[26] (Fig. 122-12).

Extensor mechanism malalignment or patellar implant malposition may lead to reoperation. Re-surfacing of only the lateral patellar facet often results in an asymmetric patellar cut with a tilted patella (Fig. 122-13). The tilted patella will lead to abnormal stresses on the implant with wear and loosening (Fig. 122-14). Insufficient patellar bone

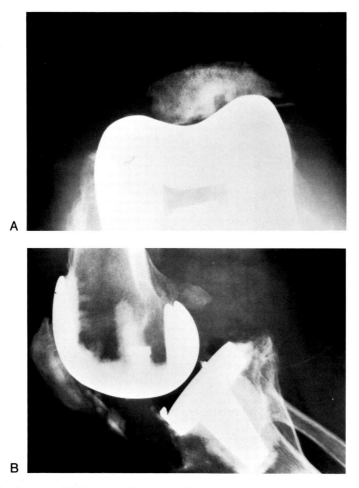

Fig. 122-14. **(A)** Merchant, and **(B)** lateral radiographs of loose patellar implant from asymmetric patellar bone cut. A fracture of the central peg of the patellar implant remains securely cemented.

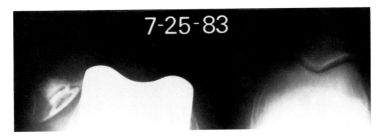

Fig. 122-15. Dislocated patella from failure to balance extensor mechanism.

resection will result in a patella that is too thick. The associated anterior displacement of the extensor mechanism will limit motion. Excessive patellar bone resection will result in a potentially weak structure due to loss of the posterior cortical layer predisposing to fracture. Inadequate balancing of the extensor mechanism will lead to patellar subluxation and dislocation with severe impairment in function (Fig. 122-15). Patellar dislocation also results from component malrotation and trauma.[54]

FAILURE MODES

The most frequent mode of failure in total knee arthroplasty has been implant loosening.[1,11,13–15,22,23,33,35,39,42,60,69,71,82,84,88] In our initial experience with 5,643 total knee arthroplasties performed between 1970 and 1980, 330 subsequently required revision for an incidence of 5.8 percent.[69] Most of these initial arthroplasties were early designs, such as the geometric or polycentric resurfacing prostheses or GUEPAR or Walldius hinges. Loosening was the most frequent mode of failure followed by instability, abnormal axial alignment, and improper component orientation.[69] Other causes of failure include patellar problems, implant or bone fractures, fibrous ankylosis, and unexplained pain.

Implant loosening is multifactorial and relates to poor implant design, excessive stress by the patient, and incorrect surgical technique. Instability results from failure of surgical technique or choice of a prosthesis with inadequate inherent constraint for the patient. Abnormal alignment results from errors in surgical technique or incomplete preoperative evaluation of femoral or tibial deformities. Improper component orientation arises from surgical technique errors. Patellar problems may be pain, instability, implant loosening, or fracture. Patellar pain may result from failure to resurface a diseased patella.[79] Patellar instability results from excessive valgus alignment, component malposition, or inadequate extensor mechanism balancing. Patellar implant loosening relates to incorrect patellar implant position, abnormal patellar tracking, or insecure initial fixation. Patellar fracture may occur with or without patellar resurfacing and results from maltracking, avascularity, excessive bone resection, or a large patellar fixation peg and is most frequent in knees with more than 100 degrees of flexion.[76,81] Implant breakage results from poor design, excessive stress by the patient, or errors in surgical technique resulting in high stress levels on the component. Bone fracture results from stress concentration by implants, errors in implant placement, or trauma.[53,68]

INDICATIONS AND CONTRAINDICATIONS FOR REVISION

The indication for revision total knee arthroplasty is failure from any of the previously described mechanisms. A prerequisite for considering revision arthroplasty must be a clear understanding of the failure mechanism or mechanisms. Failure to understand the reason or reasons for failure of the initial arthroplasty will allow repetition of these errors at the time of revision. An intelligent, cooperative patient who will follow ad-

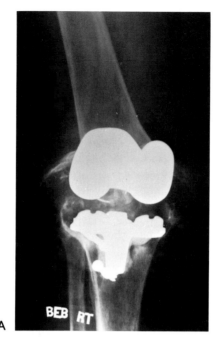

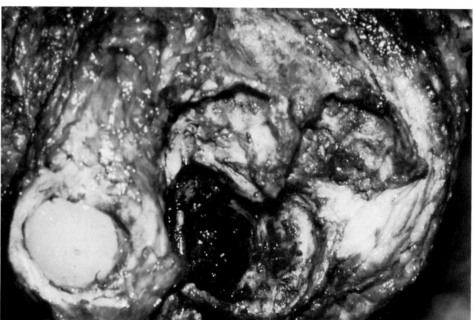

Fig. 122-16. **(A)** AP radiograph, and **(B)** operative photograph of osteolysis around loose total knee arthroplasty. *(Figure continues.)*

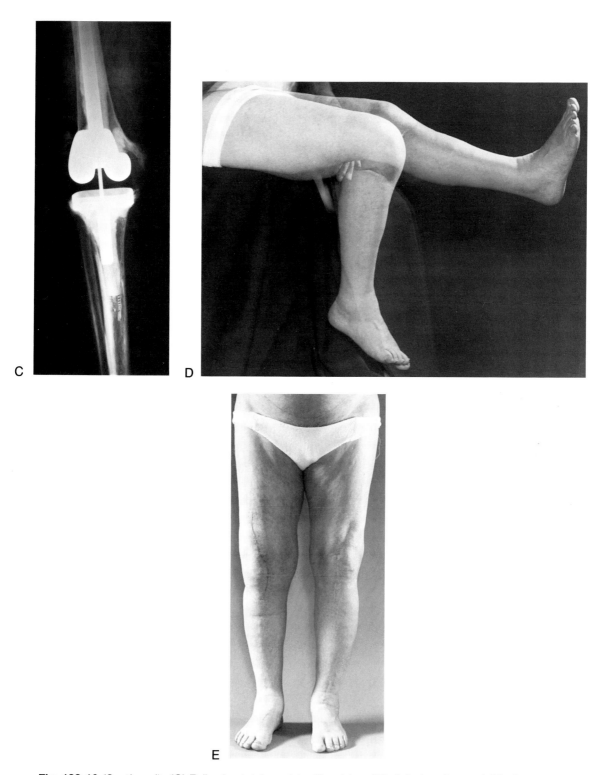

Fig. 122-16 *(Continued).* **(C)** Following total condylar III revision, **(D)** clinical motion, and **(E)** alignment.

vised levels of restriction of activity and who will follow the rehabilitation program is essential. Mechanical loosening should be treated early before osteolysis and bone resorption occur (Fig. 122-16). Ligamentous instability should be treated initially by nonoperative measures of muscle strengthening and bracing. If these measures are ineffective, revision should be considered.

Contraindications to revision are a noncompliant patient, vigorous demands in a young patient, severe soft tissue deficiencies, and pain of indeterminate etiology. The noncompliant patient will abuse the arthroplasty or will fail to follow the rehabilitation program, leading to an unsatisfactory result. The young, vigorous patient with single joint disease, especially if employed in a laboring occupation, is best served by arthrodesis. Severe soft tissue deficiencies, such as an absent or paralyzed extensor mechanism, longstanding patellar tendon avulsion, or inadequate soft tissue coverage of the knee, are extremely difficult problems to correct. The patient with pain of indeterminate etiology will often continue to have pain following revision and may continue to have pain following arthrodesis. Relative contraindications are obesity, severe bone loss, and severe instability. The patient with mild subjective disability from any reason is best treated nonoperatively.

EVALUATION

Evaluation of the failed total knee arthroplasty begins with a definition of the reason or reasons for failure. Definition of the reasons for failure will permit correction of the deficiencies and prevent their recurrence. Septic failure must always be considered in the differential diagnosis of pain or loosening. Sepsis with a virulent organism is easily diagnosed. However, a low virulence or anaerobic organism may present with minimal systemic and local symptoms. The only findings can be pain or pain and implant loosening. Progressive osteolysis at the bone-cement interface and periosteal reaction are highly suggestive of sepsis. Radiographs may only demonstrate progressive implant loosen-

ing without signs of bone destruction or early in the course of infection may be normal. Differential technetium 99m methylene diphosphonate (Tc 99m MDP) and gallium citrate (Ga 67) or indium (In 111) scans may be helpful in diagnosis.[61,66] Aspriation of the knee is helpful in defining infection when positive but a negative aspiration does not preclude the presence of sepsis. Aspiration will reveal positive cultures in the presence of infection in approximately 60 percent of patients.[61] Routine hematologic tests, such as white blood cell (WBC) count and erythrocyte sedimentation rate (ESR), may be normal but the ESR is usually elevated in long standing infections.[61]

Loosening is best defined by a progression of lucent lines on sequential radiographs. A complete lucent line of 2 mm or greater in width, progression of lucent lines, or a shift in implant position are highly suggestive of loosening if consistent radiographic technique has been used[72,73] (Fig. 122-17). Radiographic technique is extremely important. A 1-mm lucent line adjacent to a metal-backed tibial component can be obliterated by as little as 5 degrees of rotation or knee flexion.[50] Loosening frequently corresponds with technical errors in implant positioning or alignment. Technetium 99m methylene diphosphonate bone scans often show intense uptake adjacent to a loose component.[73]

The integrity and mobility of the soft tissues must be assessed. Instability may be evident on radiographs showing tibial subluxation or dislocation (Fig. 122-18). Instability may be in the coronal or sagittal plane. Stability must be assessed by a careful physical examination. Varus-valgus stability must be assessed throughout the range of motion not just in extension. AP stability should be assessed throughout a range of motion. The integrity of the collateral ligaments and extensor mechanism must be evaluated as their presence or absence will affect prosthetic choice as well as the ability to salvage the implant.

The quality and quantity of the remaining bone stock must be determined from a careful review of the radiographs. Bone loss may be central or peripheral and may be symmetric or asymmetric. Femoral bone loss is usually symmetric and involves the distal and posterior bone from the femur. The extent of bone loss will influence the need for an augmented prosthesis rather than a

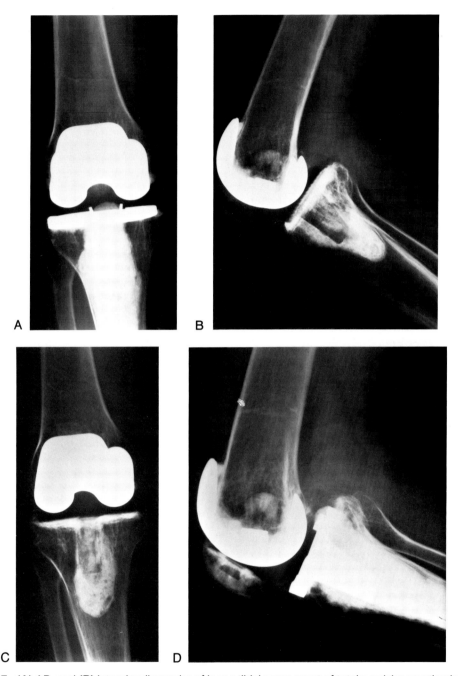

Fig. 122-17. **(A)** AP, and **(B)** lateral radiographs of loose tibial component of total condylar prosthesis. **(C)** AP, and **(D)** lateral radiographs 5 years after revision with metal-backed tibial component.

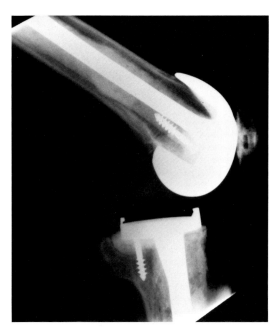

Fig. 122-18. Posterior tibial subluxation of a kinematic stabilizer revision prosthesis due to instability in flexion.

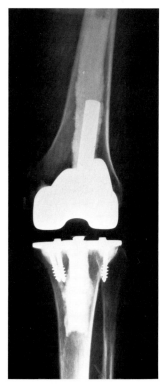

Fig. 122-19. Central tibial defect from geometric prosthesis revised to porous-coated anatomic revision total knee arthroplasty treated by screws and cement.

standard implant. Tibial bone loss that is central may be treated by bone grafting or filling of the defect with cement reinforced with screws or wire mesh (Fig. 122-19). In the case of a peripheral defect without an intact cortical rim, cement filling is inadequate, and a custom component may be required.

REVISION TECHNIQUE

The principles of revision total knee arthroplasty are the same as a primary procedure. There must be correct limb alignment, proper component orientation, and soft tissue balance providing stability throughout a range of motion. The problems inherent with revision surgery are bone loss, the previous bone-cement interface, and soft tissue scarring.

Surgical exposure can be difficult in revision surgery. Extensive scarring may be present. The collateral ligaments and extensor mechanism must be preserved for optimal function. Previous surgical incisions should be used whenever feasible to prevent areas of skin necrosis between the old and new incisions (Fig. 122-20). If flaps must be elevated because of less than ideally placed previous incisions, they should be full thickness comprising skin and subcutaneous tissue in a single layer to maintain the blood supply to the skin (Fig. 122-21). Surgical exposure should commence with restoration of the suprapatellar pouch, and medial and lateral gutters to permit eversion of the patella and knee flexion.[38] In some instances, a tight extensor mechanism may not permit eversion of the patella without the risk of patellar tendon avulsion. In these instances, turndown of the extensor mechanism is preferrable to the risk of patellar tendon rupture. A V-Y release of the extensor mechanism may be used, or a full turndown of the patella may be required[18,75] (Fig. 122-22). In order to regain motion, extensive scar, especially in the posterior capsule, should be excised.

Implant removal can be relatively easy in the case of a loose implant, and an osteotome may be sufficient (Fig. 122-23). In the case of a securely

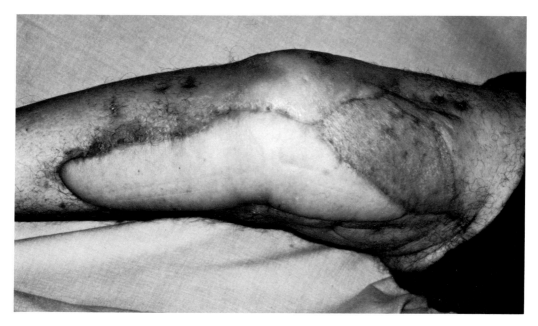

Fig. 122-20. Skin necrosis with subsequent infection, resulting in arthrodesis and free flap for wound coverage due to failure to use existing incision.

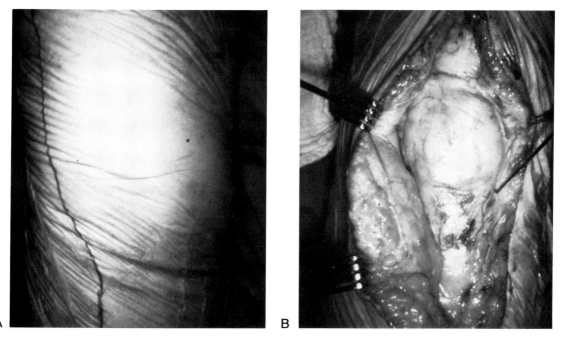

Fig. 122-21. **(A)** Previous lateral parapatellar skin incision for unicompartmental replacement. **(B)** Elevation of full-thickness flap for revision through old skin incision with anteromedial fascial incision.

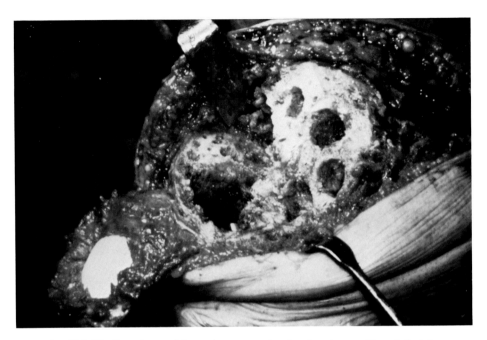

Fig. 122-22. Turndown of the extensor mechanism in a knee with patella infra.

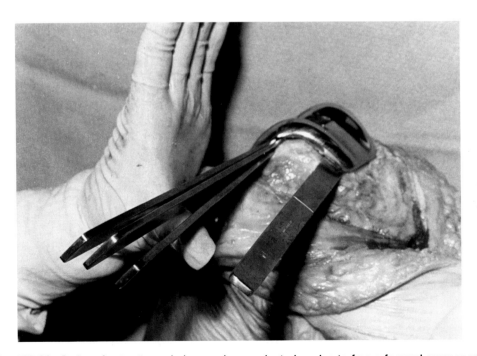

Fig. 122-23. Series of osteotomes being used as graduated wedge to free a femoral component.

Fig. 122-24. Securely fixed femoral component. **(A)** Midas Rex dissection at the prosthesis-cement interface. **(B)** Following dissection. **(C)** After removal of component.

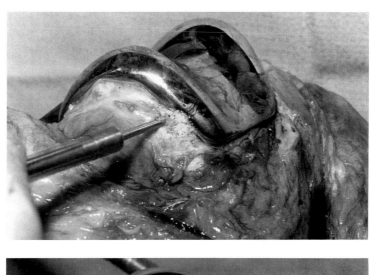

A

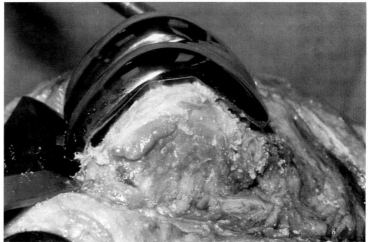

B

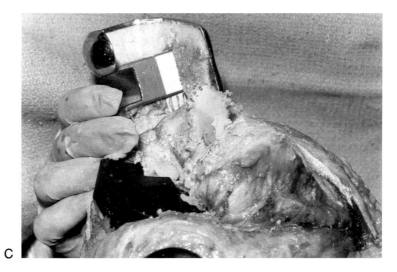

C

fixed implant, a high-speed cutting instrument such as the Midas Rex is invaluable. Dissection should be performed at the implant-cement interface to avoid damage to bone stock (Fig. 122-24). Initial management of a metal backed tibial component that is securely fixed to bone should be by dissection at the bone-cement interface. Once the tibial plateau portion of the prosthesis has been freed, longitudinal traction should be applied to the prosthesis. If the implant remains securely fixed by the intramedullary stem, the tibial plateau portion of the prosthesis should be sectioned with a diamond saw to permit access to the intramedullary stem (Fig. 122-25). The stem can be mobilized by dissection at the prosthesis-cement interface. The underlying cement can then be removed with a combination of osteotomes and the Midas Rex. It is preferable to leave some remaining securely fixed cement than sacrifice bone stock by overly vigorous cement removal provided there is no evidence of infection.

Once the implant and cement have been removed, a fibrous tissue membrane will remain at the bone-cement interface (Fig. 122-26). This membrane must be removed to allow apposition between the new cement and bone. Residual fragments of fibrous tissue and cement can be best identified by debridement with a high speed pulsating lavage. Areas of sclerotic bone can be better penetrated by cement by making several small drill holes (Fig. 122-27).

Selection of the appropriate revision implant is critical. The least constrained implant appropriate for the patient's soft tissues should be utilized. Hinge-type prostheses have a high failure rate.[1,3] In revision surgery, a hinged implant provides less satisfactory results than does a less constrained prosthesis.[3,11] Satisfactory results are more frequently obtained with an unconstrained than with unlinked or linked hinge.[15] Using acturarial techniques, a longer duration of implant function was estimated for resurfacing than for constrained implants[69] (Fig. 122-28). Current condylar designs are the implant of choice for the patient with intact collateral ligaments and minimal loss of bone stock.[11,39] In the patient with instability or loss of bone stock, a stemmed implant with further inherent constraint will be required (Fig. 122-29). A stemmed implant will permit fixation away from an area of bone deficiency in the metaphysis of either

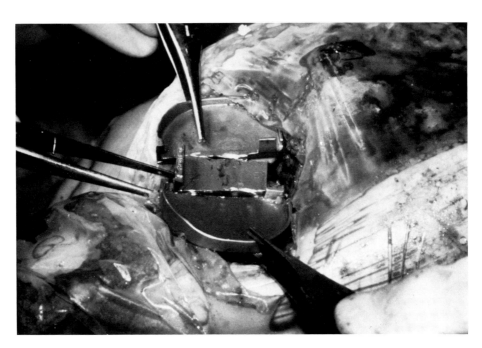

Fig. 122-25. Transection of the tibial plateau of an anametric prosthesis to allow access to the intramedullary stem for removal.

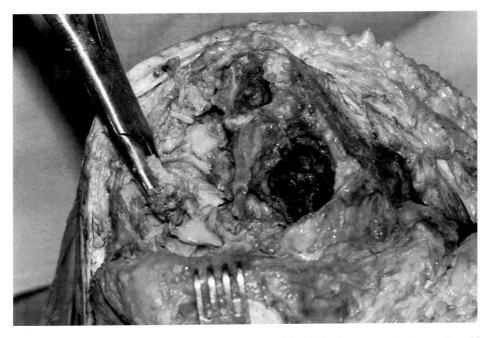

Fig. 122-26. Fibrous tissue membrane adjacent to tibia remaining following removal of cement and implant.

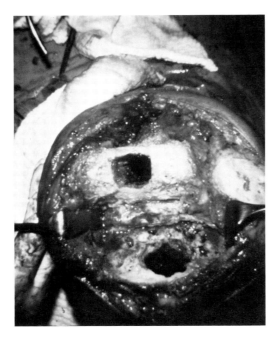

Fig. 122-27. Cement can better penetrate sclerotic bone by preparation with several small drill holes.

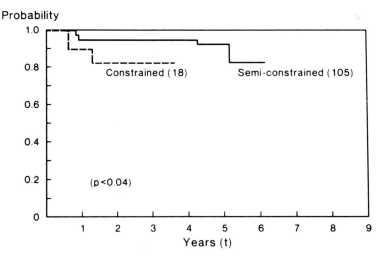

Fig. 122-28. Implant survival for current design resurfacing compared with constrained implants. (From Rand,[69] with permission.)

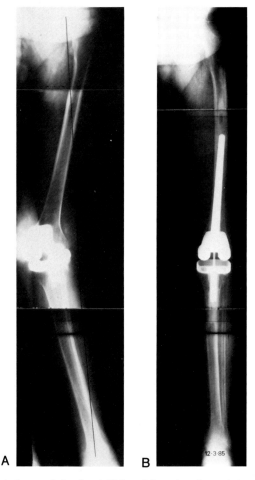

Fig. 122-29. (A) AP radiograph 1 year following initial revision showing rotatory malposition, excess valgus, instability, and chronic patellar dislocation. **(B)** Following long-stemmed total condylar III revision.

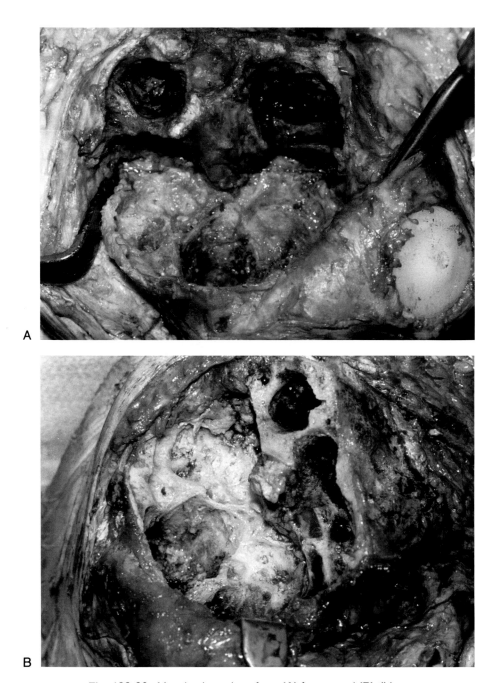

Fig. 122-30. Massive bone loss from **(A)** femur, and **(B)** tibia.

the femur or tibia. The use of a long-stem will decrease the load on the cancellous bone and will transmit load more directly to cortical bone.[6] Finite element analysis suggests that marked stress shielding occurs along the entire length of the intramedullary stem, which may adversely affect long-term fixation.[9] Therefore, the stem length should be only long enough to achieve adequate fixation. Prostheses with central stabilizing pegs are useful in the patient with an absent posterior cruciate and will provide increased stability in many patients, obviating the need for a hinged design. A rotating hinge implant should be reserved for those individuals with an absent collateral ligament and severe bone loss when stability cannot be achieved with a less constrained implant. Results with one rotating hinge design provided only 55 percent satisfactory results in revision surgery.[67]

Bone loss can be dealt with by four mechanisms: (1) cement with or without reinforcement, (2) bone grafting, (3) augmented prostheses, and (4) shift of the implant away from the bone defect. Optimum loading across a tibial implant occurs in the presence of tibial component-cortical rim contact.[9] At the very least, coverage of the tibia should be as complete as possible. In the case of a central defect,

load transfer will occur around the periphery of the component and along the intramedullary stem. Therefore, the presence of an isolated central defect of small or moderate size can be easily dealt with by filling with bone grafts or cement and stress bypassed by the intramedullary stem. In the case of massive central bone deficiency on the tibia or femur, implant fixation will be severely compromised (Fig. 122-30). A long-stemmed implant to achieve fixation in intact diaphyseal bone is indicated. The central defect may be bulk filled with cement or extensively bone grafted, or a custom component with augmentation can be used[78] (Fig. 122-31). The optimal approach in these circumstances is unclear, but bulk cement filling should be avoided whenever feasible and bone grafting with component augmentation would be our current procedure of choice.

In the case of an asymmetric peripheral bone defect on the tibia, additional bone resection to the level of the defect is undesirable because of the decreasing strength of the tibial bone.[36] In vitro, a custom augmented prosthesis will provide the best loading characteristics followed by a metal wedge with the poorest results occurring with cement filling alone[12] (Fig. 122-32). Shifting of the implant

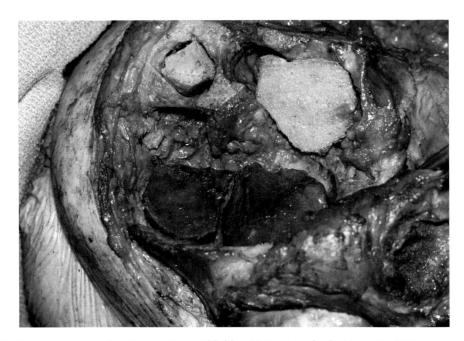

Fig. 122-31. Appearance of patient in Figure 122-30, with bone grafts fashioned to fill the bone defects.

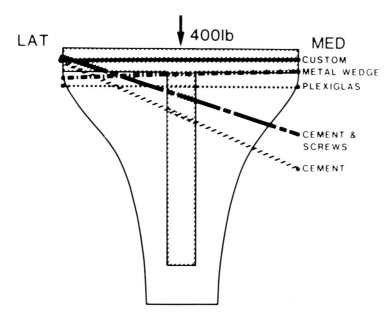

Fig. 122-32. In vitro deflections of a tibial component with various types of support for an asymmetric peripheral defect. (From Brooks,[12] with permission.)

away from the side of the tibial defect with or without cement filling of a defect that is less than 50 percent of the tibial surface, has provided satisfactory results without loosening in 63 knees followed for 3 to 8 years.[51] Bone grafting can be used for structural replacement of lost bone (Fig. 122-33). If successful incorporation of the bone graft occurs, lost bone stock will be replaced. Unfortunately, bone graft incorporation does not always occur and if it does occur some resorption and settling of the graft may occur leaving a portion of the implant unsupported. Autogenous bone is preferable to allograft and rigid fixation with screws should be used.[89] The proximal site of contact between the tibia and graft should be sealed to prevent cement intrusion at the time of placement of the tibial component. Sealing of the graft-tibial interface can be performed with an initial small quantity of cement or by gelfoam (Fig. 122-34). Bone grafting of 24 large tibial defects with a follow-up of 3 to 6 years was successful in 22 cases.[21] Failure in two cases resulted from residual limb malalignment in one and from failure to prepare a vascular bone bed in the other case.[21]

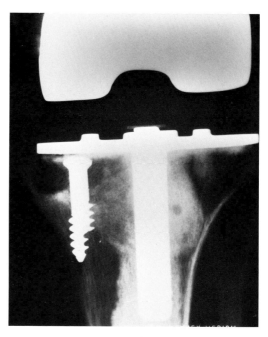

Fig. 122-33. AP radiograph of bone graft 1 year after porous-coated anatomic revision total knee arthroplasty.

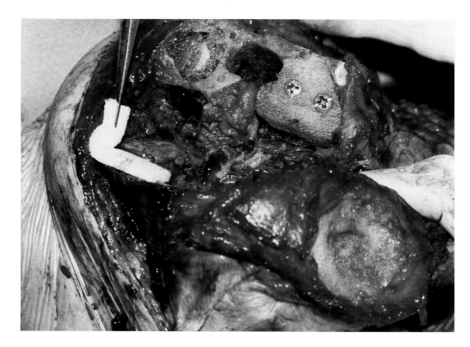

Fig. 122-34. Sealing of interface between bone graft and host bone with gelfoam to prevent cement intrusion between the graft and host bone.

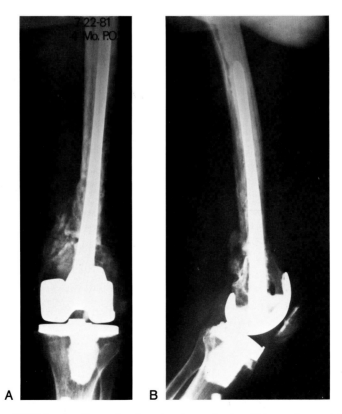

Fig. 122-35. **(A)** AP, and **(B)** lateral radiographs of custom long-stemmed kinematic condylar prosthesis used to bridge supracondylar fracture.

Femoral bone loss is best managed by the use of a prosthesis with distal and posterior augmentation. The augmented implant will maintain the correct level of the joint line and proper collateral ligament kinematics. In severe cases of bone loss proximal to the collateral ligaments, the soft tissue attachments of the ligaments are usually present on a thin shell of bone. In this instance, the joint line must be maintained with an augmented prosthesis with a long stem for fixation. The underlying metaphyseal bone defects should be filled with bone grafts for structural support.

The patient with a fracture in the supracondylar area or proximal metaphysis of the tibia with nonunion presents a difficult bone loss problem. In these instances, bone stock in the metaphysis is often insufficient for internal fixation devices. Revision with a custom long-stemmed component to act as an intramedullary rod across the defect combined with bone grafting is a viable technique (Fig. 122-35). The advantage of this approach is that it maintains soft tissue attachments to the metaphyseal fragment.

Once the decision regarding the choice of an implant has been made, trial fitting of the prosthesis should be performed. Although instrumentation systems are available for some revision prostheses, revision surgery requires frequent trial reduction and assessment, since bony landmarks are deficient, and fixation for cutting jigs is frequently ab-

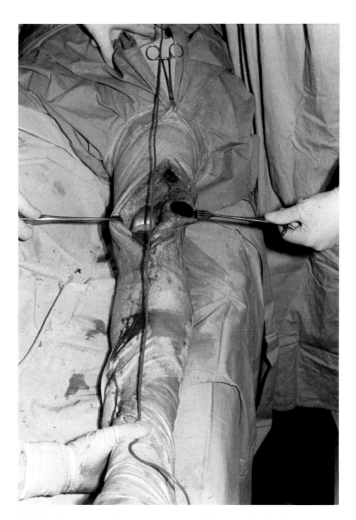

Fig. 122-36. Intraoperative assessment of the mechanical axis of the limb.

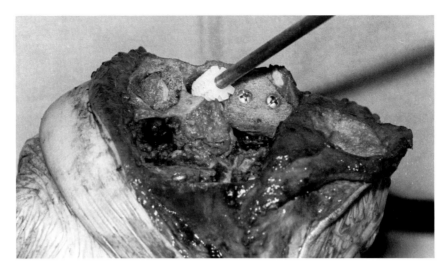

Fig. 122-37. Cement restricter to plug intramedullary canal.

sent. On the femoral side, the revision implant should replace the lost bone to the original anatomical level both distally and posteriorly. Rotational alignment is best assessed by the femoral epicondyles. A valgus alignment of 5 to 7 degrees on the distal femoral cut is usually sufficient to maintain a correct mechanical axis of the limb. On the tibial side, the tibial component should be placed per-

pendicular to the mechanical axis of the tibia and a thick enough component should be used to restore the normal joint line and stability. Rotational placement of the tibial component should be with the center of the implant along the medial aspect of the tibial tuberosity. With the trial implants in place, there should be adequate bone apposition, stability in the coronal and sagittal planes throughout a

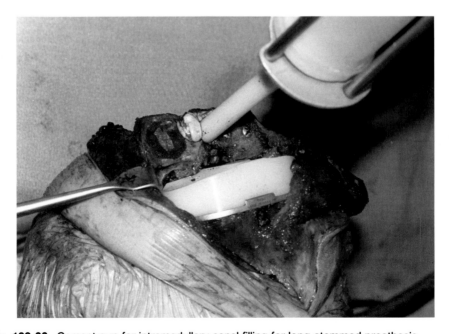

Fig. 122-38. Cement gun for intramedullary canal filling for long-stemmed prosthesis.

range of motion, and a correct mechanical axis of the limb (Fig. 122-36).

Once a satisfactory trial reduction has been achieved, a decision must be made regarding implant fixation. Cement or cementless fixation may be used. If cement fixation is selected, the cement is used early with a cement gun to permit penetration into the drill holes in sclerotic bone. If the intramedullary stems of the implant are to be cemented, the intramedullary canal is plugged (Fig. 122-37) and the cement gun (Fig. 122-38) is used to achieve local cement filling similar to total hip arthroplasty. The tibial and patellar components are cemented, followed by trial fitting of the femur and extension of the knee. This technique permits pressurization of the tibial component and will ensure full extension of the knee. Once these components are secure, a similar technique is used for the femoral component. It is preferable to leave some securely fixed cement than to jeopardize bone stock by its removal since the new cement will bond to the old cement.[29]

Cementless fixation is a potential technique in revision surgery. Cementless fixation relies on the use of intramedullary stems for initial fixation in the presence of bone loss while extensive bone grafting of the metaphyseal areas is performed. A porous ingrowth surface may be used, but a press fitting of either the condylar portion of the implant or the stem must be achieved for initial fixation.

AUTHOR'S PREFERRED TECHNIQUE

The technique of revision will vary with the failure mechanism, patient age, diagnosis, and implant type. Septic failure and its salvage are covered in Chapter 168. Therefore, only salvage of aseptic knees will be reviewed. Salvage in the physiologically older patient will be with a cemented implant. In the younger patient, cementless revision can be considered. Cementless primary and revision procedures have only a short follow-up, and the duration of function of these implants compared with cemented prostheses is unknown. In spite of only short-term results, cementless revision potentially has the advantage of restoring rather than sacrificing further bone stock, making subsequent salvage possible. The type of revision procedure is largely dependent on the previous implant, quantity of remaining bone stock, and integrity of the collateral ligaments.

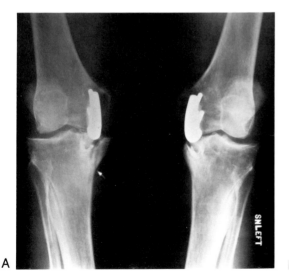
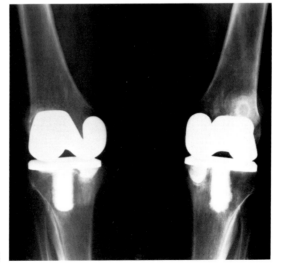

Fig. 122-39. **(A)** AP radiograph of loose tibial components of unicompartmental polycentric total knee arthroplasty. Stress fracture of the medial tibial plateau (arrow). **(B)** AP radiograph 5 years after revision to cruciate condylar total knee arthroplasty.

MINIMAL BONE LOSS

Revision of a knee with minimal loss of bone stock is only slightly more difficult than a primary total knee arthroplasty. Examples of this type of patient would be a failed unicompartmental prosthesis, failed polycentric prosthesis, or condylar implant with minimal bone resection (Fig. 122-39). In these cases with intact collateral ligaments and often a functioning posterior cruciate ligament, a standard condylar type of resurfacing implant without stems will suffice. The technique will consist of routine exposure through the old anteromedial incision, followed by implant removal. Standard total knee instrumentation can generally be used with correction of the bone cuts to provide correct limb alignment and component orientation. The implant used for revision in this group of patients would be a kinematic condylar, cruciate condylar, or total condylar prosthesis. Trial reduction of the components is performed to confirm soft tissue balance. Standard cement technique is used.

MODERATE BONE LOSS

Revision of a knee with moderate bone loss, but functioning collateral ligaments presents the problems of implant fixation and posterior cruciate substitution in most cases, since the posterior cruciate is usually absent. Examples would be a condylar prosthesis with osteolysis, spherocentric, variable axis, or similar prosthesis. Standard exposure and implant removal techniques are used. Minimal additional bone resection should be performed in these patients. The only additional bone removal should be to correct the plane of the femoral or tibial cuts or the chamfer for the femoral component. Bone grafting should be used to fill defects and restore lost bone rather than resection of bone to the base of the defect. A prosthesis with an intramedullary stem will frequently be required to achieve fixation in intact healthy bone and stress relieve deficient areas in the metaphysis. A porous-coated anatomic (PCA) revision or kinematic stabilizer revision implant would be our prosthesis of choice (Fig. 122-40). Both implants have sufficient

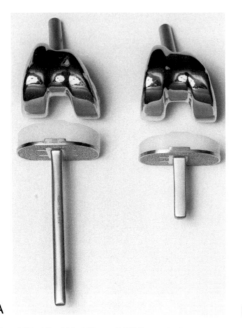
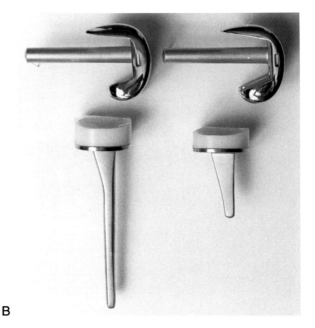

A   B

Fig. 122-40. (A) AP, and **(B)** lateral photographs of porous-coated anatomic revision standard and augmented prosthesis. *(Figure continues.)*

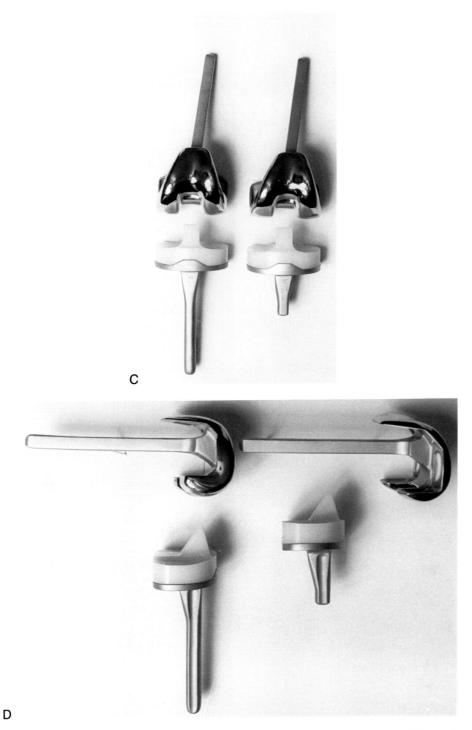

C

D

Fig. 122-40 *(Continued).* **(C)** AP, and **(D)** lateral photographs of standard and augmented kinematic stabilizer revision prosthesis.

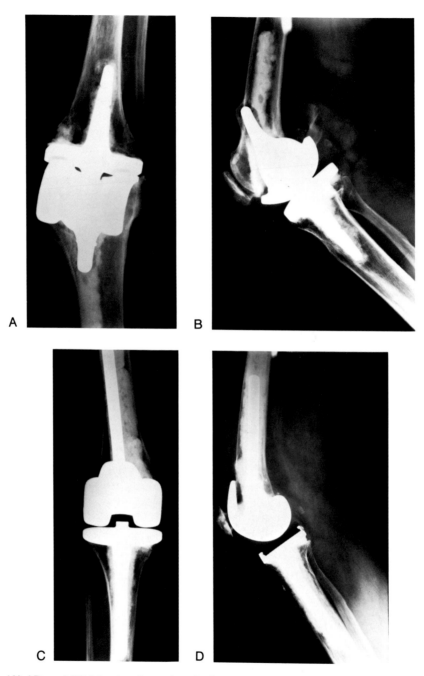

Fig. 122-41. (A) AP, and **(B)** lateral radiographs of a loose spherocentric prosthesis. **(C)** AP, and **(D)** lateral radiographs 1 year following revision to a kinematic stabilizer revision prosthesis.

intramedullary stems for fixation on both the femoral and tibial sides and can be obtained with longer stems as custom-made prostheses. The advantage of these two designs is that the femoral component is available with or without distal and posterior augmentation. The augmented version of the kinematic stabilizer revision is 5 mm and in the PCA revision is 4 mm thicker than the nonaugmented implant. The augmentation on the femur allows compensation for femoral bone loss, which maintains the axis of rotation of the knee and appropriate collateral ligament tensions (Fig. 122-41). Augmentation on the femoral side will maintain the position of the joint line and minimize problems of patellar impingement against the tibia, which would otherwise occur if only a thick tibial component were used. The PCA revision has the advantages of generous chamfer cuts, which permit good implant-bone apposition in instances of femoral bone loss. The PCA tibial component cannot be augmented and lacks a central stabilizing peg for posterior cruciate substitution. The kinematic stabilizer revision tibia has a central stabilizing peg, and metal wedges can be cemented to the tibial component to compensate for bone defects[12] (Fig. 122-6C). The kinematic stabilizer tibial compo-

nents are slightly smaller in area than the PCA revision and may not provide complete coverage of the tibia in a large individual. Instrumentation exists for both implants, but frequent trial reduction is recommended.

Cement fixation of the intramedullary stems is usually required, plugging of the intramedullary canal with bone or a commercially available bone plug is used to restrict and pressurize the cement. Pulsatile lavage of the femoral and tibial canals is utilized followed by a cement gun to introduce the cement. Separate cementing of the tibial and femoral components is recommended with trial reduction of the femur and knee extension at the time of tibial component implantation.

MASSIVE BONE LOSS

The problems of massive bone loss occur following hinged prostheses, multiple revisions, or massive osteolysis from longstanding loose implants. There are often significant problems with the soft

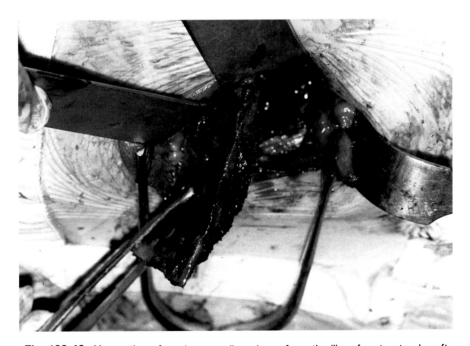

Fig. 122-42. Harvesting of corticocancellous bone from the ilium for structural graft.

tissues and the collateral ligaments may be absent. The same problems exist as in the patient with moderate bone loss but are more extensive. In these instances, a long-stemmed prosthesis will be required to achieve implant fixation. Augmentation for the distal femur and proximal tibia may be required. A central peg for posterior cruciate substitution will be necessary. A constrained articulating geometry may be required. In some instances, a rotating hinge-type prosthesis will be necessary. Exposure and implant removal will be the same as previously described only more difficult. Extreme care must be exercised to preserve all remaining bone stock. Bone grafting will usually be required. If autogenous bone is to be used, posterior iliac crest bone should be harvested prior to beginning the knee-revision procedure. Large corticocancellous pieces consisting of the outer table of the ilium and underlying cancellous bone can be used for structural support (Fig. 122-42). If allograft bone is used, femoral heads removed at the time of total hip arthroplasty can provide good structural grafts.

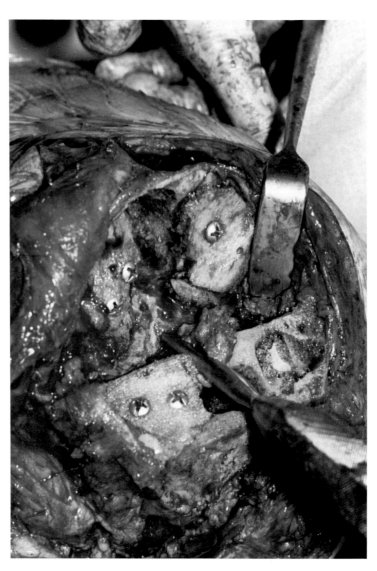

Fig. 122-43. Screw fixation of bone grafts.

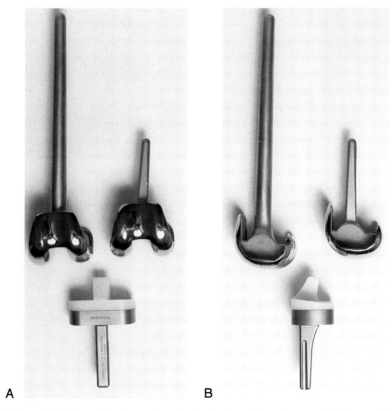

Fig. 122-44. (A) AP, and **(B)** lateral photographs of standard and long-stemmed total condylar III prosthesis.

Once the implant and cement have been removed, minimal bone cuts should be performed to correct limb alignment and component position. Bone grafts should either be cut, so that they can be rigidly press fit into a defect or fixed with screws (Fig. 122-43).

A total condylar III implant (Fig. 122-44) has proved most useful in these patients. The large intramedullary stems can be either press fit or cemented depending upon the quality of fixation. The articular geometry provides stability as does the large central peg. The large femoral stem will permit placement of the articulating portion of the implant at the chosen level yet provide adequate fixation (see Fig. 122-16). Any resultant gap can be filled with structural bone graft. Frequent trial reduction is necessary to achieve appropriate positioning and stability. In the rare instance in which this prosthesis provides inadequate stability, due to an absent collateral ligament, a rotating hinge may

be required. Cement techniques and bone preparation are similar to the patient with moderate bone loss.

CEMENTLESS REVISION

Cementless revision remains an unproven but potentially valuable technique. This technique is used in the physiologically young patient and in the older patient with massive bone loss after multiple revision procedures. These patients will generally require bone grafting, and autogenous bone is recommended. In the case of massive bone loss, autogenous and allograft bone will be required. Bone grafts should be harvested before beginning knee revision as described under Marked Bone Loss.

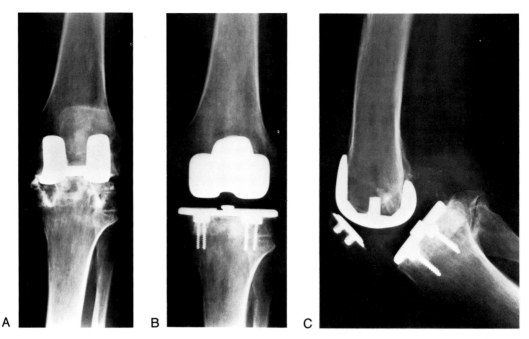

Fig. 122-45. (A) AP radiograph of loose geometric total knee arthroplasty. **(B)** AP radiograph. **(C)** Lateral radiograph following revision to cementless Miller-Galante total knee arthroplasty.

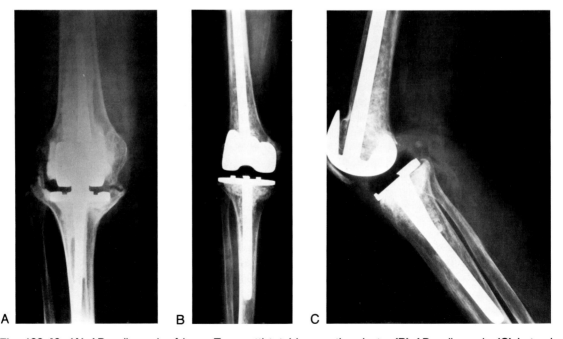

Fig. 122-46. (A) AP radiograph of loose Tavernetti total knee arthroplasty. **(B)** AP radiograph. **(C)** Lateral radiograph following cementless long-stemmed porous-coated anatomic revision and bone grafting.

Prosthetic choice will depend upon the extent of bone loss. In the case of minimal bone loss such as a failed unicompartmental or resurfacing implant, a resurfacing prosthesis such as a PCA or Miller-Galante implant may suffice (Fig. 122-45). In the case of moderate bone loss, the PCA revision implant is selected. A porous-coated stem should not be placed cementless as bone ingrowth into the stem could lead to stress shielding and late implant failure.[8] Therefore, either the resurfacing tibial plateau or a smooth tibial stem should used. In the case of massive bone loss, long smooth stems will be required for fixation with the area of ingrowth limited to the distal condylar portion of the prosthesis. A custom long-stemmed PCA revision is used with appropriately sized stems to provide a press fit in the femur and tibia for initial stability (Fig. 122-46). Extensive autogenous and allograft bone is placed within the medullary canal. The bone is prepared in a bone mill to provide particles of bone 0.5 cm in diameter. Autogenous cancellous bone is placed about the ingrowth portion of the prosthesis. This technique is not viable if a collateral ligament is absent and a more constrained central stabilized peg or hinge is required. Initial implant

stability must be achieved throughout a range of motion or cement fixation will be required. The technique of implant placement must ensure excellent apposition between the implant and bone with gaps less than 1 mm.

PATELLA

In any revision procedure, the patella may or may not present a problem. If a patellar implant has not been previously used, patellar resurfacing is performed. Patellar resurfacing appears to improve knee function during stair climbing activity. If a previously placed patellar button is secure, the patella is not cut asymmetrically, and the polyethylene is not severely deformed, the patellar implant is not disturbed. Most patellar implants are symmetric dome-shaped devices and will articulate reasonably well with most femoral designs, since hypertrophy of soft tissues occurs around the periphery of the patella after resurfacing. In the case of a loose patellar implant, an asymmetrically cut

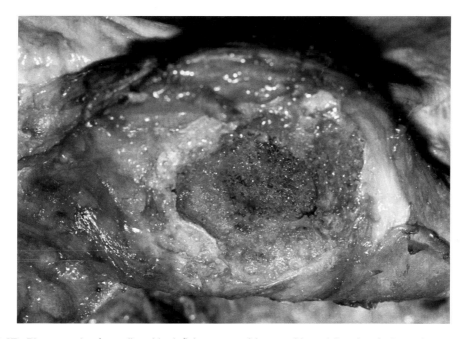

Fig. 122-47. Photograph of patella with deficient central bone with peripheral soft tissue hypertrophy after removal of loose patellar implant.

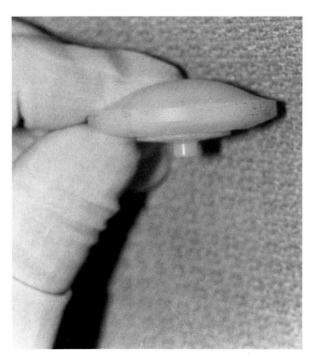

Fig. 122-48. Photograph of prototype biconvex patellar button. (Courtesy of Ramon Gustilo, M.D., Minneapolis, and Richards Medical Corporation, Memphis.)

patellar bone, or erosion of the polyethlene exposing metal backing, the patellar implant should be revised with correction of bone cuts. The problem of patellar bone loss can be significant. Most cemented patellar implant designs have a central stabilizing peg for fixation. In the event of revision, there will be a substantial central defect (Fig. 122-47). The use of a design with three peripheral pegs will provide fixation in remaining bone stock. In the case of severe bone loss with only a concave shell of bone remaining, currently available patellar implants will be inadequate. A biconvex patellar implant is needed for these patients (Fig. 122-48).

recovery room and increased 10 degrees/day until 90 degrees of flexion is achieved. CPM is continued until the patient maintains 90 degrees of flexion in physical therapy. Ambulation is begun on the third postoperative day once the drainage tubes have been removed. Weight hearing as tolerated with two crutches is encouraged for cemented implants, including those with bone grafts. Crutches are maintained for 8 weeks until the extensor mechanism has healed and the quadriceps strengthened. Isometric quadriceps strengthening is encouraged in the perioperative period to eliminate any extensor lag. Quadriceps strengthening is continued until 10 kg of weight can be lifted isometrically. Progression to a cane is usually possible, once the quadriceps has been rehabilitated.

There are three exceptions to the usual rehabilitation protocol. The cementless revision will have a period of touch weight bearing from 4 to 16 weeks, depending on the extent of bone grafting required. Once consolidation of the bone graft is evident, progressive weight bearing is begun. The patient who requires a turndown of the extensor mechanism must be protected from active quadriceps use during the first 2 months following surgery. Passive motion is begun with the CPM 3 to 4 days following surgery as well as active flexion. Only passive extension and no quadriceps strengthening are allowed for 8 weeks. A knee immobilizer is used during ambulation or a hinged knee brace with the hinges locked (Fig. 122-49). If wound drainage occurs, motion is terminated until drainage ceases. If extensive soft tissue releases are required with complete release of a collateral ligament at the time of revision, a hinged knee brace is used to control varus-valgus forces. A polyaxial knee hinge with locks is preferred. The brace can be unlocked for controlled motion but is locked for ambulation. The brace is worn for 8 weeks.

REHABILITATION

Rehabilitation following revision is similar to a primary total knee arthroplasty in most patients. Continuous passive motion (CPM) is begun in the

RESULTS OF REVISION

The results of revision surgery depend upon the type of implant and the criteria used for a satisfactory result. Unfortunately, standard criteria or

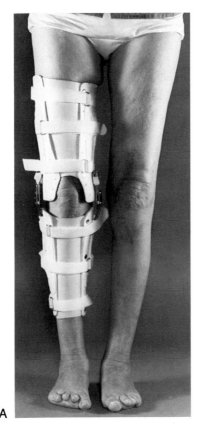

A

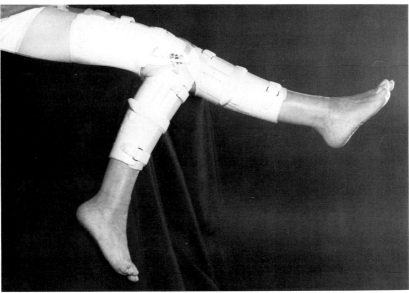

B

Fig. 122-49. Hinged knee brace used during rehabilitation to protect extensor mechanism or collateral ligaments.

knee scoring systems have not been used, making comparison of data difficult. The initial experience with revision procedures was salvage of early resurfacing designs such as a polycentric or geometric prosthesis with either a similar design or a fixed-hinged implant. A review of 30 failed implants revealed best results with a total condylar and worst results with a GUEPAR hinge.[11] A series of 17 revisions using the GUEPAR or Herbert hinge designs, failed to achieve adequate pain relief in 41 percent of cases.[31] In another short-term follow-up, four of five revisions using hinged prostheses were satisfactory.[1] A review of 68 spherocentric prostheses for revision with a 2- to 8-year follow-up revealed complications in 24 knees.[41] Of 73 revisions with a variety of implant types used for salvage, satisfactory results were achieved in 30 percent.[16,35] A subsequent report by the same authors of 78 revisions revealed 37 percent satisfactory results.[15] They noted a correlation between the results and implant constraint. Satisfactory results were achieved in 48 percent with a semiconstrained prosthesis, 24 percent with an unlinked hinge, and 21 percent with a fixed hinge prosthesis.[15] A review of 100 revisions followed for 3.7 years using early resurfacing or fixed-hinge designs, achieved pain relief in 86 cases.[88] Five of seven revisions with the UCI prosthesis were satisfactory at a short follow-up of 6 months.[22] A review of the Mayo Clinic experience with 427 revision procedures with a follow-up of 3.7 years using a variety of implant designs achieved satisfactory results in 60 percent of first revisions, in 52 percent of second revisions, and in 50 percent after three revisions.[13,60,69] Using actuarial statistical analysis technique, the probability of implant survival (function) was better for newer semiconstrained condylar implants than more constrained stabilized prostheses (Fig. 122-25). Of 103 revisions with unspecified implant designs, 35 percent were failures (14.6 percent pain, 20.4 percent limited motion).[23] Seventy-eight of 100 revisions with various implants achieved pain relief.[42] Therefore, the results of revision with early prosthetic designs were not optimal, with 30 to 80 percent satisfactory. Better results were achieved with resurfacing than with constrained designs.

More recent series of revision procedures have used condylar knee designs. Satisfactory results were achieved in 27 of 67 revisions (58 total condylar prostheses).[30] In a review of 170 revisions with a 2-year follow-up, 156 were improved.[83] In another report by the same investigator, 53 of 65 knees followed for 33 months were improved.[82] A 2-year follow-up of 116 revisions using condylar prostheses achieved 80 percent satisfactory results.[33] Satisfactory results were achieved in 89 percent of 72 revisions using mostly posterior stabilized prostheses.[39] A 5-year follow-up of 51 revisions using a condylar prosthesis have shown satisfactory results in 76 percent.[63] Therefore, the results of current revision procedures with condylar implant designs are better than earlier series and the results are maintained for at least 5 years.

COMPLICATIONS

Complications following revision surgery are of the same type as following primary total knee arthroplasty. Loosening and infection are the two most serious problems. Other problems such as patellar instability, malalignment, instability, patellar tendon avulsion, and bone fracture occur but are largely related to technical errors at the time of revision. The reasons for these problems have been discussed in the section on surgical technique.

Lucent lines at the bone-cement interface following revision are frequent. The significance of these findings, however, remains unclear. Schneider et al[72] stated that no specific radiographic width is indicative of loosening. Progression of lucent lines in width and extent as well as a shift in implant position are indicative of loosening.[72,73] In 427 revisions, lucent lines were observed about 86 percent and progression of lucent lines in 36 percent of cases.[69] Five of 68 spherocentric revisions demonstrated radiographic loosening, but none was subsequently revised for this complication.[41] Radiolucent lines were found in 63 percent of 100 revisions with unspecified implant types.[42] Two-thirds of 67 revisions had radiolucent lines in one series.[28] Sixty-five percent of 170 condylar knees in one series and 60 percent of 65 knees in another series by the same group had lucent lines, usually under the medial or lateral tibial plateau.[82,83] An 84 percent incidence of radiolucent lines was present in 116 condylar revisions.[33] Insall and Dethmers[39] stated that the lucent lines reflect the difficulty in achieving cement penetration of sclerotic bone that has formed adjacent to the previously loose components and the radiolucent lines do not progress or represent loosening. In a 5-year follow-up of 54 condylar revisions, lucent lines were identified in 28 percent and were progressive in 23 percent of cases.[63] There were two loose implants at 5 years.[63] In summary, lucent lines are frequent following revision. Progression of lucent lines or a shift in component position is suggestive of loosening.

The incidence of deep infection following revision depends on the implant type and duration of follow-up. The incidence of deep sepsis has been 10 to 11 percent in a series of 73 revisions with various implant types.[15,16,35] In 427 revisions with various prostheses, the infection rate was 2.1 percent.[69] In other series, the infection rate has been 1 percent,[42] 1.5 percent,[28] and 3 percent.[23] The highest infection rate reported has been with the use of the kinematic rotating hinge at 16 percent.[67] There were no deep infections in 54 condylar revisions followed for 5 years by the same group of surgeons.[63] Therefore, the incidence of infection appears to be slightly increased over primary total

knee arthroplasty and occurs with increased frequency with hinged type prostheses.

FUTURE OF REVISION SURGERY

The future of revision surgery will consist of improved patient selection, better surgical technique, and improved implant designs. Modular total knee prostheses are being developed that will improve fitting of the implant to the patient in the operating room. Modular designs will permit selection of various stem lengths, metal wedge augmentation for the tibia and femur, and varying degrees of implant constraint. These features may avoid the need for most custom implant designs which have been needed for revision in the past.[33] The use of custom implants has achieved good to excellent results in 85 percent of first revisions and in 71 percent of second revisions in a series of 21 knees.[79]

The long-term results of use of cementless knees for revision in young patients remains unknown. The potential advantages are preservation or restoration of lost bone stock and hopefully a decreased incidence of late loosening. Cementless long-

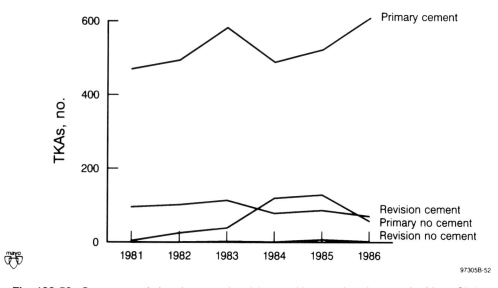

Fig. 122-50. Current trends in primary and revision total knee arthroplasty at the Mayo Clinic.

stemmed prostheses with proximal defect filling with cement achieved 91 percent satisfactory pain relief in 53 revisions followed for 18 months.[7] A cementless noningrowth-stemmed prosthesis provided satisfactory results in 17 of 17 patients, of which three were revisions.[25] Our preliminary experience with cementless revision of nine knees provided good to excellent results in seven of eight patients followed.[69] Our current technique in total knee arthroplasty continues to be primarily cement fixation (Fig. 122-50).

SUMMARY

Failure of total knee arthroplasty results from improper patient selection, poor implant design, or errors in surgical technique. Revision arthroplasty is best performed with the least constrained implant possible. The principles of correct limb alignment, proper component orientation, and soft tissue balance must be followed. Using these principles and a condylar-type implant, a success rate of 75 to 90 percent should be possible, with an infection rate only slightly higher than primary surgery.

REFERENCES

1. Ahlberg A, Lunden A: Secondary operations after knee joint replacement. Clin Orthop 156:170, 1981
2. Audell RA, Cracchiolo A: The use of implants with polyethylene peg fixation in total knee arthroplasty. p. 179. In Rand JA, Dorr L (eds): Total Arthroplasty of the Knee. Aspen Systems, Rockville, MD, 1986
3. Bargar WL, Cracchiolo A, Amstutz HC: Results with the constrained total knee prosthesis in treating severely disabled patients and patients with failed total knee replacements. J Bone Joint Surg 62A:504, 1980
4. Bargren JH, Blaha JD, Freeman MAR: Alignment in total knee arthroplasty. Clin Orthop 173:178, 1983
5. Bargren JH, Day WH, Freeman MAR, Swanson SAV: Mechanical tests on the tibial components of non-hinged knee prostheses. J Bone Joint Surg 60B:256, 1978
6. Bartel DL, Burstein AH, Santavicca EA, Insall JN: Performance of the tibial component in total knee replacement. J Bone Joint Surg 64A:1026, 1982
7. Bertin KC, Freeman MAR, Samuelson KM, et al: Stemmed revision arthroplasty for aseptic loosening of total knee replacement. J Bone Joint Surg 67B:242, 1985
8. Bobyn JD, Cameron HU, Abdullar D, et al: Biologic fixation and bone modeling with an unconstrained canine total knee prosthesis. Clin Orthop 166:301, 1982
9. Bourne BB, Finlay JB: The influence of tibial component intramedullary stems and implant-cortex contact on the strain distribution of the proximal tibia following total knee arthroplasty. Clin Orthop 208:95, 1986
10. Bourne RB, Goodfellow JW, O'Conner JJ: A functional analysis of various knee arthroplasties. Orthop Trans 2:164, 1978 (abst)
11. Brady TA, Ranawat C, Kettlekamp DB, Rapp GF: Salvage of the failed total knee arthroplasty. Orthop Trans 1:101, 1977 (abst)
12. Brooks PJ, Walker PS, Scott RD: Tibial component fixation in deficient tibial bone stock. Clin Orthop 184:302, 1984
13. Bryan RS, Rand JA: Revision total knee arthroplasty. Clin Orthop 170:116, 1982
14. Bryan RS, Rand JA: Indications, results, and complications of revision total knee arthroplasty for mechanical failure. p. 249. In Ranawat CS (ed): Total Condylar Knee Arthroplasty. Springer-Verlag, New York, 1985
15. Cameron HU, Hunter GA: Failure in total knee arthroplasty. Clin Orthop 170:141, 1982
16. Cameron HU, Hunter GA, Welsh RP, Bailey WH: Revision of total knee replacement. Can J Surg 24:418, 1981
17. Colley J, Cameron HU, Freeman MAR, Swanson SAV: Loosening of the femoral component in surface replacement of the knee. Arch Orthop Traum Surg 92:31, 1978
18. Coonse KD, Adams JD: A new operative approach to the knee joint. Surg Gynecol Obstet 77:344, 1943
19. Dorr LD, Boiardo RA: Technical considerations in total knee arthroplasty. Clin Orthop 205:5, 1986
20. Dorr LD, Conaty JP, Schreiber R, et al: Technical factors that influence mechanical loosening of total knee arthroplasty. p. 121. In Dorr LD (ed): The Knee. Presented at the First Scientific Meeting of the Knee Society. University Park Press, Baltimore, 1985

21. Dorr LD, Ranawat CS, Sculco TA, et al: Bone graft for tibial defects in total knee arthroplasty. Clin Orthop 205:153, 1986

22. Ducheyne P, Kagan A, Lacy JA: Failure of total knee arthroplasty due to loosening and deformation of the tibial component. J Bone Joint Surg 60A:384, 1978

23. Dupont JA, Campbell ED, Lumsden RM: Total knee arthroplasty revisions. Orthop Trans 4:321, 1980 (abst)

24. Ewald FC, Jacobs MA, Miegel RE, et al: Kinematic total knee replacement. J Bone Joint Surg 66A:1032, 1984

25. Ewald FC, Walker PS, Poss R, et al: Uncemented press-fit total knee replacement. p. 173. In Rand JA, Dorr LD (eds): Total Arthroplasty of the Knee. Proceedings of the Knee Society. Aspen Systems, Rockville, MD, 1986

26. Figgie HE, Davy DT, Heiple KG, Hart RT: Load-bearing capacity of the tibial component of the total condylar knee prosthesis. Clin Orthop 183:288, 1984

27. Figgie HE, Goldberg VM, Heiple KG, et al: The influence of tibial-patellofemoral location on function of the knee in patients with the posterior stabilized condylar knee prosthesis. J Bone Joint Surg 68A:1035, 1986

28. Goldberg VM, Sachs BL: The results and complications of revision total knee arthroplasty. Orthop Trans 7:547, 1983 (abst)

29. Greenwald AS, Norten NC, Wilde AH: Points in the technique of recementing in the revision of an implant arthroplasty. J Bone Joint Surg 60B:107, 1978

30. Grimer RJ, Karpinski MRK, Ewards AN: The long-term results of Stanmore total knee replacements. J Bone Joint Surg 66B:55, 1984

31. Gross MS, Jaffe WL, Weinger EB: GUEPAR hinge knee arthroplasty: a five year follow-up. Orthop Trans 6:437, 1982 (abst)

32. Haemmerle J, Bartel D, Chao E: Mechanical analysis of polycentric tibial tract loosening. Presented at the Joint Applied Mechanics, Fluids Engineering, and Bioengineering Conference, New Haven, CT, June 15–17, 1977

33. Hood RW, Insall JN: Total knee revision arthroplasty: indications, surgical techniques, and results. Orthop Trans 5:412, 1981

34. Hungerford DS, Krackow KA: Total joint arthroplasty of the knee. Clin Orthop 192:23, 1985

35. Hunter GA, Cameron HV, Welsh RP, Bailey WH: The natural history of the failed knee replacement. Orthop Trans 4:389, 1980

36. Hvid I, Hansen SL: Cancellous bone strength patterns at the proximal tibial epiphysis. Orthop Trans 9:262, 1985 (abst)

37. Insall JN: Total knee replacement. p. 587. In Insall JN (ed): Surgery of the Knee. Churchill Livingstone, New York, 1984

38. Insall JN: Revision of total knee replacement. p. 290. In American Academy of Orthopaedic Surgeons Instructional Course Lectures. Vol. 35. CV Mosby, St. Louis, 1986

39. Insall JN, Dethmers DA: Revision of total knee arthroplasty. Clin Orthop 170:123, 1982

40. Insall JN, Kelly M: The total condylar prosthesis. Clin Orthop 205:43, 1986

41. Kaufer H, Matthews LS: Revision total knee arthroplasty: indications and contraindications. p. 297. In American Academy of Orthopaedic Surgeons Instructional Course Lectures. Vol. 35. CV Mosby, St. Louis, 1986

42. Kim L, Finerman G: Results of revisions for aseptic failed knee arthroplasties. Orthop Trans 7:535, 1983

43. King TV, Scott RD: Femoral component loosening in total knee arthroplasty. Clin Orthop 194:285, 1985

44. Krug WH, Johnson J, Nahon D, et al: An evaluation of the dimensions and strength of the proximal tibia in relation to the coverage of knee implants. Orthop Trans 8:218, 1984 (abst)

45. Laskin RS: Alignment of total knee components. Orthopedics 7:62, 1984

46. Lew WD, Lewis JL: The effect of knee-prosthesis geometry on cruciate ligament mechanics during flexion. J Bone Joint Surg 64A:734, 1982

47. Lewallen DG, Bryan RS, Peterson LFA: Polycentric total knee arthroplasty. 66A:1211, 1984

48. Lewis JL, Askew MJ, Jaycox DP: A comparative evaluation of tibial component designs of total knee prostheses. J Bone Joint Surg 64A:129, 1982

49. Lotke PA, Ecker ML: Influence of positioning of prosthesis in total knee replacement. J Bone Joint Surg 59A:77, 1977

50. Lotke PA, Windsor R, Ecker ML, Cella J: Long-term results after total condylar knee replacements: significance of radiolucent lines. Orthop Trans 8:398, 1984

51. Lotke PA, Wong R, Ecker M: The management of large tibial defects in primary total knee replacement. Orthop Trans 9:425, 1983 (abst)

52. Mendes DG, Brandon D, Galor LS, Roffman M: Breakage of the metal tray in total knee replacement. Orthopedics 7:860, 1984

53. Merkel KD, Johnson EW: Supracondylar fracture of the femur after total knee arthroplasty. J Bone Joint Surg 68A:29, 1986

54. Merkow RL, Soudry M, Insall JN: Patellar dislocation following total knee replacement. J Bone Joint Surg 67A:1321, 1985

55. Merritt P, Conaty JP, Dorr LD: Effect of soft tissue releases on results of total knee replacement. p. 25. In Rand JA, Dorr LD (eds): Total Arthroplasty of the Knee. Proceedings of the Knee Society. Aspen Systems, Rockville, MD, 1986

56. Mochizuki RM, Schurman DJ: Patellar complications following total knee arthroplasty. J Bone Joint Surg 61A:879, 1979

57. Muller JO, Chao EYS, Coventry MB: Analysis of mechanical failure in the geometric total knee. Presented at the Joint Applied Mechanics, Fluids Engineering, and Bioengineering Conference, New Haven, CT, June 15–17, 1977

58. Nogi J, Caldwell JW, Kauzlarich JJ, Thompson RC: Load testing of geometric and polycentric total knee replacements. Clin Orthop 114:235, 1976

59. Ranawat CS, Johanson NA, Rimnac CM, et al: Retrieval analysis of porous-coated components for total knee arthroplasty: a report of two cases. Clin Orthop 209:244, 1986

60. Rand JA, Bryan RS: Revision after total knee arthroplasty. Orthop Clin North Am 13:201, 1982

61. Rand JA, Bryan RS: Reimplantation for the salvage of an infected total knee arthroplasty. J Bone Joint Surg 65A:1081, 1983

62. Rand JA, Bryan RS: Alignment in porous coated anatomic total knee arthroplasty. p. 111. In Dorr LD (ed): The Knee. Proceedings of the First Scientific Meeting of the Knee Society. University Park Press, Baltimore, 1985

63. Rand JA, Bryan RS: Condylar revision total knee arthroplasty. J Bone Joint Surg 70A:738, 1988

64. Rand JA, Bryan RS: Porous ingrowth total knee revision. p. 169. In Scott WN: Total Knee Revision Arthroplasty. Grune & Stratton, Orlando, FL, 1987

65. Rand JA, Bryan RS, Chao EYS, Ilstrup DM: A comparison of cement versus cementless fixation in porous coated anatomic total knee arthroplasty. p. 195. In Rand JA, Dorr LD (eds): Total Arthroplasty of the Knee. Aspen Systems, Rockville, MD, 1986

66. Rand JA, Bryan RS, Morrey BF, Westholm F: Management of infected total knee arthroplasty. Clin Orthop 205:75, 1986

67. Rand JA, Chao EYS, Stauffer RN: Kinematic rotating hinge total knee arthroplasty. J Bone Joint Surg 69A:489, 1987

68. Rand JA, Coventry MB: Stress fracture after total knee arthroplasty. J Bone Joint Surg 62A:226, 1980

69. Rand JA, Peterson LFA, Bryan RS, Ilstrup DM: Revision total knee arthroplasty. p. 305. In American Academy of Orthopaedic Surgeons Instructional Course Lectures. Vol. 35. CV Mosby, St. Louis, 1986

70. Reilly D, Walker PS, Ben-Dov M, Ewald FC: Effects of tibial components on load transfer in the upper tibia. Clin Orthop 165:273, 1982

71. Samuelson KM, Freeman MAR, Day WH: Salvage of failed total knee replacements: is a hinge necessary? Orthop Trans 4:98, 1980

72. Schneider R, Abenavoli AM, Soudry M, Insall JN: Failure of total condylar knee replacement. Radiology 152:309, 1984

73. Schneider R, Soudry M: Radiographic and scintigraphic evaluation of total knee arthroplasty. Clin Orthop 205:108, 1986

74. Scott RD, Ewald FC, Walker PS: Fracture of the metallic tibial tray following total knee replacement. J Bone Joint Surg 66A:780, 1984

75. Scott RD, Siliski JM: The use of a modified V-Y quadricepsplasty during total knee replacement to gain exposure and improve flexion in the ankylosed knee. Orthopedics 8:45, 1985

76. Scott RD, Turnoff N, Ewald FC: Stress fracture of the patella following duopatellar total knee arthroplasty with patellar resurfacing. Clin Orthop 170:147, 1982

77. Sculco TP: Technique of revision of total knee arthroplasty. p. 238. In Ranawat CS (ed): Total Condylar Knee Arthroplasty. Springer-Verlag, New York, 1985

78. Soudry M, Bizazzi R, Mestriner L, Insall JN: Custom made total knee arthroplasty. Orthop Trans 10:234, 1986

79. Soudry M, Mestriner L, Binazzi R, Insall JN: Total knee replacement without patellar resurfacing. Orthop Trans 8:399, 1984

80. Tew M, Waugh W: Tibiofemoral alignment and the results of knee replacement. J Bone Joint Surg 67B:551, 1985

81. Thompson FM, Hood RW, Insall JN: Patellar fractures in total knee arthroplasty. Orthop Trans 3:490, 1981 (abst)

82. Thornhill TS, Dalziel RW, Sledge CB: Alternatives to arthrodesis for the failed total knee arthroplasty. Clin Orthop 170:131, 1982

83. Thornhill TS, Hood RW, Bath NJ, et al: Knee revision in failed non-infected total knee arthroplasties: the Robert Breck Brigham Hospital and Hospital for Special Surgery Experience. Orthop Trans 6:36, 1982

84. Turner RH: Revision of total knee replacement implants: surgical techniques and available implants. Orthop Trans 4:89, 1980 (abst)

85. Walker PS: Revision of total knee arthroplasty: Design of knee prostheses for bone loss and instability. p. 229. In Ranawat CS (ed): Total Condylar Knee Arthroplasty. Springer-Verlag, New York, 1985

86. Walker PS, Greene D, Reilly D, et al: Fixation of tibial components of knee prostheses. J Bone Joint Surg 63A:258, 1981

87. Walker PS, Hsieh HM: Conformity in condylar replacement knee prostheses. J Bone Joint Surg 59B:222, 1977

88. Wertzberger KL, Bryan RS: Analysis of failed total knee arthroplasty excluding infection, undergoing reoperation. Orthop Trans 3:265, 1979 (abst)

89. Windsor RE, Insall JN, Sculco TP: Bone grafting of tibial defects in primary and revision total knee arthroplasty. Clin Orthop 205:132, 1986

Arthrodesis 123

Arthrodesis of the Knee Joint

James A. Rand
Richard S. Bryan
Mark P. Broderson

HISTORICAL ASPECTS

Arthrodesis of the knee joint is an old operation with applications and techniques that have changed with the passage of time. Cleveland[19] credits a Professor Albert with the first fusion of an unstable knee following poliomyelitis on July 10, 1878. Only 30 cases were reported from 1878 to 1920, indicating a lack of popular acceptance. Hibbs, in 1911, reported a new technique in which he fashioned a bed of cancellous bone from the anterior surfaces of the tibia and femur and embedded the patella (with its cartilage removed) into this bed.[51] The cruciate ligaments were not disturbed. This technique was later modified to include removal of the menisci and of all the articular cartilage. Cleveland, in 1932, reported on 90 fusions using the Hibbs technique for unstable or flail knees[19] with an incidence of nonunion of only 2.2 percent and 91 percent patient satisfaction. Cleveland[19] found a fracture incidence of 13.5 percent in the extremity with the fused knee joint.[19] He found that the result was less satisfactory in patients younger than 13 years of age.

Key described a compression technique using two Steinmann pins and turnbuckles.[64] He left these in place 8 weeks and kept the patient in bed. They were then removed, a cast was applied, and crutches were used for 8 weeks. Of his five patients, four had union and one died of sepsis. Key, apparently in 1937, described a second method for knees with bone loss using a graft from the tibial crest, with which he impaled both femur and tibia.[65]

Toumey reported on 199 patients with tuberculosis of the knee treated by a Hibbs arthrodesis and followed up for more than 1 year.[109] All but three patients had achieved fusion; however, the three that developed sinuses required amputation. One of the complications of arthrodesis in these young patients was epiphyseal slip, occurring in 19 of the patients. Hatt, in 1940 and 1943, used a centrally placed graft across the epiphyses and joint in 21 patients (ages 4 to 14 years) without growth arrest.[49]

Charnley, in 1948, popularized the compression method of arthrodesis (Fig. 123-1) with a report on 15 patients, some of whom had clinical union in 2 weeks.[15] He stressed that the compression must appose good flat cancellous surfaces. The same year, Chapchal described an intramedullary nail for fixation.[14] Morris and Mosiman compared knees treated by compression with knees treated without compression[80] (most by two crossed pins). They found compression superior. Charnley and Baker, in 1952, reported a further series of 67 knees treated with compression and noted that 74 percent had solid union clinically at 4 weeks, when the pins were removed.[17] Charnley considered the absence of shearing primarily responsible for only two failed fusions.

Fett and Zorn in 1953 modified the apparatus to use four pins.[33] The method became so standardized that Charnley and Lowe, in 1958, reported 171 cases, with a success rate of 98.8 percent.[18] Charnley's protocol used 100 pounds (45.4 kg) of compression for 4 weeks, with the limb supported

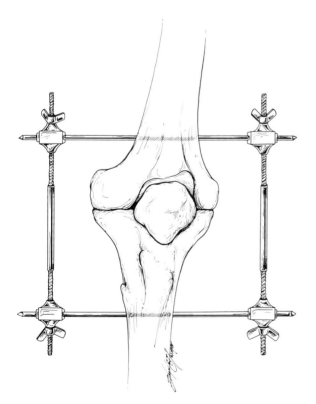

Fig. 123-1. Charnley single-pin compression clamp.

in a Thomas splint. The pins were then removed, and a plaster cast was applied for 4 more weeks, with ambulation permitted.

Stewart and Bland, in 1958, reported 37 patients successfully fused by compression arthrodesis compared with 50 of 61 treated by other techniques.[104] They strongly favored compression.

Moore and Smillie, in 1959, reported the results of 126 arthrodeses in 116 patients above 14 years of age.[78] Their method used a massive graft in 44 patients, Brittain grafts in 5, crossed pins in 32, and compression in 35. Only one patient in their series had nonunion. These investigators stressed that nearly full extension should be the position of fusion, especially in children, because a flexion deformity tends to develop with growth. They pointed out that in extension the tibial tubercle is lateral to the patellofemoral groove and that placing the two in a direct line causes the foot to be in internal rotation, handicapping gait. Unexpectedly, varus-valgus varied in their patients from 17 degrees valgus to 11 degrees varus, without much effect on function.

Charnley, in 1960, addressed the problem of function in these patients and stated that they can put on their shoes and socks (because their hips gain motion) and that they can get up from a chair and the floor, even with bilateral arthrodeses of the knee.[16] Their main handicap is the inability to use public transportation or to attend the theater or other events, where the unbendable leg would obstruct their movement. Of 171 patients, only two had failed results. Six patients had pin-tract infections, five had thromboses, four had supracondylar fractures, two had sepsis, two had broken pins, one had a temporary peroneal palsy, and one had a draining sinus.

Mazet and Urist, in 1960, reported 12 patients treated with standard femoral length intramedullary nails and noted fusion in 10 patients.[74] They reported that fracture of the femur through the hole of entry of the nail in the femur was the major complication of this method. To obviate fracture, the technique was changed to drilling from the knee proximally into the femur and out the anterior cortex at the angle of flexion desired at the knee. A short incision was made over the drill, and the nail followed the drill back to the knee, where it was then driven into the tibia.

Mazzetti studied the effect of the angle of immobilization on energy expenditure in normal subjects compared with patients who had fused knees.[75] He found that immobilization in normal knees increased the expenditure of energy, especially at 45 degrees of flexion. At 0 to 20 degrees of flexion, he found that energy expenditure did not increase and that shortening had little effect. Lucas and Murray, in 1961, used dual 8-inch plates at right angles and achieved union in 18 of 18 knees.[70]

Crenshaw, in 1963, strongly favored compression but did not advise it in children under 10 years of age.[22] He cautioned that bracing for several years is necessary in children in order to prevent epiphyseal slip. For position, he advised 10 degrees of flexion in adults and full extension in children.

Green et al., in 1967, suggested that the type of patient had changed; they divided their 142 patients seen from 1937 to 1965 into three groups.[42] In group 1 (1937 to 1947), 77 percent were patients with tuberculosis or poliomyelitis, whereas in group 3 (1957 to 1965), only 18 percent had these diseases. They reported their results both by technique and by disease. Of 54 patients with Hibbs-type procedures, 19 percent had fusion, and of the 24 with Hibbs-type procedures in which internal fixation was added, all obtained fusion. Internal fixation alone was successful in 94 percent of 16 patients, and compression alone was successful in 85 percent of 20 patients. Fusion was obtained in 83 percent of patients with tuberculosis, 100 percent of patients with poliomyelitis, 93 percent of patients with posttraumatic arthritic knees, 100 percent of patients with osteoarthritic knees, 91 percent of patients with rheumatoid arthritis, and 67 percent of patients with neuropathic joints. Their patients with arthrodesis avoided public transportation and found it difficult to get in and out of cars but could drive a car. They attended theater infrequently and had problems with housework.

Salenius and Kivilaakso, in 1968, reported on 106 patients and found that the Charnley-Key method was best, with only three nonunions after 53 such procedures.[97] Potter, in 1969, described a unique method of inserting an intramedullary nail.[88] He first inserted the nail down the tibia and then measured the insertion distance. He windowed the distal tibia and removed the nail. The nail was reinserted through the tibial window and driven up across the knee at the chosen angle.

Nelson and Evarts, in 1971, added failed arthroplasty to the list of indications for fusion.[81] They favored an angle of 20 degrees in females and 5 to 10 degrees in males and preferred the Charnley-Key method. The Charcot knee remained a problem to most orthopedists. Drennan and Maylahn, in 1971, found 151 attempts at fusion in Charcot knees recorded in the literature, with a success rate of 55 percent.[25] They used intramedullary nails and an extensive synovectomy-debridement and achieved fusion in 9 of 10 patients; the tenth patient died before treatment was complete. Drennan and Maylahn found 10 cases reported by four other investigators in which fusion after synovectomy was successful; they stressed that bone must be resected to good bleeding cancellous bone and that all scarred capsule, synovium, and heterotopic debris be removed.

Brattström and Brattström, in 1971, followed 43 patients for 7 years and found that 11 loaded the fused leg more than 70 percent, 4 loaded from 60 to 70 percent, and 8 loaded the legs equally.[8] Only 3 of the 43 put most of their weight on the movable leg. Cloutier and Fortin, in an effort to eliminate stressing of the femur, used a long Küntscher nail extending from the hip across the knee and augmented by two staples at the knee.[20] They obtained fusion in all nine patients, including three who had Charcot knees in which synovectomy was not performed.

Frymoyer and Hoaglund, in 1974, claimed that the knees of children should be fused in extension and braced to protect the epiphyses.[39] They summarized the types and numbers of patients described in the literature as 186 (22.5 percent) with paralysis, 178 (21.5 percent) with tuberculosis, 160 (19.3 percent) with rheumatoid arthritis, 151 (18.3 percent) with Charcot knees, 73 (8.9 percent) with osteoarthritis, 59 (7.1 percent) with infection, and 20 (2.4 percent) with miscellaneous problems. They believed that the indications for arthrodesis were: (1) conditions in which the patient cannot or will not cooperate in a rehabilitation program for arthroplasty, such as neurotrophic joints (due to neurosyphilis, congenital indifference to pain, diabetes, syringomyelia, peripheral nerve lesions, or Riley-Day syndrome); (2) infections; (3) failed arthroplasty; (4) paralyzed or muscularly insufficient limbs; (5) rheumatoid arthritis; and (6) neoplasms requiring knee resection.

Siller, in 1975, stressed that, before the advent of total knee arthroplasty, most arthrodeses were performed for relief of pain, sepsis, or instability and that, after total knee arthroplasty was introduced, most were salvage procedures after a failed total knee with or without sepsis or, in a few cases, in knees not amenable to arthroplasty.[101] In a series of 41 patients, Siller noted many complications and complaints. Eighteen patients had back pain, which he considered attributable to abnormal gait. Siller noted two types of gait: an excessive pelvic rise despite shortening in those fused in extension and a side swing of the leg *au fauchent* in those fused in flexion. Fifteen patients had persistent knee pain and six had fractures at various levels of the affected extremity.

Therefore, the classic indications for knee arthrodesis have included infection, tumor, severe ligamentous instability, paralysis, severe bone loss, and neuropathic arthropathy.[8,19,24,25,33,37,39,50–52,81,101,109] Recently, failure of total knee arthroplasty has been added to this list.[5,11,26,31,34,43,46,47,63,67,69,85,91,96,107,108,110–112,118] Relative contraindications to arthrodesis include ipsilateral ankle or hip disease, severe segmental bone loss, contralateral leg amputation, and bilateral knee disease.[16] It is interesting that Charnley noted 11 patients who were satisfied with a bilateral knee arthrodesis.[16]

Failure of total knee arthroplasty generally has been from mechanical loosening with older implant designs and from infection, regardless of the implant type. Although instability, implant setting, bone fracture, prosthesis fracture, and extensor mechanism dysfunction have been responsible for arthroplasty failure, these reasons are infrequent with current implant designs, careful surgical technique, and appropriate patient selection.

Infection has remained a major unsolved problem. The infection rate in large series of total knee arthroplasties has ranged from a low of 1 percent with a resurfacing prosthesis to as high as 16.0 percent with a kinematic rotating hinge.[57,95] At the Mayo Clinic (1970 to 1983), 7,308 total knee arthroplasties were performed with an overall infection rate of 1.51 percent.[91]

The etiology of prosthetic infection and the alternatives for management have been delineated in several recent reviews.[87,93,94,107,108] Host factors, surgical technique, and local tissue response to foreign materials are all important determinants of sepsis.[91]

Regardless of the technique of salvage chosen, the objectives for management of the infected total knee arthroplasty remain the same. There must be eradication of the infection, limb salvage, preservation of all bone stock to permit whatever reconstruction procedure is chosen, and maintenance of a functional extremity. Eradication of the infection is the first priority. An infected arthroplasty can lead to generalized sepsis and a fatal outcome. Surgical debridement remains the mainstay of therapy. Systemic antibiotics alone are rarely of value.[57,99]

A variety of options are available for management of the infected total knee arthroplasty. Early surgical debridement following the onset of infection may occasionally salvage a prosthesis.[93,118] Reimplantation appears most valuable when used for a low-virulence micro-organism and when performed as a delayed technique.[37,49,57,85,90,98] Resection arthroplasty in our experience has proved unpredictable and frequently requires the use of a brace for support.[32,53,112] Amputation should be reserved for those patients with life-threatening sepsis and/or sepsis combined with massive bone loss. Arthrodesis provides the potential of a painless stable base of support but at the expense of knee motion.

PROBLEMS WITH ARTHRODESIS FOLLOWING TOTAL KNEE ARTHROPLASTY

The problems inherent with arthrodesis as a salvage for the failed total knee arthroplasty are those of bone loss, shortening, and gait disturbance.[47,75] If infection is also present, one has the additional problems of soft tissue management and eradication of the infection. Hankin and co-workers have experimentally studied the quantity of bone re-

Table 123-1. Limb Shortening

Investigators	Shortening (cm)
Brodersen et al.[11]	6.4
Fahmy[31]	3.8
Harris and Frochlich[48]	5
Knutson et al.[67]	4
Poss et al.[87]	5.7
Rand[91]	3.3 (1–10)
Thornhill et al.[108]	6.2
Vahvanen[110]	3–7.5

maining for arthrodesis following a variety of failed total knee arthroplasties.[47] The least bone was sacrificed by a polycentric, and the most with a Walldius hinge. The largest interface remained following a Townley prosthesis. However, once additional bone was removed to permit knee arthrodesis, the total quantity of bone removed varied only 55 ml among the various prosthetic types.[47] Shortening ranged from 3.0 to 3.5 cm.[47] In clinical studies, shortening has ranged from a low of 3 cm to as much as 10 cm[92,110] (Table 123-1).

TECHNIQUES OF ARTHRODESIS FOLLOWING A FAILED TOTAL KNEE ARTHROPLASTY

A variety of techniques have been used in primary knee arthrodesis, including intramedullary nails, plates, pins, and external fixation.[6–8,14–17,43,49,64,65,70,74,80,82,88,97,104] Broderson and colleagues achieved a successful arthrodesis following a failed total knee arthroplasty in 39 of 45 using external fixation compared to two of three with crossed pins, one of two with a plate, and one of three with a cast alone.[11] The importance of adequate fixation has been recognized. Hankin and associates have found an improved success rate of arthrodesis using a two-pin rather than a single-pin Charnley clamp.[47] Similar results were reported by Knutson et al., with 25 of 43 arthrodeses being successful with multiple pin fixation compared with 11 of 36 with a single-pin Charnley clamp.[67] External fixation is advantageous in managing the

infected arthroplasty because it permits wound management; does minimal damage to the bone vascularity, which has already been compromised by the previous prosthesis and cement; and permits the application of compression across the bone surfaces.[15–17,64,80,96,104] The disadvantages of external fixation are those of possible pin-tract infection, neurovascular injury during pin insertion, and difficulty in providing anteroposterior (AP) stability.[15–17,64,80,96,104] Several investigators have studied the bending stiffness of a variety of external fixation devices.[10,36,66,76] Regardless of the device chosen, with uniplanar pin fixation there is poor rigidity in the AP bending mode. Consequently, several workers have included anterior half-pins to help control these forces.[12,34,66,67] A successful result using biplanar external fixation has been reported in six of seven knees,[12] four of four knees,[34] and five of 11 knees.[67] A comparison of uniplanar to biplanar external fixation found union in six of six with biplanar external fixation compared with 31 of 37 with uniplanar pin fixation.[96]

A recent review of 28 arthrodeses using a biplanar Ace-Fischer apparatus for salvage of a failed total knee arthroplasty demonstrated a success rate of 68 percent.[92] The biomechanical stability of the frame was affected by pin placement but was not significant in determining the result. The single most important factor in determining bone union was the extent of bone loss.[92] The success rate of arthrodeses following a constrained implant of 43 percent and following a resurfacing implant of 84 percent was no better than results previously reported by our clinic using older external fixators with uniplanar pins.[11,92]

Intramedullary arthrodesis as a salvage for the failed total knee arthroplasty has been used by several investigators.[31,48,63,67,68,107,115] The procedure is best performed in two stages.[63,107,115] Initially, the implant is removed, the wound debrided, and the infection resolved. Once arrest of the infection has been confirmed, arthrodesis with a long intramedullary nail from the greater trochanter to the distal tibia is performed.[63] Some workers have recommended no external support,[63] while others have suggested additional support for rotational control, including a Charnley clamp[31,48] or brace.[68] Complications of this technique have included nail migration, fatigue fracture of the tibia at the end of the nail, and reactivation of infection.[31,63] Overall, intramedullary arthrodeses have proved successful in 42 or 45 cases.[63,68,115]

CURRENT PRACTICE IN ARTHRODESIS

Indications

Arthrodesis is rarely considered as a primary treatment modality but is indicated in patients who are not candidates for total knee arthroplasty. Examples of this situation would be a knee destroyed by tuberculosis or other infection still actively present.[1] A tumor involving the knee may be amenable to special custom knee replacements, but if the quadriceps muscle is excised along with the tumor, arthrodesis is preferred. A similar situation associated with destruction of both knee and quadriceps may be found in the explosion fractures of the distal femur, and again arthrodesis is the more advisable procedure.[3]

Paralysis of any type is rare as an indication for arthrodesis, and most patients would rather have a brace with a lock than an arthrodesed knee. Nonetheless, arthrodesis can be done in the patient who is unable or unwilling to use a brace or to keep it in repair.[4] Also, in some of the poorer Third World nations, braces may not be available. Patients with limited intelligence may present such an indication in the presence of paralysis in order to prevent self-injury. Muscular insufficiency due to trauma, tumor, or paralysis may not always be an indication for arthrodesis because bracing often will stabilize the knee in walking and permit bending when the patient is seated.

Neurotrophic joints due to diabetes, neurosyphilis, congenital indifference to pain, amyotrophic lateral sclerosis, peripheral nerve lesions, or Riley-Day syndrome usually are best treated with arthrodesis. Occasionally, in joints with milder and more stable conditions, total knee arthroplasty may be indicated, but the prognosis in these situations must be guarded, and the risk of arthrodesis, which is difficult to achieve in these conditions, is even greater than usual after arthroplasty.

Rheumatoid arthritis is now rarely an indication for arthrodesis, but in the neglected patient, deformity may be so extreme that arthrodesis may be the only possible salvage. This is especially true in the juvenile rheumatoid patient whose extreme deformity is associated with tiny bones and abnormal shortened muscles and tendons.

The most frequent indication for arthrodesis is failure of total knee arthroplasty, usually from infection. Less frequent indications are failure of upper tibial osteotomy, severe loss of proximal tibial bone, and pronounced ligamentous instability. In these situations, arthrodesis may be more reasonable than a hinged replacement, with its increased risk of infection and loosening.

Severe ligamentous instability by itself is not an indication for arthrodesis because such instability can almost always be corrected by the proper knee implant and soft tissue releases; however, in the patient with chronic skin ulceration or chronic urinary infection, severe instability may be an indication for arthrodesis. Similarly, occupation and age may alter the approach to the damaged knee, in that no knee replacement currently used will permit heavy manual labor to be performed regularly for many years without failing.[10]

Contraindications

Bilateral knee disease has been considered both an indication and a contraindication for arthrodesis. The argument has been that by stabilizing one knee the other is spared and thus is less likely to fail after total knee arthroplasty. Exactly the opposite argument has also been advanced; that is, fusion of one knee with arthroplasty of the second creates more stress, hence greater likelihood of failure of the arthroplasty. We prefer bilateral total knee arthroplasty in such patients, but there may be an exceptional situation in which unilateral fusion is indicated.

Destruction of the ankle or hip creates problems and is a contraindication to arthrodesis of the knee until it has been corrected. Severe segmental bone loss may make arthrodesis unattainable. Amputation or a severe deformity due to congenital anomaly of the contralateral limb is a contraindication to arthrodesis of the knee. A patient's height is not a contraindication to arthrodesis, although a short person with arthrodesis of the knee incurs less impairment of function and activity than does a tall person.

Technique

In our group practice, we have found a significant difference in the fusion rate between the minimally constrained arthroplasties and hinges. We therefore prefer to alter our technique in accordance with the degree of bone loss.

Minimal Bone Loss

Minimal bone loss that occurs after upper tibial osteotomy or a MacIntosh prosthesis lends itself to the standard Charnley-Key compression fusion. A long parapatellar or straight anteromedial or transverse incision may be used, depending on the scars already present. Any foreign bodies present are excised, and the opposing tibial and femoral surfaces are flattened to bleeding cancellous bone. When the knee surfaces are in apposition, the knee should be in 10 to 15 degrees of flexion and in 5 to 8 degrees of valgus. In a child, the knee should be in complete extension.

The patella may be enucleated and used as multiple bone grafts or may be freshened to cancellous bone on its undersurface and fixed to the tibia and femur in a fashioned bed crossing the joint line anteriorly. The quadriceps and patellar tendons should not be destroyed needlessly, as later circumstances might permit revision to an arthroplasty. An external fixation apparatus is used to apply compression and rigid fixation, maintaining constant bony contact between the two surfaces.

Infection may preclude the insertion of bone grafts at one operation. If the wound cannot be debrided to excellent bleeding tissue and bone, the wound should be packed open and the patient should return in 2 to 4 days for insertion of the fixation apparatus and grafts, if they appear to be needed. Grafts are rarely necessary in this group.

The application of plaster over the apparatus or the addition of anterior pins enhances the fixation. In most cases, the pins are left in place for 8 to 10 weeks, after which a cylinder cast is used until fusion is achieved.

Mild to Moderate Bone Loss

Mild to moderate bone loss after failure of a resurfacing arthroplasty presents few additional difficulties, and the same essential protocol is followed. Removal of the prostheses and cement without destruction of bone is a measure of the skill of the surgeon. We have found it easiest to use power saws, such as the Midas Rex, to cut through the anchoring stems of either polyethylene or metal, and to remove the cement from beneath the metallic components.

Once the components have been removed, the cement can be removed using any of the commercially available cement chippers or small osteotomes. If the components are loose, removal is easier, and the flanges are surrounded by a fibrous membrane with hard cortical bone beneath. If the components are not loose, the bone surrounding the flanges is cancellous, and some bone is usually lost during the removal. Generally, debridement is more extensive than in cases with minimal bone loss because of the scarring. We try to preserve the quadriceps and patellar tendons and collateral ligaments, but the entire synovium, much of the capsule, and the cruciates are excised.

The major difference in the fashioning of the arthroplasties is that, instead of removing bone to form two flat surfaces, the surfaces lend themselves to an interdigitation technique (Fig. 123-2). Most of the surfaces have bony projections in the region of the tibial spines, with deep troughs or plateaus on either side. The femoral condyles are deficient but may be fashioned to absorb the trident-shaped tibia. The fit is often enhanced by using the patella as a bone graft crossing the joint. In most cases, excellent bony apposition can be attained; consequently, rigid fixation can be achieved with compression. We have had few failures of arthrodesis in this group, whether infection was present or not.

Moderate to Severe Bone Loss

Prostheses responsible for moderate to severe bone loss include revision prostheses with intramedullary stems and hinge devices. These prostheses require the removal of bone from the anterior, distal, and posterior femur and upper tibia with a deep central tibial peg hole that, with failure, results in the loss of most of the cancellous bone of the

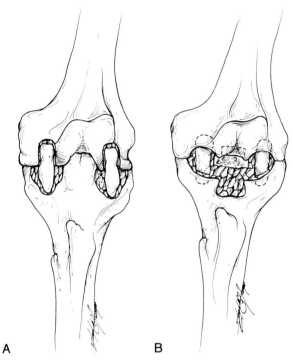

Fig. 123-2. Artist's conception of arthrodesis after failure of **(A)** polycentric and **(B)** geometric total knee.

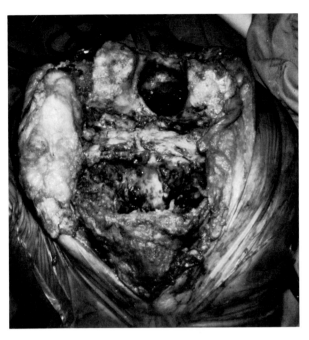

Fig. 123-3. Small rim of cortical bone remaining following removal of a total knee arthroplasty with an intramedullary stem.

upper tibia (Fig. 123-3). This is particularly true with infection if a pressure cement technique was used because the cancellous surface both superiorly and centrally is impregnated with methyl methacrylate and must be removed.

In the presence of infection, all diseased tissue must be excised. Excision involves the surface of the bone as well as the scarred capsular tissues. With the loosening that is usually present, there is additional loss of bone adjacent to the components, and the amount of bone loss depends on the configuration of the component. Thus, stems add greatly to bone loss, either with or without infection. With infection, the cement in the medullary canal, whether loose or not, must be removed, which may greatly weaken the bone, leaving little strength to afford secure compression and fixation.

If infection is not present, loosening alone may result in considerable loss of bone by the sandpaper-like abrasive action of the cement, perhaps augmented by a foreign-body reaction. If the prostheses are not loose, removal may produce a fracture, which often results in the loss of a large amount of bone. Salvage in these circumstances requires rigid biplanar external fixation if infected or a long intramedulary nail extending from the greater trochanter to the distal tibia if infection is absent. Cancellous bone grafting about the periphery of the arthrodesis is required. Thus, the amount of bone actually lost with any given type of knee replacement may vary considerably, and the technique used to arthrodese the knee also must vary.

AUTHORS' PREFERRED TECHNIQUE

A careful technique of arthrodesis is essential. Adequate bone apposition is key. Ideally, there should be healthy vascular cancellous bone opposed to healthy vascular cancellous bone.

The technique for knee arthrodesis using external fixation consists of four basic steps: (1) removal of the prosthesis, (2) preparation of the bony bed, (3) application of the external fixator, and (4) bone grafting if necessary. The surgical approach should use preexisting surgical incisions whenever feasible to prevent areas of skin necrosis between the old and new incisions. A longitudinal anteromedial approach is ideal. Removal of the implant may be relatively easy if it is loose. However, in the case of a secure component, a high-speed cutting instrument such as a Midas Rex has proved invaluable in removal. Dissection should be made in the plane between the prosthesis and cement to prevent loss of bone stock. In the case of metal-backed components, it may occasionally be necessary to transect the metal component in order to remove it without damage to the bone. All cement, both from the surface of the bone as well as from an intramedullary location, should be removed. Retained cement can act as a stress riser as well as a source for residual sepsis in the future. An interposed fibrous membrane will be present at the bone-cement interface, and this as well as any infected granulation tissue must be completely removed. A high-speed pulsating lavage should be used to prepare the bone surfaces, as this will permit identification of

any retained fragments of cement or fibrous membrane.

Correct alignment consists of a correct mechanical axis with the knee in slight flexion, but no more than 20 degrees of flexion. Alignment can be best determined by placing a radiographic marker over the hip preoperatively. This will permit definition of the mechanical axis of the limb intraoperatively by palpating the previously placed radiographic marker as well as the center of the ankle (Fig. 123-4). The mechanical axis should extend from the center of the femoral head to the center of the ankle and pass through the center of the knee.

Standard total knee arthroplasty instrumentation is very helpful in preparing the bony bed as well as alignment. In order to obtain healthy vascular cancellous bone, 2 to 3 mm of the proximal tibia as well as the distal femur should be resected. A tibial cutting guide is used to make a transverse cut on the tibia in both the coronal and sagittal planes, removing 2 mm of bone. This may leave some residual defects that can be bone grafted but should leave a stable peripheral cortical rim.

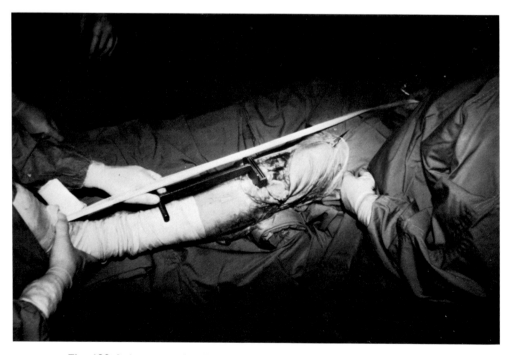

Fig. 123-4. Intraoperative determination of the mechanical axis of the limb.

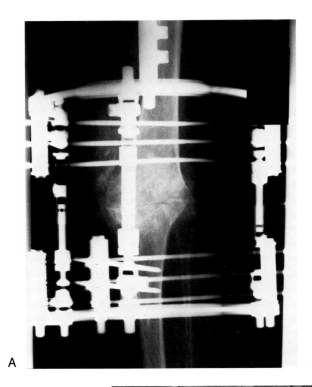
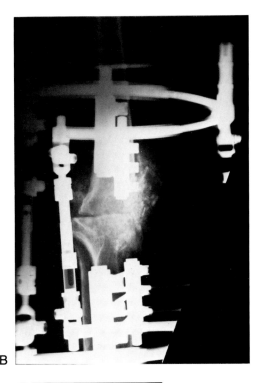

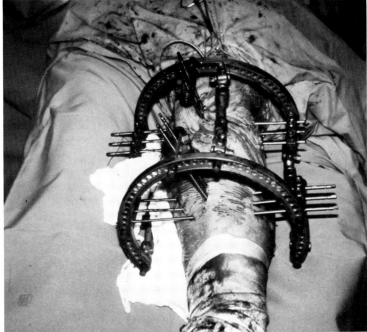

Fig. 123-5. (A) AP and **(B)** lateral radiographs. **(C)** Clinical appearance following arthrodesis with a biplanar Ace-Fischer apparatus.

The knee is placed in the proper degree of flexion and alignment; using a distal femoral cutting guide, an osteotomy of the distal femur is performed. Approximately 2 to 3 mm of bone is removed from the distal femur in order to expose a healthy vascular cancellous bed. The bone ends are then approximated and should be stable with correct alignment.

The external fixator may be applied. Three transfixing pins are used in the distal femur and three pins in the proximal tibia, all with a threaded central portion. A 5-mm titanium pin is best, as it provides the greatest rigidity of fixation. The femoral pins are placed from the medial side and the tibial pins from the lateral side to prevent impingement on neurovascular structures. The Ace-Fischer apparatus employs a cannula for pin placement through the soft tissues to bone. The central obturator is removed and the hole for the pin predrilled. This minimizes thermal necrosis of the bone and subsequent pin-tract problems.[35,106] All pins should be parallel. In order to prevent tethering of the soft tissues by the pins, traction should be applied to the soft tissues at the time of pin insertion.

After the pins have been placed, the semicircular rings are attached to the pins; three connecting bars are used to join the two rings. One connecting bar is placed anteriorly in the midline and the other two posteriorly. The rings should be placed such that they extend posterior to the pin sites to permit the connecting bars to be placed posterior to the axis of the limb. The three connecting bars are then compressed. Only hand tightening is required to obtain a considerable amount of force; some plastic deformation of the pins will be seen. Once the apparatus has been assembled, alignment should again be checked. Some AP instability will remain before application of the anterior pins. Two anterior half-pins are placed in the distal femur and two in the proximal tibia and connected to the semicircular rings. In the case of a hinged prosthesis, there will be poor bone stock, and the anterior half-pins should be placed on the outside of the ring. In the case of a resurfacing prosthesis, the anterior half-pins may be placed on the inside of the ring (Fig. 123-5).

Bone grafting may now be performed. If there has been extensive loss of intramedulary bone, as in the case of a hinged prosthesis, cancellous bone grafting about the periphery of the arthrodesis should be performed (Fig. 123-6). A combination of autogenous iliac cancellous bone and allograft bone from the bone bank are finely ground in a bone mill. In the case of a resurfacing prosthesis with remaining small bony defects, bone grafting may not need to be performed or may be very limited. The patella can be used as a source of bone graft to fill small defects in the proximal tibia or distal femur before application of the external fixator.

Suction drains are placed in the wound, and the wound is closed in the routine manner. A bulky Robert Jones dressing is used for the first 4 to 5

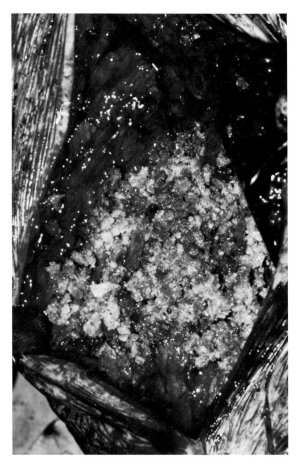

Fig. 123-6. Peripheral placement of combined autogenous iliac and homogeneous bone graft about the arthrodesis site.

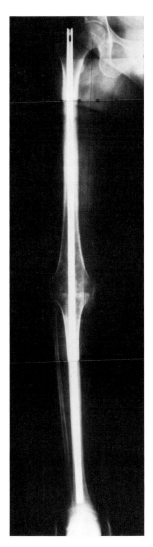

Fig. 123-7. AP radiograph following Küntscher nail and bone graft.

failed arthrodesis with quiescent sepsis, a long intramedullary nail will provide rigid fixation, even in the presence of substantial loss of bone from the metaphysis (Fig. 123-7). Careful preoperative planning is required to assess the correct length and diameter of the nail. A full-length radiograph of the limb with a magnification marker permits determination of nail length (Fig. 123-8). The nail should extend from the greater trochanter to the distal tibial metaphysis. Lateral radiographs of the femur and tibia are essential to evaluate any sagittal plane bowing. The use of a marker or an intramedullary nail of known size adjacent to the limb permits correction for variations in radiographic magnification. The limiting size for the nail will be dependent on the isthmus of the tibia and not the femur. Generally, a 10- to 12-mm diameter nail is

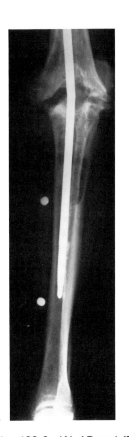
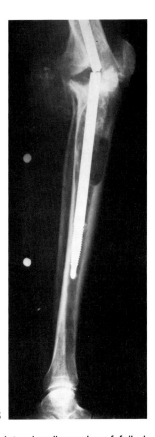

A   B

Fig. 123-8. (A) AP and **(B)** lateral radiographs of failed intramedullary arthrodesis performed with a 9-mm Schneider rod without bone grafting. A radiographic marker for magnification is adjacent to the tibia.

days, after which it may be removed and routine pin site care begun.

The fixation devices must be kept in as long as possible, as healing is slow. We prefer at least 10 weeks with the external fixation but have left the device in as long as 6 months with proper pin site care. A cylinder cast is then worn for 2 to 4 months, and bracing is used until the arthrodesis is solid. Since there may be 2 to 3 cm or shortening, a shoe lift is often required.

In the case of a nonseptic failed prosthesis or a

used. It is wise to have available a nail 1 mm larger and one 1 mm smaller than the predicted nail size. Although a variety of nail configurations are available, the Küntscher type has been reliable and easy to use.

The knee is first explored through the preexisting incision. Debridement of all scar tissue and pathologic evaluation of tissue for infection should be performed. A small quantity of bone is resected from the distal femur and proximal tibia to expose a healthy vascular bed. Alignment of the limb to permit bone apposition requires a tibiofemoral angle of near 0 degrees and thus differs from the alignment attempted with an external fixator. Progressive intramedullary reaming of the tibia over a standard guide wire is performed until firm contact with cortical bone is encountered in the isthmus. A standard-length intramedullary nail is used to evaluate the fit in the tibia. The size of the nail used is usually the same size as the last reamer. If too tight a fit of the nail in the tibia is attempted, the arthrodesis site will distract during the final portion of insertion of the long nail. Once the size of the tibial reaming is determined, the femur is reamed retrograde from the knee as well as from the hip over a guide wire. Reaming is performed only to the size of the tibia. The AP curvature of the femur will provide three-point fixation of the nail in the femur.

Once the femur and tibia have been prepared for the nail, a combination of autogenous iliac cancellous bone and allograft bone is prepared similar to that described for external fixation. Bone grafting is indicated in knees with loss of bone stock to allow union prior to fatigue failure of the nail (see Fig. 123-8). A portion of the bone graft is placed peripherally about the posterior aspect of the arthrodesis site before reduction of the arthrodesis since that area will not be accessible once the intramedullary nail is in place. The intramedullary nail is then placed from the greater trochanter to the knee. The arthrodesis is reduced and the nail driven into the tibia. An image intensifier is very helpful during this portion of the procedure. Correct rotation of the limb must be maintained. Finally, the remaining bone graft is placed about the anterior, medial, and lateral periphery of the arthrodesis site, and the wound is closed. A Robert Jones dressing is used for the first week followed by a long-leg cast with a pelvic band to control rotation until the arthrodesis is solid.

POSTOPERATIVE CARE

Postoperative care depends on the problem for which arthrodesis was performed. If infection is present, systemic antibiotics based on culture reports are administered intravenously for 4 weeks. Additional oral antibiotics are administered for a variable period of time. The antibiotic regimen chosen should be bacteriocidal and should achieve adequate bone and soft tissue concentrations; therapy is monitored according to serum antibiotic levels.[11]

Time to Union

The time to arthrodesis following the failed total knee arthroplasty varies considerable and depends on the prosthesis type and extent of previous surgery. The time to arthrodesis has ranged from a low of 2.5 months following a resurfacing prosthesis to 22 months with a hinged arthroplasty.[25,108] Our technique is to maintain external fixation for 2 to 4 months, until bone union is believed to be occurring, followed by a cylinder cast for 2 to 4 months. Additional bracing may be required until the arthrodesis is solid. It is often difficult to determine when bone union has occurred; tomography is of value in this determination.

RESULTS

The results of arthrodesis of the knee for the failed total knee arthroplasty vary considerably in the literature.[5,11,23,46,52,67,84,98,110] The results following a resurfacing prosthesis are generally better than those following a hinged arthroplasty (Tables 123-2 to 123-4). The success rate in the literature

Table 123-2. Knee Arthrodesis: Resurfacing Prostheses

Investigators	Year	No. of Attempted Arthrodeses	Technique	No. of Successful Unions
Petty et al.[84]	1975	8	External fixation	6
Gunsten and MacKenzie[45]	1976	6	Unspecified	6
Evanski et al.[29]	1976	3	Unspecified	2
Bargren et al.[4]	1976	2	Unspecified	1
Marmor[72]	1976	4	Unspecified	4
Skolnick et al.[102]	1976	15	External fixation	15
Skolnick and Brand[103]	1976	6	External fixation	6
Brodersen et al.[11]	1979	36	Various	29
Vahvanen[110]	1979	7	External fixation	4
Insall et al.[56]	1979	2	External fixation	2
Insall et al.[58]	1979	2	Unspecified	2
Moreland et al.[79]	1979	1	Unspecified	1
Cracchiolo et al.[21]	1979	2	Unspecified	2
Goldberg and Henderson[41]	1980	5	Unspecified	5
Mallory et al.[71]	1982	1	Unspecified	1
Thornhill et al.[108]	1982	5	External fixation	4
Hunter et al.[54]	1982	4	Unspecified	3
Eftekhar[27]	1983	4	Unspecified	4
Insall et al.[55]	1983	1	Unspecified	1
Moller and Goldberg[77]	1983	2	Unspecified	2
Rothacker and Cabanela[96]	1983	19	External fixation	18
Rand and Bryan[90]	1983	4	External fixation	4
Fidler[34]	1983	3	Biplanar external fixation	3
Wade and Denham[111]	1984	15	External fixation	8
Knutson et al.[66]	1984	21	External fixation	8
Knutson et al.[66]	1984	21	Biplanar external fixation	14
Knutson et al.[67]	1984	3	IM nail	3
Knutson et al.[68]	1985	2	IM nail	2
Knutson et al.[68]	1985	3	External fixation	3
Walker et al.[113]	1986	6	Unspecified	6
Wiedel[115]	1986	10	External fixation	8
Rand et al.[92]	1986	19	Biplanar external fixation	16
Total		242		193 (80%)

Table 123-3. Knee Arthrodesis: Various Prostheses

Investigators	Year	No. of Attempted Arthrodeses	Technique	No. of Successful Unions
Hageman et al.[46]	1978	14	External fixation	9
Lortat-Jacob et al.[69]	1979	4	Biplanar external fixation	4
Salvati and Insall[99]	1980	14	External fixation	4
Stinchfield et al.[105]	1980	3	External fixation	3
Shea et al.[100]	1981	24	External fixation	5
Goldberg and Hardy[40]	1981	13	Unspecified	9
Ahlberg and Lunden[1]	1981	3	Unspecified	2
Cameron and Hunter[13]	1982	11	Unspecified	6
Woods et al.[118]	1983	16	Unspecified	16
Kaufer et al.[63]	1983	18	IM nail	18
Bigliani et al.[5]	1983	20	Electrical coils	17
Knutson et al.[64]	1984	4	Unspecified	1
Fahmy[31]	1984	5	IM nail and Charnley	5
Freeman et al.[85]	1985	16	Unspecified	10
Rand[93]	1986	27	Unspecified	20
Rand[91]	1986	120	Unspecified	95
Johnson and Bannister[59]	1986	12	External fixation	6
Grogan et al.[44]	1986	5	Unspecified	5
Total		329		235 (71%)

Table 123-4. Knee Arthrodesis: Constrained Prostheses

Investigators	Year	No. of Attempted Arthrodeses	Technique	No. of Successful Unions
Walldius[114]	1960	5	Unspecified	5
Young[119]	1963	7	Unspecified	7
Jones[60]	1960	3	Unspecified	2
Jones[61]	1973	9	External fixation	8
Phillips and Taylor[86]	1975	2	Unspecified	2
Deburge and Guepar[23]	1976	10	Unspecified	3
Wilson and Venters[117]	1976	2	Unspecified	2
Engelbrecht et al.[28]	1976	2	External fixation	2
Attenborough[2]	1978	3	Unspecified	3
Jones et al.[62]	1979	3	Unspecified	1
Brodersen et al.[11]	1979	9	Various	5
Vahvanen[110]	1979	1	External fixation	0
Barger et al.[3]	1980	1	Unspecified	1
Hui and Fitzgerald[53]	1980	3	Unspecified	2
Wilson et al.[116]	1980	1	Unspecified	1
Phillips and Mears[85]	1980	1	External fixation	1
Thornhill et al.[108]	1982	4	External fixation	2
Fidler[34]	1983	1	Biplanar external fixation	1
Rothacker and Cabanela[96]	1983	10	External fixation	7
Rand and Bryan[90]	1983	1	External fixation	0
Walker and Schruman[112]	1984	1	Unspecified	1
Wade and Denham[111]	1984	23	External fixation	11
Knutson[67]	1984	15	External fixation	3
Knutson[67]	1984	22	Biplanar external fixation	11
Knutson[67]	1984	2	IM nail	2
Knutson[68]	1985	4	IM nail	3
Knutson[68]	1985	4	External fixation	2
Ewald et al.[30]	1985	6	Unspecified	3
Harris and Frochlich[48]	1985	6	IM nail	5
Wiedel[115]	1986	5	IM nail	4
Rand	1986	7	Biplanar external fixation	2
Total		186		102 (55%)

is 55 percent of 186 constrained, 80 percent of 242 resurfacing, 71 percent of 329 mixed prostheses, or 70 percent of 756 attempts at arthrodesis. This must be compared with a 95 to 98 percent success rate for primary compression arthrodesis of the knee.[15-17]

COMPLICATIONS

The complications associated with compression arthrodesis of the knee for the failed total knee arthroplasty are those related to the technique, such as pin-tract infection, neurovascular injury, and malalignment, which should be preventable, and the complications of ipsilateral limb fracture and failure of arthrodesis. Minor pin-tract inflammation and drainage are not infrequent, but serious pin-tract infections are infrequent.[12] Complications in our recent review affected 36 percent of 28 cases treated with biplanar external fixation.[92] Complications consisted of delayed wound healing (1 case), femoral artery laceration (1 case), pin-site sepsis (3 cases), pin-site fracture (2 cases), and recurrent local sepsis (2 cases).[92] In 20 cases, of which 7 were treated by external fixation and the remainder by intramedullary nails, fracture occurred in 4 cases, nail migration in 2 cases, delayed wound healing in 1 case, and recurrent infection in 5 cases.[68] In a multicenter study of 91 cases, complications consisted of pin breakage (2 cases), pin loosening (10 cases), pin-site infection (3 cases), sepsis (6 cases), delayed wound healing (2 cases), tibial fracture (1 case), peroneal palsy (1 case), intramedullary nail migration (1 case), and tibial shaft penetration by an intramedullary nail (1 case).[67]

Pin-tract problems can be minimized by the use of predrilling of the pins as well as adequate soft tissue releases adjacent to the pin sites.[35,42,73] Pins should not be placed through areas of retained and presumably infected cement. All cement and foreign material should be removed to minimize the risk of recurrent sepsis.[67,92] Ipsilateral limb fracture complicates 10 to 15 percent of patients following arthrodesis and probably reflects a long lever arm acting at the fracture site.[106] Stress risers, such as pin tracts either with or without the pin in place, as well as retained fragments of cement may be contributing factors. An intramedullary nail used for arthrodesis should extend into the distal tibia to prevent acting as a stress riser.[63]

The most frequent complication is that of failure of arthrodesis. The etiology of failure has generally been that of bone loss, persistent sepsis, or repeated manipulation leading to loss of bone apposition.[12] The importance of bone loss contributing to pseudarthrosis has been emphasized by several investigators.[5,11,46,67,89] The importance of bone loss in influencing union is reflected in the higher success rate of arthrodesis following a resurfacing compared with constrained implant. Bone loss was the single most important factor influencing union

using biplanar external fixation for arthrodesis.[92] In an attempt to offset the effects of bone loss, bone grafting has been used, including patella, femoral condyles, iliac, sliding grafts, and allografts.[25,48,67,92,110,115] Union was obtained in 22 of 37 treated with bone graft compared with 30 of 62 without bone grafts.[67] Ten of 12 knees treated with bone grafts compared with 11 of 16 without bone grafts united.[92] Although these differences are not statistically significant, the results do not reflect that the knees with the largest defects were bone grafted. Bone grafting is best performed with combined iliac and allograft bone placed about the periphery of the arthrodesis.[89] Bone grafting is best done for arthrodeses with less than 70 percent bone apposition.[92]

The functional results of failed knee arthrodeses are often poor. Of 20 failed arthrodeses, 4 patients had pain, 11 were limited in walking ability, and 6 were not satisfied[84] compared with 39 united arthrodeses with two painful, 7 with limited walking ability, and 1 not satisfied.[66] Of 29 knees of which 5 united and 24 did not, one-half of the patients were satisfied.[100] Of 11 nonunions, 5 were painful compared with 1 of 10 with union.[91] By contrast, 5 of 6 knees with nonunion were painless.[59]

Salvage techniques for the failed arthrodesis in-

Table 123-5. Repeat Arthrodesis

Investigators	Year	N	Technique	Union
Bigliani et al.[5]	1983	20	Electrical coils	17
Goldberg and Hardy[40]	1981	1	Unspecified	1
Knutson et al.[68]	1985	1	Bone graft	1
		2	IM nail	2
		1	External fixation and bone graft	1
		1	IM nail and bone graft	1
Rand[89]	1986	29	External fixation	8
		4	Electrical coils	2
		3	Bone graft	1
		2	Plate and bone graft	1
Rand[92]	1987	3	Electrical coils	0
		1	Electrical coils and bone graft	1
		1	Dual plates	1
Vahvanen[110]	1979	2	Bone graft	0
		2	External fixation	1
		1	Dual plates	1
Wade and Denham[111]	1984	2	External fixation	2
Woods et al.[118]	1983	1	Bone graft	1

clude bone grafting alone, bone grafting combined with a repeat course of external fixation, internal fixation with a plate or intramedullary nail, and/or electrical stimulation. Internal fixation is best performed once there is no longer evidence of active sepsis.

Repeat attempts at arthrodesis have resulted in union in 42 of 75 (56 percent) cases reported in the literature[3,40,68,91,92,110,111,118] (Table 123-5). The success rate for each repeat attempt at arthrodesis is approximately 50 percent through four attempts.[91] The most successful techniques have been intramedullary nailing (100 percent), electrical stimulation (77 percent), and plate fixation (75 percent) (Table 123-5).

patients have had draining sinuses subsequent to such treatment at other institutions. We have noted also that many of the patients with failed arthrodeses and healed infection seem to function fairly well with bracing and with only mild pain, but there is, in our opinion, much better function in the patient with successful arthrodesis. This is particularly true for the obese woman whose leg configuration does not lend itself to brace control of an unstable pseudarthrosis. Nevertheless, repeated attempts at bone grafting, electrical stimulation, plating, and so forth may all fail in these desperate circumstances. In these situations, amputation should be considered.

DISCUSSION

More patients are being seen with infected hinge-type total knees in whom other types of total knees were performed with perhaps one or two revisions. In these patients especially, bone loss is extreme, and the tibia and femur at the knee level may consist of two different-sized circles of sclerotic bone immersed in scar tissue. Just as Drennan et al. found in the Charcot knee that the scarred tissues and sclerotic bone must be excised, we believe that in the failed multiply revised total knee arthroplasty with infection, all the scar tissue must be excised and debrided to bleeding bone, if fusion is to be obtained.[25] The problem is that there is often already shortening of 5 cm or more simply by removal of the prostheses and cement and that further removal of bone (1) shortens the extremity to the extent that a massive shoe lift must be used, and (2) makes skin closure extremely difficult, if not impossible. We have had very few patients in whom the infection could be suppressed permanently with retention of the prosthesis if the infection was well established before the diagnosis could be made.

Particularly when associated with loosening of the stems, the use of antibiotic therapy, with or without surgical debridement, did not seem to be effective in a lasting suppression, and many of our

SUMMARY

Arthrodesis of the knee joint has existed as a primary mode of treatment for certain infections, such as tuberculosis, for severe destruction as in neuropathies, and for instability subsequent to poliomyelitis or other such causes. Its secondary use has been as a salvage procedure after debridements, osteotomy, or arthroplasty have failed. The use of arthrodesis has changed because of the early success of low-friction total knee arthroplasty. The procedure is now used after repeated revisions of knee arthroplasty have failed or after infection of a total knee arthroplasty. Rarely is it used primarily in knees unsuitable for total knee arthroplasty.

Therefore, we recommend thorough excision of all scarred and infected tissues with careful contouring of the bone ends to ensure adequate bone apposition. Cancellous bone grafts placed about the periphery of the arthrodesis should be considered in the case of loss of bone stock to improve the surfaces for bone apposition. In the presence of sepsis, rigid biplanar external fixation should be done to obtain a compression arthrodesis combined with prolonged immobilization. In the absence of infection or quiescent sepsis, a long intramedullary nail provides the best fixation. Unfortunately, some patients will remain who require permanent bracing.

Intramedullary Knee Arthrodesis Using a Curved Nail

Herbert Kaufer

Larry S. Matthews

Although primary knee arthrodesis for nonneuropathic disease is successful in nearly 100 percent of cases,[125] currently most knee-fusion operations are performed for salvage of failed total knee arthroplasty.[122,123] In this very challenging population, knee fusion in the best of hands has yielded 70 to 80 percent successful bony arthrodesis, when performed for septic failure of minimally constrained resurfacing prostheses and has yielded only 50 to 60 percent successful bony arthrodesis when used for salvage of infection of the more constrained devices with medullary stems.[121] For sterile failure of the multiply revised total knee or for septic failure of a knee prosthesis, knee fusion is considered by most to be the ultimate knee-salvage procedure.[123,124]

Recent experience with intramedullary arthrodesis of the knee using a curved intramedullary nail, extending from the trochanter across the knee, and into the distal tibial metaphysis has resulted in secure bony arthrodesis in all 34 limbs, in which it was used. The 34 successful arthrodeses included 11 primary arthrodesis performed for gross post-traumatic instability of the knee. Of these, 2 were neuropathic, 2 had osteogenesis imperfecta, and 1 had paralytic instability secondary to poliomyelitis residual paralysis. Four arthrodeses were performed following resection of malignant tumors at the knee (3 femoral, 1 tibial). In these cases, autogenous fibular and iliac bone graft was used to span a resection gap of 13 to 17 cm (Fig. 123-9). Six were performed for sterile failure of multiply revised total knee arthroplasties (2 total condylar, 1 PCA, 1 geometric, 1 UCI, and 1 spherocentric). Fifteen were performed for salvage of septic failure of a total knee prosthesis: 3 spherocentric (Fig. 123-10), 1 Walldius, 2 GUEPAR, 1 Bechtol, 2 Herbert, 2 total condylar, 1 geometric, 1 Marmor, 2 Townley. All have secure bony arthrodesis and excellent weight bearing function. Except for the tumor resections, which were kept non-weight bearing on crutches for 3 to 6 months postoperatively, all other intramedullary arthrodesis patients started unrestricted weight bearing, within the

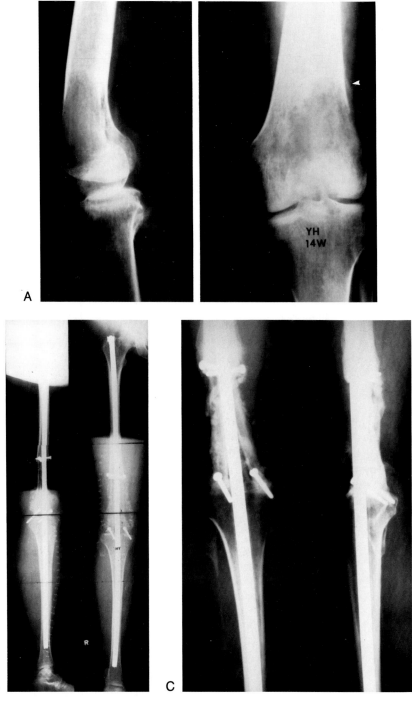

Fig. 123-9. Resection-arthrodesis for aggressive giant cell tumor of the distal femur. **(A)** Large distal femoral lytic lesion, 14 weeks following onset of symptoms. Note the Codman's triangle at the lateral femoral cortex (arrow). **(B)** Immediate postoperative radiograph. A 15-cm resection gap is bridged by two segments of autogenous fibula fixed with screws at either end and augmented by autogenous iliac bone graft. Note the distal end of the nail extending into the distal tibial metaphysis. **(C)** Two years following resection-arthrodesis, the grafts have incorporated, the fusion is secure.

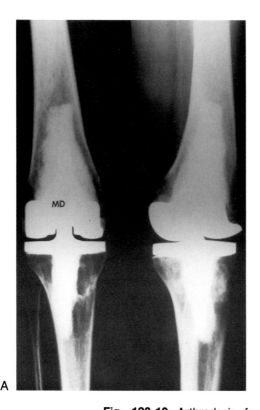

A

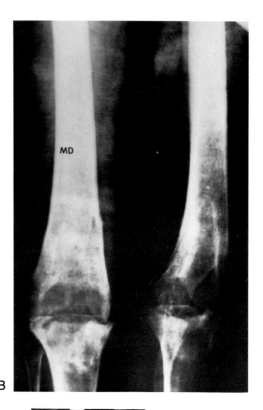

B

Fig. 123-10. Arthrodesis for chronic infection of a spherocentric knee prosthesis. **(A)** Chronic pain 3 years following spherocentric arthroplasty, persistent knee effusion is culture positive for *Staphylococcus aureus.* Note the zone of osteosporosis surrounding the femoral cement. **(B)** Following debridement that included removal of the prosthesis and all cement, the limb is immobilized in a long leg plaster cast, and full weight bearing as tolerated is encouraged. **(C)** Intraoperative radiograph, demonstrating the medullary nail, passing the tibial isthmus. Note the large empty cavity within the proximal tibial metaphysis and the distal femoral metaphysis. *(Figure continues.)*

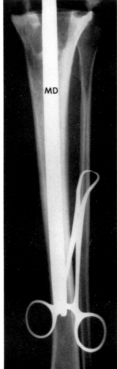

C

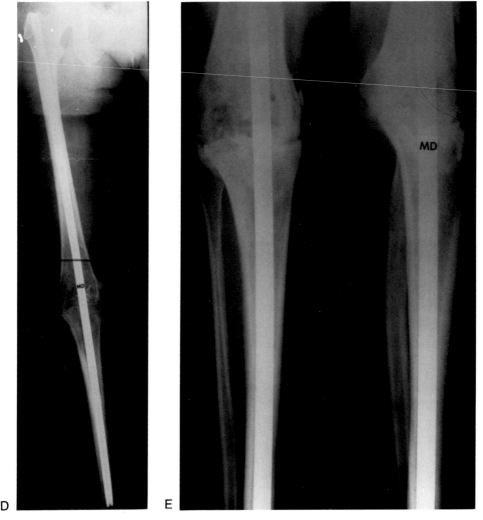

D   E

Fig. 123-10 *(Continued).* **(D)** One-year following arthrodesis. Note excellent alignment of the limb and changes suggesting secure bony arthrodesis. The trochanteric wire fixing the eye of the nail to the trochanter is intended to prevent nail migration. **(E)** Three years postoperative. The arthrodesis is secure. Note the effect of osteoplasty of the anterior proximal tibial metaphysis performed in order to permit tension-free soft tissue closure.

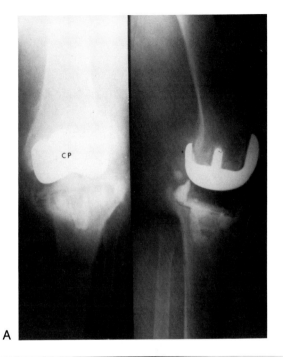

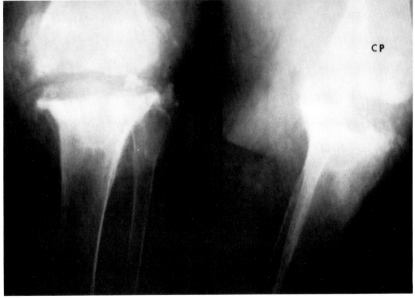

Fig. 123-11. Arthrodesis for salvage of an infected condylar total knee. **(A)** Condylar knee prosthesis with chronic drainage, culture positive for *Proteus mirabilis*. **(B)** Three months following debridement with removal of prosthesis and cement. The wound is healed and dry with no inflammatory signs. *(Figure continues.)*

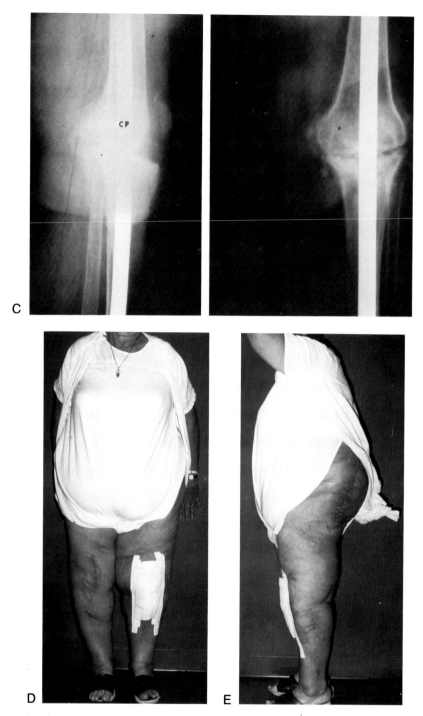

C

D

E

Fig. 123-11 *(Continued).* **(C)** Early postoperative radiographs of the arthrodesis knee. Note relative anterior displacement of the proximal tibial metaphysis. If this displacement leads to an excessively tight skin closure, the problem can be solved by osteoplastic resection of the anterior proximal tibial metaphysis **(E)**. **(D)** Front view of this 320-pound patient on her sixth postoperative day, bearing weight on the arthrodesed limb without restriction. Note the desirable degree of valgus alignment of the arthrodesed left knee, produced by insertion of the intramedullary nail with its convexity directed anterior medially. **(E)** Lateral view demonstrates the recent gluteal wound, and a desirable degree of flexion posture at the knee produced by insertion of the nail with its convexity directed anterior medially. The patient is able to bear weight without restriction on the sixth postoperative day, with no cast, brace, splint, or other external support.

first postoperative week (Fig. 123-11). No external immobilization, cast or brace, was used postoperatively in any patient.

OPERATIVE PREPARATION

Because the procedure requires an intramedullary nail extending from the trochanter across the knee into the distal tibial mataphysis, it should not be performed in any knee with active sepsis. Therefore, if one is attempting arthrodesis for salvage of an infected total knee prosthesis, the fusion is at least a two-stage procedure. The first stage consists of complete debridement and removal of the prosthesis, cement, and all devitalized tissue. Debridement should be conservative. While all devitalized tissue should be removed and a complete synovectomy performed, infected but viable scar and bone with good blood supply should not be removed. Following complete debridement, depending on the condition of the wound, it is either closed or packed open and immobilized in a well-fitted plaster cast, maintaining the proximal tibia in an end-on relationship to the distal femur, keeping the limb aligned in 7 to 10 degrees of valgus and 20 degrees of flexion at the knee (Figs. 123-10, 123-11).

One week later, the patient is returned to the operating room for redebridement and closure. Because poor condition of the wound made either primary or delayed primary closure unwise, 7 of the 34 knees were allowed to heal by secondary intent.

The second-stage intramedullary arthrodesis should be performed only after the infection has been controlled, with elimination of all active inflammation and drainage. The debridement wound should be securely healed and dry. In this group of patients, the briefest interval between debridement and intramedullary arthrodesis was 10 weeks, the longest was 14 months. During the interval between debridement and intramedullary arthrodesis, the patients are permitted and encouraged to ambulate ad lib, bearing full weight on the operated limb. In order to minimize postresection instability, prolonged cast immobilization is desirable. The period of cast-supported full weight bearing should be at least 6 months. Following cast removal, continued full weight bearing, if necessary with the support of a splint or brace, is encouraged.[120] Of the 31 infected total knee prostheses treated by systemic antibiotics and debridement, followed by ad lib ambulation with cast support, active sepsis was eliminated in all but 2. Sixteen patients in whom infection was eliminated found that their function with the resection arthroplasty was satisfactory. In these patients, secondary arthrodesis was not advised and was not done. They continue to function satisfactorily on their resection knee arthroplasty. The second-stage intramedullary arthrodesis is reserved for those patients who find their resection arthroplasty unsatisfactory. Fifteen patients in whom the infection had been eliminated found that, because of excessive instability, the resection arthroplasty was not adequate for their needs. These 15 patients had a successful intramedullary arthrodesis performed by the technique to be described.

TECHNIQUE

Either general or spinal anesthesia is acceptable. The patient should be positioned on the operating table in the lateral position, with the affected side up. Pads or other devices to keep the patient in lateral position should not be used. The patient should be positioned free so that he or she can be rolled into supine position, to facilitate access to the distal femur, proximal tibia and the anterior aspect of the knee. Full lateral position permits access to the gluteal region for insertion and driving of the intramedullary nail.

Skin preparation should include the full circumference of the proximal third of the leg, the knee, and the entire thigh, as well as of the trochanteric and gluteal regions. The entire lower extremity should be draped free. A sterile tourniquet should be used at midthigh level so that the intraarticular portion of the operation to be done under tourniquet control in a bloodless field. Following skin preparation and draping, the patient is rolled from the full lateral position to the supine position. The tourniquet is inflated. Depending on the location of prior surgical scars, the knee is exposed through either a medial or lateral parapatellar incision. Intraarticular adhesions are usually dense and extensive. They are sharply divided. The knee is mobilized to permit complete inspection of the distal femur, proximal tibia, and patella surfaces. If any occult abscess or other evidence of persistent sepsis is found, repeat debridement rather than arthrodesis is performed. One proceeds to the planned intramedullary arthrodesis only if complete and thorough inspection of the knee region is not suspicious of persistent infection. All fibrous scar separating the distal femur and proximal tibia is excised. Any fibrous scar within the medullary potion of the femur or tibia should be completely excised. If the infected prosthesis was a large device with intramedullary stems, the end of the femur and of the tibia are likely to resemble the bell end of a trumpet, permitting contact of only a peripheral rim of bone when the tibia and femur are approximated. The peripheral rim of contact is perfectly adequate for reliable fusion. There is no need to resect bone in order to eliminate the empty trumpet ends, nor is there any need to fill the empty trumpet end, with bone graft (Fig. 123-10). Because of the superb fixation provided by the intramedullary nail, peripheral contact of the hollow metaphysis of the femur and tibia is all that is necessary for prompt and secure bony arthrodesis, by the intramedullary fixation arthrodesis technique.

Having demonstrated that there is no occult infection, one may proceed with mobilization of the proximal tibia and the distal femur, which should include subperiosteal exposure of at least 1 inch of the full circumference of the proximal tibia and distal femur. Circumferential subperiosteal exposure of the distal femur and proximal tibia must be obtained in order to permit close approximation of the bone ends. The tibial medullary canal should be reamed first, because the diameter of the tibial medullary canal is less than that of the femur. Any nail that the tibia can accommodate will certainly be accommodated by the femur. The opposite, however, is not true; since the femoral medullary cavity has a larger diameter than that of the tibia, the femur could be reamed to a nail size too large for the tibia to accommodate. For this reason, the tibial medullary canal is prepared first. The medullary cavity of the tibia is located with an awl or currette. Guide pins should be passed through the mid-diaphysis of the tibia into the distal tibial metaphysis; if there is any doubt about the location of the guide pin, it should be confirmed by two plane radiographs. Flexible reamers are passed over the guide pin, and reaming is extended down into the distal tibial metaphysis.

A curved intramedullary nail with a single radius of curvature is used. Nails of this description are available from all commercial suppliers. Curve mismatch among the nail, the tibia, and the femur is relied on in order to gain optimal torsional control. Nails of less than 13-mm diameter are to be avoided, if possible. If one is planning to use a Küntscher nail, the tibia should be reamed 0.5 to 1 mm larger than the diameter of the nail, and the femur should be reamed 1 to 2 mm larger than the diameter of the nail. Once reaming of the tibia has been completed, one should plan to use a Küntscher nail 0.5 mm smaller than the largest diameter reamer that has passed the length of the tibia. The femur should be reamed to a diameter 1 mm greater than the largest reamer that has passed through the isthmus of the tibia.

The medullary canal from the distal end of the femur is located with an awl or currette. A guide pin is then placed from its distal end into the medullary canal of the femur and beyond the femoral isthmus. Because the femur of most adults is longer than available flexible reamers, in order to fully ream its entire length, it is necessary to ream the femur from both its distal and trochanteric ends. Reaming starts distally and continues proximately beyond the isthmus, to a diameter 1 mm greater than the largest diameter reamer that has passed beyond the isthmus of the tibia. This portion of the operation is done under tourniquet control.

The patient is rolled from a supine to a lateral position. The usual surgical approach through the buttock to the piriformis fossa is made. The piriformis fossa is exposed and perforated with a quarter-inch drill. A guide pin is inserted through this hole and then down into the medullary cavity of the femur, until it is visualized in the distal femoral medullary cavity. The proximal portion of the femur is then reamed over this guide pin, using flexible medullary reamers passed from the piriformis fossa down beyond the femoral isthmus. The largest reamer used should be 1 mm larger than the largest-diameter reamer that has passed beyond the isthmus of the tibia. Thus, the femur will have been reamed 1.5 mm larger than the selected nail.

The length of the femur from the piriformis fossa to its distal articular end is measured, as is the length of the tibia from its proximal articular end to the distal tibial metastasis. The sum of these two measurements is the length of nail to be used. Curved 75-cm Küntscher nails are available from all manufacturers. One such nail in each diameter, from 12 through 18 mm, should be available. A nail with a diameter 0.5 mm less than the largest reamer that has passed beyond the isthmus of the tibia is selected and cut to length, using a sterile hacksaw. I prefer to cut off the eye end of the nail, leaving the tapered end undisturbed in order to facilitate nail insertion. After cutting off the eye end of the nail to the desired length, metal burrs on the cut end should be removed with a file. Using a ¼ metal cutting drill, a hole should be drilled adjacent to the end of the nail; this hole will accommodate the hook fitting on the Küntscher nail extraction device and facilitate nail removal, should it become necessary. After the nail has been selected, cut to length, and a new nail eye created with a ¼ metal-cutting drill, the nail is placed over the guide pin and driven from proximal to distal down the entire length of the femur, until it appears at the distal articular end of the femur. The convexity of the curve of the nail should be directed anteromedially relative to the femur. In this rotational orientation, the nails curve will give the arthrodesed limb a desirable degree of flexion and valgus at the knee (see Fig. 123-11). If the nail is inserted so that its convexity matches the anterolateral convexity of the femur, the arthrodesed limb will have the appearance of flexion and varus at the knee. If necessary, the femur should be reamed an addition 0.5 to 1 mm in order to allow the nail to be inserted with the convexity of the nail directed anteromedially relative to the femur. The nail should be driven 2 to 3 cm beyond the end of the femur. The reamed medullary cavity of the proximal tibia is then reduced over the protruding end of the nail, and the tibia is brought into extension, in order to align its medullary canal with the nail. The nail is then driven down the length of the tibia, beyond its

isthmus and into its distal metaphysis (see Fig. 123-10).

In order to prevent proximal migration of the nail, it is wise to pass a loop of 18-gauge stainless steel wire through the eye of the nail and through a drill hole in the greater trochanter. After the nail has been fully inserted, the 18-gauge stainless steel wire loop should be twisted tight and the excess removed (Fig. 123-12). Prior to routine use of a trochanteric wire, several cases of proximal nail migration with gluteal irritation were observed.

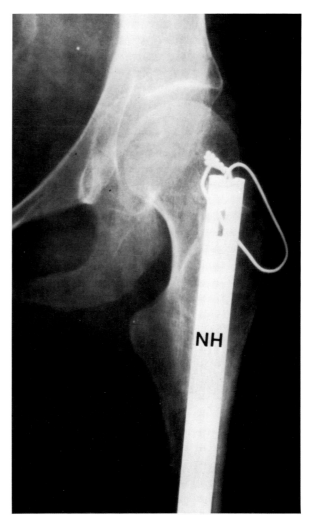

Fig. 123-12. An 18-gauge stainless steel wire passed through the eye of the nail and a drill hole in the greater trochanter effectively prevent nail migration.

This problem has been eliminated by routine use of supplemental trochanteric wire fixation at the completion of nail insertion. In our early experience with this technique, several intramedullary arthrodeses were done, using nails that ended at or near the tibial isthmus. These patients experienced postoperative pain and an intense remodeling response of the tibia coinciding with the distal end of the nail. In 4 patients, a fatigue fracture developed at this location. In one patient, the fracture displaced and went on to a nonunion. This problem of symptoms associated with tibial remodeling and fatigue fracture at the distal end of the nail has been totally eliminated by routine use of a longer nail that extends beyond the isthmus, into the distal tibial metaphysis.

When reducing the tibia over the protruding end of the nail, it is important to see that there is an appropriate amount of external tibial rotation relative to the femur. One must take care that the proximal tibia is kept in contact with the distal femur as the nail is being inserted. There is a tendency for the knee to be distracted and for the tibia to separate from the femur as the nail is being driven beyond the tibial isthmus. Once the nail has been fully inserted, there will be complete stability at the knee, in all directions, including torsion. There is no need for any supplementary fixation, such as staples, screws, and plates (Figs. 123-10, 123-11).

In a normal limb, the medullary cavity of the tibia is somewhat posterior to that of the femur. Insertion of a transarticular intramedullary nail displaces the proximal metaphysis of the tibia in an anterior direction (Fig. 123-11), making it difficult to close the soft tissues over the now prominent, anteriorly displaced, proximal tibial metaphysis. If one encounters this problem, it is best solved by resecting the anterior prominence of the proximal tibial metaphysis (see Fig. 123-10E). The quantity of anterior proximal tibial metaphysis resected should be sufficient to allow tension free soft tissue closure. If the resected autogenous cancellous bone from the anterior proximal tibial metaphysis is used for bone graft, it is best placed at the periphery of the knee, between bone and soft tissue, rather than within the metaphyseal cavities of the femur and tibia. Despite impressively large metaphyseal cavities (Fig. 123-10C) with or without supplemental peripheral bone graft from the prox-

imal tibia, secure bony arthrodesis has occurred in all knees treated by intramedullary arthrodesis.

Following closure of the knee and gluteal wounds, a light dry sterile dressing is applied. No cast, brace, splint, or other external support is used. The patient is encouraged to begin weight bearing ad lib as soon as possible. All patients treated by this technique were able to bear full weight, without restriction, within the first postoperative week (Fig. 123-11D,E). Functional arthrodesis occurs immediately. The patient walks "on the nail" until arthrodesis occurs. All patients have a functional fusion. It is often difficult to determine from clinical evaluation and radiographs exactly when arthrodesis occurs. In some patients, with the nail still in situ, it may be difficult to be certain that bony fusion has occurred. The four patients who had their nails removed all have confirmed solid bony fusion. Shortening averaged 3.5 cm (range 2 to 8 cm).

COMPLICATIONS

Five patients experienced reactivation of their previous infection; however, in spite of active infection, prompt secure arthrodesis occurred in all five. The infection eventually came under control, with cessation of drainage in four of the five patients. Eight of the 15 patients complained of discomfort at the distal end of the intramedullary nail, which lasted 6 to 9 months. Pain in these patients was associated with an intense periosteal response of the tibial shaft at the distal end of the nail, resulting in hypertrophy of bone, adjacent to the end of the nail. In one patient, a displaced fracture developed through the tibia and periosteal new bone at the distal end of the nail, which went on to nonunion. This was successfully treated by replacing the nail with a longer one that crossed the tibial fracture site. Five patients experienced proximal migration of the rod, and sufficient gluteal symptoms to warrant reinsertion of the Küntscher nail, which resulted in clearing of the gluteal symptoms. In one patient, postoperative palsy of the tibial and peri-neal nerve developed, probably due to a malfunction of the pneumatic tourniquet.

The problem with this operation is its duration, which varies from 2½ hours for an arthrodesis of the knee with posttraumatic instability to nearly 6 hours for arthrodesis of the knee associated with a tumor resection. Blood loss varied from 800 to 2700 cc. The advantage of intramedullary arthrodesis of the knee is that a very high proportion of attempts result in successful bony fusion (100 percent in our experience). Casts, braces, percutaneous pins, and external fixators are avoided entirely (Fig. 123-11). All patients are capable of unrestricted full weight bearing immediately postoperatively. Our experience has demonstrated that, except for fusion associated with tumor resection, there is no need for either supplemental bone graft, electrical stimulation, or external fixation in order to achieve reliable arthrodesis of the knee. Even when attempting fusion after infected failure of a relatively large intramedullary knee joint prosthesis, our successful fusion rate has been 100 percent. Maintaining a stable relationship between the periphery of the proximal tibia and distal femur is sufficient to induce prompt secure bone union and to permit immediate unrestricted full weight bearing. There is simply no need to fill the empty cavity of the trumpet ends of distal femur and proximal tibia or to eliminate them by resection, which would result in unacceptable shortening.

On the basis of this experience, we believe that except for those patients with a proximal femoral prosthesis on the ipsilateral side, intramedullary arthrodesis of the knee is the procedure of choice for all patients in whom knee arthrodesis is indicated. In our opinion, the advantages of immediate full weight bearing without external appliances and a 100 percent probability of successful fusion, far exceed the disadvantages of a relatively difficult and time-consuming operative procedure. The Küntscher cloverleaf type of intramedullary nail is preferred over a more rigid tubular nail, such as the Sampson nail, because the cloverleaf type of open section nail is (1) strong enough (no nail failure in our cases), (2) far easier to insert, and (3) much more forgiving because its greater flexibility lets it accommodate to the curve mismatch between the bones and the nail, with much less chance of nail jamming or bone fracture.

REFERENCES

Arthrodesis of the Knee Joint

1. Ahlberg A, Lunden A: Secondary operations after knee joint replacement. Clin Orthop 156:170, 1981
2. Attenborough CG: The Attenborough total knee replacement. J Bone Joint Surg 60B:320, 1978
3. Barger WL, Cracchiolo A, Amstutz HC: Results with the constrained total knee prosthesis in treating severely disabled patients and patients with failed total knee replacements. J Bone Joint Surg 62A:504, 1980
4. Bargren JH, Freeman MAR, Swanson SAV, Todd RC: ICLH arthroplasty in the treatment of arthritic knee. Clin Orthop 120:65, 1976
5. Bigliani LU, Rosenwasser MP, Caulo N, et al: The use of pulsing electromagnetic fields to achieve arthrodesis of the knee following failed total knee arthroplasty. J Bone Joint Surg 65A:480, 1983
6. Bosworth DM: Knee fusion by the use of a three-flanged nail. J Bone Joint Surg 28:550, 1946
7. Brashear HR: The value of the intramedullary nail for knee fusion particularly for the Charcot joint. Am J Surg 87:64, 1954
8. Brattström H, Brattström J: Long-term results in knee arthrodesis in rheumatoid arthritis. Acta Rheum Scand 17:86, 1971
9. Brause BD: Infected total knee replacement. Orthop Clin North Am 13:245, 1982
10. Briggs BT, Chao EYS: The mechanical performance of the standard Hoffmann-Vidal external fixation apparatus. J Bone Joint Surg 64A:566, 1982
11. Broderson MP, Fitzgerald RH, Peterson LFA, et al: Arthrodesis of the knee following failed total knee arthroplasty. J Bone Joint Surg 61A:181, 1979
12. Brooker AF Jr, Hansen NM Jr: The biplane frame. Clin Orthop 160:163, 1981
13. Cameron HV, Hunter GA: Failure in total knee arthroplasty. Clin Orthop 170:141, 1982
14. Chapchal G: Intramedullary pinning for arthrodesis of the knee joint. J Bone Joint Surg 30:734, 1948
15. Charnley J: Positive pressure in arthrodesis of the knee joint. J Bone Joint Surg 30B:478, 1948
16. Charnley J: Arthrodesis of the knee. Clin Orthop 18:37, 1960
17. Charnley J, Baker SL: Compression arthrodesis of the knee. A clinical and histological study. J Bone Joint Surg 34B:187, 1952

18. Charnley J, Lowe HG: A study of the end-results of compression arthrodesis of the knee. J Bone Joint Surg 40B:633, 1958

19. Cleveland M: Operative fusion of the unstable or flail knee due to anterior poliomyelitis: a study of the late results. J Bone Joint Surg 14:525, 1932

20. Cloutier JM, Fortin R: Arthrodèse du genou avec un long clou de Küntscher. Union Med Can 101:1842, 1972

21. Cracchiolo A, Benson M, Finerman GAM, et al: A prospective comparative clinical analysis of the first generation knee replacements. Clin Orthop 145:37, 1978

22. Crenshaw AH: Campbell's Operative Orthopaedics. p. 981, 4th Ed. CV Mosby, St. Louis, 1963

23. Deburge A, and GUEPAR: GUEPAR hinge prosthesis. Clin Orthop 120:47, 1976

24. Dee R: The case for arthrodesis of the knee. Orthop Clin North Am 10(1):249, 1979

25. Drennan DB, Maylahn DJ: Important factors in achieving arthrodesis of the Charcot knee. J Bone Joint Surg 53A:1180, 1971

26. Drinker H, Potter TA, Turner RH, Thomas WH: Arthrodesis for failed knee arthroplasty. Orthop Trans 13(3):302, 1979

27. Eftekhar NS: Total knee replacement arthroplasty. J Bone Joint Surg 65A:293, 1983

28. Engelbrecht E, Siegel A, Rottger J, Buchholz HW: Statistics of total knee replacement: partial and total knee replacement, design St. Georg. Clin Orthop 120:54, 1976

29. Evanski PM, Waugh JR, Onofrio CF, Anzel SH: UCI knee replacement. Clin Orthop 120:33, 1976

30. Ewald F, Christie M, Thomas W, et al: Salvage of infected metal to metal hinge total knee replacement. Orthop Trans 9:424, 1985

31. Fahmy NRM: A technique for difficult arthrodesis of the knee. J Bone Joint Surg 66B:367, 1984

32. Falahee MH, Kaufer H, Matthews LS: Resection arthroplasty of the infected total knee arthroplasty. Presented at the American Academy of Orthopaedic Surgeons, Las Vegas, 1985

33. Fett HC, Zorn EL: Compression arthrodesis of the knee. J Bone Joint Surg 35:172, 1953

34. Fidler MW: Knee arthrodesis following prosthesis removal. Use of the Wagner apparatus. J Bone Joint Surg 65B:29, 1983

35. Fischer DA: The Hoffman external fixator: Technique of application in external fixation. p. 393. In Brooker AF, Edwards CC (eds): External Fixation: The Current State of the Art. Williams & Wilkins, Baltimore, 1979

36. Fischer DA: Skeletal stabilization with a multiplane external fixation device. Clin Orthop 180:50, 1983

37. Freeman MAR, Charnley J: Arthrodesis. p. 142. In Freeman MAR (ed): Arthritis of the Knee: Clinical Features and Surgical Management. Springer-Verlag, Berlin, 1980

38. Freeman MAR, Sudlow RA, Casewell MW, Radcliff SS: The management of infected total knee replacements. J Bone Joint Surg 67B:764, 1985

39. Frymoyer JW, Hoaglund FT: The role of arthrodesis in reconstruction of the knee. Clin Orthop 101:82, 1974

40. Goldberg VM, Hardy P: The treatment and outcome of the infected total knee arthroplasty. Orthop Trans 5:467, 1981

41. Goldberg VM, Henderson BT: The Freeman-Swanson ICLH total knee arthroplasty. J Bone Joint Surg 62A:1338, 1980

42. Green DP, Parkes JC II, Stinchfield FE: Arthrodesis of the knee: a follow-up study. J Bone Joint Surg 49A:1065, 1967

43. Griend RV: Arthrodesis of the knee with intramedullary fixation. Clin Orthop 181:146, 1983

44. Grogan TJ, Darcy F, Rollins J, Amstutz HC: Deep sepsis following total knee arthroplasty. J Bone Joint Surg 68A:226, 1986

45. Gunston FH, MacKenzie RI: Complications of polycentric knee arthroplasty. Clin Orthop 120:11, 1976

46. Hageman WF, Woods GW, Tullos HG: Arthrodesis in failed total knee replacement. J Bone Joint Surg 60A:790, 1978

47. Hankin F, Louis KW, Matthews LS: The effect of total knee arthroplasty prosthesis design on the potential for salvage arthrodesis: measurements of volumes, lengths, and trabecular bone contact areas. Clin Orthop 155:52, 1981

48. Harris CM, Frochlich J: Knee fusion with intramedullary rods for failed total knee arthroplasty. Clin Orthop 197:209, 1985

49. Hatt RN: The central bone graft in joint arthrodesis. Arch Surg 46:664, 1943

50. Henderson MS, Fortin HJ: Tuberculosis of the knee joint in the adult. J Bone Joint Surg 9:700, 1927

51. Hibbs RA: An operation for stiffening the knee joint with report of cases from the service of the New York Orthopedic Hospital. Ann Surg 53:404, 1911

52. Hibbs RA: The treatment of tuberculosis of the

joints of the lower extremities by oeprative fusion. J Bone Joint Surg 12:749, 1930

53. Hui FC, Fitzgerald RH: Hinged total knee arthroplasty. J Bone Joint Surg 62A:513, 1980

54. Hunter JA, Zorra AA, Scullion JE, et al: The geometric knee replacement in polyarthritis. J Bone Joint Surg 64B:95, 1982

55. Insall JN, Hood RW, Flawn LB, Sullivan DJ: The total condylar knee prosthesis in gonarthrosis. J Bone Joint Surg 65A:619, 1983

56. Insall J, Scott WN, Ranawat CS: The total condylar knee prosthesis. J Bone Joint Surg 61A:173, 1979

57. Insall JN, Thompson FM, Brause BD: Two-stage reimplantation for the salvage of infected total knee arthroplasty. J Bone Joint Surg 65A:1087, 1983

58. Insall J, Tria AJ, Scott WR: The total condylar knee prosthesis. Clin Orthop 145:68, 1979

59. Johnson DP, Bannister GC: The outcome of infected arthroplasty of the knee. J Bone Joint Surg 68B:289, 1986

60. Jones GB: Arthroplasty of the knee by the Walldius prosthesis. J Bone Joint Surg 50B:505, 1968

61. Jones GB: Total knee replacement — the Walldius hinge. Clin Orthop 94:50, 1973

62. Jones EC, Insall JN, Inglis AE, Ranawat CS: GUEPAR knee arthroplasty: results and late complications. Clin Orthop 140:145, 1979

63. Kaufer H, Irvine G, Matthews C: Intramedullary arthrodesis of the knee. Orthop Trans 7:547, 1983

64. Key JA: Positive pressure in arthrodesis for tuberculosis of the knee joint. South Med J 25:909, 1932

65. Key JA: Arthrodesis of the knee with a large central autogenous bone peg. South Med J 30:574, 1937

66. Knutson K, Bodelind B, Lidgren L: Stability of external fixators used for knee arthrodesis after failed knee arthroplasty. Clin Orthop 186:90, 1984

67. Knutson K, Hovelius L, Lindstrand A, Lidgren L: Arthrodesis after failed knee arthroplasty. Clin Orthop 191:202, 1984

68. Knutson K, Lindstrand A, Lidgren L: Arthrodesis for failed knee arthroplasty. J Bone Joint Surg 67B:47, 1985

69. Lortat-Jacob A, Lelong P, Benoit J, Ramadier JO: Arthrodesis of the knee after removal of infected knee prostheses. Orthop Trans 3:29, 1979

70. Lucas DB, Murray WR: Arthrodesis of the knee by double plating. J Bone Joint Surg 43A:795, 1961

71. Mallory TH, Smalley D, Danyi J: Townley anatomic total knee arthroplasty using total tibial component with cruciate release. Clin Orthop 169:197, 1982

72. Marmor L: The modular knee. Clin Orthop 120:86, 1976

73. Matthews LS, Green CA, Goldstein SA: The thermal effects of skeletal fixation-pin insertion in bone. J Bone Joint Surg 66A:1077, 1984

74. Mazet R Jr, Urist MR: Arthrodesis of the knee with intramedullary nail fixation. Clin Orthop 18:43, 1960

75. Mazzetti RF: Effect of immobilization of the knee on energy expenditure during walking. J Bone Joint Surg 42:533, 1960

76. McCoy MT, Kasman RA, Chao EYS: Comparison of mechanical performance in four types of external fixators. Clin Orthop 180:23, 1983

77. Moller H, Goldberg VM: The results and problems of the posterior stabilized total condylar prosthesis. Orthop Trans 7:420, 1983

78. Moore FH, Smillie IS: Arthrodesis of the knee joint. Clin Orthop 13:215, 1959

79. Moreland JR, Thomas RJ, Freeman MAR: ICLH replacement of the knee. Clin Orthop 145:47, 1979

80. Morris HD, Mosiman RS: Arthrodesis of the knee. A comparison of the compression method with the non-compression method. J Bone Joint Surg 33A:982, 1951

81. Nelson CL, Evarts CM: Arthroplasty and arthrodesis of the knee joint. Orthop Clin North Am 2(1):245, 1971

82. Nesse L: Arthrodesis of the knee using two plates. Acta Orthop Scand 49:636, 1978

83. Papineau LJ: L'excision-greffe avec fermeture retardée délibérée dans l'ostéomyélite chronique. Nouv Presse Med 2:2753, 1973

84. Petty W, Bryan RS, Coventry MB, Peterson LFA: Infection after total knee arthroplasty. Orthop Clin North Am 6:1005, 1975

85. Phillips HT, Mears DC: Knee fusion with external skeletal fixation after an infected hinge prosthesis. A case report. Clin Orthop 151:147, 1980

86. Phillips H, Taylor JG: The Walldius hinge arthroplasty. J Bone Joint Surg 57B:59, 1975

87. Poss R, Thornhill TS, Ewald FC, et al: Factors influencing the incidence and outcome of infection following total joint arthroplasty. Clin Orthop 182:117, 1984

88. Potter TA: Fusion of the destroyed arthritic knee. Compression arthrodesis versus intramedullary rod technique. Surg Clin North Am 49:939, 1969

89. Rand JA: Arthrodesis of the knee for the failed total knee arthroplasty. p. 277. In American Academy

of Orthopaedic Surgeons. Instructional Course Lectures. Vol. 35. CV Mosby, St. Louis, 1986

90. Rand JA, Bryan RS: Reimplantation for the salvage of an infected total knee arthroplasty. J Bone Joint Surg 65A:1081, 1983

91. Rand JA, Bryan RS: The outcome of failed knee arthrodesis following total knee arthroplasty. Clin Orthop 205:86, 1986

92. Rand JA, Bryan RS, Chao EYS: Arthrodesis of the knee for salvage of the failed total knee arthroplasty using the Ace Fischer apparatus. J Bone Joint Surg 69A:39, 1987

93. Rand JA, Bryan RS, Morrey BF, Westholm F: Management of infected total knee arthroplasty. Clin Orthop 205:75, 1986

94. Rand JA, Morrey BF, Bryan RS: Management of infected total joint arthroplasty. Orthop Clin North Am 15:491, 1984

95. Rand JA, Stauffer RN, Chao EYS: Kinematic rotating hinge total knee arthroplasty. Orthop Trans 9:424, 1985

96. Rothacker GW, Cabanela ME: External fixation for arthrodesis of the knee and ankle. Clin Orthop 180:101, 1983

97. Salenius P, Kivilaakso R: Follow-up examination of a series of arthrodeses of the knee joint. Acta Orthop Scand 39:91, 1968

98. Salvati EA, Braun BD, Chekofsky KM, Wilson PD: Reimplantation in infection: an elevan year experience. Orthop Trans 5:370, 1981

99. Salvati EA, Insall JN: The management of sepsis in total knee replacement. p. 49. In Savastano AA (ed): Total Knee Replacement. Appleton & Lange, E. Norwalk, CT, 1980

100. Shea G, Wynn J, Arden GP: A study of the results of the removal of total knee prostheses. J Bone Joint Surg 63B:287, 1981

101. Siller TN: Arthrodesis in the treatment of degenerative arthritis of the knee. p. 203. In Cruess RL, Mitchell NS (eds): Surgical Management of Degenerative Arthritis of the Lower Limb. Lea & Febiger, Philadelphia, 1975

102. Skolnick MD, Bryan RS, Peterson LFA, et al: Polycentric total knee arthroplasty. J Bone Joint Surg 58A:743, 1976

103. Skolnick MD, Coventry MB, Ilstrup DM: Geometric total knee arthroplasty. J Bone Joint Surg 58A:749, 1976

104. Stewart MB, Bland WC: Compression in arthrodesis. A comparative study of methods of fusion of the knee in ninety-three cases. J Bone Joint Surg 40A:585, 1958

105. Stinchfield FE, Bigliani LU, Neu HC, et al: Late hematogenous infections of total joint replacements. J Bone Joint Surg 62A:1345, 1980

106. Stoltz MR, Ganz R: Fracture after arthrodesis of the hip and knee. Clin Orthop 115:117, 1976

107. Stulberg SD: Arthrodesis in failed total knee replacements. Orthop Clin North Am 13:213, 1982

108. Thornhill TS, Dalziel RW, Sledge CB: Alternatives to arthrodesis for the failed total knee arthroplasty. Clin Orthop 170:131, 1982

109. Toumey JW: Knee joint tuberculosis: two hundred twenty-two patients treated by operative fusion. Surg Gynecol Obstet 68:1029, 1939

110. Vahvanen V: Arthrodesis in failed knee replacement in eight rheumatoid patients. Ann Chir Gynaecol 68:57, 1979

111. Wade PJF, Denham RA: Arthrodesis of the knee after failed knee replacement. J Bone Joint Surg 66B:362, 1984

112. Walker RH, Schruman DJ: Management of infected total knee replacements. Clin Orthop 186:81, 1984

113. Walker SJ, Sharma P, Parr N, Cavendish ME: The long-term results of the Liverpool Mark II knee prosthesis. J Bone Joint surg 68B:111, 1986

114. Walldius B: Arthroplasty of the knee using an endoprosthesis. Acta Orthop Scand 30:137, 1960

115. Wiedel JD: Arthrodesis for the failed total knee replacement. Compl Orthop p. 7, 1986

116. Wilson FC, Fajgunbaum DM, Venters GC: Results of knee replacement with the Walldius and Geometric prostheses. J Bone Joint Surg 62A:497, 1980

117. Wilson FC, Venters GC: Results of knee replacement with the Walldius prosthesis. Clin Orthop 120:39, 1976

118. Woods CW, Lioberger DR, Tullis HS: Failed total knee arthroplasty. Clin Orthop 173:184, 1983

119. Young HH: Use of a hinged vitallium prosthesis for arthroplasty of the knee. J Bone Joint Surg 45A:1627, 1963

Intramedullary Knee Arthrodesis Using a Curved Nail

120. Brodersen MP, Fitzgerald RH Jr, Peterson LFA, et al: Arthrodesis of the knee following failed total knee arthroplasty. J Bone Joint Surg 61A:181, 1979

121. Falahee MH, Matthews LS, Kaufer H: Resection arthroplasty as a salvage procedure for a knee with

infection after a total arthroplasty. J Bone Joint Surg 69A:1013, 1987

122. Hagemann WF, Woods GW, Tullos HS: Arthrodesis in failed total knee replacement. J Bone Joint Surg 60A:790, 1978

123. Nelson CL, Evarts CM: Arthroplasty and arthrodesis of the knee joint. Orthop Clin North Am 2:245, 1971

124. Salvati EA, Insall JN: The management of sepsis in total knee replacement. p. 55. In Savastano AA (ed): Total Knee Replacement. Appleton & Lange, E. Norwalk, CT, 1980

125. Stewart MJ, Bland WG: Compression in arthrodesis: A comparative study of methods of fusion of the knee in ninety-three cases. J Bone Joint Surg 40A:585, 1958

Biologic Resurfacing of the Knee

124

Peter J. Brooks
David J. Zukor
Allan E. Gross

It has long been a goal of the medical profession to replace injured or diseased organs and parts with healthy ones. History, literature, and art have recorded such efforts for at least 2,000 years. It has only been during the past few decades, however, that tissue and organ transplantation has become a reality.

Interest in bone and joint transplantation has developed gradually as a result of various events. The first heterotopic bone autograft was performed by Merrem in 1809 to replace a portion of a dog's skull.[10] Macewen in 1881[16] and Lexer in 1908[14] described a series of human bone and joint transplants and in 1925 Lexer[15] reported successful results in 50 percent. Over the next 30 years, relatively little regarding bone transplantation was published, until Herndon and Chase[8] reported on their experiments in 1952.

The 1960s saw rapid growth in the fields of immunology and transplantation. Developments in bone and cartilage allografts were stimulated by successes with kidney transplants. Large clinical series were reported by Ottolenghi,[19] Volkov and Imamaliev,[27,28] and Parrish[20] during the 1970s. The availability of tissue increased as the public became more aware of the benefits of organ donation and transplantation. The American Association of Tissue Banks was established to set standards for tissue procurement and storage.

The clinical need for osteochondral allografts has grown as chemotherapy and a better understanding of malignant bone tumors led to an increase in limb-sparing resections. Mankin's review of his experience with bone allografts brought this concept to new prominence.[17]

At the same time, allograft availability improved with the emergence of several large bone banks. Research into allograft biology and healing was being carried out at several centers.[1,5,7,12,23]

Another factor in the emergence of allografts in orthopaedic surgery has been the increasing number of failed total joint replacements. The accompanying loss of bone stock may be the indication for most allografts performed in the coming decade.

The bone and cartilage transplantation program at our institution has four major arms. Frozen large-fragment grafts are used for skeletal reconstruction following tumor excision. Frozen femoral heads, and segments of hemipelvis, femur, and tibia are used during revision arthroplasty procedures. Allografts are made available to orthopaedic surgeons in other communities for a variety of indications. Finally, fresh small-fragment allografts are used to resurface damaged joints.

This chapter deals with fresh small-fragment osteochondral allografts performed for resurfacing of the damaged knee. The aspects of patient selection, biology, immunology, and biomechanics are discussed and in many ways are applicable to allografts performed elsewhere in the skeleton and for other indications.

PATIENT SELECTION AND SURGICAL INDICATIONS

When fresh osteochondral allografts were first performed in Toronto in 1972, the indications were not well defined. As a result, the procedure was performed for a variety of conditions, including trauma, osteoarthritis, osteochondritis dissecans, and osteonecrosis.

Following a review of our first 100 cases,[18] in which the best results were found in the posttraumatic group, the procedure has been performed mainly in cases of traumatic bone and cartilage loss. Osteochondritis dissecans remains a relative indication, particularly for large weight-bearing lesions. Osteoarthritis and osteonecrosis are at best relative indications for fresh small-fragment allografts. Encouraged by the high percentage of successful results in young posttraumatic cases, we have continued to perform about 20 fresh small-fragment allografts each year for this indication. This is a group of high-demand patients for whom no conventional prosthetic resurfacing procedure is advisable.

Malalignment of the extremity is often present as a result of the depressed plateau or condyle. It is important not to insert the allograft into a compartment that is under compression because of deformity. The indications, timing, and techniques of corrective osteotomy are discussed below.

Range of motion is typically limited in these patients, but is usually improved postoperatively by the combination of restored joint congruity and the opportunity to carry out debridement. Limitation of knee motion may be considered a relative indication, rather than a contraindication, to this procedure.

Our early experience also indicated that results were best when only one side of one compartment was replaced. Thus, it is advisable to perform such surgery before the onset of degenerative changes in the opposing articular surface. Therefore, the potential for development of degenerative arthritis should be recognized, and resurfacing should be undertaken prior to destruction of the entire compartment.

Finally, these procedures do not sacrifice bone stock, but rather restore it. Thus, any future surgery that may become necessary will not have been compromised but in fact will probably be made less complicated by the previous allograft and restoration of bone stock.

DONOR SELECTION

All fresh osteochondral allografts are taken from donors who have already meet the criteria set forth by the American Association of Tissue Banks.* In Toronto, the Multiple Organ Retrieval and Exchange Program has been instrumental in coordinating the activities of all the appropriate parties. No donor may have evidence of bacterial infection, slow virus disease, malignancy (with the possible exception of primary nonmetastasizing central

---

*American Association of Tissue Banks, 12111 Parklawn Drive, Rockville, MD 20852.

nervous system tumors), arthritis, connective tissue or metabolic bone disease, toxic drug ingestion, parenteral drug abuse, or death from unknown causes. Jaundice, hepatitis, or syphilis also rule out organ donation. Acquired immune deficiency syndrome (AIDS) or evidence of previous exposure also makes donation impossible. Major blunt or penetrating trauma, compound fractures, or gross soft tissue injury predispose to contamination.

Laboratory tests for hepatitis, syphilis, human immunodeficiency virus (HIV) antibodies, and three sets of blood cultures are drawn. Prolonged intubation, tracheostomy, indwelling Foley catheters, or hemodynamic monitoring lines in place for more than 48 hours pose a risk of bacteremia, which may be masked by antibiotics. For the purpose of fresh osteochondral allografts, the ideal donor is an adult under 30 years old who meets the criteria outlined above.

GRAFT PROCUREMENT

All tissue for transplantation is obtained under sterile operating room conditions. The skin is prepared and the extremity draped as for a surgical procedure. Sterile precautions are observed throughout. Ventilatory and hemodynamic support is unnecessary and is discontinued after other organs are harvested.

Longitudinal incisions are made. Areas of soft tissue injury or venipuncture are avoided. The bones are exposed subperiosteally, and as much soft tissue as possible is removed while the bone is still in the cadaver. Short lengths of tendon or ligament are left intact where these will aid in the reconstruction.

Bones may be disarticulated at either end and removed intact. For the purposes of knee allografts the joint and capsule are removed intact. The femoral and tibial diaphyses are sectioned with an oscillating saw above and below the joint. The quadriceps tendon is divided, entering the suprapatellar pouch. Muscles are removed, but the ligaments,

capsule, and tendon stumps remain. Cultures are obtained by swabs of the joint and medullary canal. Small specimens of medullary cancellous bone are also sent for culture.

The knee is placed in a large metal cannister containing 1 L of lactated Ringer's solution, cefazolin (1 g), and bacitracin (50,000 units). The container is closed, sealed with adhesive plastic, and placed in a sterile plastic bag. It is refrigerated for use as a fresh allograft at 4°C for up to 24 hours, but usually less than 12 hours.

Stored or cryopreserved cartilage has not been used for small-fragment grafts in our series. We believe that cartilage viability is better when the allograft has not been frozen. However, the decision to harvest fresh osteochondral segments for rapid transplantation has resulted in difficult logistic problems requiring coordination and planning.

By using fresh osteochondral allografts harvested within 12 hours of the death of the donor and implanted within 12 hours of the harvest, we are transplanting viable cartilage. This has been confirmed by routine histology and electron microscopy in our long-term follow-up studies,[6,9] and more recently by autoradiography.

Those segments of bone and joint that are not to be used as fresh allografts are cultured and wrapped in three plastic bags, followed by a surgical towel. This is labeled with the donor identification number and a description of the graft within. No cryopreservatives are employed. The allografts are then placed in a freezer and stored at −70°C to be used for the other aspects of our transplant program. Appropriate records are maintained for incoming and outgoing allografts.

Patients who are candidates for fresh osteochondral resurfacing procedures are told that they will be notified when a suitable allograft becomes available. We generally have a waiting list of fewer than 10 patients. Once patients are notified, they must immediately make arrangements for hospital admission. We have been able to perform fresh transplantation on patients from any part of the continent within 12 to 24 hours of graft procurement. Patients who are not readily available by telephone have rented electronic paging devices for this purpose. No attempt is made to match the donor and recipient immunologically.

SURGICAL TECHNIQUE

The usual fresh osteochondral allograft is unipolar and unicompartmental (e.g., a lateral tibial plateau, or a medial femoral condyle). Bipolar allografts have been associated with less favorable results.

Preoperative evaluation includes routine radiographic views of the knee as well as a full-length standing orthoradiograph to assess alignment. Tomograms may also be helpful. The size, shape, and location of the allograft can be judged preoperatively.

If realignment is necessary, the decision as to where to perform the correction is made, taking into account the predominant location of the deformity and the slope of the joint line on the standing roentgenogram.

When realignment is required through the same bone that requires the allograft, the osteotomy is carried out several months in advance. This ensures

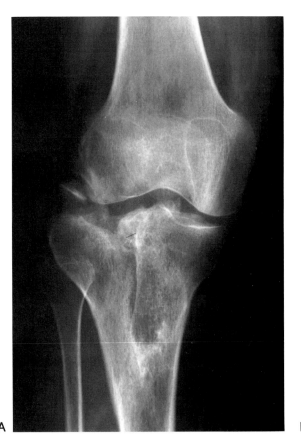
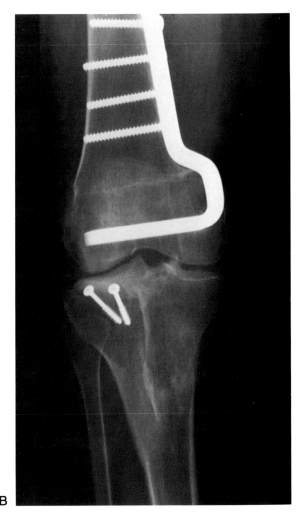

A   B

Fig. 124-1. (A) A 32-year-old woman with malunion of a tibial plateau fracture, 21 months after open reduction and internal fixation. **(B)** Same patient as Figure A 2 years after fresh lateral tibial plateau allograft, with simultaneous distal femoral varus osteotomy.

a well-vascularized bed for the allograft. For example, a proximal tibial osteotomy would not be carried out at the same time as a tibial plateau allograft.

If realignment is to be carried out through the bone opposite that of the allograft, both procedures are carried out at once. For instance, a distal femoral varus osteotomy may be performed at the same time as a lateral tibial plateau allograft in a patient with late posttraumatic depression of the lateral tibial plateau and a valgus knee (Fig. 124-1). Likewise, a proximal tibial valgus osteotomy may

be performed simultaneously with a medial femoral condyle allograft (Fig. 124-2).

Our goal is to realign the knee so that the transplanted cartilage is not subject to excessive loading as a result of an abnormal biomechanical axis. Realignment is carried out by osteotomy and not by relying on the height of the allograft. In general we aim for 0 degrees femoral tibial axis following varus osteotomy and for 10 degrees valgus following valgus osteotomy. This results in the biomechanical axis passing through the nonallografted compartment.

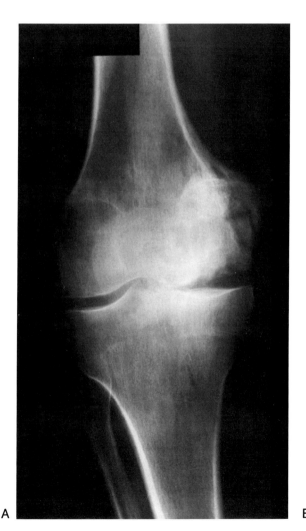
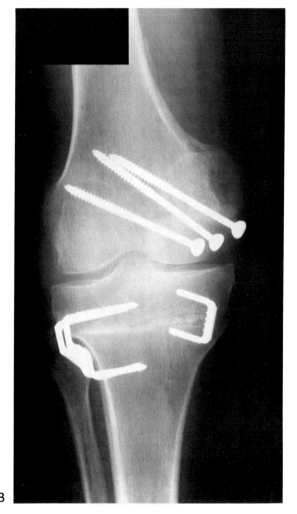

A   B

Fig. 124-2. (A) A 21-year-old man 15 months after a motorcycle accident with fracture of the medial femoral condyle. Open reduction and internal fixation had been performed. **(B)** Same patient as Figure A 18 months after fresh medial femoral condyle allograft, with simultaneous valgus proximal tibial osteotomy.

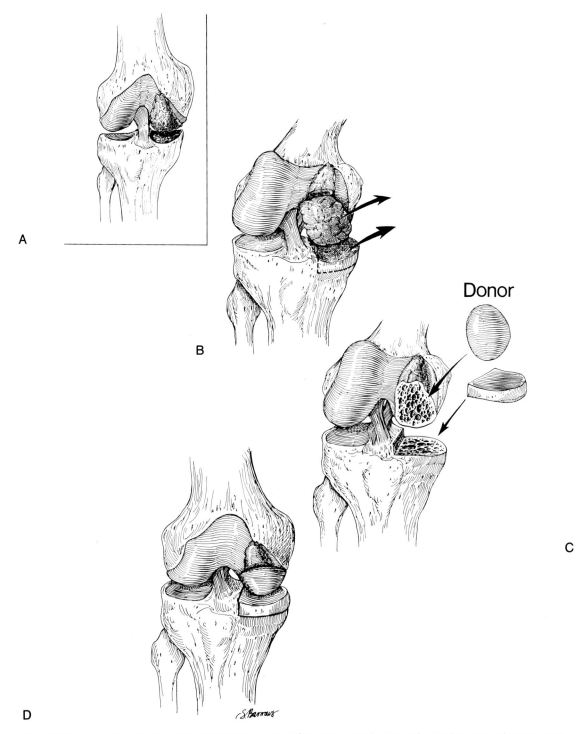

Fig. 124-3. Technique for combined tibial plateau and femoral condyle allograft. **(A)** Diagram of degenerative arthritis femoral condyle and tibial plateau. **(B)** Outline for segment of tibial plateau to be excised. Diseased portion of femoral condyle has been excised. **(C)** Prepared areas of condyle and plateau to be replaced with prepared grafts. **(D)** Allografts in place. Screw fixation not shown.

Whenever possible, surgery is performed using a straight midline incision. Both allograft and osteotomy can be performed through a single incision. The involved compartment is examined and debrided. Meniscal tears are trimmed. The damaged condyle or plateau is resected down to healthy cancellous bone and the defect is squared off to allow for proper fit of the graft. Sclerotic bone that remains may be drilled to enhance healing.

The appropriate thickness of graft fits snugly into the defect but is not under excessive pressure. For adequate strength, it should be at least 1 cm thick. Soft tissue releases may be necessary for long-standing deformity, but the graft itself does not achieve the correction of malalignment. A stable interference fit is achieved and is supplemented by cancellous screws.

When the meniscus is absent or extensively damaged, a meniscal allograft is performed. In the case of a tibial plateau, the donor meniscus simply remains attached to the allograft. In femoral condyle allografts, a free meniscal transplant is required.

The technique for combined tibial plateau/femoral condyle allograft is illustrated in Figure 124-3, but this is now rarely performed.

POSTOPERATIVE CARE

All patients are placed on continuous passive motion (CPM) in the recovery room. This is thought to benefit chondrocyte nutrition and aid in early rehabilitation. We have modified a standard CPM machine to permit adjustment for varus or valgus, allowing correction to be maintained and preventing excessive loading of the graft. Quadriceps-setting and isometric exercises are begun immediately.

Ambulation is encouraged from the first postoperative day. Patients are initially fitted with a polypropylene splint molded into varus or valgus as the situation demands. No weight bearing is permitted until a custom-made ischial weight-bearing caliper is obtained, usually at 3 to 4 weeks. Patients are discharged when independently ambulatory, and outpatient physiotherapy is arranged. The patient is allowed to ambulate without aids after becoming accustomed to the long-leg brace, which is worn for 1 year.

Union of the allograft is usually complete by 3 months, and creeping substitution is well under way by 1 year. Complete remodeling occurs over 2 to 3 years or even more.[18]

IMMUNOLOGY OF OSTEOCHONDRAL ALLOGRAFTS

Fresh osteochondral allografts are immunogenic.[13] The various sources of immunogenicity include all the organic constituents of the tissue. No evidence exists to implicate hydroxyapatite or other inorganic minerals in an immune response.

The major source of antigenicity is the marrow cell population. Here, cell-surface elements of the blood group and major histocompatibility system induce immune responses. These cells, together with passenger leukocytes, are inevitably transplanted with the allograft and cannot be removed by mechanical or other means.[4]

Other sources of immunogenicity are the articular cartilage proteoglycans[3,21] and possibly collagen[26] as well as the surface antigens of fibrous, endothelial, adipose, and neural tissue present in the allograft.

Our technique involves the transplantation of fresh bone and cartilage, both of which are immunogenic. Frozen allografts evoke a less intense response, while freeze-dried allografts show a marked reduction in immunogenicity.[4] Both techniques, however, result in decreased chondrocyte survival compared with fresh allografts. Cryopreservatives, such as glycerol or dimethylsulfoxide (DMSO), are thought to improve chondrocyte viability, but, in our opinion, not to the level expected with fresh transplantation.[24,25]

While experimental studies continue to elucidate the intensity and characteristics of the immune response to osteochondral allografts, there is considerable debate as to its biological significance.[1,2,22]

Against the background of this debate is the apparent lack of clinical significance of the observed immune responses. No investigators have correlated an immune response with adverse clinical effects. Generally satisfactory results are the rule, and failures appear to be related more to mechanical factors, infections, or technical complications.

This is in striking contrast to the observed effects of graft rejection in other organ systems. The explanation for this apparent inconsistency is related to the basic biology of bone healing.

Bone is one of the very few tissues in the body that, when injured, restores itself to its preinjury morphology. Bone heals with bone. Most other tissues heal by modulation or migration of fibroblasts, in turn producing a scar bearing little or no histologic resemblance to the parent tissue.

In the case of allotransplantation of heart, kidney, skin, or other organs, healing and rejection are opposites and are mutually exclusive. The sequence of vascular cuffing, thrombosis, necrosis, infiltration of immunocompetent cells, and phagocytosis is followed by fibroblast proliferation and ultimately scar formation.

Bone allografts similarly undergo vascular invasion and destruction by cutting cones of vascular buds and osteoclasts. The allograft acts as a scaffold for the advancing margin of osteoblastic activity as new bone is laid down on dead trabeculae. Eventually, the entire allograft may be replaced by host bone, over a period of months or years. In effect, the process of healing of bone allograft is difficult to distinguish from rejection. The biologic processes that occur following autografts and allografts of bone differ in rate and intensity but are fundamentally the same. In our series of fresh osteochondral allografts, no attempt was made to match blood type or histocompatibility antigens. No adverse effects of the resulting immune response could be identified.

Articular cartilage accompanying the allograft is also composed of many potentially immunogenic components. However, in spite of the presence of significant quantities of proteoglycans, collagen, and chondrocytes, the cartilage is immunologically privileged, and the immunologic load is small. The vast majority of cells are immunologically isolated. Both afferent and efferent arms of the immunologic response are thwarted by the dense matrix and by the absence of blood vessels or lymphatics.

Our own experimental work demonstrated that exposed chondrocytes were immunogenic but, if protected by a healthy matrix, were isolated from the host immunocompetent system.[12] We also showed that fresh bone was immunogenic, but so was frozen bone, although less so.[11] We concluded that the marginally decreased immunogenicity gained by freezing was outweighed by the death of the chondrocytes and opted to use fresh grafts.

Thus, in spite of experimental and clinical studies clearly showing that an immune response follows osteochondral allografting, the biology is such that adverse effects do not seem to occur. In our series, mechanical factors appeared to far outweigh any possible immune factors.

CLINICAL RESULTS

Fresh osteochondral allografts for biologic resurfacing of the knee have been performed at our institution since 1972. Initially, the indications were broad and included osteoarthritis, osteonecrosis (steroid-induced or spontaneous), osteochondritis dissecans, and posttraumatic joint surface defects.

The first 100 patients were reviewed in 1985.[18] Results were best (75 percent successful) in young patients with posttraumatic defects. Less encouraging results occurred in osteoarthritis (42 percent), osteonecrosis (27 percent), and osteochondritis dissecans (25 percent) (Fig. 124-4). The latter group was thought to reflect patient noncompliance to some extent.

Following this review, the emphasis has been on resurfacing for posttraumatic defects. We recently reviewed the 85 fresh osteochondral allografts for traumatic defects performed between 1972 and 1985.[29] Fifty-five of these were resurfacing procedures of the knee, with more than 1 year follow-up (average follow up 4.3 years).

Thirty-three involved a tibial plateau — five medial and 28 lateral. Seventeen were femoral condyle allografts, eight medial, and nine lateral. Four were bipolar unicompartmental (both femoral condyle and matching tibial plateau) (Fig. 3). One was a patellar resurfacing.

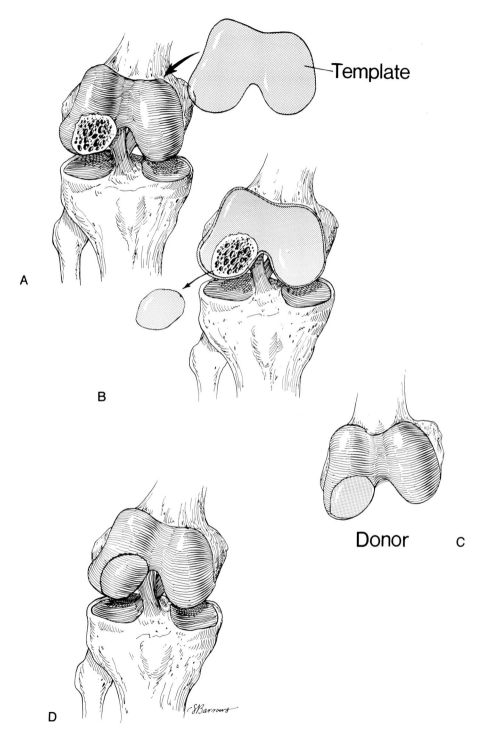

Fig. 124-4. Technique for allograft for osteochondritis dissecans. **(A)** Defect after debridement: template for condyles. **(B)** Template in position; pattern of the defect has been cut. **(C)** Pattern placed over donor condyle. **(D)** Donor graft press-fitted into position. Screw fixation not shown.

Twenty realignment osteotomies were carried out in 19 patients. Ten of these were distal femoral varus osteotomies, two were distal femoral valgus osteotomies. High tibial osteotomies were performed in eight patients, valgus in seven, and varus in one. Nine of the 20 osteotomies were carried out prior to, or simultaneous with, the resurfacing procedure. Recently, this practice has increased in frequency.

Menisci were transplanted along with the tibial plateau in 26 patients. In two other patients, free meniscal allografts were performed at the time of femoral condyle transplantation.

Patients were rated by a modified Hospital for Special Surgery (HSS) scoring system.[18] Results were judged successful if the final rating was 75 points or more or if the final score was at least 10 points higher than preoperatively. Failures were those with any decrease in the rating score or those requiring salvage surgery.

Overall, 42 of the 55 knee-resurfacing procedures (76 percent) were successful. These had an average preoperative score of 66.5 (range 31 to 93) and an average postoperative score of 91 (range 68 to 100). All 17 femoral condyle replacements were successful, as were four of the five medial plateau allografts, 21 out of 28 lateral plateau replacements, and the single patellar allograft. All four bipolar grafts failed. Postoperative radiographic assessment demonstrated that virtually all grafts settled by 1 to 3 mm. Most did not collapse further. Fifteen grafts showed total loss of height of 4 to 5 mm, and two resorbed completely.

Assessment of alignment by full-length standing radiographs revealed three failures in 16 well-aligned patients. Two of the three failures had achieved correction by virtue of the allograft height. Six failures occurred in the 26 patients whose alignment was suboptimal. Optimal alignment was that in which the biomechanical axis (center of femoral head to center of ankle) passed through the nonallografted compartment.

Those patients who had realignment osteotomies tended to do well (79 percent successful). Our tendency now is toward more liberal use of osteotomy to unload the allograft.

The complication rate was 11 percent. There were no overt failures of fixation or fit. There were no infections, documented deep venous throm-boses, or pulmonary emboli. Three patients required knee manipulations for stiffness prior to our routine use of CPM. Included were one wound hematoma, one intraoperative patellar tendon rupture, and three postoperative pulmonary complications. Four patients required revision surgery. These included three total knee arthroplasties and one arthrodesis.

CONCLUSIONS

Fresh osteochondral allografts for biologic resurfacing of the knee continues to be an important part of our surgical armamentarium. Patient selection, graft procurement, and surgical technique must be careful and exacting.

The ideal patient for this procedure is one with a posttraumatic defect of a femoral condyle or tibial plateau. Bipolar grafts should be avoided. The procedure is ideally suited to the young high-demand patient precisely because it is for these patients that no prosthetic option is advisable. The operation should be avoided in cases in which significant degenerative arthritis has supervened, and in older or low-demand patients for whom prosthetic arthroplasty is preferred.

Malalignment should be corrected by osteotomy prior to, or simultaneous with, the allograft procedure. Osteotomy may only be carried out simultaneously if it may be performed on the opposite side of the knee as the allograft (e.g., distal femoral varus osteotomy with lateral tibial plateau allograft). The graft itself should not be used to correct alignment.

Allografts should be obtained fresh from skeletally mature donors under the age of 30 and transplanted within 12 to 24 hours. We do not use frozen or cryopreserved grafts for this procedure. We believe that the cartilage is immunoprivileged, and the immune response to the transplanted bone has not proved deleterious. Rather, the potential for chondrocyte viability outweighs any immunologic or logistic advantage to the use of frozen or freeze-dried allografts. Patients must be prepared for admission for surgery with only a few hours notice.

Mechanical factors appear to have the greatest bearing on clinical outcome. Grafts should be well matched for size and shape. There should be a stable press fit prior to supplemental screw fixation. Bone thickness of the allograft should not be less than one centimeter to prevent stress fracture. Alignment should be judged on full-length standing roentgenograms, and the final mechanical axis should not pass through the allograft, but should rather be shifted to the intact compartment, by osteotomy if necessary. If there is any doubt, it is better to perform the osteotomy than to risk excessive forces on the allograft. Meniscal allografts should be included whenever a tibial plateau allograft is performed and the host meniscus is significantly damaged or absent.

REFERENCES

1. Burchardt H, Glewczewskie FP, Enneking WF: Allogeneic segmental fibular transplant in azathioprine-immunosuppressed dogs. J Bone Joint Surg 59A:881, 1977
2. Esses SI, Halloran P, Langer F, et al: The effect of the immune response on healing of bone allografts. Trans Orthop Res Soc 5:246, 1981
3. Friedlaender GE, Ladenbauer-Belles I, Chrisman OD: Cartilage matrix components as antigenic agents in an osteoarthritic model. Trans Orthop Res Soc 5:170, 1980
4. Friedlaender GE, Mankin HJ, Langer F: Immunology of osteochondral allografts: background and general considerations. p. 133. In Friedlander GE, Mankin HJ, Sell KW (eds): Osteochondral Allografts: Biology, Banking and Clinical Applications. Little, Brown, Boston, 1983
5. Glimcher MJ, Kato F, Ninomiya S, et al: The biology of bone healing and the repair of autograft, allograft and xenograft metatarsal-phalangeal joint transplants in rabbits. p. 2. In Friedlaender GE, Mankin HJ, Sell KW (eds): Osteochondral Allografts: Biology, Banking and Clinical Applications. Little, Brown, Boston, 1983
6. Gross AE, Kandel RA, Ganel A, et al: Analysis of the histopathology of failed fresh osteochondral allografts. Presented at the fifty-first Annual Meeting of the American Academy of Orthopaedic Surgeons, Atlanta, Georgia, February 1984
7. Heiple KG, Chase SW, Herndon CH: A comparative study of the healing process following different types of bone transplantation. J Bone Joint Surg 45A:1593, 1963
8. Herndon CH, Chase SW: Experimental Studies in the transplantation of whole joints. J Bone Joint Surg 34A:564, 1952
9. Kandel RA, Gross AE, Ganel A, et al: Histopathology of failed osteoarticular shell allografts. Clin Orthop 197:103, 1985
10. Kountz SL: Autotransplantation. p. 564. In Sabiston DC (ed): Textbook of Surgery. 11th Ed. WB Saunders, Philadelphia, 1977
11. Langer F, Czitrom A, Pritzker KP, Gross AE: The Immunogenicity of fresh and frozen allogenic bone. J Bone Joint Surg 57A:216, 1975
12. Langer F, Gross AE: Immunogenicity of allograft articular cartilage. J Bone Joint Surg 56A:297, 1974
13. Langer F, Gross AE, West M, Urovitz EP: The immunogenicity of allograft knee joint transplants. Clin Orthop 132:157, 1978
14. Lexer E: Die Verwendung der freien Knochenplastik nebst versuchen uber Gelenkversteifung und Gelenktransplantatum. Arch Klin Chir 86:939, 1908
15. Lexer E: Joint transplantation and arthroplasty. Surg Gynecol Obstet 40:782, 1925
16. Macewen W: Observations concerning transplantation of bone: illustrated by a case of interhuman osseous transplantation, whereby over two-thirds of the shaft of a humerus was restored. Proc R Soc Lond 32:232, 1881
17. Mankin HJ, Doppelt SH, Sullivan TR, Tomford WW: Osteoarticular and intercalary allograft transplantation in the management of malignant tumors of bone. Cancer 50:613, 1982
18. McDermott AGP, Langer F, Pritzker KPH, Gross AE: Fresh small-fragment osteochondral allografts. Long-term follow-up study on the first 100 cases. Clin Orthop 197:96, 1985
19. Ottolenghi CE: Massive osteo and osteoarticular bone grafts: technique and results of 62 cases. Clin Orthop 87:156, 1972
20. Parrish FF: Allograft replacement of all or part of the end of a long bone following excision of a tumor: report of 21 cases. J Bone Joint Surg 55A:1, 1972
21. Poole AR, Reiner A, Choi H: Immunological studies of proteoglycan subunit from bovine and human cartilages. Trans Orthop Res Soc 4:162, 1979
22. Schachar NS et al: A feline model for the study of frozen osteoarticular allograft. I. Quantitative assessment of cartilage viability and bone healing. Trans Orthop Res Soc 3:130, 1978

23. Schachar NS, Henry WB, Wadsworth, P et al: Fate of massive osteochondral allograft in a feline model. p. 81. In Friedlaender GE, Mankin HJ, Sell KW (eds): Osteochondral Allografts: Biology, Banking and Clincial Application. Little, Brown, Boston, 1983

24. Tomford WW, Fredericks GR, Mankin HJ: Cryopreservation of isolated chondrocytes. Trans Orthop Res Soc 6:100, 1981

25. Tomford WW, Fredericks GR, Mankin HJ: Cryopreservation of intact articular cartilage. Trans Orthop Res Soc 7:276, 1982

26. Trentham DE, Townes AS, Kang AH: Humeral and cellular sensitivity to collagen in type II collagen-induced arthritis in rats. J Clin Invest 61:89, 1978

27. Volkov M: Allotransplantation of joints. J Bone Joint Surg 52B:49, 1970

28. Volkov MV, Imamaliev AS: Use of allogenous articular bone implants as substitutes for autotransplants in adult patients. Clin Orthop 114:192, 1976

29. Zukor DJ, Paitich B, Oakeshott RD, et al: Reconstruction of post-traumatic articular surface defects using fresh, small-fragment osteochondral allografts. Presented at the Eighth Combined Meeting of the Orthopaedic Association of the English Speaking World, Washington, DC, May 1987

Section 8

THE TIBIA AND ANKLE

Robert E. Leach

Section Editor

Introduction

Robert E. Leach

This section on the tibia and ankle deals with many of the problems that an orthopaedic surgeon commonly encounters. The majority of the operations described are performed for conditions resulting from trauma to the leg.

Operative procedures are presented in detail in this section, as we recognize that a major portion of an orthopaedic surgeon's practice will involve the lower leg. Although the authors have each presented their procedure of choice in their chapter, we realize that each author retains a bias for a particular procedure that reflects his own teaching and experience. The reader must study each procedure and temper this input with his or her own teaching and experience when choosing that procedure best suited for an individual patient and a particular condition.

No topic in this section is more important than the treatment of tibial fractures. Dr. Michael Chapman, a well-known authority in the field of lower extremity trauma, presents a number of options for the handling of simple and complex tibial fractures. It is important for the reader to understand the principles that underlie the treatment methods and not simply adopt a cookbook approach. The treatment modes described by Dr. Chapman are well accepted. His use of internal fixation for severe tibial fractures complicated by extensive soft tissue injury follows basic precepts and has enabled him to deal effectively with many badly traumatized limbs. The section on malunion and nonunion of tibial fractures is authored by Drs. Sigvard Hansen, Allan Bach, and Steven Benirschke. They present up-to-date methods of handling infected and noninfected nonunions of the tibia and show how to correct a malunion. They have also given us some interesting information concerning the use of the Ilizarov apparatus and its possible use in complex problems of the lower extremity.

Drs. David Segal and Isadore Yablon believe that the best results in displaced ankle fractures result from open reduction and rigid internal fixation plus early weight bearing. Their experience at the University and Boston City hospitals provides the background for this work, and the long-term results of this treatment program appear to justify their basic treatment concepts. Other ankle operations, including arthrotomy and arthrodesis, are well presented by Dr. Richard Stauffer of the Mayo Clinic. Based upon his experience and that of other members of the Clinic, he believes that total ankle replacements are much less successful than total knee or total hip replacements, and that it is an operation rarely indicated.

Drs. Robert Leach and Anthony Schepsis briefly describe several conservative treatment methods for patients with ankle sprains and make a case for open surgical repair in specific patients with acute ankle injuries. Secondary reconstruction of the lateral ankle ligaments is a well-accepted procedure, and several of the established methods are detailed. A short section is included on compartment syndromes of the lower extremity in an attempt to delineate the anterior and posterior compartment syndromes and the deep medial tibial syndrome, ofttimes known to athletes as "shin splints."

The most difficult chapter in this section deals with soft tissue surgery and tendon repairs of the lower leg. Drs. John Elstrom and Arsen Pankovich have completely rewritten this chapter, and they describe the surgical treatment of an acute Achilles tendon rupture and present several methods of repair. They detail many of the soft tissue procedures for a variety of conditions that involve the lower leg. Other procedures involving the lower leg, and not covered here, may be described in chapters in Section 9.

Fractures of the Tibial and Fibular Shafts

125

Michael W. Chapman

The tibia and fibula occupy a unique place in orthopaedic trauma surgery, since they are two of the most frequently fractured long bones. In this age of vehicular accidents, the tibia and fibula are frequently subjected to high-energy trauma. The tibia has poor soft tissue coverage and a poor blood supply. Because of this, severe injury, particularly if combined with inadequate or inappropriate treatment, can lead to severe complications and major disability.

Fracture treatment and patient expectations have changed considerably since the era before World War II. As is evidenced in Speed's textbook on fractures and dislocations, published in 1942,[196] and in Wilson's *Management of Fractures and Dislocations*, published in 1938,[223] a nonunion rate of up to 20 percent, a 4 percent incidence of amputations, and even deaths from isolated fractures of the tibia and fibula were described. The prognosis in open fractures was even worse with up to a 10 percent incidence of chronic infection, a 15 percent incidence of nonunion, and 5 percent incidence of amputations.

Excellent results have been reported using nonsurgical and surgical methods. In spite of this, considerable controversy exists about the role of early internal fixation of tibial fractures, as reflected by the voluminous literature on these fractures. This chapter contains 225 references that represent a review of the English literature alone; a totally comprehensive review is not presented.

Recent authors, whether advocating surgical or nonsurgical treatment, emphasize the need for early restoration of function to prevent muscle atrophy and loss of joint motion and to avoid the osteoporosis and dystrophy of prolonged disuse.

Closed treatment has been advocated by many investigators.[7, 8, 16, 21, 27, 28, 33-35, 37, 45, 50-54, 56, 64, 87, 99, 100, 103, 105, 116, 121, 122, 133, 152, 161, 162, 177-180, 186, 216-219]

Sarmiento,[180] reporting on a 10-year experience with 482 tibial fractures using closed reduction and functional bracing, had only two nonunions, a union rate of 99 percent with no infections in closed fractures. The average healing time was 14.5 weeks. The average shortening was 6.4 mm with 88 percent having shortening less than 4.1 mm. Because unacceptable shortening tended to occur in open fractures and in those with severe displacement, he advocated pins in plaster for no longer than 3 weeks in this group. Ninety-one percent of the patients had less than 5 degrees of angulatory deformity. Although joint range of motion was not consistently recorded, he believed that permanent limitation of motion had not been encountered. Nicoll[161,162] reported union without deformity and good functional results in 97 percent of 674 cases treated conservatively. Nicoll stated that it is difficult to imagine that these results could be improved by routine internal fixation. He emphasized that the "personality" of the fracture must be taken into account. He gave five special indications for primary internal fixation: (1) open fractures with a skin problem requiring complicated plastic surgery, (2) associated fracture of the femur or other associated major injury, (3) paraplegia with sensory loss, (4) displaced segmental fractures, and (5) fractures with a gap of greater than 1 cm due to bone loss.

Müller[155,156] and his associates[151,157,158,175] are the strongest advocates of primary internal fixation of tibial fractures using open reduction and interfragmentary lag screw and compression plate fixation.

Ruedi et al.,[175] in a study of 334 closed and 101 open fractures treated with dynamic compression plates, reported good to very good functional results in 98 percent of the closed cases. The closed fractures had a 6 percent rate of complications, including three cases of osteomyelitis, three fixation failures, 10 delayed unions, three nonunions, and one refracture. In the open fractures 88 percent achieved a good to very good functional end result. A 32 percent incidence of complications included a 12 percent infection rate and 7 percent incidence of nonunion. These results are comparable to those of Sarmiento[180,181] and Nicoll,[161,162] although it is not really possible to compare the functional end results; their excellence is the justification used by Rüedi and Müller for internal fixation. Many other investigators[5,6,9,14,18,19,30,39-42,61, 68,69,74,77,80,81,88,89,95,96,102,109,110,117,119,124,127-132,134, 138,140-142,144,145,147,154,165,166,167,171,173,182,183,184,187- 192,198,201,203,205,208,211,212,214,220,222,224,225] also discuss internal fixation of tibial fractures. None of the previous investigators reports results as good as those of Rüedi et al. Burwell,[30] in 181 fractures of the tibia fixed with Burns or Venable plates, had an infection rate of 6.6 percent, a nonunion rate of 4.4 percent, and associated loss of joint motion in 22

percent. Olerud and Karlström,[165] using AO plates in 135 tibial fractures, experienced complications in 19 percent but rated 90 percent as having a good functional end result. In a review of 470 tibial shaft fractures, Smith[192] concluded that delayed internal fixation produced fewer complications. Of 180 closed fractures treated with early internal fixation, infection occurred in 6.6 percent and delayed union in 30 percent. In 78 cases treated 1 to 3 weeks after injury the infection rate was essentially unchanged at 6.4 percent, however, the delayed union rate fell to 16.6 percent.

Intramedullary nailing, particularly when done using closed technique, has fewer complications than plate fixation. Lottes,[131] using his triflanged nail in 837 fractures, reported infections in only 0.9 percent of 330 closed fractures and 7.3 percent of 204 open fractures, with an overall nonunion rate of 2.3 percent.

Similar favorable results have been reported by d'Aubigne et al.,[13] Bayne et al.,[17] Böhler,[20] Sedlin et al,[184] Solheim et al.,[190,191] Velazco et al.,[211] and Zucmann and Maurer.[225]

Sisk,[64] reporting on the recent experience of the Campbell Clinic as compared with that previously reported by Boyd et al.,[22-26] noted a decrease in the rate of nonunion of the tibia. He attributed this in part to the fact that almost all tibial shaft fractures at the Campbell Clinic are now treated with closed methods.

Comparing the efficacy of operative and nonoperative methods is difficult since most series do not take into account the "personality" of the fracture, as described by Nicoll.[162] Nicoll found that a number of factors worsen the prognosis: (1) wide initial displacement, (2) comminution, (3) presence of infection, and (4) the presence of severe soft tissue injury. Prognosis was not influenced by level of the fracture, whether the fibula was fractured, and the age of the patient (in adults). Hoaglund and States[99] found the prognosis to be related to whether the fracture was due to high-energy trauma or low-energy trauma. High-energy trauma was caused by vehicular accidents and crush injuries whereas low-energy injuries were due to accidents such as falls on ice or while skiing. High-energy injuries accounted for 90 percent of the open fractures and required an average of 6 months to heal. Low-energy fractures required only 4 months to heal. In addition, these investigators found that decreased contact between the fracture ends prolonged the time to union.

External fixation using multiple percutaneous transfixing pins attached to a rigid external frame has recently gained popularity, particularly for the treatment of severe open fractures and very unstable or comminuted closed fractures. Edge and Denham,[62] Edwards et al.,[66] Evans et al.,[75] Karlström and Olerud,[111,112,164] Rezaian,[172] and Shaar et al.[182,185] discuss the use of external fixation and most investigators[3,63,113,115,209,210,213] report on results with the Videl-Adrey modification of the Hoffman device. External fixators are relatively simple to apply compared with open reduction and internal fixation. They permit anatomic reduction of many fractures and can provide rigid fixation. They provide wide access to the extremity for observation, wound care, and plastic reconstructive procedures. When used in type III open fractures (see Fracture Classification) they have fewer complications than with internal fixation. The major complications associated with their use is pin-tract infection and delayed union, which can be minimized by proper technique.

As in all aspects of trauma, tibial fractures cannot be treated successfully with only one approach or simple set of rules. The surgeon must individualize the treatment of each fracture, taking into account its personality and the patient. The surgeon must be prepared and competent to use functional methods of closed treatment, external fixation, and techniques of internal fixation, including intramedullary rods, interfragmentary screws, and plates. When using functional weight-bearing casts and braces such as those advocated by Sarmiento, one can expect 90 percent of fractures of the shaft of the tibia to go on to union with insignificant shortening, angulation, or functional limitation. In closed fractures with severe initial displacement or severe comminution, early measures to control position, such as an external fixator, may be necessary. In suitable fractures not controllable by closed means, intramedullary rodding, preferably by closed technique, provides excellent stability and early function with a low complication rate. In those closed fractures with unacceptable position after closed treatment which are not suitable for intramedullary fixation (such as a long spiral frac-

ture in the distal third) in patients in whom an anatomic reduction is deemed to be necessary, open reduction and screw and/or plate fixation may be indicated. This occasion should occur only rarely.

In open fractures of the tibia, early reestablishment of stability is essential to optimize soft tissue healing and prevent infection. This is discussed in detail under the section on open fractures of the tibia.

The situations under which internal fixation or external fixators are most strongly indicated are (1) type III open fractures in which limb salvage justifies these techniques; (2) shaft fractures with an associated intra-articular component necessitating internal fixation; (3) fractures with a gap due to bone loss; (4) fractures with a compartment syndrome requiring fasciotomy; (5) those fractures with an associated vascular injury in which fracture instability threatens the repair; (6) the mutilated limb with either a severe ligamentous injury of the knee or an associated ipsilateral femur fracture; and (7) segmental fractures with a displaced central fragment.

ANATOMIC CONSIDERATIONS

The anatomy of the leg makes the tibia particularly susceptible to open fracture; its entire medial border is covered only by skin and a thin layer of subcutaneous fat. Fractures of the tibia are accompanied by a high incidence of neurovascular injuries and are not infrequently complicated by the compartment syndrome; therefore, the surgeon must be familiar with the anatomy of these structures. The following brief discussion of the anatomy of the leg provides a background for the surgical approaches to be described later in this chapter. Interested readers should consult standard textbooks on anatomy for greater detail.

The anatomy of the tibia and fibula is perhaps best appreciated as illustrated in Figures 125-1 to 125-3, which are cross-sections in the proximal, middle, and distal thirds of the leg. The neurovascular structures entering the leg are at highest risk in the proximal third. The popliteal artery, from a

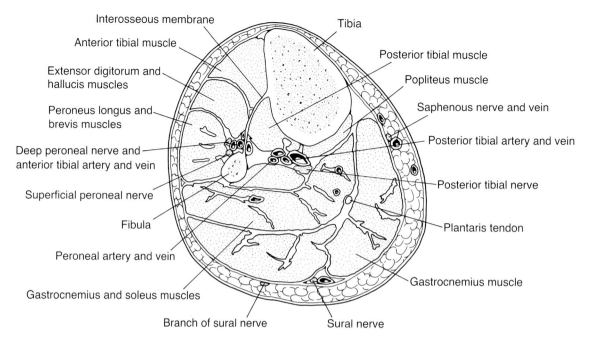

Fig. 125-1. Cross-section in the proximal third of the leg, about 2.5 cm below the tibial tubercle. The popliteal muscle still appears in this section The peroneal and posterior tibial neurovascular bundles are still together and lie deep to the soleus separated from the tibia by the tibialis posterior muscle. The deep and superficial peroneal nerves and their accompanying arteries are still gathered together and hug the fibula and interosseous membrane. (Modified from Eychleshmer,[75a] with permission.)

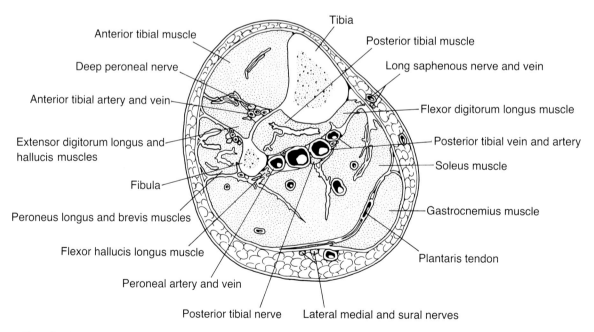

Fig. 125-2. Cross-section through the middle one-third of the leg. All the muscles controlling the ankle and foot have now appeared, except for the inconsequential peroneus tertius, and the origin of the flexor hallucis longus is just appearing. The large posterior tibial neurovascular bundle is seen sandwiched between the deep posterior and superficial posterior compartments and the anterior tibial vessels still lie against the anterior aspect of the interosseous membrane. (Modified from Eychleshmer,[75a] with permission.)

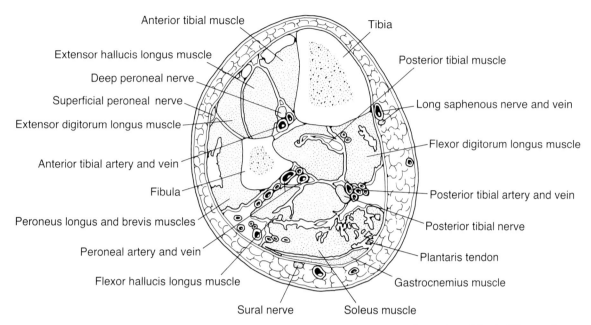

Fig. 125-3. Cross-section through the distal third of the leg that begins to show formation of the Achilles tendon; the soleus muscle belly is now becoming quite small. The route to the posterior aspect of the tibia anterior to the muscles of the deep posterior compartment on the medial side is evident. From the lateral side the fibula, interosseous membrane, and tibia can be completely exposed by dissecting along the posterior aspect of the peroneal compartment. Once the fibula is contacted stay against the bone and the interosseous membrane. Note the sharp right-angle curve necessary on reaching the most medial extent of the fibula to avoid entering the muscle belly of the tibialis posterior . Through this posterolateral approach the tibial neurovascular bundle is well protected by the muscles of the deep posterior compartment. (Modified from Eychleshmer,[75a] with permission.)

midline position between the medial and lateral heads of the gastrocnemius muscle behind the knee, sweeps somewhat laterally and then branches into the anterior tibial, posterior tibial, and peroneal arteries. This occurs after the artery has passed anterior to and beneath the soleus muscle bridge. These three arteries enter the anterior, posterior, and lateral compartments, respectively. This branching tethers the artery at this point. Therefore, traction injuries to the artery at or slightly above the trifurcation are common. The sciatic nerve lies lateral to the popliteal artery and has already divided into its posterior tibial and common peroneal components above the knee. As the popliteal artery enters the leg, the posterior tibial nerve supplying the posterior compartment of the leg continues with the posterior tibial artery to enter the posterior compartment. The common peroneal nerve, having passed from posterior and

medial to the biceps tendon proximal to the knee, then curves around the lateral aspect of the neck of the fibula and splits into its deep (anterior-tibial) and superficial peroneal branches, which enter the anterior tibial and lateral peroneal compartments, respectively. The common peroneal nerve is tethered at this point as it passes on a subcutaneous route, hugging the neck of the fibula. Here it is easily subject to injury by either external impingement from a cast, inappropriate retraction during surgery, or the major displacement that may occur during a fracture. In the proximal quarter of the leg, deep against the ligamentous and osseous structures, these three arteries and three nerves join up to pass distalward together into the leg. In the proximal third of the leg, one encounters muscles originating from the distal femur, including both heads of the gastrocnemius and the popliteal muscles. In the middle third of the leg, the relationships between the neurovascular bundles and the bone are well established, and one encounters the major bulk of the muscles of the leg. In the anterior compartment, arranged as illustrated in Figure 125-2, one finds the anterior tibial, extensor hallucis longus, extensor digitorum longus, and peroneus tertius muscles. The anterior tibial artery and nerve travel at the level of the interosseous membrane and come to lie deep against the tibial shaft in its distal third. In the lateral compartment are found the peroneus longus and brevis muscles and in the middle third of this compartment the sensory portion of the superficial peroneal nerve is still subfascial. The posterior tibial compartment contains a superficial and deep portion; the superficial contains the soleus and the heads of the gastrocnemius muscles. The deep posterior compartment contains the posterior tibial, flexor hallucis longus, and flexor digitorum longus muscles. The posterior tibial artery and nerve, protected by the flexor hallucis longus and soleus muscles, lies on the posterior aspect of the flexor digitorum and tibialis posterior muscles throughout the shaft region of the tibia. In the distal third of the leg most of these muscles have become tendons.

Of importance is the well-developed and tight deep fascia incorporating all four compartments of the leg, particularly the anterior tibial compartment. This makes the muscles and nerves of the leg particularly susceptible to ischemic damage from increased intracompartmental pressure. (See Ch. 131.) Note in Figures 125-1 to 125-3, the intermuscular intervals and dissection planes between the compartments supplied by different nerves through which the tibia can be safely approached from anterior, posteromedial, and posterolateral aspects.

The blood supply to the tibial shaft comes from the nutrient artery, metaphyseal vessels, and periosteal vessels, particularly at ligamentous attachments. Where muscle originates directly from the tibia, throughout the majority of the shaft, few vessels penetrate the outer cortex and the majority of the blood supply (90 percent of the overall thickness of the cortex) is from the nutrient arteries of the medullary canal. The nutrient artery to the tibia is derived from the posterior tibial artery and enters the posterolateral cortex just below the oblique line on the tibia made by the origin of the

soleus muscle. As seen in Figure 125-4, this artery divides into three ascending and one major descending branch. Preservation of the nutrient endosteal blood supply to the tibia plays a major role in the healing of fractures of the tibia; however, damage to this blood supply does result in reversal of the normal centrifugal flow of blood through the tibia to a centripetal flow from the perosteum. When a fracture interrupts the endosteal blood supply, or when intramedullary nailing has been used, preservation of the soft tissue attachments of the tibia is critical. The combination of plate fixation and intramedullary nailing is particularly problematic because it devascularizes the entire cortex. The tibia is particularly susceptible to avascular necrosis at the junction between the middle and distal thirds since, at this point, the nutrient artery has become smaller and the perforating vessels passing from the distal tibia proximally are likewise small. It is unfortunate that most open fractures of the tibia tend to occur at this junction.

LEFT TIBIA- POSTERIOR VIEW

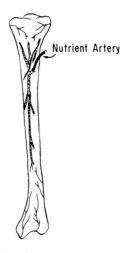

Nutrient Artery

Fig. 125-4. Intramedullary blood supply to the tibia. The nutrient artery to the tibia, which is the largest in the body, is derived from the posterior tibial artery. It has three ascending and one descending branch. Other branches enter at the ligamentous attachments, particularly at the ends of the bone.[141,160]

SURGICAL APPROACHES TO THE TIBIAL AND FIBULAR SHAFTS

Atraumatic soft tissue technique is as vital in surgery of the shaft of the tibia as it is in surgery of the tendons and nerves of the hand. Successful surgery in this area requires meticulous attention to the soft tissues.

Anterior Approach

The simplest, most utilitarian, and most commonly used approach to the tibia is the anterior approach. The lack of muscle coverage over the anterior aspect of the tibia and the tenuous blood supply to the skin in this area makes this simple exposure the most dangerous approach because inappropriate technique can easily result in skin sloughs with secondary infection. Open wounds of the tibia commonly occur on the anterior surface due to direct and indirect trauma, therefore this approach is most frequently used for debridement of open fractures. The presence of poor quality skin often makes this approach inadvisable.

If at all possible, the anterior skin incision should not be made directly over the subcutaneous border of the tibia. An anterolateral incision can be made approximately 5 to 10 mm lateral to the tibia (Fig. 125-5). An incision in this location lies over muscle and, if of sufficient length, permits easy access to the subcutaneous border of the tibia and exposure of the lateral border, which is the surface of choice for placement of a compression plate. The posterior tibial artery is not at risk in this exposure. This incision can be extended proximally for exposure of the knee joint or the tibial plateaus. It can be extended into a lateral or median parapatellar incision or can be curved gently along the origin of the anterior compartment muscles over to the fibular head and then proximally along the biceps tendon. This incision can also be extended distally in a medial midline or lateral curvilinear fashion to expose various aspects of the distal tibia and ankle joint.

The skin incision is carried directly through the subcutaneous fat and deep fascia. Undermining is done at either a subfascial or subperiosteal level to preserve the blood supply to the skin. Gentle re-

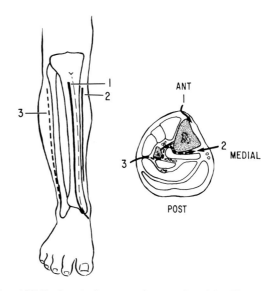

Fig. 125-5. Surgical approaches to the tibia. These approaches are described in detail in the text. (1) The anteromedial approach to the tibia utilizing its subcutaneous border. (2) The posteromedial approach to the tibia. (3) The posterolateral approach to the fibula, interosseous membrane, and tibia.

traction with hand-held retractors is superior to self-retaining retractors in protecting the fragile skin in this area. Exposure of the anterior surface of the tibia is accomplished by subperiosteal or extraperiosteal dissection with a periosteal elevator and retraction should be with Bennett or Hohman retractors to avoid injury to the skin. In plate fixation, the plate is best placed on the lateral border of the tibia. Dissection along the subcutaneous border of the tibia should be avoided if at all possible. On occasion the interosseous membrane must be exposed. This can be accomplished by subperiosteal dissection deep along the lateral border of the tibia until the interosseous membrane is reached. Perforation of the membrane is avoided by using a periosteal elevator along the anterior aspect of the membrane. The path of the anterior tibial artery and nerve, as illustrated in Figures 125-1 to 125-3, should be kept in mind to avoid injury to this vessel.

Posteromedial Approach

The basic mechanics of the posteromedial approach are identical to the anterolateral. The skin incision is illustrated in Figure 125-5. In the subcutaneous tissue, one must take care to avoid injury to the saphenous vein and long saphenous nerve. When the tibia is reached, dissection should be kept against the bone in a subperiosteal manner. The posterior tibial artery and nerve in this approach are protected by the muscle bellies of the flexor hallucis and posterior tibial muscles. For this approach the leg is best rotated externally at the hip and the knee flexed to bring the operated leg across the uninvolved leg, giving the surgeon a downward view. This approach is quite adequate for posterior bone grafting of the tibia but is difficult to use for internal fixation because it is difficult to retract laterally the large muscle mass posterior to the tibia. Access for instruments used to place screws is limited. In severe fractures of the tibia in which the condition of the anterior compartment and anterior tibia do not permit surgery, this approach provides an alternative.

Posterolateral Approach

Harmon,[93] and subsequently Jones and Barnett[108] and Hanson and Eppright,[91] described the posterolateral approach to the tibia and demonstrated its effectiveness. The major advantage of this approach is that it allows combined exposure of the fibula, interosseous membrane, and tibia and, in addition, goes through the largest muscle mass of the leg. The soft tissue coverage of the tibia in this approach is nearly always intact even with severe trauma or chronic osteomyelitis. This approach is most useful for bone grafting procedures and, although internal fixation can be applied through this approach, the exposure is not optimal. This approach requires the patient to be positioned in the lateral decubitus or prone position on the operating table. As in the anterior incisions, this incision is extensile. The route of this approach is illustrated in Figure 125-5. The deep fascia is incised just posterior to the intermuscular septum behind the peroneal compartment. Dissection is carried posterior to the peroneal muscles and along the posterior aspect of their compartment. The surgeon should hug these muscle bellies closely and dissection into muscle should be avoided. Once the fibula is reached, dissection remains against the fibula but is not subperiosteal, since this will carry one anterior

to the interosseous membrane and risk injury to the anterior tibial vessels and nerve. Once the interosseous membrane is gained, blunt dissection should be carried out with an elevator across the membrane to the tibia. Dissection can then be carried subperiosteally to expose the tibia. In nonunions and in cases of osteomyelitis, normal dissection planes will be distorted, and identification of the interosseous membrane may not be possible. It may be necessary to expose the posterior tibial artery and nerve both proximally and distally and then follow them into the involved area to avoid injuring them. To avoid working in a deep hole, and to avoid excessive soft tissue retraction, it is very important to use an incision of sufficient length, usually at least 20 cm.

Approaches to the Fibula

Although sometimes difficult to palpate in heavily muscled or fat limbs, the lateral border of the fibula remains subcutaneous throughout its length. An incision over the subcutaneous border, anterior to the peroneal muscles, can be carried directly down to the fibula and the entire fibular shaft can then be exposed by subperiosteal dissection. This approach is useful in fibular osteotomy and in resecting the fibular shaft for either decompression of the leg or when the fibular shaft is used as a bone graft. Proximally, Henry's approach is necessary to avoid injury to the common peroneal nerve and its branches.

MECHANISMS OF INJURY

As described by Hoaglund and States,[99] probably the most important prognostic factor in fractures of the tibia is the amount of energy absorbed by the tibia and soft tissues at the time of injury. High-energy fractures have been shown to have a worse prognosis than low-energy fractures. The higher the strain rate, the more energy the bone can absorb until fracture. When fracture occurs, the higher energy absorbed produces more extensive comminution. Indirect injuries, such as seen in skiing injuries, are generally low-energy injuries and show simple patterns; such as the spiral or long oblique fractures seen in Figure 125-6. Direct trauma, as occurs in motor vehicle accidents and gunshot wounds, produces high-energy injuries resulting in more open wounds, more extensive soft tissue damage, and more bone displacement and comminution, as seen in Figure 125-7.

Open fractures from handguns are generally low-velocity wounds, depending on how much energy is absorbed by the tibia on impact of the missile. Gunshot wounds from magnum pistols may be high velocity if a substantial portion of their force is absorbed. All military weapon, rifle, and shotgun wounds should be regarded as high velocity.

Fibular shaft fractures generally occur in con-

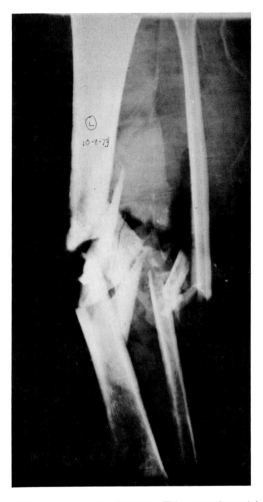

Fig. 125-7. High-energy fracture. This comminuted fracture of the tibia with wide displacement of the tibia from the fibula indicating severe soft tissue trauma is characteristic of the high-energy fractures associated with motorcycle and motor vehicle accidents.

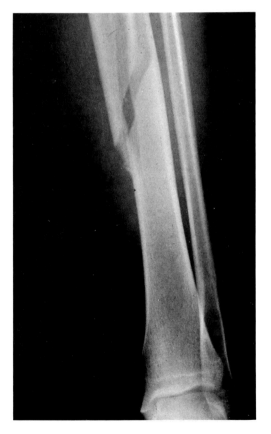

Fig. 125-6. Low-energy fracture. This long spiral fracture is typical of a low-energy torsional injury such as those commonly seen in association with skiing.

junction with tibia fractures. The absence of a fibular fracture is more common in children and in adults is generally an indication of a low-energy injury. Wide separation between the tibia and fibula is associated with disruption of the interosseous membrane and is indicative of instability, which makes management difficult (see Fig. 125-7).

Tibial shaft fractures are commonly associated with fractures of either the tibial plateau or plafond. Plateau injuries are usually due to motor vehicle or pedestrian accidents, whereas tibial plafond injuries are usually due to falls from a height or sudden deceleration. Commonly, both are high-velocity injuries.

It is important to think of a fracture in terms of a high-velocity or low-velocity injury. This has direct implications on the risks of fixation and to what degree wounds must be debrided. These issues are addressed below.

FRACTURE CLASSIFICATION

Fracture classifications are of value only if they help the surgeon choose the method of treatment or define the prognosis better. One might wish for a classification that would define when an open reduction is indicated and what type; I know of no fracture classification that permits this. Judgment about the need for internal fixation is a very complex process that must take into account the nature of the fracture, associated injuries, and the patient. The identical fracture in a 22-year-old professional football player, a 72-year-old woman, or a paraplegic may be treated in entirely different manners.

Precision and completeness in describing fractures permit better classification and help to clarify one's thinking about the fracture. The precise anatomic location of the fracture, the position and pattern of the fracture lines, and the position and dis-

placement of the fracture fragments should be noted. This becomes critically important when one is planning for rigid internal fixation. The configuration of the internal fixation to be used should be determined before surgery. The presence of comminution and whether the fracture is open or closed are obviously of great importance.

Ellis,[70-73] Weissman et al.,[218,219] Nicoll,[161,162] and Leach's[126] modification of Ellis' classification all grade tibial fractures according to severity and indicate the prognosis from this. None of these classifications permits absolute decisions regarding treatment. These investigators use a combination of various factors, such as the presence of comminution, presence of an open wound, presence of displacement, and/or angulation, and to use them to formulate classifications in three general categories: minor, moderate, and severe. The general prognosis for these three categories of injury are indicated in Table 125-1.

In determining open fracture wound management and prognosis, a useful classification is that of Gustilo and Anderson.[85] They classify open fractures according to the severity of the wound, mechanism of injury, and degree of contamination. A type I open fracture has a clean wound with minimal soft tissue injury, generally less than 1 cm in length, which represents a low-energy inside-to-outside fracture. A type II open fracture is more severe, more likely to be due to direct trauma producing an outside-to-inside wound, and has some

Table 125–1. Classification of Severity of Tibial Fractures

		Investigators			Time to Union (Weeks)	Delayed Union (%)
Severity	Factors	Ellis[70-73]	Weissman et al.[219]	Nicoll[161]		
Minor	Displacement	Undisplaced	20% width of tibia	Little or none	10	2[71]–9[a]
	Angulation	None	Less than 10°	Little or none		
	Comminution	None	None	None		
	Wound	Closed or minor type I	—	None		
Moderate	Displacement	Total	20–40% width of tibia	—	15	11[b]
	Angulation	Moderate	—	—		
	Comminution	Small	10–30°	—		
	Wound	Type I or low-grade type II	—	—		
Major	Displacement	Complete	>50% of shaft	Severe	23	30–55[b]
	Angulation	Severe	—	Severe		60[c]
	Communition	Major	—	—		
	Wound	Severe type II or III	—	Type III		

[a] From Murray et al.[159]
[b] From Ellis.[71]
[c] From Nicholl.[161]

deep contamination and muscle injury. The wound is more than 1 cm long. A type III wound is grossly contaminated, a high-velocity injury with significant muscle damage, and the wounds are generally longer than 5 cm. Included in this category are segmental fractures, open fractures occurring in a farmyard, high-velocity gunshot wounds, shotgun wounds, and injuries associated with vascular injuries. I would add to this any tibial fracture sustained when a motorcyclist or pedestrian is struck by a moving automobile. Type III open fractures are subdivided into types A, B, and C. In type IIIA, the amount of periosteal and muscle stripping from bone is miminal to moderate and soft tissue reconstructive flaps are rarely necessary to achieve closure. In type IIIB, extensive soft tissue and periosteal loss has occurred, and coverage of bone generally requires plastic reconstructive surgery. Type C is a type III fracture with a vascular injury requiring repair. The prognosis for infections in these open fracture types is indicated in Table 125-2. Most authorities, including Chapman and Mahoney,[38,39] Rittman et al.,[173] Patzakis et al.,[168] and Gustilo and Anderson,[85] agree that all Type III wounds require extensive and meticulous irrigation and debridement and that they should always be left open.

There is a disagreement about the management of type I and II wounds. However, Gustilo and Anderson have shown that type I wounds can be closed primarily with a low infection rate. A type I wound should never be closed when the contamination is severe. The risk of gas gangrene and tetanus should be kept in mind. As type I wounds are quite small, they usually do not require closure and heal quickly by secondary intention. Management of type II wounds requires good surgical judgement. There is little question that the safest approach is to leave all type II wounds open.[146]

Table 125–2. Infection Rate in Open Fractures

Wound Type	Infection Rate (%)
I	$0^{85}-1.9^a$
II	$-8^{°39}$
III	$9.9^{85}-41^°$
Overall	$2.4^{85}-10.6^°$

[a] Internal fixation used.
Data from Chapman et al.[39]

TREATMENT

Closed Fractures

Nonsurgical methods are generally the treatment of choice in tibial shaft fractures. Methods available include skeletal traction using a distal tibial or calcaneal pin, plaster immobilization using a long-leg or short-leg cast or splints, external skeletal fixation using pins above and below incorporated into plaster, and external fixation. Closed reduction and temporary or permanent fixation at the fracture site with percutaneous Kirschner (K)-wires or wire loops have also been described.

Open reduction can be performed without the use of internal fixation but I know of no authority who would advise that today since the risk of open reduction without the advantages of stable fixation is not rational. Internal fixation can be divided into four types: interfragmentary screw or wire fixation, plate fixation, circlage wiring, and intramedullary nailing. Parham bands or similar devices, although advocated in the past, should be avoided because of adverse effects on bone circulation.

Initial Treatment

Neither closed nor open treatment will achieve optimal results if the initial care of the fracture in the emergency department does not prevent further injury to the soft tissues and further contamination of open wounds, minimize edema, and protect neurovascular structures.

The injured leg is gently restored to grossly normal alignment using gentle traction. Hemorrhage is controlled with a compression dressing and a long-leg, well-padded, radiolucent splint should be applied. The neurovascular status of the limb is assessed and recorded. Anteroposterior (AP) and lateral radiographs that include the knee and ankle are then obtained. While waiting for definitive care the patient is kept supine and the limb elevated 10 cm above the level of the heart. Wound care is discussed under Open Fractures.

Methods of Closed Treatment

Traction treatment of tibia fractures was popularized by Böhler[21] and is used in many parts of the world. It usually is not the definitive method of treatment but is used to obtain initial stabilization and alignment. After a week or so, the traction is discontinued and a cast is applied. In the English-speaking world, traction is rarely used for the treatment of fractures of the tibia because overdistraction can lead to delayed or nonunion. The primary indication for early skeletal traction is the presence of severe soft tissue injury, which contraindicates application of immediate internal fixation, an external fixator, or a circumferential plaster cast. Traction is most useful in overcoming unacceptable overriding and shortening that is not correctable by closed reduction. With the advent of modern external fixators, the indications for skeletal traction for fractures of the tibia have nearly disappeared.

If there is some possibility of subsequent internal fixation, careful technique must be used in the application of skeletal traction to minimize the risk of pin-tract infection. To avoid pulling across the ankle and subtalar joints and to eliminate the complications of pin loosening that are frequent in the calcaneus, I prefer to use a K-wire placed in the tibial metaphysis approximately 1 to 2.5 cm above the tibial plafond. This requires a large K-wire bow to reach around the heel. The pin is inserted anterior to the fibula. Movement of the K-wire along its axis is avoided by placing 2 × 2 dressings between the skin and the K-wire bow, as illustrated in Figure 125-8. A calcaneal pin is used only when fractures of the tibial plafond are being treated or a subsequent incision for open reduction will pass through the area of a distal tibial pin.

Closed Reduction and Cast Immobilization

Closed reduction and application of a plaster cast is the most commonly used method for treating fractures of the tibia and fibula. Plaster casts can be used for non-weight-bearing treatment or early weight bearing, as popularized by Dehne,[50-53] Brown,[27] and Sarmiento.[177-180] These are very different methods with different indications. I prefer immediate weight bearing and delay it only when shortening cannot be controlled. Immediate

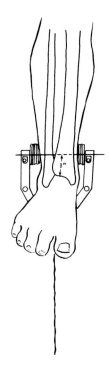

Fig. 125-8. Distal tibial K-wire traction. A 0.062-inch K-wire is placed transversely through the metaphysis of the tibia from lateral to medial just anterior to the fibula approximately 2.5 cm above the ankle joint. Use smooth wires because threaded wires often break. Place a stack of 2 × 2 sterile gauze sponges over the K-wire on both sides. Then place a large K-wire bow that will extend around the heel without impinging upon the skin to hold the 2 × 2s firmly against the skin. The 2 × 2s act as spacers and prevent migration of the K-wire in the tibia. Antiseptics about the pin site or on the 2 × 2s are unnecessary. The K-wire should be kept tight, to avoid bending the wire.

weight-bearing cast technique is as demanding and exacting as any form of internal fixation for fractures of the tibia, if not more so. As with open reduction and internal fixation, the best results in difficult fractures are obtained only by masters of the technique who follow their patients closely and who are willing to modify or change casts frequently to maintain anatomic reduction. The surgeon should strive for an anatomic rather than an "acceptable" reduction. Because plaster cast treatment is the most frequently indicated technique for fractures of the tibia, it deserves description here.

In displaced fractures, closed reduction is best obtained using gentle traction. With good premedication and a cooperative patient this can often be achieved without an anesthetic. If a first attempt is unsuccessful, a regional or general anesthetic is indicated, to avoid patient discomfort and excessive soft tissue handling. The patient is placed in a supine position on a treatment table with a hydraulic lift. The limb with the fractured tibia is abducted at the hip and supported in the midthigh by a well-padded board or crutch slipped under the table

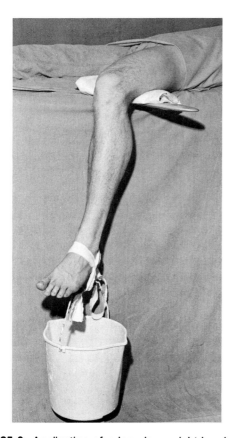

Fig. 125-9. Application of a long leg weight-bearing and Sarmiento weight-bearing plaster cast (Figs. 125-9 to 125-12). Closed reduction and cast application can often be done without an anesthetic if the patient is well-medicated and cooperative. Otherwise, a regional or general anesthesia should be used. The limb with the fractured tibia is positioned as illustrated. The crutch or board should be well-padded. Use a bucket filled with the appropriate amount of water or the surgeon can use one foot in the bandage to apply gentle traction to stabilize the limb.

pad, as illustrated in Figure 125-9. The knee is flexed to 90 degrees. A removable ankle traction bandage is applied, as illustrated in Figure 125-10. Traction is applied through this bandage either by applying one's foot to a sling attached to the ankle traction bandage or by filling with water a bucket attached to the ankle bandage strap. This traction should be used only to stabilize the fracture and achieve alignment. Excessive traction should be avoided. This method permits the surgeon to control and stabilize the limb and frees both hands for manipulation of the fracture and application of the cast. The attitude of the foot and rotation is best controlled by an assistant holding on to the forefoot.

The short-leg portion of the cast is applied first; the toes are covered to the base of the toenails and the cast is carried up to the midportion of the patella so that adequate plaster is present for molding against the condyles of the tibia proximally. Cast padding is applied two layers thick, without wrinkles. A third layer is placed over bony prominences and about the tibial plateaus. Using water at approximately 72°F, the plaster is then applied. In the average adult male leg, one 10-cm and three 15-cm rolls are required. All the plaster is wet simultaneously and applied rapidly to ensure a strong cast. The 10-cm roll is used to cover the foot to just above the malleoli. Each roll is thoroughly rubbed in as it is applied. The first 15-cm roll is begun on the foot. As the plaster is carried proximally, all tucks are taken over the posterior calf to avoid any irregularities in the plaster over the subcutaneous border of the tibia. The plaster is carried as high as the flexed knee will allow. After all the plaster is applied, it is thoroughly rubbed in, then, the molding, which is the most important part of the procedure, is carried out. The cast is carefully molded to restore the normal longitudinal and transverse arches of the foot and molded firmly against the entire anterior surface of the tibia. Anterior molding will cause the cast to bulge somewhat posteriorly above the Achilles tendon, giving it room to function. It should be carefully molded about the malleoli. As the plaster begins to set, the base of the palm is molded along the entire length of the subcutaneous border of the tibia to produce a flat surface against which the tibia can be pushed from posteriorly. The cast is then molded into a

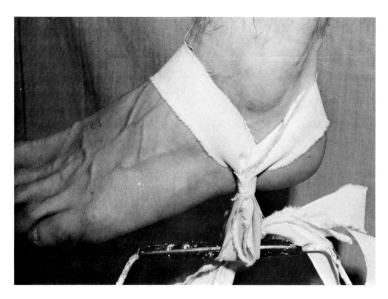

Fig. 125-10. Removable ankle-traction bandage. This bandage is applied with 2.5-cm-wide strips of muslin doubled over. The doubled-over strips should be at least 65 cm in length, so that they can be easily tied to a bucket or set of weights beneath the foot. One strip is placed over the instep and another over the heel, and they are taped together with 12-mm tape, level with the bottom of the foot as illustrated. A thin layer of petroleum jelly applied to the skin (underneath each strip) eases removal. The junctions of the two strips should be located directly below the malleoli. Sufficient traction is applied to stabilize the fracture and achieve alignment. Excessive traction should be avoided unless pins in plaster are to be used.

triangular shape by running the base of the palm in a longitudinal fashion over the soft tissues of the anterior compartment. This produces a slight anterior ridge in the plaster, decompressing the prominent anterior border of the tibia. As the plaster begins to become firm, it is molded against the proximal third of the calf posteriorly to push the tibia forward in the cast against its previously molded and now reasonably firm smooth anterior border. As the most proximal portion of the cast begins to set the plaster is then carefully molded to fit the medial and lateral flares of the tibia. Note that this molding is similar to that used for a total contact prosthesis, however, no particular effort is made to create a patellar shelf. It is now well known that this is not a major area of weight bearing and can be a source of pressure problems.

After the short-leg section is completed, the ankle traction bandage is removed by cutting the tape (Fig. 125-10) that holds the two bandages together. The muslin straps are then cut off as short as possible on the medial side and are withdrawn from the lateral side. A small amount of Vaseline or K-Y

jelly placed on the skin immediately beneath the straps at the time of application facilitates removal. These straps must never be left in the cast because they may cause pressure sores. The hole in the bottom of the cast is padded and sealed with plaster.

When the cast has set sufficiently to permit handling, the knee is straightened by lifting the leg with a hand beneath the fracture site and placing the foot against the assistant's chest. The proximal portion of this cast is then trimmed to produce a snug fit and avoid any sharp edges. Two layers of padding are then applied snuggly to the thigh and are wrapped above the prominence of the greater trochanter. Sufficient room is allowed medially to prevent groin impingement. Three to four 15-cm rolls are required for the average size man. These are then wetted simultaneously and applied smoothly. The full width of one roll should overlap between the two halves of the cast to assure good adhesion. The principles of fitting of a total contact quadralateral socket are then employed to mold the upper half of the cast. The plaster is carefully molded from anterior to posterior to produce a close fit about the medial and lateral epicondyles of the femur. The cast should be molded in above the epicondyles so that it is narrower in the medial-to-lateral diameter than at the knee. This will cause bulging of the plaster in the anteroposterior plane, allowing room for the patellar and hamstring tendons to function. As this begins to set, molding is carried up the thigh in the form of a quadralateral socket. The surgeon's hip can be used to mold the plaster over the trochanter and the hands are used to flatten the cast over the femoral triangle.

This produces a close fit about the anterior and lateral aspects of the cast and bulges the plaster to allow room for the function of the adductor and hamstring tendons. After the plaster has set, the edges about the toes and upper rim of the cast should be trimmed and padded with whatever technique the surgeon prefers. Either a walker or a

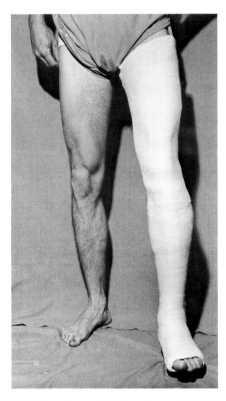

Fig. 125-11. Long-leg weight-bearing cast. Note the anatomic molding of this cast. It fits closely about the malleoli, is triangular in its midsection and fits closely about the tibial and femoral condyles. The thigh section is molded as a quadrilateral socket.

walking shoe can then be applied. The completed cast is illustrated in Figure 125-11.

In acute tibial shaft fractures, hospitalization and elevation of the extremities are usually mandatory. The cast as well as the soft padding should be prophylactically cut along the anterior surface and then spread as needed to accompany swelling. Most often, the cast need not be spread at all, and this does not interfere with subsequent function of the cast. If spreading is necessary, the cast can be enlarged symmetrically through the single split. As the swelling decreases, it can subsequently be reclosed and sealed with a single layer of plaster to be as functional as if it had not been split. I prefer this single split to bivalving the cast because it maintains the integrity of the cast and provides more uniform decompression of the leg.

The patient should be encouraged to be up and bearing weight as tolerated within 1 to 2 days. The usual patient requires at least 3 to 4 weeks to achieve full, unsupported weight bearing. A program of isometric exercises for all muscle groups immobilized in the cast should be instituted and undertaken on a daily basis. At approximately 4 to 6 weeks, the cast can be changed, final alignment achieved, and a Sarmiento-type weight-bearing plaster, as illustrated in Figure 125-12, applied.

Fracture Bracing

The techniques of fracture bracing popularized by Sarmiento are very useful in the treatment of fractures of the tibial shaft and are generally applied after initial treatment with a plaster cast, as described above. Fracture braces can be custom-fabricated and are also available as "off the shelf"prefabricated devices. The description of this technique is beyond the purview of this text.[177-180] An example of a cast brace is illustrated in Figure 125-13.

Indications for Open Reduction of Closed Fractures

The most common indication for internal fixation of a shaft fracture of the tibia is when the fracture occurs in conjunction with an intra-articular fracture at the ankle or knee. Fixation of the articular fracture may also require fixation of the shaft to obtain adequate stability for early functional treat-

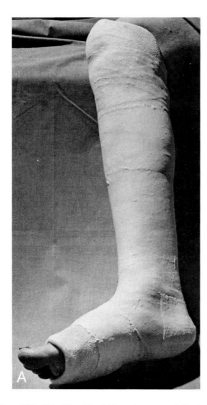
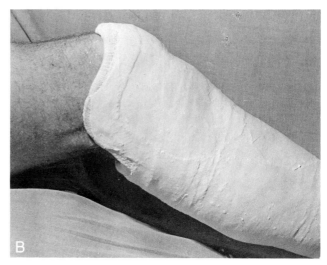

Fig. 125-12. Modified Sarmiento weight-bearing cast. The cast is applied below the knee as described in the text for the long-leg cast. At the knee the plaster is carried well above the patellar tendon and carefully molded to the lateral femoral condyles and patella. The upper edge of the cast is then trimmed as illustrated. I prefer to leave the cast above the patella and femoral epicondyles as in a PTS prosthetic suspension. This provides a better hold and avoids patellar impingement. The cast is cut out posteriorly to allow as much flexion as the surgeon wants the patient to have. Early in treatment, one may choose to limit flexion to 45 degrees; this can be gradually cut down to permit full flexion as fracture stability progresses.

ment. In isolated shaft fractures, the usual indication is inability to achieve adequate alignment and sufficient length by closed methods. Another indication is when fractures of the tibial shaft are associated with fractures of the femur, producing a "floating knee." The "floating knee," however, can be managed by internal fixation of the femur and external immobilization of the tibia, provided the fracture is not so unstable or so close to the knee that early knee motion is not possible. For internal fixation to be considered, the fracture must not be so comminuted that stable internal fixation cannot be achieved and the soft tissues should permit safe internal fixation. When displacement of the fracture is present, in particular shortening, internal fixation should not be delayed much beyond 2

weeks, or restoration of normal anatomy may become quite difficult due to early soft tissue healing and contracture.

Certain fracture configurations are predictably difficult to manage by plaster immobilization alone. If the surgeon chooses to not use some form of external fixation then internal fixation may be indicated. The most common configurations (Fig. 125-14) are transverse or short oblique fractures in the midshaft area of both bones with marked initial displacement, particularly with diastasis between the tibia and fibula indicating a rupture of the interosseous membrane. Segmental fractures are difficult to treat closed, and delayed union is quite common. Fractures at the junction of the middle and distal thirds of the tibia or in the distal third of

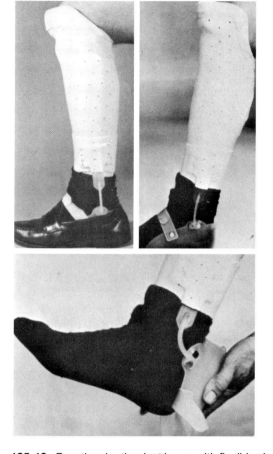

Fig. 125-13. Functional orthoplast brace with flexible plastic insert. (From Sarmiento,[180] with permission.)

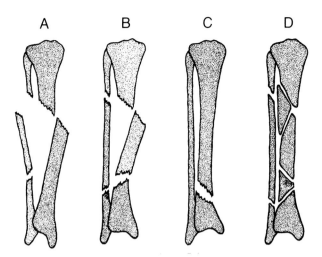

Fig. 125-14. Unstable tibial fractures. These fracture patterns tend to be unstable or to have a high incidence of complications. **(A)** The short oblique or transverse fracture with wide initial displacement with evidence of interruption of the interosseous membrane. These are difficult to control in plaster and angulation or shortening is not uncommon. **(B)** A segmental fracture with displacement where nonunion is frequent. **(C)** An oblique fracture at the junction of the middle and distal one-third of the tibia with an intact fibula where varus angulation and/or delayed union due to the intact fibula is not infrequent. All types of severely comminuted fractures of the tibia **(D)** present problems because they are associated with severe soft tissue injury, and delayed or nonunion with angulation is not infrequent.

the tibia, particularly with an intact fibula, frequently develop varus angulation, which is difficult to control by plaster casts alone. Extremely comminuted fractures may also be difficult to treat closed; however, these are usually not suitable for internal fixation and external fixation is usually indicated.

If open fasciotomies are required for a compartment syndrome, some[137] investigators find that internal fixation at the time of fasciotomy is indicated to permit optimal treatment of the soft tissues. External fixation can also be used. In view of the condition of the soft tissues, this may represent a better choice. The specific indications for each type of internal fixation are discussed under the specific technique.

Contraindications to internal fixation of closed fractures are excessive swelling, poor condition of the skin, and the presence of significant infection elsewhere in the body.

Open Fractures

Immediate internal fixation of open fractures of the shaft of the tibia generally has a higher risk of infection and other complications than does external fixation. An exception is a type I open fracture, where the same indications as in closed fractures can be used. With current external fixation techniques, the need for internal fixation has diminished considerably.

The usual indication for internal fixation of open fractures is a severe type III or type II open fracture where management of the soft tissues is not possible by external fixation and where limb salvage requires immediate stabilization of the bone to optimize treatment of the soft tissues. Rigid stabilization of the fracture, whether by external or internal means, may lower the infection rate and contribute to soft tissue healing.[173]

Intra-articular fractures should almost always be internally fixed and an associated shaft component may also require rigid fixation. An alternative approach is to use limited internal fixation for the articular component of the fracture and external fixation for the metaphyseal component. If necessary, the external fixation can be converted to plate fixation at a later time, when the soft tissues are in better condition.

Vascular injuries caused by the bone may require internal fixation to protect the vascular repair, although this is rare in the tibia due to the presence of three major vessels. Internal fixation is usually necessary in implantation of amputated legs.

For a more complete discussion of this controversial subject the reader is referred to Chapman,[38] Chapman and Mahoney,[39] Rittmann et al.,[173] and others.[94,221]

SURGICAL TECHNIQUE

Pins in Plaster

With the advent of external fixators, the indications for pins in plaster have lessened; however, the simplicity of the technique and low cost make it widely used particularly in third world countries.

I prefer to use three bicortical pins, one distal to the fracture site and two proximal. With this technique, it is not necessary to use a long-leg cast and early knee rehabilitation is possible. Occasionally, the distal pin may not be necessary and in these cases early partial weight bearing can be instituted if good fracture contact is present. I prefer to use stout threaded pins, such as 8-mm threaded Steinmann pins. Smooth Steinmann pins work as well, but loosening occurs more frequently.

The distal pin is placed in the metaphysis of the tibia about 2.5 cm proximal to the ankle joint and can also be placed through the calcaneus. Proximally, a transverse pin is placed slightly distal to the tibial tubercle and a second pin is placed at right angles to the subcutaneous border of the tibia slightly distal to the other pin. It is drilled through both the near and far cortex, but the posterior cortex is penetrated no more than 6 mm and only the near side of the pin protrudes, as shown in Figure 125-15. This arrangement of pins proximally gives excellent fixation, prevents rotation of the proximal fragment about the single transverse pin, avoids muscle tie down, and simplifies application and subsequently removal of the plaster from about the pins.

A formal surgical preparation of the limb is done first. A stab wound somewhat smaller than the overall diameter of the pin is made with a #11 blade to ensure a snug fit of the skin about the pin.

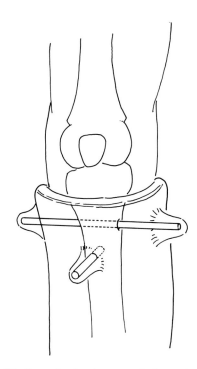

Fig. 125-15. Two-pins-in-plaster technique. A transverse through-and-through Steinmann pin is placed somewhat distal to the tibial tubercle. A second Steinmann pin is driven from the medial subcutaneous border of the tibia through the posterior cortex, but not penetrating the soft tissues. These are then incorporated into a short-leg cast. These three protruding pins provide good fixation and ease of plaster application and removal. (From Chapman,[38a] with permission.)

Great care must be taken in placing the pins to avoid distortion of the skin. If any occurs, the skin must be incised to relieve tension to prevent skin necrosis. The larger wound can then be closed about the pin with a single interrupted 5-0 nylon suture. The pins should be inserted with a hand-powered drill at slow speeds to avoid overheating and bone necrosis. These pins should be placed at the maximum bicortical diameter of the tibia; the solid cortical bone of the anterior crest should be avoided.

Reduction is obtained by placing the limb in traction with the limb flexed 90 degrees over the side of the table, as described under Closed Reduction. The pins can also be placed in a Roger Anderson apparatus or in the Steinmann pin-holding devices of the various orthopaedic tables. The latter devices permit a nearly anatomic reduction and hold it while the plaster is being applied. A single layer of dry, sterile dressing is placed about the pin wounds, and the plaster cast is applied. No padding should be placed over the pins, and they should be incorporated directly into the plaster. At least 5 cm of pin is left protruding from the skin and incorporated solidly into the plaster. If necessary, the final position can be obtained by wedging the cast after the plaster has set.

Removal of the plaster from about these pins at the time of cast removal is facilitated by running the cast saw directly alongside the pin in a longitudinal fashion along the shaft. This divides the plaster about the pin, which can then be pulled away from the pin.

Interfragmentary Screw Fixation

When screws and plates are to be used to fix a tibial shaft fracture, the most important component of the fixation is interfragmentary compression obtained through the use of interfragmentary lag screws. Except in a pure transverse fracture of the tibia, the primary fixation to be obtained should always be with interfragmentary lag screws, using the techniques advocated by the AO group. The stresses across the fracture then usually need to be neutralized by application of a plate. Because interfragmentary screws play a primary role; this technique is described first.

The interfragmentary compression achieved with lag screws produces static compression. This increases the intimacy of contact and friction between the fragments, thereby better neutralizing the stresses to which the fracture site will be subjected during healing. To achieve interfragmentary compression, the screw must not have purchase on the cortex nearest to the head of the screw. This is most easily obtained through the use of the lag screws illustrated in Figure 125-16, where the shaft of the screw adjacent to the head is not threaded. This type of screw has a disadvantage in cortical bone: the smaller diameter of the unthreaded shaft makes it difficult to remove with-

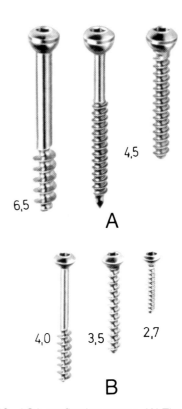

Fig. 125-16. AO bone fixation screws. **(A)** The three types of screws available in the large fragment set. On the left is a 6.5-mm cancellous screw and on the right is a 4.5-mm cortical screw. The screw in the middle is a cortical screw with no threads on the portion of the shaft adjacent to the screw head; thus, it can be used as a lag screw. **(B)** The comparable screws in the small fragment set measuring 4.0 mm, 3.5 mm, and 2.7 mm in diameter. A new 3.5-mm cortical screw that has a finer thread is now available as well. (Modified from Müller,[157] with permission.)

out screw breakage after the fracture is healed. For this reason, cortical screws should be used in cortical bone; they should function as lag screws by overdrilling the near cortex. The screw hole in the near cortex is called the gliding hole: the screw is permitted to glide in this hole; the hole in the far cortex is called the threaded hole because the threads gain purchase here. The application of these screws is described below; however, the lag screw technique can also be applied through the holes of the plate and is described in the section on plating. The following techniques are described for a standard 4.5-mm AO cortical screw. For smaller bones, these techniques can be applied using the 3.5-mm and 2.7-mm screws.

Preoperative planning is important. The surgeon should radiograph the opposite normal leg and draw on the radiograph the configuration of the fracture to be fixed. One should also draw in the fixation to be used. The surgical team will then be properly prepared for the procedure and less time will be spent making decisions while the wound is open.

In general, the holes for interfragmentary lag

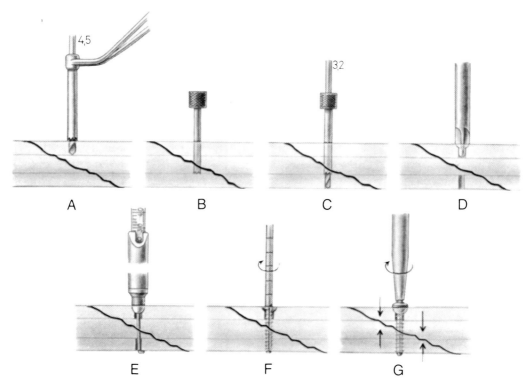

Fig. 125-17. Lag screw fixation technique. **(A)** The fracture is anatomically reduced and securely held with a bone-holding forceps. The gliding hold is drilled using a 4.5-mm drill bit placed through a 4.5-mm tap sleeve used as a drill guide and to protect the soft tissues. In this example the screw is place at right angles to the longitudinal axis of the bone. **(B)** A 58-mm drill sleeve with an outside diameter of 4.5 mm and an inside diameter of 3.5 mm is then inserted into the previously drilled hole and pushed in until its end abuts on the opposite cortex. This provides perfect centering of the drill bit, even when oblique holes are being drilled. **(C)** The threaded hole is then drilled with a 3.2-mm drill bit. **(D)** To avoid a stress riser effect on the cortex, a recess for the screw head is then cut with the countersink. **(E)** A depth gauge is then used to determine the proper length screw. **(F)** A short 4.5-mm tap placed through a tap sleeve (not illustrated) is then used to cut the thread in the threaded hole. **(G)** A 4.5-mm cortex screw of the proper length is then inserted with the screw driver. If more than one screw is to be used, the screw is only lightly tightened and final tightening is done sequentially after all screws have been placed. The lag effect across the fracture line can be seen as the screw is tightened. (From Müller,[157] with permission.)

screws should be drilled before reduction of the fracture. This permits optimal localization of the screws in the tips of the fracture fragments. For a screw to provide optimal fixation, it must be placed at right angles to the fracture surfaces at the particular area along the length of the fracture it is being applied. This means, for example, that in a long spiral fracture, the screws will be at differing angles at different areas of the fracture. In very simple oblique and spiral fractures, the fracture can first be reduced and then the interfragmentary screws placed, while the reduction of the fracture is held with bone-reduction forceps. It is difficult, however, to obtain optimal placement of the screws using this technique, but for purposes of illustration this technique is discussed first.

As noted in Figure 125-17, the fracture is reduced anatomically; in this case, the fracture line is sufficiently short for a single lag screw. The correct angle of the screw to the cortex is a compromise. When a screw is placed at 90 degrees to the cortex rather than to the fracture site, increased compression at the fracture site occurs with axial loading, but optimal interfragmentary compression is not possible. If the screw is placed at right angles to the fracture site, compression across the fracture is optimal. However, distraction occurs with vertical loading. Therefore, in most cases a compromise between these two angles is chosen. In the short oblique fracture in this example, the screw will be placed at right angles to the cortex to provide optimal stability under vertical loading. A 4.5-mm tap sleeve is used as a drill guide to gain purchase on the cortex and determine the inclination of the screw. Through this, a 4.5-mm drill point is used to make a hole in the near cortex. Next, a 58-mm-long drill sleeve with an outside diameter of 4.5 mm and an inside diameter of 3.2 mm is placed into the drill hole and pushed in until its serrated end abuts the opposite cortex. This ensures that the hole in the opposite cortex will be perfectly centered. The hole to be threaded in the opposite cortex is then drilled using a 3.2-drill point. A recess for the screwhead is cut with the countersink in the near cortex. The screw length is then determined by measuring with a large-fragment depth gauge. The soft tissues are protected with a tap sleeve while the opposite·cortex is threaded using the short 4.5-mm tap. The appropriate length 4.5-mm cortical

screw can then be inserted. If more than one screw is to be used, the first is only lightly tightened and then all the screws are completely tightened one after the other.

Two other methods of inserting this same lag screw can be employed. These provide more accurate placement of the screw and are useful when it is difficult to visualize the opposite cortex or when one wishes to use minimal soft tissue dissection. These are the "inside-out-technique" and the "threaded-hole-first technique."

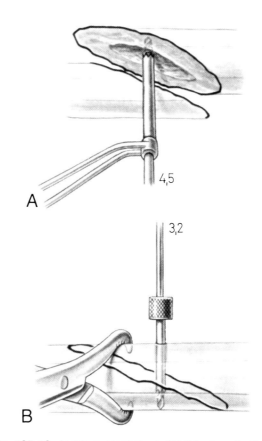

Fig. 125-18. Inside-out technique. **(A)** Prior to reduction of the fracture, a 4.5-mm hole is drilled from inside the intramedullary canal in the tip of the spike of the fragment most available to the surgeon in the wound. By drilling this hole from the inside outward, perfect localization of the hole in the center of the tip of the fragment can be achieved. A 4.5-mm tap sleeve is used as a drill guide. **(B)** The fracture is then reduced and held with a bone-reduction forceps, and the 58-mm drill sleeve is slipped into the predrilled gliding hole and the procedure is then carried as outlined in Fig. 125-17. (Modified from Müller, with permission.[157])

In the inside-out technique, the gliding hole is drilled first, but from the inside of the fracture to the outside. As seen in Figure 125-18, the 4.5-mm tap sleeve is centered in the opening of one of the fragments, sufficient distance back from the tip of the fragment to assure good purchase of the screw with no risk of fracture to the tip of the fragment. After this hole is drilled, the fracture is reduced and held with bone-reduction forceps. The 58-mm drill sleeve is then slipped into the gliding hole and the technique proceeds as described.

In the threaded-hole-first technique, a 3.2-mm hole is drilled in the tip of the opposite fragment through the middle of the bony spike; the screw should be kept at the appropriate angulation for the fracture. As shown in Figure 125-19, a pointed drill guide is then slipped into the threaded hole, and the fracture is reduced. A 4.5-mm tap sleeve inserted into the sleeve of the pointed drill guide can be used to help hold the reduction as well as serve as the drill guide for the gliding hole. It is also usually necessary to hold the reduction with a bone-reduction forceps. Once the gliding hole has been drilled, the near cortex is countersunk, the threaded hole tapped, and the screw placed, as in the first sequence.

In the typical spiral fracture, as seen in Figure 125-20, screws also can be used if the fracture line is at least twice as long as the diameter of the tibia at the level of the fracture. In most cases, however, a neutralization plate is necessary to protect the fracture. Note that the screws follow the spiral of

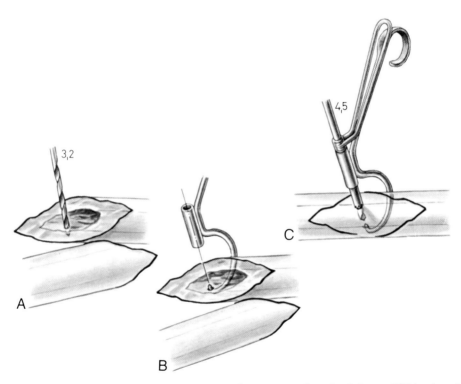

Fig. 125-19. Threaded-hole-first technique. **(A)** With the fracture unreduced, a 3.2-mm drill bit, placed through a tap sleeve (not illustrated), is used to make a hole in the center of the tip of the fragment on the deep side from the surgeon. This technique assures accurate centering of the drill hole and makes soft tissue dissection on the opposite side of this fragment unnecessary. **(B)** The pointed drill guide is then inserted into the hole, and the fracture is reduced. **(C)** The fracture is reduced and held with a reduction clamp and a 4.5-mm tap sleeve inserted into the sleeve of the pointed drill guide serves as the drill guide for the 4.5-mm drill bit and in addition, helps secure the fracture reduction. A 4.5-mm drill bit is then used to make the gliding hole. This ensures centering and coaxial drilling of the gliding hole. The fixation is then completed as illustrated in Fig. 125-17. (From Müller,[157] with permission.)

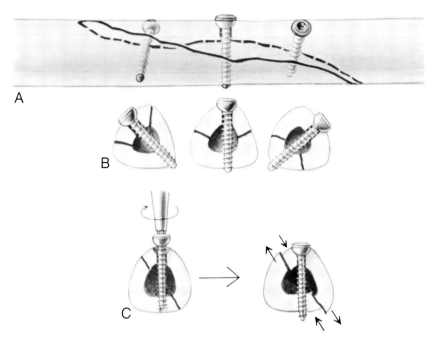

Fig. 125-20. Screw fixation of a spiral fracture. The direction of the screws must follow the spiral of the fracture if they are to provide optimal interfragmentary compression. The screws are inserted more or less at right angles to the long axis of the tibia. **(A)** Staggering of the screw heads is seen on the surface of the bone. **(B)** In these cross-sectional views, the screws can be seen to pass precisely through the middle of the opposite cortex at right angles to the fracture plane. **(C)** If the threaded hole is not properly placed, tightening of the screw will tend to displace the fracture fragments. (From Müller,[157] with permission.)

the fracture and are always at right angles to the fracture surfaces and to the long axis of the tibia. If the screw is not properly oriented (Fig. 125-20C), the fracture will displace when the screw is tightened.

These techniques become more critical as the fracture becomes more comminuted, such as in a fracture with a simple butterfly fragment (Fig. 125-21). In this case, proper placement of the threaded hole in the pointed end of the butterfly

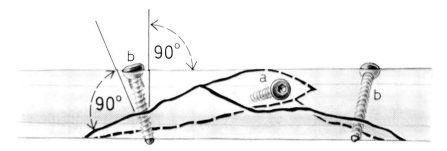

Fig. 125-21. Fixation of a simple butterfly fracture. In this example, screw *(a)* connects the two main fragments. Screws *(b)* secure the butterfly fragment to the main fragments proximally and distally. Note that screws *(b)* are placed such that they bisect the angle formed by perpendiculars to the fracture plane and to the long axis of the tibia. After all three screws have been placed, sequential tightening can be used to secure the fracture. (From Müller,[157] with permission.)

fragment is critical for absolute stability; therefore, either inside-out or threaded-hold first technique should be used. Note that screws A and C secure the butterfly fragment to the two main fragments and screw B secures the two main fragments together. In this technique, the AO group strongly emphasizes delicate surgical technique with maximum preservation of soft tissue attachments to the bone fragments. For this reason, dissection is not done subperiosteally but extraperiosteally, with minimal stripping of the bone fragments.

Plate Fixation

Plate fixation of tibial fractures remains controversial. Routine interfragmentary screw and plate fixation of tibial shaft fractures is advocated by the AO group as the optimal method for obtaining primary bone union and early restoration of function and is practiced particularly in Switzerland and Germany. In North America, routine use of closed techniques, preferably with early functional weight bearing, is advocated as the treatment of choice, as this avoids the complications of surgery.

Plates can function as static compression plates, dynamic compression (tension band) plates, neutralization plates, or buttress plates. With static compression, the tensile prestressing of the plate results in axial compression of the fracture. A transverse fracture of the tibia diaphysis is the best indication for the static compression plate. In the tibia, a single compression plate should never be used without a lag screw inserted obliquely across the fracture. A dynamic compression plate involves placement of the plate along the tension side of the

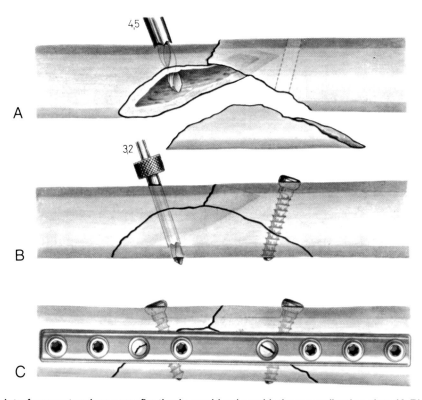

Fig. 125-22. Interfragmentary lag screw fixation in combination with the neutralization plate **(A,B)**. The fracture is first assembled and fixed with interfragmentary lag screws in the usual fashion **(C)**. A neutralization plate is then placed at approximately right angles to the interfragmentary screws and, in this case, a round hole plate is utilized. I now use only the dynamic compression plate. Note that the holes directly over the fracture sites are not filled with screws. For ideal fixation perhaps one additional screw hole could have been used on the left side of the bone in the illustration. (From Müller,[157] with permission.)

fracture. This should result in neutralization of all tensile forces acting across the fracture line. In the classic instance of a pseudarthrosis, this would be applied to the lateral surface of the tibia. The most common function of a plate in the tibia is protection of lag screw fixation by application of a contoured neutralization plate. A plate serves a buttress function when it protects the cortex or a cancellous bone graft from collapsing. In the shaft of the tibia, a buttress plate is most commonly used to bridge a diaphyseal defect which has been filled with bone graft. This is my most common indication for a plate, as I do not routinely plate closed fractures. A narrow or broad dynamic compression plate is used with 4.5-mm cortical screws.

For fractures of the shaft of the tibia, it is always necessary to conform the plate to the shape of the tibia, particularly in torsion. This is done by first applying a malleable template to the bone and using this as a guide to shape the plate with bending irons and a bending press. Figure 125-22 illustrates the application of a round-hole narrow plate as a neutralization plate on a fracture with a butterfly fragment fixed with interfragmentary screws. Note that the holes over the fracture site are not filled with screws and that the plate has been placed at approximately right angles to the plane of the interfragmentary screws.

In transverse or short oblique fractures of the tibia, static compression all of the way across the fracture is improved by slightly prebending the plate (Fig. 125-23). A bicortical screw engaging both cortices is placed in the hole nearest the fracture site on the end opposite the tension device. The tension device is then attached using a unicortical screw. Note that the plate has been placed such that the cortex to be slid toward the fracture line engages the axilla formed by the plate and the fragment to which it is fixed. An eight-hole plate is recommended in which three screws are placed bicortically and the end screw is placed unicortically. The minimum number of cortices on each side of the fracture necessary for good fixation is five, requiring two bicortical and one unicortical screw. When tension is applied, uniform compression across the fracture site is achieved by the prebend placed in the plate. Once tension has been applied, the next cortical screw is inserted in the hole, one hole away from the fracture site. This

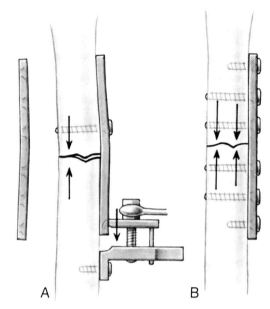

Fig. 125-23. Static compression. To achieve optimal compression across the fracture site, particularly on the cortex opposite the plate, it is necessary to overbend the plate slightly in its middle **(A)**. The plate is fixed to the bone with one screw; the hook of the tension device is then hooked through the hole of the plate and the tension device fixed to the bone. As the screw of the tension device is turned, the fracture surface comes under compression. With further tension, the plate straightens and both the bone and plate become straight. In final configuration **(B)** the whole fracture surface is under compression and there is no longer gaping in any part of the fracture. (From Müller,[157] with permission.)

permits subsequent insertion of a interfragmentary bone screw (Fig. 125-24).

The dynamic compression plate offers some advantages because angulation of the screw is possible. Optimum interfragmentary compression can be obtained when a screw angle of less than 20 degrees is used; however, up to 30 degrees is possible through the holes of the AO dynamic compression plate.

When used with the dynamic compression plate, provisional placement of the interfragmentary lag screw first is possible and usually advisable. In this case, the screw is placed by making the gliding hole first (Fig. 125-25). The fracture is reduced, the plate applied to the fracture surface, and a drill sleeve placed through the plate and the gliding

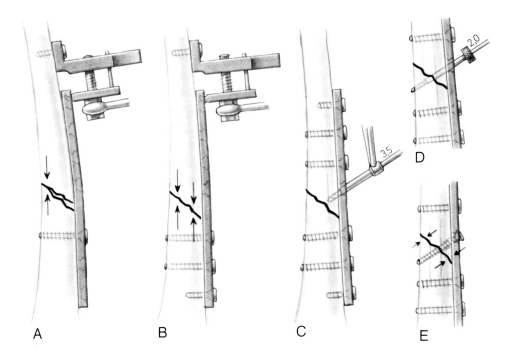

Fig. 125-24. Fixation of an oblique fracture of the tibia with a compression plate and interfragmentary lag screw. **(A,B)** The fracture is fixed. **(C)** The screws on the tension device side of the fracture are then placed, with the exception of the screw hole closest to the fracture line. A 4.5-mm tap sleeve is used as a drill guide and is directed to place the screw at right angles to the fracture. A 4.5-mm drill point is then used to make the gliding hole first **(D)**. The 58-mm drill sleeve is then inserted into the hole, and the hole is drilled and screw placed resulting in the final configuration **(E)**. (From Müller,[157] with permission.)

hole. A self-centering reduction forceps is then used to hold the fracture and plates reduced while a neutral drill guide is used to place the first screw in the fragment opposite the interfragmentary screw. With this screw in place, a load drill guide is used to place a loaded screw. Tightening of this screw results in compression across the fracture. A drill sleeve is then reinserted into the previously drilled hole and the interfragmentary screw fixation is obtained using the usual technique. The remaining screws are then placed using the neutral drill guide resulting in the final configuration illustrated in Figure 125-26.

Postoperative Care

If rigid fixation has been obtained in a reliable patient, postoperative protection in a cast or splints is not necessary. A dry sterile dressing is applied and the leg elevated 10 cm above the heart until the postoperative risk of swelling has passed. Ac-

tive assistive subtalar, ankle, and knee range-of-motion and isometric muscle exercises are begun under supervision of a physical therapist as soon as the patient's comfort permits. Non-weight bearing walking with crutches is permitted until fracture union is evident on radiographs. Partial weight-bearing is often possible by 6 to 8 weeks and full weight bearing by 16 to 24 weeks after fracture fixation. An Allgöwer patton bottom brace is often useful in achieving earlier walking.

Intramedullary Nailing

Intramedullary nailing of the tibia is not as popular as for fractures of the femur, probably because closed techniques work so well in the tibia. Closed intramedullary nailing is preferable to open nailing due to the higher incidence of infection and nonunion in the latter. Initial reamed intramedullary nailing of open fractures is usually contraindicated,

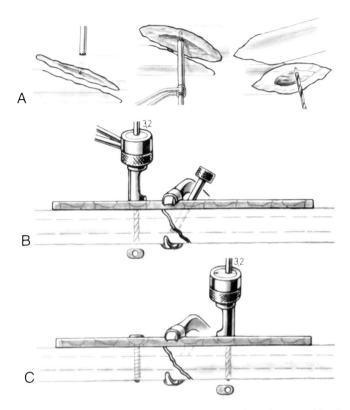

Fig. 125-25. Axial compression fixation with the dynamic compression plate combined with interfragmentary compression. In short oblique fractures rigidity can be considerably improved by the introduction of a lag screw through the plate. **(A)** Prior to reduction, the gliding hole is placed first in the fragment nearest the surgeon. **(B)** The fracture is then reduced and the plate applied to the surface of the bone with a 58-mm drill sleeve inserted through the previously drilled hole to help locate the plate. With the assembly firmly held by bone-reduction forceps, the neutral drill guide is used to make a 3.2-mm drill hole in the fragment opposite the intrafragmentary screw. **(C)** A load drill guide (Gold) is then used to place another 3.2-mm hole in the screw hole adjacent to the screw hole, which will be used for interfragmentary compression. (Modified from Müller, with permission.[157])

although delayed closed nailing after successful delayed primary closure of the wound is acceptable. Nonreamed nails, such as Lottes nails and Ender pins, have regained acceptance during the past few years for immediate fixation of open fractures. Results comparable to those using external fixators have been reported.[138,145,147,167,184] Except in rare circumstances, intramedullary nailing of the tibia should be undertaken using closed techniques rather than open reduction of the fracture. Emphasis is given to this technique.

Lottes popularized intramedullary nailing of the tibia and his nail remains the most frequently used device in the United States. The Küntscher nail is also commonly used, and a modified version of it has been popularized by the AO group. More recently, Ender pins have been advocated by Pankovich for tibial fractures.[167]

The preoperative preparation for all three of these techniques is identical. It is important to maintain full length of the tibia and preliminary treatment in traction through a pin in the calcaneus may be necessary. All three techniques are best carried out with the patient on an orthopaedic fracture table. The nail should be inserted using closed technique under fluoroscopic control. The patient is placed on the operating table, as illustrated in Figure 125-27. The best support device under the knee is the Lottes knee saddle. It provides the best distribution of pressure about the knee and helps

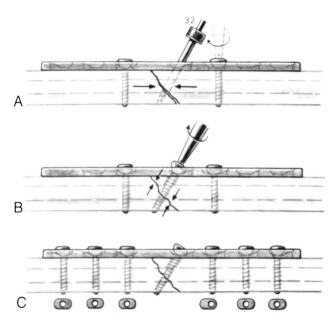

Fig. 125-26. (A) Axial compression is achieved by tightening the screw in the loaded hole. A 58-mm drill sleeve is then placed in the gliding hole as illustrated, and a 3.2-mm drill point is used to place the threaded hole in the opposite cortex. **(B)** As this screw is tightened, interfragmentary compression is achieved. **(C)** The remainder of the screws are placed with a neutral drill guide. Some authorities would prefer a nine-hole plate in which the end screws would be unicortical. (From Müller,[157] with permission.)

prevent injury to neurovascular structures. The foot is placed in a foot holder, and the knee is flexed to at least 90 degrees. The other limb is placed in abduction so that AP and lateral views with a fluoroscope can be obtained without difficulty. The entire shaft of the tibia and knee is then prepared in the usual manner and draped so that the anterior half of the knee and entire tibia is available to the surgeon. I prefer to apply sheets above and below and cover the entire tibia with adhesive clear plastic drape so that it is visible and available for direct manipulation. Preliminary closed reduction is obtained under fluoroscopic control.

AO Intramedullary Nailing

A vertical incision approximately 5 cm in length is placed directly over the patellar tendon. The tendon is split and access to the cortex of the tibia is gained just superior to the tibial tubercle and in front of the fat pad of the knee (Fig. 125-28). Some surgeons prefer to enter just medial to the patellar tendon. An awl is then used to penetrate the cortex

of the tibia. Care is taken to stay in the longitudinal axis of the tibia. A 3.2-mm guide pin is then slid into the proximal fragment and, with closed manipulation, is passed across the fracture site into the distal fragment and subsequently to the subchondral bone of the distal tibia. Care is taken that the guide pin is in the central portion of the distal tibia on both the AP and lateral views. If reduction of the fracture is difficult an 8- or 9-mm intramedullary nail can be slid into the proximal fragment and used as a lever to help reduce the fracture. By measuring the length of guide pin remaining outside the tibia and by comparing it with another guide pin of like length, the proper length nail can be determined. For maximum fixation, it is generally advisable to drive the nail to within 1 cm of the plafond of the tibia and to the subchondral bone in distal fractures. Using flexible reamers driven with a high-torque power reamer, the tibia is then reamed up to the appropriate size rod. In general, once good cortical contact with the reamer is obtained, the canal should be enlarged an additional 2 mm. In the AO system, the reamer size should match the rod

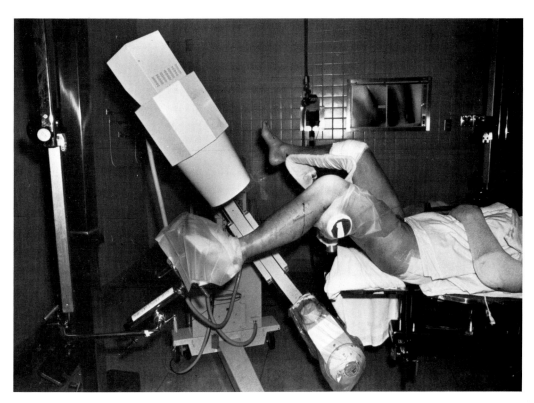

Fig. 125-27. Closed intramedullary nailing of the tibia. The patient is placed on an orthopaedic table (I prefer the Chick-Langren table) and the procedure is performed with the aid of a fluoroscope with an image intensifier and disk recorder. The patient is placed supine and the knee is bent to an angle of somewhat more than 90 degrees over a large, well-padded bolster placed beneath the knee. Care is taken to avoid injury to the peroneal nerve. Traction is usually applied through a foot holder, but can also be applied through a traction pin in either the os calcis or distal tibial metaphysis. If a tibial metaphyseal pin is used care must be taken when the nail is driven home to avoid hitting the pin. We normally use the foot piece. Proper rotation should be ensured. (From Chapman,[38a] with permission.)

size to be used, however, it is always wise to confirm the size of the rod as compared with the reamer by testing both in a go-no-go guide. Reaming should be done throughout the isthmus of the tibia and not in the cancellous bone of the distal metaphysis. Once reaming has been completed, the rod can be driven. The driving assembly is assembled, as illustrated in Figure 125-29. The most common error is directing the rod too far posteriorly, resulting in either posterior penetration of the cortex or comminution. This can be avoided by driving under fluoroscopic control with careful technique (Fig. 125-30). During reaming and driving, the traction on the extremity should have been

released to avoid prolonged tension on the soft tissues and to provide impaction when the nail is driven. This ensures optimal interfragmentary contact, which gives rotational stability and better fixation. The rod should be left with its proximal end flush with the proximal cortex of the tibia. For additional rotational stability, the ledge wires of Herzog and a proximal screw through the nail can be used. The insertion site is copiously irrigated with sterile saline to remove all bone fragments and is closed in the usual fashion. A typical fracture is seen in Figure 125-31. For a more detailed description of this technique the reader is referred to the AO manual.[157]

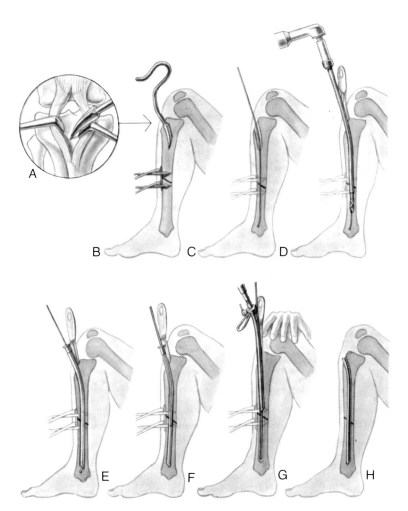

Fig. 125-28. Intramedullary nailing of the tibia. **(A)** A longitudinal incision is made over the patellar tendon. The patellar tendon is split and an awl used to perforate the cortex above the tibia tubercle. **(B)** Keep the awl in the long axis of the tibia to avoid penetrating the posterior cortex. **(C)** The fracture is reduced, and a 3 mm reaming guide with curved tip pointing forwards is placed across the fracture site and down to the subchondral bone of the distal tibia. Proper location of the reaming guide is confirmed with the fluoroscope. **(D)** A tissue protector is placed and the entire isthmus area of the tibia is reamed in 0.5-mm increments until the canal has been enlarged 2 mm larger than the normal canal diameter. **(E)** When reaming is completed, the plastic medullary tube is inserted over the reaming guide, it is removed, and the 4-mm nail guide is inserted through the medullary tube **(F)**. **(G)** The medullary tube is removed and the appropriately sized tibial nail is driven. The nail should move easily with each drive of the ram and its progress checked frequently with the fluoroscope. Once into the distal fragment, the nail guide can be removed, the fracture impacted, and the nail driven home so that the top of the nail is flush with the cortex **(H)**. (Modified from Müller, with permission.[157])

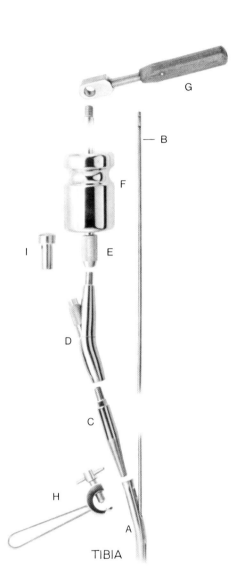

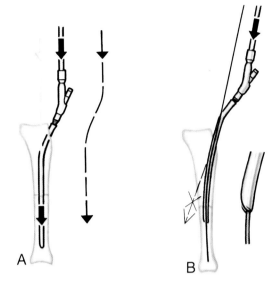

Fig. 125-30. **(A)** The curved driving piece makes it possible to drive the nail in the long axis of the nail and tibia. The driving assembly, the 4-mm nail guide, and the tapered tip of the nail are all designed to prevent posterior penetration of the cortex of the tibia and ensure smooth driving of the nail across the fracture line. **(B)** In spite of this, the surgeon must be careful to avoid impingement of the nail on the proximal portion of the distal fragment during driving and a concerted effort must be made to keep the nail in the long axis of the tibia. (From Müller,[157] with permission.)

Fig. 125-29. AO instrumentation for insertion of the tibial intramedullary nail. **(A)** The intramedullary nail. **(B)** A 4-mm nail guide. **(C)** The threaded bolt which is twisted into the proximal portion of the nail. **(D)** The curved driving piece is attached to the conical bolt, tightening the knurled nut. **(E)** The cannulated weight guide rod is then attached. **(F)** The ram is placed on the guide rod. **(G)** The flexible grip is then attached to the guide rod. **(H)** The guide handle is attached to the nail and permits the nail to be held to control rotation during insertion. **(I)** A driving head can be inserted onto the curved driving piece **(D)** if the ram is not to be used. (Modified from Müller, with permission.[157])

Postoperative Care

The postoperative regimen is as described for screw and plate fixation, except that immediate full weight bearing is desirable in many fractures. The intramedullary rod is a load-sharing device. If the fracture is in the middle two-thirds of the diaphysis, is short oblique or transverse, and is free of comminution, full weight bearing is possible without risk of shortening. External protection is usually unnecessary. Using crutches, most patients will achieve full unprotected weight bearing by 3 to 6 weeks. In unstable fractures, delayed weight bearing or protection in a splint or cast may be necessary.

Locked Intramedullary Nailing

Since the last edition of this book, reamed intramedullary nails with the capacity for crosslocking have become popular. They are indicated when-

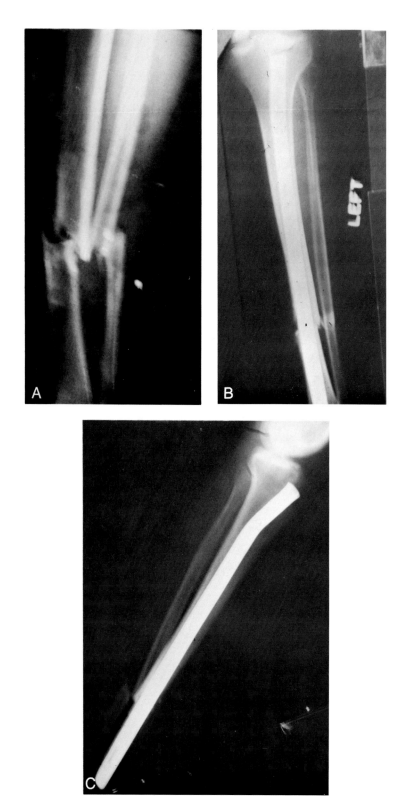

Fig. 125-31. Intramedullary nailing of the tibia. **(A)** Preoperative anteroposterior radiograph of a fracture of the tibia and fibula. **(B)** Postoperative radiograph showing AO intramedullary rod in position. **(C)** Lateral view of **(B)**. (Courtesy of Lorraine J. Day, M.D., San Francisco, CA.)

ever a nonlocked intramedullary nail will not provide sufficient stability, and it is undesirable to augment fixation with a long-leg cast. All the unstable fracture patterns illustrated in Figure 125-14 are indications for locked nailing. Dynamic nailing, that is, locking only one end of the nail, is indicated when the fracture pattern is stable but either the proximal or distal fragment is too short to gain adequate fixation with the nail alone. Static locking, that is, placing cross-screws at both ends of the nail, is indicated in any fracture pattern in which shortening or malrotation is a significant risk. My experience is limited to the Grosse-Kempf nail, which is the most popular in North America. Several other interlocking nails have just come on the market that in principle are essentially identical to the Grosse-Kempf nail.

With the exception of the instrumentation for driving the nail, the procedure is identical to that just described for the AO reamed intramedullary nail. After the nail has been driven into place, crosslocking is performed. A jig (Fig. 125-32) is used for proximal crosslocking. Because the jig is very short and the distance from the attachment of the jig to the proximal hole in the nail short, crosslocking is simple and reliable. Follow the manufacturer's directions carefully. The jig must be mounted onto the nail before it is driven completely into the tibia, as this makes mounting the jig easier. Once the nail is in satisfactory position, the drill sleeves are placed in the jig and the skin is marked to place the incision precisely. After subperiosteal exposure of the bone, the drill sleeve is slid down to bone and the tibia is drilled through the nail with the appropriately sized drill, and the screw is placed. It is important to confirm the accuracy of placement with the fluoroscope. We have not found the distal crosslocking guides in the Grosse-Kempf system sufficiently reliable to merit their use. Crosslocking with free hand technique is

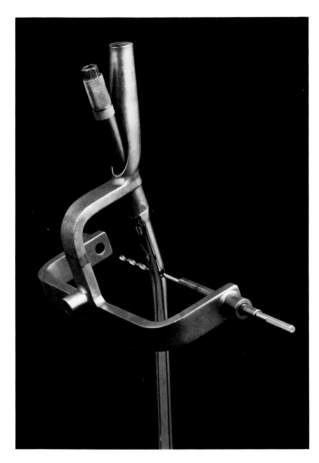

Fig. 125-32. Grosse-Kempf tibial nail with drill point in place through proximal crosslocking guide.

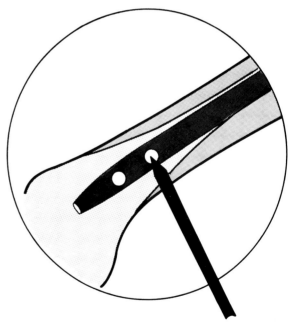

Fig. 125-33. Lateral fluoroscopic view showing perfect superimposition of the distal crosslocking holes of a locking intramedullary nail. A hand-held guide is centered over the proximal hole (From Chapman,[38a] with permission.)

advised. The fluoroscope is brought into the lateral position and the distal crosslocking holes of the nail visualized. The fluoroscope must be precisely aligned with the hole to be crosslocked such that the two holes in the rod are perfectly superimposed, are perfectly round, and are precisely in the middle of the fluoroscope field (see Fig. 125-33). A short incision is made and the bone exposed. A long-handled awl is brought into the operative field, with care taken to keep the surgeon's hand out of the direct beam of the fluoroscope. The tip of the awl is placed precisely in the center of the hole in the rod as visualized on the fluoroscope. It is then tilted up into direct alignment with the fluoroscope tube. While maintaining this alignment, the awl is driven into the bone. If the bone is fairly soft, the awl can be driven down to the hole in the nail. If it is hard, the appropriately sized drill point is brought in and the rod drilled through, with the drill point kept precisely aligned with the head of the fluoroscope. The drill point is left in place and the power source removed, and it is verified on the fluoroscope that the drill point is through the rod. Finally, the correct length screw is placed and it is verified on the fluoroscope that crosslocking has been accurately performed (Fig. 125-34).

Postoperative Care

Dynamically locked rods with stable configurations usually permit early weight bearing without external protection using crutches. Patients are allowed to progress to full weight bearing as tolerated. If the fracture pattern is unstable but dynamically locked, immobilization in a functional brace with early weight bearing is usually possible. It is not advisable to bear weight, prior to bone union, on fractures requiring static locking, as screw or rod breakage may occur. I advise partial weight bearing with crutches with no external immobilization until 12 weeks. If adequate healing is seen, the rod can then be dynamized by removing the distal screws and weight bearing can begin with or without an orthosis depending upon the stability of the fracture. The stability of fixation with interlocking is excellent, and a rehabilitation program of joint range-of-motion and muscle strengthening exercises is an important part of the treatment program.

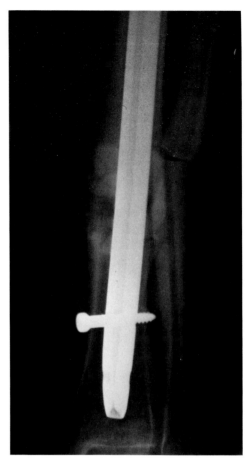

Fig. 125-34. Anteroposterior radiograph of the left tibia. Osteotomy with distally crosslocked Grosse-Kempf nail in place.

Lottes Nailing

Using closed technique and the Lottes nail, the patient is treated preoperatively and placed on the fracture table as described for the AO tibial nailing. The skin incision is made in the longitudinal axis of the leg and is placed one finger-breadth medial to the tibial tubercle and extended proximally to the level of the knee joint. The medial metaphysis of the tibia is exposed in the lower 2.5 cm of this wound and the knee joint is not violated. A 9.5-mm drill is then used to perforate the metaphyseal cortex on the medial side of the tibial tubercle. A Küntscher awl can be used as well. Once the cortex is perforated, it is extremely important to swing the drilling hand toward the knee to place the drill in the longitudinal axis of the tibia. Proper position can be verified with the fluoroscope. The most common error in this technique is to perforate the posterior cortex of the tibia. When the Lottes nail is driven through an improperly placed drill hole, it is nearly impossible to avoid driving the nail out the back of the tibia. Improper alignment of the drill hole can result in the upper fragment splitting and also in the nail bending, producing recurvatum. To avoid injury to the skin and soft tissues, it is helpful to use a metal shield in the proximal portion of the incision. The placement of this drill hole is illustrated in Figure 125-35.

The length of nail should have been determined preoperatively using a tape ruler to measure the distance from the medial malleolus to the tibial tubercle. A nail should be selected that comes to within 2 cm of the tibial plafond. This can be veri-

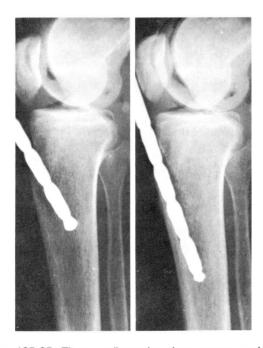

Fig. 125-35. These radiographs show proper and improper placement of the drill bit for a Lottes nail. On the left the drill is angulated too posteriorly and, if drilling is continued in this plane, perforation of the posterior cortex will occur. On the right, the drill has been pressed against the knee to keep the long axis of the drill within the canal of the tibia. (From Lottes,[128a] with permission.)

fied on the operating room table by picking a nail of the appropriate size and laying it along side the tibia. Reaming is not necessary, and the nail is driven without a guide pin. The largest diameter that will pass through the isthmus without jamming should be used. This can be determined preoperatively by measuring the patient's radiograph. The driver is attached to the nail and the tip of the nail is then inserted into the drill hole with its anterior fin pointing forward. The surgeon should then depress the driver toward the knee to drive the nail parallel to the anteromedial border of the tibia. The nail needs to be pressed into the skin over the knee. The nail is driven under fluoroscopic control and any errors in alignment corrected. When the nail is driven home, the driver should strike the cortex, leaving sufficient thread available for extraction. As the nail is driven into the distal fragment, the traction is released to impact the bone fragments and obtain better rotational control.

Preoperative traction to achieve adequate length in the fracture will usually make alignment easy. If alignment cannot be achieved by closed means and the surgeon can justify the risk of opening the fracture, a small incision can be made over the subcutaneous border of the tibia and the fracture manipulated to facilitate passing the nail across the fracture site.

To enhance union and encourage impaction at the fracture site, Lottes now routinely sections the fibula at the time of original nailing before insertion of the nail to facilitate manipulation of the fracture, particularly where the fracture is at the junction of the middle and distal thirds.

In unstable fractures, plating of the fibula prevents shortening and provides fairly good rotational control. Plating of the fibula increases the risk of nonunion of the tibia, and bone grafting may be necessary. We reserve this technique for open fractures (Fig. 125-36).

Postoperative Care

Lottes nails provide less stable fixation than the AO Küntscher nail, particularly in rotation. Lottes routinely elevates the patient's leg until swelling has dissipated, begins early rehabilitation, and then applies a long-leg cast. In stable configurations he

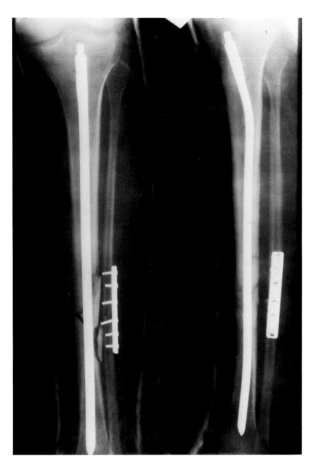

Fig. 125-36. Unstable type I open fracture of the tibia and fibula stabilized with a Lottes nail and a plate on the fibula to prevent shortening and help control rotation. A bone graft may be necessary. (From Chapman,[38a] with permission.)

permits the patient to begin immediate weight bearing. After 6 weeks, the cast is removed and unrestricted weight bearing, with the assistance of crutches if necessary, is permitted.

Ender Pinning of Tibial Fractures

Pankovich[167] and others[138,147] have popularized the use of Ender pin fixation for tibial fractures. Its advantages are that the pins are inserted percutaneously; reaming is not necessary; the small diameter of the nails interferes minimally with intramedullary blood supply; and the procedure can be performed rather quickly, has a minimal infection rate, and is suitable for patients with multiple inju-

ries for whom immediate fixation under adverse circumstances is desirable. The disadvantages are that the fixation with Ender pins is unstable and perfect alignment is often not achieved, external protection is always necessary, and the technique is less suitable for fractures in the distal third.

See the work of Pankovich[167] for a description of his technique, which differs somewhat from that described here. The preoperative preparation and setup and preparation of the patient in the operating room are identical to that described for Lottes and AO nails.

The nails are inserted proximally to distally through the medial and lateral metaphysis of the tibia. A 2.5-cm incision is made longitudinally over the medial subcutaneous border of the metaphysis of the tibia and either a 6-mm drill or Küntscher awl is used to perforate the proximal cortex approximately 2.5 cm beneath the joint line of the knee. A 3.5-mm Ender nail of sufficient length to reach to the subchondral bone of the distal tibia is then inserted with the Ender nail driver. Under direct fluoroscopic control, this nail is then passed down the proximal fragment, across the fracture site, and into medial side of the distal fragment. A second pin is inserted from the lateral side using a similar approach. It is usually necessary to split the muscles of the anterior compartment somewhat to localize the insertion point for the nail. If the reduction is not perfect, it is occasionally necessary first to pass a nail through the medial side and use it to reduce the fracture while a second nail is passed either from the medial or lateral side. Although one nail will provide some fixation, ideal fixation requires at least two nails and on occasion three (Fig. 125-37).

Postoperative Care

Postoperatively, the patient should be protected in a long-leg plaster cast although it is usually possible to change this to a cast brace with a hinged knee and hinged ankle early. In pure transverse or short oblique fractures weight bearing can be begun immediately. However, if the fracture configuration will permit shortening, weight bearing should be delayed. Protection with a cast or cast brace is usually necessary for approximately 6 weeks, after which time sufficient stability is present that the patient can be left free. If there is any question, a

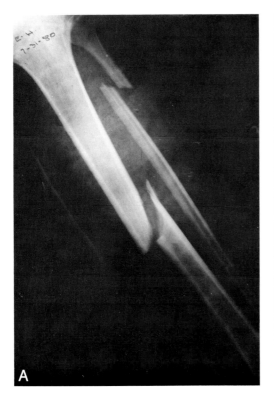

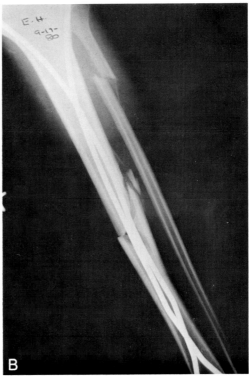

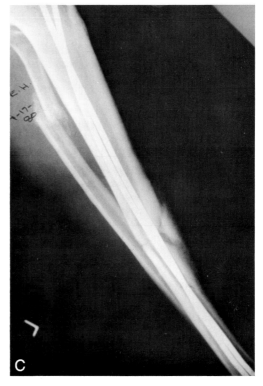

Fig. 125-37. Ender nailing of the tibia. **(A)** Anteroposterior radiograph showing oblique midshaft fracture of the tibia with associated fracture of the fibula. **(B)** Because of difficulties in controlling length, fixation was performed as shown in this anteroposterior radiograph. **(C)** Lateral view of **(B)**. (Courtesy of Frederick Pollack, M.D., Chicago.)

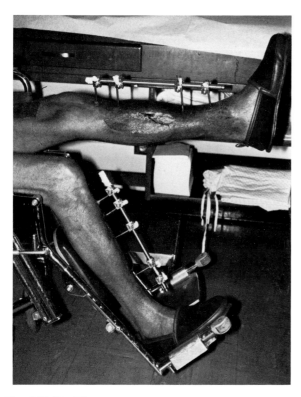

Fig. 125-38. Bilateral single-plane half-pin AO external fixators. (From Chapman,[38a] with permission.)

cast brace can be continued beyond 6 weeks, as this permits excellent function.

This technique should be undertaken with care in older patients whose tibiae are osteoporotic because the pins will not infrequently crush the metaphyseal cortical bone of the tibia and drop into the intramedullary canal. This risks penetration into the knee joint and loss of fixation.

External Fixation

External fixation for fractures of the tibia has been popular since the latter part of the nineteenth century. The development of more versatile and rigid frames that provide excellent stabilization has led to renewed interest in the advantages of external fixation. Popular external fixation devices are Vidal's modification of the Hoffmann frame, the AO external fixator, and the Roger Anderson frame, which have been the most widely used fixators in the United States. Many other types are now available. The advantage of external fixators is that they eliminate the necessity for a circumferential plaster cast when a cast is either contraindicated or impractical and they often provide anatomic reduction.

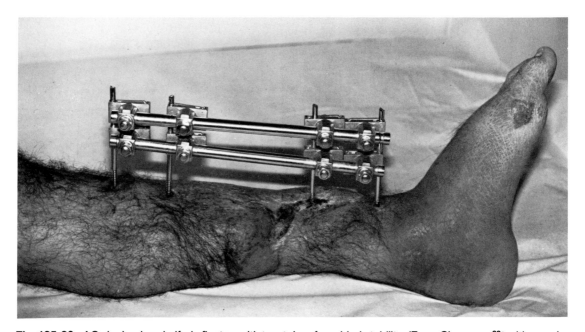

Fig. 125-39. AO single-plane half-pin fixator, with two tubes for added stability. (From Chapman,[38a] with permission.)

External fixators are most easily classified into those based on full pins and those using only half pins. Nearly all systems currently available have been modified for use with either full pins or half pins. The classic full-pin frame is the Hoffmann frame (see Fig. 125-46). At publication of the last edition, this was the standard frame in use. Since then, half-pin frames, as exemplified by the AO fixator (Fig. 125-38), are most widely used.[82] Half-pin fixators can achieve adequate stability approaching that of the full-pin frames. Half-pin frames vastly improve the versatility of pin location, avoid tie down of tendon units, and minimize the risk of injury to neurovascular structures. Half-pin fixators can be constructed in many different configurations, but three basic patterns are most frequently used. Figure 125-39 shows a single anterior plane fixator, with double tubes mounted on the pins for increased stability. A more stable configuration uses two half-pin frames (Fig. 125-40) and an even more stable configuration uses a full-pin frame, attached to an anterior half-pin frame (Fig. 125-41). The latter is known as a delta frame.

The most frequent indication for an external fixator is an open fracture of the tibia and fibula. Any fracture accompanied by a vascular injury in which bone instability may threaten the repair, or a fracture accompanied by a compartment syndrome, is also a strong indication. Severely comminuted and unstable closed fractures not suitable for traditional internal fixation or casts or traction immobilization are also an indication. External fixation may be used to augment the stability achieved with minimal internal fixation.

Any closed or open fracture of the tibia that is relatively stable and unaccompanied by severe soft tissue damage and that is treatable by traditional means is a relative contraindication to the use of external fixation. The risk of pin-tract infection, soft tissue tiedown, and injury to neurovascular structures must be offset by the advantages to be gained.

Surgical Technique

Fixators are applied in the operating room. Strict sterile technique is required, and the placement of multiple pins generally requires a regional or general anesthetic.

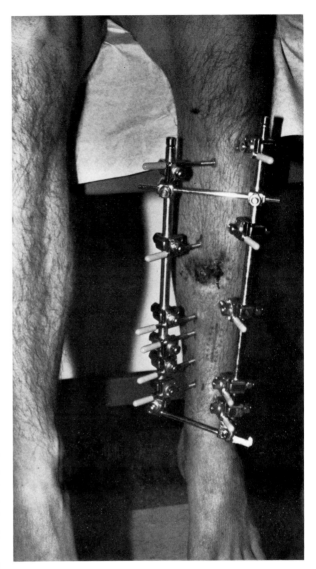

Fig. 125-40. AO biplanar external fixator. (From Chapman,[38a] with permission.)

Preoperative planning is important to avoid difficulties with the fixator. The locations of the pins is drawn on the radiograph. If the surgeon is unfamiliar with the equipment the fixator is preassembled to match the drawing to ascertain that the components available will permit the planned approach. Pin location is critical to avoid tying down tendons or muscles and to avoid injury to neurovascular bundles. It is beyond the scope of this chapter to present more detail of the anatomy of the leg rela-

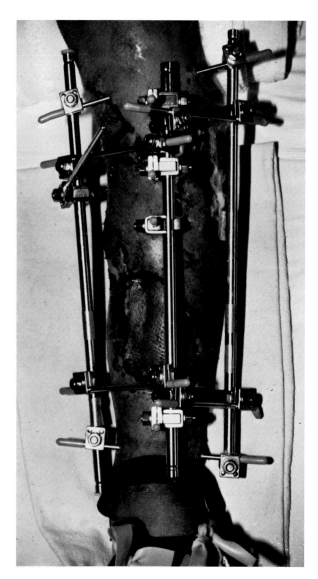

Fig. 125-41. AO delta configuration external fixator. (From Chapman,[38a] with permission.)

tive to pin placement than already provided. See the excellent description by Greene.[82] This text is mandatory reading for anybody using external fixators. A few general comments are in order. In the tibia, all pins are inserted through the subcutaneous border of the tibia first. It is verified that there is no tension on the skin. It is preferable to place the pin through intact skin. In the proximal quarter of the tibia, pins placed in the transverse axis are quite safe. Those placed in the sagittal plane risk injuring

the neurovascular bundle posteriorly and caution is necessary. Moving from proximal to distal, in the next quarter, pins placed in the usual locations do not threaten neurovascular bundles unless the pin penetrates too deeply posteriorly. One should be cautious with pins penetrating from the medial side at 30 degrees to the sagittal plane, as the anterior tibial neurovascular bundle is at risk. In the next most distal quarter, straight transverse pins are reasonably safe; however, pins entering at an angle on the subcutaneous border threaten the anterior tibial neurovascular bundle and straight anterior to posterior is safer. In the distal quarter, the anterior tibial artery and nerve lie on the lateral border of the tibia and pass from posterior to anterior exiting into the dorsal compartment of the foot. Transverse pins in the proximal portion of this compartment are contraindicated because of the high risk of injury to this neurovascular bundle. Full transverse pins are best placed in the proximal and distal one-fifth of the tibia, if needed.

AO Half-Pin Single-plane Fixator

The following technique is generic to the application of any single-plane fixator. With a single-frame fixator, I prefer to place the frame at right angles to the subcutaneous surface of the tibia, in its anterior portion, avoiding the thick cortical bone of the anterior ridge of the tibia. If two half-pin frames are to be used, I place the first frame about 1 cm posterior to the anterior ridge of the tibia and close to the sagittal plane and the second 1 cm anterior to the posterior border of the tibia in the frontal plane. The angle between these two frames should be between 60 and 90 degrees. For the purposes of this description, it assumed that the fracture is transverse and mid-diaphyseal. The first pin is placed just distal to the tibial tubercle. Good-quality cortical bone is present in this region. Proximal to the tubercle, the cortical bone is not of sufficient thickness to give an adequate purchase for a half-pin. To place this pin, a drill sleeve is used and predrilling is done with a 3.5-mm drill bit for a 5-mm fixation pin. The drill point is cooled with saline. An appropriate-length fixation pin is inserted using hand power. Proper length is verified on the fluoroscope. A preliminary reduction of the fracture is performed, making certain that rotation

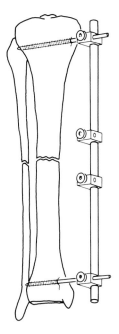

Fig. 125-42. Initial step in the application of a single-plane fixator. See text for details. (From Chapman,[38a] with permission.)

is correct. A second fixation pin is inserted 3 to 4 cm proximal from the ankle joint. Four universal clamps are assembled on the appropriate length tube and the two outer clamps are secured to the fixation pins (Fig. 125-42). Then the fracture is reduced as anatomically as possible. The inner two universal clamps are secured loosely to the fixator tube, the drill sleeves placed through the universal clamp, and the next two pins placed. These are placed through good-quality skin approximately 2.5 to 5 cm away from the fracture site. Pin length is verified by fluoroscopy. Then all pins are slightly loosened, final reduction achieved, the tube placed approximately 2.5 cm from the surface of the skin, and all the universal clamps secured. During this maneuver, it is desirable to introduce compression across the fracture site in stable fracture patterns. This can be done by hand or with the compressor in the AO system. Finally, to minimize the chances of pin loosening, eccentric forces are introduced between the proximal and distal pin sets. This can be achieved by loosening one of the proximal universal pin clamps and then slightly distracting the pin away from its partner and resecuring the clamp. A

similar maneuver is carried out distally. The final configuration is illustrated in Figure 125-43. For biplanar frames, this process is then repeated; however, since the fracture is already anatomically reduced and under compression, application is much simpler. The two frames are then cross-connected at two points near their ends with connecting rods. The delta frame is used when sufficient stability cannot be obtained with the biplanar frame or when there is extensive comminution with many segmental pieces. In this situation, it is often easier to first place a transverse pin in the proximal fragment and in the distal fragment. Connect these with medial and lateral longitudinal tube. This simple fixator can then be used to distract the fracture and obtain preliminary alignment prior to application of the anterior frame.

Hoffman Fixator: Quadrilateral

For best stability, the minimum number of pins in a cluster is three. They are placed close to the fracture without entering the fracture itself or other fracture lines. The constraints of the frame will dictate the distance separating the components. The most commonly used pin is a transfixing pin that goes through and through. Half pins are available for special applications.

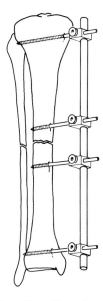

Fig. 125-43. Final configuration of a single-plane fixator. See text for details. (From Chapman,[38a] with permission.)

The pin closest to the fracture site is placed first. All pins are predrilled with a drill point somewhat smaller than the diameter of the pins. The first pin can be placed freehand and should be at right angles to the long axis of the tibia in all planes. A skin incision with a #15 blade facilitates entry of the pin and prevents skin necrosis due to skin tension about the pin. The initial drill hole is made with power equipment but low speed should be used and the drill point cooled to avoid thermal necrosis of bone. The first fixation pin is then placed using a brace and bit. The pin should always be driven by hand. Even with predrilling and hand power, it is important to avoid overheating of the pins. After the first pin has been placed, the pin guide is placed over the pin and the appropriate pin distribution is selected. For the average tibial fracture, pins driven through the holes marked 1, 3, and 5 will provide appropriate pin spacing (Fig. 125-44). It is important to place the pin closest to

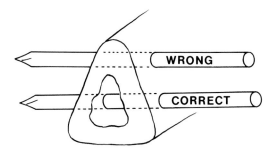

Fig. 125-45. Pin placement. Pins should be placed through the middle of the medullary canal. The anterior cortex should be avoided.

the fracture first and the pin farthest from the fracture site second, so that the intervening pins will be in the proper location. Proper location of the pins on a cross-sectional view is seen in Figure 125-45. A common error is to place the pins too anteriorly through solid cortical bone rather than through the

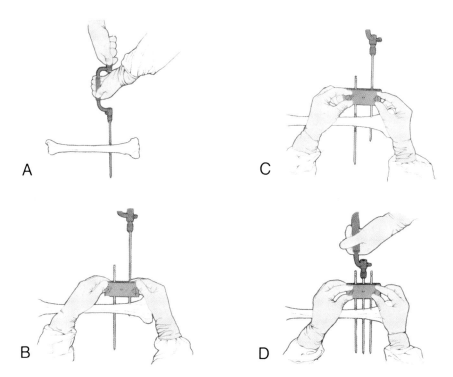

Fig. 125-44. **(A)** The initial pin is driven nearest to the fracture site. The pin guide is then used to place the other pins. The holes marked 1, 3, and 5 will usually provide appropriate pin spacing. **(B)** The pin guide is placed over the initial pin using hole #1. Pin 5 should be placed to assure that all three pins will be properly located. **(C)** As the threads of the pin contact the guide it must be opened. **(D)** The third pin is placed in hole #3. (Courtesy of Howmedica Inc.)

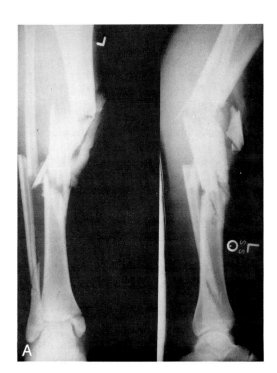

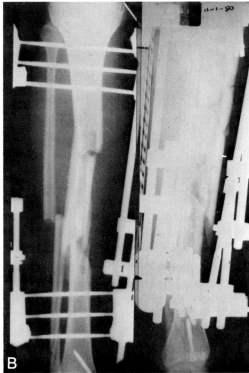

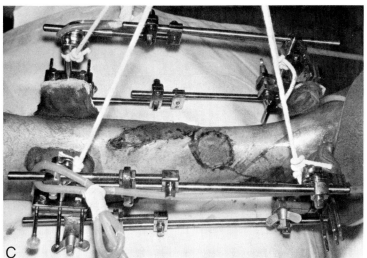

Fig. 125-46. Hoffmann external fixation. **(A)** This open comminuted fracture of the tibia and fibula in a 28-year-old motorcyclist was treated with irrigation, debridement, and application of an external fixator, and the wounds were left open. **(B)** These AP and lateral radiographs show the initial reduction, which was improved later. **(C)** These skin grafts were applied 5 days after injury to achieve wound closure and are shown here at 18 days after injury. The external fixation suspended by rope from an overhead bed frame and a dorsiflexion foot support are shown (photograph of another patient).

intramedullary canal. This results in overheating of the bone and a higher incidence of necrosis. As previously discussed, awareness of the location of neurovascular bundles is important to avoid injury to these structures. Inadvertent perforation of soft tissues posterior to the tibia is particularly dangerous. After the placement of a group of pins above and below the fracture site, universal ball joints with rods (pin clamps) are attached to the pins. These should be applied as close to the limb as possible without contacting the skin and permitting adequate space for swelling. The ball joints are placed in line with each other, as this will facilitate manipulation of the frame and fracture. One set of adjustable connecting rods can now be placed and the universal joints left loose. Stop clips make assembly of the frame easier. The fracture is reduced and the nuts tightened to maintain reduction. The second set of connecting rods can then be applied. If the fracture is transverse or a short, oblique compression across the fracture should always be applied. This greatly enhances mechanical stability of the fracture site. After final adjustment of the frame, all the pin entry sites should be checked and skin incisions made to relieve any tension. A complete Hoffmann fixator is shown in Figure 125-46.

A light sterile dressing is then applied about the pin entry sites. If significant swelling is anticipated, bulk cotton can be placed in and about the frame and the entire frame and extremity then wrapped with bias-cut stockinette to apply compression. A dorsiflexion foot support should be applied immediately since the foot tends to hang in equinus in the frame and a heel cord contracture can develop very quickly. This should be an elastic-type support so that the patient can begin early ankle motion. When the transfixing pins are placed, the foot should be dorsiflexed to avoid tieing down the musculotendinous units in equinus.

Postoperative Care

Elevation of the extremity 10 cm above the heart helps prevent edema. Immediate range-of-motion exercises of the ankle, joints of the foot, and knee, as well as isometric exercises of uninvolved muscle groups are usually possible. To avoid pin-tract infection, good pin care is necessary. Because most of the patients are discharged with external fixation devices in place, while under nursing supervision in the hospital, they should be taught how to carry out pin care. The pin sites are cleaned daily with a betadine swab to remove all crusts. This permits drainage and prevents creation of a closed space, which can become infected. In most cases only a day dressing is necessary. A topical antibiotic ointment about the pins may be helpful. If the fixator has been placed in compression, partial weight bearing with crutches is usually possible.

Management of Complications

Pin-tract infection is the most frequent complication, with a rate of less than 5 percent, although up to a 40 percent infection rate was reported in earlier series. This is usually due to improper insertion technique. If infection occurs but the pin is stable, and the infection is limited to the soft tissues, incision and drainage of the soft tissues about the pin site, leaving the pin in place, will suffice. If radiologic or clinical evidence of loosening of the pin is evident, another pin should be placed in a separate location, and the infected pin should be removed.

The distraction imposed by the usual fixator configuration, when left in place for more than 6 weeks, has a high correlation with delayed union. Proper postoperative management of external fixator frames is important to avoid delayed union and malunion. In cases in which good bone apposition is present, delayed union is avoided by allowing early weight bearing and by making the external fixation configuration progressively more flexible. If the fracture site can be placed under compression and the frame is stable, it may be possible to begin partial weight bearing immediately and to progress to full weight bearing using crutches for protection. If insufficient instability can be achieved to permit weight bearing in the frame, removal of the frame at 6 to 8 weeks and application of a functional weight-bearing cast or brace may be the best approach. To avoid malunion, however, at the time of frame removal, the fracture must have enough stability to prevent both shortening and manual translation of the fracture. In fractures with defects or with extensive comminution, early bone grafting should be considered. As the fracture heals, it is desirable to allow progressive weight bearing through the bone by gradually changing the configuration of the frame to make it more flexible. In a single-bar frame, this can be achieved by moving the bar farther away from the skin. In rigid frames, such as a biplanar or delta frame, one plane at a time is removed until it is reduced to a single-plane frame. Joint range-of-motion and muscle-strengthening muscle exercises are important throughout the healing period. At frame removal, I apply a functional brace in all cases to avoid unexpected angulation of the fracture.

As an alternative regimen, some surgeons prefer to use external fixators to stabilize the limb for soft tissue treatment and then convert to internal fixation early. This conversion occurs as soon as the soft tissue wounds have healed and the major risk of infection has passed. The pin sites must be dry and sealed prior to internal fixation. This is achieved by removing the frame and placing the limb in a cast for 10 to 20 days prior to fixation. In my opinion, the safest procedure following external fixation is closed unreamed intramedullary nailing with Lottes nails or Ender pins. Additional stability can be achieved by plating the fibula. Reamed nails are satisfactory in closed fractures but, in my opinion, are contraindicated in open fractures. Plate fixation may occasionally be indicated but carries the highest risk of all the types of internal fixation following external fixation. For more details on this decision-making process, see the algorithm in Figure 125-49.

COMPLICATIONS

Tibial and fibular fractures can be followed by many complications, usually attributable to the nature of the fracture but which can also be due to treatment. The most common acute complications are infection, loss of skin and soft tissues, neurovascular injury, compartment syndrome, and amputation. Later complications are delayed union, nonunion, infected nonunion, malunion, joint stiffness,[141d] traumatic arthritis, sympathetic dystrophy, refracture, and late amputation. Systemic complications such as fat embolism can also occur but are beyond the scope of this chapter.

Infection

Infection is most commonly due to an open fracture, although it occasionally occurs as an early complication of internal fixation.[46] Infection can also present late, and acute infection can become chronic osteomyelitis. *Staphylococcus aureus* and *Streptococcus* still remain the most common infecting organisms. However, patients with open wounds who are in a hospital for prolonged periods, particularly if on antibiotics, not infrequently develop gram-negative infections such as pseudomonas. Acute infection, particularly with an abscess, requires early incision and drainage and thorough debridement and irrigation to remove all infected and nonviable tissue. Cultures, both anaerobic and aerobic should be taken and an appropriate regimen of high-dose intravenous antibiotics instituted. In most cases, 3 weeks of treatment is necessary, and occasionally 6 weeks is required. Afterward, prolonged oral antibiotics are necessary in some cases. Infection is usually fairly easy to control if fracture union is present. If fracture union is not present, nonunion frequently ensues, leading to an infected nonunion.

Management of infected nonunions is a complex problem. Clearing of the infection, although desirable, is not a necessary prerequisite to obtaining union, and in fact, bone union facilitates treatment of the infection.[91,107,108,172]

After the acute phase of treatment has passed, if the fracture does not have internal fixation appliances in place and is unstable, achievement of stability is necessary for successful treatment. In some cases, this can be obtained with early weight bearing in either a long-leg or Sarmiento cast such as has been used so successfully by military surgeons in recent wars. Instability, particularly with segmental loss or severe soft tissue problems, almost always requires the use of an external fixation device. An external fixator provides excellent stability, can be used to achieve proper alignment, and bone grafting or other reconstructive procedures can be done with the fixator in place until union occurs.

If infection occurs with plate and screw fixation in place, they are left in place if they are stable. They facilitate management of the infection. Secondary bone grafting may be necessary to achieve union. If an infected intramedullary rod is loose, removal of the rod and debridement of the intramedullary canal by reaming. Stabilization of the fracture with an external fixator. Some surgeons would inset a new rod. I do not do this often in the tibia.

Occasionally, after subsidence of the acute infection internal fixation to achieve stability may be necessary again to obtain bone union. With bone union, infection often spontaneously subsides. Other operative procedures to treat infected nonunions will be discussed under nonunions.

Delayed Union

The average time to union in Sarmiento's hands is approximately 16 weeks plus or minus 4 weeks. Thus, a routine closed fracture that does not show osseous union by 20 weeks can be regarded as a delayed union. Nicoll confirms this criterion. Delayed union of the tibia is a common complication and the incidence has been reported to be from 1 to 17 percent.[4,65,98,161,173,175,176,180,219]

Souter[195] advises routine cancellous bone grafting of tibia fractures that are not united and are mobile at 12 to 16 weeks. Although most delayed unions will go on to union without bone grafting, I would agree with Souter that a substantial number of delayed unions do go on to nonunion and prolonged immobilization is often necessary to achieve union without bone grafting. Prolonged immobilization results in higher incidence of, and more permanent effect from, joint stiffness, muscle atrophy, and osteoporosis and significantly delays the patient's return to work. I would advise that a fracture which demonstrates significant clinical instability, particularly if the fracture can be translated and crepitus produced, as opposed to just elastic bending, be bone grafted, and, if necessary, internally fixed. Certainly by 20 weeks, any fracture that remains mobile merits surgical intervention. Fractures that are clinically stable but have a persistent fracture line can be managed by func-

tional bracing, which permits full foot and ankle function. Eventual union will occur in most cases.

A pernicious and not often recognized cause of delayed union is early union of the fibular shaft fracture or presence of an intact fibula, which prevents settling in the tibia fracture. This is particularly true in fractures in the distal third of the tibia. Early resection of a portion of the fibula with continued treatment in a weight bearing plaster cast has been successful.[55,76,194]

For the stable delayed union of more than 20 weeks, which is in good alignment, the treatment of choice is onlay bone grafting without taking the fracture down.[169,170]

Nonunion

Nonunion of a fracture of the tibia is that point at which no further progress toward union is expected without external intervention. Considerable information on the treatment of nonunion is available to the reader.[1,10,12,22,24–26,60,78,79,92,100,135,139,159,175,193,201,207,217]

Nonunions can be classified into three categories: hypertrophic, atrophic, and those with large segmental defects. Hypertrophic nonunions are characterized by exuberant callus about the nonunion site producing an "elephant's foot" or "mushroom callus." These nonunions retain substantial biologic capability of healing, are generally due to instability, and respond well to rigid internal fixation (Fig. 125-47). Atrophic nonunions show minimal callus and have tapered and atrophic bone ends, and the medullary canal is sealed with dense sclerotic bone. These fractures have minimal biologic potential for union and usually require bone grafting in addition to stabilization.

The precise role of electrical stimulation for treatment of nonunion of various long bones is still a matter of debate. Its popularity stems from the fact that it is noninvasive. To some extent, electrical stimulation seems to be most useful in those fractures that also respond well to other techniques, such as rigid internal fixation and bone grafting. It is probable that the next 5 years will permit us a more accurate judgment of when electrical stimulation will be most helpful. In the tibia,

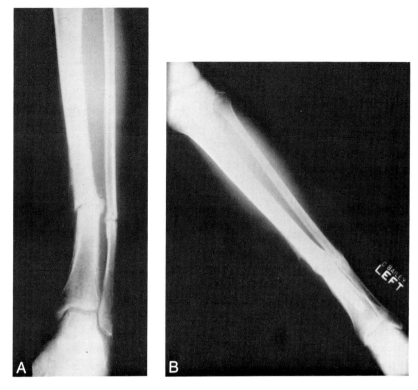

Fig. 125-47. **(A)** This nonunion of the tibia occurred in a 27-year-old sky diver after 13 months of immobilization in plaster casts. **(B)** The nonunion was treated with an AO intramedullary nail using closed technique. It united within 12 weeks of nailing during which time he bore full weight without a cast or brace.

success rates of up to 85 percent have been reported.

Most nonunions are due to the type of fracture. Type III open fractures of the tibia with severe displacement, soft tissue injury, and compromise of blood supply are most likely to not heal. Infection, distraction due to inappropriate traction or external fixation, inadequate external immobilization, inadequate internal fixation, and delayed weight bearing are also causes of nonunion.

The most common type of nonunion is one in acceptable alignment with a stable fibrous union. These are best treated with a Phemister-type onlay cancellous bone graft.[107,108,120,150,215] The graft is most successful when laid along the lateral or posterior surface of the tibia. An anterior or posterior lateral approach can be used. I prefer the postero lateral approach because wound complications are

fewer and optimal position of the graft can be achieved. The fracture site should not be taken down. The fibula, interosseous membrane, and tibia well above and below the fracture site should be exposed. The tibia is roughened with an osteotome; petals of bone can be turned across the nonunion. A large mass of cancellous bone is then laid along the posterior surface of the tibia, across the interosseous membrane, and along the fibula, creating a local synostosis. This is an excellent approach for infected nonunions of the tibia draining anteriorly. After the acute postoperative period, patients with this bone graft can be permitted to walk in a weight-bearing plaster.

If gross motion or significant angulation is present, an osteotomy and internal fixation or application of an external fixator must be considered. In suitable fractures, an intramedullary nail, which

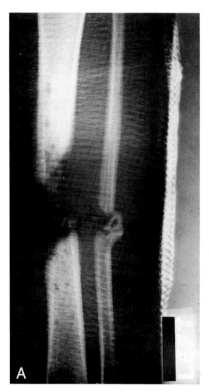

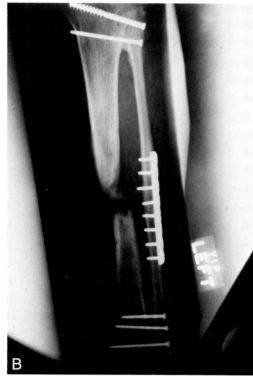

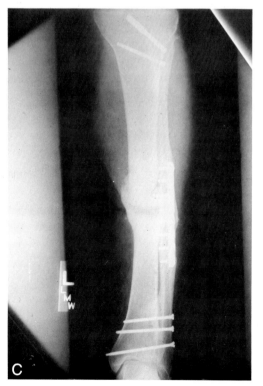

Fig. 125-48. Proximal and distal synostosis as treatment for nonunion of the tibia. **(A)** AP radiograph showing the tibia and fibula of a 38-year-old carpenter 13 months after having sustained severe Type III open fractures of the tibia and fibula when he was struck by a car. He lost 7.25 cm of middiaphysis with severe soft tissue loss. At this point he had an unstable leg with a low-grade infection and a small draining fistula anteriorly. **(B)** The fibula was exposed through posterolateral incisions. The midshaft nonunion of the fibula was stabilized with a compression plate and a cancellous bone graft was applied. A distal and proximal tibiofibular synostosis was accomplished with screws and bone graft as depicted on this AP radiograph taken 3 months postoperatively. Note the early evidence of spontaneous bridging of the defect in the tibia. **(C)** The patient was kept in a weight-bearing brace and spontaneous union of the tibia occurred by 1 year after the synostosis surgery. Note the hypertrophy of the fibula.

permits immediate weight bearing, is the procedure of choice,[125] but plates and screws are often necessary (Fig. 125-37B).

A segmental diaphyseal defect in the tibia has been treated by most surgeons with proximal and distal synostosis between the tibia and fibula,[43,90,143,150] transfer of the fibula to the tibia,[31,32,36,49,104] or direct massive bridging of the defect.[23] Proximal and distal synostosis using lag screws, augmented by cancellous bone graft with postoperative weight bearing and a brace, has been successful[149] (Fig. 125-48).

Malunion

Malunion of a tibial shaft fracture is difficult to define and is dependent on the limb and the patient in which it occurs. *Malunion* is perhaps an inappropriate word in that healing of a fracture in a nonanatomic position is not necessarily a bad union, as the word implies. Although cosmetic deformity may be of major concern to some patients, unacceptable position of the bones at the time of union is better described in functional terms.

Shortening is the most common problem. Shortening resulting in a leg-length discrepancy of greater than 15 mm is frequently symptomatic and may require a lift. Shortening should be kept under 1 cm. Varus or valgus angulation of greater than 10 degrees is undesirable, although angulation up to and slightly over 10 degrees is often not noticed by the patient. Angulation over 10 degrees is thought by some to lead to early arthritis in the ankle joint, although there is insufficient evidence to prove this. Recurvatum is less well tolerated than any anterior bowing. Up to 10 degrees of recurvatum is acceptable. More than 15 degrees is often cosmetically and functionally unacceptable. Anterior bowing of up to 10 degrees is seldom of functional significance, although cosmetic considerations may make this unacceptable. Rotatory malalignment is better compensated for by the patient than varus – valgus angulation. Internal rotation of more than 5 degrees is often noticeable and over 10 degrees is usually unacceptable. External rotation is better tolerated. External rotation of more than 10 to 15 degrees is usually noticeable, and more than 15 degrees may create functional problems. With conservative care, nonanatomic alignment at the time

of union is common, but functional or cosmetic disability from this is unusual. Osteotomy is rarely necessary. Careful follow-up and early intervention will prevent the vast majority of unacceptable malunions.

Neurovascular Injuries

Injuries to nerves and arteries can be confused because vascular injuries may present with loss of sensation and apparent muscle paresis.

The most common nerve injury is a stretch palsy of the common peroneal nerve where it courses about the neck of the fibula and splits into its superficial and deep branches. A careful neurologic examination at the time of initial evaluation, recorded in the medical records, is important to document whether treatment has caused a nerve palsy. Partial palsy of the common peroneal nerve usually improves but complete palsy has a poor prognosis. Exploration is rarely necessary. However, if palpation of the sheath of the nerve at the fibular neck reveals a hematoma, decompression may occasionally be necessary. On rare occasions, the peroneal nerve becomes trapped in a high fibular fracture. A persistently unreduced fracture of the neck of the fibula, accompanied by a peroneal palsy, should lead to suspicion of this.

When circumferential immobilization such as casts is applied, patients should be checked frequently to be certain that peroneal palsies do not occur. With the earliest sign of decreased sensation in the first web space or weakness of the extensor hallucis longus, the cast should be univalved, all padding cut, and the cast windowed over the common peroneal nerve.

Vascular injuries in association with fractures of the tibia are not uncommon, but they are usually in the proximal third of the leg in the region of the trifurcation.[44,47,97,106,197] Significant injury in the area of the trifurcation may deprive the leg of all its blood supply; therefore, early diagnosis and arterial repair are of ultimate importance. Survival of the limb generally requires restoration of blood flow within 8 hours of injury. Absent pulses without evidence of circulatory impairment are not always an indication for an arteriogram, however, a cool or pale extremity with decreased sensation generally is an indication for one. If there is any question in the surgeon's mind, arteriography should be done. Reduction of the fracture by closed manipulation often relieves distortion of the vessels with restoration of circulation in the limb and should always precede arteriography. If vascular repair becomes necessary, it is generally advisable to repair the vessel before treating the fracture because restoration of blood flow to the limb is of utmost importance. Once arterial repair is completed, some form of fracture stabilization, either internal or external fixation, is indicated, although Connelly[44] has shown that internal fixation is not absolutely necessary to protect vascular repairs.

Amputation

In most surgeons' hands, a type IIIC open fracture of the tibia has an amputation rate of at least 50 percent. The decision to salvage a severely injured leg with vascular injury is difficult. Most commonly, we salvage limbs that should be immediately amputated. It is unfair to the patient to invest 2 or more years to salvage a limb that subsequently requires amputation because it is not functional and is painful. Lange and associates[123] provided guidelines for early amputation.

Absolute indications are type IIIC open fractures with a vascular injury requiring repair in which the posterior tibial nerve is transected, and type IIIC open fractures due to crush with a vascular injury requiring repair when the warm ischemia time is greater than 6 hours. Relative indications are serious associated polytrauma, anticipated prolonged course for reconstruction, or severe ipsilateral foot trauma.

Early amputation must be considered if one of the absolute indications and two or three of the relative indications are present. Often, this decision is made at the time of a "second look" surgery following the initial debridement and after a thorough discussion with both the patient and family.

Fatigue Fractures

Stress fractures of the tibia and fibula occur in young active people such as athletes,[57–59,114] ballet dancers,[29] and military recruits,[153] whose lower extremities are subject to repeated, prolonged activity. More detail on stress fractures is given in the excellent monograph of Morris and Blickenstaff,[153] who studied 700 military recruits. In this group 17 percent of the fractures occurred in the tibia and only 1 percent in the fibula. The site of the fractures varies according to the activity. The majority in their study occurred in the tibia at the junction of its middle and upper thirds and involved predominantly the posteromedial aspect. In young athletes, these fractures occur in the metaphyseal area at the junction of the middle and distal thirds, while in ballet dancers most fractures were found to occur in the middle third of the tibia. Fatigue fractures of the distal third of the fibula are common at the top of the boot in skiers wearing rigid high boots.

There is usually no history of acute injury and these fractures are frequently confused with a compartment syndrome involving the anterior compartment, "shin splints," and tendinitis. The patient usually experiences insidious low-level pain in the leg coincidental with and aggravated by activity. The symptoms gradually worsen, so that the patient experiences pain even at rest and at night. Acute fracture through the fatigued area may, on rare occasions, occur with minor trauma.

On physical examination, the most important finding is localized tenderness of the bone accompanied by swelling and thickening of the soft tissues in the area.

Roentgenograms within the first 2 to 4 weeks of onset are frequently normal. The best method of early diagnosis is a technetium bone scan. When a fracture appears on radiography, it typically shows a soft periosteal reaction with some bony sclerosis. A fracture line may not be seen, although a narrow transverse radiolucent line involving one or more cortices may occur.

The treatment is varied according to the patient's involvement. Complete immobilization is contraindicated because the osteoporotic process in stress fractures may continue and prolong recovery. The aggravating activity is discontinued or markedly decreased and the patient placed on protective weight bearing with crutches. Occasionally, a cast may be necessary for a short period of time, but weight bearing should be continued. Healing generally requires 6 to 10 weeks. Return to the aggravating activity must be slow and should generally be modified to prevent recurrence of fracture.

FRACTURES OF THE FIBULA

Fibula shaft fractures in the absence of ankle involvement are usually due to direct trauma and most frequently occur from the same violence that causes a tibial shaft fracture and thus most commonly accompany tibial fractures. Fracture of the shaft of the fibula accompanying a tibial fracture requires no special treatment other than that described for fractures of the tibia.

Isolated fractures of the fibular shaft are generally due to direct violence. Findings include local tenderness and swelling. Pain with walking may be minimal. When treating fibular shaft fractures it is important to always look for occult involvement of the ankle joint.

Treatment varies depending on the symptoms. Often a soft dressing and weight bearing, as tolerated, with crutches suffices. Most fractures, however, are quite painful and require a long-leg cast for the first 2 to 3 weeks. This can then be cut down to a short-leg walking cast. Most of these fractures are stable by 6 weeks and external immobilization can be discontinued. Complications from isolated fractures of the fibula are extremely rare and uneventful union can be expected in the majority of cases.

AUTHOR'S PREFERRED METHODS AND RATIONALE

The decision-making process for the treatment of fractures of the tibia and fibula is complex, involving many factors. An overall picture of my approach is illustrated in Figure 125-49, an algorithm for the treatment of tibial fractures.

I treat closed stable fractures of the tibial shaft, where the initial shortening does not exceed 1 cm, with closed reduction, application of a long-leg weight-bearing cast, and then full weight bearing as tolerated. In most cases, at 6 weeks I convert the long-leg cast to a Sarmiento cast or a cast brace and order continued weight bearing until union occurs.

I try to mobilize the ankle with an ankle hinge by 12 weeks.

In closed fractures of the tibia and fibula with shortening over 1 cm or an unacceptable reduction using closed means, I prefer to use closed reduction with closed intramedullary nailing with a reamed nail. I use a Grosse-Kempf nail with crosslocking as needed. When closed intramedullary nailing is contraindicated, I will occasionally stabilize a closed fracture with a single-plane AO fixator. On rare occasions, in a long oblique or spiral fracture not controllable by closed means, I use interfragmentary screw fixation. I will almost never use compression plate fixation for a closed fracture of the tibia or fibula.

I treat open fractures with either external fixation or immediate nailing with a Lottes nail. If the fracture is unstable, additional stability to prevent shortening and malrotation is achieved by plating the fibula. The latter usually requires postoperative protection in a weight-bearing cast for approximately 6 weeks. A study is under way at the University of California, Davis, Medical Center to compare these two techniques. In an unpublished series, there were few differences between the two groups of patients. Because of the ease of using the Lottes nail and plate on the fibula, particularly from the patient's viewpoint, I tend to lean slightly in favor of that approach. Others have had good experience with this approach on open fractures of the tibia.[209] I seldom use plate and screw fixation for fractures of the mid diaphysis of the tibia. In metaphyseal regions, particularly where there is intra-articular involvement, I do not hesitate to use a plate with screws, as external fixators in this location often require bridging a normal joint. I have not found limited internal fixation particularly advantageous when combined with external fixators, with a few rare exceptions. When there is a free-floating intercalary butterfly or larger fragment, it is often useful to use limited screw fixation to stabilize the butterfly fragment to the proximal and distal fragments, rather than using additional pins with the external fixator.

Finally, I believe it is essential to prevent delayed union and nonunion of the tibia. Whenever there is substantial comminution, a high-energy injury, or any bone loss, I routinely bone-graft the fracture with autogenous cancellous iliac bone. In

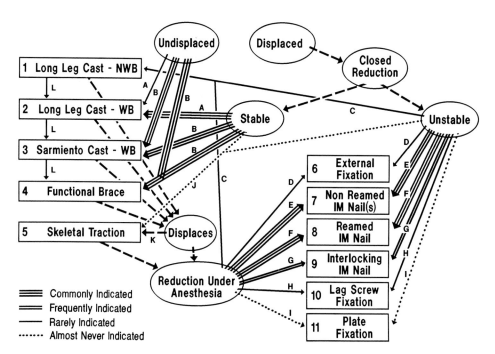

Fig. 125-49. Algorithm for treatment of fractures of the tibia and fibula. Slight modifications may be necessary for open fractures, but the basic schema applies. Comments on each modality or decision as denoted by letters or numbers are as follows: *A,* Proximal fractures. *B,* Middle and distal one-third fractures. *C,* Where alignment is less critical or surgery is contraindicated. *D,* Primary indication is in unstable, open fractures. Also used when internal fixation is impossible or undesirable. *E,* When fracture will be stable with a nonreamed nail. Useful as primary stabilization in open fractures as an alternative to external fixation. *F,* Where large nail required for stability. Contraindicated in most open fractures because of the risk of infection. *G,* Used when communication requires interlocking to achieve stability. *H,* Rarely indicated, particularly alone. Fracture must be spiral or oblique with a length three times the width of the diaphysis. Most common indication is a fracture of the distal third with an intact fibula. *I,* Almost never indicated in a shaft fracture unless required to stabilize an associated metaphyseal or intra-articular fracture. *J, K,* Rarely indicated. Used for temporary immobilization to treat severe soft-tissue injury when surgery is not possible or external fixation is not indicated. May be used to maintain length when internal fixation is anticipated. *L,* Movement from *1* to *4* is the usual progression in nonoperative treatment. I usually start at *2.* Stable fractures usually reach *3* or *4* by 4 to 6 weeks; unstable fractures usually require 8 to 12 weeks to reach the same stage. *5,* when removed, may need *3, 4, 6, 7, 8,* or *9.* *6,* When removed, will usually need *3* or *4* and may need *7, 8,* or *9.* (*NWB,* Non-weight bearing; *IM,* Intramedullary; *WB,* Weight bearing.) (From Chapman,[38a] with permission.)

closed fractures, the decision to bone graft is usually made at about 12 weeks and is dependent on the stability of the fracture and amount of callus. If no callus is seen, and the fracture remains unstable, bone grafting is usually indicated as the chances of the fracture going to a nonunion are close to 50 percent. In open fractures, grades I and II, in which the soft tissues are in good condition and there is no

evidence of infection, I will most often graft at the time of delayed primary closure. In more severe wounds, I prefer to wait for complete healing and perform bone grafting between 6 and 10 weeks after fracture.

No matter what approach is employed, I try to begin early range-of-motion exercise of all noninvolved joints and institute exercise for all muscles.

REFERENCES

1. Abbott LC: The use of iliac bone in the treatment of ununited fractures. American Academy of Orthopaedic Surgeons Instructional Course Lectures. Vol. 2. JW Edwards, Ann Arbor, 1944
2. Adler JB, Shaftan GW, Rabinowitz JG, et al: Treatment of tibial fractures. J Trauma 2:59, 1962
3. Aho AJ, Nieminen SJ, Nylamo EI: External fixation by Hoffman-Vidal-Adrey osteotaxis for severe tibial fractures. Clin Orthop 181:154, 1983
4. Albert M: Delayed union in fractures of the tibia and fibula. J Bone Joint Surg 26:566, 1944
5. Alms M: Medullary nailing for fractures of the shaft of the tibia. J Bone Joint Surg 44B:328, 1962
6. Anderson LD: Compression plate fixation and the effect of different types of internal fixation on fracture healing. J Bone Joint Surg 47A:191, 1965
7. Anderson LD, Hutchins WC: Fractures of the tibia and fibula treated with casts and transfixing pins. South Med J 59:1026, 1966
8. Anderson LD, Hutchins WC, Wright PE, et al: Fractures of the tibia and fibula treated by casts and transfixing pins. Clin Orthop 105:179, 1974
9. Anderson MK, McDonald K, Stephens JG: A study of the effect of open and closed treatment on rate of healing and complications in fractures of the tibial shaft. J Trauma 1:290, 1961
10. d'Aubigne RM: Surgical treatment of non-union of long bones. J Bone Joint Surg 31A:256, 1949
11. d'Aubigne RM: Infection in the treatment of ununited fractures. Clin Orthop 43:77, 1965
12. d'Aubigne RM, Maurer P: Traitment des pseudarthroses graves de jambe. Mem Acad Chir 85:673, 1959
13. d'Aubigne RM, Maurer P, Zucman J, et al: Blind intramedullary nailing for tibial fractures. Clin Orthop 105:267, 1974
14. Batten RL, Donaldson LJ, Aldridge MJ: Experience with the A-O method in the treatment of 142 cases of fresh fracture of the tibial shaft treated in the U.K. Ing 10:108, 1978
15. Bauer CH, Edwards P: Fracture of the shaft of the tibia. Incidence of complications as a function of age and sex. Acta Orthop Scand 36:95, 103, 1965–1966
16. Bauer G, Edwards PO, Widmark PH: Shaft fractures of the tibia. Etiology of poor results in a consecutive series of 173 fractures. Acta Chir Scand 124:386, 1962
17. Bayne LG, Morris H, Wickstrom J: Evaluation of intermedullary fixation of the tibia with the Lottes nail. South Med J 53:1429, 1960
18. Bergentz SE, Thureborn E: Shaft fractures of the lower leg: open versus closed reduction. Analysis of a twenty-year series. Acta Chir Scand 114:235, 1957
19. Blockey NJ: The value of rigid fixation in the treatment of fractures of the adult tibial shaft. J Bone Joint Surg 38B:518, 1956
20. Böhler J: Treatment of non-union of the tibia with closed and semiclosed intramedullary nailing. Clin Orthop 43:92, 1965
21. Böhler L: The Treatment of Fractures, English Ed. 5. Grune & Stratton, New York, 1956–1958
22. Boyd HB: The treatment of difficult and unusual non-unions. With special reference to the bridging of defects. J Bone Joint Surg 25A:535, 1943
23. Boyd HB: Non-union of the shafts of long bones. Postgrad Med J 36:315, 1964
24. Boyd HB, Anderson LD, Johnston DS: Changing concepts in the treatment of non-union. Clin Orthop 43:37, 1965
25. Boyd HB, Lipinski SW: Causes and treatment of non-union of the shafts of the long bones, with a review of 741 patients. American Academy of Orthopaedic Surgeons Instructional Course Lectures. Vol. 17. CV Mosby, St. Louis, 1960
26. Boyd HB, Lipinski SW, Wiley JH: Observations of non-union of the shafts of the long bones with a statistical analysis of 842 patients. J Bone Joint Surg 43A:159, 1961
27. Brown PW, Urban JG: Early weight-bearing treatment of open fractures of the tibia. J Bone Joint Surg 51A:59, 1969
28. Burkhalter WE, Protzman R: The tibial shaft fracture. J Trauma, 15:785, 1975
29. Burrows HJ: Fatigue infraction of the middle of the tibia in ballet dancers. J Bone Joint Surg 38B:83, 1956
30. Burwell HN: Plate fixation of tibial shaft fractures —a survey of 181 injuries. J Bone Joint Surg 53B:258, 1971
31. Campbell WC: Transference of the fibula as an adjunct to free bone graft in tibial deficiency. Report of three cases. Am J Orthop Surg 1:625, 1919
32. Carnesale PL, Guerrieri AG: Fibula transplant for loss of substance of tibia: Report of a case. J Bone Joint Surg 37A:204, 1955
33. Carpenter EB: Management of fractures of the shaft of the tibia and fibula. J Bone Joint Surg 48A:1640, 1966
34. Carpenter EB, Butterworth JF III: The conserva-

tive treatment of shaft fractures of the tibia and fibula. South Med J 50:1209, 1957

35. Carpenter EB, Dobbie MM, Sewers CF: Fractures of the shaft of the tibia and fibula. Comparative end results from various types of treatment in a teaching hospital. Arch Surg 64:443, 1952

36. Carrell WB: Transplantation of fibula in the same leg. J Bone Joint Surg 41A:807, 1938

37. Cave EF (ed): Fractures and Other Injuries. Chicago, Year Book Medical Publishers, 1958

38. Chapman MW: Immediate internal fixation in open fractures. Orthop Clin North Am 11:579, 1980

38a. Chapman MW: Fractures of the tibia and fibula. In Chapman MW, Madison M (eds): Operative Orthopaedics. JB Lippincott, Philadelphia, 1988

39. Chapman MW, Mahoney M: The role of internal fixation in the management of open fractures. Clin Orthop 138:120, 1979

40. Chrisman OD, Snook GA: The problem of refracture of the tibia. Clin Orthop 60:217, 1968

41. Claffey T: Open fractures of the tibia. J Bone Joint Surg 42B:407, 1960

42. Clancey GJ, Hansen ST Jr: Open fractures of the tibia. J Bone Joint Surg 60A:118, 1978

43. Companacci M, Zanolli S: Double tibiofibular synostosis for nonunion and delayed union of the tibia. J Bone Joint Surg 48A:44, 1966

44. Connolly JF, Whittaker D, Williams E: Femoral and tibial fractures combined with injuries to the femoral or popliteal artery. J Bone Joint Surg 53A:56, 1971

45. Conwell HE, Reynolds FC: Management of Fractures, Dislocations, and Sprains, ed. 7. St. Louis, CV Mosby, 1961

46. Copeland CX Jr, Enneking WF: Incidence of osteomyelitis in compound fractures. Am Surg 31:156, 1956

47. Crellin RQ, Tsapogas MJC: Traumatic aneurysm of the anterior tibial artery. Report of a case. J Bone Joint Surg 45B:133, 1963

48. Davis AG: Fibular substitution for tibial defects. J Bone Joint Surg 26:229, 1944

49. deCosta GIB, Kumar N: Early weight bearing in the treatment of fractures of the tibia. Injury 11:123, 1970

50. Dehne E: Treatment of fractures of the tibial shaft. Clin Orthop 66:159, 1969

51. Dehne E: Ambulatory treatment of the fractured tibia. Clin Orthop 105:192, 1974

52. Dehne E, Deffer PA, Hall RN, et al: The natural history of the fractured tibia. Surg Clin North Am 41:1495, 1961

53. Dehne E, Metz CW, Deffer PA: Nonoperative treatment of the fractured tibia by immediate weight bearing. J Trauma 1:514, 1961

54. Delbet P: Methode de traitement des fractures de jambes. Ann Clin Chev 5, 1916

55. DeLee JC, Heckman JD, Lewis AG: Partial fibulectomy for ununited fractures of the tibia. J Bone Joint Surg 63A:1390, 1981

56. DePalma A: The Management of Fractures and Dislocations, ed. 2. WB Saunders, Philadelphia, 1970

57. Devas MB: Stress fractures of the tibia in athletes or "shin soreness." J Bone Joint Surg 40B:227, 1958

58. Devas MB: Shin splints or stress fractures of the metacarpal bone in horses and shin soreness or stress fractures of the tibia in man. J Bone Joint Surg 49B:310, 1967

59. Devas MB, Sweetman R: Stress fractures of the fibula—a review of fifty cases in athletes. J Bone Joint Surg 38B:818, 1956

60. Dunlop K, Wirzalis EF: Two-stage transplant for persistent nonunion with gross loss of tibia—a report of five cases. Milit Surg 107:356, 1950

61. Dunn AW: Displaced tibial shaft fractures: A comparison of treatment methods. So Med J 69:37, 1976

62. Edge AJ, Denham RA: The portsmouth method of external fixation of complicated tibial fractures. Injury 11:13, 1979

63. Edge AJ, Denham RA: External fixation for complicated tibial fractures. J Bone Joint Surg 63B:92, 1981

64. Edmonson AS, Crenshaw AL (eds): Campbell's Operative Orthopaedics, ed. 6. St. Louis, CV Mosby, 1980

65. Edwards CC, Jaworski MF, Solana J, et al: Management of compound tibial fractures using external fixation. Am Surg 45:190, 1979

66. Edwards P: Fracture of the shaft of the tibia: 492 consecutive cases in adults. Importance of soft tissue injury. Acta Orthop Scand (Suppl. 76), 1965

67. Edwards P, Baver G, Widmark PH: The time of disability following fracture of the shaft of the tibia. Acta Orthop Scand 40:501, 1969

68. Eggers GWN: Indications and operative technique for open reduction and internal fixation of fractures of the shafts of the tibia and fibula. Surg Clin North Am 41:1515, 1961

69. Eggers GWN, Shindler TO, Pomerat CM: The influence of the contact-compression factor on osteogenesis in surgical fractures. J Bone Joint Surg 31A:693, 1949

70. Ellis H: A Study of Some Factors Affecting Prog-

nosis Following Tibial Shaft Fractures. Bodleian Library, Oxford, 1956

71. Ellis H: Disabilities after tibial shaft fractures. J Bone Joint Surg 40B:190, 1958

72. Ellis H: The speed of healing after fracture of the tibial shaft. J Bone Joint Surg 40B:42, 1958

73. Ellis J: Treatment of fractures of the tibial shaft. J Bone Joint Surg 46B:371, 1954

74. Evans EB, Eggers GWN: Internal fixation of the fibula in fractures of both bones of the leg. JAMA 169:321, 1959

75. Evans GA, Bang RL, Cornah MS, et al: The value of the Hoffmann skeletal fixation in the management of cross leg flaps, particularly those injuries complicated by open fractures of the tibia. Injury 11:110, 1979

75a. Eychleshmer AC, Schoemaker DW: A Cross Section Anatomy. Appleton & Lange, East Norwalk, CT, 1970

76. Fernandez-Palazzi F: Fibular resection in delayed union of tibial fractures. Acta Orthop Scand 40:105, 1969

77. Fisher WD, Hamblen DL: Problems and pitfalls of compression fixation of long bone fractures: A review of results and complications. Injury 10:99,1978

78. Flanagan JJ, Burem HS: Reconstruction of defects of the tibia and femur with opposing massive grafts from the affected bone. J Bone Joint Surg 29:587, 1947

79. Forbes DB: Subcortical iliac bone grafts in fracture of the tibia. J Bone Joint Surg 43B:672, 1961

80. Gallinaro P, Crova M, Denicolai F: Complications in 64 open fractures of the tibia. Injury 5:157, 1973

81. Ganosa ACL, Carruiterro J, Rogers S: Straight nails in tibial fractures. Techniques and reports of thirty cases. J Bone Joint Surg 49A:280, 1967

82. Gershuni DH, Halma G: The AO external skeletal fixator in the treatment of severe tibial fractures. J Trauma 23:986, 1983

83. Green SA: Complications of External Fixation: Causes, Prevention, and Treatment. Charles C Thomas, Springfield, IL, 1981

84. Greenbaum E, O'Loughlin BJ: Value of delayed filming in the anterior tibial compartment syndrome secondary to trauma. Radiology 93:373, 1969

85. Gustilo RB, Anderson JT: Prevention of infection in the treatment of 1025 open fractures of long bones. J Bone Joint Surg 58A:453, 1976

86. Gustilo RB, Simpson L, Nixon R, et al: Analysis of 511 open fractures. Clin Orthop 66:148, 1969

87. Haines JF, Williams EA, Hargadon EJ, Davies DRA: Is conservative treatment of displaced tibial shaft fractures justified? J Bone Joint Surg 66B:84,1984

88. Hampton OP Jr, Holt EP Jr: The present status of intramedullary nailing of fractures of the tibia. Am J Surg 93:597, 1957

89. Hamza KN, Dunkerley GE, Murray CMM: Fractures of the tibia: A report on fifty patients treated by intramedullary nailing. J Bone Joint Surg 53B:696, 1971

90. Hand FM: Crisscross tibiofibular graft for nonunion of the tibia. Clin Orthop 1:154, 1953

91. Hanson LW, Eppright RH: Posterior bone grafting of the tibia for nonunion. A review of twenty-four cases. J Bone Joint Surg 48A:27, 1966

92. Harkins HM, Phemister DB: Simplified technique of onlay grafts. For all ununited fractures in acceptable position. JAMA 109:1501, 1937

93. Harman PH: A simplified approach to the posterotibia for bone grafting and fibular transferral. J Bone Joint Surg 27:496, 1945

94. Harvey JP Jr: Management of open tibial fractures. Clin Orthop 105:154, 1974

95. Hassenhuttl K: The treatment of unstable fractures of the tibia and fibula with flexible medullary wires. J Bone Joint Surg 63A:921, 1981

96. Hedenberg I, Pompeius R: Shaft fractures of the lower leg. Comparing the early results of open and closed treatment in 120 cases. Acta Chir Scand 118:339, 1960

97. Hedrick DW, Hawkins FB, Townley CO: Primary arterial injury complicating extremity fractures. J Bone Joint Surg 29:738, 1947

98. Hjelmsted A: Fractures of the tibial shaft. A study of primary and late results in 105 cases. Acta Chir Scand 121:511, 1961

99. Hoaglund FT, States JD: Factors influencing the rate of healing in tibial shaft fractures. Surg Gynecol Obstet 124:71,1967

100. Hoderman WD: Results following conservative treatment of fractures of the tibial shaft. Am J Surg 98:593, 1959

101. Holden CEA: Bone grafts in the treatment of delayed union of tibial shaft fractures. Injury 4:175, 1972

102. Holstad HA: Primary osteosynthesis versus conservative treatment of compound fractures of long tubular bones. J Oslo City Hosp 12:225, 1962

103. Hughston JC, Whatley GS, Bearden JM: Tibia fractures. South Med J 62:931, 1969

104. Huntington TW: Case of bone transference. Use of

a segment of fibula to supply a defect in the tibia. Ann Surg 41:249, 1905

105. Jackson RW, Macnab I: Fractures of the shaft of the tibia. A clinical and experimental study. Am J Surg 97:543, 1959

106. Jeffery CC: Spasm of the posterior tibial artery after injury. J Bone Joint Surg 45B:223, 1963

107. Jones KG: Treatment of infected non-union of the tibia through the posterolateral approach. Clin Orthop 43:103, 1965

108. Jones KG, Barnett HC: Cancellous bone grafting for non-union of the tibia through the posterolateral approach. J Bone Joint Surg 37A:1250, 1955

109. Karaiharju EO, Alho A, Niemissen J: The results of operative and non-operative management of tibial fractures. Injury 7:47, 1975

110. Karlstrom G, Olerud S: Fractures of the tibial shaft: A critical evaluation of treatment alternatives. Clin Orthop 105:82, 1974

111. Karlstrom G, Olerud S: Percutaneous pin fixation of open tibial fractures: Double-frame anchorage using the Vidal-Adrey method. J Bone Joint Surg 57A:915, 1975

112. Karlstrom G, Olerud S: Stable external fixation of open tibial fractures a report of five years of experience with the Vidal-Adrey double-frame method. Orthop Rev 6:25, 1977

113. Karlstrom G, Olerud S: External fixation of severe open tibial fractures with the Hoffmann frame. Clin Orthop 180:68, 1983

114. Kelly RP, Murphy FE: Fatigue fractures of the tibia. South Med J 44:290, 1951

115. Kimmel RB: Results of treatment using the Hoffmann external fixator for fractures of the tibial diaphysis. J Trauma 22:960, 1982

116. Kratochvil BL, Premer RF: The Delbet splint: A report of three cases. Clin Orthop 36:151, 1964

117. Kristensen KD: Tibial shaft fractures. Acta Orthop Scand 50:593, 1979

118. Kunkel WG, Lynn RB: The anterior tibial compartment syndrome. Can J Surg 1:212, 1958

119. Lam SJ: The place of delayed internal fixation in the treatment of fractures of the long bone. J Bone Joint Surg 46B:393, 1964

120. Lamb RH: Posterolateral bone graft for nonunion of the tibia. Clin Orthop 64:114, 1969

121. Landoff GA: A comparative study of methods of treatment of diaphyseal fractures of the leg. Acta Orthop Scand 18:37, 1948

122. Langard O, Bo O: Segmental tibial shaft fractures. Acta Orthop Scand 47:354, 1976

123. Lange RH, Bach AW, Hansen ST Jr, Johansen KH: Open tibial fractures with associated vascular injuries: prognosis for limb salvage. J Trauma 25:203, 1985

124. Laurence M, Freeman MAR, Swanson SAV: Engineering considerations in the internal fixation of fractures of the tibial shaft. J Bone Joint Surg 51B:754, 1969

125. Laurent LE, Langenskiold A: Osteosynthesis with a thick medullary nail in non-union of long bones. Acta Orthop Scand 38:341, 1967

126. Leach RE: A means of stabilizing comminuted distal tibial fractures. J Trauma 4:722, 1964

127. Lottes JO: Intramedullary fixation for fractures of shaft of tibia. South Med J 45:407, 1952

128. Lottes JO: Blind nailing technique for insertion of the triflange medullary nail. JAMA 155:1039, 1954

128a. Lottes JO: Medullary nailing of the tibia with the triflange nail. JAMA 155:1039, 1954

129. Lottes JO: Intramedullay nailing of the tibia. American Academy of Orthopaedic Surgeons Instructional Course Lectures, Vol. 15. JW Edwards, Ann Arbor, 1958

130. Lottes JO: Treatment of delayed or non-union fractures of the tibia by medullary nail. Clin Orthop 43:111, 1965

131. Lottes JO: Medullary nailing of the tibia with the triflange nail. Clin Orthop 105:253, 1974

132. Lottes JO, Hill LJ, Key JA: Closed reduction, plate fixation and medullary nailing of fractures of both bones of the leg. J Bone Joint Surg 34A:861, 1952

133. Lucas K, Todd C: Closed adult tibial shaft fractures. J Bone Joint Surg 55B:878, 1973

134. Macnab I: Blood supply of the tibia. J Bone Joint Surg [B] 39:799, 1957

135. Marmor L: How to treat the infected ununited fracture of the tibia. Am J Surg 113:475, 1967

136. Marshall DV: Three-side plate fixation for fractures of the femoral and tibial shafts. J Bone Joint Surg 40A:323, 1958

137. Matsen FA III: Compartmental Syndromes. Grune and Stratton, New York, 1980

138. Mayer L, Werbie T, Schwab JP, Johnson RP: The use of Ender nails in fractures of the tibial shaft. J Bone Joint Surg 67A:446, 1985

139. McCarroll HR: The surgical management of ununited fractures of the tibia. JAMA 175:578, 1961

140. McCormack MP, Carr M: Alms technique of Kuntscher nailing for fractures of the tibia. J Bone Joint Surg 47B:586, 1965

141. McLaughlin HL: On the operative treatment of tibial fractures. Surg Clin North Am 41:1489, 1961

142. McLaughlin HL, Gaston SR, Neer CS et al: Open

reduction and internal fixation of fractures of the long bones. J Bone Joint Surg 31A:94, 1949

143. McMaster PE, Hohl M: Tibiofibular cross-peg grafting. J Bone Joint Surg 47A:1146, 1965

144. McNeur JC: The management of open skeletal trauma with particular reference to internal fixation. J Bone Joint Surg 52B:54, 1970

145. Melis GC, Sotgiu F, Lepori M, Guido P: Intramedullary nailing in segmental tibial fractures. J Bone Joint Surg 68A:1310, 1981

146. Mendes JE, Cabral AT, Lima C: Open fractures of the tibia. Clin Orthop 156:98, 1981

147. Merianos P, Cambouridis P, Smyrnis P: The treatment of 143 tibial shaft fractures by Ender's nailing and early weight-bearing. J Bone Joint Surg 67B:576, 1985

148. Merriam WF, Porter KM: Hindfoot disability after a tibial shaft fracture treated by internal fixation. J Bone Joint Surg 65B:326, 1983

149. Milch H: Tibiofibular synostosis for non-union of the tibia. Surgery 27:770, 1950

150. Miller W, Jetter GL, Frank GR: Posterior bone grafts in nonunion of fractures of the shafts of the tibia: A review of 27 cases. South Med J 62:1254, 1969

151. Moed BR, Morawa LG, Pedersen HE: Screw fixation of closed oblique and spiral fractures of the tibial shaft. Clin Orthop 177:196, 1983

152. Moore ST, Storts RA, Spencer JD: Fractures of the tibial shaft in adults: A ten year survey of such fractures. South Med J 55:1178, 1962

153. Morris JM, Blickenstaff LD: Fatigue Fractures — A Clinical Study. Charles C Thomas, Springfield, Ill, 1967

154. Mortiz JR, Saviers G, Earle AS, et al: Spiral fractures of the tibia: Long term results of Parham band fixation. J Trauma 2:147, 1962

155. Müller ME: Internal fixation for fresh fractures and for nonunion. Proc Soc Med 56:455, 1963

156. Müller ME: Treatment of nonunions by compression. Clin Orthop 43:83, 1965

157. Müller ME, Allgöwer M, Schneider R, et al: Manual of Internal Fixation, ed 2. Springer-Verlag, New York, 1979

158. Müller ME, Allgöwer M, Willenegger H: Technique of Internal Fixation of Fractures. Springer-Verlag, New York, 1965

159. Murray WR, Lucas DB, Inman VT: Treatment of nonunion of fractures of the long bones by the two-plate method. J Bone Joint Surg 46A:1027, 1964

160. Nelson G, Kelly P, Paterson L, et al: Blood supply of the human tibia. J Bone Joint Surg 42A:625, 1960

161. Nicoll EA: Fractures of the tibial shaft. A survey of 705 cases. J Bone Joint Surg 46B:373, 1964

162. Nicoll EA: Closed and open management of tibial fractures. Clin Orthop 105:144, 1974

163. Nonnemann HC, Blariza G: The application of the Maatz-spreading-nail in operative treatment of distal tibial fractures. J Trauma 16:604, 1976

164. Olerud S: Treatment of fractures by the Vidal-Adrey method. Acta Orthop Scand 44:516, 1973

165. Olerud S, Karlstrom G: Tibial fractures treated by A-O compression osteosynthesis: experiences from a five year material. Acta Orthop Scand [Suppl.] 140:1, 1972

166. Onnerfalt R: Fracture of the tibial shaft treated by primary operation and early weight bearing. Acta Orthop Scand [Suppl.] 171:59, 1978

167. Pankovich AM, Tarabishy I, Yelda S: Flexible intramedullary nailing of tibial-shaft fractures. Clin Orthop 160:185, 1981

168. Patzakis MJ, Harvey JP, Ivler D: The role of antibiotics in the management of open fractures. J Bone Joint Surg 56A:532, 1974

169. Phemister DB: Splint grafts in the treatment of delayed and nonunion of fractures. Surg Gynecol Obstet 52:376, 1931

170. Phemister DB: Treatment of ununited fractures by onlay bone grafts without screw or tie fixation and without breaking down of the fibrous union. J Bone Joint Surg 29:946, 1947

171. Ratliff AHC: Fractures of femur and tibia in same limb. J Bone Joint Surg 47B:586, 1965

172. Rezaian SM: A new external fixation device for treatment of complicated fractures of the leg. Injury 9:17, 1977

173. Rittmann WW, Schibli M, Matter P, et al: Open fractures — long term results in 200 consecutive cases. Clin Orthop 138:132, 1979

174. Rombouts L, Cuypers L: Follow-up of A-O osteosyntheses of tibia fractures. Acta Orthop Belg 43:43, 1977

175. Ruedi T, Webb JK, Allgower M: Experience with the dynamic compression plate (DCP) in 418 recent fractures of the tibial shaft. Injury 7:252, 1976

176. Sakellarides HT, Freeman PA, Grant BD: Delayed union and nonunion of tibial shaft fractures. A review of 100 cases. J Bone Joint Surg 46A:557, 1964

177. Sarmiento A: A functional below-the-knee cast for tibial fractures. J Bone Joint Surg 49A:855, 1967

178. Sarmiento A: A functional below-the-knee brace for tibial fractures. J Bone Joint Surg 52A:295, 1970

179. Sarmiento A: Functional bracing of tibial and femoral shaft fractures. Clin Orthop 82:2, 1972

180. Sarmiento A: Functional bracing of tibial fractures. Clin Orthop 105:202, 1974

181. Sarmiento A, Sobol PA, Sewhoy AL, et al: Prefabricated functional braces for the treatment of fractures of the tibial diaphysis. J Bone Joint Surg 66A:1328, 1984

182. Schatzker J: Compression in the surgical treatment of fractures of the tibia. Clin Orthop 105:220, 1974

183. Scudese VA, Dirotte A, Gialenella J: Tibial shaft fractures: Percutaneous multiple pin fixation, short leg cast and immediate weight bearing. Clin Orthop 72:271, 1970

184. Sedlin ED, Zitner DT: The Lottes nail in the closed treatment of tibial fractures. Clin Orthop 192:185, 1985

185. Shaar CM, Krenz FP Jr, Jones DT: Fractures of the tibia and fibula-treatment with the Stader reduction and fixation splint. Surg Clin North Am 23:599, 1943

186. Shands AR, Raney RB: Handbook of Orthopaedic Surgery. CV Mosby, St. Louis, 1967

187. Skelley JW, Hardy AE: Results of bone grafts in the treatment of tibial fractures. Clin Orthop 158:108, 1981

188. Sladek EC, Kopta JA: Management of open fractures of the tibial shaft. South Med J 70:662, 1977

189. Slatis P, Rokkanen P: Closed intramedullary nailing of tibial shaft fractures. Acta Orthop Scand 38:88, 1967

190. Solheim K, Bo O: Intramedullary nailing of tibial shaft fractures. Acta Orthop Scand 44:323, 1973

191. Solheim K, Bo O, Langard O: Tibial shaft fractures treated with intramedullary nailing. J Trauma 17:223, 1977

192. Smith JEM: Results of early and delayed internal fixation for tibial shaft fractures. A review of 470 fractures. J Bone Joint Surg 56B:469, 1974

193. Smith WD, Evans JP: Anterior bone grafts in tibial shaft fractures: a review of 32 cases. Okl State Med Assoc J 68:469, 1975

194. Sorenson KH: Treatment of delayed union and nonunion of the tibia by fibular resection. Acta Orthop Scand 40:92, 1969

195. Souter WA: Autogenous cancellous strip grafts in the treatment of delayed union of long bone fractures. J Bone Joint Surg 51:63, 1969

196. Speed K: A Textbook of Fractures and Dislocations. Philadelphia, Lea & Febiger, 1928

197. Stein AH Jr: Arterial injury in orthopaedic surgery. J Bone Joint Surg 38A:669, 1956

198. Stephens JG, Andersen MM: An analysis of open and closed treatment of fractures of the tibial shaft. Canad J Surg 4:65, 1960

199. Straub LR: Brace management in complicated fractures of the tibia. Surg Clin North Am 41:1579, 1961

200. Strobel CJ, Indeck W: Fractures of the tibia. An analysis of treatment at Minneapolis General Hospital. Minn Med 43:469, 1960

201. Thompson JEM: Nonunion and malunion of fractures of the lower extremity treated by medullary fixation. Clin Orthop 2:142, 1953

202. Torok G, Serfati A: Treatment of fractures of the tibial shaft. Harefuah 63:467, 1962

203. Trieta J, Cavadias AX: Vascular change caused by the Kuntscher type of nailing. J Bone Joint Surg 37B:492, 1955

204. Tucker JT, Watkins FP, Carpenter EB: Conservative treatment of fractures of the shaft of the tibia. JAMA 178:802, 1961

205. Thunold J, Varhaug JE, Bjerkeset T: Tibial shaft fractures treated by rigid internal fixation: The early results in a 4-year series. Injury 7:125, 1975

206. Urist MR: End result observations influencing treatment of fractures of shaft of tibia. JAMA 159:1088, 1955

207. Urist MR, Mazet R Jr, McLean FC: The pathogenesis and treatment of delayed union and non-union. A survey of eighty-five ununited fractures of the shaft of the tibia and one hundred control cases with similar injuries. J Bone Joint Surg 36A:931, 1954

208. Van Der Linden W, Larsson L: Plate fixation versus conservative treatment of tibia shaft fractures. J Bone Joint Surg 61A:873, 1979

209. Velazco A, Fleming LL: Open fractures of the tibia treated by the Hoffmann external fixator. Clin Orthop 180:125, 1983

210. Velazco A, Fleming LL, Nahai F: Soft-tissue reconstruction of the leg associated with the use of the Hoffmann external fixator. J Trauma 23:1052, 1983

211. Velazco A, Whitesides TE Jr, Fleming LL: Open fractures of the tibia treated with the Lottes nail. J Bone Joint Surg 65A:879, 1983

212. Veliskakis KP: Primary internal fixation in open fractures of the tibial shaft. The problem of wound healing. J Bone Joint Surg 41B:342, 1959

213. Vidal J, Buscayret C, Connes H et al: Guidelines for treatment of open fractures and infected pseudarthroses by external fixation. Clin Orthop 180:83, 1983

214. Wade PA, Campbell RD Jr: Open versus closed

methods in treating fractures of the leg. Am J Surg 95:599, 1958

215. Wagner JG: Anterolateral approach in bone grafting for ununited fractures of the tibia. Am J Surg 73:282, 1947

216. Watson-Jones R: Fractures and Joint Injuries, ed. 4. Williams & Wilkins, Baltimore, vol. 1, 1952, vol. 2, 1955

217. Watson-Jones R, Coltart WD: Slow union of fractures. With a study of 804 fractures of the shafts of the tibia and femur. Br J Surg 30:260, 1942

218. Weissman SO, Herold HZ: Treatment of tibial shaft fractures. A review of 103 cases. Harefuah 63:462, 1962

219. Weissman SL, Herold HA, Engelberg M: Fractures of the middle two-thirds of the tibial shaft. Results of treatment without internal fixation in 140 consecutive cases. J Bone Joint Surg 48A:257, 1966

220. White EW, Radley TJ, Earley NN: Screw stabilization in fractures of the tibial shaft. J Bone Joint Surg 35A:749, 1953

221. Widenfolk B, Ponten B, Karlstrom G: Open fractures of the shaft of the tibia: Analysis of wound and fracture treatment. Injury 11:136, 1979

222. Wiggins H, Bundens W, Park B: Complications following open reduction and plating of fractures of the tibia. Am J Surg 86:273, 1953

223. Wilson PD: Management of Fractures and Dislocations. JB Lippincott, Philadelphia, 1938

224. Zucmann J, Maurer P: Primary medullary nailing of the tibia for fractures of the shaft in adults. Injury 2:84, 1970

225. Zucmann J, Maurer P: Two-level fractures of the tibia. J Bone Joint Surg 51B:686, 1969

Delayed Union, Nonunion, and Malunion of the Tibial Shaft

126

Stephen K. Benirschke
Allan W. Bach
Sigvard T. Hansen, Jr.

Nonunion of the tibial shaft is a common problem in orthopaedic traumatology, and the open tibial fracture could properly be termed an "unsolved" fracture. The high incidence of auto and motorcycle accidents, as well as the increasing popularity of sports such as hang gliding and mountain climbing, has made the severe open tibial fracture a common injury. Under favorable circumstances a closed fracture of the tibial shaft will heal without surgical intervention. In contrast, high rates of nonunion have been reported in several series of open fractures of the tibial shaft [7,14,25,44]; almost half of these cases were infected nonunions. Although simple methods of treatment such as immobilization with a long-leg cast, as suggested by Watson-Jones,[61] or cast immobilization with early weight bearing, as advocated by Dehne,[19] can yield high rates of union, nonunion of the open tibial fracture is still a significant problem, and malunion is common.

The definition of a tibial nonunion is arbitrary. Tibial fractures have been termed *delayed unions* if stability, or at least some evidence of callus formation, has not been achieved at 16 to 20 weeks.[43]

The term *nonunion* is often reserved for those fractures that have not healed after 9 months of adequate treatment. These tibial fractures frustrate both the orthopaedist and the patient. Rather than be limited by a definition of nonunion that involves a set time frame, it may be more useful either to decide on indications for altering treatment or to establish a fixed time to change treatment if at that point the fracture shows no progress toward union after use of the initial method. Surgical intervention may be indicated at 4 to 6 months[5,43] after injury if a tibia is not healing or healed. It is our opinion that a decision to change treatment should be made between 16 and 20 weeks if healing is not evident from some callus on radiography or stability on clinical testing. In this instance, a nonunion, or a delayed union, may be predicted, and a change in treatment is probably justified. The rationale for this approach is arguable, but it is our belief that very prolonged immobilization of the leg or modified use of the foot and leg produces significant long-term disability and that the risk:benefit ratio of intervention after this number of weeks begins to swing in favor of some method of hastening union.

FACTORS CONTRIBUTING TO NONUNION OF THE TIBIA

The most important factors affecting the healing of tibial shaft fractures relate to the regional anatomy, particularly the blood supply, of the tibia. The tibial shaft is an essentially straight bone for which tension or compression loading is not significantly different on the medial and lateral sides. The cross section of the tibial shaft is roughly triangular; the lateral and posterior surfaces are covered by muscles, but the anteromedial surface is covered by a very small amount of soft tissue (periosteum, subcutaneous tissue, fat, and skin).

The anatomy of the tibial blood supply has been described in great detail.[36,44,50,59] Four systems of vessels, exist in the tibia: the nutrient, periosteal, metaphyseal, and epiphyseal systems. Of these, the nutrient and periosteal systems are of greatest importance in tibial shaft fractures. The nutrient artery system originates from the posterior tibial artery. This vessel penetrates the posterior tibial cortex just distal to the soleal line and immediately divides into ascending and descending branches. The nutrient system is the major supplier for the endosteal vessels, which, according to Rhinelander,[50] supply the internal two-thirds of the cortical bone. Obviously, any fracture of the tibial shaft will destroy much of the endosteal blood supply to one portion of the bone. Destruction of this endosteal supply is more extensive when the fracture is in the middle one-third of the tibia than when the fracture occurs in the distal third.[36] However, the incidence of tibial nonunion seems to be fairly evenly divided between the middle, proximal, and distal thirds of the shaft.[45]

The anterior tibial artery contributes to much of the periosteal blood supply. The segmental vessels contributing to the periosteal network originate from the posterolateral aspect of the leg. Many vessels penetrate the tibia at the attachment of the interosseous membrane and through the posterior periosteum. The supply to the anteromedial periosteum is segmental and easily destroyed. The metaphyseal and epiphyseal vessels supply the proximal and distal portions of the tibia but are of secondary importance in shaft fractures. Thus with tibial shaft fractures that involve stripping of periosteum, it is inevitable that some cortical bone will become avascular.

The severity of injury, or amount of energy absorption, and the degree of related vascular disruption influence the development of a nonunion. In general, the greater the severity of injury, the higher the incidence of nonunion. The fracture pattern is a good indication of the amount of energy dissipated in the soft tissue and bone.[21] Low-energy injuries such as skiing fractures usually produce a fairly simple spiral or oblique fracture pattern. High-energy injuries associated with automobile accidents are usually caused by a combination of bending, rotational, and axial loading forces, and a great deal of comminution is frequently present. Segmental or severely comminuted fractures are prone to nonunion.

Examples of Energy Absorption

Fall from sidewalk	100 ft-lb
Skiing injury	300–500 ft-lb
Gunshot wound	2,000 ft-lb
Bumper injury, 20 mph	100,000 ft-lb

The amount of soft tissue injury also influences the course of bone healing. Closed fractures, which are usually less severe injuries with less stripping of blood supply, have a much lower incidence of nonunion than do open fractures. The higher rate of nonunion with open fractures may also be secondary to the periosteal tube destruction and lack of "fracture hematoma" in these fractures.[35] The incidence of nonunion, and especially infected nonunion, increases with the severity of open fractures.[19]

A logical classification of open fractures divides them into three groups. Grade I open fractures involve small wounds, frequently but not necessarily generated from within the limb involved, and radiographs should show a low-energy fracture pattern. Soft-tissue injury and periosteal stripping are minimal. These fractures should heal at nearly the same rate as closed fractures.

Grade II open fractures have more severe soft tissue injury, some visible contamination, and more periosteal stripping; damage to soft tissues can be expected. Radiographs should show a slightly higher energy fracture pattern and/or more displacement at the fracture site. Secondarily, there is more potential for vascular dysfunction and necrotic bone. These fractures will tend to heal more slowly, since bone ends must be revascularized before good healing can progress, and they are more prone to delayed union or nonunion and to infection than are grade I fractures. Whatever treatment is applied to these fractures must take into account the more significant generalized instability and the likelihood of prolonged healing time. More stabilization of the area will be needed to encourage revascularization and soft tissue healing.

Grade III soft tissue injuries include a large range of fractures, up to traumatic near amputation, and may include gross contamination, large wounds, and significant obvious damage to muscle and other soft tissues; often there is vascular, nerve tendon, and skin disruption and/or loss. Gustilo has subdivided grade III injuries into IIIa, IIIb, and IIIc based on the extent of soft tissue involvement. Tscherne has developed a similar system, numbering the injuries 3, 4, and 5.

A Gustilo grade IIIc (Tscherne grade 4) soft tissue injury has the same characteristics as a simple grade IIIa injury, but in addition there is an associated major neural or arterial (inflow) injury. Once this has been documented by visualization of the injured vessel or nerve, the risk of possible amputation increases dramatically. If all goes well in the reconstructive effort, the patient may still be left with cold intolerance, pain, hypesthesia, or dysesthesia. These sequelae often result in a below-knee amputation as a salvage procedure.

Grade IIIa, IIIb, and IIIc soft tissue injuries frequently give radiographs showing a very high energy absorptive fracture pattern with comminution or segmentation. There is often cortical bone loss, or there may be cortical fragments in the wound, which are significantly or totally stripped of their soft tissue attachments. Up to 50 percent of grade III injuries progress to nonunion and very frequently become infected.

As with fractures of other bones, certain modes of treatment appear to discourage union of tibial shaft fractures. Foremost among these is distraction; the patient's compliance with a complicated treatment program will also influence the rate of tibial healing.

The result of the treatment of tibial shaft fractures, for closed and open injuries, has frequently been shortening. This is due to the alignment achieved by closed means or to bone loss resulting from avascular fracture fragments. Most patients can tolerate shortening of up to 2 cm without much morbidity (i.e., excessive lift or gait modification). Limb length inequality greater than 2 cm becomes a separate problem, often frustrating for physician and patient. Therefore, in our treatment of tibial fractures, the ideal would be to have a minimum of shortening, proper alignment, and good knee, ankle, and subtalar motion following treatment.

Dehne[19] and Brown and Urban[11] found that early weight bearing stimulates fracture healing in the tibia. Using this method they had success with a series of 63 open fractures. Sarmiento and Latta believe that if weight bearing is delayed more than 6 weeks with cast treatment of tibial fractures, the incidence of nonunion increases significantly.[55]

In addition to local factors, general patient factors may contribute to healing of the tibia. The patient's age and nutritional status, the presence of premorbid diseases such as diabetes, and the type and severity of any other injuries will influence the course of healing. More problems with tibial healing and a high incidence of nonunion are found in multiply injured patients, who have often sustained other long bone fractures. Such problems will be compounded if multiply injured patients are not treated for their markedly increased nutritional needs, much as is the case with burn patients.

CLASSIFICATION OF TIBIAL NONUNIONS

Numerous methods of treatment for tibial nonunions exist, and some classification of the various types of nonunions is necessary for developing a rational treatment program based on an appropriate method of treatment of each type.

Two important factors in the classification of nonunions are the expected vascularity of the fracture site and the presence or absence of infection. A true synovial pseudarthrosis should be recognized and treated differently from other nonunions. This distinction is especially pertinent when treatment by electrical stimulation is considered.[5]

The vascularity of the bone ends at the nonunion site is a major determinant of whether a nonunion

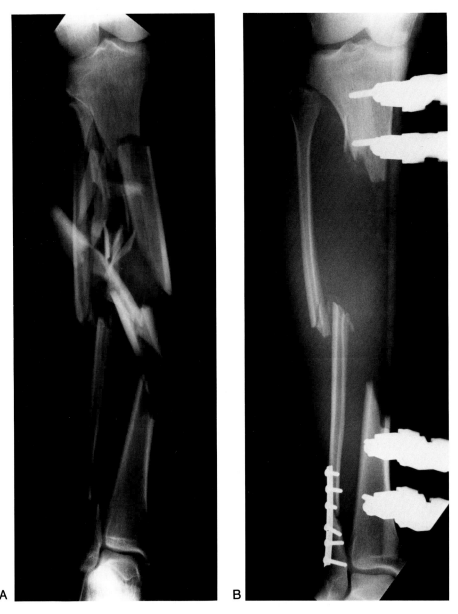

A   B

Fig. 126-1. (A) The initial AP radiograph of a 22-year-old man's grade IIIB open right tibia fracture. **(B)** The limb is 2 cm short (overlapping fibula) with a 19-cm segmental defect after external fixation with a unilateral half pin frame and debridement of all devitalized bone and soft tissues. *(Figure continues.)*

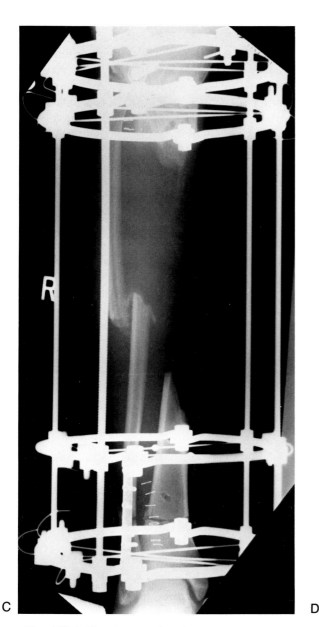

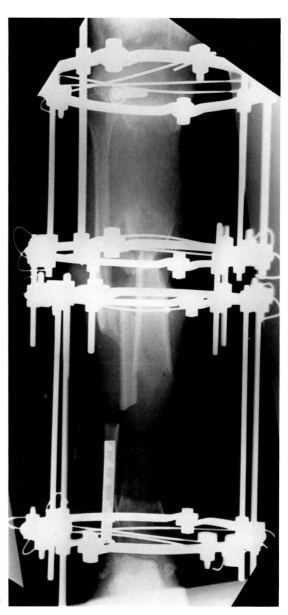

Fig. 126-1 *(Continued)*. **(C)** After changing to a circumferential Ilizarov external fixator, proximal and distal corticotomies were performed to initiate bidirectional osseous transport of proximal and distal metaphyseal segments. **(D)** Transportation has been completed and limb lengths equalized after fibular osteotomy. Note the maturing regenerate bone seen between rings 1 and 2, and rings 3 and 4. Compare the position of the bidirectionally transported osseous projectiles attached to the middle two rings in both 1C and 1D.

falls into the so-called hypertrophic or atrophic classifications. A hypertrophic nonunion, often termed the "elephant foot" nonunion, is characterized by flaring, rather dense bone ends. The gap is only a few millimeters wide, but the bone has made an obvious attempt to produce callus and heal. The bone ends are generally well vascularized, at least initially. Occasionally, however, if multiple surgical attempts have been made to treat the initial hypertrophic nonunion, this large amount of bone may be hypovascular. In this case the "elephant foot" portion of the bone may be quite inactive.[56]

In contrast, atrophic nonunions are characterized by tapered osteopenic bone ends. Bone vascularity may be deficient in these fractures, although some other lack of stimulation may be causing the lack of bone healing. Most infected nonunions are also atrophic.

Nonunions can be classified in several ways based on infection[12]: they may be noninfected, previously infected, or currently infected, with either a nonvirulent or virulent infection. Previously infected nonunions are those with a history of infection but that are clinically free of infection at the time of treatment. The radiographic appearance of these nonunions is also an important factor in classification. Any significant bony defect that limits the choices for managing the nonunion must be noted.

Infected nonunions represent a great problem. These frequently involve poorly vascularized bone, bony defects and often present challenging soft tissue problems. In the past it was believed that eradication of the infection was necessary before bone healing procedures could be started. However, eradicating an infection with an unstable tibial shaft is frequently difficult or impossible. Infected fractures are much easier to resolve when the tibial nonunion is stabilized.

The Swiss AO group considers the primary goal in these infected fractures to be the consolidation of the nonunion and the secondary goal to be eradication of the infection itself. They have proved that a bone can heal in the presence of an infection.[40]

GA Ilizarov from Kurgan, USSR, developed a method of transosseous bone synthesis in 1952 that has only recently been tested in the West, beginning in Italy in 1980. Ilizarov has reported that with use of external fixation with transosseous wires loaded in tension, together with a corticotomy, previously ununited, infected fractures have rapidly healed (Fig. 126-1). The corticotomy involves a technique in which the cortex of the metaphysis is cut without disturbing the intramedullary cancellous bone. In the case of an infected nonunion, the fracture is debrided to clean edges, and the metaphyseal segment is transported down the limb by wires attached to the external frame. At a rate of 1 mm/day in a rhythm of four distractions per day the segment is moved, with formation of a column of bone behind the corticotomized segment. No additional bone grafting has been necessary, with weight bearing encouraged from the outset. The Ilizarov method may prove to be an excellent method for addressing difficult nonunion and shortening problems of the tibia provided there is good patient compliance and adherence to the techniques described. Other devices besides that of Ilizarov are being tested that use the same principle of corticotomy and slow transportation of a live segment across a bony defect. Reggazoni in Basel and others in Europe are attempting to develop better equipment and/or modifications of existing equipment to use this seemingly sound principle.

An alternative device is a combination of the AO tubular frame and the Weber threaded frame, which looks very promising and more familiar.

SKIN AND SOFT TISSUE COVERAGE WITH TIBIAL NON-UNION

Severe open tibial fractures that proceed to nonunion present particular soft tissue problems. In these fractures the anteromedial surface to the tibia is frequently exposed, with no soft tissue covering the cortical bone. Split-thickness skin grafts will "take" on periosteum but not on cortical bone. Decortication and/or drilling of a tibia in an attempt to encourage a better granulation tissue have been used with open tibial fractures. Although these procedures may be useful, they can diminish the bony stability and remove necessary bone stock. Bipedicle skin flaps may be useful to cover relatively small areas, but care must be taken not to cause necrosis of more skin. The use of local muscle and myocutaneous transfers for open tibial fractures has been discussed by Ger.[24] These procedures help bring vascularity to the area of a nonunion and eradicate dead space. The medial heads of the gastrocnemius and the soleus muscles have been used to cover the tibia in the proximal and middle third areas. The muscle belly of the flexor digitorum longus can be rotated anteriorly in the junction of the middle third and distal third regions. Because of its segmental blood supply, the lower portion of the soleus from a distally based flap can be used to cover defects over the distal third of the tibia, but this procedure is not easily performed.

Since large defects are not always treated adequately by these local rotation flaps, cross-leg flaps or distal pedicle flaps can also be used. However, the use of cross-leg flaps involves both legs for a considerable time and presents technical difficulties. Cross-leg flaps injure the contralateral leg significantly and are cosmetically unacceptable or at least undesirable. We find very rare indications for this procedure.

The recent use of microvascular anastomosis for composite tissue transfer now opens up more possibilities for the treatment of large soft tissue defects.[2,39] Free cutaneous and myocutaneous grafts can be used to cover these defects. La Rossa has outlined the principles for these grafting procedures.[34] The timing of the procedure is not critical, but it is important that the wound be clean, as documented by quantitative wound cultures. Exposed bone is not a problem if it is clean and viable. Adequate debridement is necessary, and bone stabilization is essential.

NONSURGICAL TREATMENT

Immobilization

Most tibial shaft fractures, even open fractures,[11] will heal if immobilized properly and for a sufficient time. Casting for periods of more than 1 year has been advocated. However, such prolonged im-

mobilization may cause significant morbidity. Patients may lose considerable time from productive work and may find it difficult to return to work at all. Residual foot and ankle stiffness is common after prolonged immobilization.[57] Muscle atrophy and knee stiffness can also be problems. Prolonged cast treatment for nonunions may lead to excessive shortening or unacceptable angulatory or rotational deformities. Aside from these drawbacks, however, prolonged cast treatment is quite safe and can be combined with bone grafting procedures.

Some patients with stable nonunions of the tibia may function well with patellar-tendon-bearing braces or casts. Sarmiento and Latta[55] have shown that healing can take place when such braces are used, and this method at least relieves the knee of secondary effects from immobilization. This mode of treatment can be used in the patient who does not desire or cannot undergo surgery for treatment of a tibial nonunion.

Electrical Stimulation

The use of electrical stimulation as a treatment for nonunited fracture has expanded greatly since Fredenburg reported successful treatment of a medial malleolar pseudarthrosis with electrical stimulation in 1971.[10] Two methods of electrical stimulation, the noninvasive inductive technique and invasive direct current stimulation, have been developed.

Bassett et al. have obtained healing in 87 percent of tibial nonunions with the use of externally applied coils.[5] An asymmetric pulsing electromagnetic field is used to induce a current in the bone. This method requires precise application of the external coils, use of the coils (plugged into a wall outlet) for 12 to 16 hours per day, and no weight bearing until there are radiographic signs of healing. This method is contraindicated with synovial (true) pseudarthrosis or when the gap between the bone fragments is greater than 1 cm. Good patient cooperation is required. No stress can be applied to the bone while the treatment is being carried out, and therefore no correction of angulatory or rotatory malunion can be performed. The rate of healing in patients who have undergone many previous procedures for treatment of tibial nonunions is impressive with this method. Infected nonunions can be treated successfully with electromagnetic fields. Also, the presence of internal fixation devices made of 316L stainless steel or cobalt–chromium alloys does not interfere with electromagnetic coil use.

Brighton et al. have used implantable direct-current cathodes to stimulate healing of nonunions.[10] The current is applied constantly through four cathodes at a level of 20 amp. Weight bearing is contraindicated by this method, usually for 12 to 16 weeks. In Brighton's series, 84 percent of patients with tibial nonunions experienced healing of their fractures. As with externally applied coils, this system is ineffective with synovial pseudarthrosis or when large gaps are present at the fracture site. Metal interference is not a factor with this method.

The exact mechanism of bone healing by electrical stimulation is not completely understood. The effect of the current at low voltage may be to lower tissue oxygen tension and produce a more favorable environment for bone growth. Low tissue oxygen is found in the bone–cartilage junction of the growth plate and in fracture callus, and in vitro bone growth has been stimulated by low oxygen environments. Other cellular mechanisms may be present, including changes in the level of cyclic AMP.[10]

Electrical stimulation offers an important adjunct to treatment of nonunions both in infected pseudarthroses and in situations where good anatomic alignment of the tibia can be maintained with a cast. This method prolongs joint immobilization and increases muscle atrophy because a long leg non-weight-bearing cast is required. In many cases, however, this disadvantage may be of minor importance.

SURGICAL TREATMENT

Bone Grafting

Bone grafting of nonunions of long bones has been standard treatment for several decades. Numerous methods of bone grafting are used and have been reviewed by Abbott et al.[1] and others.[9,38,49]

Bassett[4] has emphasized factors important to the success of bone grafting. Treatment of nonunions requires altering the biologic or mechanical environment of the fracture site. The only method that attempts to alter both factors in one procedure is cortical grafting with fixation. However, this method is now rarely used because cortical bone provides poor stimulation of the fracture site. Cancellous grafting, with its higher osteogenic potential, is advocated and is frequently successful.

In general, bone grafting is indicated for most atrophic nonunions, either infected or noninfected. Elmslie stated that interposed tissue did not have to be removed from a nonunion site.[13] Phemister's principles of bone grafting are therefore still in use.[48]

Fibrous tissue should not be removed from the nonunion site because this tissue adds some stability. The radiolucent zone at the nonunion site will ossify spontaneously if the graft bridging the area has stabilized the bone adequately. However, removal of necrotic bone and infected granulation tissue may be necessary in septic cases, and these may therefore fall into a completely different treatment group.

The bone graft may directly stimulate the osteogenic potential of the cells at the nonunion site. Bone grafts can be used in certain infected cases if they can be inserted through normal tissue at a distance from the septic area.[28] For example, in clearly localized anterior infection, a posterolateral bone graft could be applied without the graft communicating with the infected area, and stabilization could be obtained before the infected area is cleaned out.

Posterolateral Bone Grafting

Posterolateral bone grafting of the tibial shaft is a well-accepted method for treating nonunion. High rates of union have been obtained in both clean and infected cases. Freeland and Mutz reported a 100 percent union rate in a series of 23 infected tibial nonunions.[22] The success rate of the posterolateral bone grafting can be expected to be 80 to 90 percent, with union occurring within 5 to 7 months after operation.[25,28,49] Posterolateral bone grafting is usually performed to effect union of the tibia. However, if the defects in the tibia are large, this method can be used to gain cross-union to the fibula and thereby bridge these defects.[42]

Malposition of the tibia is not affected by bone grafting. This malposition may contribute to some failures of posterolateral bone grafting because angulation produces an abnormal compression and tension side in the tibia.

The technique of posterolateral bone grafting requires exposure between the lateral and posterior compartments of the leg. This exposure is simple in the middle and distal thirds of the tibial shaft but becomes difficult in the most proximal area of the shaft. A medial approach to expose the posterior tibial cortex is advocated for proximal fractures. When the posterolateral approach is used, the musculature of the deep posterior compartment is reflected off the interosseous membrane and posterior tibia and is retracted medially to expose the posterior tibial cortex. The peroneal and posterior tibial artery and nerve can adhere to scar tissue, and care must be taken to avoid injuring them. Cancellous bone is applied in strips over the posterior tibial cortex and, if desired, may also be continued over onto the fibula. Weight bearing immediately after bone grafting is advocated by some authors,[22] while others defer it for at least 6 weeks.[49] This delay is theoretically to allow vascularization of the bone graft and to host bed healing. We believe that the decision to start weight bearing with posterolateral bone grafting must be based on the inherent stability and alignment at the nonunion site. In the better aligned and more stable fractures, earlier weight bearing may be allowed. Posterolateral bone grafting is often done in the presence of anterior drainage or internal fixation devices (Fig. 126-2).

Subcortical Bone Grafting

In 1939 Dunn advocated the use of subcortical elevation for the treatment of nonunion.[20] Judet and Patel have described the method of "soft tissue

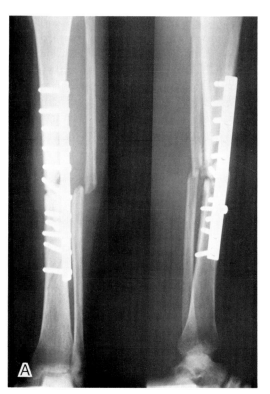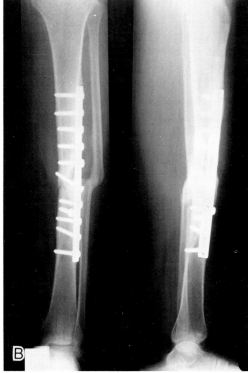

Fig. 126-2. A 24-year-old woman with a comminuted grade II open tibia fracture from an auto accident. **(A)** Three months after the injury. The fracture had been immediately plated and a flexor digitorum longus pedicle graft used to cover the bone. There is resorption at the fracture site and mild drainage. The plate is not loose. **(B)** Nine months after a posterolateral bone graft, the tibia has united and the drainage has diminished.

pediculated bone grafting" for the treatment of nonunion.[30] This method involves careful shingling of 1-mm-thick cortical bone fragments off the tibial cortex. The soft tissue attachments are carefully preserved. This dissection is carried around at least two-thirds of the bone circumference, and no additional graft material is used. Judet reported a 92 percent union rate with this method in a series of more than 1,000 cases. Charnley advocated the combination of subcortical shingling with cancellous bone grafting.[13] Rokkanen and Slatis had a 96 percent success rate using this combined method for treating tibial nonunions.[51]

Authors' Preferred Technique for Posterolateral Grafting

Our preferred method is a very useful procedure in the middle and distal thirds of the tibia only, because the approach more proximally is too complex; it is simpler to approach this area medially if similar bone grafting is to be done there.

For posterolateral bone grafting the patient is positioned midway between lateral and prone, which allows easy access to the posterolateral portion of the affected leg and the ipsilateral posterior iliac crest. We prefer the posterior crest because there is almost always more volume and more reliable bone available, but in patients who are more heavily boned, the anterior crest may be used. In this case we tend to use the inner surface only and do not strip the abductor muscles from the outer side.

Once the patient is positioned, the approach for posterolateral grafting begins with a rather long, linear incision placed fairly well posterior to the fibula (Fig. 126-3). A long incision facilitates exposure, and one must be careful to find the proper natural interval between the lateral and posterior muscle compartments. The posteromedial surface of the fibula is exposed, and the dissection is carried across the posterior surface of the interosseous membrane into the back of the tibia. The posterior surface of the tibia is then exposed to at least 5 cm above and below the pseudarthrosis. The posterotibial cortex is exposed by subcortical shingling, as previously described by Judet and Patel.[30] Strips of corticocancellous or cancellous bone are used and laid across the full length of the exposed posterior

tibia. Also, we frequently choose to decorticate the posterior portion of the fibula and encourage a cross-union, particularly in the middle third.

If a tourniquet is used, it is deflated prior to wound closure, and after a few minutes of compression in the wound, the wound is carefully inspected to ensure that no major vessels have been damaged. Suction wound drainage is used for up to 48 hours, along with slight elevation of the leg and a compressive dressing. The time to weight bearing varies depending on several factors, including the inherent stability of the fracture, the shape of the leg, the amount of stabilization to be expected by a well-applied cast, and the agility of the patient. Most patients will be bearing weight in either a long leg or perhaps a well-molded short leg cast for more distal fractures by approximately 6 weeks postsurgery.

Our criteria for fibular osteotomy, which might be needed at the time of a posterolateral bone graft, merit discussion here. If the fibula provides a fair amount of stability (by having united or by not being broken at the site of tibial nonunion), we like to take advantage of the stability it provides. However, if it seems to be causing some distraction at the tibial fracture site or if the tibia is drifting uncontrollably into varus because of the intact fibula, we would recommend a fibular osteotomy. We believe this is best done by an oblique osteotomy at a level near the tibial fracture site. The obliquity of the osteotomy will allow the fibula to shorten, and the varus position of the tibia could be appropriately straightened. At the same time it will probably heal again. If the fibular osteotomy is not done at a level very close to the tibial fracture, we believe that the spanning fibular segment near the fracture continues to provide distraction through its interosseous membrane attachments and may not allow a good correction of the angulation at the appropriate site.

Open Cancellous Bone Grafting

Matti first described the use of cancellous chip bone grafting for the treatment of nonunions.[37] Burri has discussed the open cancellous grafting technique, or Papineau-type grafts, in much detail.[12] This method is helpful in treating nonunions with open anterior defects.

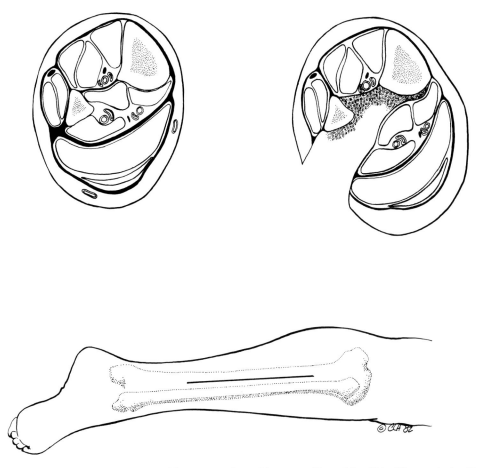

Fig. 126-3. A semiprone position is used for posterolateral bone grafting of the tibia. The posterior iliac crest serves as the donor site. A long skin incision just posterior to the fibula allows exposure between the lateral and posterior compartments. The interval between the deep and superficial posterior muscle compartments should not be entered. Cross-union, particularly in middle third nonunions, is stimulated by decortication and grafting around the fibula.

With open, infected, unstable nonunions, this method is often combined with external fixation.[46,61] Infection is first controlled with debridement, external fixator stabilization, and open irrigation techniques. When all dead tissue has been removed and good nutrition is established at the fracture site, the defect will form a granulation bed and then will be ready for the open grafting. We have also used this technique with good success in the appropriate salvage case.

The open cancellous method is useful in the treatment of infected nonunions from which all dead tissue has been removed and in which a bed of granulation tissue is obtained. The cancellous chips are initially quite resistant to infection and will survive if incorporated in granulation tissue within 2 weeks. A layer of cancellous bone about 1 cm deep is applied in the defect on top of a granulation bed and is not disturbed. A dressing of fine mesh gauze or silk is applied directly over the graft, and the area is then splinted. After several days the dressing can be removed, and wet to dry dressings of saline-soaked fine mesh gauze are applied to the open wound. A process called ''gardening'' is then performed as the top layer of cancellous bone becomes necrotic. This is performed sparingly, as one is waiting for the underlying cancellous bone to be revascularized by the granulation tissue growing up into and incorporating it. Thicker layers of cancellous bone will usually not incorporate fully, and even in the 1-cm thick grafts, the most superficial 1 or 2 mm may be lost eventually.

One problem occurring with the Papineau technique has been refracture through the grafted area. The inherent strength of an open cancellous graft may take much longer to develop in comparison with that of more rapidly revascularized bone grafts (i.e., cancellous grafts under muscle). Therefore, we recommend that the patient be protected with external devices (casts or braces) until the graft has radiographically incorporated.

Free Vascularized Bone Grafting

Microsurgical techniques have brought advances in the treatment of large soft tissue defects. Equally exciting is the use of free vascularized bone grafts in tibial nonunions with large defects. Fibular, iliac crest, and rib grafts can be transferred with their surrounding vessels and revascularized by anastomosis of these vessels with the tibial vessels. Weiland et al.[62] and Taylor and Watson[59] have reported success with these methods. These procedures are time consuming, technically difficult, and not without morbidity at the donor sites and risks at the operative site. Inspection of the local blood supply must show an available major vessel, and thus careful analysis and preparation must be made before transfer. Use of these techniques, however, may save the time eventually required for the revascularization of conventional grafts and may offer an alternative to amputation in severe cases.

Cortical Bone Grafting

Cortical bone grafts have been used in long bone fractures by Boyd,[9] and Albee has used them in the form of sliding bone grafts in tibial nonunions.[3] In investigating the Albee sliding grafts, Holden found that they required a longer time to unite and were associated with a higher incidence of nonunion, graft fracture, and infection than were cancellous grafts.[27] All cortical grafts have these same problems. Their use is not advocated by us or in general by others.

Stable Fixation

Fixation of fractures is now more commonly termed *stable* than *rigid* because almost no fixation device is found to be totally rigid. Stable fixation, however, implies a method that attempts to prevent motion at the fracture site during all normal loading. Use of stable fixation devices for the treatment of tibial diaphyseal healing problems has become well accepted. Compression plates, either with or without intrafragmental screw fixation and external fixators, have advocates, and both devices are classified as stable fixation devices.[5,47,52,56] An intramedullary nail may provide rather stable fixation when used with reaming,[7,33] but this device could be referred to more accurately as an internal splint. Plates and external fixators may also be used in combination, as may external fixators and intrafragmental screws. Finally, cancellous bone grafting may be used in addition to stable fixation or internal splinting. Stable fixation has been used in the treatment of both infected and noninfected nonunions and pseudarthroses and also in osteotomies for malunion.

Treatment by stable fixation requires careful timing at two points. The first is in deciding when intervention is needed (determining that the original treatment will not lead to bone union or at least not within an acceptable time). This decision will be based on judgment, but one rule of thumb is that if no change or progress toward healing is apparent during the 8 weeks after an initial 8 weeks, intervention might be considered. The second point at which timing is important is in determining whether the soft tissues are stabilized enough to tolerate a surgical insult without the risk of infection and whether the bone has regained optimal blood supply. For example, in a grade II or III open fracture with considerable stripping of periosteum and blood supply to bone, there is little use in repeated intervention until the bone has been revascularized. Therefore, a treating surgeon who judges that stripping and vascular destruction have been considerable would wait longer to intervene surgically than if this damage had been minimal and there were evidence that persistent motion was a greater problem than inadequate blood supply.

To maintain optimal nutrition at the fracture site, stable fixation devices must be applied with the least possible disruption of the more critical blood supply. Treatment of the nonunion by stable fixation must take into account the problems caused by the initial injury, including the extent of damage to soft tissue coverage, as well as the effects of any treatment carried out previously. Karlström and Olerud found that tibial nonunions treated initially by compression plating could be safely treated secondarily with reaming and an intramedullary nailing if time was allowed for the periosteal blood supply to recover.[31] In these cases the bone must have been surrounded by adequate soft tissues, from which it could derive this blood supply.

Compression Plating of Tibial Nonunions

Danis[17] and Muller[43] have advocated compression plating in the treatment of closed tibial nonunions. A recent discussion by Schatzker[56] outlines well the principles underlying this method. The success rate with these devices as the sole treatment method has been high in hypertrophic nonunions. With atrophic nonunions, however, bone grafting is usually a necessary adjunct.

Compression plating is of greatest benefit in malpositioned nonunions, primarily those with an angulatory deformity. The plate is affixed to the tension side of the tibia, and when placed under heavy tension with an external tension device, the plate tends to realign the fracture (Fig. 126-4). Because of the resistance to the tensile forces, the plate provides superb stability, which tends to foster primary union. Bone exposure by decortication[40] may be beneficial in these cases. This decortication effect may offset the partial disadvantage of the external exposure and disruption of some of the periosteal blood supply. Osteotomy of the fibula may be necessary when rotational, valgus angulation, or shortening problems must be corrected (Fig. 126-5). Indeed, sometimes if there is heavy callus, a small wedge in the apex of a tibial malunion may be necessary, but this malunion should be slightly undercorrected by the wedge itself, allowing the plate to provide the final straightening by strong compression.

Plating is especially useful when joint stiffness is a problem. When a plate is used, knee, ankle, and foot motion can be quickly resumed without jeopardizing stability at the nonunion site. Fixation

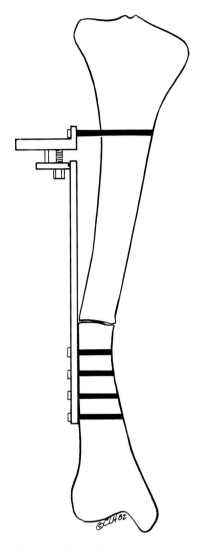

Fig. 126-4. A tension band plate used to straighten an angulated nonunion is always placed on the convex side of the bone. Angulatory deformity cannot always be corrected by this method alone.

with compression plates should be quite rigid; however, compression plates are still load-bearing devices, and weight bearing on the extremity must be minimized or delayed until adequate union is achieved.

An infected nonunion is a possible complication of primary plate fixation of a tibial fracture, and, unfortunately this complication is common.[23,57] Since the most likely cause of bone necrosis is the stripping at the initial fracture, the risk of infection

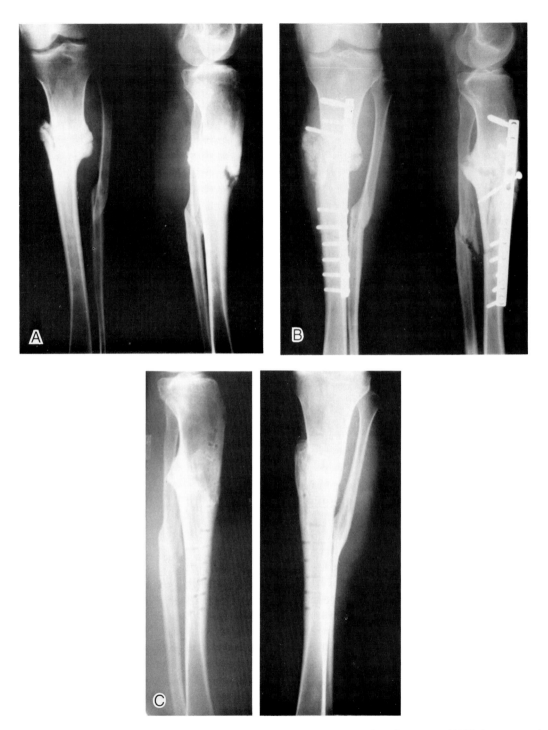

Fig. 126-5. A 37-year-old man with an open tibia fracture treated in a cast for 12 months. **(A)** Eighteen months after injury there is slight motion at the fracture site. **(B)** Tibia was lengthened 12 mm after fibular osteotomy and use of a Küntscher distractor. A fracture through a distractor pin hole necessitated a longer plate. **(C)** One year later the tibia was well healed, and the plate was removed.

can be reduced if plating is applied at the appropriate time, when the bone has regained its blood supply from the periosteal tissues.

In the treatment of an infected nonunion that has been plated, the utility of the original fixation device is controversial. If the plate is still providing very stable fixation, it may best be left in place. Bone debridement, bone grafting, and electrical stimulation can all be done with the plate in place. The internal fixation device must be removed, however, if it is not providing stability. This lack of stability may be evidenced by broken screws, resorption around a screw or plate, breaking of the plate, or obvious malposition. At this point, if at all possible and after any obvious dead tissue has been debrided, the bone should be restabilized. This stabilization can be achieved with a plate, but an external fixator is more commonly used.

Compression plates are of limited value in infected nonunions. If used at all, they must be applied by those very skilled in this procedure. The amount of exposure required to apply a plate may further devascularize the bone ends in cases in which the critical blood supply is already tenuous. If compression plating is to be used for primary treatment of an infected nonunion, the infection must first be well controlled. Meyers et al. have described an open irrigation treatment to accomplish this goal.[40] Closed suction irrigation methods have also been used, but in general they have not been as successful in the tibia as in some other areas.[41] Subcortical dissection, or "shingling," has been advocated by several authors to limit the amount of bone devascularized when a compression plate is applied. The efficacy of this method is as yet unproven.

External Fixation Devices

Numerous external fixators are now used in the treatment of tibial fractures. The Vidal-Audry modification of Hoffmann's frame has gained wide acceptance and is the most elegant. Olerud and Karlström have popularized its use in Scandinavia.[32,46] The rigidity gained with this device can be quite exceptional.[29] On the other hand, numerous other frames used expertly can provide all the stability needed. The use of external fixation devices requires as much skill and care as the use of internal fixation devices and probably requires more day-to-day follow-up.

The success of the external frame device in the treatment of open fresh fractures of the tibia has led to its use in nonunions. This device can be especially useful in an infected nonunion, since it can be placed away from the infected site so that the site itself can be debrided and treated without disruption from the application of a stabilizing device. For example, one might use this device to prepare for an open cancellous grafting, since there is little risk that its application will devascularize the important portion of the bone near the fracture site.

The use of external frames has several drawbacks, however. Excellent care must be taken of pin tracts to avoid infection, and the pins may begin to loosen before they have provided the long-term stability sometimes needed. In some cases the pins will stay firm in the bone for several months, but frequently they will loosen within 8 to 12 weeks. Specially made new pins and more precise methods of applying them seem to be neutralizing this problem. A second drawback is that the anterior compartment musculature can be damaged or affixed to the tibia by the pins. The anterior tibial artery may also be injured. Placement of the pins almost entirely through the subcutaneous surface can help prevent this damage. A further disadvantage of external frames is that malalignment cannot always be corrected perfectly.

Our preferred method for applying external frames is to use half-pin units placed through the anteromedial surface of the leg when possible (Fig. 126-6). The choice of frame type (Hoffmann, Anderson, AO, etc.) is less important than the method of application. The pin tracts should be predrilled, and large pins (at least 4.5 mm) are used. Threaded pins are used in metaphyseal bone, and either threaded or smooth pins may be used in cortical bone. Stability is greatly improved if two half-pin frames are applied in different planes. Ideally, the pins will be placed so that the fracture site can be compressed, and fibular osteotomy may be necessary. However, we frequently use this method when infection, loss of bone stock, or both, exist, in which cases compression is not possible. In these fractures we use the frame to stabilize the bone while infection is being eradicated and the bone ends revascularized. Cancellous bone grafting, ei-

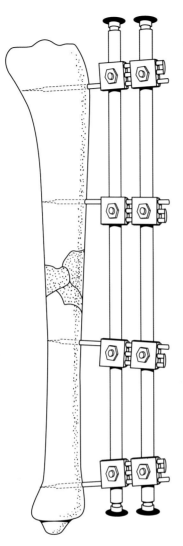

Fig. 126-6. External fixation devices are useful in stabilizing and applying compression to infected nonunions. Half-pin units are preferred over transfixion pins, which penetrate the anterior compartment musculature. Double single-bar units are used to increase rigidity greatly.

ther open or posterolateral, usually accompanies the application of the external fixation for nonunions. As soon as stability of the tibia is obtained, we remove the external fixator and apply a long leg weight-bearing cast (Fig. 126-7).

Many external fixation devices are on the market, and their evolution continues. The reader is referred to the excellent practical work of Behrens.[6]

Intramedullary Nailing

A further operative method of treating tibial malunions and nonunions, intramedullary nailing, is also useful for treating noninfected pseudarthoses. Küntscher,[33] Muller and Thomas,[42] and Böhler[7] have all used reamed intramedullary nails. Lottes has employed unreamed nails in both fresh fractures and nonunions of the tibia.[35]

Unreamed closed intramedullary nailing can be a relatively simple procedure provided that the bone is well aligned. Open osteotomy may be necessary to gain reduction, and this procedure increases the risk of infection and prolongs the healing time. Fibular osteotomy or short segmental fibular resection may be helpful in reducing any malalignment and allowing impaction. Unreamed nails do not provide stable fixation because they provide poor rotational control and are obviously a form of internal splinting. In nonunions, scarring in the soft tissue sometimes prevents excessive motion, and aligning the bone even with an unreamed nail so that it has good function and impaction may provide sufficient stability for union.

However, because it provides stimulation of the fracture site by reaming as well as added nail width and stabilization, intramedullary nailing with pre-reamed Küntscher nails is our preferred treatment for most noninfected delayed unions and nonunions of the tibia. It is also our preferred method for fixation of osteotomies for malunion in the middle third area of the tibia (Fig. 126-8). Our success rate in both applications is approximately 95 percent.[16]

By far the most important principle in the use of this technique is that because reaming of the tibia destroys the intramedullary blood supply, it must not be performed until the external blood supply from periosteum and other surrounding soft tissues has been entirely reestablished. A previously fractured tibia is likely to have established most of its blood supply from an external source. Almost any fracture will create an interruption of the main interosseous artery to the distal fragment, causing the external blood supply to be enhanced. Although the time required for this external blood supply to develop is not yet clearly known, it is our impression that a minimum of 4 to 6 weeks is necessary. With more violent stripping or damage to the

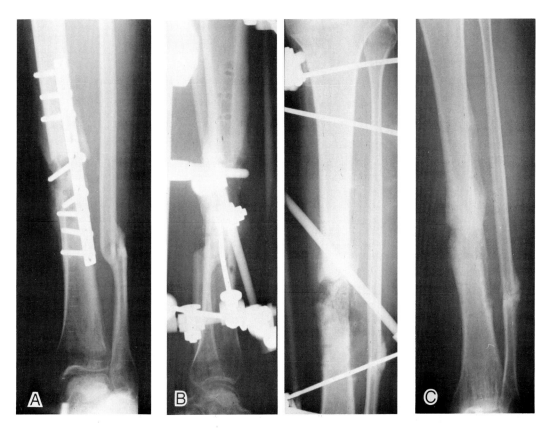

Fig. 126-7. A 40-year-old man involved in a motorcycle accident sustained a grade III open tibia fracture and a severe ipsilateral grade III open femur fracture. **(A)** Five months after injury and plate fixation, the patient had an infected nonunion. The plate was loose. **(B)** AP and lateral radiographs after plate removal, debridement, application of external fixator, and delayed open cancellous bone graft. **(C)** Five months after bone grafting the fracture is healed. There is no drainage.

external tissues, a longer time should be allowed before reaming and nailing the tibia.

The second principle for the use of intramedullary nailing is that the fracture pattern must be fairly stable and the fracture must be in the middle of the tibia. Some would say that the fracture should be confined to the middle third. Because of the broad flare of the upper portion of the tibia, better control is gained by an intramedullary nail in the middle and slightly toward the distal end than in the proximal end.

The major advantage of intramedullary nailing, once the criteria for blood supply, fracture pattern, and level of fracture have been met, is that it offers fully functional postoperative treatment. We generally advocate the use of a walking cast for a short time to provide external soft tissue support. With the ideal situation of a fairly stable fracture in the middle portion of the shaft, the patient can be free of all external support fairly quickly and can bear full weight while healing progresses. This treatment is ideal for maintenance and rehabilitation of the joints and other soft tissues, particularly in the foot. Full weight bearing is possible because an intramedullary nail is a weight-sharing device that allows most of the stress to be borne by the bone. The stress on the tibia not only seems to stimulate union but also prevents the cancellization or weakening of the bone caused by stress protection. Furthermore, the device itself is unlikely to fracture because it bears only a small portion of the load.

For intramedullary nailing of the tibia, we use

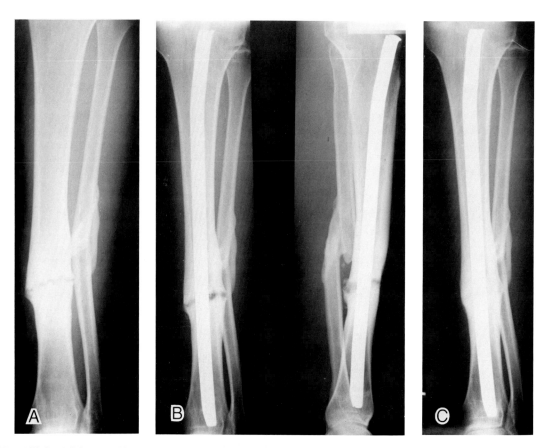

Fig. 126-8. A 24-year-old man sustained a grade II open tibia fracture. **(A)** Two years after fracture, the patient's tibia is 23 mm short, and there is slight motion at nonunion site. Ambulation is slightly painful. No drainage or other signs of infection are present. **(B)** Closed intramedullary nailing with reaming performed. **(C)** Six months after intramedullary nailing, the tibia is healed and the patient is without pain.

the standard Küntscher technique with minor modifications. Placing the patient supine on the fracture table allows the tibia to be raised in a fairly horizontal position but with 90 degrees of flexion at the knee. Positioning must allow clear anteroposterior (AP) and lateral visualization of the tibia with the image intensifier (Fig. 126-9). A transverse incision at the midpoint of the patellar tendon yields good exposure for the starting point of the nail. Care should be taken to minimize the trauma to the superior skin flap while reaming and driving the nail. Access to the starting point (Fig. 126-10) is usually possible by retraction of the patellar tendon laterally. A vertical skin incision may be employed, but may result in a disfiguring scar, which is of special concern for women. Splitting the

tendon is preferred by some and is perfectly acceptable. The tibia is opened with an awl in the smooth, sloping area of the bone just behind the patellar tendon attachment and just in front of the fat pad that is external to the knee joint.

In the tibia, especially in nonunion with hypertrophic and or dense bone, one must be extremely careful not to cause heat necrosis of bone. This is aggravated by dull reamers, progressing by 1-mm rather than 0.5-mm increments. The worst mistake is to perform an open osteotomy under tourniquet and then leave the tourniquet in place while reaming. This removes the circulation cooling of the bone and increases thermal damage and necrosis inside the bone, which can be virtually full-thickness at times and can lead to very prolonged heal-

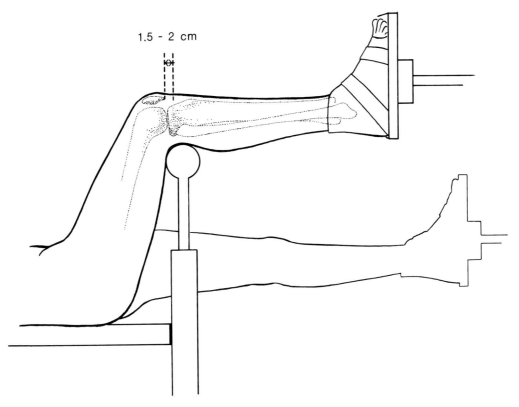

1.5 - 2 cm

Fig. 126-9. Lower-extremity position for intramedullary nailing of tibia. The lower leg is parallel to the floor. The C-arm image intensifier was rotated about both legs to obtain AP and lateral views. The knee must be flexed at least 70 degrees (ideally 90 degrees).

ing or even to loss of large bone segments with infection, even in closed fractures.

A sharp hand reamer is usually required to transect an intramedullary plug of fibrous tissue or callus. It can be difficult to keep the reamer aligned properly so that this opening does not fall too far posterior in the tibia. It is wise to have available some slightly bent, very sharp, stout guide wires to drive across this area in the proper position, which must be monitored closely with the image intensifier.

After the area has been opened up, reaming can proceed over the usual bulb-tipped reaming guide until a fairly large nail can be inserted. We use larger nails in nonunions than in fresh fractures because in nonunions the external portion of the tibia is well vascularized and the bone usually is not brittle. Smaller nails must be used in fresh fractures, where reaming can be risky because the bone is brittle and/or not well vascularized from external sources and if hairline splits are present. For nonunions we tend to use intramedullary nails with a diameter of 11 to 12 mm in women or small men and 13 to 14 mm in men or larger women; we use even larger nails in older osteoporotic bone with large canals. The nail must be measured very accurately so that it extends from the insertion site just above the tibial tubercle to the old metaphyseal scar above the ankle joint.

Intramedullary nailing is relatively easy in fractures that have been previously treated with an unreamed nail or with a plate and screws, where the medullary canal is in perfect alignment. On occasion, reamed nailing may even follow the use of an external fixator, although the risk of infection may be high if there have been any pin-tract problems (Fig. 126-11). When the fracture has been treated nonsurgically, which is often the case, the

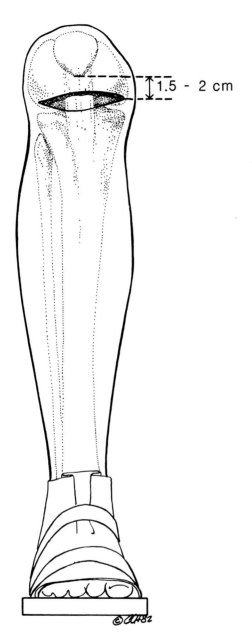

1.5 - 2 cm

Fig. 126-10. Skin incision for intramedullary nailing of the tibia. The patellar tendon is exposed through a transverse incision. The tendon is usually split longitudinally to gain access to the correct starting point. Variation in the shape of the proximal tibia may necessitate starting *medial* to the tendon.

medullary canal may not be in alignment. In this case a very limited open procedure may be required to remove some hypertrophic bone or fibrous tissue and to align the canal (Fig. 126-12). If there has been some loss of length and the fibula has healed, we frequently find that it should be osteotomized by removing a small portion of the bone, generally very near the level of the tibial fracture. The fractured ends of the tibia may then collapse and impact together. This procedure may also be needed if an angulatory correction must be made in the tibia (Fig. 126-13). On the other hand, if a fairly marked angulatory correction is needed and if the fracture is not close to the center of the bone, ideal alignment frequently cannot be achieved with an intramedullary nail. In this case the correction would be made with a compression plate and screws; again a wedge would be removed at the apex of the angulation as with a nonunion. If the malunion is either too proximal or too distal or if there is a rotational component, a compression plate and screws would give a more satisfactory result.

A particularly dysfunctional malunion in the tibia is one in the region of only 2.52 to 7.56 cm above the ankle joint where there has been a hyperextension deformity. This deformity brings the weight-bearing line of the tibia posterior to the dome of the talus and causes significant discomfort and gait abnormality. Also, significant varus or valgus angulation may occur, with varus angulation being more difficult to adjust to, probably because the range of motion of the subtalar joint allows compensation for more valgus than varus angulation. We believe that valgus malunions of more than 10 to 12 degrees and varus malunions of more than 5 to 7 degrees warrant realignment to protect both the ankle and knee joints. The closer the malunion is to the distal tibia, the more the ankle joint appears to be adversely affected.

In summary, for malunions in the middle shaft of the tibia without significant rotary abnormality, we would use the intramedullary nail, which allows excellent functional aftertreatment. A small incision can be made to remove a wedge at the apex, and the tibia can be aligned and reamed in a standard manner. For malunions in the metaphyseal areas or toward the upper end of the shaft and for those with rotational abnormalities, a compression

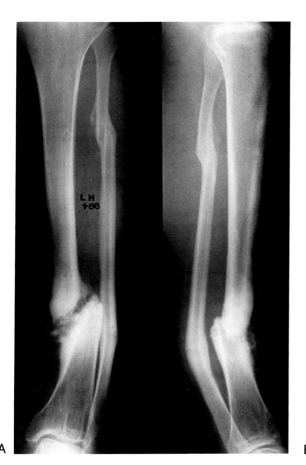 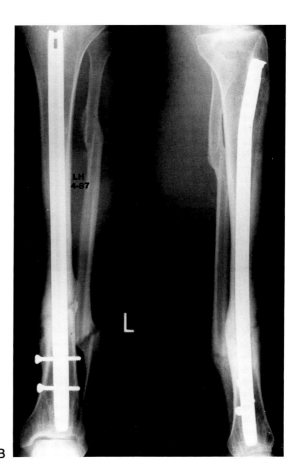

A   B

Fig. 126-11. (A) A 30-year-old-man with a previous grade II open fracture of the distal tibia and fibula, which was treated first with external fixation and cast, in which he drifted into varus and extension and shortening position with nonunion. Soft tissues were well healed, and the foot was normal. **(B)** The patient was treated with a reamed, distal locked intramedullary nail. A small incision was made to loosen the fracture site and to perform an osteotomy in the fibula. The nailing was done using intramedullary osteotomes and hand reamers to get across the medullary plugs, and a distractor was placed for realignment, resulting in a central position. It progressed to solid union, but note the slight residual extension, which is unfortunately common, but of minor consequence, when using this technique. The distal locking screws add significant stability to these relatively distal fractures. If done very carefully, they allow treatment of fractures up to 2 cm more distal than this. However, control of alignment becomes progressively more difficult, and, compression plating on the side of the apex of the malunion is recommended in the area near the metaphysis.

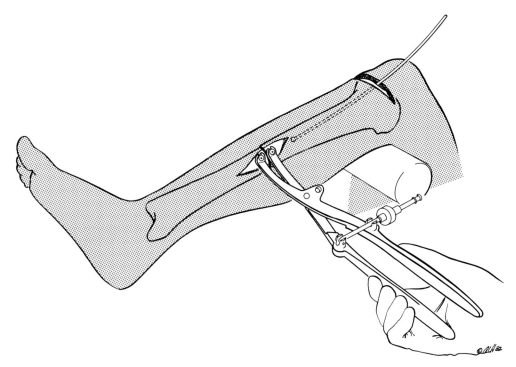

Fig. 126-12. A large pelvic reduction forceps is used to hold the reduction for intramedullary nailing for a tibial nonunion. Transverse screws placed in the tibia *anterior* to the medullary canal allow attachment of the forceps. The reduction is held by the assistant as reaming and nailing progress.

plate and screws provide the most anatomic correction. For malunions very near the ankle or near the knee, combinations of devices using special T-plates, L-plates, cloverleaf plates, and occasionally long cancellous screws are needed to give perfect correction.

CONCLUSION

High-energy and open fractures of the tibia, which are all too common in our modern, fast-moving society, continue to present extremely challenging problems to the orthopaedic traumatologist. In our very large series of multiply injured patients, our general protocol is immediate internal fixation of long bone fractures, especially in open wounds. This treatment proves to be very safe for all fractures in all bones except the tibia. With

tibial fractures, we still have a significant incidence of delayed union, nonunion, and infection. If any one factor can be singled out as most important, it would be the status of the blood supply to the dense cortical bone. This blood supply is virtually always disrupted to some degree in a high-energy injury, and an open fracture presents the added problems of contamination and disruption of the protective soft tissues. If one keeps in mind that the major goal early in the course of treatment is restoration and protection of soft tissues along with their blood supply, one can carefully design secondary procedures that can be very successful in the treatment of delayed union, nonunion, and even infected fractures. Different fixation techniques and grafting methods will be appropriate for different types of fractures, and various combinations can be used. Although intramedullary nailing is the most functional treatment, its use is limited to fractures in the middle portion of the tibial shaft, relatively stable fractures, and those that have reestablished an external blood supply, so that the reaming away of the

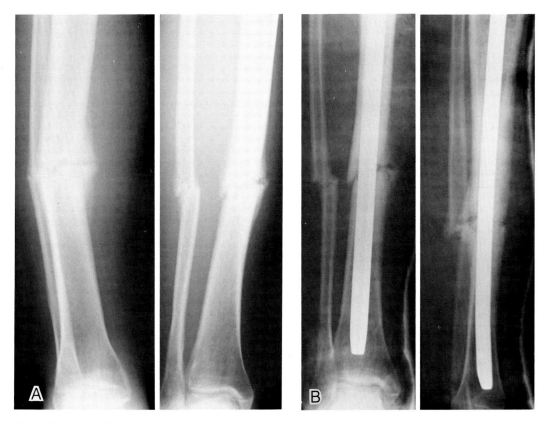

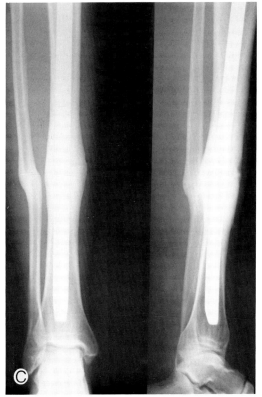

Fig. 126-13. A 32-year-old man experienced a closed tibia fracture, which had not healed after 9 months of immobilization. **(A)** Posterior angulation of 15 degrees at the fracture site. **(B)** Intramedullary nailing with a fibular and tibial osteotomy. Closed reduction of the posterior angulation was not possible. **(C)** The fracture is well healed 10 months after surgery.

internal blood supply is not devastating and does not cause massive necrosis of bone. When internal fixation is adopted, very careful soft tissue technique must be used to maintain the blood supply to the bone as completely as possible. This supply in a previously fractured tibia has been derived primarily from the external tissues in the early postinjury period. Finally, the tibia must eventually be anatomically restored very close to its proper length, rotation, and angulation to render a patient fully functional.

REFERENCES

1. Abbott LE, Schottstaedt EP, Saunders JB, et al: The evaluation of cortical and cancellous bone as grafting material. J Bone Joint Surg 29A:381, 1947
2. Acland R, Smith P: Microvascular surgical techniques used to provide skin cover over an ununited tibial fracture. J Bone Joint Surg 58B:471, 1976
3. Albee FH: Principles of the treatment of nonunion of fractures. Surg Gynecol Obstet 51:389, 1930
4. Bassett CAL: Clinical implication of cell functions in bone grafting. Clin Orthop 87:49, 1972
5. Bassett CAL, Mitchell SN, Gaston BR: Treatment of ununited tibial diaphyseal fractures with pulsing magnetic fields. J Bone Joint Surg 63A:511, 1981
6. Behrens F: External skeletal fixation. In Murray DG (ed): American Academy of Orthopaedic Surgeons Instructional Course Lectures, Vol. 30. CV Mosby, St. Louis, 1981
7. Böhler J: Treatment of nonunion of the tibia with closed and semiclosed intramedullary nailing. Clin Orthop 43:93, 1965
8. Boyd HB: The treatment of difficult and unusual nonunions. With special reference to the bridging of defects. J Bone Joint Surg 25:535, 1943
9. Boyd HB: Nonunion of shafts of long bones with a statistic of 842 patients. J Bone Joint Surg 43A:159, 1961
10. Brighton CT, Fredenburg DZB, Mitchell EL, et al: Treatment of nonunion with constant direct current. Clin Orthop 124:106, 1977
11. Brown PA, Urban JG: Early weight bearing treatment of open fractures of the tibia. An end result of 63 cases. J Bone Joint Surg 51A:59, 1969
12. Burri C: Post-traumatic Osteomyelitis. Hans Huber, Bern, 1975
13. Charnley J: The Closed Treatment of Common Fractures. 3rd Ed. Churchill Livingstone, Edinburgh, 1972
14. Christensen NO: Küntscher intramedullary reaming and nail fixation for nonunion of fractures of the femur and the tibia. J Bone Joint Surg 55B:312, 1973
15. Clancy GJ, Hansen ST: Open fractures of the tibia. A review of 102 cases. J Bone Joint Surg 60A:118, 1978
16. Clancy GJ, Winquist RA, Hansen ST: Nonunion of the tibia treated with Küntscher intramedullary nailing. Clin Orthop 167:191, 1982
17. Danis R: Théorie et Pratique de l'Ostiosynthèse. Masson, Paris, 1949
18. DeHaas DG, Watson J, Morrison OM: Noninvasive treatment of nonunited fractures of the tibia using electrical stimulation. J Bone Joint Surg 62B:465, 1980
19. Dehne E: The weight bearing principle in treatment of lower extremity fractures, 1885–1972. J Trauma 12:539, 1972
20. Dunn N: Treatment of ununited fractures. Br Med J 2:221, 1939
21. Frankel VH, Burstein AH: Orthopaedic Biomechanics. Lea & Febiger, Philadelphia, 1970
22. Freeland AE, Mutz SB: Posterior bone grafting for infected ununited fracture of the tibia. J Bone Joint Surg 58A:653, 1976
23. Fisher WD, Hamblen DL: Problems and pitfalls of compression fixation of long bone fractures. A review of results and complications. Injury 10:99, 1978
24. Ger R: Muscle transposition for treatment and prevention of chronic post-traumatic osteomyelitis of the tibia. J Bone Joint Surg 59A:784, 1977
25. Hansen LW: Posterior bone grafting of the tibia for nonunion. J Bone Joint Surg 48A:27, 1966
26. Hoaglund FT, States JD: Factors in influencing the rate of healing in tibial shaft fractures. Surg Gynecol Obstet 124:71, 1967
27. Holden CEA: Bone-grafts in the treatment of delayed union of tibial shaft fractures. Injury 4:175, 1972
28. Jones K: Treatment of infected nonunion of the tibia through the posterolateral approach. Clin Orthop 43:103, 1965
29. Jorgensen TE: Measurements of stability of crural fractures treated with Hoffman osteolaxis. Acta Orthop Scand 43:207, 1972
30. Judet R, Patel A: Muscle pedicle bone grafting of long bones by osteoperoseal decortication. Clin Orthop 87:7, 1972

31. Karlström G, Olerud S: Fractures of the tibial shaft: a critical evaluation of treatment alternatives. Clin Orthop 105:82, 1974
32. Karlström G, Olerud S: Secondary internal fixation. Acta Orthop Scand, suppl., 175:1, 1979
33. Küntscher G: The Practice of Intramedullary Nailing. Charles C Thomas, Springfield, IL, 1967
34. LaRossa D, Mellissinos E, Matthews D, et al: The use of microvascular free skin muscle flaps in management of avulsion injuries of the lower leg. J Trauma 20:545, 1980
35. Lottes JO: Treatment of delayed or nonunion fractures of the tibia by a medullary nail. Clin Orthop 43:111, 1965
36. Macnab I, DeHaas WG: The role of periosteal blood supply in the healing of fractures of the tibia. Clin Orthop 105:27, 1974
37. Matti H: Über freie Transplantationen von Knochenspongiosa. Langenbecks Arch Chir 168:236, 1932
38. McCarrol HR: Surgical management of tibial nonunions. JAMA 175:578, 1961
39. McConnell CM, Hyland WT, Neale HW: Microvascular free groin flap for soft tissue coverage of the extremities. J Trauma 20:593, 1980
40. Meyers S, Weiland AJ, Willene G, et al: The treatment of infected nonunion of fractures and long bones. J Bone Joint Surg 57A:836, 1975
41. Michelinakis E: Treatment of chronic osteomyelitis with the continuous irrigation suction method. Acta Orthop Scand 43:25, 1972
42. Milch H: Tibio-fibular synostosis for nonunion of the tibia. Surgery 27:770, 1950
43. Müller ME, Thomas RJ: Treatment of nonunion in fractures of long bones. Clin Orthop 43:141, 1965
44. Nelson GE, Kelly PJ, Peterson LFA, et al: Blood supply of the human tibia. J Bone Joint Surg 42A:625, 1960
45. Nicoll EA: Fractures of the tibial shaft. J Bone Joint Surg 46B:373, 1964
46. Olerud S: Treatment of fractures by the Vidal–Aorey method. Acta Orthop Scand 44:516, 1973
47. Parker B: Two-plate fixation for nonunion. Injury 5:291, 1974
48. Phemister OB: Treatment of ununited fractures by only bone grafts without screw fixation or tie fixation and without breaking down of the fibrous union. J Bone Joint Surg 29:946, 1947
49. Reckling FW, Waters CH: Treatment of nonunions by posterolateral cortical cancellous bone grafting. J Bone Joint Surg 62A:936, 1980
50. Rhinelander FW: Tibial blood supply in relation to fracture healing. Clin Orthop 105:34, 1974
51. Rokkanen P, Slatis P: Subcortical cancellous bone grafting in the treatment of delayed union of tibia shaft fractures. J Trauma 12:1075, 1973
52. Rosen H: Compression treatment of long bone pseudarthrosis. Clin Orthop 138:157, 1979
53. Rosenthal RE: Nonunion in open tibial fractures. J Bone Joint Surg 59A:244, 1977
54. Sakellarides HT, Freeman PA, Grant BD: Delayed union and nonunion of tibial shaft fractures. A review of 100 cases. J Bone Joint Surg 46A:557, 1964
55. Sarmiento A, Latta LL: Functional bracing in the management of tibial fractures: the intact fibula. In Moore T (ed): Symposium on Trauma to the Leg and Its Sequelae. American Academy of Orthopaedic Surgeons Instructional Course Lectures. Vol. 30. CV Mosby, St. Louis, 1981
56. Schatzker J: Results of compression plating of closed nonunion of the tibia. In Moore T (ed): Symposium of Trauma to the Leg and Its Sequelae. American Academy of Orthopaedic Surgeons Instructional Course Lectures. CV Mosby, St. Louis, 1981
57. Smith JEM: Results of early and delayed internal fixation for tibial shaft fractures. J Bone Joint Surg 56B:469, 1974
58. Solheim K, Vaagem S: Delayed union and nonunion of fractures. Clinical experience with the ASIF method. J Trauma 13:121, 1973
59. Taylor GI, Watson N: One-stage repair of compound leg defects with free revascularized flaps of groin skin and iliac bone. Plast Reconstr Surg 61:494, 1978
60. Trueta J: Blood supply and the rate of healing of tibial fractures. Clin Orthop 105:11, 1974
61. Watson-Jones R: Injuries to the leg. In Wilson JN (ed): Fractures and Joint Injuries. Churchill Livingstone, Edinburgh, 1976
62. Weiland AJ, Kleinert HE, Kute JE, et al: Free vascularized bone grafts in surgery of the upper extremity. J Hand Surg 4:129, 1979
63. Widenfalk B, Ponten B, Karlström G: Open fractures of the shaft of the tibia. Analysis of wound and fracture treatment. Injury 11:136, 1979

Ankle Fractures

127

Isadore G. Yablon
David Segal

Ankle fractures are common injuries that may vary in severity from an undisplaced incomplete fracture of the malleolus to a severely comminuted injury involving the weight-bearing surface of the tibial plafond with ligament disruption. In contrast with long-bone injuries, severe comminution or displacement is not always associated with high-energy trauma. Many of these injuries will occur as a result of rotational stresses, with the weight of the body acting as the offending force. This is understandable, since the ankle bears up to five times the body weight. It is the most congruous joint of the lower extremity, bound by the distal end of the tibia and medial malleolus medially and the distal end of the fibula and lateral malleolus laterally, with the talus positioned between them. The axis of motion of the ankle joint passes through the distal limits of the medial and lateral malleoli, creating a complex hinge motion, with dorsiflexion accompanied by external rotation and plantar flexion by internal rotation.

The stability of the ankle is provided by the configuration of the mortise and by additional ligamentous structures (Figs. 127-1 to 127-3). The syndesmotic ligaments include the anterior and posterior tibiofibular ligaments, the inferior transverse ligament, and the interosseous ligament, the latter being the distal expansion of the interosseous membrane. These syndesmotic ligaments hold the distal tibia and fibula in close contact and allow for slight rotation of the distal fibula, thereby increasing the width of the mortise during dorsiflexion. Additional stability is provided by the deltoid ligament on the medial aspect, consisting of a superficial and deep portion, and by the fibular collateral ligaments on the lateral side, which include the anterior and posterior talofibular, calcaneofibular, and calcaneal ligaments. These latter ligaments are most frequently involved in sprains of the ankle.

The pathomechanics of ankle fractures were described in detail by Lauge-Hansen[16] (Table 127-1).

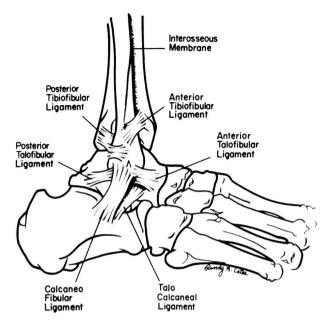

Fig. 127-1. The syndesmotic ligament stabilizes the distal tibiofibular articulation. A second distinct group is the fibular collateral ligaments, which include the anterior and posterior talofibular ligament, and the talocalcaneal and the calcaneofibular ligaments.

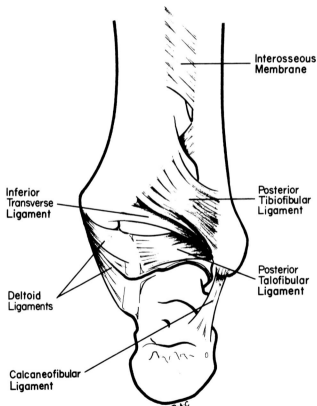

Fig. 127-2. The posterior aspect of the distal part of the tibiofibular articulation illustrates the interosseous membrane, the posterior tibiofibular ligament, and distally the inferior transverse ligaments, which are all part of the syndesmotic ligaments.

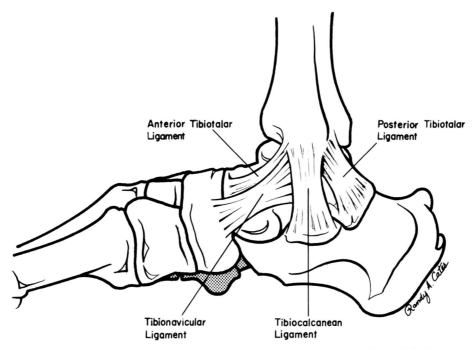

Fig. 127-3. On the medial side of the ankle joint, the deltoid ligament provides stability with its four components: the anterior tibiotalar, the tibionavicular, the tibiocalcaneal, and the posterior tibiotalar ligaments.

On the basis of his experimental work, Lauge-Hansen demonstrated that the type of fracture depended on the position of the forefoot, the direction of force, and the direction of rotation of the ankle on the foot. He observed five different fracture patterns. Each pattern was subclassified into stages; as the force continued to act, the severity of the injury was increased. Thus, with the forefoot in supination and with an external rotatory force of the foot on the ankle the first structure to fail was the anterior tibiofibular ligament followed by an oblique or short spiral fracture of the lateral malleolus. As the force continued, the posterior lip of the tibia was fractured, and finally a fracture of the medial malleolus occurred or the deltoid ligament was torn (Fig. 127-4). With the foot in supination and with a medially directed force, a transverse fracture of the lateral malleolus or tear of the fibular collateral ligaments was observed followed by a vertical fracture of the medial malleolus at the level of the joint (Fig. 127-5). When the forefoot was held in pronation and an external rotatory force applied, the first structure to fail was the medial malleolus or deltoid ligament. As the injury progressed, there was a disruption of the anterior tibiofibular ligament and interosseous membrane, a short oblique fracture of the fibula 8 cm or more proximal to the lateral malleolus, and a disruption of the posterior tibiofibular ligament and fracture of the posterior lip of the tibia. These injuries are characterized by a diastasis of the tibiofibular joint (Fig. 127-6). With the forefoot in pronation and with a force directed laterally, the medial malleolus was fractured or the deltoid ligament was torn. This was followed by a disruption of the anterior and posterior tibiofibular ligaments with the subsequent development of an oblique fracture of the lateral malleolus in which there was comminution of the lateral cortex. This fracture is horizontal when viewed on the lateral radiograph (Fig. 127-7). When the forefoot was in pronation and the ankle forcefully dorsiflexed, as in axial loading of the tibia, the medial malleolus was fractured, followed by fracture of the tibial plafond. The amount of comminution is determined by the magnitude of the force. With further progression, a fracture of

**Table 127-1. Classification of Ankle Injuries
According to Lauge-Hansen**[a]

		Description
Supination-eversion		
Stage		
	1	Disruption of anterior tibiofibular ligament
	2	Oblique or short spiral fracture of lateral malleolus
	3	Fractured posterior lip of tibia
	4	Fractured medial malleolus or tear of deltoid ligament
Supination-adduction		
Stage		
	1	Transverse fracture of lateral malleolus or tear of fibular collateral ligaments
	2	Vertical fracture of medial malleolus at joint level
Pronation-eversion		
Stage		
	1	Fracture of medial malleolus or tear of deltoid ligament
	2	Disruption of anterior tibiofibular ligament and interosseous membrane
	3	Short oblique fracture of fibula ≥8 cm proximal to lateral malleolus
	4	Disruption of posterior tibiofibular ligament and fracture of posterior lip of tibia
Pronation-abduction		
Stage		
	1	Fracture of medial malleolus or tear of deltoid ligament
	2	Disruption of anterior and posterior tibiofibular ligaments
	3	Oblique fracture of lateral malleolus with comminution of the lateral cortex; fracture horizontal on the lateral view
Pronation-dorsiflexion		
Stage		
	1	Fracture of medial malleolus
	2	Fracture of tibial plafond
	3	Fracture of posterior lip of tibia
	4	High transverse or oblique fracture of fibula

[a] The terms supination and pronation refer to the position of the forefoot. Adduction and abduction describe the direction of the force. Eversion and inversion designate the direction of rotation of the ankle on the foot.

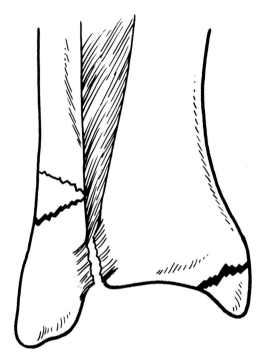

Fig. 127-4. Supination-eversion injury according to the Lauge-Hansen classification.

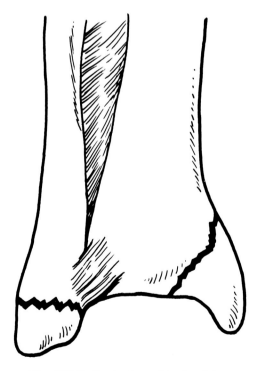

Fig. 127-5. Supination-adduction injury.

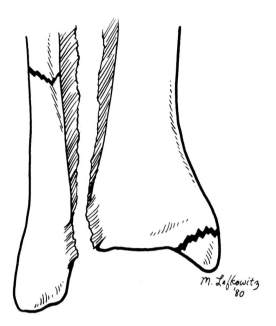

Fig. 127-6. Pronation-eversion fracture.

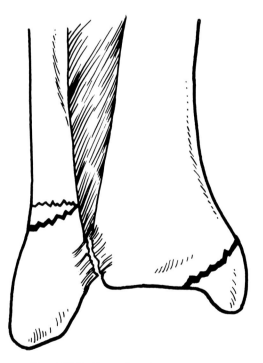

Fig. 127-7. Pronation-abduction injury.

the posterior lip of the tibia was noted, followed by a high transverse or oblique fracture of the fibula.

The ultimate aim in treating ankle fractures should be to achieve anatomic reduction in order to restore normal function. Despite controversy regarding the best method of treatment, the literature confirms that excellent long-term results are obtained only when an anatomic reduction is achieved. Any residual talar displacement or instability will predispose to late degenerative changes.[4,5,7,18] It is therefore appropriate to consider the radiologic criteria that determine the accuracy of the reduction.

One of the earliest methods[1,3,7] involved the measuring of the joint space between the talus and the tibial plafond (Fig. 127-8). Residual talar displacement should be suspected, if any of these measurements is greater than 2 mm. The problem with this method is that all three measurements cannot be obtained in a single view. A routine anteroposterior (AP) projection of the ankle in which the x-ray beam is parallel to the inner surface of the medial malleolus cannot show the space be-

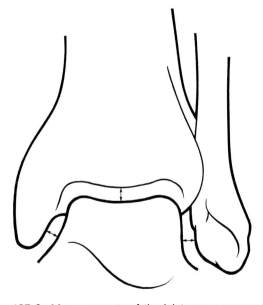

Fig. 127-8. Measurements of the joint space among the medial, lateral, and tibial plafond surfaces and the corresponding articulating surfaces of the talus. Measurements should be within 2 mm or less of difference, indicating no talar displacement.

tween the talus and the lateral malleolus (Fig. 127-9). Similarly, in the mortise or internal oblique view in which the ankle is internally rotated to 20 degrees, the x-ray beam will be parallel to the inner surface of the lateral malleolus, but not to the medial one (Fig. 127-10). It is therefore recommended that if this method is to be used, both **AP** and mortise projections should be obtained.

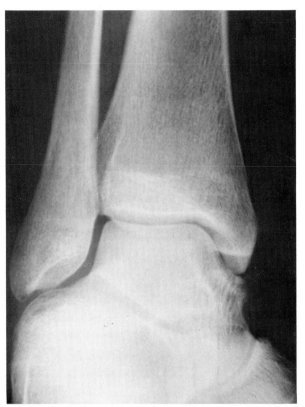

Fig. 127-10. Mortise view projection of the ankle in Fig. 127-9. The central beam is parallel to the inner surface of the lateral malleolus and the measurement between the opposing surfaces of the lateral malleolus and the talus equals that between the plafond and the dome of the talus.

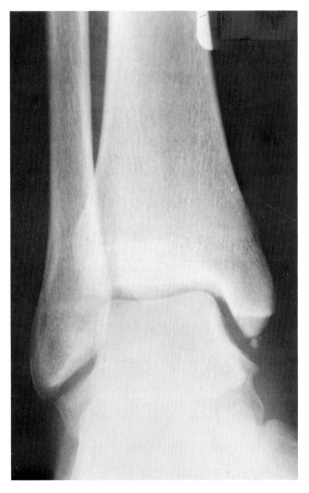

Fig. 127-9. AP projection of injured ankle. Note that the central radiograph beam is parallel to the inner surface of the medial malleolus and corresponding articulating surface of the talus. The distance between the inner surface of the medial malleolus and corresponding articulating surface of the talus equals that between the tibial plafond and the talus.

In our opinion, the most accurate method with which to evaluate the quality of the reduction was described by Joy et al.[13] A vertical line is drawn down the center of the tibia on the standard **AP** view (Fig. 127-11) and should pass through the center of the talus. If not, a talar shift has occurred, indicating that the talus is being displaced either medially or laterally. The amount of displacement is represented by the distance between the midline of the tibia and the midline of the talus and should not exceed 0.5 mm. On the lateral projection, a vertical line along the middle of the tibia should pass through the most superior part of the dome of the talus (Fig. 127-12). If it does not, an anterior or

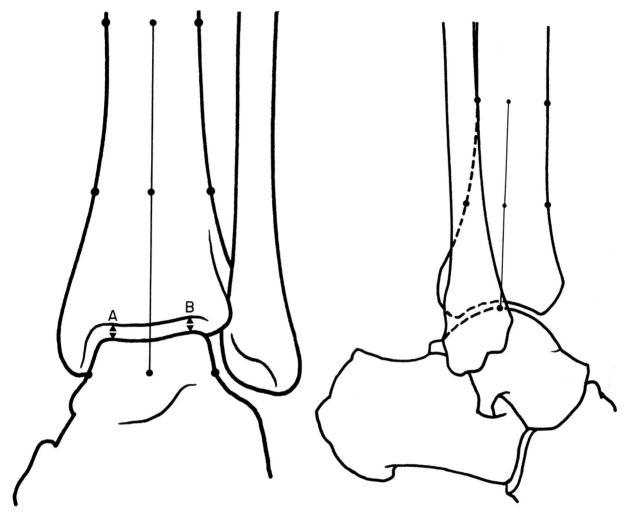

Fig. 127-11. Measurements of the talar tilt and talar displacement. The distance between the talar dome and the tibial plafond should not be greater than 0.5 mm when measured at the medial **(A)** and lateral **(B)** sides of the ankle joint. The central midline of the tibia should transect the middle of the dome of the talus.

Fig. 127-12. Lateral drawing of the ankle joint in a true lateral projection. The dome of the talus will appear as a single line and the most superior part of the dome is transected by the midline of the tibia.

posterior displacement of the talus exists. Talar tilt is evaluated by measuring the distance between the articular surfaces of the tibia and talus in the medial and lateral parts of the joint on the AP view (Fig. 127-11). The difference between these two measurements should not be greater than 0.5 mm.

From a practical point of view, it may sometimes be somewhat difficult in obtaining such precise radiographics, especially if the ankle is immobilized in a cast. In such instances, it has been our policy to accept a reduction in which the medial or lateral malleolus has a residual displacement of not greater than 2 mm. This also applies to the posterior lip of the tibia (posterior malleolus) if it involves 20 percent or more of the articulating surface. Table 127-2 may be helpful in this regard.

Table 127-2. Radiologic Criteria in Assessing Reduction

	Good	Fair	Poor
Lateral malleolus	Anatomic alignment of ≤ 1 mm of displacement in any direction[a]	2–5-mm displacement	Displacement > 5 mm in direction
	Mortise widening ≤ 0.5 mm	Mortise widening ≤ 2 mm	Mortise widening > 2 mm
	Talar tilt ≤ 0.5 mm	Talar tilt ≤ 1.0 mm	Talar tilt > 1.0 mm
	Fractures at or above plafond	Fractures at or above plafond	Angulation rotation and displacement > 5
	≤ 2-mm displacement in any direction	2–5-mm displacement	
	Mortise widening ≤ 0.5 mm	Mortise widening ≤ 2 mm	Mortise widening > 2 mm
Medial malleolus	Talar tilt ≤ 0.5 mm	Talar tilt ≤ 1.0 mm	Talar tilt > 1.0 mm
	Fractures distal to plafond	Fractures distal to plafond	
	< 2-mm displacement laterally[b]	≥ 2-mm displacement laterally	
	May be up to 5-mm displacement in any other place	≥ 5-mm displacement in any other place	
	Marginal and posterior lip fragments ≤ 25% of articular surface	Posterior lip fragment ≤ 25% of articulating surface	Posterior lip fragment > 25% of articulating surface
Posterior malleolus	Proximal displacement < 2 mm	Proximal displacement 2–5 mm	Proximal displacement > 5 mm
	Mortise widening ≤ 0.5 mm	Mortise widening ≤ 2 mm	Mortise widening > 2 mm
	Talar tilt ≤ 0.5 mm	Talar tilt ≤ 1.0 mm	Talar tilt > 1.0 mm
Talus	Talar displacement in any direction ≤ 0.5 mm	Talar displacement ≤ 2 mm	Talar displacement > 2 mm
	Talar tilt ≤ 0.5 mm	Talar tilt ≤ 1.0 mm	Talar tilt > 1.0 mm

[a] In isolated fractures of the lateral malleolus in which no ligaments are torn, ≤ 4 mm of displacement is acceptable.
[b] Lateral displacement may cause impingement, with subsequent degenerative arthritis between the medial malleolus and talus.

TREATMENT OPTIONS

Ankle fractures may be treated either by manipulation and immobilization or by open reduction and internal fixation. Closed reduction and plaster immobilization should be reserved for stable fractures, whereas unstable fractures should be treated by open reduction and internal fixation. Stable injuries include isolated fractures of the medial and lateral malleolus when no ligaments are torn and fractures of the anterior and posterior lip of the tibia involving less than 20 percent of the articular surface. Unstable injuries are those in which there is 2 mm or more displacement of the talus or lateral malleolus or if a talar tilt exists as determined radiologically by the above-described method.

A closed reduction should be performed under general or spinal anesthesia to ensure good muscular relaxation. It is helpful to flex the knee over the end of the operating table. Manual traction is applied along the longitudinal axis of the leg to bring the fragments out to length, following which a corrective force is applied to reduce the fracture. The Lauge-Hansen classification is useful in this regard because, the surgeon who is aware of the forces that caused the injury is better equipped to reduce the fracture by reversing them. For example, a supination-eversion injury is denoted radiographically by an oblique or short spinal fracture of the lateral malleolus just above the joint and a transverse fracture of the lateral malleolus at or below the level of the joint. Reduction is achieved by pronating the forefoot and forcibly internally rotating the foot on the ankle. The same reasoning applies to fractures caused by other forces. If a reduction has been obtained, a short-leg cast is applied and molded to maintain the corrective force. Intraoperative radiographs are obtained and, if these are satisfactory, the knee is brought out to 15 degrees of flexion and the cast extended to the groin. Repeat radiographs should be obtained at 48 hours and at 2-week intervals, until 6 weeks have elapsed, to detect any loss of position. The patient is ambulating during this time but does not bear weight on the affected extremity.

If the position of the fracture is maintained, a short-leg cast is applied at 6 weeks; the patient commences touch-down ambulation still using crutches. The cast must be changed if it becomes too loose or is excessively constricting. These fractures generally show evidence of union at 10 weeks. The cast is then removed, an elastic bandage applied, and range-of-motion exercises with graduated weight bearing instituted.

If intraoperative radiographs after the first manipulation show that the fracture has not been reduced, a further attempt might be undertaken. If this attempt fails to achieve a satisfactory result, the surgeon must decide whether to continue with repeated manipulations or to proceed with an open reduction and internal fixation.

If it is elected to treat ankle fractures by manipulation and immobilization, postreduction radiographs must be of good quality, and close attention must be paid to the position of the fragments, since some detail may be obscured by the plaster cast. It is crucial to pay particular attention to the lateral malleolus. It was previously demonstrated that the talus faithfully follows the displacement plane of the lateral malleolus.[35] If the lateral malleolus remains incompletely reduced, the talus will also be incompletely reduced. It is possible to reposition the talus anatomically with force despite an incomplete reduction of the lateral malleolus. In such instances, the lateral ligaments are stretched to permit reduction of the talus.[36] When external immobilization is discontinued, the talus remains potentially unstable and may thereby predispose to late degenerative changes. The surgeon who accepts a reduction in which the talus appears reduced but for which the lateral malleolus is displaced more than 2 mm must also accept the possibility that late degenerative arthritis may occur.

In the presence of marked swelling, it may not be possible to achieve anatomic reduction; the surgeon may prefer to accept an incomplete reduction and immobilize the extremity in a long-leg cast or posterior splint with elevation for 48 hours, until swelling subsides. Repeat manipulation at this time has a better chance of success. The same principle prevails if an open reduction is contemplated. Edema is the enemy of wound healing and should be treated before the ankle is opened. The condition of the skin must also be considered. Surgery should not be performed on patients with blisters or open contaminated wounds that have been present for more than 12 hours. In such instances, it is advisable to treat the soft tissues and do an open reduction when the skin has healed, even if surgery is performed as late as 3 weeks after the injury. This is preferable to operating in the presence of suboptimal conditions and risking infection. Surgery is not recommended in the presence of established infection. In these cases, it is better to treat the infection by debridement and appropriate antibiotic therapy and to apply the plates and screws when the acute phase of the infection has been brought under control.

In rare cases, the skin is so damaged that neither cast immobilization nor open reduction is possible. The displaced ankle may be reduced by manipulation and the position of the talus secured with a Steinmann pin drilled through the plantar aspect of the calcaneum, traversing the talus, and entering the tibial shaft. Alternatively, an external fixator may be used. Steinmann pins are passed transversely through the tibia and talus or other bones of the foot and attached to outriggers to prevent shortening and rotation. Although these methods may not afford a complete reposition, this can be achieved at a later date.

AUTHORS' PREFERRED METHOD

It has been said that the quintessence of fracture treatment would be to wish the fragments into place, hold them there by moral suasion, and send the patient on about his business while the fracture heals. While this ideal has as yet not been achieved, open reduction accompanied by internal fixation and early ambulation comes closer to fulfilling this aim than any other available method. The only advantages that closed reduction offer are the avoidance of a scar and possible infection. The disadvantages are related to the difficulty in obtaining anatomic reduction, maintaining that reduction, and achieving repeated manipulations and cast changes, prolonged immobilization, non-weight bearing, postreduction edema, and postreduction stiffness, which may often prevent the ankle from regaining a full range of motion.[2,7,24] Unless anatomic reduction is achieved, there will be a significant incidence of late posttraumatic degenerative arthritis.[5,11,20,25,33] Ramsey and Hamilton[26] demonstrated that 1 mm of lateral displacement of the talus causes a 42 percent reduction in the tibiotalar articulation. Because of the inverse relationship between pressure and surface area, as the surface area decreases, the pressure applied will increase, and this undoubtedly plays a major role in the development of degenerative arthritis.

With appropriate internal fixation of ankle fractures, early range-of-motion exercises and weight bearing may be instituted and cast immobilization avoided. Thus, the advantages of achieving predictable results by open reduction and of permitting early function and weight bearing far outweigh the apparent advantages of a closed reduction.

OPERATIVE TECHNIQUE

Surgery of ankle fractures should achieve anatomic restoration and secure fixation of the fragments, resulting in early postoperative function. Thus, in a bimalleolar fracture, both malleoli should be fixed. Similarly, in an injury involving a tear of the deltoid ligament and fracture of the lateral malleolus, the deltoid ligament should be repaired and the lateral malleolus immobilized with a plate. Fractures of the anterior or posterior lip of the tibia involving more than 20 percent of the articular surface should be reduced and held with a screw.[4,6,14] Injuries involving a rupture of the interosseous membrane resulting in a diastasis should be reduced by inserting a screw through the fibula into the tibia.

OPEN FRACTURES

The principles regarding the management of open fractures have been well documented by Gustilo and Anderson.[10] Type 1 and 2 wounds require early debridement under a general anesthetic. If this can be achieved within 8 hours, open reduction and internal fixation, which is described below, may be performed if the fracture is unstable. A cephalosporin should be started intravenously prior to the debridement and continued for 24 to 48 hours. If the wound has been present for more than 8 hours, is clean, and there is no sign of infection, internal fixation may be done within 5 days, and the wound can be closed.

Type 3 wounds are an entirely different situation because the incidence of infection is much higher. These must be considered emergencies; patients should be taken to the operating room as soon as their general condition permits. A cephalosporin and an aminoglycoside antibiotic are given intravenously at surgery and meticulous debridement and irrigation carried out. It is mandatory that the wound be left open and the patient returned to the operating room within 24 hours for repeat debridement, under general anesthesia. Antibiotics are continued for approximately 2 to 3 days. It is inadvisable to continue antibiotics for a prolonged period of time, since this may lead to a superinfection with the emergence of resistant organisms that may become quite difficult to control. If no infection occurs, the fracture may be internally fixed and the wound closed within 5 to 7 days.

If a type 3 wound becomes infected, it is necessary to perform a complete and thorough incision and drainage. Cultures are obtained and the appropriate antibiotic given intravenously. A repeat debridement is recommended within 24 hours and may have to be repeated at regular intervals, until the acute phase of the infection is brought under control. This usually occurs within 5 to 7 days, at which time internal fixation may be accomplished and the wound closed. The indications for internal fixation and wound closure are as follows. The patient should be free of systemic signs of infection. There should be no chills, fever, and restlessness, no purulent drainage, and no redness or swelling of the wound. Bacterial cultures may not be negative at this time but as long as these conditions are met and appropriate antibiotic coverage maintained, internal fixation may be done and the wound closed. Even if it is not possible to close the wound, the surgeon should fix the fracture. Rittman et al.[27] and Rosen[28] provided impressive results that the plating of an infected fracture does not adversely affect healing and may even help to control the infection.

It is desirable to close the wound directly; if this cannot be achieved, however, closure by whatever means available should be attempted. In some instances, it may not be possible to achieve coverage at this time because of massive soft tissue loss. For these cases, internal fixation may still be done and the wound covered with sterile dressings. The hardware may be removed in 6 to 8 weeks, when there is sufficient union to continue immobilization either in an external fixator or in a cast. Fractures can and do heal in the presence of infection, and the functional result will be far better if an anatomic position is obtained.

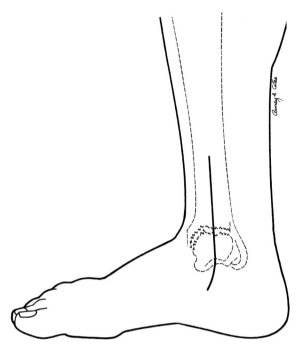

Fig. 127-13. Fractured medial malleolus. The skin incision is placed halfway between the anterior and posterior borders and is curved slightly at the distal part.

FRACTURES OF THE MEDIAL MALLEOLUS

A 10-cm incision is placed midway between the anterior and posterior borders of the medial malleolus and is carried down to the periosteum, developing full-thickness subcutaneous flaps (Figs. 127-13, 127-14). Often the displaced fragment will have some periosteum or fibrous tissue interpositioned. The interpositioned tissue and clots are removed, but stripping of the periosteum is limited to that affording visualization of the fracture site. The next step is to identify the anterior inferior part of the medial malleolus. Occasionally, this will require dissecting the capsule from the distal tibia as it inserts into the medial malleolus. The joint is irrigated and inspected and bony or cartilaginous fragments removed. Reduction of the medial malleolus can be achieved accurately only by means of two-plane visualization of the fracture (Fig.

127-15). One plane is the junction of the medial malleolus and the anterior portion of the distal tibia. The other plane is the interdigitation of the distal tibia and medial malleolus at the medial aspect. This method of reduction will ensure accurate repositioning and has proved quite reliable. The medial malleolus is secured either with two screws or with one screw and a Kirshner (K-) wire (Fig. 127-16). This prevents rotation of the distal fragment, which can occur if only one screw is used. The screw has the advantage of adding compression to the fixation, thereby reducing the incidence of nonunion. Small fragments that cannot be fixed can be safely excised, especially if they are distal to the tibial plafond. Figure-of-eight or tension-band fixation of the medial malleolus is rarely indicated. The tension-band principle does not apply to either the medial or lateral malleolus, since joint motion occurs in a plane parallel to the malleoli rather than perpendicular to them, a prerequisite whenever tension band fixation is used.

If the medial malleolus is fractured at its tip and

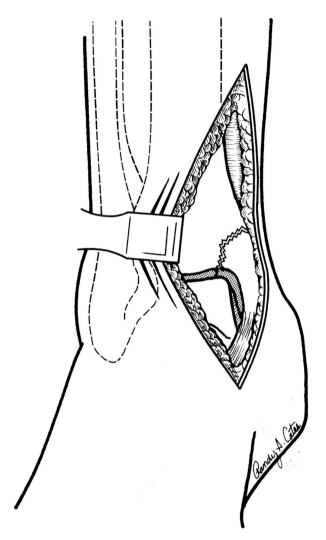

Fig. 127-14. The incision is carried down to the fracture site without developing subcutaneous flaps. Occasionally, the capsule has to be dissected off the distal tibial malleolar junction to enable alignment of the fracture in two planes.

the fragments are too small to be secured with a screw or K-wire, the fragments may be excised. If the deltoid ligament cannot be reattached to the remaining medial malleolus, it is sutured to the surrounding soft tissues. Medial stability will not be jeopardized as long as part of the medial malleolus extends beyond the tibial plafond to provide medial buttressing.

On the rare occasions in which the fracture of the medial malleolus extends proximally and posteriorly to include a significant portion of the tibial

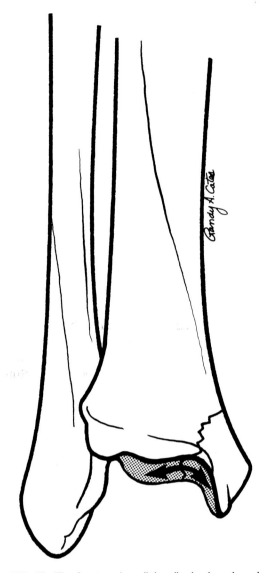

Fig. 127-15. The fractured medial malleolus is reduced and aligned in two planes. The anteromedial alignment at the distal tibial malleolar junction is illustrated by the arrow. The second plane of alignment is along the fractured site, where the interdigitation of the fragments takes place along the medial side of the distal tibia.

plafond, the surgical incision is extended more proximally. Occasionally, such large fragments must be fixed with a buttress plate because of comminution at the junction of the fragment and the distal tibia to avoid collapse and varus deformity of the ankle.

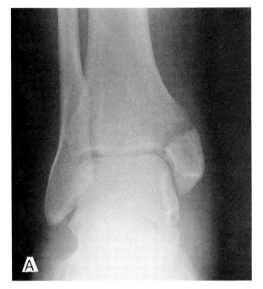 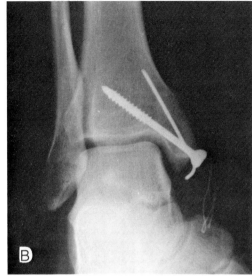

Fig. 127-16. Isolated fracture of the medial malleolus **(A)** and following anatomical reduction **(B)**. It was transfixed with a malleolar screw and a Kirschner wire. The malleolar screw allows compression of the fragments and the additional K-wire will prevent rotation of the distal fragment.

TEARS OF THE DELTOID LIGAMENT

Isolated tears of the deltoid ligament are extremely rare. They may occur in lateral dislocations of the talus not associated with fractures of the malleoli. Most deltoid tears occur in conjunction with ankle fractures in which the lateral malleolus or the distal fibula is fractured. Repair of the deltoid ligament is indicated when injuries involving the lateral malleolus or syndesmotic ligaments are also present. The incision begins at the joint level and extends distally, curving slightly anteriorly for about 4 cm. The subcutaneous tissues and superficial fascia are incised in line with the incision, and the deep part of the deltoid ligament anterior to the posterior tibial tendon is identified. The deltoid ligament may be torn through its substance or avulsed from its origin at the medial malleolus or, more frequently, from its insertion into the talus. In the latter instance, the talus must be temporarily displaced laterally to permit placement of the suture into the remnant portion of the deltoid ligament on the talus. This is impossible if the talus is in its anatomic position. The joint is irrigated and all

debris removed. The torn ends of the deltoid are approximated and sutures inserted but are tied only at the conclusion of the surgical procedure, after the lateral malleolus has been reduced, to avoid inadvertent disruption of the repair.

FRACTURES OF THE DISTAL FIBULA AND LATERAL MALLEOLUS

The incision is placed midway between the anterior and posterior borders of the fibula, extending 5 cm proximal to the fracture and to the tip of the lateral malleolus (Fig. 127-17). By sharp dissection, the incision is carried down through the soft tissues, until the periosteum is identified. At the proximal aspect of the incision, one should avoid the cutaneous branch of the lateral peroneal nerve. The periosteum is incised at the fracture, but stripping is limited to the fracture site. The distal fragment is pulled distally and internally rotated (Fig. 127-18). To ensure an anatomical reduction, the fracture should be visualized in the lateral and pos-

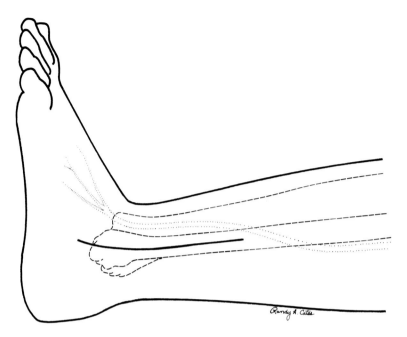

Fig. 127-17. The skin incision along the lateral malleolus is placed halfway between the anterior and posterior borders of the distal fibula and curved slightly at its distal end. At the proximal part of the illustration, the lateral branch of the peroneal nerve is demonstrated. If the incision has to be carried more proximally, frequently this branch is inadvertently cut.

terior planes (Fig. 127-19). The reduced fragments are held in position with a small self-locking bone clamp (Fig. 127-20). A five- to six-hole plate is used to transfix the fragments (Fig. 127-21). The screws should avoid purchasing on small fragments and should be engaged in the intact portion of the proximal and distal fibula. The distal fibula and lateral malleolus differ significantly among individuals; therefore, the plate may require bending to conform to the shape of the fibula. Both lateral and medial cortices should be drilled, but the screws placed at the level below the plafond should be 2 mm shorter than the original measurement to ensure that they will not protrude into the articulating surfaces of the talus. In addition, by aiming the screws slightly posteriorly, the chances are that less of the articular cartilage will be damaged during the drilling. Even if the distal fragment can hold only one or two screws, this will suffice, since the distal portion of the plate acts as a buttress and will provide adequate stability against lateral displacement.

Both Sherman and ASIF plates, 3 mm in thick-ness, have been routinely employed. Conventional self-tapping screws are used in conjunction with a Sherman plate and 4.5-mm cortical screws, which require tapping before insertion are used in conjunction with the ASIF plate. Interfragmentary screws without the use of a plate may afford anatomic reduction of the fractured lateral malleolus, but the fixation is not strong enough to permit early motion and weight bearing. The one exception in which interfragmentary screws may be used is a long noncomminuted fracture of the lateral malleolus, in which the length of the fracture is equal to or greater than twice the width of the fibula.

The use of circlage wires or intramedullary rods to stabilize the lateral malleolus is contraindicated if early motion and weight bearing are to be instituted. These devices do not prevent shortening or rotation of the fragments and may lead to malunion. In the presence of marked comminution, they provide insufficient fixation. Recently, a tapered, tri-flanged, V-shaped malleable intramedullary nail was described to fix the lateral malleolus.[22] This yielded good results in the hands of the investiga-

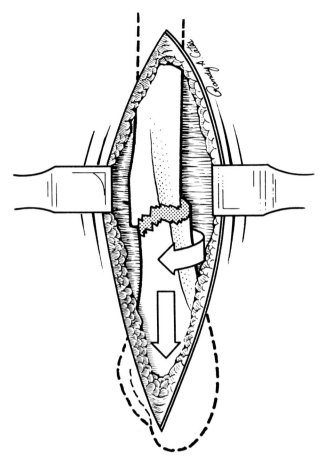

Fig. 127-18. Reduction of fractured lateral malleolus is achieved by applying a force to the distal fragment in the direction of the arrows. The fractured lateral malleolus is pulled distally and internally rotated to achieve anatomic reduction.

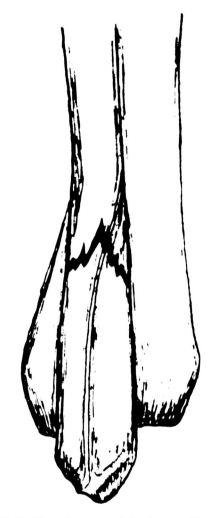

Fig. 127-19. The alignment of the fractured lateral malleolus has to be anatomically in two planes. The posterolateral and anterior surfaces of the fragments must interdigitate accurately. (From Segal,[31] with permission.)

tors, but to date we have had no experience with this method.

During surgery, the distal part of the peroneus tertius originating from the anterior edge of the distal fibula should be gently elevated and the anterior tibiofibular ligament visualized throughout its length. A torn anterior tibiofibular ligament should always alert the surgeon to the possibility of other torn syndesmotic ligaments. This ligament represents the first line of defense, and it is the only ligament that can be visualized adequately at surgery. Manually pulling the distal fibula laterally in the presence of intact syndesmotic ligaments is impossible. However, if the fibula can be pulled later-

ally, it is an indication of a diastasis. In addition to reconstructing the distal fibula, the surgeon should stabilize the distal tibiofibular joint with a transfixation screw (vide infra). In the rare case of marked comminution of the fibula, rather than using longer plates and more extensive surgery, the proximal and distal fibular fragments may be secured by screws into the lateral cortex of the tibia. In this way, the lateral cortex of the tibia is used as a stabilizing structure. This method is also helpful in the presence of severe osteoporosis, when the purchase of the screws in the fibula is not firm. The

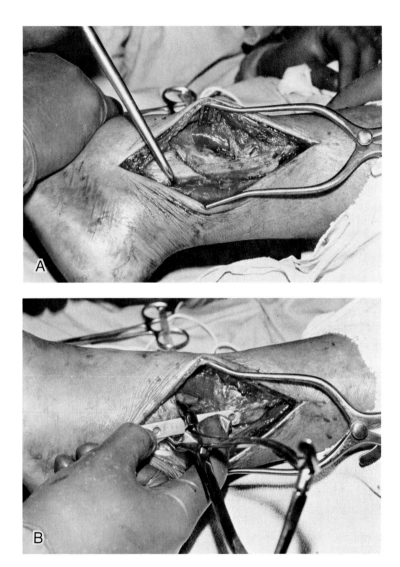

Fig. 127-20. (A) Reduction of fracture of the lateral malleolus. A unicortical hole has been drilled into the posterior fragment and a bone hook has been inserted. The distal fragment is being pulled distally and the foot is internally rotated to achieve a reduction. **(B)** The reduced lateral malleolus is firmly held with a self-locking bone clamp. This allows the surgeon to apply the plate while maintaining the reduction.

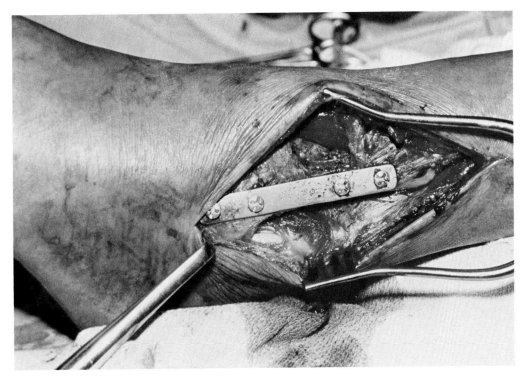

Fig. 127-21. The plate has been applied, securely fixing the lateral malleolus.

syndesmotic screw is removed within 10 to 12 weeks.

ANKLE INSTABILITY ASSOCIATED WITH FRACTURE OF THE FIBULAR SHAFT

These injuries are often misleading because the only radiologic sign is often that of a fracture of the fibular shaft. It is tempting to treat these as minor injuries. However, isolated fractures of the lateral malleolus or fibular shaft do occur, and these are stable only if no ligaments are torn. The surgeon must therefore ascertain the extent of these injuries. The whole of the fibular shaft should be palpated on physical examination. Tenderness anywhere along the shaft warrants additional radiographs, since the initial films may miss the fracture if only the ankle region has been examined. Tenderness along the medial aspect of the ankle or over the anterior tibiofibular ligament should alert the examining physician to a tear of the deltoid or anterior tibiofibular ligament. It may be necessary to obtain inversion stress films under local anesthesia to demonstrate a diastasis and talar displacement if any of these ligaments are torn.

Such injuries are generally caused by external rotation forces. In the first stage, there is a fracture of the medial malleolus or a tear of the deltoid ligament, followed by a rupture of the anterior tibiofibular ligament and a tear of the interosseous membrane. This will result in a diastasis. As the force continues to act, the fibula finally fractures. If the fracture is situated in the lower diaphysis, it is called a Dupuytren[8] fracture (Fig. 127-22); if it is located in the proximal one-third of the diaphysis or at the neck of the fibula, it is called a Maisonneuve[21] fracture (Fig. 127-23). The importance of fractures of the fibular shaft is that they are usually associated with severe ligamentous disruption involving the interosseous membrane, resulting in a

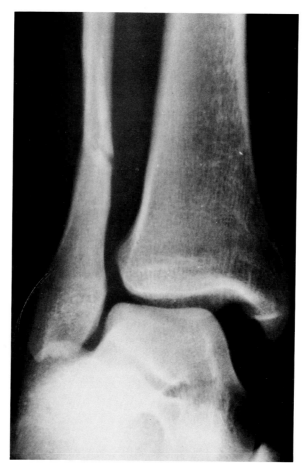

Fig. 127-22. Dupuytren fracture. The talus is displaced laterally, there is a diastasis, the medial malleolus has been fractured, and there is a fracture of the distal shaft of the fibula.

diastasis between the tibia and fibula rendering these fractures very unstable.

The fracture of the fibular shaft is treated as described using a four- or five-hole plate. However, because of the diastasis, this must be reduced and can most readily be accomplished by inserting a screw across the fibula into the tibia through one of the holes in the plate (Fig. 127-24). The screw maintains reduction of the syndesmotic joint, therefore, a cortical screw is adequate; only rarely is it necessary to overdrill the fibula in order to apply a compressive force. The syndesmotic screw should be removed under local anesthesia 10 to 12 weeks after insertion.

Fractures occurring more proximally along the fibular shaft may be stabilized with a small four-hole plate. Shortening of the fibula or malrotation, regardless of where it occurs along the fibular shaft, must be anatomically reduced to prevent an adverse effect on the function of the ankle. One must differentiate between these injuries and isolated fractures of the fibular shaft which do not involve tears of ligaments or fractures of the medial malleolus. Attention should be paid to the common peroneal nerve, which crosses the lateral aspect of the fibula in this area. In proximal fibular shaft fractures it is preferable to use a separate syndesmotic screw distally since the more proximal the position of the screw, the greater the fulcrum of the distal fibula, which may cause an angular deformity.

Fractures at the fibular neck are not amenable to plate fixation. In this instance, since most of the

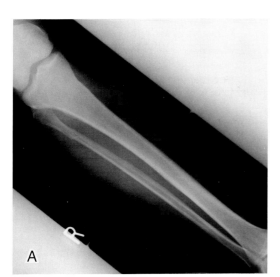
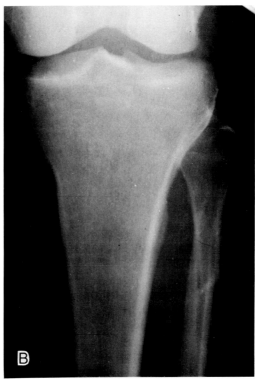

Fig. 127-23. **(A)** Maisonneuve fracture. Note that the fibular fracture would have been missed if the whole length of the fibula had not been included in the radiograph. **(B)** Close-up of the fracture of the proximal fibula.

fibular shaft is intact, it is necessary only to treat the diastasis using one or two syndesmotic screws.

FRACTURES OF THE POSTERIOR TIBIAL LIP

The posterior tibial lip is frequently avulsed by the capsule, the posterior inferior transverse ligament, or direct impingement of the talus when the tibia is forcibly displaced forward. Small avulsion fragments need not be treated surgically and may be left alone, provided the talus is in its anatomic position. However, when the posterior lip of the tibia involves 20 percent or more of the articulating surface, anatomic reduction should be done and the severity of the fracture upgraded, as this is considered an injury of the tibial plafond.

Posterior lip fractures involving 20 percent or more of the tibial plafond rarely occur as isolated injuries but occur in conjunction with fractures of the medial or lateral malleoli. Because the posterior part of the distal tibia protrudes slightly more laterally than medially, surgical exposure of the posterior lip may be facilitated through a lateral incision (Fig. 127-25).

The medial or lateral malleolus should be stabilized before an attempt is made to reduce the posterior lip because, by first reducing the medial or lateral malleolus, the posterior lip fragment is very often aligned with the tibial plafond. It is impossible to visualize the articulating surfaces of the posterior lip fracture without removing the distal portion of the fibula. The peroneal and Achilles

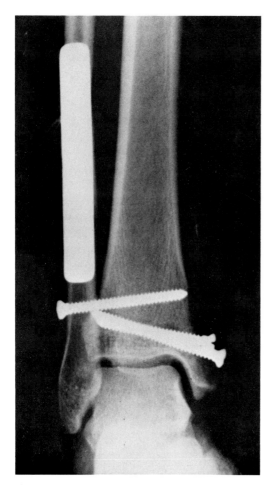

Fig. 127-24. Dupuytren fracture that has been anatomically reduced and securely fixed.

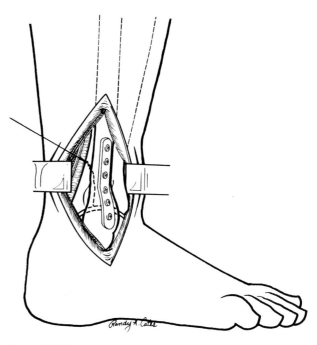

Fig. 127-25. Posterior lip fracture associated with fractured lateral malleolus. If the lateral malleolar fracture is reduced and stabilized, reduction of the posterior lip fragment will usually occur. Minor adjustments are carried out by adjusting the posterior lip at its junction with the distal tibia as demonstrated by the arrow. Only single-plane visualization is possible in posterior lip fractures.

tendons are retracted to permit identification of the fracture site. Manipulation of the fragment with a small periosteal elevator or bone hook with the foot in plantar flexion will generally reposition the fracture. The reduction can be verified by observing the alignment of the fragment on the posterior tibial surface. A K-wire is inserted from an anterior to posterior direction to engage the fragment, and the position is verified radiologically. If it is satisfactory, a stab wound is made on the anterior aspect of the distal tibia and a lag screw inserted from an anterior to posterior fragment (Fig. 127-26). If left unreduced, these fractures will cause incongruity of the articulating surface of the tibia and will result in degenerative arthritis.

FRACTURES OF THE ANTERIOR LIP OF TIBIA

These fractures are less common than those involving the posterior lip and may present as an avulsion of the anterior margin of the tibia caused by the capsule and associated with forced plantar flexion. They may also present as fractures of the anterior articular surface. Those that are displaced and that involve more than 20 percent of the articular surface will require open reduction and internal fixation. The smaller fragments do not require surgical treatment.

The fracture is approached through an anterolateral incision, and the extensor tendons are retracted laterally, exposing the anterior tibia. The

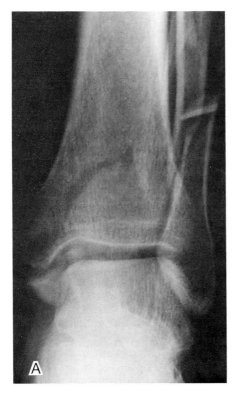

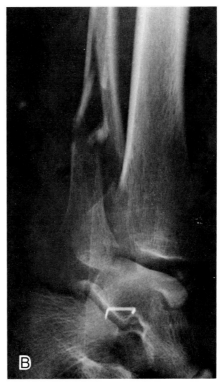

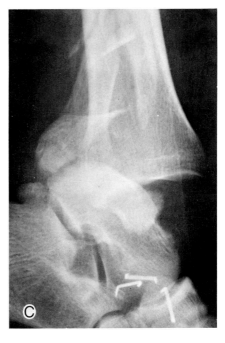

Fig. 127-26. Preoperative and postoperative radiographs of a fractured posterior lip of the tibia in association with a fractured medial and lateral malleolus. **(A)** AP view. **(B)** Oblique. **(C)** Lateral projection of the injury. The oblique radiograph is helpful in evaluating the size of the posterior fragment and its location, whether it be more medially or laterally. *(Figure continues.)*

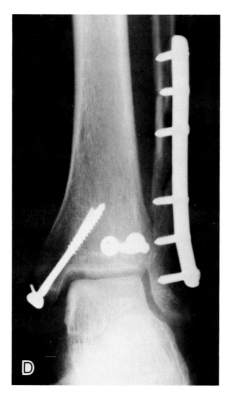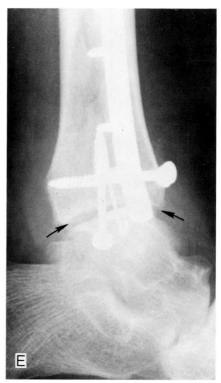

Fig. 127-26 *(Continued).* **(D,E)** Postoperative radiographs of the same fracture. After the medial and lateral malleolus is reduced and stabilized, the posterior lip fragment is reduced and transfixed with two lag screws introduced in an anteroposterior direction through stab wounds.

fragment is manipulated with a bone hook or a towel clamp and brought into position. Because of the exposure, the fracture can be visualized in two planes; thus, the surgeon can be more certain of the reduction. The fragment is fixed with a screw inserted anteriorly, which engages the posterior tibial cortex. Intraoperative radiographs should be obtained routinely.

POSTOPERATIVE MANAGEMENT

Traditionally, it was advocated that a short-leg or long-leg cast be applied after internal fixation of ankle fractures and that weight bearing be restricted for the first 6 weeks. Thereafter, graduated weight bearing was permitted until union oc-

curred, provided that the reduction was maintained. Following the removal of the cast, physical therapy was instituted to help the patient regain motion and strength.

We have departed from this traditional approach because we have been convinced that rigid internal fixation of the medial malleolus and plate fixation of the lateral malleolus provide sufficient immobilization for the safe institution of early range of motion and weight bearing. This applies to all fractures, with the exception of those injuries involving the tibial plafond and anterior and posterior tibial lip fractures involving more than 20 percent of the articular surface.

We have instituted early weight bearing in more than 200 fractures and have not experienced any instances of fixation failure or displacement of the fracture. What we did observe was a much faster return of normal function and strength and a very significant decrease in the number of patients complaining of postoperative pain, swelling, and stiffness. Biomechanical studies performed in our laboratory[31] demonstrated that the fibula bears only 10 to 15 percent of the body weight, which is not sufficient to displace the lateral malleolus if it is fixed with a plate. Larger forces were seen to act on the lateral malleolus with external rotation; if motion in this plane can be prevented, the patient may safely commence early weight bearing.

Postoperative care commences with the elevation of the treated ankle. This is mandatory if

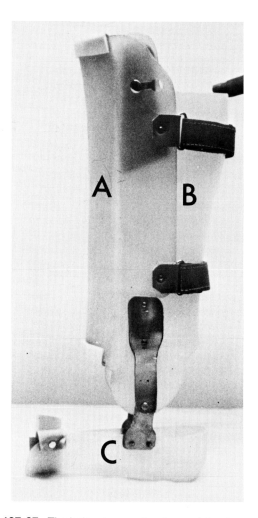

Fig. 127-27. The below-knee orthosis consists of an anterior shell **(A)** attached via a keyhole slot and two Velcro straps to the posterior shell **(B)**. The foot piece **(C)** is attached with rigid hinges to the posterior shell. (From Segal,[31] with permission.)

edema and wound complications are to be avoided. The extremity is suspended from an overhead frame so that the level of the ankle is always above the level of the heart. A short-leg cast is applied; this is bivalved 48 hours postoperatively, and dorsiflexion exercises are started. The leg is splinted in the bivalved cast and elevated between exercise periods. A custom-made below-knee orthosis is then obtained (Fig. 127-27). This consists of an anterior shell, a posterior shell, and a foot piece fitted with rigid hinges to permit dorsiflexion and plantar flexion but no rotation. Thus the patient may begin to ambulate in the orthosis as early as the fourth or fifth postoperative day. Most patients can bear full weight without pain by 10 to 14 days and can discontinue using crutches. The orthosis is worn continuously for the first 6 weeks, after which it is used during the day only for an additional 6 weeks. Throughout this period, the patient is encouraged to continue with active plantar flexion and dorsiflexion exercises. We recommend the removal of the plate and screws in patients 50 years of age or younger when union is solid, usually about 6 months after surgery.

Because fractures of the anterior and posterior lip of the tibia involving more than 20 percent are intraarticular, we believe that weight bearing should be avoided until union has occurred. However, the fixation as described is sufficiently rigid that postoperative plaster immobilization may be discontinued. The patient may walk using crutches and follows a strict program of dorsiflexion and plantar flexion exercises. Muscle tone is maintained and stiffness and swelling avoided.

FRACTURES OF THE TIBIAL PLAFOND

These fractures involve the distal articulating surface of the tibia and are potentially disabling because they disrupt the surface against which the talus articulates. The generally poor prognosis of these fractures has been radically altered by the work of Maale and Seligson[19] and Ruedi and Allgower,[29,30] who have shown that open reduction and anatomic fixation of the fragments can offer a much better prognosis, allows the patient an opportunity to regain normal joint motion and decreases the incidence of traumatic arthritis.

Although many classifications of these fractures have been described, perhaps the most useful is that of Ruedi and Allgower.[29] Type 1 injuries are cleavage fractures of the distal tibia, usually involving the medial malleolus and the metaphysis, with no major disruption of the articular surface of the tibia itself. Type 2 fractures are those in which there is significant disruption of the joint surface with large fragments but no comminution. Type 3 fractures involve impaction and comminution of the distal tibia.

NONSURGICAL TREATMENT

Fractures of the tibial plafond involving less than 20 percent of the articulating surface or in which the fractures are displaced less than 2 mm may be treated nonoperatively. There are circumstances in which the surgeon may decide not to intervene surgically and to treat the patient with early range of motion and delayed weight bearing. One such occasion involves a markedly comminuted plafond injury considered by the surgeon to be beyond reconstruction and appears on radiographs as "a bag of bones." It must be emphasized, however, that such injuries are rare and that most plafond fractures can be anatomically reduced and fixed if adequate exposure is obtained and if the surgical principles to be described are followed. Other situations include peripheral vascular disease, diabetes, and a plafond fracture associated with paralysis.

The patient should be hospitalized for elevation, ice application, and observation of the neurovascular condition. Swelling is occasionally associated with a compartment syndrome or with ischemic changes of the skin necessitating a surgical release. Elevation and immobilization in a well-padded cast or posterior splint with icing will usually reduce the swelling within a period of 5 to 7 days. At this stage, active dorsiflexion and plantar flexion are encouraged. An ankle brace with rigid hinges permitting motion in the sagittal plane is prescribed, but weight bearing is delayed for 3 months or until bony union occurs.

A modification of the nonsurgical treatment is traction through the os calcis. There are circumstances in which a comminuted plafond injury is not displaced beyond the 2 mm and in which the articulating surfaces are properly aligned. Because of the possibility that active range of motion may displace some of the fragments traction is applied through a Steinman pin inserted in the os calcis. By applying traction that counteracts the muscle pull, range of motion can be permitted. As healing proceeds active range of motion is modified to active assisted range of motion with the patient using an ace bandage to aid in dorsiflexion of the ankle joint. Weight bearing is postponed until there is bony union, usually within 3 months.

SURGICAL TREATMENT OF FRACTURES INVOLVING THE TIBIAL PLAFOND

Plafond injuries are caused by a force driving the talus into the distal tibia. The direction of the vertical drive of the talus depends on whether the foot is in plantar flexion or in dorsiflexion. In the former, more of the central and anterior portions of the plafond will be injured; in the latter, the thrust of the force will damage the central and/or posterior portions of the distal articulating surface of the tibia. Every plafond injury is associated with one of the following: a fracture of the distal shaft of the tibia, a fracture of the distal tibia and fibular shaft, or a disruption of the syndesmotic ligaments.

In analyzing the fracture, the following radiologic features should be evaluated:

1. Is the fibula intact or is it fractured? Is it comminuted? An intact fibula gives the surgeon a reliable landmark against which to reconstruct the tibial plafond. It is more difficult to do so when the surgeon is dealing with a comminuted fracture of the distal fibula. In such a case, the land-

marks are less obvious, and the length of the fibula must be reestablished before reducing the plafond.

2. Is there a free fragment or a fracture involving the lateral part of the distal tibia? This is the keystone in reconstructing the articular surface of the plafond. The lateral part of the tibial plafond is also usually impacted and displaced proximally. It must be reduced to its normal length; otherwise, the talus will assume a valgus position, which will result in early and severe degenerative arthritis. (Figs. 127-28, 127-29).

3. Is there a concomitant fracture of the distal tibial shaft, associated with shortening? Whenever this occurs, surgical reduction must include fixation of the distal shaft as well; otherwise, the plafond cannot be stabilized. The surgeon must plan the reduction of the distal shaft and the tibial plafond and properly use the plates and screws to stabilize both components.

4. What is the condition of the soft tissues and the neurovascular status of the extremity? Plafond injury can be compared with an "explosion" of the distal tibia, with immediate onset of severe swelling. It may sometimes be necessary to perform an acute fasciotomy of the leg to avoid muscle necrosis. In most instances, surgery must be postponed from 5 to 7 days. During that time, the leg should be continuously elevated,

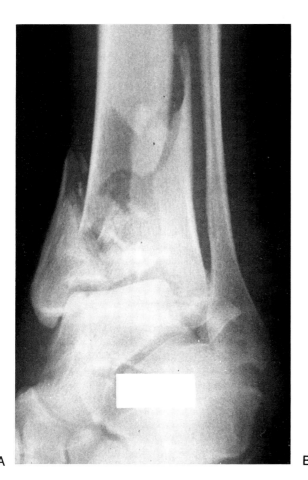
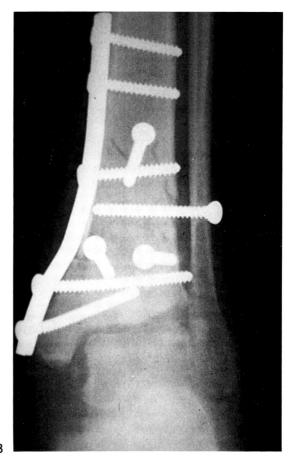

A   B

Fig. 127-28. **(A)** AP radiograph showing displaced fracture of tibial plafond. **(B)** Open reduction with buttress plates and screws did not completely reduce the lateral plafond fragment. Degenerative arthritis is the likely sequela with incomplete reduction.

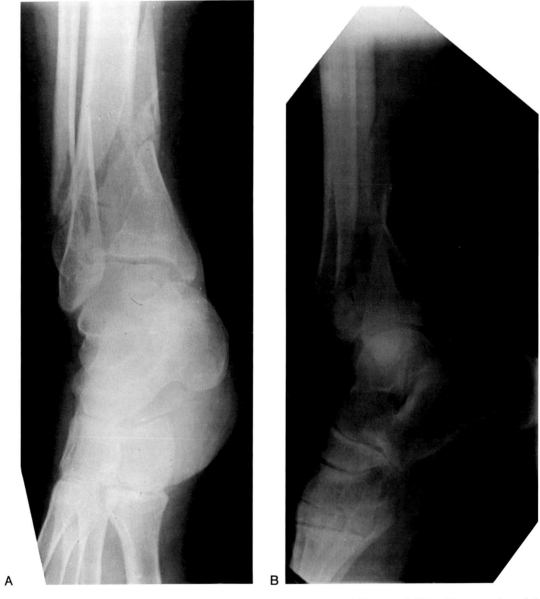

A   B

Fig. 127-29. (A,B) AP and lateral radiographs show fracture of distal fibula and tibia with extension of the fracture into the tibial plafond. *(Figure continues.)*

iced, and immobilized in either a well-padded cast or a posterior splint. Rarely can these patients be brought to the operating room before swelling ensues because associated injuries are common; by the time these are properly evaluated, the edema has developed. If surgery is performed under less than optimal conditions, the surgeon may face a dilemma at the termination of the operation. He will probably be unable to close the incision and should be prepared to do either a delayed primary closure or skin grafting. In addition, the incidence of postoperative infection is significantly increased.

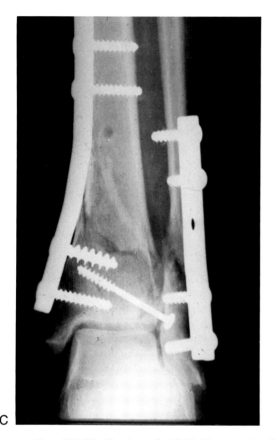

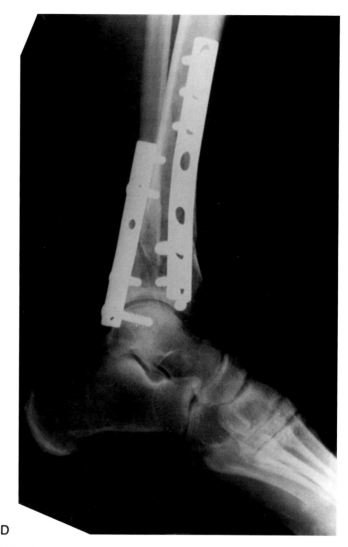

C   D

Fig. 127-29 *(Continued)*. **(C,D)** Plate on the fibula plus buttress plate on tibia and interfragmentary screw reestablishes proper anatomy.

The principles established many years ago by Ruedi and Allgower[29] are valid and should be followed:

1. The fibula must be brought out to length. It then acts as a landmark permitting anatomic reduction of the plafond.
2. Displaced fragments of the tibial plafond should be reduced and aligned anatomically, held temporarily with K-wires, and ultimately firmly fixed with screws, followed by the application of

one or more neutralizing plates to add stability to the distal tibia and to the reconstructed tibial plafond.[17]

Finally, bone grafting is an essential part of the surgery. Adequate amounts of cancellous bone should be harvested from the iliac crest and inserted into the defects remaining after the impacted fragments are reduced. Inadequate grafting is associated with nonunion, pain, and ultimate loss of position.

SURGICAL PROCEDURE

Surgery is performed through one or two incisions; occasionally, a third is required. The anterolateral incision is the most important. It enables the surgeon to address the displaced lateral part of the tibial plafond. If the incision is long enough, the surgeon can also reach the anterior surface of the fibula by subcutaneous dissection.

In the presence of severe fibular comminution, a separate incision must be made directly over the lateral aspect of the fibula. Establishing correct fibular length is the first step in the surgical treatment of these fractures. The second step in the reconstruction involves anatomic reduction of the distal tibial shaft. Whenever a fracture of the plafond is associated with a spiral or displaced fracture of the distal tibia that extends to the plafond, the surgeon must reduce the distal tibia before addressing the plafond fracture itself. The tibia can be held in its reduced position with K-wires or with interfragmentary screws. The neutralizing plate should extend proximally enough to include the shaft above the fracture.

Following this, attention is directed toward reduction of the displaced lateral fragment of the plafond. Through the anterolateral incision, the surgeon exposes the tibial plafond and will find that the lateral fragment is displaced proximally; its articulating surface may be rotated and comminuted. This lateral fragment should be brought down to its anatomic location at the level of the remaining tibial plafond. It is temporarily held in place with K-wires. The lateral fragment is the keystone to the reduction; when in doubt, intraoperative radiographs should be obtained to ensure its anatomic position. Other fragments of the tibial plafond or a fractured medial malleolus are then reduced anatomically and fixed with compression screws. A third incision may be required over the medial side of the ankle. This is necessary when the fracture extends to the medial malleolus or involves the posteromedial part of the plafond.

Prior to replacing the K-wires with screws and plates, a bone graft is added to fill the defects created by the reduction. It is important to use cancellous bone and to avoid as much as possible the use of cortical struts. Tightly packed bone grafts will add to the stability of the reduced plafond.

K-wires are replaced with permanent interfragmentary 4.5-mm cortical screws and small fragment screws where necessary. However, a neutralizing plate (spoon shape, T or L, or clover leaf) should be used as a neutralizing support to bypass the small fragments and anchor the plafond to the distal tibia. The length of the plate must be sufficient to anchor the plafond to the intact portion of the tibial shaft (Fig. 127-29).

It is crucial that special care and attention be given at the time of surgery to the small bony fragments and to the soft tissue attachments. Fractures along the anterior surface of the distal tibia can be lifted out as "windows" to facilitate easier reduction of the articular surfaces. In doing so one should preserve the soft tissue attachment and close the window at the end of the surgery. Many displaced fragments of the plafond itself have no soft tissue attachments but, being metaphyseal bone, they will probably unite.

The tourniquet should be released before closure of the wound and during surgery, if the elapsed time is more than 90 minutes. At least one suction drain is inserted along the major incision (the anterolateral one), and the leg is immobilized in a well-padded short-leg cast, elevated, and ice applied immediately in the recovery room.

POSTOPERATIVE CARE

The circulation should be watched carefully and frequently on the day of surgery. When in doubt, the cast should be bivalved, leaving the leg immobilized in the posterior splint. A constricting soft tissue dressing should be cut as well. Within 5 to 7 days, as swelling subsides and as wound healing proceeds, the patient is instructed in active dorsiflexion and plantar flexion exercises. Reliable patients can be discharged in a below-knee orthosis with instructions to actively move the ankle. It is important that, upon discharge, the patient be able to bring the ankle at least to the neutral position and preferably to a few degrees of dorsiflexion. The unreliable patient is best discharged in a short-leg cast applied under sedation with the ankle in a neutral or 5 to 10 degrees of dorsiflexion. No weight bearing is allowed for at least 3 months or until bony union can be confirmed radiologically.

COMPLICATIONS

Malunion

Lateral Malleolus

The most common cause of malunion of the lateral malleolus is incomplete reduction obtained by a closed manipulation. In unstable fractures, the talus will follow displacement of the lateral malleolus. As the talus moves into place during the reduction, the lateral malleolus impinges on the proximal fibular fragment, frequently preventing further reduction of the lateral malleolus. The talus may be forced into place, but this can only occur at the expense of the fibular collateral ligaments, which are stretched. This results in a radiograph in which the position of the talus may appear satisfactory but, because of the incomplete reduction of the lateral malleolus and the stretching of the fibular collateral ligament, the talus remains potentially unstable, which may cause pain and late degenerative changes. The lateral malleolus is shortened and is almost always in some degree of external rotation, as seen on good-quality lateral radiographs (Fig. 127-30).

If symptoms persist to the point where they interfere with the patient's activities, the anatomy must be restored. Surgery may be undertaken at any time after the original injury, provided there is no radiologic evidence of severe degenerative arthritis of the ankle. This is best done by exposing the fracture site and performing an osteotomy through the original fracture. The plane and direction of the osteotomy can best be determined by

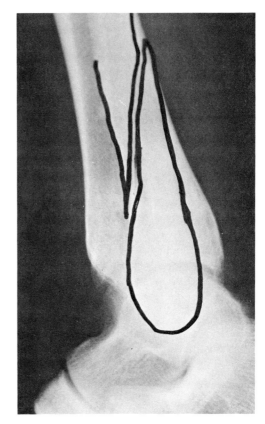

Fig. 127-30. Lateral radiograph of malunion of the lateral malleolus, which is shortened and in some external rotation.

careful study of lateral preoperative radiographs, which indicate the malalignment of the lateral malleolus. After the osteotomy is complete, the anterior tibiofibular joint should be exposed and cleaned of scar and fibrous tissue. A unicortical hole is then drilled in the posterior aspect of the distal portion of the lateral malleolus into which is inserted a bone hook. The lateral malleolus is then pulled distally and is internally rotated to restore the integrity of the anterior tibiofibular joint so that the fibula articulates perfectly with the fibular notch on the tibia (Fig. 127-31). The lateral malleolus is held in a corrected position with a four- or five-hole plate (Fig. 127-32). A slight gap may be present at the osteotomy site, but this generally fills in with bone. If the gap is more than 3 mm, it may be packed with autogenous bone obtained locally.

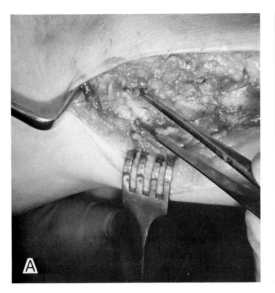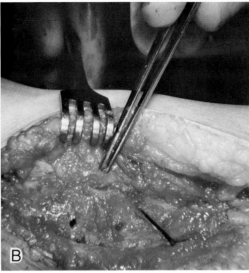

Fig. 127-31. (A) Intraoperative photographs showing the widening of the distal tibiofibular joint *(arrows)* due to the shortening and external rotation of the lateral malleolus. The interosseous space is widened as denoted by the periosteal elevator, and the anterior tibiofibular ligament is attenuated. **(B)** Intraoperative photographs. The lateral malleolus has been osteotomized. The bone hook has pulled the lateral malleolus distally and into internal rotation thereby reducing the subluxation of the anterior tibiofibular joint *(arrows)*.

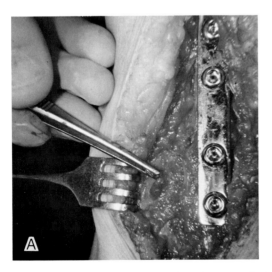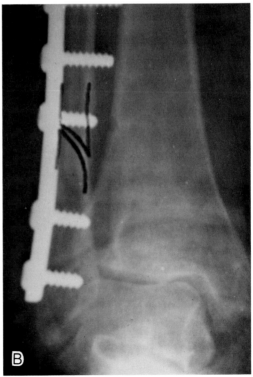

Fig. 127-32. (A) A five-hole plate has been applied to the lateral malleolus to maintain the correction. **(B)** Postoperative radiograph. The lateral malleolus has been lengthened. A small gap exists at the osteotomy site but will ultimately heal.

Medial Malleolus

Malunion of the medial malleolus also results from either an incomplete closed reduction or a failure to observe the fracture in two planes during open reduction. Because the talus is wider anteriorly, impingement of the medial malleolus will occur during dorsiflexion, which will result in pain and degenerative changes in this area (Fig. 127-33).

Treatment consists of osteomizing the medial malleolus through the original fracture and obtaining anatomic reduction. The fragment should be rigidly fixed with a malleolar screw and K-wire. If an avulsion fracture has united in an unsatisfactory position such that it abuts against the medial aspect of the talus and causes symptoms, the fragment may be exised.

Posterior Malleolus

Malunion is significant only if the fragment is more than 20 percent of the articular surface. The malunited fragment must be approached under direct vision, since it is necessary first to osteomize the fracture and then to reduce it anatomically. Good-quality preoperative radiographs are necessary to indicate the extent of the fragment.

The best visualization will be obtained by using the Gatelier[9] approach. The skin incision is identical to that described for treatment of the lateral malleolus. The distal fibula is identified and osteotomized about 6 cm proximal to the tip of the lateral malleolus. With sharp dissection, the fibula is freed from the interosseous membrane and ligament and from the anterior and posterior tibiofibular ligaments and turned distally on itself, leaving the fibular collateral ligaments intact. This will now bring the whole of the lateral aspect of the tibia into view. The malunited fragment is osteotomized and pulled into anatomic position with a bone hook. A K-wire is now inserted to transfix the fragment, and intraoperative radiographs are obtained. If these are satisfactory, fixation is augmented with a compression screw inserted through the posterior fragment into the anterior aspect of the tibia. The K-wire is cut and bent on itself to prevent migration.

The fibula is then fixed with a five-hole plate. Two screws are inserted into the proximal fibula and three into the distal fragment. The most distal screw must also enter the tibia to prevent diastasis, since the syndesmotic ligaments were divided in making the exposure.

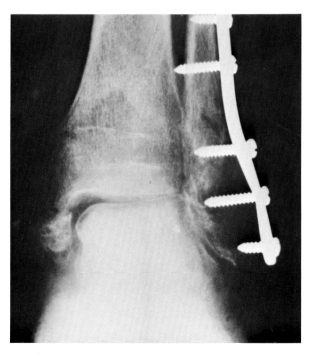

Fig. 127-33. Malunion of the medial malleolus. Note medial joint space narrowing.

Nonunion

The literature confirms that the rate of nonunion is significantly higher in those fractures treated conservatively. Most of the results reported are for the medial malleolus and can be as high as 15 percent.[12,15,20,23,34] Figures for nonunion of the medial malleolus treated after rigid internal fixation are not readily available but appear to be less than 1 percent. Nonunion of the lateral malleolus is far less frequent than that of the medial malleolus. Klossner[15] lists an incidence of about 1 percent and Sneppen[32] found it to be 5 percent following conservative treatment. There are no reliable data to indicate the rate of nonunion after rigid internal fixation.

The nonunion should be visualized using the usual exposures and cleared of all soft tissue. The ends of the fractures are freshened, and rigid internal fixation is achieved by a screw and K-wire for the medial malleolus and a plate for the lateral malleolus. A rectangular slot is then created across the fracture site, which is filled with a corticocancellous bone graft obtained locally from the tibia.

Distal Tibiofibular Synostosis

As the ankle mortise widens during dorsiflexion, movement of the fibula is necessary to accommodate the talus. This takes place by external fibular rotation and vertical excursion of the fibula during normal weight bearing.[6] Thus, widening of the mortise must occur during dorsiflexion or this will be severely restricted. This concept is well recognized during surgical reconstruction of ankle fractures associated with syndesmotic tears. In such cases, the syndesmotic screw is inserted and tightened, with the ankle held in dorsiflexion. It has been our experience that in some severe ankle fractures associated with significant soft tissue injury, bony synostosis will develop at the distal tibiofibular joint. This may restrict dorsiflexion of the injured ankle. To avoid this complication, the ankle must be immobilized in as much dorsiflexion as possible. However, if surgical stabilization is used, dorsiflexion exercises are started early after the injury, and physiologic dorsiflexion (beyond 10 degrees) will be present in most instances despite immobilization of the distal tibiofibular joint. Figure 127-34A demonstrates 2-year follow-up of an open comminuted ankle fracture that resulted in a synostosis of the distal tibiofibular joint. Figure 127-34B shows the dorsiflexion present in the same patient indicating that despite the occurrence of a synostosis functional dorsiflexion may still be present.

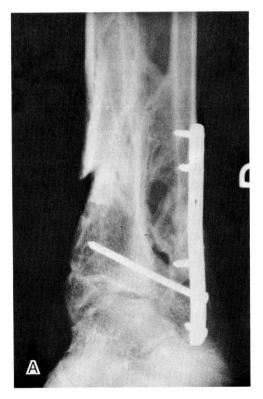 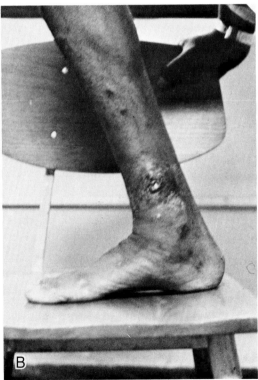

Fig. 127-34. (A) Comminuted fracture of distal tibia with a bimalleolar component 2 years after open reduction and internal fixation. A marked tibiofibular synostosis has occurred. **(B)** Same patient demonstrating 12 degrees of dorsiflexion.

Wound Dehiscence

Application of a plate on a subcutaneous bone such as the fibula should not cause undue complications if the principles of postoperative management as described are followed. One should pay particular attention to wound closure and perform a meticulous apposition of the subcutaneous tissues before closing the skin. Equally important is the prevention of postoperative edema, which is the enemy of wound healing. The best way to avoid this is to elevate the extremity such that the level of the ankle is always above the level of the heart by suspending the leg in a sling attached to an overhead frame. Thus, the use of pillows or elevation of the foot of the bed is insufficient. Elevation should be continued for about 5 days, and the patient must be instructed to begin active dorsiflexion and plantar flexion of the ankle. If carefully followed, these measures will promote uneventful wound healing.

Infection

For reasons that are not well understood, the ankle appears to be less susceptible to infection than most other areas of the body. Should infection occur, however, it is necessary to follow the recommendations described earlier. The wound should be opened in the operating room and a complete debridement performed. If the plate and screws are not loose and are doing their job, they should be left in situ and should not be removed. Cultures are obtained and appropriate intravenous antibiotic therapy started. The wound should be inspected; if it looks clean, it may be closed within 5 to 7 days. Intravenous antibiotics should be maintained for approximately 6 weeks. If drainage persists, the wound should be packed open and the hardware removed when the fracture has united. This may take anywhere from 6 to 12 weeks to occur. The question of antibiotic therapy throughout this time has not yet been settled. If the wound is still draining after a 6-week course of antibiotics, we discontinue the antimicrobial agents and allow the wound to drain to the exterior. Because union may be delayed, full weight bearing is not permitted. When union has occurred, the patient is readmitted to hospital, cultures are obtained, intravenous antibi-

otics are reinstituted, and the hardware is removed. The wound is debrided and can usually be closed within 5 to 7 days.

REFERENCES

1. Bonnin JG: Injuries to the Ankle. Hafner, Darien, CT, 1970
2. Braunstein PW, Wade PA: Treatment of unstable fractures of the ankle. Ann Surg 149:217, 1959
3. Burns BH: Diastasis of the inferior tibiofibular joint. Proc R Soc Med 36:330, 1943
4. Burwell NH, Charnley AD: The treatment of displaced fractures of the ankle by rigid internal fixation and early joint movement. J Bone Joint Surg 47B:634, 1965
5. Cedell CA: Supination-outward rotation injuries of the ankle. A clinical and roentgenological study with special reference to the operative treatment. Acta Orthop Scand 110(suppl):1967
6. Close JR: Some applications of the functional anatomy of the ankle joint. J Bone Joint Surg 38:761, 1956
7. Denham RA: Internal fixation for unstable ankle fractures. J Bone Joint Surg 46B:206, 1964
8. Dupuytren G: Mémoir sur la fracture de l'extrémité intérieure du pérone, les luxatrous et les accidents qui en vont la suite. Annu Med Chir Hop Hosp Civ Paris 1:1, 1819
9. Gatelier J: The juxaretroperoneal route in the operative treatment of fractures of malleolus with posterior marginal fragment. Surg Gynecol Obstet 52:67, 1931
10. Gustilo RB, Anderson JT: Prevention of infection in the treatment of one thousand twenty five open fractures of long bones. J Bone Joint Surg 58A:453, 1976
11. Iselin M, DeVellis H: La primaute du pérone dans les fractures du cou-de-pied. Mem Acad Chir 87:399, 1961
12. Jones WC, Neal EG, Surgery of the fracture of the medial malleolus. South Med J 55:1054, 1952
13. Joy G, Patzakis MJ, Harvey JP: Precise evaluation of the reduction of severe ankle fractures. J Bone Joint Surg 43:971, 1974
14. Kleiger B: The treatment of oblique fractures of the fibula. J Bone Joint Surg 43:971, 1961
15. Klossner O: Late results of operative and non-opera-

tive treatment of severe ankle fractures. Acta Chir Scand 293(suppl):1962

16. Lauge-Hansen N: Fractures of the ankle. II. Combined exploration-surgical and exploration roentgenologic investigation. Arch Surg 60:957, 1950

17. Leach RE: Fractures of the tibial plafond. p. 88. In American Academy of Orthopaedic Surgeons Instructional Course Lectures. Vol. 28., CV Mosby, St. Louis, 1979

18. Lee HG, Horan RB: Internal fixation in injuries of the ankle. Surg Gynecol Obstet 76:493, 1943

19. Maale R, Seligson D: Distal tibial plafond fracture. Orthopedics 3:517, 1980

20. Magnusson R: On the late results in non-operated cases of malleolar fractures. Clinical-roentgenological-statistical study. I. Fractures by external rotation. Acta Chir Scand 84(suppl):1944

21. Maisonneuve JG: Recherches sur la fracture du pérone. Arch Gen Med 1:165, 1940

22. McLennan JG, Ungersma JA: A new approach to the treatment of ankle fractures: The Inyo nail. Clin Orthop 213:125, 1986

23. Mendelsohn MA: Non-union of malleolar fractures of the ankle. Clin Orthop 42:103, 1965

24. Philips RS, Balmer GA, Monk CJE: The external rotation fracture of the fibular malleolus. Br J Surg 56:801, 1969

25. Picaud AJ: Reflexions à propos d'un traitement chirurgical simple des fractures récentes de la cheville. Rev Chir Orthop 39:570, 1953

26. Ramsey PL, Hamilton W: Changes in the tibio-talar area of contact caused by lateral talar shift. J Bone Joint Surg 58A:356, 1976

27. Rittman WW, Schibli M, Matter P, et al: Open fractures: long term results in two hundred consecutive cases. Clin Orthop 138:132, 1979

28. Rosen H: Compression treatment of long bone pseudarthroses. Clin Orthop 138:154, 1979

29. Ruedi TP, Allgower M: Fractures of the lower end of the tibia into the ankle joint: results nine years after open reduction and internal fixation. Injury 5:130, 1973

30. Ruedi TP, Allgower M: The operative treatment of intra-articular fractures of the lower end of the tibia. Clin Orthop 138:105, 1979

31. Segal D: Ankle fractures—Internal fixation. II. p. 81. In American Academy of Orthopedic Surgeons Instructional Course Lectures. Vol. 28. CV Mosby, St. Louis, 1979

32. Sneppen O: Non-union of malleolar fractures of the ankle. Clin Orthop 42:103, 1965

33. Solonen KA, Lauttamus L: Operative treatment of ankle fractures. Acta Orthop Scand 39:223, 1968

34. Wilson FC, Skilbred AL: Long-term results in the treatment of displaced bi-malleolar fractures. J Bone Joint Surg 48A:1065, 1966

35. Yablon IG, Wasilewski S: Management of unstable ankle fractures. Bateman J, Trott A (eds): The Foot and Ankle. Thieme-Stratton, New York, 1980

36. Yablon IG, Heller FG, Shouse L: The key role of the lateral malleolus in displaced fractures of the ankle. J Bone Joint Surg 59A:169, 1977

Richard N. Stauffer

OSTEOCHONDRAL FRACTURES OF THE TALAR DOME (OSTEOCHONDRITIS DISSECANS AND TRANSCHONDRAL FRACTURES)

General Statement of the Problem

Many misconceptions and controversies persist regarding osteochondral fractures of the talus. Confusion as to the etiology, treatment, and prognosis of this lesion has perhaps been perpetuated by its unfortunate designation as "osteochondritis dissecans." This term, literally translated, implies separation of an inflammatory lesion of cartilage and bone, and has no relevance to the actual pathophysiology of the condition. The term has been ascribed to Koenig,[18] who described loose bodies in the knee joint, due to spontaneous necrosis of bone, in 1888. Kappis,[17] in 1922, used the term applied to similar lesions in the ankle. Although uncommon, the disease process has been reported in cases involving the elbow, hip, and first metatarsophalangeal joints. The uncertainty as to preferred treatment — watchful expectancy, immobilization, internal fixtion, or excision of the osteochondral fragment — is due to the designation "osteochondritis dissecans" (which shrouds the disease in the cloak of a mysterious or unknown process), and a differing prognosis, depending on site and degree of involvement. Also, various mechanical and biologic factors result in a somewhat different behavior from one joint to another.

Osteochondral fractures of the talar dome are relatively uncommon. However, they probably occur much more commonly than clinically recognized because radiographic identification may be subtle and radiographs may not even be taken because the trauma may seem insignificant. In one large series, osteochondral fractures of the knee accounted for 82 percent of cases, while the ankle was involved in 4 percent.[21] Other sites were also uncommon (elbow, 6 percent; hip 2 percent). Osteochondral fractures account for only about 14 percent of all fractures involving the talus,[22] or about 0.09 percent of fractures of all bones.[3,10]

Contrary to the lesion involving the knee, osteochondral talar fractures do not show a male predilection in most nonmilitary series. The right ankle is involved with slightly greater frequency than the left. Although the talar lesion may occur at any age,

3861

it most often affects adolescents and young adults, with a peak incidence in the third decade. This coincides with the age of peak incidence of all limb fractures[10] (when femoral neck fractures are excluded).

Talar osteochondral fractures may involve either the medial or lateral prominence, although mid-dome fractures have been reported rarely. The medial lesion tends to be located more posteriorly; frequently it involves more depth of subchondral bone than does the lateral lesion, which is in the anterior or middle third of the talar convexity and generally appears as a shallow, "flake" fracture (Fig. 128-1). The medial site is the most common, accounting variously for 56 to 85 percent.[3,21,25] Concurrent medial and lateral lesions have been occasionally reported.[5,21] The fractures tend to involve a circular-to-ovoid segment of the talar surface, 0.5 to 1.5 cm in diameter. Histologic examination of the fracture fragment reveals viable articular cartilage over necrotic trabecular bone, covered on the inferior surface by fibrous or fibrocartilaginous tissue, typical of a pseudarthrosis.

Clinically, patients with osteochondral talar fractures present with complaints of pain, "catching" with motion, swelling, and instability, most often following an inversion injury to the ankle. All too frequently, patients seek medical attention because of persistent symptoms of a "mild ankle sprain" that occurred weeks or months previously. The symptoms may also occasionally arise spontaneously with no recognized, antecedent trauma, hence the confusion regarding the nature and etiology of the lesion.

The role of trauma in the etiology of these talar dome lesions is now well recognized. Alexander and Lichtman[1] demonstrated significant ankle trauma in 92 percent and Canale and Belding[5] in 80 percent of their reported cases. It is suggested that the arbitrary and opaque term, osteochondritis dissecans, be discarded. A number of investigators had suggested that the talar lesions were due to trauma, but it remained for Berndt and Harty[3] to publish their definite study in 1959 in which they produced experimental evidence of a traumatic origin. They termed the lesions *transchondral talar fractures* and classified them according to a spectrum of severity (Fig. 128-2). This classification has relevance for treatment and prognosis.

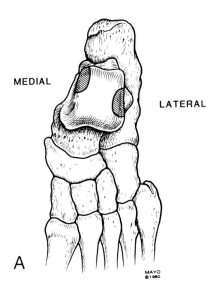

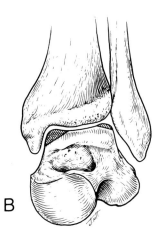

Fig. 128-1. Location of osteochondral fractures of talus. **(A)** Dorsal view of talar fractures. Note the posterior location of medial lesion and mid- to anterior location of lateral lesion. **(B)** Frontal view of talar fractures. Lateral lesion tends to be more shallow than medial lesion. (By permission of Mayo Foundation.)

According to Berndt and Hardy, the stage I lesion represents a compression of the medial (and, uncommonly, the lateral) talar dome, caused by an inversion stress with sparing of the lateral ankle ligaments. The articular cartilage remains intact while the underlying bony trabeculae fracture and buckle. Because of the well-known vulnerable ability of the intraosseous vascular supply of the talus, these bony fractures do not heal but become avas-

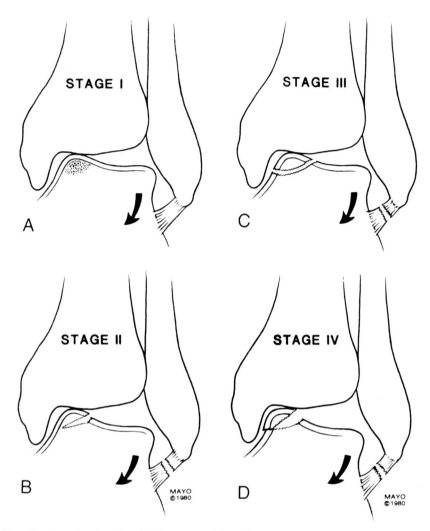

Fig. 128-2. Classification of osteochondral fractures of the talus, according to Berndt and Harty. **(A)** Stage I: an impact or cyclic compression fracture of the talar dome; lateral ligaments remain intact. Articular cartilage remains intact and viable while underlying trabecular bone becomes necrotic. **(B)** Stage II: an incomplete fracture of bone and cartilage with rupture of lateral ligaments. **(C)** Stage III: complete osteochondral fracture with fragment undisplaced from its bed. **(D)** Stage IV: complete osteochondral fracture with displacement of fragment within the ankle joint. (By permission of Mayo Foundation.)

cular and necrotic. These stage I osteochondral fractures often do not have a convincing history of trauma and have contributed to the mystery of "osteochondritis dissecans" (Fig. 128-3). We suggest that this lesion may be caused by a single-impact compression due to inversion injury or by cyclic compression loading due to repeated subclinical talar inversions. The repetitive compression loads exceed the physiologic healing capacity of the

bone and necrosis ensues. The resulting lesion could be thought of as a compression, fatigue fracture. This sort of repeated, painless inversion episode might readily occur in persons with lax ankle ligaments. This relationship is suggested by the case report of Davis.[7]

Stage II lesions represent incomplete fracture of both articular cartilage and subchondral bone, with injury to the lateral ankle ligaments. Either medial

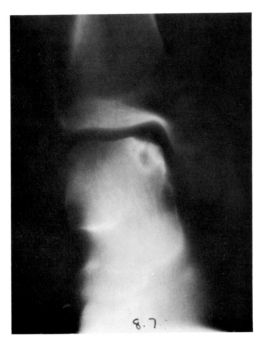

Fig. 128-3. Anteroposterior tomogram of stage I lesion of medial talar dome in 25-year-old woman with no history of recognized ankle trauma.

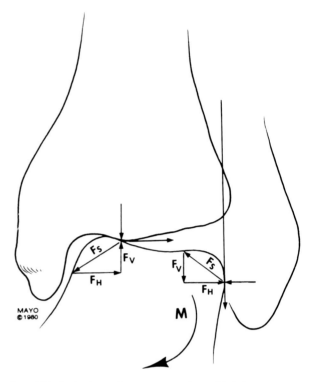

Fig. 128-4. An inversion stress on the ankle joint creates a moment of force *(M)*, which can be resolved along coordinate axes as a vertical (F_V) and a horizontal force (F_H). The resultant of these two forces is a shear force (F_S), along which the talar dome fracture occurs. (By permission of Mayo Foundation.)

or lateral portions of the talar dome may be involved. Berndt and Harty convincingly suggest that the medial lesion is produced by compression against the tibial plafond with ankle inversion in plantar flexion, while the lateral lesion is produced by compression against the lateral malleolus with ankle inversion in dorsiflexion. This would explain the posterior location of the medial fracture and the more anterior location of the lateral fracture.

Stage III lesions include a complete fracture of articular cartilage and/or bone with no displacement of the fragment from its bed. Figure 128-4 indicates the resolution of forces acting on the talar dome during application of an inversion force (moment of force, M). The fracture occurs along the line of the shear force component (F_s). Whether the medial or lateral aspect of the dome is involved may depend on whether the ankle is in a plantar- or dorsiflexed position. Since the ultimate shear stress of cartilage is greater than that of bone, the articular cartilage may momentarily deform but remain intact while the underlying bone fractures (Fig. 128-5A). This produces a stage II or III lesion. If the magnitude of the resultant shear stress is greater than the ultimate strength or *both* articular cartilage and bone a complete lesion is produced (Fig. 128-5B), and is apt to displace from its bed, producing a stage IV lesion.

Treatment

A great deal of confusion exists regarding treatment for these talar lesions. We recently saw a patient with a grade I medial osteochondral fracture who was evaluated by three different surgeons all of whom made a diagnosis of "osteochondritis dissecans" and advised three entirely different methods of treatment. This confusion is probably due to uncertainty about the etiology and nature of the problem. If one accepts that the lesion,

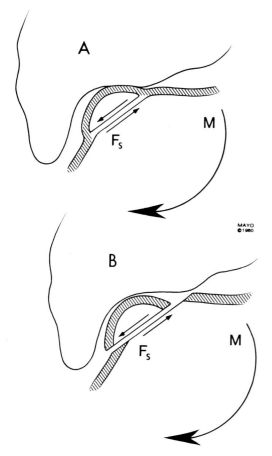

Fig. 128-5. The articular cartilage may remain intact or may be fractured along with the subchondral bone in stage II or III lesions, depending on whether **(A)** The shear stress is greater than the ultimate strength of bone, but less than that of cartilage; or **(B)** The shear stress is greater than the ultimate strength of both cartilage and bone. (By permission of Mayo Foundation.)

whether medial or lateral, represents a shearing fracture of bone (and cartilage), the basic principles of fracture management can be employed.

The first step in treatment is the diagnosis. Many osteochondral talar fractures are missed at first presentation, either because radiographs of a routine ankle "sprain" are not taken, or because the talar fracture is overlooked. All ankle "sprains" deserve a radiographic evaluation. An attitude of expectancy and awareness of the possibility of the lesion is necessary since the fracture may represent

a very subtle finding, particularly on the initial anteroposterior, mortise, and lateral ankle films. Frequently, an oblique radiograph is necessary to show the fracture to best advantage (particularly because the medial lesion tends to be located well posterior). Tomograms of the talus are then advised for demonstrating the location and extent of the lesion.

A conservative, or nonsurgical, approach to treatment of type I or II talar osteochondral fractures seems justified by long-term clinical studies. With an average follow-up of 7 years, 7 of 11 patients in the series of Lindholm et al.,[21] were asymptomatic. Several studies have indicated that the lesion may show radiographic failure to heal over a long period of follow-up but that this is not incompatible with a successful outcome and an asymptomatic ankle.[21,33] Degenerative changes in the ankle joint appear in a small percentage of both surgically and nonsurgically treated cases. These changes are generally mild and are progressive in only a very few. Progressive degenerative changes were noted in only 5 of 41 patients in the series of Roden et al.[33]

Those cases with complete separation of the osteocartilaginous fragment do require surgical treatment. Canale and Belding[5] have outlined the following rational approach to treatment, with which we concur:

Stage I lesions
Stage II lesions $\Big\}$ nonsurgical treatment
Stage III
  medial lesions   nonoperative treatment initially, then surgical treatment only if symptoms persist

Stage III
  lateral lesions $\Big\}$ surgical treatment
Stage IV lesion

Pettine and Morrey[30] found that delay in treatment is one of the important prognostic elements. Delay of more than 12 months in surgical treatment resulted in less satisfactory outcome. These workers also recommended surgical treatment of medial stage III lesions, which is contrary to the above treatment plan.

Arthrotomy and Fragment Excision

As implied above, it is not unusual to see an apparently undisplaced stage **III** fracture subsequently become displaced and require surgical removal. Careful periodic follow-up is required regardless of the treatment method employed. The nonsurgical regimen advised is cast immobilization for 8 weeks (4 weeks in a non-weight-bearing and 4 weeks in a walking cast). Surgical treatment consists of excision of the osteochondral fragment with curettage and drilling (multiple small-diameter drill holes about 5 mm deep) of the bony base of the talar defect. Care should be taken to excise the cartilage margins at an angle of 90 degrees to the articular surface and not to undermine or bevel the margins. This "quarry effect" (as opposed to "puddle effect") may lead to better clot retention in the defect and subsequent metaplasia to fibrocartilage with the potential for reconstitution of the articular surface. Postoperative cast immobilization for 8

weeks is recommended. Alexander and Lichtman[1] found that the optimum result following surgical treatment may not be reached for 18 months (and that there was little likelihood of long-term decline in result after 18 months).

Surgical exposure of the lateral talar osteochondral fracture is not difficult, due to the usual anterior location of the lesion and the more posterior position of the lateral malleolus. A slightly oblique vertical incision over the anterolateral aspect of the ankle, with division of the transverse crural retinaculum just medial to the peroneus tertius tendon, and plantar flexion of the ankle, allows very adequate exposure of the lateral lesion (Fig. 128-6).

Since the medial lesion is generally in the middle to posterior portion of the talar dome, it is frequently inaccessible without a careful osteotomy of the medial malleolus (Fig. 128-7). A slightly curved vertical incision is made over the middle aspect of the medial malleolus. Subperiosteal dissection of the malleolus is performed. A drill hole is placed through the malleolus into the metaphysis

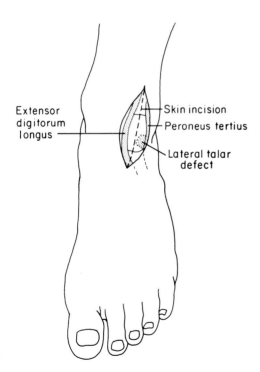

Fig. 128-6. Anterolateral approach to lateral (and anterior) talar osteochondral fracture; vertical skin incision and deep dissection between tendons of peroneus tertius (lateral) and extensor digitorum longus (medial).

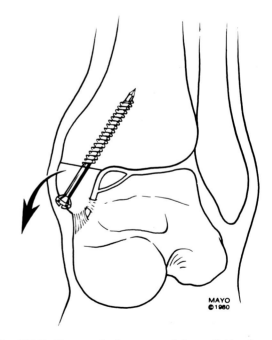

Fig. 128-7. Transmalleolar approach to medial (and posterior) talar osteochondral fracture. (By permission of Mayo Foundation.)

of the distal tibia, with care taken to avoid the joint surface. The hole is tapped and a malleolar screw is inserted. The screw is then removed and an osteotomy made across the malleolus at the level of the joint with a thin-bladed oscillating saw. The malleolus is retracted distally, hinging on the intact medial ligaments. The ankle is everted, exposing the medial talar fracture. Once joint inspection, fragment removal, and curettage are completed, the malleolus is anatomically reduced and held in place by reinsertion of the malleolar screw. Compression afforded by the cancellous threads on the screw generally gives good resistance to torsion of the malleolus and makes supplemental fixation unnecessary.

Postoperative Management

A modified Robert Jones compression dressing with a stirrup plaster splint is applied and the leg is elevated in bed for about 4 days. Crutch walking with touch weight bearing is then begun. At about 10 days the compression dressing is removed and a short-leg walking cast is applied for 8 weeks. Progressive weight bearing is then allowed over the next 4 to 6 weeks.

Arthrotomy and Fragment Fixation

Internal fixation of the talar fracture fragment is generally not advisable or possible, due to the small size and avascular necrotic nature of the fragment. However, in cases in which the fragment is unusually large (e.g., greater than 2 cm), it may be internally fixed with small screws or bone pegs countersunk through the articular cartilage. The fibrous tissue bed should be thoroughly curetted before the fragment is replaced and fixed. Non-weight bearing should be maintained for 10 to 12 weeks to permit revascularization of the fragment. We have no personal experience with this method of treatment.[30] Pettine and Morrey report success in only two of five cases of attempted fragment fixation.

It is hoped that a better understanding of the true nature, etiology, and pathomechanics of these talar dome injuries will result in the formulation of more logical treatment plans and less confusion for both patient and physician.

DEGENERATIVE ANKLE JOINT DISEASE

General Statement of the Problem

Although degenerative disease involving the ankle joint is distinctly less common than similar problems at the hip and knee joints, it is nonetheless an equally disabling condition. Also, current treatment options are possibly not as satisfying as those available for other joints. A brief review of our experience over the past 10 years indicates that of all cases of disabling degenerative disease of the major lower extremity joints, only about 6 percent involved the ankle. Intrinsic, or so-called primary degenerative disease, so common in the hip and knee, is extremely rare in the ankle. On the basis of studies of ankle mechanics over the past decade, we have concluded that the ankle is an inherently stable, kinematically simple (relative to other lower extremity joints) joint which bears tremendous compression forces[36] with relative ease because of a large weight bearing surface area.[40]

Trauma is the underlying etiologic agent in virtually all cases of ankle joint degenerative disease. We have personally seen only two patients (out of more than 300) with disabling ankle degeneration who did not give a convincing history of past fracture or recurrent ankle ligament injuries. Because of the posttraumatic nature of this problem patients tend to present at a considerably younger age than those with hip or knee problems. Figure 128-8 indicates a bimodal age distribution with posttraumatic degenerative disease following ankle fracture (with a slightly increased incidence in males) reaching a peak in the fourth decade and following recurrent sprains (with slight female predisposition) peaking in the sixth decade.

The common factor underlying degenerative disease following ankle fracture is an imperfect reduction or a less than perfect anatomic restoration of the form and function of the ankle mortise. Imperfect reduction of ankle fractures may be categorized as having the following three etiologies, only the first of which is generally *not* under the control of the treating physician:

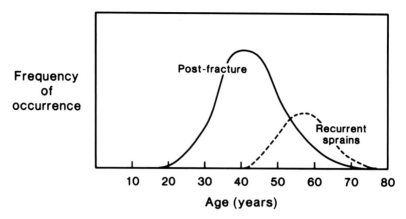

Fig. 128-8. Bimodal age distribution of posttraumatic degenerative disease of the ankle.

1. Complete loss of portions of the articular surface, as may occur especially with open, or vertical compression to ankle fractures
2. Residual subluxation of the talus (most often lateral subluxation)
3. Rotary malunion of the lateral maleolus

Ramsey and Hamilton[31] showed that even 1-mm lateral subluxation of the talus reduces the weight-bearing surface area of the tibiotalar joint by about 40 percent. Since a compressive force of more than five times body weight acts across the ankle during normal level walking[40] *any* residual subluxation greatly increased the "unit load" or pressure on the joint and exceeds the biologic load-bearing capacity of articular cartilage. Both of the first two factors listed above result in a rapidly progressive degeneration of the ankle joint, which generally becomes disabling within 3 to 5 years of the injury. The third factor results in a certain, but more delayed and insidious, degenerative process which often is not manifest as significant disability until 5 to 10 years after fracture. Perfect reduction of an eversion, lateral-rotation-type ankle fracture by either open or closed methods is difficult. The importance of anatomic reduction of the resulting spiral fracture of the lateral malleolus has perhaps not been recognized in the past. Attention has been focused instead on restoring the mortise in frontal plane projection. Lambert[19] demonstrated that the talofibular joint bears about one-sixth of the compression load acting across the ankle. Even mild rotary malunion of the lateral malleolus therefore

results in articular incongruity and subsequent degeneration, beginning in the weight-bearing talofibular compartment of the joint, and eventually involving the tibiotalar compartment.

Treatment

Ankle Arthrotomy and Debridement

Arthrotomy and debridement of the ankle joint are most commonly performed in conjunction with synovectomy for such disease processes as synovial chondromatosis, septic arthritis, and rheumatoid arthritis. Description of the technique of synovectomy is included in the discussion of rheumatoid arthritis in this chapter.

Arthrotomy and debridement of the degenerative ankle joint are most often considered in the presence of apparent impingement of anterior marginal osteophytes on the tibia and talus. Patients not uncommonly present with complaints of limitation of motion of the ankle, generalized ache, and a sharp pain during the latter portion of stance phase of gait; their radiographs show anterior osteophyte formation. It is tempting to consider arthrotomy and excision of the osteophytes. However, when there are accompanying significant degenerative changes involving the rest of the joint the procedure is of little, if any, value. Excision of the anterior osteophytes in this common instance represents a needless meddlesome operation.

However, in carefully selected cases in which the ankle is free of degenerative changes on radiographs, arthrotomy and excision of the impinging osteophytes may be quite beneficial (Fig. 128-9). These anterior marginal osteophytes have been termed hurdler's spurs because they are often seen in athletes and are presumably due to repetitive dorsiflexion injury. O'Donohue[28] makes a distinction between the nature of the isolated osteophytes in the athlete and those accompanying generalized degenerative ankle joint disease. Clearly, both represent a biologic repair process; in the former case, an attempted repair of a repetitive isolated injury, and in the latter an abortive attempt at repair of a generalized degenerative process.

Surgical Technique

An anteromedial surgical approach is advised for arthrotomy and debridement (Fig. 128-10). A slightly oblique, vertical skin incision is followed by division of the cruciate crural retinaculum, just lateral to the anterior tibial tendon. This tendon is retracted slightly medially and the extensor hallucis longus tendon retracted laterally. The incision is carried straight down to the periosteum of the tibia, talus, and anterior capsule of the ankle joint. Exposure to the entire anterior aspect of the ankle joint is gained by subperiosteal and subcapsular, medial and lateral dissection. The neurovascular bundle lies laterally, beneath the extensor digitorum longus tendons, and is well protected by this subperiosteal approach. The osteophytes apparent on the lateral radiographs generally represent a ridge of hypertrophic bone and cartilage along the opposing, anterior margins of the articular surfaces of tibia and talus. These ridges are divided with a curved osteotome and are removed (along with any loose osteochondral fragments), to restore the contour of the opposing articular sur-

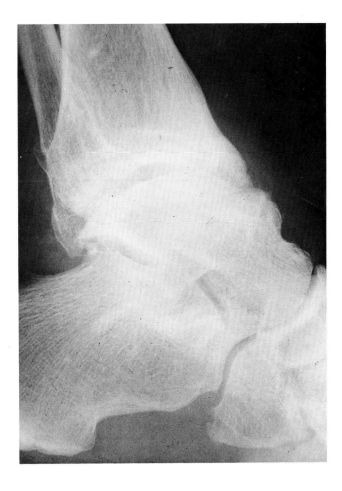

Fig. 128-9. Lateral ankle radiograph of a 28-year-old former world-class hurdler and professional football player. Note that the ankle is relatively free of degenerative changes with the exception of the marginal anterior tibial and talar osteophytes. Arthrotomy and excision of the osteophytes relieved pain, increased range of ankle dorsiflexion, and extended the patient's professional athletic career another 5 years. His ankle joint was still free of degenerative disease at the last follow-up, 11 years later.

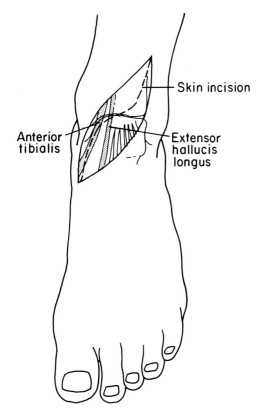

Skin incision

Anterior tibialis

Extensor hallucis longus

Fig. 128-10. Anteromedial approach for arthrotomy and debridement of the ankle joint; slightly curvilinear skin incision (dashed line), proximal-lateral to distal-medial, and deep dissection between tendons of anterior tibialis (medial) and extensor hallucis longus (lateral).

faces. An improved range of dorsiflexion should be obvious at once. Cast immobilization should be maintained for 3 weeks to allow for soft tissue healing. Active range-of motion ankle exercises are then instituted, combined with progressive weight bearing on crutches for another 3 weeks.

Ankle Arthrodesis

Arthrodesis of the tibiotalar joint has been a well-accepted and commonly performed surgical procedure and has been used to treat severe ankle joint disability since it was first described in 1878. Currently there is disagreement, not as to the utility of the procedure, but as to whether ankle arthrodesis is the optimum long-term solution to the problem of the painful ankle joint. A number of recent retrospective studies of the clinical results

following ankle arthrodesis present surprisingly consistent findings: a pseudarthrosis rate of 10 to 20 percent and a satisfactory clinical result in about two-thirds of cases.[12,16,20,26,27] The controversy surrounds interpretation of these results. One group claims that the results indicate that ankle arthrodesis is a satisfactory procedure, while another believes that a two-thirds success rate is not "good enough."

The advantages of ankle arthrodesis include the following:

1. A permanently stable joint is achieved. Once tibiotalar fusion occurs, it is subject to subsequent mechanical failure.
2. A relatively normal gait is possible. Mazur et al.[24] and Buck et al.[4] have demonstrated that with a solid, unilateral ankle fusion, compensatory mechanisms in the ipsilateral knee and contralateral ankle provide a near-normal gait pattern. Clinical experience indicates that many patients with an ankle fused in optimum position (neutral in both sagittal and coronal planes) walk without any perceptible limp, except when they are fatigued, or when they walk rapidly or attempt to run.

The disadvantages of ankle arthrodesis are as follows:

1. Three to 12 months of cast immobilization (5.5 months average in reported series)
2. A pseudarthrosis rate of 10 to 20 percent
3. Subsequent long-term degenerative changes in subtalar and midtarsal joints

This last point is still being debated. Jackson[15] showed that, contrary to accepted teaching, there is not necessarily a compensatory increase in midtarsal motion subsequent to ankle arthrodesis. In their series of patients with ankle fusion, roughly one-third showed normal midtarsal motion, one-third had less than normal, and one-third more than normal motion. Radiographic degenerative changes in the midtarsal joints were very common but were not necessarily correlated with clinical symptoms. All their patients had reduced subtalar joint motion. In a study of 21 patients examined at the University of Iowa, 8 to 33 years (average 16 years) after ankle arthrodesis, we found that all patients lost subtalar joint motion and 17 of the 21 had pain when walking on uneven surfaces.[2] Figure 128-11 is a graphic example of the degenerative process can occur in distal joints following ankle arthrodesis.

Notwithstanding these problems, for the relatively youthful active person with disabling posttraumatic degenerative disease, ankle arthrodesis remains the most efficacious surgical treatment available. Total ankle joint replacement, as its present state of development, does not offer a consistently satisfactory solution in this situation.

Indications for ankle arthrodesis include posttraumatic degenerative disease, secondary to fracture, recurrent sprains, or avascular necrosis of the talus; septic arthritis; neurologic disease with imbalance of muscular forces across the ankle joint; and Charcot's arthropathy.

Contraindications to ankle arthrodesis are relative rather than absolute. Factors that weigh against arthrodesis include established significant degenerative changes in subtalar and midtarsal joints, rheumatoid arthritis, and bilateral ankle joint disease.

Surgical Technique

A wide variety of techniques to accomplish ankle arthrodesis have been described. These include various combinations of anterior, posterior, lateral, and medial approaches, with and without bone grafting (sliding, dowel, or iliac crest bone blocks), with and without internal fixation, with and without external compression. The literature has been well summarized by White[39] who found 22 different techniques espoused by various authors. Regardless of the specific procedure used, the final position of the fused joint is critical. A number of studies have indicted that a hindfoot position of neutral in three planes is desirable (i.e., 0 degrees of flexion-extension, varus-valgus, and rotation). Previously a position of 10 to 15 degrees of plantar flexion was advised, especially in women to allow for wearing high-heeled shoes. However, ankle fusion in plantar flexion may result in greater dorsiflexion through the midtarsal joint. This joint appears to accommodate more plantar flexion than dorsiflexion motion from the neutral position. Thus a fused ankle in plantar flexion may result in increased stress on the midtarsal joint and more rapid appearance of degenerative changes. In seeking the neutral position for arthrodesis it is better to err on the side of slight ankle dorsiflexion than plantar flexion. Also, the result of our follow-up study indicates that a slight valgus hindfoot position is more compatible with a good result than is varus position.[2]

We have used three different techniques to achieve ankle arthrodesis, the choice depending on the preoperative situation. External fixation/compression is used in all three techniques and appears to reduce the time necessary for achieving solid arthrodesis to about 4 months. A variety of these external fixation/compression devices are currently available, using both bicortical and unicortical fixation pins.

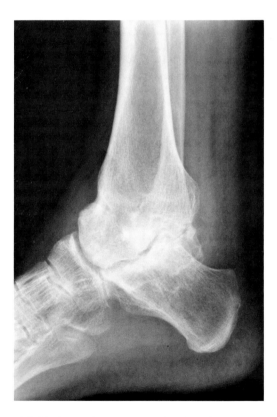

Fig. 128-11. Lateral radiograph of a 46-year-old man who underwent an ankle fusion 8 years previously for posttraumatic degenerative disease. At follow-up, he had pain when walking on any uneven surface, due to the rather severe subtalar and midtarsal degenerative changes.

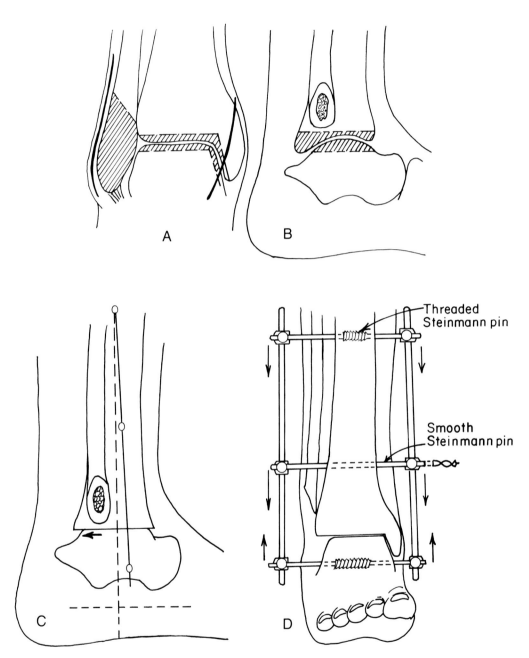

Fig. 128-12. Lateral compression ankle arthrodesis technique. **(A)** Lateral (primary) and anteromedial (second-ary) skin incisions (dark lines) with bone resections indicated. **(B)** Resection of distal fibula and exposure of lateral ankle joint. Parallel saw cuts in tibia and dome of talus indicated. **(C)** After completion of saw cuts, the talus is displaced posteriorly, position is checked, and pins for compression apparatus are placed in tibia and talus. **(D)** Application of Roger-Anderson compression device. *(Figure continues.)*

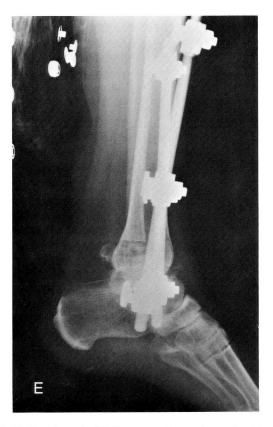 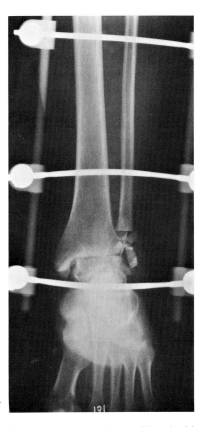

Fig. 128-12 *(Continued).* **(E)** Postoperative radiographs. The fibular bone has been "minced" and added to the lateral side of the ankle joint in this case; probably an unnecessary step.

Lateral Approach with Compression

The lateral approach is preferred when no significant varus-valgus ankle deformity exists and represents a modification of previously described transfibular techniques.[12] (Fig. 128-12). The sagittal plane position of the ankle is under direct vision, which facilitates a neutral flexion angle.

A longitudinal skin incision approximately 10 cm long is made directly over the lateral malleolus. The distal portion of the incision is curved slightly anteriorly.

The fibula is obliquely osteotomized with an oscillating saw at a level just above the level of the tibiotalar joint (4 to 5 cm proximal to the tip of the lateral malleolus) and the distal fibula is subperiosteally exposed and excised. With subperiosteal excision of the fibula, damage to the peroneal tendons is avoided and the peroneal sheath and retinaculum

are preserved. Subsequent dislocations of the peroneal tendons have not been a problem.

Subperiosteal stripping of the tibia and joint capsule is carefully extended anteriorly and posteriorly using a periosteal elevator. Chandler self-retaining retractors are then inserted to protect the soft tissues.

A cut is made through the distal tibia, just above the level of concavity of the joint, with a reciprocating saw. This cut should be perpendicular to the long axis of the tibia in both sagittal and coronal planes. The depth of cut should extend to the level of the medial corner of the ankle mortise. Tibial bone distal to the cut is then removed.

The ankle is then held in exactly neutral flexion and a second saw cut is made, through the dome of the talus, parallel to the tibial cut, and the talar bone removed. No more than about 1-cm shortening of the limb should result.

Generally, a second, short anteromedial incision is necessary. The horizontal saw cut in the tibia is completed through this incision, and the articular surfaces of the medial malleolus and medial talus are excised. This removes the deep portion of the deltoid ligament and allows the talus to be displaced upward and posteriorly to appose the tibial surface.

If the bony surfaces of the tibia and talus are well apposed, the ankle is in neutral position, and the talus is displaced posteriorly, the compression device may then be applied.

We prefer to use the Roger Anderson compression device. The distal and proximal pins are threaded to prevent slippage. The distal pins should be placed slightly anterior to the neutral axis of the arthrodesis surface. The clasps and side bars are applied and, while an assistant holds the

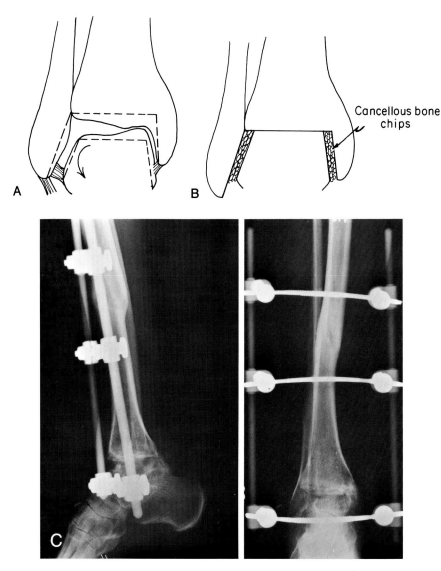

Fig. 128-13. Anterior compression ankle arthrodesis technique. **(A)** Exposure of the anterior aspect of the ankle by anteromedial skin incision (Fig. 128-11) and parallel saw cuts in tibia and talus indicated. **(B)** Completed saw cuts in sagittal plane. **(C)** Postoperative radiograph.

foot in desired position, a third intermediate pin (we use Crowe-tip pins to prevent bone necrosis) is drilled through one clasp, the tibia, and the opposite clasp. Manual compression is then applied evenly across the ankle and the clasps tightened with a wrench.

Anterior Approach with Compression

The anterior approach is especially helpful in the presence of a varus or valgus deformity (Fig. 128-13). We also use this exposure for septic arthritis because more complete synovectomy and debridement is possible than with the lateral approach.

A slightly curvilinear incision is made over the anterior aspect of the ankle (as in Fig. 128-11). The interval is deepened through the extensor retinaculum between the anterior tibial tendon, medially, and the extensor hallucis longus tendon, laterally. The anterior capsule and tibial periosteum are stripped medially and laterally. Chandler retractors are slipped around the malleoli.

The saw cut through the distal tibia must be made perpendicular to the long axis of the tibia in the coronal plane to correct hindfoot deformity. Care must be taken as the flare of the anterior aspect of the distal tibia may cause the cut to be tilted anteriorly. The saw cut must be made perpendicular to the long axis of the tibia in the sagittal plane as well.

Tibial bone distal to the saw cut is excised. The hindfoot is then held in neutral position in both sagittal and coronal planes and a saw cut through the talar dome is made exactly parallel to the tibial cut. No more than 1 cm of limb shortening need result due to the bone resection. The articular surfaces of the malleoli and the medial and lateral surfaces of the talus are excised.

The talus is displaced upward and slightly posteriorly and held in this position while the compression device is applied, as described previously for the lateral approach.

Modified Chuinard Arthrodesis with Compression

The modified technique (originally described by Chuinard and Peterson[6] to be used in children with open distal tibial epiphysis) is useful in preventing limb shortening due to bone resection during ankle arthrodesis (Fig. 128-14). This technique has proved particularly useful as a salvage for failed total ankle arthroplasty.

An anteromedial approach to the ankle joint is used, as illustrated in Figure 128-10. Bone is resected from the tibia and talus (or the prosthetic ankle joint is removed and the bony surfaces thoroughly curetted of all cement and fibrous tissue).

The ipsilateral anterior iliac crest is exposed subperiosteally, and a full-thickness block of bone is removed, about 3 fingerbreadths behind the anterior superior iliac spine (the thickest portion of the crest). This full-thickness block need measure no more than 2.5 cm wide $\times$ 2.5 cm high. The curved superior margins of bone block generally must be shaved or tailored slightly, to provide a proper fit of the block within the ankle mortise and to achieve proper neutral position of the hindfoot. We do not believe that drilling this cortical bone will have any effect in facilitating vascularization of the graft.

This block of cortical bone serves primarily as a spacer. It will probably retain a dense sclerotic appearance on the radiograph for several years and should not be relied on to participate in the fusion process to a significant degree. As much cancellous bone as possible is removed from the iliac crest, using gouges or curettes. This cancellous bone is packed posteriorly, medially, laterally, and anteriorly within the ankle mortise and about the spacer block of cortical bone. The compression apparatus is then applied, as previously described (Fig. 128-12C,D).

Postoperative Management

We have used the same postoperative regimen for all three of these ankle arthrodesis techniques. Postoperatively a below-knee Robert Jones dressing with a posterior plaster splint is applied. The limb is elevated in bed for 3 days to prevent swelling. After 9 to 10 days, the sutures are removed and a below-knee, non-weight-bearing cast is applied, incorporating the compression apparatus. At 8 weeks, the cast and compression apparatus are removed (a brief general anesthetic is recommended). A short-leg walking cast is applied.

At 16 weeks, the walking cast is removed. If the arthrodesis appears solid clinically and radiographically, a **SACH** heel and rocker-bottom sole are ap-

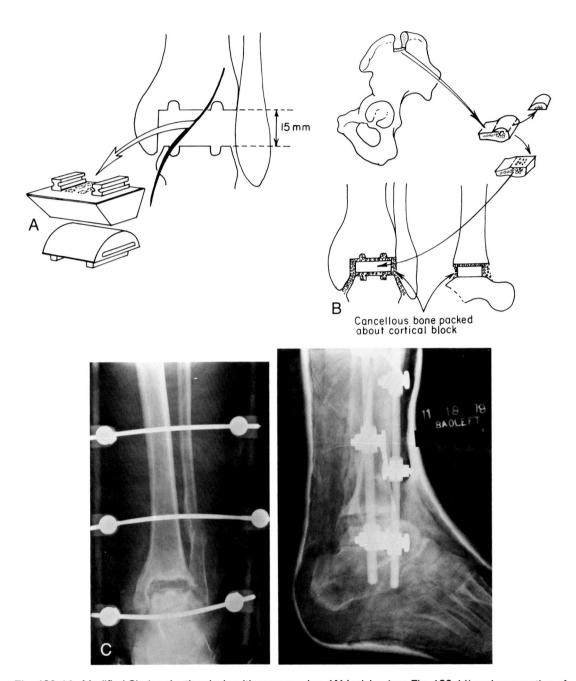

Fig. 128-14. Modified Chuinard arthrodesis with compression. **(A)** Incision (see Fig. 128-11) and preparation of ankle-joint mortise (removal of prosthetic components and curettage of bony surfaces). **(B)** Removal and insertion of anterior iliac crest cortical bone block and cancellous bone. Application of Roger-Anderson compression device as in Figure 128-13C. **(C)** Postoperative roentgenograms of modified Chuinard ankle arthrodesis.

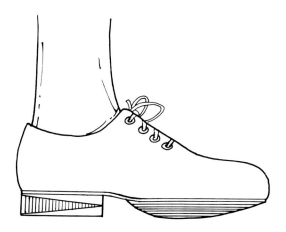

Fig. 128-15. Shoe with SACH-type heel insert of cushion material and rocker-bottom sole.

plied to the patient's shoe (Fig. 128-15). We recommend that these appliances be worn permanently to reduce the impact at heel strike and to reduce the dorsiflexion moment across the midtarsal joints during the latter portion of stance phase (which may contribute to subsequent degenerative disease).

Total Ankle Replacement

A wide variety of total ankle joint replacement prostheses are currently available. They vary in geometry and mechanical design from congruent to noncongruent bearing surfaces and from fully constrained to totally unconstrained types. Most investigators have found that clinical results with total ankle replacement in relatively youthful active persons with posttraumatic degenerative disease are not consistently satisfactory[6,11,34,37] (no better than 60 percent good results even over the short term). It is only in the elderly less active patient

(over 60 to 65 years of age) with degenerative disease, who places much less physical demand on the lower extremity, that total ankle replacement has an indication (see Table 128-1).

The chief indication for total ankle replacement, at the present state of development, appears to be in people with disabling ankle joint disease due to rheumatoid arthritis.

RHEUMATOID ARTHRITIS

General Statement of the Problem

Rheumatoid arthritis is an inflammatory connective tissue disease of unknown etiology that disables and incapacitates millions of people. It is a systemic disease (except for those uncommon cases of apparently monoarticular disease) that involves all connective tissue structures, and all joints of the body, at least to some degree. When considering disability due to rheumatoid involvement of the ankle joint, one must consider the status of the remainder of the individual's musculoskeletal system and the effect of the ankle disease on his overall functional capacity. The joints of the lower extremity should be considered as a multilinkage system with interdependent function. Impairment of one link (i.e., articulation) in the system requires a compensatory change in function of the other links. Mazur[24] and Buck et al.[4] have demonstrated that loss of motion in the ankle joint results in compensatory motion in the ipsilateral knee and contralateral ankle. These altered motion patterns undoubtedly also mandate altered load configurations through these joints. The person with purely monoarticular ankle joint disease, such as posttraumatic degenerative disease, may be able to tolerate these compensatory joint mechanisms with negligible effect, whereas the rheumatoid patient, with disease of all other joints, cannot. Therefore, the treating physician must bear in mind the effect of the diseased ankle joint on the remainder of the musculoskeletal system, as well as the effects of a proposed treatment plan.

On the basis of a large clinical experience with

Table 128-1. Results of Total Ankle Replacement According to Diagnostic Category

Diagnosis	Clinical Results (No. of Ankles)			
	Good	Fair	Poor	Total
Posttraumatic degenerative disease				59
Under 60 years of age	23	11	8	
Over 60 years of age	13	4	0	
Rheumatoid arthritis	38	1	4	43
				102

rheumatoid treatment in Sweden, Tillman[38] found that 60 percent of all rheumatoid patients have clinically obvious involvement of the ankle joint. Between 20 and 30 percent of all rheumatoid surgery involves the hindfoot and ankle. Although a number of different foot configurations may be encountered, a pes planovalgus deformity is by far the most common (87 percent in Tillman's series[38]). The typical valgus, pronated foot results from both altered dynamic and static loading of the rheumatoid foot and static loading of the rheumatoid foot and loss of constraint systems. The hindfoot collapses into valgus because of altered inertial forces due to gait aberrations and an increased valgus movement acting across the ankle joint (due to valgus deformity of diseased knee joints and a widened gait base). Loss of active muscular constraint on the hind- and midfoot results from tenosynovitis of the posterior tibial and peroneal tendons. Passive ligamentous constraint is lost due to degradation of articular cartilage, direct rheumatoid involvement of connective tissues (with resulting change in rheologic properties), and distention and stretching due to synovial hyperplasia and joint effusions. Degenerative joint disease then becomes superimposed on the inflammatory changes.

Rheumatoid involvement and deformity of the ankle joint tend to occur late in the disease process and generally follow involvement of the tarsal joints. It is often clinically difficult to distinguish between a hindfoot deformity due to the ankle joint and that due to subtalar joint disease. The latter is more common. However, because of the altered extrinsic loads and the intrinsic involvement of the tibiofibular ligaments, not infrequently roentgenograms will reveal a lateral migration of the fibula, widening of the ankle mortise, and a resulting lateral tilt of the talus (Fig. 128-16). A typical clinical symptom complex of weight-bearing anterolateral pain (due to talofibular impingement or impaction) and posteromedial pain (due to stretching of the inflamed posterior tibial tendon) often results.

Treatment

Medical management with rest and anti-inflammatory drugs is the mainstay of treatment of rheumatoid arthritis. Nonsurgical treatment of the

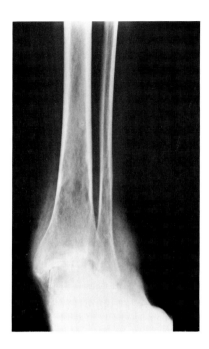

Fig. 128-16. Anteroposterior radiograph of rheumatoid ankle showing diastasis or widening of the joint mortise and lateral tilt of the talus.

rheumatoid hindfoot with various orthotic devices is commonly advised. The use of the UC-BL molded orthotic shoe insert[14] often provides gratifying relief of pain and disability. This device gives static support for the collapsed, plan-ovalgus hind- and midfoot. We also frequently advise a SACH-type insert of cushion material in the heel, with or without a 5-mm medial heel wedge and a rocker-bottom sole on the shoe (Fig. 128-15). The rocker on the sole enables the patient to roll over the foot during the mid- to late portion of stance phase of gait, reduces the amount of dorsiflexion motion required, and thereby reduces stress on both the ankle and midtarsal joints.

Because of the multiple joint involvement and because a prolonged period of cast immobilization is poorly tolerated, ankle arthrodesis for rheumatoid arthritis is ill-advised and is not described in this section.

Synovectomy

Surgical synovectomy of the rheumatoid ankle joint has not been used with the same enthusiasm in the United States as in the Scandinavian countries.

However, it does appear to be an effective treatment method in carefully selected patients. Synovectomy should be thought of as essentially a prophylactic, rather than a reconstructive, surgical procedure. The inflammatory and superimposed degenerative destruction in the joint are irreversible. Removal of the diseased synovium and pannus tissue may halt or slow the inexorable progression of rheumatoid joint destruction. However, there is a definite tendency for loss of motion and stiffness of a joint following synovectomy, and it has been demonstrated that the diseased synovium tends to regenerate in a variable period,[29,33] often to the preoperative status within 1 to 3 years. Synovectomy is no substitute for good medical management. We believe that surgical synovectomy is indicated in the rheumatoid patient with significant clinical synovitis of the ankle, when

1. Good medical management of the disease has failed and the ankle joint synovitis is relatively isolated
   AND
2. There is radiographic evidence of significant sparing of ankle joint articular cartilage.

Synovectomy is contraindicated in those patients who

1. Have not had adequate medical management or those who are experiencing a generalized florid, inflammatory stage of the disease with multiple joint synovitis
   OR
2. Have advanced destruction of the ankle joint with superimposed degenerative changes

Surgical Technique

All portions of the ankle joint are, unfortunately, not accessible by one surgical exposure. Either anteromedial or anterolateral exposures are commonly used. Some investigators have advocated a transverse skin incision directly across the anterior aspect of the ankle joint. This incision is parallel to the primary lines of skin tension, results in significant interruption of venous circulation, and endangers the small sensory cutaneous branches of the anterior tibial nerve. Generally, we find the anterolateral approach most useful. The largest accumu-

lation of hyperplastic synovial tissue tends to be at the anterolateral aspect of the joint, and this approach allows easier access to the talofibular and tibiofibular joints. We use a slightly oblique skin incision (Fig. 128-6). The retinaculum is divided vertically between the peroneus tertius tendon laterally and the long toe extensor tendons medially. The joint capsule is entered in the same plane and hyperplastic synovium is sharply excised from the anterior capsule, dissecting as far medially as possible. Synovial tissue and rheumatoid granulation tissue are removed with rongeur and curette from the articular surfaces of the tibiotalar, talofibular, and recess of the tibiofibular joint. Plantarflexion of the ankle facilitates this. The very real danger of delayed wound healing and slough of the atrophic rheumatoid skin demands careful skin retraction and soft tissue handling.

Postoperative Care

A Robert Jones compression dressing with a stirrup plaster splint is applied. The foot is elevated in bed for 4 days. Then the patient is gradually mobilized on crutches with touch weight bearing. The compression dressing is replaced by an Ace bandage at 7 days and gentle, active range-of-motion exercises are instituted, with emphasis on regaining dorsiflexion motion. Skin sutures are generally not removed until 14 days postoperatively and full weight bearing is allowed by 6 weeks.

Total Ankle Joint Replacement

Prosthetic replacement of the ankle joint has been advocated and developed as a means of alleviating pain, as well as preserving joint motion, particularly in patients with concomitant disease of the joints proximal and distal to the tibiotalar joint, in whom arthrodesis appears ill-advised. Clinical experience with total ankle prostheses has been gathered over the past 13 years. Investigators have developed a number of different types of prostheses varying in configuration from congruent- to noncongruent-bearing surfaces, and in mechanical properties from constrained to totally unconstrained. All types currently in use have some advantages and some definite shortcomings. Total ankle replacement as a generic category of devices must still be considered in the developmental stage.

Our experience in development and clinical trial has been with a totally constrained total ankle prosthesis (Fig. 128-17). This prosthesis, consisting of a concave polyethylene tibial component and a convex Vitallium talar component, has a weight-bearing surface with a radius of curvature of 2.1 cm and a surface weight-bearing area of 13 cm². Both values are consistent with those of the normal ankle joint. The arc described by the articulating surfaces allows a theoretical range of motion of 30 degrees (adequate for the 24 to 27 degrees of flexion-extension normally used for level walking, but less than adequate to allow the 56 degrees normally used for descending stairs.[9,35]

The totally congruent, totally constrained design of this prosthesis permits resistance to impact torsional forces very near that of the normal, unaltered ankle joint.[23,37] This confers less risk of malleolar fracture or ankle ligament injury than might occur with other, less constrained, devices. How-

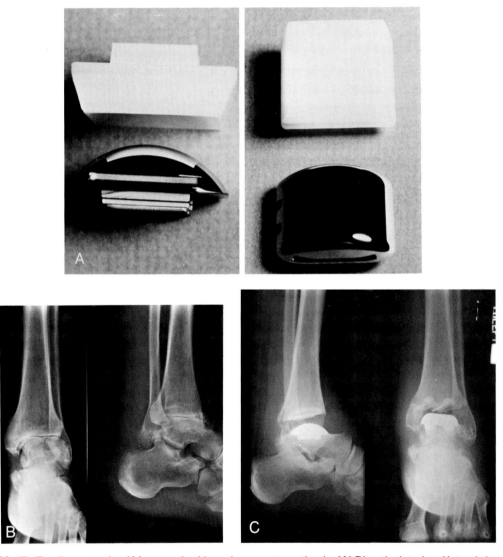

Fig. 128-17. Totally constrained Mayo total ankle replacement prosthesis. **(A)** Disarticulated and lateral views of prosthetic components. **(B)** Preoperative radiographs. **(C)** Postoperative radiographs.

ever, the design constraint also means that much more repetitive torsional stress is transferred to the bone-prosthesis interface and might result in an increased incidence of prosthetic component loosening. To date, we have confirmed definite prosthesis loosening in 7 percent of cases.[38] This represents a minimum incidence, and we suspect that many patients, particularly youthful, active individuals with posttraumatic degenerative disease who have only fair, or poor, pain relief, may have prosthetic loosening. Modifications of the prosthesis are under consideration. A semiconstrained design seems ideal. This has been accomplished in the past by using a talar component with a somewhat smaller radius of curvature than the convex tibial component. However, this results in a markedly reduced weight-bearing area and may lead to gently increased deformation and/or wear of the polyethylene component. We have plotted the axial load across the ankle against motion during stance phase of gait (Fig. 128-18). Maximum compression load (of greater than five times body weight) occurs between about 60 and 90 percent of stance phase, during which the ankle is in maxi-

mum dorsiflexion. Therefore, if the talar component is constructed with maximum width anteriorly and tapered posteriorly, maximum surface area is preserved where needed for distributing maximum load. However, some "slop" or rotation is allowed in neutral and plantarflexed position to relieve torque transmitted to the prosthesis-bone interface. This posterior tapering is also precisely the shape of the anatomic talar dome.

One of the chief complications, or identifiable reasons for continued pain, has been persistent bony impingement, most commonly at the talofibular joint. This joint bears about one-sixth of the total axial load across the ankle,[19] and is not altered by the design of this prosthesis. Continued anterolateral ankle pain has required reoperation to excise this talofibular impingement in several cases.

On the basis of clinical follow-up studies (Table 128-1), we recommend the following indications for total ankle arthroplasty:

1. Rheumatoid arthritis
2. Posttraumatic degenerative ankle joint disease in elderly (over 65 years) persons

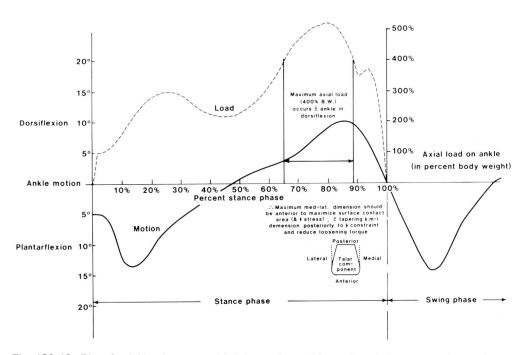

Fig. 128-18. Plot of axial load across ankle joint against ankle motion, during stance phase of gait.

Contraindications include the following:

1. Active or recent ankle joint sepsis
2. Neurologic disease with muscular imbalance across the ankle joint
3. Charcot's arthropathy
4. Posttraumatic degenerative disease in relatively youthful, active persons

Surgical Technique

A slightly curved anterior skin incision is used and the extensor retinaculum divided between the anterior tibial tendon medially and the extensor hallucis longus tendon laterally (see Fig. 128-10). The capsule synovium and tibial periosteum are incised vertically and subperiosteal dissection is carried out both medially and laterally over the malleoli. Self-retaining retractors are then inserted behind the malleoli. Careful skin retraction is mandatory.

The amount of tibial and talar bone to be removed is determined by using a spacer block of the same width and thickness as the articulated prosthetic components (Fig. 128-19A). After marking, a transverse saw cut is made with a reciprocating saw in the distal tibia. This cut must be made perpendicular to the long axis of the tibia in both sagittal and coronal planes. The articular surface of the medial malleolus is removed by a vertical saw cut. Care must be taken to avoid removing too much bone from the isthmus of the medial malleolus, to avoid a fracture. A screw may be placed in the medial malleolus. However, this is generally unnecessary if the proper sized prosthesis is chosen and care is taken in cutting and resecting the minimum amount of bone necessary.

At this point the talus is positioned in exactly neutral position for flexion-extension and varus-valgus, the spacer block is used to mark the talus, and a cut is made across the talar dome precisely parallel to the tibial cut (Fig. 128-19B). The spacer block should then be inserted easily into the ankle joint and the position of the hindfoot checked with the spacer in place.

The trial prosthetic components without anchoring fins are then inserted (Fig. 128-19C). The components are shifted anteriorly and posteriorly while the ankle is flexed and extended to find the proper location (center of rotation), where ankle motion is smooth and there is no hinging open of the components. This anteroposterior position is then marked for future reference. The prosthetic components should not contact the articular surface of the fibula because of the relative motion (rotation) that occurs between tibia and fibula.

These trial components are removed, and slots are prepared in the tibial and talar surfaces with a double-bladed rasp (Fig. 128-19D). In the presence of hard, sclerotic bone a saw may occasionally be needed to complete cutting of the slots, once they are marked by the rasp.

The actual prosthetic components are then inserted for a trial fit (Fig. 128-19E). Position and motion are checked. At this point, it is critically important to excise any impinging osteophytes from the remaining talofibular joint laterally. This can be accomplished using a thin osteotome. The anterior talofibular ligament must be preserved. The bony surfaces are then thoroughly cleaned with a Water-Pik using sterile saline solution, the prosthetic components are cemented in place separately (tibial component first), using "one-half batch" of polymethylmethacrylate for each component. Only a very small amount of polymethylmethacrylate is used to avoid extrusion of cement posteriorly. Should this occur, a separate posterior medial incision may be necessary to remove the cement. Even a small amount of cement extruded posteriorly could cause mechanical irritation of the extensor tendons and neurovascular structures, as well as a mechanical block to plantar flexion of the ankle.

The thigh tourniquet is then released, hemostatis accomplished, and the wound closed in layers (with at least a portion of the extensor retinaculum repaired) over one medium suction drain. A modified, short-leg, Robert Jones compression dressing with a stirrup plaster splint is applied.

Postoperative Care

Broad-spectrum antibiotic coverage is started the evening before surgery and continued intraoperatively and for 48 hours postoperatively. The suction drain is removed 24 hours following surgery. The leg is continuously elevated in bed for 48 hours and then the patient is allowed up in a chair for brief periods. At 5 days postoperatively the

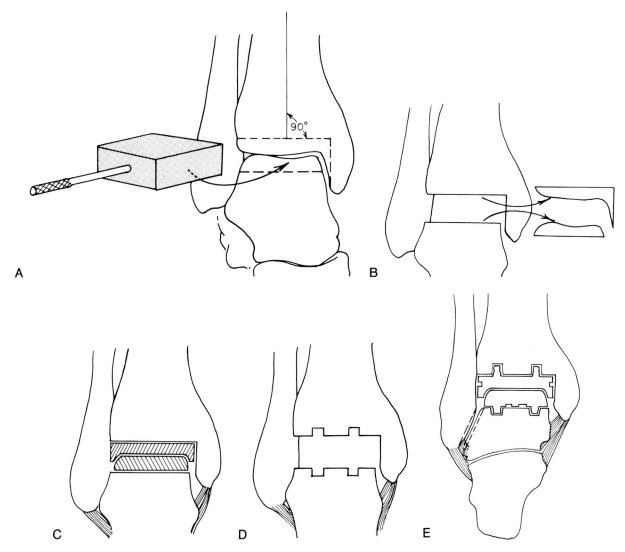

Fig. 128-19. Technique for Mayo total ankle arthroplasty. **(A)** Use of spacer block to mark bone to be resected from tibial and talar surfaces. **(B)** Bone resected from tibia and talus. Remaining bony surfaces must be exactly parallel when ankle is in neutral position in both sagittal and coronal planes. **(C)** Trial components (without anchoring fins) in place. **(D)** Slots cut in tibial and talar surfaces. **(E)** Trial insertion of prosthetic components. Impinging bone of talofibular joint is excised.

Robert Jones dressing is removed and replaced by an Ace bandage. The patient is encouraged to begin gentle active range-of-motion ankle exercises with emphasis on gaining dorsiflexion. On the sixth postoperative day the patient is started on gait training with crutches and "touch only" weight bearing on the operated extremity. The sutures are removed on the twelfth to fourteenth postopera-

tive day, and the patient is discharged from the hospital as soon as comfortable, independent ambulation is achieved (generally by the fourteenth postoperative day).

Patients return for outpatient evaluation 8 weeks after surgery. Anteroposterior and lateral ankle radiographs are evaluated and graduated weight bearing with a cane is usually advised.

REFERENCES

1. Alexander AH, Lichtman DM: Surgical treatment of transchondral talar-dome fractures (osteochondritis dissecans). J Bone Joint Surg 62A:646, 1980
2. Assenmacher DB, Stauffer RN: Long-term results of ankle arthrodesis. Paper presented at AMA Meeting, New York, 1973
3. Berndt AL, Harty M: Transchondral fractures (osteochondritis dissecans) of the talus. J Bone Joint Surg 41A:988, 1959
4. Buck PG, Stauffer RN, Laughman RK, et al: Influence of position of ankle and knee motion. Trans Orthop Res Soc 7:129, 1982
5. Canale TS, Belding RH: Osteochondral lesions of the talus. J Bone Joint Surg 62A:97, 1980
6. Chuinard EG, Peterson RE: Distraction-compression bone graft arthrodesis of the ankle. A method especially applicable in children. J Bone Joint Surg 45A:481, 1963
7. Davis MW: Bilateral talar osteochondritis dissecans with lax ligaments. Report of a case. J Bone Joint Surg 52A:168, 1970
8. Demottaz JD, Mazur JM, Thomas WH, et al: Clinical study of total ankle replacement with gait analysis. A preliminary report. J Bone Joint Surg 61A:976, 1979
9. Fitzgerald E, Chao EY, Hoffman RR: Goniometric measurement of ankle motion — A method for clinical evaluation. Trans 23rd Orthop Res Soc 2:43, 1977
10. Garraway WM, Stauffer RN, Kurland LT, et al: Limb fractures in a defined population. I. Frequency and distribution. Mayo Clin Proc 54:701, 1979
11. Groth FE, Shen GS, Fagan PJ: The Oregon ankle: A total ankle designed to replace all three articular surfaces. Orthop Trans 1:86, 1977 (abst)
12. Horowitz T: The use of the transfibular approach in arthrodesis of the ankle joint. Am J Surg 55:550, 1942
13. Huckel JR, Fuller J: Arthrodesis of the ankle. p. 156. In Bateman JE (ed): Foot Science (American Orthopedic Foot Society). WB Saunders, Philadelphia, 1976
14. Inman VT: UC-BL shoe insert: Biomechanical considerations. Bull Prosthet Res 10:130, 1969
15. Jackson A: Tarsal hypermobility after ankle fusion — fact or fiction? J Bone Joint Surg 61B:470, 1979
16. Johnson EW Jr, Boseker EH: Arthrodesis of the ankle. Arch Surg 97:766, 1968
17. Kappis M: Weitere Beiträge zur traumatisch-mechanischen Entstebung der "spontanen" Knorpelabloösungen (sogen. Osteochondritis, Dissecans). Dtsch Z Chir 171:13, 1922
18. Koenig: Uber freie Köyser in den Gelenken. Dtsch Z Chir 27:90, 1888
19. Lambert, JL: The weight-bearing function of the fibula: a strain-gauge study. J Bone Joint Surg 53A:507, 1971
20. Lance EM, Pauel A, Patterson R Jr, et al: Arthrodesis of the ankle: a follow-up study. J Bone Joint Surg 53A:1030, 1971 (abst)
21. Lindholm TS, Osterman K, Vankka E: Osteochondritis Dissecans of elbow, ankle and hip. Clin Orthop 148:245, 1980
22. Lipscomb PR: Ghormley RK: Old and new fractures and fracture-dislocations of the astrogalus. Surg Clin North Am 23:995, 1943
23. Matejczyk MB, Greenwald AS, Block JD: Ankle implant systems: laboratory evaluation and clinical correlation. Trans 25th Orthop Res Soc 4:114, 1979
24. Mazur JM, Schwartz E, Simon SR: Ankle arthrodesis: long-term follow-up with gait analysis. J Bone Joint Surg 61A:964, 1979
25. McCullough CJ, Venugopal V: Osteochondritis dissecans of the talus. Clin Orthop 144:264, 1979
26. Morrey BF, Weideman GP: Complications and long-term results of ankle arthrodesis following trauma. J Bone Joint Surg 62A:777, 1980
27. Morris HD, Herrick RT: Ankle arthrodesis. p. 136. In Bateman JE (ed): Foot Science (American Orthopedic Foot Society). WB Saunders, Philadelphia, 1976
28. O'Donohue DH: Impingement exostoses of the talus and tibia. J Bone Joint Surg 39A:835, 1957
29. Patzakis MJ, Mills DM, Bartholomew BH, et al: A visual, histological and enzymatic study of regenerative rheumatoid synovium in the synovectomized knee. J Bone Joint Surg 55A:287, 1973
30. Pettine KA, Morrey BF: Osteochondial fractures of the talus: a long-term follow-up. J Bone Joint Surg 69B:89, 1987
31. Ramsey PL, Hamilton W: Changes in tibiotalar area of contact caused by lateral talar shift. J Bone Surg 58A:356, 1976
32. Ranawat CS, Straub LR, Fryberg R, et al: A study of regenerating synovium after synovectomy of the knee in rheumatoid arthritis. Arthritis Rheum 14:117, 1971
33. Roden S, Tillegard P, Unander-Sharin L: Osteochondritis dissecans and similar lesions of the talus. Acta Orthop Scand 23:51, 1953

34. Samuelson KM, Tuke MA, Freeman MAR: A replacement arthroplasty for the three articular surfaces of the ankle utilizing a posterior approach. J Bone Joint Surg 59B:376, 1977

35. Stauffer RN, Chao EYS: Torsional stability of Mayo Total Ankle Arthroplasty. Trans 25th Orthop Res Soc 4:112, 1979

36. Stauffer RN, Chao EYS, Brewster RC: Force and motion analysis of the normal, diseased and prosthetic ankle joint. Clin Orthop 127:189, 1977

37. Stauffer RN, Segal NM: Total ankle arthroplasty: Four years' experience. Clin Orthop 160:217, 1981

38. Tillman K: The Rheumatoid Foot. Georg Thieme, Stuttgart, 1979

39. White AA III: A precision posterior ankle fusion. Clin Orthop 98:239, 1974

40. Wynarsky GT, Greenwald AS, Matejczyk MB: Pressure distributions across the articular cartilage surfaces of the ankle joint. Trans 24th Annual ORS, Vol. 3; p. 90, 1978

Acute Injuries to Ligaments of the Ankle

129

Robert E. Leach
Anthony A. Schepsis

Acute ligamentous injuries of the ankle are a common cause of disability. Most of these injuries occur on the lateral side of the ankle and can be treated nonsurgically.[12,15,17,21,36] While isolated lateral ligamentous injuries are common, isolated medial ligamentous injuries are uncommon. Medial ligamentous injuries are usually associated with a fracture of the distal fibula or with tibiofibular interosseous ligament tears. Total disruption of the medial and lateral ligamentous complex is rare but may occur with a subluxation or dislocation of the talus and be unrecognized because of a spontaneous reduction of the talus into the ankle mortise.

ANATOMY OF THE LATERAL SIDE

The articular capsule of the ankle joint can be divided into an anterior and posterior segment. The anterior part attaches proximally to the anterior portion of the distal tibia, superior to its articular surface and distally to the talus anterior to its articular surface. It attaches to the border of the articular surface of both malleoli. The posterior capsule, thinner than the anterior capsule, consists mostly of transverse fibers that blend with the transverse tibiofibular ligament. Distally, it attaches to the talus posterior to its superior articular facet and laterally to the depression on the medial surface of the lateral malleolus.

On the lateral side of the ankle, there are two major ligamentous groups, those that bind the talus and the calcaneus to the fibula and those that hold the tibia firmly to the fibula (Fig. 129-1). The three lateral ankle joint ligaments are (1) the anterior talofibular ligament, which is intracapsular and extends from the anterior border of the distal fibula to the lateral neck of the talus; (2) the calcaneofibular ligament, which is extracapsular and runs from the inferior aspect of the lateral malleolus to the lateral aspect of the calcaneus; and (3) the posterior talofibular ligament extending from the distal fossa of the fibula to the lateral tubercle on the posterior portion of the talus. The posterior talofibular ligament is the strongest of the three. The anterior

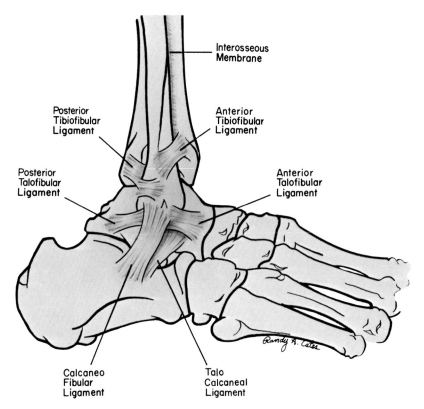

Fig. 129-1. Lateral ligamentous complex of the ankle, including the distal tibiofibular ligaments.

talofibular ligament, while broader than the others, is the weakest. One other ligament that may produce local pain but can be helpful in secondary reconstructions of the lateral ligaments is the talocalcaneal, which blends with the anterior talofibular ligament. It originates from the talus and extends to the calcaneus, attaching adjacent to the distal attachment of the calcaneofibular ligament.

The ligaments between the distal tibia and the fibula are short, strong, and less frequently torn than the ankle ligaments. Anterior and posterior inferior tibiofibular ligaments go from the anterior and posterior lips of the fibular groove on the distal tibia to the anterior and posterior aspects of the adjacent fibula. The strong inferior transverse ligament runs from the posterior aspect of the distal articular tip of the tibia to the distal fibula. The interosseous ligament, the strongest of the tibiofibular ligaments, attaches to the adjacent surfaces of the tibia and fibula, going from above the ankle joint to slightly below the fibular neck.

ANATOMY OF THE MEDIAL SIDE

The anatomy of the medial ligaments of the ankle is less complicated than that of the lateral side. The deltoid ligament (medial collateral ligament of the ankle) is a thick, strong, fan-shaped ligament with a superficial and a deep portion (Fig. 129-2). Superficially, there are four elements, which include the anterior tibiotalar, tibionavicular, tibiocalcaneal, and the posterior tibiotalar portion. These superficial fibers fan down from the medial malleolus to attach as a continuous sheath to the tarsal bones. The more important part of the ligament, the deep portion, attaches to the undersurface of the medial malleolus near its tip and runs more horizontally than the superficial fibers to attach to the medial surface of the talus. If this portion is torn and not repaired, it may lead to chronic symptoms on the medial side.

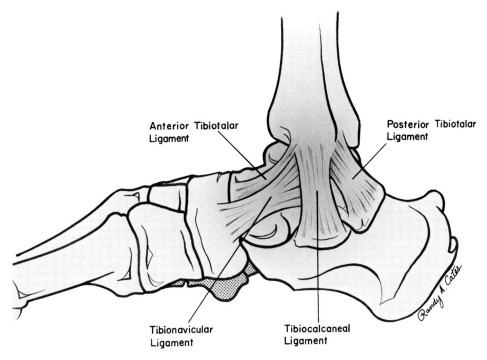

Fig. 129-2. Medial ligamentous complex of the ankle (deltoid ligament).

OPERATIVE REPAIR OF LIGAMENT INJURIES

Indications

The majority of acute lateral ligamentous injuries should be treated conservatively.[32] The usual injury will consist of a partial tear of the anterior talofibular ligament that does not require operative intervention. If there is a total disruption of the lateral ligamentous complex, including the anterior talofibular, calcaneofibular and the posterior talofibular ligaments, most authorities[3,8,16,26,44,47,51] agree that this is an indication for operative repair. Making the diagnosis presents a problem. If there is tenderness in the area of all three ligaments and if, on attempted inversion of the foot, it becomes obvious that the ankle will subluxate out of the mortise, the diagnosis is easy. In other instances, the history may indicate a momentary dislocation of the talus with a total disrup-tion of the ankle ligaments (Fig. 129-3). In such an instance, operative repair should be done.[50]

The more important diagnostic dilemma is when we believe there is a disruption of the anterior talofibular ligament and a partial or complete tear of the calcaneofibular ligament. Local tenderness over the ligaments, abnormal inversion of the ankle and foot, and an anterior drawer sign of the talus are primary physical signs of major damage (Fig. 129-4). A positive ankle arthrogram[49] demonstrates that there has been damage to the ligaments and capsule but does not indicate its extent (Fig. 129-4, 129-5). A tenogram of the peroneal tendons[2,14,54] showing extravasation of dye from the peroneal tendon sheath indicates a tear of the calcaneofibular ligament. Authorities agree that when this tear occurs, the anterior talofibular ligament has already been disrupted. Stress roentgenograms are difficult to obtain in the usual emergency room setting with local anesthesia. With good relaxation, if stress films show a tilt of 10 degrees more on the injured side than on the uninjured side, operative repair of the ligaments should be considered. A

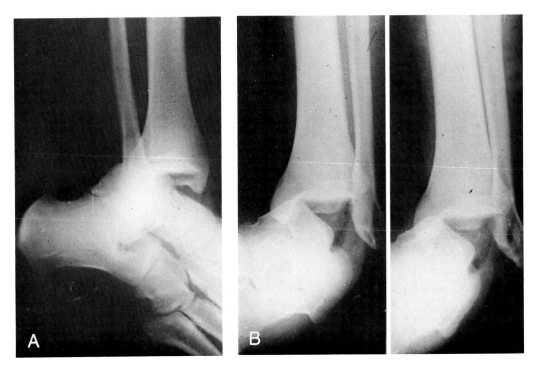

Fig. 129-3. (A) Lateral ankle radiograph showing posterior dislocation of the talus, which demonstrates total disruption of the ankle ligaments and capsule. **(B)** Anteroposterior radiograph of the same ankle showing total disruption of the lateral ligaments.

talar osteochondral fracture demonstrated on roentgenograms is another reason for operative intervention (Fig. 129-6).

Bröstrom[5a-5e] in his classic works, stated that the best results in patients with torn anterior talofibular and calcaneofibular ligaments were those repaired operatively. However, he further states that because there are so many of these ankle injuries, he would restrict his primary repairs to the young, athletic person who requires a perfect ankle. We thus have the dual dilemma of making the diagnosis that two ligaments are torn and deciding if, in that particular person, operative repair is indicated. We agree with Bröstrom[5a-5e] that operative repair of the lateral ligaments of the ankle should be restricted to very athletic people who require an excellent ankle and in whom we are sure that both the anterior talofibular and calcaneofibular ligaments are torn. A positive anterior drawer sign and an osteochondral fracture are further reasons for operative intervention.

Contraindications

Major contraindications to open repair of ankle ligaments would include vascular insufficiency and an open wound that could not be adequately cleansed. Generally, severe open wounds occurring with ankle ligamentous injuries are rare. Most patients in whom one would consider surgery are young and are not likely to have vascular insufficiency or local skin problems. Thus, the major contraindication is if the treating surgeon believes that operative intervention is not the best treatment for that particular patient and injury.

Other Treatment Options

Several options must be considered in determining the treatment of acute ligamentous injuries of the ankle. The first option is the choice between operative and nonoperative management, particu-

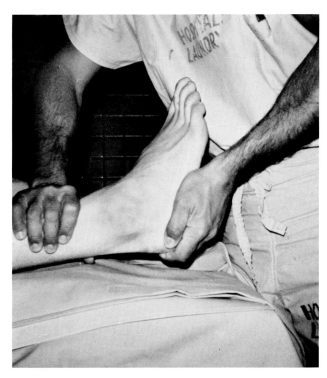

Fig. 129-4. Clinical examination demonstrating an anterior drawer test. The ankle is in slight plantar flexion to unlock the anterior talar dome.

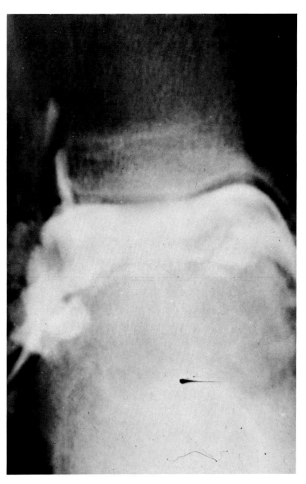

Fig. 129-5. Arthrogram of the ankle with extravasation of the contrast material laterally, indicating a tear of the lateral ligaments and capsule.

larly when dealing with double ligamentous tears. Several basic nonoperative treatment plans can be employed. The ankle can be immobilized 3 to 6 weeks until partial or full healing of the ligaments has occurred, after which the rehabilitation process begins. Another option is to cast the ankle for 7 to 10 days to relieve pain and then to begin mobilization with protection while recognizing the soft tissue healing has not yet occurred. Protection is then provided with some type of strapping or bracing to permit dorsiflexion and plantar flexion but prevent any inversion or rotational force that would stress the healing ligaments. This allows the patient to become ambulatory and begin rehabilitation earlier while still allowing for ligamentous healing. This concept of protected mobilization can also be employed without using a cast. In such cases, either a splint, brace, or adhesive strapping is used, which can be removed to apply ice; early range-of-motion and very light resistive exercises can then be started. The patient uses crutches dur-

ing the early protective weight-bearing period, a compression bandage, elevation, and intermittent icing, until swelling is under control. This is followed by mobilization with adequate protection for the next 7 to 14 days. This method has proved very effective, particularly in treating young athletes who have access to continued care.

The decision as to whether to operate on patients with severe ligamentous injuries is controversial. Several recent prospective and retrospective studies have studied comparable groups of patients treated with surgical repair and casting versus cast immobilization alone.[12,15,24,26,36,54] Most of these studies indicate that there is no significant benefit

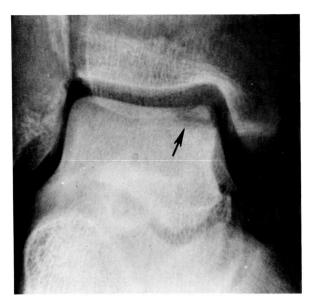

Fig. 129-6. Late osteochondral fracture of the lateral talar dome. This may be an indication for operative intervention.

for surgical management over the nonsurgical management. However, most of these series include patients with only single ligament tears. Bröstrom's[5a-5e] earlier study indicates that surgical repair would give the very best results in a young athlete. We do not have comparable studies for surgery versus early protective mobilization.

Acute Operative Repair of the Lateral Ligaments

If the decision has been made to operate on acutely injured ligaments, the concept is simple. We want to suture the disrupted structures which usually include the anterior capsule, anterior talofibular ligament, calcaneofibular ligament, and sometimes the posterior talofibular ligament. This latter structure is difficult to reach and may not be possible to suture.

The skin incision is started on the lateral aspect of

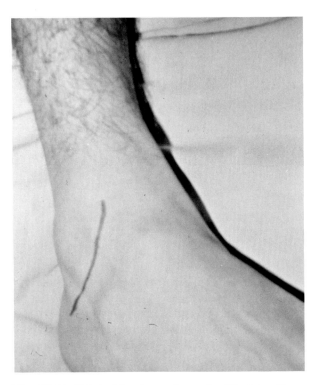

Fig. 129-7. Skin incision for acute repair of the lateral ligaments.

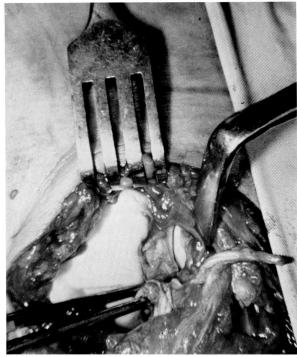

Fig. 129-8. Intraoperative photograph of acutely torn anterior talofibular ligament. The forceps are holding the portion of the ligament attached to the fibula. Note the capsular disruption.

the ankle joint above the tibial plafond curving distally and laterally past the tip of the distal fibula (Fig. 129-7). This allows easy access to the anterior talofibular and calcaneofibular ligaments. In the subcutaneous dissection, on must be careful to look for lateral branches of the superficial peroneal nerve and, distally, the sural nerve. Because of soft tissue hemorrhage, it may be difficult to identify the fibers of the anterior capsule and the anterior talofibular ligament which is intracapsular. We have seen injuries so severe that the peroneus tertius muscle was avulsed on the lower tibia and, with resultant edema and hemorrhage, was difficult to identify. The anterior talofibular ligament is usually torn in its middle or close to the fibular attachment (Fig. 129-8). Once the ankle joint is opened, it is inspected and lavaged, and a search is made for any osteochondral fragments or articular damage (Fig. 129-9). To view the calcaneofibular ligament, the peroneal tendon sheath must be opened and the tendons dislocated. With forced inversion, we can usually see the torn or intact posterior talofibu-

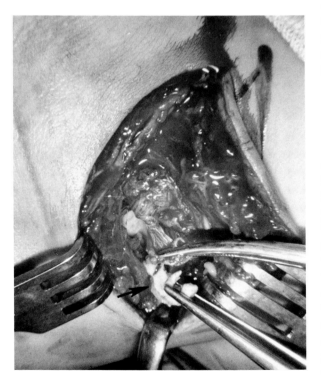

Fig. 129-9. Intraoperative photograph of acute tear of lateral ligaments with loose osteochondral fragment *(arrow)*.

lar ligament. We find it difficult to repair this short, strong ligament. However, if the other two ligaments are anatomically repaired, this posterior ligament seems to heal when the ends are in proximity or perhaps the other two ligaments are strong enough to effect ankle stability.

We repair the anterior capsule, anterior talofibular ligament, and calcaneofibular ligament with nonabsorbable sutures. Because of severe tearing of these ligaments, it may be difficult to put in more than approximating sutures, but if the ligaments are kept in close proximity, they heal well. In the few instances of severe disruption of the anterior talofibular ligament with little left to suture, one may dissect the talocalcaneal ligament off the calcaneus and use it to reinforce the anterior repair. If the anterior talofibular ligament has pulled a small bony fragment off the fibula, excise that fragment and attach the ligament to soft tissues on the fibula.

After sutures are placed, they are tied with the foot in slight eversion and neutral dorsiflexion. When a tear of the medial ligaments is being repaired, these sutures should be placed and the medial and lateral sutures tied together. Following this, the peroneal tendons are replaced and that sheath closed. A subcutaneous type closure is accomplished, and we use either a subcuticular or running skin sutures.

Postoperative Care

We apply a short-leg cast with the foot in neutral dorsiflexion and slight eversion. Because of soft-tissue swelling, this cast may have to be bivalved in the first 24 hours, in which case a new cast is applied 2 days after surgery. The extremity is elevated for at least 24 hours and then the patient is allowed to begin gradual ambulation without weight bearing. We do not allow weight bearing for the first 2 weeks, but then apply a cast boot and encourage partial weight bearing with crutches for the next 4 weeks. The cast is removed 6 weeks after surgery and the patient starts a program of active and active-assistive plantar flexion and dorsiflexion, but no inversion or eversion is allowed for another 2 weeks. Swelling may be a problem, and we recommend compression of the limb and intermittent elevation while allowing partial weight bearing with crutches. Eight weeks after surgery, the patient begins active inversion and eversion and goes on to more vigorous exercises, including stretching of the posterior ankle structures. At 10 weeks, the patient does resistive exercises for all muscle units of the lower leg, and the program is then individualized depending on the patient's progress. We try to restore proprioceptive sense[19] to the ankle by having patients do various types of agility drills germane to the particular sporting activity they do. Once the patient walks without a limp, we allow the patient to jog and then to go on to running and finally to cutting. Once that is accomplished, the patient is allowed to return to full sporting activities. We generally protect the ankle with some type of strapping during the first full season after an acute injury.

ACUTE MEDIAL LIGAMENTOUS INJURIES

Most deltoid ligament injuries occur in conjunction with a fracture of the distal fibula (Fig. 129-10), a tearing of the tibiofibular ligament, or a total disruption of the ankle ligaments. In this section, we do not discuss deltoid ligament tears associated with fibular fractures but discuss disruption of the medial ankle ligaments occurring with severe lateral ankle ligamentous injuries and that occurring, rarely, as an isolated injury. In examining a patient with a deltoid ligament injury one must be sure that there is no fibular fracture proximally (Fig. 129-11) or distally or damage to the tibiofibu-

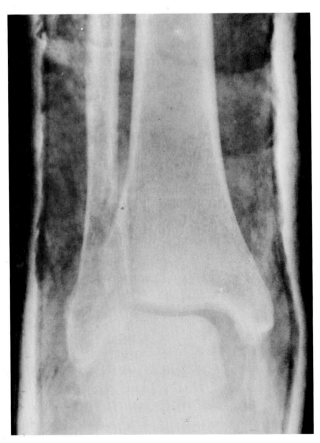

Fig. 129-10. Spiral oblique fracture of the distal fibula associated with lateral talar subluxation, denoting tear of the deltoid ligament.

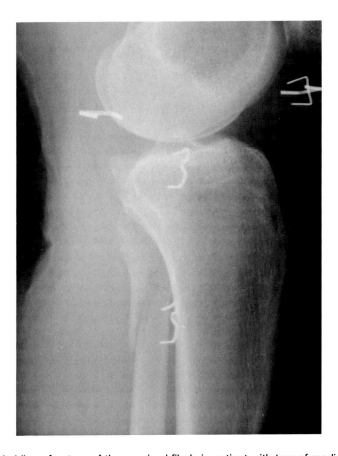

Fig. 129-11. Spiral oblique fracture of the proximal fibula in patient with tear of medial ankle ligaments.

lar ligaments. If a mortise view of the ankle shows any lateral subluxation, operative intervention for the deltoid injury and other associated injuries should be considered.

Indications

Acute repair of deltoid ligament injuries would be indicated for instances of total disruption of the medial and lateral ankle ligaments or when there is obvious lateral talar subluxation as well as deltoid ligament injury. The major question concerning treatment is whether we can expect a better long-term result from operative repair or nonoperative treatment. The decision as to whether to operate on the deltoid ligament is sometimes less difficult because the injury is so often associated with major lateral ligamentous tears or fibular fractures and

the actual operative intervention on the medial side is comparatively easy.

Operative Repair

To repair the deltoid ligament acutely, the incision is started above and lateral to the medial malleolus curving distally and medially. The long saphenous vein must be protected. The superficial fibers of the deltoid ligament spread out in a fan shape from the medial malleolus to the talus, navicular, and os calcis. The deep fibers are more posterior and on the undersurface of the medial malleolus and extend to the talus. The superficial portion of the deltoid is identified and incised to find the deep fibers. Once all portions of the deltoid ligament have been seen, the joint itself is inspected.

The deep fibers can be repaired by end-to-end repair with a strong absorbable suture. With the superficial portion, it may be difficult to do more than approximate it with interrupted mattress sutures. If the ligament is torn from the bone, it is reattached to soft tissue remnants or through drill holes in the medial malleolus. While the sutures are being tied it must be ascertained that the talus has been replaced near the medial malleolus and that there is no residual lateral subluxation. The sutures may then be tied and closure accomplished in the usual manner. The postoperative course for tears of the medial ligaments would be same as for repairs of the lateral ligaments.

Complications

Complications of acute repairs of the lateral and medial ligaments of the ankle are relatively uncommon. Infection may occur but is rare. Skin sloughs may happen particularly on the lateral side if the incision is carried inferiorly and posteriorly. Sloughs usually will heal, but one should be careful to identify all potential bleeders during the dissection to stop any posttourniquet hemorrhage and subsequent increased postoperative swelling. The sural nerve may cross the operative field, particularly at the lower part of the lateral incision and can be inadvertently lacerated, caught in a suture, or compressed by a cast. Postoperative swelling and, occasionally, thrombophlebitis may be seen and in several patients we have seen a sympathetic dystrophy. This is more common if the patient does not begin weight bearing in the cast. We encourage full weight bearing at 2 weeks. The resultant dystrophic complications may be catastrophic in the occasional patient and early weight bearing and aggressive rehabilitation after cast removal are essential.

Results

The results of acute repair of lateral ligaments of the ankle are quite good. Most patients will have a stable ankle with dorsiflexion ranging from 10 to 20 degrees above neutral and normal plantar flexion. In some, there may be slight excessive inversion. Most people are able to return to a full athletic

life. However, it takes about 6 months for the ligaments to be normal and we believe that the ankle should be protected with some external strapping method during the first athletic season.

TREATMENT OF TIBIOFIBULAR LIGAMENTOUS INJURIES

Damage to the tibiofibular ligamentous complex usually occurs as a result of external rotation to the foot or ankle, commonly with the foot in the supi-

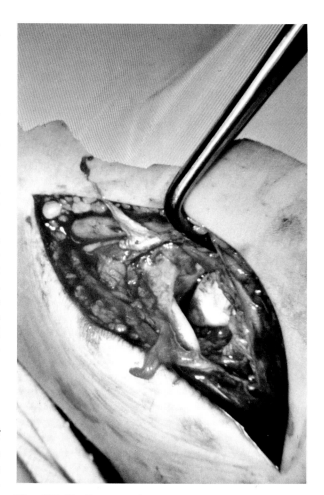

Fig. 129-12. Rupture of medial deltoid ligament with increased clear space between talus and medial malleolus.

nated position. With the exception of a Tillaux fracture, when the anterior inferior tibiofibular ligament avulses a fragment from the tibia, most injuries to the tibiofibular ligaments can be treated nonoperatively. However, this injury combined with a medial ligamentous (Figs. 129-12, 129-13) or bony injury that produces a lateral subluxation of the talus will require surgery. This necessitates a repair of the medial structures and the use of one or two screws going from the fibula to the tibia, to reduce and maintain the tibiofibular syndesmosis (Fig. 129-14).

We treat the usual instance of damage to the tibiofibular ligament with minimal or no medial ligamentous injury nonoperatively. Sometimes a partial tear of the anterior inferior tibiofibular liga-

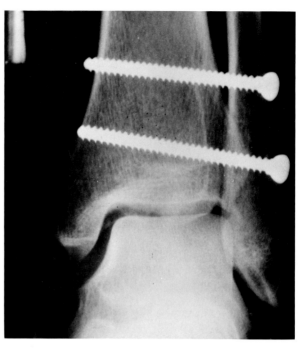

Fig. 129-14. Diastasis of the distal tibiofibular syndesmosis reduced with the screws.

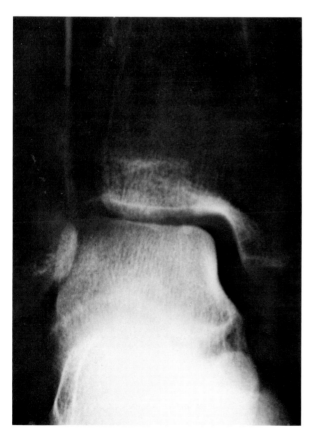

Fig. 129-13. Diastasis of the distal tibiofibular syndesmosis with lateral subluxation of the talus indicating tear of the deltoid ligament as well as the tibiofibular ligamentous complex.

ment is seen in association with lateral ligament injuries; the rehabilitation period is slightly prolonged in these patients. Tenderness is noted in the tissues between the distal tibia and fibula, and external rotation of the ankle causes pain in the region of the tibiofibular ligaments. When associated with a medial injury and there is a question of the severity of the injury to the syndesmosis, a stress radiograph with the foot in abduction and external rotation may be helpful in deciding between a surgical and nonsurgical approach. Bone scanning[35] was recently reported to be helpful in diagnosing acute ligamentous diastasis.

In most situations, we apply a compression dressing to the patient's foot and ankle, which permits slight dorsiflexion and plantar flexion but no inversion or eversion. This program is similar to our conservative treatment of acute lateral ligament injuries. In our experience, the pain felt by patients with tears of the tibiofibular ligaments has been greater than one would expect on the basis of the physical findings, such as swelling or local ecchymosis. Accordingly, patients bear partial weight with crutches and ankle support for a longer time than they would for the usual lateral ligamentous injuries. Foot dorsiflexion usually requires a longer period of time to return to these cases. Patients should not be allowed to return to active athletics until local tenderness has completely disappeared, which may take 6 weeks or more. If there is an associated medial injury, but no lateral subluxation on radiography plus a negative stress radiograph, cast immobilization may be considered, as long as one has not missed a total disruption of a medial ligamentous complex or a medial malleolus fracture, which could cause lateral subluxation of the talus; the recovery from injury to the tibiofibular ligamentous complex should be complete.

CHRONIC LATERAL INSTABILITY

Considering the number of people who have acute injuries of the lateral ligaments of the ankle, the number of patients who complain of late chronic lateral instability is relatively insignificant.[18] However, as our population becomes increasingly more active and particularly as people continue to enjoy long-term athletic endeavors, we are seeing more patients who complain of chronic lateral instability.[46] In contrast with chronic instability of the knee, which responds only moderately well to secondary surgical procedures, chronic lateral ankle instability responds surprisingly well to operative procedures.

Indications

Most patients with chronic lateral instability will complain that their ankle gives out or rolls over or that they have recurrent pain on the lateral side after athletic activities. If, on physical examination, such a person has a positive anterior drawer sign and increased inversion (Fig. 129-15) compared with the normal ankle or to what the examiner interprets as being normal, he is a potential candidate for secondary reconstruction of the lateral liga-

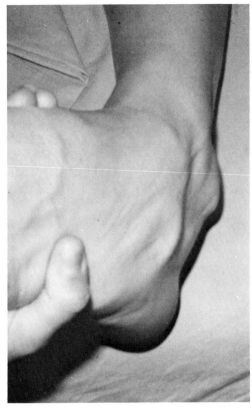

Fig. 129-15. Patient with chronic lateral ligament instability demonstrating abnormal inversion.

ments.[1] The anterior drawer sign is an indication that the anterior talofibular ligament is lax,[33] whereas abnormal inversion shows laxity of the anterior talofibular and the calcaneofibular ligaments and possibly of the subtalar joint.[4] Although one can usually decide whether a patient needs surgery based on the history and the physical examination, stress radiographs showing the degree of talar tilt in the ankle mortise can be very helpful. There is some disagreement as to how much talar tilt is abnormal but most authorities agree that 10 degrees more (Figs. 129-16, 129-17) on the symptomatic side compared with the asymptomatic is significant.[9,10,29,30,43] Stress radiographs can also be done in the lateral position to view the antero posterior drawer sign (Fig. 129-18).[33] Arthrograms of the ankle are less helpful in chronic instability than in acute injuries to the ankle.[49]

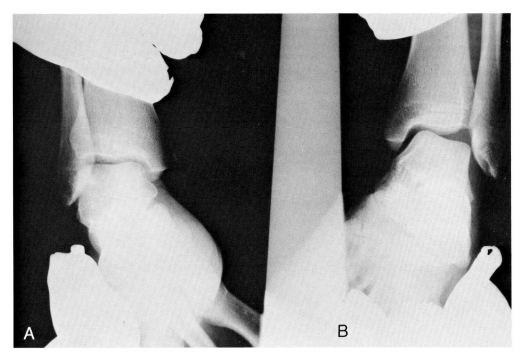

Fig. 129-16. Stress radiographs demonstrating **(A)** normal talar tilt of the uninjured right ankle compared with **(B)** abnormally increased talar tilt of the left (symptomatic) ankle.

Contraindications

Few older people need secondary ankle surgery; thus, there would be relatively few patients with major circulation problems. Some young diabetics could have ankle problems, and one must evaluate the skin-healing potential since lateral incisions below the fibula are apt to heal slowly, even in patients with normal vascular supply. Should secondary ligamentous reconstruction be performed in people who have chronic degenerative disease of the ankle thought to be secondary to ligamentous laxity? Studies by Harrington[22] appear to show that secondary repair of the ankle ligaments can help to stabilize the degenerative changes and secondary surgery is worthwhile. Thus, there are few contraindications to secondary surgery.

Conservative Treatment

Several measures can be taken to improve the functional capacity in patients with chronic ankle instability, although they are often of limited effec-

tiveness. Ankle-taping techniques for athletic activities that involve pivoting or jumping have some effectiveness in restricting abnormal tibiotalar and subtalar motion. However, taping quickly loses much of its restrictive benefits as the tape loosens, which can occur as quickly as 10 minutes after application. Laced ankle braces with rigid side stays have been shown to be almost as effective as taping. High-top shoes or sneakers and lateral heel wedges can also be helpful, particularly if there are symptoms of instability with activities of daily living and walking on uneven ground.

Exercises are prescribed to increase the strength and decrease the reaction time of the surrounding musculature, particularly those muscles that dorsiflex or evert the foot. A program of isotonic or "partner" exercises with the use of flexible rubber tubing or against the manual resistance of a partner is used to strengthen the dorsiflexors, everters, and inverters of the foot. Toe raises can be used to strengthen the calf muscles. Ankle-exercising machines have some proven effectiveness in rehabilitating acute as well as chronic ankle injuries. Iso-

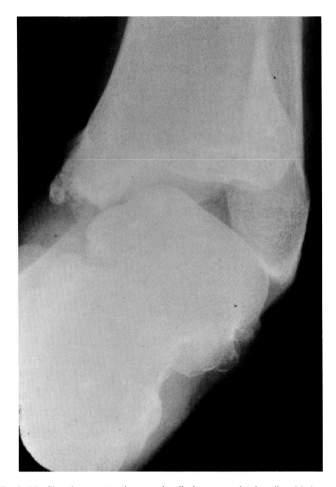

Fig. 129-17. Ankle film demonstrating markedly increased talar tilt with inversion stress.

kinetic strengthening may be helpful, particularly for dorsiflexion and plantar flexion at various speeds of resistance.

The proprioceptive and neuromuscular function of the ankle joint should also be emphasized. Improving agility and proprioceptive reaction time of the ankle, particularly the peroneals, may be helpful in avoiding some of the inversion incidents which cause pain. These helpful activities include heel and toe walking, the use of a teeter or balance board, straight and backward running, as well as running circles and figure-of-eights with taping or brace support. Since most of the problems involve athletic individuals, sport-specific agility and skill activities are also helpful. If the patient continues to have symptoms of instability, operative repair seems the only logical choice.

Operative Repair

A number of operative repairs can be performed for chronic lateral instability of the ankle, most of which have a reasonable degree of success.[6,40] St. Pierre et al[52] compared the clinical results from five difference methods of reconstruction and found that there was no statistically significant difference between them. Ninety-five percent good results were obtained with each of these procedures. The most widely used operations include the Watson-Jones,[20,23,34,42] the Evans,[13,27,28,39,53] and the Chrisman-Snook procedure.[7,8,31,41,45,49,56] The Bröstrom procedure,[5a-5e,25] more widely used in Europe, is somewhat less popular in the United States, but also has a high success rate. We have had excellent success with a modification of the Chris-

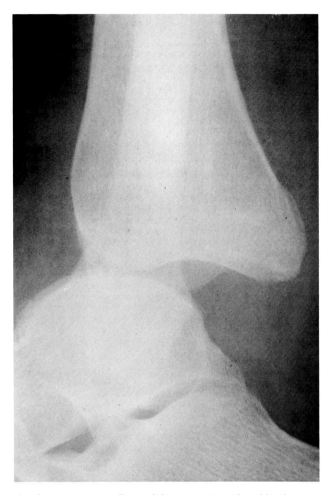

Fig. 129-18. Lateral anterior drawer stress radiograph in a symptomatic ankle, demonstrating abnormal anterior talar movement.

man-Snook reconstruction of the ankle ligaments,[31] which we describe in detail. This procedure reconstructs both the anterior talofibular and calcaneaofibular ligaments, as well as correcting any abnormal subtalar laxity, which may be a significant component of instability in these patients.

Procedure

The skin incision is started about 11 cm proximal to the distal fibula at the posterior edge of the fibular shaft (Fig. 129-19). It is extended distally behind the tip of the fibula, and curved toward the base of the fifth metatarsal. The subcutaneous tissues are dissected carefully to protect the sural nerve (Fig. 129-20), which crosses the peroneal tendon sheath below the tip of the fibula and the base of the fifth metatarsal bone. The skin is undermined over the anterior aspect of the fibula and the ankle joint to define the anterior ankle capsule and the anterior talofibular ligament. The peroneal tendon sheath is then opened from the base of the fifth metatarsal going proximally behind the fibula. The peroneus brevis tendon is identified but left in the sheath. The anterior talofibular ligament is divided transversely closer to the fibula than to the talus, leaving it attached to both the talus and the fibula. At the talar ligamentous attachment, a small area is curetted into bleeding bone to aid reattachment of the reconstructed ligament. Starting 2.5 cm proximal to the tip of the fibula, a hole is drilled through the fibula from anterior to poste-

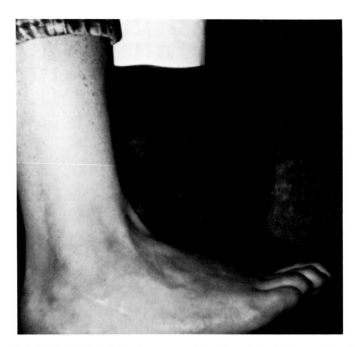

Fig. 129-19. Early healed skin incision for our modification of the Chrisman-Snook procedure.

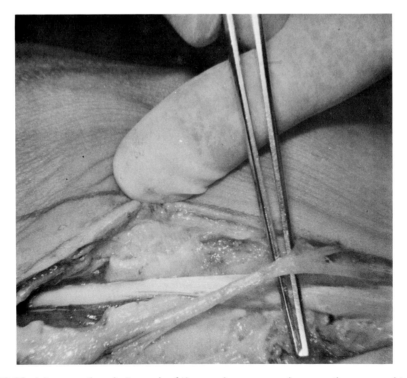

Fig. 129-20. Intraoperative photograph of the sural nerve crossing over the peroneal tendons.

rior, going from proximal to slightly distal. Using a 2.8-mm drill bit, it is gradually enlarged with drills and small curettes to make it large enough for the transplanted ligament, while care is taken to not break through the fibula laterally. The soft tissues are dissected away from the posterior aspect of the fibula to allow the transplanted tendon to pass. The original attachment of the calcaneofibular ligament is then identified and the soft tissues on the os calcis below this area are cleaned away. A small area is curetted into bleeding subcortical bone in the os calcis. The sural nerve should be observed in this area.

If the peroneus brevis tendon is small, we take the whole tendon, going as far proximal as possible. Dissecting the peroneus brevis muscle off the tendon is tedious, but a long length of tendon is needed. This dissection can be aided by using a periosteal elevator working against the grain of the muscle fibers. If the tendon is large, it may be dissected free and split in half, going from distal to proximal and left attached distally. If the whole tendon is used, the peroneus muscle belly is sutured to the peroneus longus tendon. The peroneus brevis tendon is detached proximally and brought distally. Pass the peroneus brevis tendon from distal to proximal through a small scalpel hole in the base of the anterior talofibular ligament, where it is attached to the talus. After going through the base of the talofibular ligament, the brevis tendon is passed through the hole in the fibula, using a #9 red catheter with the tendon tied into it so that it can be fed through the fibular hole (Fig. 129-21). The tendon goes through the fibula and then behind the peroneus longus tendon to the area previously curetted on the os calcis.

With the foot in neutral dorsiflexion and neutral eversion, the transplanted tendon is pulled tightly and sutured to the periosteum and adjacent tissues on the fibula as it passes through the anterior hole. With the tendon still under tension and the foot held in the same position, a small staple holds the tendon firmly to the os calcis where the bone has been previously curetted. The distal end of the transplanted tendon, if it is long enough, is led back over the peroneus longus tendon to help maintain this tendon in the tendon sheath and then sutured to the anterior aspect of the talofibular ligament (Fig. 129-22). The tendon at the base of the ante-

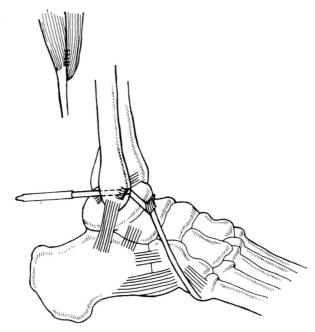

Fig. 129-21. Modified Chrisman-Snook procedures. The peroneus brevis tendon, after being detached proximally, is brought through the curetted base of the attachment of the anterior talofibular ligament on the talus and then through the drill hole in the fibula going from anterior to posterior. See text.

rior talofibular ligament is also sutured to the talofibular ligament, and we overlap the cut edges of the anterior talofibular ligament, suturing them together to reinforce our repair. The subcutaneous tissues and skin are closed in the usual manner.

Postoperative Management

We place the leg and foot in a posterior splint or short-leg cast for several days. The foot is elevated for 36 hours, and the short-leg cast may have to be bivalved because of the postoperative swelling. We keep the patient from bearing weight for the first week but, after that, the patient begins gradual weight bearing, using a cast boot with crutches and later a cane. The cast is removed 6 weeks after surgery, and the patient starts on active and active–assistive dorsiflexion and plantar-flexion exercises. The patient then gradually starts to stretch the posterior structures of the ankle. We allow patients to swim as soon as the cast is off and

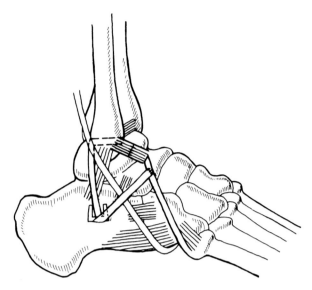

Fig. 129-22. Completed modification of the Chrisman-Snook procedure, showing the peroneus brevis passing beneath the peroneus longus after exiting from the fibula. The distal segment of the transplant has been passed over the peroneus longus and sutured to the anterior talofibular ligament and the tendon graft after being fixed with a staple to the os calcis.

encourage them to walk with a normal heel-toe gait. The patient may bicycle if so desired, to help gain strength and motion in the foot. Swelling may be a problem for the first weeks and is controlled by the use of a compression bandage and elevation. We wait 8 weeks after surgery before allowing patients to start on active inversion and eversion of the foot. At that point, the rehabilitation program is modified for each patient, depending on progress and particular needs. Agility drills are helpful in restoring normal proprioception to the extremity. Most patients will be able to return to moderate athletic activities 4 months after surgery, but will continue to improve over the next several months.

Bröstrom Operation

A curvilinear incision is made about a finger-breadth anterior to and below the lateral malleolus. The perisynovial tissue and synovial membrane are incised in the ligament free triangular region between the anterior tibiofibular and anterior talofibular ligaments, exposing the joint. The articular cartilage is carefully inspected, any intraarticular pathology is dealt with accordingly.

The anterior talofibular ligament is dissected free; all fibrotic tissue is excised in order to identify its remnants. Most commonly, the old rupture occurred within the ligament substance either in the midregion of the ligament or near its fibular attachment. If the anterior talofibular ligament has been torn in its midportion, the scar is excised and the ends imbricated with continuous nonabsorbable suture. In those cases in which the anterior talofibular ligament has ruptured near the fibular attachment with or without avulsion and bone fragments, the proximal end of the ligament is anchored to the anterior margin of the fibula with four to six solitary synthetic sutures drawn through two drill holes in the lateral malleolus (Fig. 129-23). Avulsed bone fragments are in most cases excised before suturing. If the ligament is weak or the remnants are insufficient to suture, reconstruction is performed, taking a flap from the lateral talocalcaneal ligament (Fig. 129-24). This flap is left attached distally to the talus but detached from the calcaneous and brought up to the lateral malleolus at the usual attachment of the anterior talofibular ligament. Strong synthetic suture is used through drill holes to hold the ligament in place. Occasionally, the lateral talocalcaneal ligament is used to reconstruct the anterior talofibular ligament totally when only insignificant remnants can be identified. There may be an occasional case in which avulsion of a

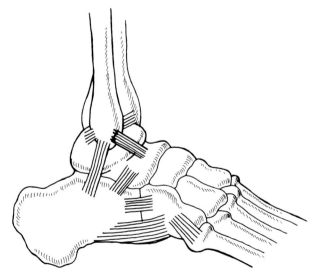

Fig. 129-23. Bröstrom procedure, reattaching the anterior talofibular ligament to the fibula through drill holes.

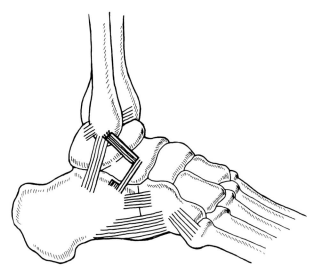

Fig. 129-24. Bröstrom procedure, using a flap of the lateral talocalcaneal ligament for reconstruction of the anterior talofibular ligament.

bone from the talus has occurred; the fragment is excised and the ligament anchored to the talus by means of four sutures through two drill holes.

The peroneal tendon sheath is opened to permit access to the calcaneo-fibular ligament. Scarring indicates injury to this ligament and if the ligament fails to tense on inversion and supination of the heel, the scar tissue between the elongated ligament ends is excised and the two ligament ends are imbricated with continuous nonabsorbable suture. Tears of the posterior talofibular ligaments are unusual and very difficult to repair.

The joint capsule, tendon sheath, and fascia are reapproximated with absorbable suture and after the skin is closed, a short-leg cast is applied with the foot at 0 degrees dorsiflexion. Ambulation with progressive weight bearing with crutches is allowed 3 to 4 days after operation. Plaster immobilization is discontinued at 3 weeks.

The Watson-Jones Procedure

The incision is made longitudinally posterior to the distal third of the fibula, curving anteriorly as it goes distally and ending about 5 cm anterior to the tip of the lateral malleolus. The subcutaneous tissues are dissected and the sural nerve looked for and protected. The peroneus brevis tendon is re-

moved from the tendon sheath and dissected from its muscle belly proximally. A good length of the peroneus brevis tendon is needed. The peroneus brevis muscle is sutured to the peroneus longus tendon.

A drill hole is made through the distal fibula, 2.5 cm above its tip, going from posterior to anterior emerging at the attachment of the anterior talofibular ligament. Another drill hole is made through the neck of the talus anterior to its articular surface and parallel to the long axis of the limb ending in the roof of the sinus tarsi. Care should be taken to make the hole medial enough that the cortex of the lateral talar neck is not broken through. The peroneus brevis tendon is passed through the fibular drill hole, going from posterior to anterior, and then through the hole in the neck of the talus going from superior to inferior. It may be necessary to curette the holes to aid passage of the brevis tendon. After passage through the neck of the talus, the tendon is brought back to the fibular malleolus at the attachment of the calcaneofibular ligament, where it is sutured to the periosteum (Fig. 129-25). Following routine closure of the wound with the foot in position, a short-leg cast is applied, which holds the foot in some eversion. Weight bearing is permitted after 2 weeks and the cast is worn for a total of 8 weeks.

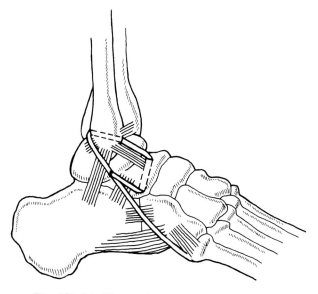

Fig. 129-25. Watson-Jones procedure. See text.

The Evans Procedure

The Evans technique reconstructs the calcaneofibular ligament. The skin approach and mobilization of the peroneus brevis tendon are performed in the same manner as for the Watson-Jones procedure. A bony tunnel is made starting at the anteroinferior tip of the lateral malleolus and emerges at the posterior aspect of the fibula about 3.2 cm proximal to the tip of the malleolus. After the tunnel is enlarged with curettes to let the tendon pass, the tendon is passed through the fibula from distal to proximal (Fig. 129-26). Under tension with the foot in neutral position and eversion, the tendon is then sutured to adjacent periosteal tissues. The peroneal tendon sheath is then closed so that there will be no dislocation of the peroneal tendons. We close the subcutaneous tissues and the skin in a routine manner.

The postoperative treatment is the same as for the Watson-Jones procedure. We apply a short-leg cast and allow the patient to bear weight 2 weeks after surgery.

The O'Phelan Procedure

The incision is made along the outer aspect of the ankle beginning approximately 16.5 cm above the lateral malleolus, extending to the tip of the mal-

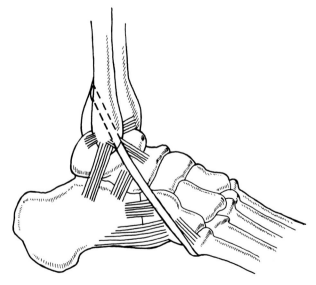

Fig. 129-26. Evans procedure passing the peroneus brevis tendon through a drill hole in the fibula.

leolus, and going forward to the insertion of the peroneus brevis tendon on the fifth metatarsal.[37] The peroneus brevis muscle and tendon are isolated and the tendon incised at the musculotendinous junction. The muscle belly is sutured directly to the peroneus longus tendon. The anterolateral aspect of the lower tibia is exposed by elevating the extensor muscles and the periosteum incised and reflected in an inverted T shape. This anterolateral aspect of the tibia is prepared for the insertion of the peroneus brevis tendon, and a staple is partially inserted approximately 1.2 cm above the articulating surface of the tibiotalar joint.

A small incision is made in the soft tissues just superior to the base of the fifth metatarsal bone and a blunt curved instrument, such as a hemostat, is directed under the soft tissue going toward the tibiotalar articulation. The peroneus brevis tendon is passed through this soft tissue canal going under the anterior talofibular ligament, which is usually stretched but intact. The brevis tendon is then brought to the anterolateral aspect of the tibia and brought underneath the staple where, with the foot held in valgus, the staple is then further inserted. This fixes the tendon directly to the bone. The periosteum is sutured to the tendon and smaller ligamentous capsular structures are sewed directly to the tendon as it passes from the base of the fifth metatarsal bone to the staple. The remaining portion of the brevis tendon is then reflected on itself and sutured to the distal portion of the remaining anterior talofibular ligament. The main portion of the peroneus brevis tendon replaces the calcaneofibular ligament. The reflected portion of this tendon reinforces the anterior talofibular ligament. The wound is closed loosely to avoid undue stress on the skin edges. The foot is held in valgus in a short-leg cast. The leg is immobilized for 6 weeks during which weight bearing is not permitted. After the cast is removed; the patient remains on crutches with partial weight bearing until foot and ankle mobility have been restored.

Complications

A possible complication of the Chrisman-Snook procedure is a small skin slough posterior to the lateral malleolus. We must go far enough posterior to be able to staple the reconstruction to the os calcis, yet still go far enough anterior to visualize completely the anterior talofibular ligament. Although we have had several small skin sloughs, we have never had a major one and all skin incisions have healed well. A second possible complication is damage to the sural nerve, which is immediately underneath the subcutaneous tissue, particularly in the distal part of the wound. Although all patients have a minor lack of inversion on the operated side compared with the unoperated side and all patients have been active; this has caused no complaints. The taking of the peroneus brevis tendon does not seem to influence foot function or prevent patients from being completely active in a variety of sports.

RESULTS

Recent literature indicates that a good success rate can be expected with any of these procedures. Lucht et al[34] reported their results with the modified Watson-Jones technique in 30 cases and achieved functional stability in all but one. However, it was noted that 15 of these patients did have pain and swelling. Hedebre et al[23] looked at 21 ankles reconstructed by the Watson-Jones technique and reported satisfactory results in 80 percent. Rijt and Evans[42] looked at the long-term results of the Watson-Jones tenodesis in 9 patients, an average of 22 years postoperatively, and found that only 3 had complete relief of symptoms with 2 satisfactory early results deteriorating with time. With clinical and radiographic examination the talar tilt was controlled more successfully than the anterior drawer.

Vainiopaa et al[53] followed up 62 Evans reconstruction for a mean of 5 years, and had excellent or good results in 87 percent of patients. Two other large clinical studies of the Evans procedure also indicated a high success rate.[28,39] Kristiansen,[27] however, looked at 18 athletic patients treated with the Evans procedure, and found that only one-third were still able to engage in athletics. One study looked at the radiographic instability of the ankle joint after the Evans repair; a high frequency of persistent anterior subluxation on stress radiographs was noted, although this did not correlate well with the functional results.[38]

Bröstrom's[5a-5e] original series of 60 ankles treated with his technique had satisfactory results in 57 cases, but length of follow-up was not made clear. Javors and Violet[25] reported good or excellent in 13 of 15 patients treated with the Bröstrom procedure. These workers emphasized that this procedure was comparable to other techniques and did not alter any normal anatomic structures. It has been shown, however, that the loss of the peroneus brevis has not resulted in any significant loss of strength or functional deficit, even in an athletic individual.

Snook and colleagues[48] looked at the long-term results of their procedure and found that 45 of 48 patients available for a follow-up, at a mean of 10 years, had excellent or good results. Two other published reports indicate a high success rate with this procedure.[41,45] Our experience with the Modified Chrisman-Snook operation has been quite favorable. It eliminates abnormal anterior drawer as well as inversion laxity. Dorsiflexion and plantar flexion return to normal, and strength returns to normal over a 6- to 9-month period. The loss of inversion has not been a problem. Although most patients return to athletic activities after about 4 months, it is about 6 months before they consider themselves back to the activity level they would like. Some athletic patients report that it is 1 year before the ankle feels normal.

CHRONIC MEDIAL LIGAMENTOUS INSTABILITY

Chronic medial instability of the ankle is uncommon and isolated disruption of the deltoid ligament is rare. Deltoid ligament damage is relatively common in association with a distal fibular fracture or disruption of the tibiofibular ligaments and syndesmosis. In the later instance, if the ankle is symptomatic there will be a lateral subluxation of the talus with scar tissue between the medial malleolus and the talus and elongation of the medial ligamentous structures (Figs. 129-27, 129-28). To correct this, one must not only operate on the medial side but also include the lateral side and either close the diastasis of the tibiofibular syndesmosis or anatomically reduce the fracture of the fibula.

Indications

The only indication for secondary reconstruction of the deltoid ligament would be symptomatic medial instability. One would expect tenderness over the deltoid ligament anterior and inferior to the medial malleolus. Lateral translation of the talus within the mortise and abnormal eversion of the foot would be evidence of medial instability. There is less written about abnormal tibiotalar tilt with medial instability than lateral instability but stress films should show abnormal talar tilt with chronic medial instability. A mortise view of the ankle showing a clear space of greater than 4 mm indicates lateral subluxation of the talus and we must look for lateral pathology along with elongation of the deltoid ligament.

Contraindications

When there is isolated damage to the deltoid ligament with chronic instability, there would be virtually no contraindications for secondary surgery other than local factors related to skin healing. With chronic lateral talar subluxation associated

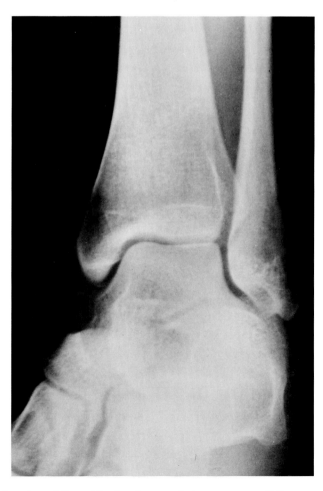

Fig. 129-27. Mortise view of the ankle showing equal clear space medially, superiorly, and laterally.

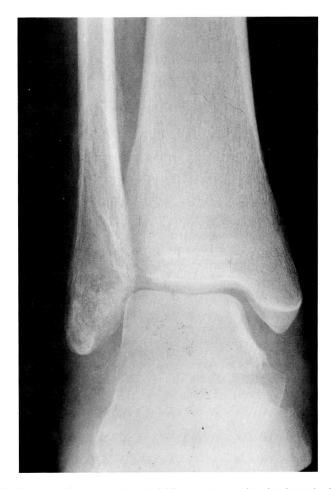

Fig. 129-28. Patient with an old deltoid ligament tear showing lateral talar shift.

with elongation of the deltoid ligament as well as lateral pathology, the lateral pathology must be corrected at the same time as secondary repair of the deltoid ligament.

Treatment Options

Other than an orthotic or ankle brace to hold the foot and ankle rigidly, there are no treatment options for chronic medial instability. Fortunately, the condition is relatively rare.

The literature reports few procedures for secondary reconstruction of the medial ligaments of the ankle. The method reported by DeVries[11] is simple but does not appear as logical as the one we present. The operative procedure by Wiltberger[55] appears reasonable, although we have had no personal experience with it. Because of this, in the several instances in which we had to reconstruct the medial ligament, we have followed the concepts of Bröstrom for the lateral side and advise a simple imbrication of the local deltoid ligamentous structures.

Operative Repair of Chronic Medial Instability

Curvilinear incision is started above the medial malleolus and extended medially and posterior below the malleolus. The saphenous vein is avoided while the entire deltoid ligament is exposed. The superficial and deep portions of the deltoid are located and the superficial deltoid ligament transected one-third of its length distal to the tibia. The deep portion of the ligament may be seen, and one must decide whether to transect it, leaving a section attached to both the talus and malleolus, or take it completely off the tibia for proximal advancement. Any fibrous tissue between the medial malleolus and talus is removed and appropriate surgery performed on the lateral side. The talus is mobilized and pushed medially. A screw may be needed through the fibula into the tibia to help hold the talus in its more medial position. The deep portion of the deltoid must be advanced proximally either to part of the remaining ligament or through drill holes in the proximal malleolus. The distal portion of the superficial deltoid can then be sutured to the undersurface of the proximal deltoid ligament in a pants-under-vest manner. If the proximal tissue is poor, the deltoid can be attached to the tibia through drill holes in the medial malleolus and lower tibia. The proximal cuff should be imbricated over the top of the distal deltoid. After closing the subcutaneous tissue and skin, we apply a long-leg or short-leg cast, depending on the surgery performed on the lateral side.

The Wiltberger and Mallory Procedure

The skin incision is made along the posterior tibial tendon behind the medial malleolus, starting about 5 cm proximal to the ankle joint and going distally to where the posterior tibial tendon attaches to the tarsus.[55] After the soft tissues are dissected, the posterior tibial tendon sheath is opened. The posterior tibial tendon is split in half longitudinally starting from its attachment to the tarsal bone and going about 4 cm proximal to the ankle. The anterior half of the tendon is detached proximally and left attached distally.

The original deltoid ligament fibers are dissected off the medial malleolus and the distal tibia. Any fibrous tissue between the medial malleolus and the talus is removed. A hole is drilled starting on the medial side of the medial malleolus above the joint and exiting through the medial malleolus distally, somewhat more laterally than its origin. This is enlarged with a curette to accept half of the tibial tendon. The detached anterior half of the posterior tibial tendon is inserted through the hole of the medial malleolus starting distally and laterally and exiting proximally and medially (Fig. 129-29).

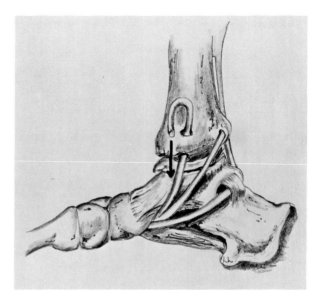

Fig. 129-29. In the Wiltberger-Mallory procedure, the anterior half of the posterior tibial tendon is passed through a drill hole on the tibia and then back on itself.

After exiting from the drill hole, the tendon is brought back distally and sutured to itself with the talus reduced against the medial malleolus and the foot inverted (Fig. 129-30). The remainder of the deltoid ligament is then resutured to the tibia more proximal either to adjacent soft tissues or through drill holes.

Postoperative Management

We keep the patient in a short-leg cast with the foot in neutral position for a total of 6 weeks. For the first 2 weeks, the patient is kept non-weight bearing and then begins to bear weight with a cast boot. After the cast is removed, the patient starts on active and active-assistive range-of-motion exercises of the ankle and gradually goes on to strengthening the muscle groups, particularly the dorsiflexors and invertors of the foot. Later, strengthening exercises extend to the plantar flexors and finally the evertors. Depending on the level of activity the patient desires, we then go on to agility exercises to restore proprioception.

Results

We have had little personal experience with late repairs of the deltoid ligament, and there are few

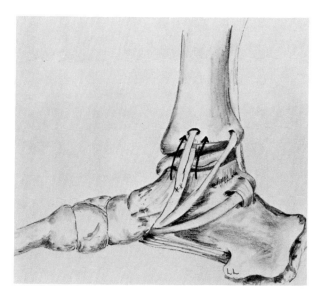

Fig. 129-30. Wiltberger-Mallory procedure. The tendon transplant has been sutured back on itself. The remainder of the deltoid ligament is reattached to the tibia *(arrows).*

published results. Chronic degeneration of the tibiotalar joint may occur from lateral subluxations of the talus. Thus, if stabilization is performed late, we can expect a poor result. If, however, the stabilization is performed early, we would expect the result to be good. In the several patients in whom we have done a direct repair as described, this appears to have been adequate. However, these patients were not high-performance athletes.

REFERENCES

1. Anderson KJ, LeCocq JF, LeCocq EA: Recurrent anterior subluxation of the ankle joint. J Bone Joint Surg 34A:853, 1952
2. Black HM, Brand RL, Eichelberger MR: An improved technique for the evaluation of ligamentous injury in severe ankle sprains. Am J Sports Med 6:276, 1978
3. Brand RL, Collins DF, Templeton T: Surgical repair of ruptured lateral ankle ligaments. Am J Sports Med 9:40, 1981
4. Brantigan JW, Pedegara RL, Lippert FG: Instability of the subtalar joint. J Bone Joint Surg 59A:321, 1977
5a. Bröstrom L: Sprained ankle. I. Anatomic lesions in recent sprains. Acta Chir Scand 128:483, 1964
5b. Bröstrom L: Sprained ankle. II. Arthrographic diagnosis of recent ligament ruptures. Acta Chir Scand 129:485, 1965
5c. Bröstrom L: Sprained ankle. III. Clinical observations in recent ligament ruptures. Acta Chir Scand 130:560, 1965
5d. Bröstrom L: Sprained ankle. IV. Surgical treatment of "chronic" ligament ruptures. Acta Chir Scand 132:551, 1966
5e. Bröstrom L: Sprained ankle. V. Treatment and prognosis in recent ruptures. Acta Chir Scand 132:537, 1966
6. Buri C, Neugebauer R: Carbon fiber replacement of the ligaments of the shoulder girdle and the treatment of lateral instability of the ankle joint. Clin Orthop 196:112, 1985
7. Chrisman OD, Snook GA: Reconstruction of lateral ligament tears of the ankle. J Bone Joint Surg 51A:904, 1969
8. Cox JS: Surgical treatment of ankle sprains. Am J Sports Med 5:250, 1977
9. Cox JS, Hewes TF: "Normal" talar tilt angle. Clin Orthop 140:37, 1979
10. Delplace J, Castaing J: Apports de l'etude radiographique du tiroir astragalien anterieur (TAR). Rev Chir Orthop 61 (suppl II):137, 1975
11. DeVries HL: Surgery of the Foot. 2nd Ed. CV Mosby, St. Louis, 1965
12. Drez D, Young JC, Waldman D, et al: Non-operative treatment of double lateral ligament tears of the ankle. Am J Sports Med 10(4):197, 1982
13. Evans DL: Recurrent instability of the ankle — a method of surgical treatment. Proc R Soc Med 66:343, 1953
14. Evans GA, Frenyo SD: The stress tenogram in the diagnosis of ruptures of the lateral ligament of the ankle. J Bone Joint Surg 61B:347, 1979
15. Evans GA, Hardcastle P, Frenyo AD: Acute rupture of the lateral ligament of the ankle. To suture or not to suture? J Bone Joint Surg 66B:209, 1984
16. Eyring EJ, Guthries WD: A surgical approach to the problem of severe lateral instability at the ankle. Clin Orthop 206:185, 1986
17. Freeman MAR: Treatment of ruptures of the lateral ligament of the ankle. J Bone Joint Surg 47B:661, 1965
18. Freeman MAR: Instability of the foot after injuries to the lateral ligaments of the ankle. J Bone Joint Surg 47B:669, 1965
19. Freeman MAR, Wyke B: Articular reflexes at the ankle joint. Br J Surg 54:990, 1967
20. Gillespie HS, Boucher P: Watson-Jones repair of lat-

eral instability of the ankle. J Bone Joint Surg 53A:920, 1971

21. Gross AE, MacIntosh DL: Injury to the lateral ligament of the ankle: a clinical study. Can J Surg 16:115, 1973

22. Harrington KD: Degenerative arthritis of the ankle secondary to long standing lateral ligamentous instability. J Bone Joint Surg 61A:354, 1979

23. Hedabre J, Johannsen A: Recurrent instability of the ankle joint. Surgical repair by the Watson-Jones method. Acta Orthop Scand 50:337, 1979

24. Homminga GN, Kluft O: Long term inversion stability of the ankle after rupture of the lateral ligaments. Neth J Surg 38(4):103, 1987

25. Javors JR, Violet JT: Correction of chronic lateral ligament instability of the ankle by use of the Brö-strom procedure. A report of 15 cases. Clin Orthop 201, 1985

26. Korkala O, Lauttamus L, Tanskanen P: Lateral ligament injuries of the ankle. Results of primary surgical treatment. Am Chir Gynaecol 71(3):161, 1982

27. Kristiansen B: Surgical treatment of ankle instability in athletes. Br J Sports Med 16(1):40, 1982

28. Lauttamus L, Korkala O, Tanskanen P: Lateral ligament injuries of the ankle. Surgical treatment of late cases. Ann Chir Gynaecol 71(3):164, 1982

29. Laurin C, Mathieu J, Levesque HP: LeSigne du titoir de la chéville. Laxité sagittale normale de la chéville. Un Med Can 102:2116, 1973

30. Laurin C, Quellet R, St. Jacques R: Talar and subtalar tilt: an experimental investigation. Can J Surg 11:270, 1968

31. Leach RE, Namiki O, Paul GR, Stockel J: Secondary reconstruction of the lateral ligaments of the ankle. Clin Orthop 160:201, 1981

32. Leonard MH: Injuries to the lateral ligaments of the ankle. J Bone Joint Surg 31A:373, 1949

33. Lindstrand A, Mortensson W: Anterior instability in the ankle joint following acute lateral sprain. Acta Radiol Diag 18:529, 1977

34. Lucht TU, Vang PS, Termangen NB: Lateral ligament reconstruction of the ankle with a modified Watson-Jones operation. Acta Orthop Scand 52(3):363, 1986

35. Marymont JV, Lynch MA, Henning CT: Acute ligamentous diastasis of the ankle without fracture. Evaluation by radionuclide imaging. Am J Sports Med 14:407, 1986

36. Niedermann B, Andersen A, Andersen SB, et al: Rupture of the lateral ligaments of the ankle: operation or plaster cast? A prospective study. Acta Orthop Scand 52:579, 1981

37. O'Phalen HE: Diagnosis and reconstruction of the ankle ligaments for lateral instability. Presented at the American Society for Sports Medicine, New Orleans, LA, 1978

38. Orava S, Jarmoa H, Weitz H, et al: Radiographic instability of the ankle joint after Evans' repair. Acta Orthop Scand 54:734, 1983

39. Ottosan L: Lateral instability of the ankle treated by a modified Evans procedure. Acta Orthop Scand 49(3):302, 1978

40. Pieron AP: Dynamic peroneus tendon transfer for repair of the unstable ankle. Can J Surg 25:672, 1982

41. Riegler HF: Reconstruction for lateral instability of the ankle. 66A:336, 1984

42. Rijt AJ, Evans GA: The long term results of Watson-Jones tenodesis. J Bone Joint Surg 66B:371, 1984

43. Rubin G, Witten M: The talar tilt angle and the fibular collateral ligament. J Bone Joint Surg 42A:311, 1969

44. Ruth CJ: The surgical treatment of injuries of the fibular collateral ligaments of the ankle. J Bone Joint Surg 43A:229, 1961

45. Savastano AA, Lowe EB Jr: Ankle sprains; surgical treatment for recurrent sprains. Report of 10 patients treated with the Chrisman-Snook modification of the Elmslie procedure. Am J Sports Med. 8(3):208, 1980

46. Seligson D, Gassman J, Page M: Ankle instability — evaluation of the lateral ligaments. Am J Sports Med 8:39, 1980

47. Settan GK, George J, Fitton JM, McMillen H: Reconstruction of the anterior talofibular ligament for the treatment of the unstable ankle. J Bone Joint Surg 61A:352, 1979

48. Snook, GA, Chrisman OD and Wilson TC: Long term results of the Chrisman-Snook operation for reconstruction of the lateral ligaments of the ankle. J Bone Joint Surg 67A:1,1-7, Jan, 1985.

49. Spiegel PK, Staples OS: Arthrography of the ankle joint: problems in diagnosis of acute lateral ligament injuries. Radiology 114:587, 1975

50. Staples OS: Result of ruptures of lateral ligaments of the ankle. Clin Orthop 85:50, 1972

51. Staples OS: Ruptures of the fibular collateral ligaments of the ankle. Result study of immediate surgical treatment. J Bone Joint Surg 57A:101, 1975

52. St Pierre R, Allman F Sr, Bassett FH, et al: A review of lateral ankle ligamentous reconstruction. Foot Ankle 3(2):114, 1982

53. Vainiopaa S, Kirves P, Laike E: Lateral instability of the ankle and results by the Evans procedure. Am J Sports Med 8:437, 1980

54. Van den Hoogenband CR, Van Moppes FI, Stapert JW, Greep JM: Clinical diagnosis, arthrography, stress examination and surgical findings after inversion trauma of the ankle. Arch Orthop Trauma Surg 103(2):115, 1984

55. Wiltberger BR, Mallory TH: A new method for the reconstruction of the deltoid ligament of the ankle. Orthop Rev 1:37, 1972

56. Windfeld P: Treatment of undue mobility of the ankle joint following severe sprains of the ankle with avulsion of the anterior and middle bands of the external ligament. Acta Chir Scand 104:229, 1954

Muscle and Tendon Surgery of the Leg

130

John A. Elstrom
Arsen M. Pankovich

TENDON RUPTURES

Acute Rupture of the Gastrocnemius Muscle

Rupture of the gastrocnemius muscle is usually the consequence of a vigorous contraction of the muscle when the knee fails to flex and the foot is dorsiflexed. Sometimes it is due to the direct blow of a sharp object on the muscle while it is in active contraction. It usually occurs in the substance of the medial head of the gastrocnemius or at the musculoaponeurotic junction.[23]

Diagnosis

A history of sudden pain and a snapping sensation in the calf is common and often occurs while the patient pushes off suddenly (tennis leg).[2,3] Initially, local tenderness medially above the musculotendinous junction, swelling, and induration in the muscle are noted. The patient is unable to walk without a limp or crutches. In a more severe case, the course of the rupture may be complicated by formation of a large tense hematoma under the crural fascia (Fig. 130-1A) and increasing pain, particularly on attempted dorsiflexion of the ankle. These signs of developing muscle ischemia in the posterior superficial compartment of the leg secondary to the hematoma[73,74,102] may be followed by an equinus contracture of the gastroc-soleus group in an extreme case. Since no major vessels or nerves pass through this compartment, no signs of sensory or circulatory insufficiency are present. Rarely, hypesthesia may occur in the distribution of the sural nerve, which passes partway through the compartment. The arteriogram usually shows no abnormalities (Fig. 130-1B). Muscle ischemia can develop in other compartments of the leg as a result of this injury.[74,102]

Treatment

For the ordinary partial tear, a short-leg cast with the foot in slight equinus and a built-up heel can be applied for 2 to 3 weeks to enable the patient to bear weight without crutches, or the patient can apply ice and start ambulation with crutches and bear partial weight with a built-up heel after 10 to

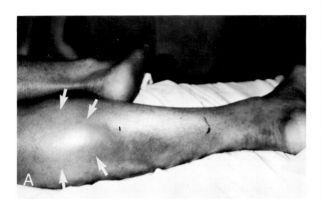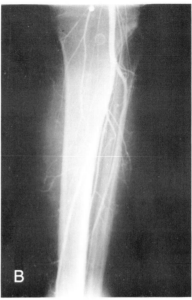

Fig. 130-1. Posterior superficial compartment syndrome. **(A)** Hematoma under the tense crural fascia. **(B)** The arteriogram is usually normal, the vessels being in the deep posterior compartment.

14 days.[97] Surgical evacuation of the tense hematoma is indicated as soon as the diagnosis of muscle ischemia is suspected.

Technique

A curvilinear incision, as long as necessary, is made over the area of swelling. The crural fascia is incised over the tense area, where the large hematoma may be apparent. Large amounts of blood coagula are then evacuated, and the cavity is thoroughly irrigated. The ruptured muscle ends are debrided if necrotic. A drainage tube is left in the cavity before the wound is closed and is removed after 24 hours. A short-leg cast with the ankle plantar flexed at 20 degrees is applied at the end of the procedure.

Postoperative Management

The short-leg cast is removed after 3 weeks and active exercises are started. Full weight bearing is allowed about 2 weeks later, when active dorsiflexion of the ankle appears to be adequate. Stretching of the posterior calf musculature and resistive strengthening are needed to complete rehabilitation.

Acute Rupture of the Achilles Tendon

A fresh rupture of the Achilles tendon commonly occurs in patients aged 30 to 50 years, and much more often in men.[38,39,50,88] A good number of patients in one study were found to have participated in sports activities in earlier years but were engaged in sedentary occupations at the time of tendon rupture.[5] Increased vascularity of the tendon during active years and subsequent decrease in vascularity have been postulated as a cause of degenerative changes found regularly in the tendon.[28] Sports requiring a vigorous push-off in pursuit of a moving object lead the list of most compendia concerning themselves with the activity responsible for this injury. Rupture can occur at any site from the musculotendinous junction to the insertion of the tendon to the os calcis, yet it is found most commonly 2 to 6 cm above the insertion. The rupture is usually complete and is only rarely partial. Rupture of the plantaris tendon is also sometimes present.

Diagnosis

The diagnosis of a rupture of the Achilles tendon is made by the history of a sudden snap in the back of the leg or ankle. Very commonly this is noted with forceful plantar flexion. In addition to local tenderness, there are four diagnostic signs on physical examination: (1) results of the Thompson-Doherty calf squeeze test[106]; (2) results of the heel resistance test; (3) the palpation of a gap; and (4) the needle test of O'Brien.[79] In the Thompson-Doherty calf squeeze test, the patient is placed prone with the knee bent 90 degrees, so that the leg is pointed toward the ceiling. When the examiner squeezes the calf muscle above the area of injury and tenderness, plantar flexion of the foot is elicited if the tendon is in continuity; if the tendon is ruptured, there is no response (Fig. 130-2). In order to perform the heel resistance test, the heel is grasped firmly and plantar flexion resisted. Resistance is easily broken when the Achilles tendon is intact but, although the intact peroneal and posterior tibial muscles can plantar flex the foot when the Achilles tendon is ruptured, they cannot do so against this resistance. A gap is usually palpable at the site of injury in the tendon when the patient is seen after complete rupture. In the needle test described by O'Brien, a 25-gauge needle is inserted at a right angle into the Achilles tendon 10 cm

proximal to the superior border of the calcaneus. The foot is then passively dorsiflexed and plantar flexed and the movement of the needle hub noted. Swiveling of the needle about its pivot point in the skin so that it points in the direction opposite to the movement of the foot indicates that the Achilles tendon is intact throughout its distal 10 cm. Absence of swiveling indicates loss of continuity of the Achilles tendon.[79] Radiography and xerography[9,108] are useful additional means of establishing the diagnosis. In our experience, the Thompson-Doherty calf squeeze test along with local tenderness and a palpable gap have been sufficient to make the diagnosis in all acute injuries.

Treatment

The treatment of acute rupture of the Achilles tendon is controversial because excellent results have been reported by surgeons using only cast immobilization and also by those who favor operative repair. It is the opinion of Pankovich that cast immobilization of the leg with the foot in a plantar flexed position[53] is an excellent method that offers the following advantages: no need for hospitaliza-

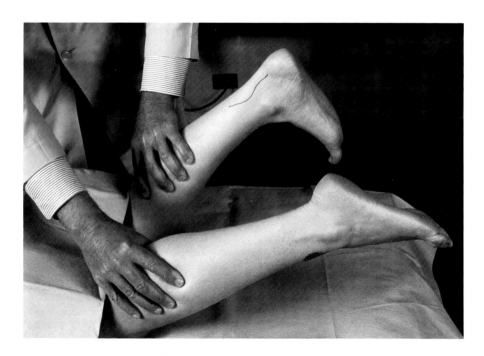

Fig. 130-2. Thompson-Doherty calf squeeze test.

tion, no risks of anesthesia, no postoperative wound complications, and earlier return to work for patients who generally regard their injury as minimal because surgery was not required.[76] Surgical repair is the choice treatment of acute rupture of the Achilles tendon, according to Elstrom. It is not difficult and provides for more exact approximation of the tendon ends. However, it still requires cast immobilization and protection of the repair for 8 to 10 weeks. Inglis and co-workers[40,41] reported 30 percent more strength and endurance and much less risk of rerupture when surgical repair was compared with plaster-cast immobilization.

Several operative techniques are used to repair the Achilles tendon. The end-to-end approximation with various types of suture material followed by cast immobilization is most commonly used. This provides better approximation than closed casting. The suture line can be reinforced by fascial flaps from the gastroc-soleus complex, by plantaris tendon, or by transfer of the peroneus brevis tendon. Occasionally direct suture of the proximal tendon end to the os calcis via a transverse drill hole is necessary. Either pull-out wires, which involve tying the suture material over a bolster on the skin surface, or a cast should generally be avoided and may increase the incidence of complications.[91] In any surgical repair, it is important to protect the sural nerve, which perforates the crural fascia at the level of the musculotendinous junction and passes subcutaneously downward on the lateral side of the Achilles tendon. The plantaris tendon passes under the crural fascia on the medial side of the Achilles tendon. It should be noted that the Achilles tendon does not have a true sheath: it is surrounded with areolar, fatty connective tissue interposed with elastic fibers. This tissue, called peritenoneum externum, merges with and penetrates the tendon.[4] Whenever possible during the dissection, this tissue should remain with the skin and subcutaneous tissues and should be carefully repaired to prevent adhesion of the tendon to the skin.

Although the prone position, general anesthesia, and a thigh tourniquet are usually used, Cetti and Christensen[15] have satisfactorily performed open repair with local anesthesia and adrenalin without a tourniquet. Even the need for postoperative cast-ing with the foot in some equinus considered by most surgeons as routine has been questioned. Marti et al.[67] start active dorsiflexion 1 week after surgery and then cast the foot at 0 degrees. Levy et al.[56] devised a technique of repair using a 4-mm Dacron (or Mersilene) suture passed through a drill hole in the calcaneal tuberosity and woven into the proximal end at the musculotendinous junction that eliminates cast immobilization altogether.

Surgical Approach

In most instances, a curvilinear incision extending from the mid calf to the os calcis should be used. The incision can be carried down either side of the Achilles tendon but should not be over the distal portion of the tendon. A curvilinear incision (Fig. 130-3A) has less tendency to contract and results in a better incisional scar.

Repair with Mersilene Strip: Pankovich and Elstrom

The Achilles tendon is exposed by a longitudinal curvilinear incision placed on the posteromedial aspect of the leg. After the skin and subcutaneous tissues have been opened, the peritenoneum is incised (Fig. 130-3B) and the site of the rupture identified. Occasionally, one of the tendon ends is folded ventrally on itself. The site of the tendon separation is not trimmed back to healthy tendon, because there may not be enough healthy tendon to approximate without requiring a special releasing incision proximally. The tendon ends usually come together without any difficulty in the fresh rupture, and the repair is carried out as follows. A 5-mm Mersilene strip (or 3-mm Dacron suture) is passed transversely through healthy tendon approximately 2.5 to 3.5 cm proximal to the ruptured surface. The suture is then passed obliquely across the tendon distally to emerge 1 to 2 mm proximal to the torn surface on the opposite side of the tendon (Fig. 130-3C). The suture is passed in a similar pattern into the distal portion of the tendon. The torn surfaces are pulled together and the suture ends are tied in a square knot. A 4-0 nylon suture is used to keep the knot in the Mersilene strip from untying. The ragged edges of the tendon ends are then brought into approximation with a few interrupted sutures of 2-0 chromic (Fig. 130-3D). The periten-

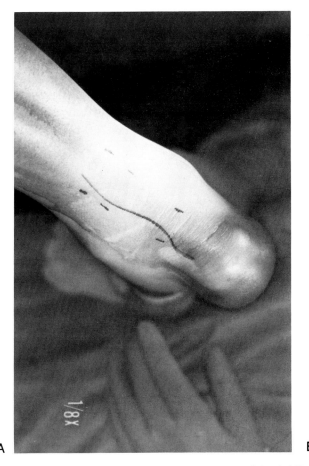
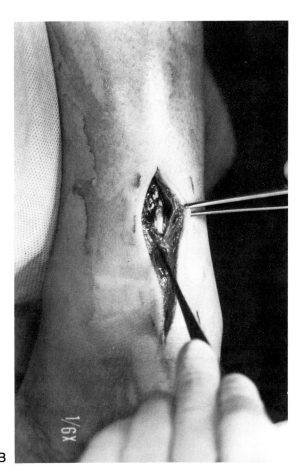

Fig. 130-3. Surgical repair of acute rupture of the Achilles tendon with Mersilene strip. **(A)** Surgical incision. **(B)** Incision of peritenoneum. *(Figure continues.)*

oneum is then closed using 4-0 chromic sutures. The subcutaneous tissue is closed using 3-0 to 4-0 subcuticular stitches, and the skin is closed with Steristrips or fine suture material. Very careful handling of the soft tissues is important to prevent complications.

When the Achilles tendon is ruptured near its insertion, the Mersilene strip may be woven through the proximal portion of the tendon and then passed through a transverse drill hole in the os calcis. This approach avoids the need for a pull-out wire and later removal of the material.

Postoperative Management A long-leg cast with the knee flexed and the foot in 20 degrees of plantar flexion is applied for 2 to 3 weeks. This is followed by a short-leg cast with the foot in 5 to 10 degrees of equinus for an additional 6 weeks. Partial weight bearing with crutches on a built-up heel is encouraged for the last 2 weeks in plaster. On removal of the plaster, the patient is placed in a short-leg double upright brace with a 90-degree dorsiflexion stop, to prevent accidental reinjury of the tendon repair; ambulation is begun with crutches. The initial exercise program consists of active dorsiflexion of the ankle and gentle manual resistance exercises against plantar flexion. Later the patient progresses to heel-cord stretching exercises done leaning forward against the wall with the heel held to the ground and progressive resistance exercises to restore calf muscle strength on a Cybex machine.

Marti et al.[67] advocate repair of the acute Achilles tendon rupture by a three-tissue bundle

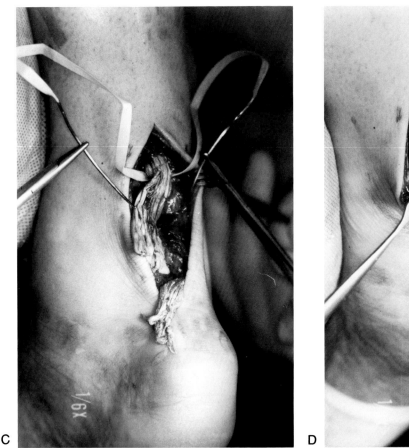
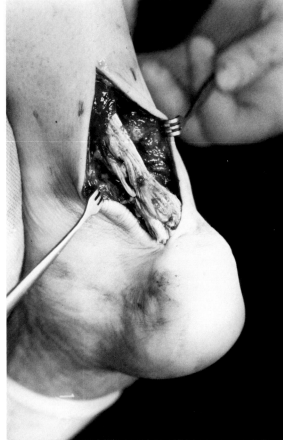

C   D

Fig. 130-3 *(Continued).* **(C)** Placement of Mersilene strip. **(D)** Completed repair.

technique and functional aftertreatment. Absorbable suture material is preferable for spontaneous healing, should wound sinuses occur. Beskin et al.[8] recently reported satisfactory results using this method with nonabsorbable suture material.

Three-Tissue Bundle Technique with Functional Aftertreatment: Weber and Marti

Surgery is performed with the patient positioned prone, a tourniquet is used, and a medial incision is made.[8,67] The disorganized fibers of the Achilles tendon are gathered into three bundles, using three continuous Bunnell sutures of Dexon or Vicryl. The three bundles are then sutured together as a "sandwich," with two bundles from one end of the repair brought around the single bundle from the opposite end of the repair in an attempt to create a minimal shortening of the tendon (Fig. 130-4). The tendon sheath and skin are closed. The ankle is immobilized in a relaxed equinus position by means of a below-knee plaster splint.

Postoperative Management The patient becomes ambulatory with crutches on the first postoperative day. Approximately 1 week after surgery, the plaster splint is removed, and gentle active dorsiflexion of the ankle is encouraged. When ankle dorsiflexion to 0 degrees or more is achieved, a below-knee walking cast with the ankle at 90 degrees is applied for 6 to 8 weeks. Progressive weight bearing is encouraged.[7] When the cast is removed, the patient starts active range of motion of the ankle and is placed on crutches with instructions to return gradually to full weight bearing over a period of 4 to 6 weeks. This technique is believed by its advocates to promote favorable tissue re-

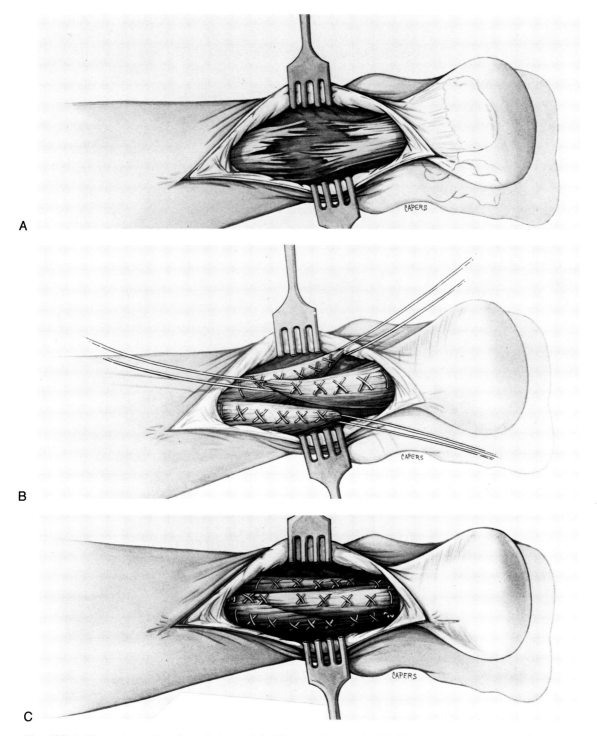

Fig. 130-4. Three tissue bundle technique of Achilles tendon repair. **(A)** Disrupted Achilles tendon fibers. **(B)** Disorganized fibers gathered into three bundles. **(C)** Reapproximation of Achilles tendon fibers. (From Beskin,[8] with permission.)

sponses by permitting early motion and functional loading of the extremity. Marti et al.[67] also advocate the three-tissue bundle technique with functional aftertreatment for management of the Achilles tendon rupture that has been neglected.

In our experience, reinforcement of the acute Achilles tendon rupture repair by local tendon or fascial flaps has seldom been necessary. These procedures are described next for those rare instances in which they may be required.

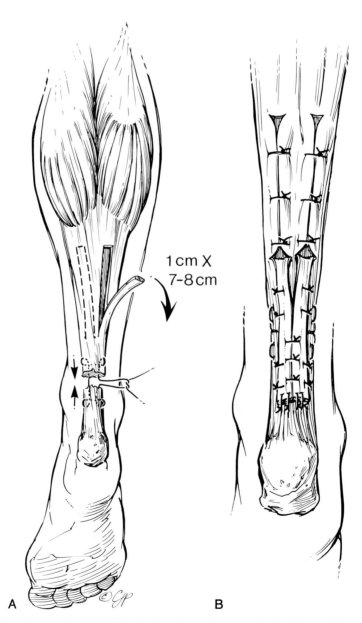

1 cm X
7-8 cm

A   B

Fig. 130-5. Repair of the ruptured Achilles tendon by reinforcement with inverted tendon strips. See text. (Modified from Lindholm,[57] with permission.)

Reinforcement with Inverted Tendon Strips: Lindholm

A posterior curvilinear incision is made, and the peritenoneum is incised longitudinally.[57] The irregular tendon ends are debrided and approximated with nonabsorbable interrupted stitches and one heavy box-type mattress suture (Fig. 130-5).

Two tendon flaps, 1 cm wide and 7 to 8 cm long, are cut from the gastrocnemius aponeurosis and the tendon, leaving them attached distally. The flaps are pulled down, twisted 180 degrees on themselves, and sutured to the distal part of the Achilles tendon and to each other. The peritenoneum is carefully sutured over the repair and the wound closed. A long-leg cast with the knee at 30 to 40 degrees of flexion and the ankle at 20 degrees of plantar flexion is applied.

Postoperative Management The long-leg cast is removed after 6 weeks, and a short walking cast is worn a further 4 weeks. A heel lift of 1 to 2 cm or a short double upright brace with a 90-degree stop to prevent further dorsiflexion is worn for 3 months.

Reinforcement with Plantaris Tendon: Lynn

The distal end of the curvilinear incision is carried down on the medial side of the Achilles tendon for a direct approach to the plantaris tendon.[63] After removal of the hematoma, the shredded ends of the tendon are sutured with interrupted stitches, without any part of the tendon being debrided. The plantaris tendon is either detached distally when intact or mobilized as needed when ruptured. Edges of the plantaris tendon are grasped with forceps and repeatedly stretched laterally until a membrane is formed. About 8 to 10 cm of this membrane is sutured around the Achilles tendon on both sides of the rupture (Fig. 130-6). The peritenoneum is sutured as far distally as possible and the wound is closed.

Postoperative Management A below knee cast with the foot at 20 degrees of plantar flexion immobilizes the repair for 5 weeks. After that, hydrotherapy is started. When the foot dorsiflexes to 90 degrees, usually at 6 weeks after surgery, a double upright brace with neutral dorsiflexion stop is worn for another 6 weeks.

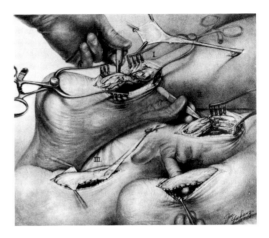

Fig. 130-6. Repair of the ruptured Achilles tendon by reinforcement with plantaris tendon. See text. (From Lynn,[63] with permission.)

Percutaneous Repair of Acute Achilles Tendon Ruptures: Ma and Griffith

Percutaneous repair of the Achilles tendon can be performed under local anesthesia without a tourniquet.[64] It is held by its advocates to minimize trauma to the tenuous blood supply of the skin overlying the heel cord, thereby reducing the risk of complications associated with open surgical repair. The patient is operated on in the prone position. The proximal portion of the ruptured Achilles tendon is palpated 2.5 cm proximal to the defect between the free ruptured ends. Using a #15 blade, stab wounds are made through the skin on the medial and lateral aspects of the tendon. After the stab wounds are made, a small curved hemostat is introduced into the wound between the subcutaneous tissue and the tendon sheath and rotated 360 degrees to free the skin and subcutaneous tissue from the tendon sheath underneath.

A #1 or 2 nonabsorbable suture 30 to 35 cm in length is used with a 7.5 cm straight needle on each end. The steps of this repair are shown in Figure 130-7.

Step 1. Starting with the lateral stab wound, the needle and suture are passed transversely through the stab wound, subcutaneous tissue, and tendon and out the medial stab wound. This creates a skin-to-skin suture that runs

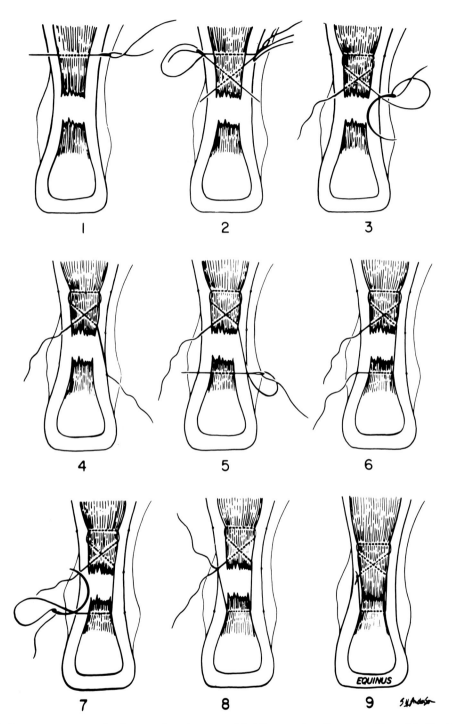

Fig. 130-7. Percutaneous repair of acute closed ruptured Achilles tendon. See text. (From Ma,[64] with permission.)

transversely lateral-to-medial through the largest anterior-to-posterior diameter of the Achilles tendon. The transversing suture is adjusted so that equal lengths of the free ends are on the medial and lateral sides of the tendon.

Step 2. The stab wounds from which the free suture ends exit are carefully enlarged with a small curved hemostat, as described above. Care is taken not to damage the suture with the hemostat. The straight needles are then inserted through the ipsilateral stab wound angulated distally 45 degrees to the long axis of the tendon and passed through the tendon then out through the skin on the contralateral side. The needles are not pulled completely through the skin, until the new skin puncture wounds are enlarged around the needle using a #15 blade and a small curved hemostat. The site of exit for the angulated needles and sutures is usually near the proximal edge of the rupture. At this point, the ends of the sutures are both pulled completely through the skin; traction is applied to both suture ends simultaneously, tightening the proximal portion of the suture. Undermining the suture with a clamp minimizes snaring of subcutaneous tissue when the suture is tightened. The straight needle on the lateral suture is replaced with a curved cutting needle.

Step 3. The curved cutting needle on the lateral suture is passed distally between the subcutaneous tissue and the tendon sheath (parallel to the tendon) and out the skin at the level of the midportion of the distal segment of the ruptured tendon about 1.25 cm distal to the rupture gap.

Step 4. The distal skin exit hole is carefully enlarged around the curved needle (before pulling the suture through the skin) with the #15 blade and a small curved hemostat, to separate the subcutaneous tissue from the tendon sheath. The suture is then pulled through the enlarged curved needle puncture hole.

Step 5. The curved needle is replaced with the straight needle on the lateral suture. The suture is then passed back through the enlarged lateral skin puncture hole and transversely through the tendon and out the skin on the medial side. At this point, the suture courses transversely through the tendon 1.25 cm distal to the rupture defect. The medial skin puncture hole is enlarged around the needle (before pulling the suture through the skin) with the #15 blade and curved hemostat.

Step 6. The suture on the medial side is pulled through the enlarged distal medial needle puncture hole and is pulled taut. This flattens the suture against the lateral aspect of both the proximal and distal segments of the tendon.

Step 7. A curved needle again replaces the straight needle on the distal medial suture, and passes the suture through the distal medial skin puncture hole proximally between the subcutaneous tissues and the tendon sheath (parallel to the tendon) and out through the enlarged medial skin puncture hole at the level of the rupture gap. Thus, two sutures exit from the skin at the middle hole on the medial aspect of the ankle.

Step 8. Traction is applied to both of the free ends of the suture in a criss-cross manner. This traction is applied while the ankle is positioned in maximum equinus, and the ends of the ruptured Achilles tendon are approximated. Once the approximation is considered complete, a surgeon's knot is tied, followed by two more knots. The suture is cut short and then pushed subcutaneously with the point of the hemostat. No skin sutures are required, since stab wounds and puncture wound enlargements are limited. The puncture wounds are covered with a dry sterile dressing.

Step 9. A non-weight-bearing short-leg cast is applied to the injured leg with the ankle in equinus. All patients are treated with a non-weight-bearing equinus short-leg cast for 4 weeks postoperatively. A short-leg equinus cast that permits weight-bearing is then applied for an additional 4 weeks. Patients are then instructed in toe-heel-raising gastrocnemius-soleus exercises and continue these for 4 weeks. Finally, patients are given heel-cord stretching exercises for an additional 4 weeks.

When performing the procedure, several points are important, including (1) tying the surgeon's knot on the medial side of the tendon (to avert sural nerve damage); (2) separating subcutaneous tissue from the tendon sheath adequately for suture passage (to avert adhesions and skin dimpling); (3) limiting the final surgeon's knot to only about two further knots (to minimize tender nodule granuloma formation about the knot); and (4) averting damage to the suture when enlarging skin puncture wounds (damaged sutures will break under tension).

We have no experience with this technique, but Ma and Griffith[64] and Rowley and Scotland[90] reported excellent results with only minor complications. There were no reruptures of repaired tendons, no wound infections, and ankle plantar flexion power was superior to closed methods. Complications consisted of one sural nerve injury, one tender nodule at the site of a surgical knot, and one skin retraction in 28 patients.

Neglected Rupture of the Achilles Tendon

When end-to-end repair of the ruptured Achilles tendon is not possible because of contraction and retraction of its parts and the intervening scar, a neglected rupture exists. The time interval between the injury and established neglected rupture may be only a few weeks, but it is usually 2 to 3 months.

Diagnosis

Diagnosis of a neglected rupture is essentially the same as for acute injuries. The patient usually remembers the time of the injury, when snapping in the leg and subsequent pain occurred. Although the patient is often able to walk, standing and walking for prolonged periods becomes difficult, tiring, and often painful.

The gaps in the tendon to be bridged are 2 to 6 cm long. Peritenoneum, hypertrophied to a thick fibrous sheath, must be carefully dissected and preserved at surgery and used to cover the repair site.

Treatment

Treatment of a neglected rupture is surgical unless contraindicated by a situation that would be prejudicial to surgical success. For situations in which the gap in the tendon cannot be bridged by mobilization of the tendon ends and direct suture, successful surgical repair has been described with tendon and fascial strips,[10,11] with plantaris and peroneus brevis tendons,[105] and by a VY sliding flap from the proximal part of the tendon.[1] The technique we recommend for the late repair or rerupture of the Achilles tendon is the VY tendinous flap of Abraham and Pankovich.[1]

VY Tendinous Flap: Abraham and Pankovich

A curvilinear incision (Fig. 130-8A) is made and the sural nerve dissected and retracted. The peritenoneum is incised longitudinally. The scar tissue in the gap is excised; the tendon ends are mobilized and trimmed. The length of the defect is measured with the knee at 30 degrees of flexion and the foot at 20 degrees of plantar flexion.

The apex of the inverted V incision is made in the middle of the musculotendinous junction. The arms of the V incision are designed to be at least 1½ times the length of the defect in the tendon to allow for suturing in a Y configuration. The incision cuts through the aponeurosis and the underlying muscle tissue along the sides of the flap (Fig. 130-8B).

The flap is now pulled distally, until the tendon ends meet, and is sometimes dissected almost as a free graft. The proximal part of the flap incision is converted to, and sutured in, a Y configuration (Fig. 130-8C). The ruptured ends are sutured with interrupted stitches. The peritenoneum is sutured over the repair site, and the wound is closed. A long-leg cast is applied with the knee at 30 degrees of flexion and the ankle at 20 degrees of plantar flexion.

Postoperative Management The long-leg cast is removed after 6 to 8 weeks; a short walking cast is then worn for 4 to 6 weeks. A heel lift of 1 to 2 cm is used for another 1 to 2 months.

Bosworth Procedure

A vertical incision is made over the posterior surface of the calf from the heel to the upper third of the leg (Fig. 130-9). After the skin and subcutaneous tissues have been divided, the Achilles tendon and the upward extension of its tendinous raphe are exposed. A 1.3-cm-wide strip of tendon is freed

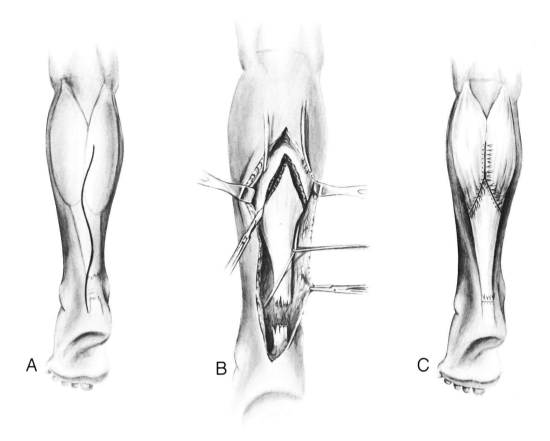

Fig. 130-8. VY tendinous flap technique in repair of the neglected rupture of the Achilles tendon. **(A)** The incision. **(B)** V incision in gastroc-soleus aponeurosis. **(C)** Y suture of the lengthened tendon. (From Abraham,[1] with permission.)

from the central portion of this raphe from above downward and left attached to the proximal end of the tendon just above the defect. This provides a section of tendinous tissue 18 to 23 cm in length. Closure of the defect left with interrupted sutures reconstitutes the lower calf muscles and the upper portion of the Achilles tendon. The strip of tendon, turned downward, is then passed transversely through the proximal end of the ruptured Achilles tendon in order to imbricate it there and to prevent it from pulling out. One or two chromic sutures should be passed through this area to fix it further. The fibrous tissue interposed between the actual tendon ends should be removed. The strip of tendon is passed transversely through the distal end of the Achilles tendon beyond the defect and then is passed through this same distal end from ventral to dorsal. It is drawn tight, and this area is sutured with chromic catgut to prevent the strip from tearing out. The strip is brought upward and is passed transversely again through the proximal end of the Achilles tendon and is drawn tight, fixed with one or two chromic sutures, and brought down and again sutured to itself. The procedure should be carried out with the foot in plantar flexion, since the calf muscles are to be drawn down as nearly into the normal position as possible. The tendon graft crossing the defect does not have sufficient strength to resist the forces imposed by the calf muscles but merely acts as a bridge of continuity of tendinous tissue between the separated ends. Following plaster encasement with the foot in plantar

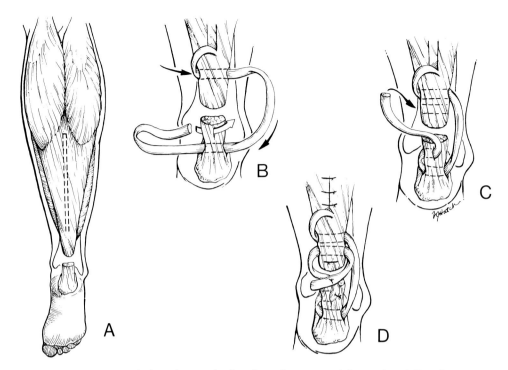

Fig. 130-9. (A-D) Bosworth technique for repair of neglected ruptures of the tendo achilles. See text. (Modified from Bosworth,[10] with permission.)

flexion and with non-weight bearing for 6 weeks, marked hypertrophy of tendinous structure occurs. Another 6 weeks is spent in gradually reestablishing weight bearing with gradual decrease in the size of this reparative tendinous mass. Full weight bearing is permitted in these patients approximately 3 months after operation.

Transfer of Peroneus Brevis Tendon

White and Kraynick[114] described the transfer of the peroneus brevis tendon to the os calcis for neglected ruptures of the Achilles tendon. A modified technique that is easily adaptable to this situation has been described by Teuffer[105] for acute ruptures of the Achilles tendon.

Technique: Modified Teuffer A curvilinear incision is carried down the lateral side of the Achilles tendon.[105] The insertion of the peroneus brevis tendon on the fifth metatarsal is exposed through a small incision, and the tendon is detached and re-

tracted proximally after the septum separating the posterior from the lateral compartment is excised.

The peritenoneum is incised longitudinally on its lateral side and the scar tissue between the ruptured tendon ends excised. The plantaris tendon is cut as far proximal as possible and used as a free graft across the gap with the foot at 20 degrees of plantar flexion. A hole large enough to permit passage of the peroneus brevis tendon is drilled transversely through the os calcis. The tendon is pulled laterally to medially and is sutured to the medial edge of the Achilles tendon as far proximal as possible (Fig. 130-10). The peritenoneum is sutured over the repair site, and the wound is closed.

Postoperative Management A long-leg cast is applied with the knee in 30 degrees of flexion and the ankle at 20 degrees of plantar flexion. The cast is removed at 6 weeks, and a short walking cast is applied for 4 to 6 weeks. An ankle-foot orthosis with a 90-degree dorsiflexion stop is worn for an additional 6 to 12 weeks.

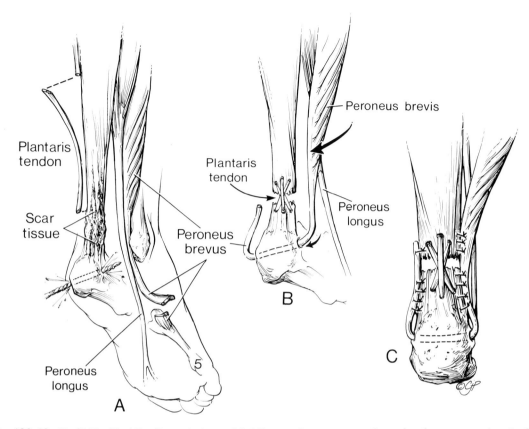

Fig. 130-10. (A-C) Modified Teuffer technique of Achilles tendon reconstruction using the peroneus brevis. See text. (Modified from Teuffer,[105] with permission.)

Results

Although the optimum results of repair of a neglected Achilles tendon rupture will take longer to achieve, and there will be about 1 cm of calf atrophy, careful physical therapy will usually result in gastroc-soleus strength of 85 percent of the uninjured side.[96] The patient should be able to lift equally off both heels.

Barnes and Hardy[6] reported good results with both the Bosworth and Abraham and Pankovich procedures in late reconstruction of the ruptured Achilles tendon. Other procedures for neglected rupture of the Achilles tendon have been described by White and Kraynick[114] and Bugg and Boyd.[12] These procedures have the disadvantage of requiring a second surgical incision and of using a free fascia lata graft that may more easily become infected in case of problems with wound healing.[67]

The reader is referred to the references at the end of this chapter for further details concerning these procedures.

Common Complications After Repair of the Achilles Tendon

Complications are best avoided. A review of published surgical complications suggests that they are more frequent after the use of pull-out suture techniques and when avascular grafts used to supplement the surgical repair. In the event of sinus formation and infection, nonabsorbable suture material may have to be removed in order to achieve wound healing. Patients with a history of local steroid injection or of systemic steroid use, diabetes, peripheral vascular disease, and unsatisfactory local skin conditions will have an increased incidence of complications, if surgical repair is attempted.

Rerupture of the Tendon

Rerupture of the tendon usually occurs 1 or 2 weeks after the cast immobilization is discontinued. Another immediate surgical repair is indicated.

Skin Necrosis

Necrosis of skin edges and infection of the wound can occur. Although this problem may be related to trauma to the skin and subcutaneous tissues during surgery, it may also result from failure to pad the incisional area sufficiently, combined with the increased heat generated by fast-setting plasters.[44,52]

Turning the casted heel into a dependent position on a pillow will not allow heat from the setting plaster to escape. For this reason, we suggest applying the short-leg portion of the cast with the patient prone and using cold water to prolong the plaster setting time. Early radical debridement of all necrotic tissue is important to prevent total necrosis of the Achilles tendon. Following debridement, the wound is left open and saline or iodine-povidine dressings are used until a clean granulating wound is achieved. Subsequent skin grafting may be necessary to prevent excessive scarring.

Scars and Adhesions of the Tendon and Skin

Scars and adhesions of the tendon and skin are a consequence of skin necrosis and infection. These complications also develop if the peritenoneum and subcutaneous tissue are not meticulously repaired. Excision of the scar and adhesions and various plastic procedures such as rotation flaps may be necessary along with cast immobilization.

Partial Rupture of the Achilles Tendon

In contrast to complete Achilles tendon rupture, partial rupture of the Achilles tendon occurs most often in persons who have continued to be physically active. The typical patient is between the ages of 19 and 30 years and is engaged in running on a hard surface. The rupture may occur from one sudden effort or gradually from repetitive trauma. The pain is localized to the Achilles tendon above the retrocalcaneal bursa and below the gastroc-soleus musculature. On physical examination, localized tenderness, thickening, and induration are the most common findings. Increased dorsiflexion, calf atrophy, and occasionally ecchymosis also occur. Partial rupture may progress to complete rupture, if loading on the tendon is not reduced.

Ljungqvist[61] defined subcutaneous partial rupture of the Achilles tendon as a tear of a varying number of fibers in the free portion of the tendon that leaves most fibers intact. Histologically, the partial rupture is characterized by devitalized tendon tissue with a frayed fibrous structure surrounded by granulation tissue that is transformed into tendonlike connective tissue.

Differential Diagnosis

Partial Achilles tendon rupture appears to merge clinically with Achilles paratendonitis. Complete Achilles tendon ruptures can be diagnosed by the absence of plantar flexion with the Thompson-Doherty calf squeeze test. Other entities to be included in the differential diagnosis include rupture of the medial head of the gastrocnemius, retrocalcaneal bursitis, stress fractures, and periostitis of the tibia and fibula.

Treatment

Initially, patients are treated conservatively with rest, physical therapy, and anti-inflammatory medications. When training is resumed, it must progress gradually; running on hard surfaces should be avoided. Conservative treatment is often unsuccessful and, when symptoms recur with increased activity, surgical treatment may be required.

Surgical Treatment

The operation is performed with the patient prone, and a tourniquet is used. A medial curvilinear incision is made from the insertion of the Achilles tendon proximal to the gastroc-soleus musculature. The peritenoneum is divided in the midline and the ruptured tendon ends are exposed. Any granulation or devitalized tissue is excised. If no pathologic changes are seen on the surface of the tendon, palpation of the tendon will usually indicate areas of abnormal consistency or thickening. A longitudinal incision of the altered portion of the tendon will usually disclose the pathologic changes. After the pathologic tissue has been excised, the defect is closed side-to-side or end-to-end with fine sutures. In some instances, localized plastic closure of the tendon defects with the use of plantaris tendon or a flap of Achilles tendon turned down after the method of Lindholm[57] will be required.

Postoperative Care Ljungqvist recommends immobilization in a short-leg plaster cast, with the foot moderately plantar flexed to reduce tension in the sutured area. The cast is changed after 3 weeks, and a new short-leg cast is applied in 10 to 15 degrees of plantar flexion for an additional 2 to 3 weeks. At this time, the cast is removed and rehabilitation started.

Denstad and Roass[20] generally have the patient start immediate range-of-motion exercises of the ankle except in those situations in which the defect after excision was great enough to require a modified Lindholm repair. In this situation, a plaster cast is applied for 6 weeks.

Complications Ljungqvist and Denstad have reported infection, hematoma, seroma, and adherent scars as isolated occurrences after surgery in more than 80 operations. The usual patient will be walking on ordinary surfaces within 6 to 8 weeks of surgery and will resume athletic training 2 to 6 months after surgery. Complete recovery may not occur, however, until 12 months after surgery. Reoperation and dissatisfaction were present in 3 of 54 of Denstad's patients. Two of Ljungqvist's 24 patients were not able to return to competitive athletics.

Acute and Chronic Rupture of the Anterior Tibialis Tendon

Rupture of the tibialis anterior tendon is rare.[22,59,70] It usually follows a minor injury in the elderly and occurs between the extensor retinaculum and the insertion of the tendon. Early disability may be slight, hence the diagnosis delayed. The patient has a feeling of instability of the ankle, weakness, and limitation of dorsiflexion in inversion; the gait is of the drop-foot type. A firm mass in the line of the tendon at the extensor retinaculum and absence of the tendon distally help confirm the loss of function as a rupture.

Treatment

Operative repair is the procedure of choice and requires sufficient exposure along the course of the tendon to mobilize the proximal end and reapproximate it distally.

Technique: Mensor and Ordway

A longitudinal curvilinear incision is begun on the dorsomedial aspect of the foot just distal to the navicular and brought proximally and anteriorly just lateral to the medial malleolus.[70] The tendon usually does not retract proximal to the superior extensor retinaculum. If the rupture is found at or near the insertion, the tendon should be fixed directly to the medial cuneiform by means of drill holes and heavy nonabsorbable suture material.

In chronic cases, there may be a gap, and tendon grafting or transfer may be necessary. The tendon of the extensor of the fifth toe may be used as the graft. The extensor hallucis longus can be used to bridge the gap by transferring its tendon to the distal portion of the tibialis anterior or its insertion. The proximal portion of the tibialis anterior can be sutured to the extensor hallucis tendon as far distally as possible. The extensor hallucis tendon would have to be sectioned with enough length to allow it to be brought out above the extensor retinaculum and rerouted along the course of the tibialis anterior tendon. The distal portion of the extensor hallucis longus is then inserted into the long extensor tendon of the second toe. To restore the gliding of the tendon, it may be necessary to incise the extensor retinaculum if the site of the tendon repair impinges on it.

Postoperative Management A short-leg cast with the foot at 90 degrees is used for 6 weeks, after which physical therapy to restore active motion is begun. Weight bearing and active use should be restricted with crutches for a total of 8 weeks. Recovery should be completed within 3 to 6 months.

Rupture of the Posterior Tibial Tendon

Rupture of the posterior tibial tendon presents a contrast with Achilles tendon rupture. This disorder appears most commonly in women beyond 50 years of age, and a specific history of injury may not be present. A noticeable disability as evidenced by a painful flat foot (Fig. 130-11) with valgus instability results. The diagnosis is made by finding weakness when testing inversion strength of the forefoot from a position of abduction and plantar flexion. A palpable contraction of the posterior tibial tendon may be felt between the navicular and the medial malleolus, if the tendon is not completely separated. Additional diagnostic features include swelling and tenderness along the course of the tendon posterior and inferior to the medial malleolus, lack of heel inversion while rising on the toes, and the inability to perform a single limb-heel rise test. [31,48,66] Posterior tibial tendon dysfunction may result not only from rupture, but also from degeneration of the tendon with elongation and from tenosynovitis. The diagnosis is frequently delayed. Treatment with arch supports, antiinflam-

matory medication, and steroid injection into the tendon sheath proves ineffective. The use of a short-leg brace with an arch support, medial heel wedge, and T-strap, although suboptimal treatment, may slow the progression of the deformity in the older sedentary patient who is willing to accept the progressive deformity rather than submit to an operation (Fig. 130-12). For most patients with suspected tears of the tendon surgical exploration should be carried out.[35] Although weight-bearing radiographs of the foot may show a valgus position of the heel with abduction of the forefoot at the midtarsal joints, radiographic examination adds little to the clinical diagnosis. Occasionally, periosteal new bone formation is seen about the medial malleolus in patients with chronic tenosynovitis. This problem may result from infection, rheumatoid arthritis, pulmonary osteoarthropathy, or pigmented villonodular synovitis.[77]

Three different situations can confront the surgeon at the time of the operation, all of which may present with the same clinical picture: (1) the posterior tibial tendon may rupture from its insertion on the navicular and first cuneiform or in mid-substance just distal to the medial malleolus; (2) there

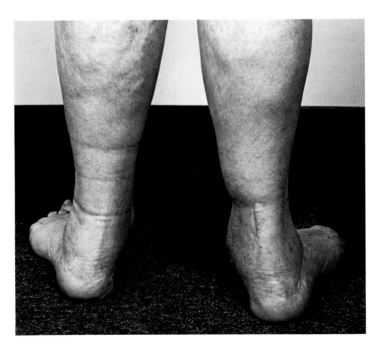

Fig. 130-11. Planovalgus deformity of both feet as the result of loss of posterior tibialis tendon function.

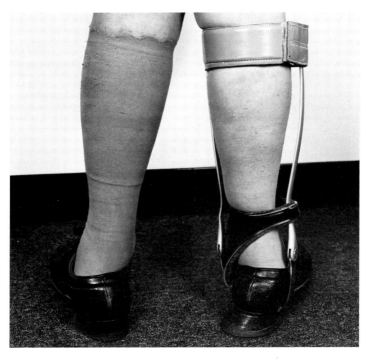

Fig. 130-12. Correction obtained with orthotic treatment of planovalgus deformity resulting from posterior tibial tendon dysfunction.

may be an in continuity tear with elongation of the tendon; and (3) there may be tenosynovitis without disruption of the tendon.

Technique

A curvilinear incision is made over the course of the posterior tibial tendon on the medial aspect of the foot and ankle extending from the first cuneiform posteriorly toward the medial malleolus and then proximally as far as required to retrieve the proximal end of the tendon. The tibialis posterior is the first structure posterior to the medial malleolus lying just ahead of the flexor digitorum longus and the posterior tibial neurovascular bundle. It is held in position behind the medial malleous by the flexor retinaculum. Below the medial malleolus, it turns forward superficial to the plantar calcaneonavicular ligament to expand and divide into bands inserting into the tuberosity of the navicular, the plantar surfaces of the three cuneiforms, and the bases of the second, third, and fourth metatarsals and cuboid bone. For those patients in whom the

insertion of the posterior tibial tendon has been disrupted, the tendon should be freed proximally to ensure that it moves freely in the tendon sheath and that the muscle exhibits normal elasticity. It is then sutured to the first cuneiform and navicular, using heavy nonabsorbable sutures through drill holes to apply the tendon to a bleeding bony surface, or may be passed through a drill hole in the bone and sutured on itself. For a clean laceration of the posterior tibial tendon proximal to the insertion, a conventional tendon repair using a Kessler or Bunnell stitch of 3-0 nylon or 3-0 Prolene should be carried out.

In the more usual situation, in which the tendon is ruptured as part of a degenerative process, there may be scarring of the tendon to the tendon sheath. A flexor digitorum longus transfer is recommended. Several different techniques using this tendon have been described.

Wrenn[116] described satisfactory results by transferring the flexor digitorum longus tendon to the posterior tibial tendon insertion. In this technique, the proximal segment of the posterior tibial tendon is sutured to the flexor digitorum longus above the medial malleolus. Mann and Thompson[66] described the details of a similar surgical technique.

Technique: Mann and Thompson

The posterior tibial tendon is exposed through an incision along the course of the tendon.[66] When opening the tendon sheath, it is important to preserve at least 2 cm of sheath beneath the medial malleolus. The tendon ends are exposed and mobilized. When exploration fails to show the tendon in the region of the medial malleolus and the navicular, the exploration is continued proximally, until the proximal end of the posterior tibial tendon is located. The flexor digitorum longus tendon is then identified in the midpart of the foot, where it crosses the flexor hallucis longus tendon. The abductor hallucis muscle is retracted plantarward. The fascia of the flexor digitorum brevis muscle is incised longitudinally and retracted plantarward. The tendon to be transferred is carefully separated from the flexor hallucis longus tendon, and its distal end is sutured to the flexor hallucis and then cut proximal to the suture line. Care must be taken in this exposure to protect the posterior tibial artery and nerve and their medial plantar branches, which cross these tendons in the foot. The proximal part of the flexor digitorum longus tendon is rerouted through the tendon sheath of the posterior tibialis and passed dorsally through a vertical drill hole in the navicular and sutured, with maximum tension, on itself. This is done with the foot in maximum plantar flexion and inversion. If scarring in the sheath of the posterior tibial tendon is too extensive to permit free gliding of the transferred flexor digitorum longus, that tendon is left in its own sheath and anchored to the navicular as described.

The transferred tendon is then augmented by suturing the proximal stump of the posterior tibial tendon to the flexor digitorum longus just distal to the musculotendinous junction.

Postoperative Management A short-leg cast with the foot inverted and plantar flexed is applied and worn for 4 weeks. This is followed by plantigrade casting of the foot for another 6 weeks. During this time, weight bearing is permitted. Following cast removal, the patient begins range-of-motion exercises to establish gliding of the transferred tendon.

These are followed by progressive manual resistance strengthening of the muscle tendon unit. Partial weight bearing with crutches is permitted using shoes with an arch support and medial heel wedge and flare.

Technique: Jahss

Jahss[42] frees the scarred elongated posterior tibialis tendon from its sheath and joins the healthy proximal and distal portions of this tendon side-to-side to the flexor digitorum longus tendon (Fig. 130-13). No tourniquet is used. A 17- to 20-cm curved skin incision is made from the navicular tuberosity proximally along the course of the tibialis posterior tendon. The tibialis posterior sheath is opened proximal to the navicular tuberosity and is followed through the scarred torn tendon area and then proximally to expose about 9 cm of normal tendon. The adjacent sheath of the flexor digitorum longus is opened, and the tendon is completely mobilized. Care is taken to avoid damage to the posterior tibial neurovascular bundle, which lies just posterior to the flexor digitorum longus.

Proximally, moderate tension is placed equally on the normal tibialis posterior tendon and the adjacent flexor digitorum longus tendon. They are sutured side to side in this area using #0 nylon. The foot is then slightly inverted and moderately plantar flexed. Moderate tension is placed simultaneously on the distal normal portion of the tibialis posterior tendon and the adjacent flexor digitorum longus tendon, and the tendons are similarly sutured side to side with #0 nylon. The tendons, including the sites of suture, are loosely covered with their available sheaths, along with local crural fascia, to provide a nonconstricting smooth pulley. It is important to close the sheaths, especially under the medial malleolus, to avoid anterior subluxation of the tendons. Subcutaneous and skin closure is done, and a short-leg cast is applied maintaining the foot in plantar flexion and mild inversion.

Postoperative Care The patient is placed on nonweight bearing crutch walking until the cast is removed 7 weeks later. Limited weight bearing is then permitted, during which time the patient gently exercises the ankle and subtalar joint. Subsequently an orthopaedic oxford shoe is worn with a

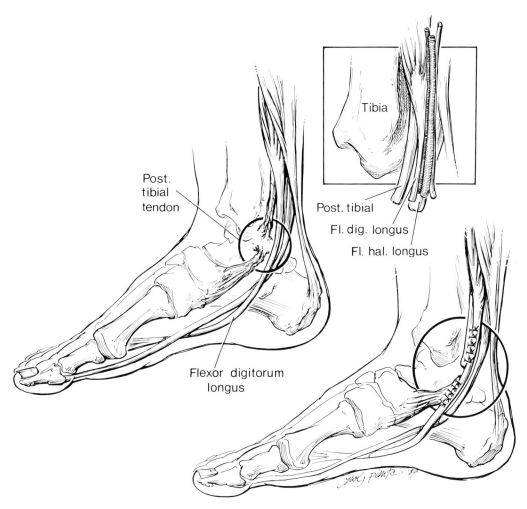

Fig. 130-13. Jahss technique of repair of spontaneous rupture of the posterior tibial tendon using flexor digitorum longus. See text.

long medial counter and a ³⁄₁₆-inch medial heel wedge.

Results

Successful surgery should eliminate pain, stop the progression of the flat-foot deformity, and restore inversion power in the hindfoot. Since the strength of the flexor digitorum longus muscle is only one-third that of the posterior tibial muscle, complete cosmetic correction of the flat-foot deformity should not be anticipated. A residual flat-foot deformity is usually present.

Goldner et al.[33] suggest that plication of the plantar calcaneonavicular ligament with nonabsorbable sutures by advancing a large distally based tongue of tissue proximally will result in a more complete correction than that obtained by tendon transfer alone.

Complications

For those patients with persistent pain and deformity following surgery double arthrodesis of the calcaneal-cuboid and talonavicular joints, subtalar, and triple arthrodesis have been recommended. For those patients who have elongation of the tendon without complete rupture, improvement has been reported following debridement, synovectomy, and division of the flexor retinaculum, thus decompressing the tendon sheath or by resection and reanastomosis of the elongated portion of the tendon.[66,107]

For the patient with an intact tendon and tenosynovitis,[115] tenosynovectomy and decompression by release of the flexor retinaculum are recommended. Care should be taken to open the flexor retinaculum at its posterior margin and to preserve its anterior portion attached to the medial malleolus. The dysfunctional posterior tibial tendon resulting in a painful flat foot should be treated by early surgical exploration and repair, if a good result is to be obtained.

TENDON LENGTHENING

Lengthening of the Achilles Tendon

Lengthening of the Achilles tendon is occasionally required to enable the heel to be brought to the floor into a better position for walking. Cozen[17] studied the effect of lengthening the Achilles tendon on the strength of the gastrocsoleus musculature. He found that strength usually improved in children. The abnormally shortened condition of the muscle fibers and of the contracted gastrocsoleus mechanism seemed to be an important factor in causing atrophy. There did not appear to be a significant difference whether a Z-type lengthening, with suture of the edges of the severed tendon, or a sliding-lengthening with partial severance of the tendon was carried out. Correction of a contracted heel cord by stretching with the use of serial plaster casts also resulted in improved strength in the gastroc-soleus musculature, which correlated with improved heel position.

White[113] and Cummins et al.[18] noted that the gastrocnemius and soleus portions of the Achilles tendon can be identified because they lie laterally and anteromedially, respectively. These workers suggest the use of this division when lengthening the tendon. However, significant variation in this anatomy makes the method unpredictable. Percutaneous lengthening is described in Section 9.

Treatment

Technique

The patient is placed in a prone position with a tourniquet around the thigh. A longitudinal lazy S incision is made on the posteromedial aspect of the ankle and is extended proximally up the leg. After the skin and subcutaneous tissues have been divided, the peritenoneum is incised longitudinally and left attached to the superficial tissues. The Achilles tendon is lengthened by one of three methods (Fig. 130-14). In the sagittal and coronal Z lengthening, a scalpel is inserted in the appropriate plane, splitting the tendon for approximately 8 cm. In the sagittal lengthening, the proximal cut usually exits laterally, and the distal cut exists medially. In the coronal plane lengthening, the proximal cut exits dorsally and the distal cut ventrally. The sectioned tendon ends are then approximated with a few interrupted sutures in the desired position. In the sliding lengthening, the incisions are determined by rotation of the fibers of the Achilles tendon. The objective is to divide one-half of the fibers proximally and the other one-half of the fibers distally. This frequently requires a transverse anteromedial incision distally near the insertion of the tendon and a transverse posteromedial incision at the proximal end of the tendon. Forceful dorsiflexion of the foot should then result in a sliding-lengthening of the partially sectioned Achilles tendon. If lengthening does not occur, palpation of the tendon will indicate a site laterally where a third transverse incision midway between the other two should be made to accomplish the lengthening. The peritenoneum and the subcutaneous tissues must be carefully sutured over the lengthened tendon, to prevent adhesions.

Postoperative Management A short-leg cast is applied with the foot in a neutral position and is worn for about 6 weeks. In instances in which the lengthening is done for a spastic neuromuscular disorder, a long-leg cast with the knee in extension may be required. Following this, range-of-motion exercises are started to establish gliding of the tendon, followed by a progressive resistance-strengthening program. Protective splinting is used for an additional period of time to prevent recurrence of the contracture.

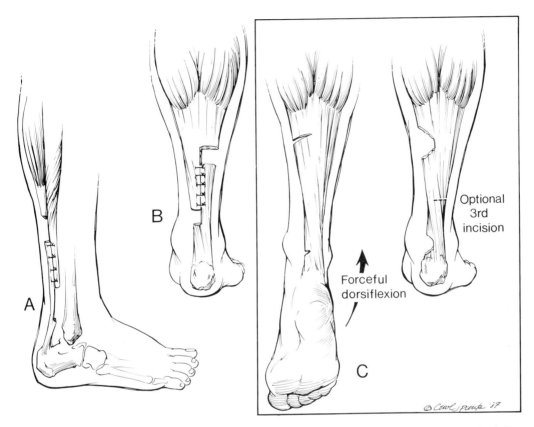

Fig. 130-14. Three methods of lengthening of the Achilles tendon. **(A)** Z-lengthening in the sagittal plane. **(B)** Z-lengthening in the coronal plane. **(C)** Sliding lengthening of the tendon by partial section and forceful dorsiflexion of the foot. See text.

Contractures of the Posterior Ankle Capsule

Contractures of the posterior ankle capsule often accompany contracture of the heel cord and are frequently seen in patients with congenital deformities of the feet, poliomyelitis, cerebral palsy, sciatic or peroneal nerve injuries, and major trauma of the leg.

Treatment

Posterior Capsulotomy

In cases of severe contracture of the ankle, it is well to divide the Achilles tendon completely and to reflect it so that the posterior capsulotomy may be carried out without hindrance. Posterior capsulotomy is carried out between the flexor hallucis longus and peroneus brevis tendons, by reflecting the flexor hallucis medially. This protects the tibial vessels and nerve that lie between the flexor hallucis longus and flexor digitorum longus from injury (Fig. 130-15).

The posterior capsule is identified and divided horizontally to the medial and lateral malleoli. Occasionally, to obtain correction of the severely contracted ankle, the following ligaments may need to be released: the posterior inferior tibiofibular, the transverse tibiofibular, the posterior talofibular, and rarely, the calcaneofibular, and the posterior portion of the deltoid ligament.

When the contracture is the result of a neurologic injury such as stroke or cerebral palsy, the foot generally is not immobilized dorsiflexed beyond a right angle. When the contracture is the result of trauma to the leg, immobilization in dorsi-

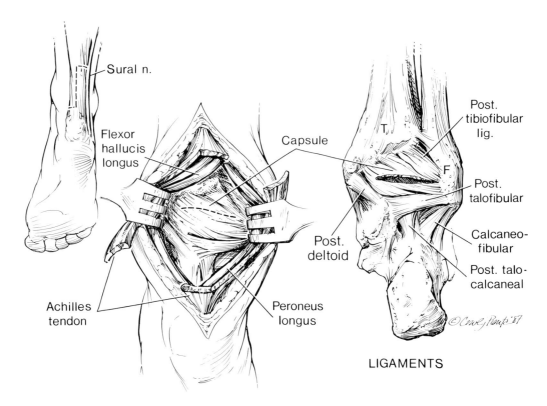

Fig. 130-15. Posterior capsulotomy of the ankle. See text.

flexion of 5 degrees is recommended. However, care must be taken not to embarrass the circulation to the skin, because a slough involving skin and even a portion of the tendon can occur. If the circulation of the skin flaps appears embarrassed, after the skin has been sutured and the tourniquet deflated with the foot in the desired position, only partial correction should be accepted. A subsequent cast change 2 weeks later, under general anesthesia, may be used to achieve further correction.

Postoperative Management A short-leg cast is applied for 6 weeks. Retentive splinting is important to prevent recurrence of the plantar flexion contracture. When scarring of the tissues on the posterior surface of the ankle has resulted from injury or previous surgical procedures, plastic repair of the involved soft tissue may be required and should be done before the contracture is corrected.

TENDON TRANSFERS

When a muscle or a muscle group acting on the foot and ankle ceases to function due either to injury or disease, a deformity may be expected from the resulting muscle imbalance. The problem may be relatively simple, as in rupture or laceration of the tendon of the tibialis posterior muscle, resulting in a flat foot. The problem may, however, be extremely complex, as in deformities resulting from anterior poliomyelitis. In such circumstances, normally functioning muscles are found along with muscles that are weakened to various degrees or are not functioning at all. Much of what we know about reestablishment of muscle power by tendon transfer has resulted from experience in treating patients with poliomyelitis.

Tendon transfer is defined as rerouting of the vector of action of a muscle-tendon unit, such that the pull of the muscle will compensate for a muscle that is functioning suboptimally. This involves a change of the point of insertion of the tendon.

When muscle imbalance occurs, every effort should be made to prevent a progressive fixed deformity by protective splinting, to prevent the overpull of active muscles. This should be combined with a physical therapy program to produce range of motion of the lost muscle function. Inconspicuous light-weight plastic orthotics may make tendon transfer unnecessary by preventing deformity, as in peroneal nerve palsy.

Principles of Tendon Transfers in the Leg and Foot

It is extremely important to keep in mind the general principles of tendon transfers in the leg and foot when doing an actual transfer.[34,35,68,79,83,84,95,101,112] Failure to do so will result in either inadequate function of the transferred muscle or a secondary deformity.

Manual Muscle Testing

Very careful manual muscle testing is essential before any tendon transfer is carried out. This should be done before and after correction of any fixed deformity because, in some instances, a muscle may appear to be functioning poorly before correction of a fixed deformity, and be quite strong following the correction. The reverse is also seen: a muscle that seems to be pulling strongly is only contracted and when the contracture is released a functional pull is not present.

Muscle Strength

The muscle to be transferred must be strong enough to carry on its new function. For example, much more power is required to provide push-off by plantar flexion of the ankle during gait, then to dorsiflex the same joint during the pickup phase. The combined push of the plantar flexor muscles create a ground reaction force that must exceed

body weight. Since one grade of motor power is usually lost with a transfer, this generally means that the weakened muscle should not be transferred. Exceptions exist, the most obvious being the benefits obtained by eliminating a deforming force or creating a weak antigravity motion to dorsiflex the ankle and foot with a grade 4 muscle. There should be adequate power in the remaining muscle, to avoid loss of function at the site from which the tendon was transferred, unless this is planned. By convention, a muscle is graded from 0 to 5:

Grade 0: No contraction
Grade 1: Palpable contraction only
Grade 2: Moves the joint but not against gravity
Grade 3: Moves a joint against gravity
Grade 4: Moves a joint against gravity and resistance
Grade 5: Normal strength

Stabilization of the Foot

With few exceptions, tendon transfers in the leg and foot must be preceded by, or combined with, stabilization of certain joints in the foot. This is quite often triple arthrodesis. Attempts to balance muscle power without stabilization of the subtalar and midtarsal joints are generally unsuccessful.[30,35,68,83,101]

Correction of Fixed Bony Deformities

Fixed bony deformities should be corrected before or, more often, at the time of tendon transfer. It is crucial to recognize these and to plan an appropriate correction. Surgical correction of fixed bony deformities and stabilization of the foot are dealt with in Section 9.

Release of Soft Tissue Contractures

Soft tissue contractures, such as those of the posterior capsule of the ankle joint or the Achilles tendon and plantar fascia, require correction either by physical therapy and retentive splinting or by surgical release before or at the time of tendon transfer.

Transfer of Antagonistic Muscles

Transfer of antagonistic muscles is often required to restore a lost function. Although good results can be expected from this type of transfer, a more lengthy and careful rehabilitation is required.

Adequate Leverage

For the muscle-tendon unit to function adequately, the tendon should be inserted at the level of the normal insertion or sometimes even distal to it.

Tendon Tension

The tension of the tendon transferred at surgery should be enough to hold the part in a slightly overcorrected position. When the patient is immobilized postoperatively, even further overcorrection should be sought to reduce any tension and consequent stretching of the transferred tendon. Failure of tendon transfers most often results from inadequate tension of the tendon, either from its laxity at surgery[100] or from postoperative stretching from inadequate immobilization. Retentive splinting to keep the transferred tendon from stretching out while strength of the muscle is restored is a crucial part of postoperative management.

Direct Line of Transfer

A direct line of transfer of a tendon is desirable so that angulations do not interfere with muscle function and so that, as angulation decreases with repeated usage, the tendon transfer does not become lax.

Preservation of Neurovascular Supply

The neurovascular supply of the transferred muscle must not be damaged while transferring the tendon. This is an important consideration, since it is usually not sufficient to redirect the tendon itself; a portion of the muscle must also be mobilized for redirection.

Prevention of Adhesions

Adhesions are prevented by careful handling of the tendon, passing it through the subcutaneous tissue or a tendon sheath. Contact of the tendon with bone or interosseous membrane should be prevented, except at the site of insertion. The tourniquet should be deflated and hemostasis carried out before wound closure. A hematoma at the operative site will result in unnecessary adhesions.

Avoidance of Ischemic Contractures

Ischemic contracture may develop if an attempt is made to suture the fascial compartments of the leg. We therefore recommend that only skin and subcutaneous tissues be closed after tendon transfer has been carried out.

Methods of Tendon Insertion

The tendon may be reattached by tendon-to-tendon, tendon-to-periosteum, or tendon-to-bone methods.[16] By far the most satisfactory method in the lower extremity is the insertion of tendon into bone, as illustrated in Figure 130-16.

The use of a pull-out wire is not recommended. It is much safer to pull a suture out in the direction of the transfer. A suture pulled out against the direction of the transfer may dislodge the transferred tendon. A wire that is kinked or crossed in a tendon frequently will break when attempts are made to remove it.

Suturing the transferred tendon to itself after passing it through bone, where possible, is the most desirable method of tendon insertion. The use of this technique is limited, however, by the size of the tendon relative to the bone. It works well for inserting the extensors of the toes into the metatarsals. A transverse drill hole is made in the metatarsal at the desired site. The tendon is prepared in such a fashion that its distal end is tapered. A suture is placed in the tendon to keep the tendon end from spreading out; the suture is then passed through the bone, followed by the tendon. The tendon is sutured on itself under maximum tension. Care must be taken that the drill hole is not so large as to weaken the structure of the bone and that it is properly positioned so that the tendon will not pull out of the bone.

In the modified pull-out suture technique, a large (6- to 8-mm) dorsal- to plantar-oriented drill hole is made in the bone. A monofilament suture of wire or heavy nylon is passed through the end of

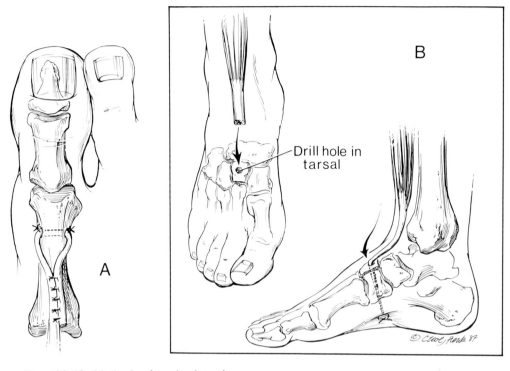

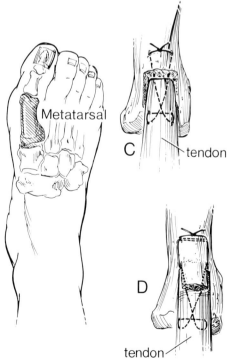

Fig. 130-16. Methods of tendon insertion. **(A)** Suturing the tendon to itself after passing it through bone. **(B)** Modified pullout suture technique. **(C)** Technique of Green. **(D)** Technique of Tachdjian. See text.

the tendon and by means of two straight needles out the plantar aspect of the foot. The tendon is then pulled into the drill hole by means of this suture which is tied over a padded button on the plantar aspect of the foot. Bredo et al.[11] recently modified this technique by making a small incision on the plantar aspect of the foot down to the plantar fascia, then passing the needles through the plantar fascia, and tying the suture under direct vision over the fascia with the foot held in the desired position. This technique is most useful when a large tendon being inserted into the tarsals or the base of a metatarsal bone.

In the Green technique, the tendon is drawn into the medullary area of a bone. A drill hole is made through the cortex into the medullary area large enough to receive the transferred tendon. The cortex distal to this hole is undermined with a curette, and two drill holes are made into this tunnel from the distal cortex. The ends of a suture in the tendon are then passed into the medulla and out the drill holes. The tendon is pulled into the medullary space and the suture tied. Adjusting tension in the tendon in this technique can be difficult. Too long a tendon will mean loss of tension; too short a tendon will mean poor fixation.

In the technique recommended by Tachdjian, an osteoperiosteal flap is created based distally. At the end of this flap, a transverse drill hole is made across the bone. The sutures that pull the tendon end beneath the flap are passed through the drill hole in opposite directions and are then tied over the bony bridge. In all these techniques, additional sutures from the surrounding periosteum to the tendon where it comes into the bone are recommended.

Secondary Deformities

After tendon transfers, secondary deformities must be anticipated.[30,112] The number of pitfalls here is immense. For example, transfer of the peroneus longus function, while leaving the tibialis anterior unopposed, causes gradual dorsiflexion of the first metatarsal bone, with a resultant dorsal bunion. Transfer of the tibialis anterior function, in the presence of active peroneus longus and toe dorsiflexors, results in claw toes and a cavus defor-

mity due to plantar flexion of the first metatarsal bone by the peroneus longus action and attempts at dorsiflexion of the foot by toe extensors. Transfer of the tibialis posterior may result in a flat foot. When one of these motor units is paralyzed, an attempt should be made to remove the deforming force to a neutral position at the time of tendon transfer.

The basic principles of tendon transfer are to stabilize the foot and to transfer the expendable motor power into the midline of the foot, either posteriorly in the case of plantar flexion insufficiency, or anteriorly in the case of dorsiflexion insufficiency.

The indications for tendon transfers in the leg and foot are neglected tendon lacerations and ruptures, peroneal nerve paralysis, muscle imbalances following stroke, sequelae of Volkmann's ischemia in the leg, sequelae of poliomyelitis, leprosy, Friedreich's ataxia, peroneal muscular atrophy, and leg muscle imbalances in cerebral palsy and myelomeningocele.

Isolated weakness of a muscle is an ideal situation for tendon transfers. Multiplicity of muscle weakness, particularly when various muscles have retained different degrees of function, poses greater problems in tendon transfer; the results of these procedures are much less certain. In this section, tendon transfers and related problems are described for common muscle weaknesses in the adult leg.

Weakness of Tibialis Anterior Muscle

The prime function of the tibialis anterior muscle is to dorsiflex the foot. It also inverts the foot and elevates the first metatarsal bone. With an isolated loss of the tibialis anterior muscle function, the continued function of the toe extensors results in claw-toe deformities, and the continued function of the peroneus longus muscle results in a tendency to a cavus foot deformity.

Paresis of Tibialis Anterior Muscle

If the function of the anterior tibialis muscle is only weakened, transfer of the extensor hallucis longus to the neck of the first metatarsal is quite satisfactory in restoring active foot dorsiflexion.[35,79,84,101] If transfer is done before a fixed cavus deformity develops, plantar fasciotomy is unnecessary. Subtalar or triple arthrodesis is not required. However, arthrodesis or tenodesis of the interphalangeal joint of the great toe is recommended. Before transfer of the tendon, any equinus contracture must be corrected by either stretching with serial casts or by release of the contracted Achilles tendon and posterior capsule. The modified Jones technique for transfer of the extensor hallucis longus is described in Section 9, Chapter 146.

Paralysis of the Anterior Tibialis Muscle

When the function of the tibialis anterior muscle is completely lost, more powerful tendon transfers must be undertaken to restore the dorsiflexion. Isolated paralysis of the tibialis anterior muscle is rare and may sometimes be seen in poliomyelitis. More commonly, the muscle is not paralyzed, but there is a neglected irreparable rupture of its tendon and equivalent functional loss.

In the presence of complete loss of function of all muscles in the anterior compartment of the leg due to paralysis of the deep peroneal nerve or the anterior compartment syndrome, a dropped foot with some cavus deformity may result. Often, after Volkmann's ischemia in the anterior compartment, tendon transfers are unnecessary because fibrosis and contractures of the muscles prevent the foot from dropping when protective splinting is applied.

When required, the dropped foot is treated by transfer of the peroneus longus to the midline of the dorsum of the foot, as recommended by Peabody[83,84] or by transfer of both peronei, as recommended by Mayer.[68] In addition triple arthrodesis or at least subtalar arthrodesis is needed.

Treatment

Transfer of the Peroneus Longus Tendon

Green[35] and Peabody,[83,84] among others, have described the procedure of transfer of the peroneus longus tendon. A longitudinal incision, 8 to 10 cm long, is made over the muscle-tendon junction of the peroneus longus muscle on the lateral aspect of the middle third of the leg (Fig. 130-17). Care must be taken to avoid injury to the superficial peroneal nerve, which passes forward between the peroneals and the extensor digitorum longus, then through the crural fascia at about the muscle-tendon junction of the peroneals, and continues subcutaneously as the medial and intermediate dorsal cutaneous nerves.

A second skin incision is made to expose the tendons of the peroneus longus and brevis muscles on the lateral aspect of the foot. The incision extends in a posterior direction from the base of the fifth metatarsal bone toward the calcaneus for 4 to 5 cm. At this level, the peroneus longus tendon passes posterior to the peroneus brevis tendon and beneath the cuboid onto the plantar aspect of the foot. The peroneus longus tendon is divided here as far distally as practical, so that enough tendon is available to permit transfer of the peroneus brevis tendon to its distal stump and thereby preserve support of the longitudinal arch and depression of the first metatarsal head (Fig. 130-17).

The peroneus longus tendon is now freed from the peroneus brevis tendon and the tendon sheath and is pulled proximally into the first incision. To avoid accidental displacement of the peroneus brevis tendon, it is better to carry this out before sectioning the peroneus brevis and reanastomosing it to the stump of the peroneus longus tendon.

An incision is made in the anterior peroneal intermuscular septum, which separates the anterior and lateral compartments of the leg. This approach permits the passage of the peroneus longus tendon into the anterior compartment.

A third longitudinal skin incision, 5 to 6 cm long, is made on the dorsum of the foot overlying the base of the second metatarsal bone. A tendon passer is directed proximally beneath the inferior and superior extensor retinacula, taking care not to injure the dorsalis pedis artery and the deep branch of the peroneal nerve, which pass also beneath these retinacula between the extensor hallucis longus and extensor digitorum longus tendons. The peroneus longus tendon is now drawn distally onto the dorsum of the foot and is fixed to the base of the second metatarsal bone or in the middle of the second cuneiform by one of the described techniques. The tendon should be inserted with enough tension

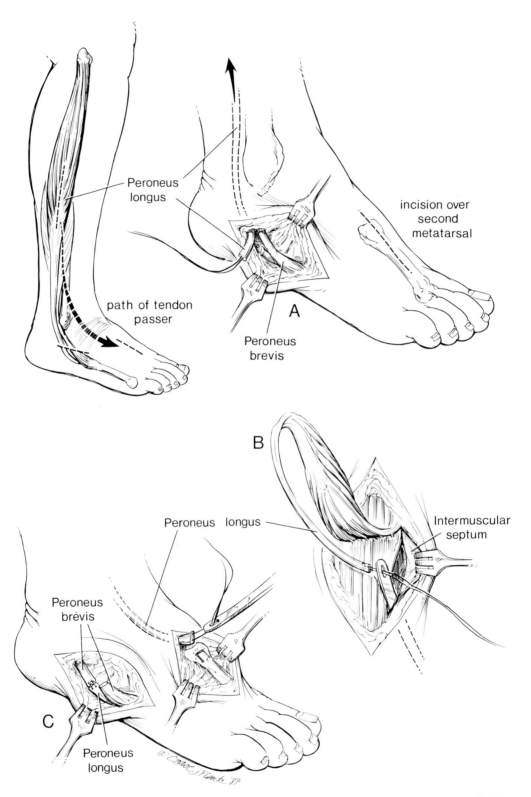

Fig. 130-17. (A-C) Transfer of the peroneus longus tendon for paralysis of the anterior tibialis muscle. See text. (Modified from Green,[35] with permission.)

to hold the ankle in 5 degrees of dorsiflexion. The peroneus longus tendon should not be transferred into the sheath and insertion of the tibialis anterior tendon because a varus deformity or even a dorsal bunion may result. The peroneus brevis tendon is cut and reanastomosed to the distal stump of the peroneus longus tendon[35] and the skin incisions are closed.

Postoperative Management The tendon transfer is protected by a short-leg cast for 4 to 5 weeks. The ankle should be in about 10 to 15 degrees of dorsiflexion to remove tension from the tendon. When the cast is removed, gentle assisted exercises are begun so that the patient will begin to use the transfer for its new function. The general principle in rehabilitation of tendon transfers is to produce the motion that was the former action of the transferred muscle while the foot is moved manually through the motion that the transfer is designed to provide. Electrical stimulation is occasionally useful in gaining control of the transfer. The peroneus longus is a more effective dorsiflexor of the foot than the peroneus brevis because of its greater excursion. In the case of transfer of the peroneus longus to restore dorsiflexion, the effort must be put into getting the tendon to function as a dorsiflexor, although it formerly functioned as a plantar flexor and evertor.

Preliminary Triple Arthrodesis

If only the peroneus longus tendon has been transferred, triple arthrodesis may be deferred if no fixed deformities require correction. With fixed deformities requiring correction or when both the peroneus longus and brevis tendons are transferred (creating mediolateral instability), triple arthrodesis should be carried out before the tendon transfer.[35,68,83,101] This may be done either several months before the tendon transfer or, ideally, at the same time.[68] This avoids the necessity of transferring tendons into osteoporotic bone resulting from the immobilization after triple arthrodesis.

Postoperative Management If triple arthrodesis has been done concomitantly, cast immobilization is continued for 8 to 12 weeks with the foot in a corrected position. A night splint is then continued for approximately 6 months, to prevent stretching of the transferred tendon.

Paralysis of the Peroneal Muscles

Now that poliomyelitis is rarely seen in the United States, instances of gross everter insufficiency resulting in varus deformity of the foot are uncommon. Isolated paralysis of the peroneal muscles might be seen rarely as a consequence of paralysis of the superficial peroneal nerve from injury, leprosy, or peroneal muscular atrophy. In these situations, the foot is inverted and weight is borne on the lateral border of the foot. A dorsal bunion is also frequently present due to the unopposed pull of the tibialis anterior muscle. Bony stabilization of the foot alone does not completely correct the varus deformity and fails to correct the dorsal bunion. Although isolated transfer of the tibialis anteriolaterad on the foot may remove the tendency for the dorsal bunion, frequently it does not balance the foot due to the presence of the tibialis posterior and the inherent difficulties of balancing the foot by tendon transfers alone.[83,84] Therefore, transfer of the tibialis anterior tendon to the midline of the foot usually must be combined with triple arthrodesis.

When there is a complete paralysis of the peroneal muscles, the anterior tibialis tendon should be transferred to the base of the third metatarsal bone. It should not be inserted further lateral because it may cause a valgus deformity.[35] The tendon is detached at the level of the talonavicular joint and withdrawn above the superior extension retinaculum. It is then redirected down the sheath of the extensor digitorum communis tendon.

Treatment

Lateral Transfer of the Tibialis Anterior Tendon

A longitudinal skin incision, 2 to 3 cm long, is made over the dorsum of the base of the first metatarsal bone and the first cuneiform where the tibialis anterior tendon is inserted. The tendon is located and divided just proximal to its insertion. At this level, the deep peroneal nerve and the dorsalis pedis artery lie lateral to the extensor hallucis longus tendon. The detached tendon is dissected proximally a short way.

The second longitudinal skin incision, 7 to 8 cm long, is made just above the superior extensor retinaculum (transverse crural ligament). The anterior tibial artery and the deep branch of the peroneal nerve are near the anterior tibial tendon in the midportion of the leg; just above the retinaculum, they pass under the tendon of the extensor hallucis longus muscle and continue on its lateral side. Care must be taken at this point to avoid damaging them when the tendon is pulled out of its sheath.

The third longitudinal skin incision, 2 to 3 cm long, is made on the dorsum of the base of the second or third metatarsal bone. Insertion of the tendon to the metatarsal provides a better lever arm than does insertion more proximally on the cuneiforms. However, tendon length may not be adequate for insertion this far distally. Care is taken to protect the dorsalis pedis artery and the deep peroneal nerve lying between the first and second metatarsals on the dorsum of the foot. This can usually be done by reflecting the extensor hallucis brevis medially and the tendons of the extensor digitorum longus laterad. A tendon passer is passed proximally within the sheath of the extensor digitorum longus tendons toward the second incision in the distal third of the leg. The sheath of the extensor digitorum longus is opened proximally, and the tibialis anterior is passed through it onto the dorsal aspect of the foot. This tibialis anterior tendon is then anchored into bone by one of the described methods with the foot at 5 degrees of dorsiflexion. All skin incisions are then closed.

Postoperative Management A short-leg cast is applied with the foot in 10 to 15 degrees of dorsiflexion. Since foot stabilization is usually carried out, the cast is removed at 12 weeks and reeducation of the transferred muscle started. The transferred tendon should be protected from stretching out by the use of a short-leg brace and a night splint for 6 months.

Combined Paresis or Paralysis of the Muscles in the Anterior and Lateral Leg Compartments

A drop-foot deformity results when, due to paralysis of the common peroneal nerve or Volkmann's ischemia of the anterior and lateral compartments, the function of the tibialis anterior, toe extensors, and peroneal muscles has been lost. This is managed by an anterior transfer of the tibialis

posterior tendon to the midline of the dorsum of the foot. The tendon is carried either around the medial border of the tibia, as advocated by Ober and Mayer, and more recently by Lipscomb and Sanchez,[60] or through the interosseous membrane as suggested by Putti and Watkins et al.[110] This is usually combined with a triple arthrodesis.

Treatment

Transfer of the Posterior Tibial Tendon Through the Interosseous Membrane: Watkins et al.

Before surgery, manual muscle testing must show that the tibialis posterior muscle is strong enough, that is, grade 4 + or better.[110] Fixed deformities, such as equinus or varus, must be corrected before the tendon is transferred. The heel of the foot must be in a neutral position, and the ankle must dorsiflex passively to at least 90 degrees.

The first incision is made on the medial border of the foot along the course of the posterior tibial tendon, from just below the medial malleolus to the medial cuneiform. The tendon is freed from its sheath and is incised distal to its primary insertion into the tuberosity of the navicular bone to add as much length as possible. It is important to avoid interfering with the spring ligament or the joint capsules on the medial border of the foot when doing this part of the procedure (Fig. 130-18) to prevent a severe drop in the medial longitudinal arch.

The second incision is made parallel and lateral to the lower third of the crest of the tibia, and the crural fascia is opened lateral to it. The anterior tibial tendon is retracted laterally along with the anterior tibial nerve and vessels to expose the interosseous membrane. The anterior tibial nerve and vessels lie deep and lateral to the anterior tibial tendon; care should be taken to protect them as the tendon is retracted. This should be accomplished without disturbing the periosteum of the tibia. The interosseous membrane is incised widely enough to allow the belly of the posterior tibial muscle to fill the interosseous space. After the opening in the interosseous membrane has been made, pressure from behind causes the muscle to bulge into the space and its tendinous portion becomes visible distally. A blunt instrument is then passed about the tendon and is pulled forward through the inter-

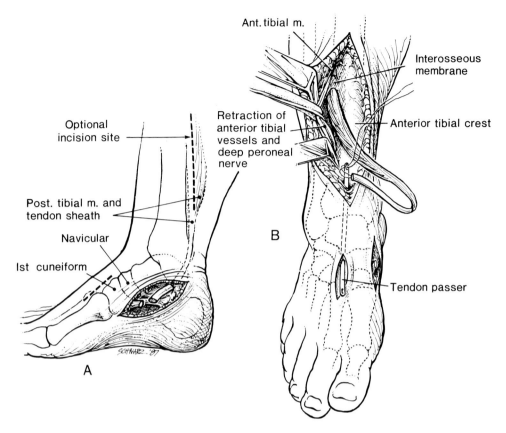

Fig. 130-18. (A,B) Transfer of the posterior tibial tendon through the interosseous membrane for paralysis of muscles in the anterior and lateral leg compartments. See text.

osseous membrane. Gentle traction on the distal end of the tendon brings more of the muscle belly into the anterior compartment (Fig. 130-18). Injury to the posterior tibial vessels and nerve lying on the posterior surface of the muscle must be avoided. If it is difficult to pull the posterior tibial tendon from the medial aspect of the ankle through the interosseous membrane, a third incision is made just posterior to the medial border of the tibia extending proximally above the metaphyseal flare. Mobilization of the tendon thus becomes easier.

The fourth incision is made on the dorsum of the foot over the desired site for insertion of the tendon, which is passed either through a subcutaneous tunnel or deep to the extensor retinaculum (Fig. 130-18). The available length of the tendon may dictate the location and method of insertion; however, the desired site of reattachment is the base of the third metatarsal.

Postoperative Management A short-leg cast with maximal dorsiflexion of the foot is applied. It is removed at 2 weeks, when skin sutures are removed. A short-leg walking cast is then applied and worn for 4 weeks. If the modified pullout suture method was used for tendon insertion, the suture is withdrawn at this time. The patient is fitted with a drop-foot brace for 3 months. Bracing is especially important when there is a strong tendency for the foot to go into equinus, thereby exerting tension on the transferred posterior tibial tendon. Muscle reeducation exercises are initiated after the cast is removed at 6 weeks.

Watkins et al.[110] performed this procedure in patients with Friedreich's ataxia, cerebral spastic paralysis, anterior poliomyelitis, congenital clubfoot, spina bifida, Charcot-Marie-Tooth disease, and common peroneal paralysis due to trauma. Triple arthrodesis was carried out prior to tendon surgery.

Recently Pinzur et al.[86] and Bredo et al.[11] described satisfactory results with transfer of the posterior tibial tendon through the interosseous membrane to the dorsum of the foot in patient's with posttraumatic paralytic peroneal foot drop without triple arthrodesis. Pinzur combined transfer of a weak or paralyzed anterior tibial tendon along with the posterior tibial tendon into the third cuneiform bone. Pinzur believed that the anterior tibial tendon would provide a static tenodesis that would restrict passive ankle equinus. At least 2 years following surgical correction, all of his nine patients walked with a heel-toe gait pattern and were able to dorsiflex their ankles past neutral against resistance. None of the patients exhibited foot deformities, and there were no significant complications.

Bredo et al.[11] modified the surgical technique. The tendon sutures are passed through a drill hole in bone to the plantar aspect of the foot; then a fourth incision is made over the plantar aspect of the foot to the plantar fascia so that the tendon sutures can be tied over the plantar fascia under direct vision. This eliminates the need for tying the suture externally over the skin or cast. Of 24 patients treated by this technique, four patients required an ankle-foot orthosis for sports and five patients had difficulty with ankle sprains. Twenty of the 24 patients had active ankle dorsiflexion to at least a neutral position with an acceptable gait. The four instances in which surgery failed are very instructive: valgus deformity of the hindfoot requiring subtalar arthrodesis, skin slough when tendon transfer was performed through compromised skin, lack of sufficient tension in the transferred tendon, and transfer of a tibialis posterior muscle weakened as the result of a complete sciatic nerve palsy.

Transfer of the Posterior Tibial Tendon Around the Medial Border of the Tibia: Ober

The first incision is made over the medial aspect of the foot along the posterior tibial tendon, which is detached from the navicular bone with a thin bone flap.[79] Care must be taken to preserve joint capsules and the spring ligament to prevent drop in the longitudinal arch (Fig. 130-19).

The second longitudinal incision, 10 to 12 cm long, is made over the junction of the posterior tibial tendon and muscle in the middle third of the leg. The tendon is drawn into the upper wound, and the muscle belly is dissected well up the tibia. The periosteum on the medial surface of the tibia is incised in an oblique direction and pushed off the bone so that the belly of the posterior tibialis muscle will be in contact with bone. The attachment of the crural fascia to the anterior tibial crest is incised and the tibialis anterior muscle retracted laterally to allow the tendon and muscle belly of the posterior tibialis muscle to enter the anterior compartment (Fig. 130-19).

The third longitudinal incision is made over the base of the third metatarsal. The posterior tibial tendon is drawn through the anterior tibial compartment such that the posterior tibial muscle is in contact with the bone surface the tibia. The distal

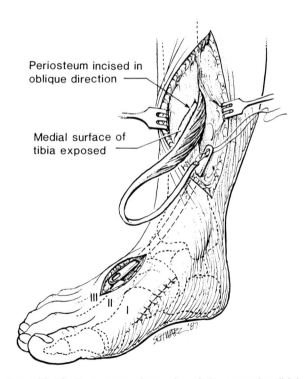

Fig. 130-19. Technique of transfer of the posterior tibial tendon around the medial border of the tibia for paralysis of muscles in the anterior and lateral leg compartments. See text.

end of the tendon is inserted into a groove in the base of the third metatarsal. Ober[79] combined this operation with a triple arthrodesis to provide mediolateral stability.

Postoperative Management The postoperative course is essentially the same as for the transfer of the posterior tibialis through the interosseous membrane.

Lipscomb and Sanchez[60] described a similar procedure for posttraumatic paralysis of the common peroneal nerve. They found that transfer of the posterior tibial tendon in a long spiral course around the medial surface of the tibia was an easier and safer surgical procedure than transfer through the interosseus membrane and that a physiologic direction of pull of the tendon is achieved. Although Ober passed the tendon through the anterior tibial sheath, they believed that it could be passed subcutaneously. The tendon was most frequently inserted into the middle cuneiform bone. Surgical stabilization of the foot by triple arthrodesis and correction of fixed equinus deformity with Achilles tendon lengthening were carried out as required during the same surgical procedure. Postoperative management was the same as for the Ober procedure.

We prefer the technique of Lipscomb and Sanchez when the posterior tibial tendon is to be transferred for a drop-foot deformity and the peroneal muscles are not available.

Results A normal posterior tibial muscle transferred for peroneal nerve palsy should provide strong dorsiflexion of the foot. However, because of limited excursion of the tendon, only 15 to 30 degrees of active ankle motion is usually obtained. This is useful range of motion for ordinary walking on a level surface and allows most patients to walk with minimal limping. These results are due to the fact that the posterior tibial tendon has an amplitude of only 2 cm of excursion whereas the dorsiflexors of the ankle have amplitudes of from 3 to 5 cm. Also, the tibialis posterior muscle is only about two-thirds the size of the tibialis anterior.

Complications When foot stabilization is not done and the transferred tendon is inserted too lateral, marked valgus results. Either the base of the third metatarsal or the middle cuneiform seems to be the ideal site for insertion of the transferred tendon. If valgus deformity develops, the tendon insertion must be repositioned more medially or a triple arthrodesis must be done; in most cases, both must be done.

Failure to estimate the strength of the tibialis posterior muscle correctly may result in its failure to function in the new position. In a rare instance, failure to estimate the strength of the gastrocsoleus group accurately could cause the posterior tibial muscle-tendon transfer to exceed the power of the calf muscles, resulting in the development of a calcaneus gait.

Finally, deficiency in posterior tibialis tendon transfer may result from the fact that, although the muscle-tendon unit can contract to provide voluntary dorsiflexion, phasic conversion of foot dorsiflexion during walking does not occur. Only careful reeducation of the muscle may resolve this problem.

Combined Transfer of the Flexor Digitorum Longus and Tibialis Posterior

Carayon et al.[14] transferred the flexor digitorum longus tendons, as well as the posterior tibialis tendon, for drop-foot deformity. These workers initially used the procedure in patients with leprosy, to avoid stabilization procedures. The procedure can be used in posttraumatic paralysis of the common peroneal nerve without triple arthrodesis.

Technique: Carayon et al. The first longitudinal incision, about 8 to 10 cm in length, is made 2 cm behind the posterior and medial border of the tibia at the lower third of the leg, ending at the tip of the medial malleolus.[14] The tendons of the tibialis posterior and flexor digitorum longus muscles are exposed and divided at the lowest possible level while the foot is maintained in plantar flexion and inversion.

The second longitudinal incision, 10 to 12 cm in length, is made 2 cm lateral to the anterior tibial crest, starting at the level of the tibial plafond and extending proximally.

The interval between the tibialis anterior and the extensor hallucis longus tendons is developed down to the interosseus membrane, which is excised as far proximally as possible. Through the interosseus membrane, the end of a curved forceps is directed along the posterior surface of the tibia. When this appears in the posterior medial incision, it is used to grasp the ends of the flexor digitorum longus and tibialis posterior tendons and bring them into the anterior compartment of the leg. Sometimes the fleshy body of one or both of these muscles extends so far distally that the muscle mass is too bulky to permit the easy gliding necessary for good function. Some of the more distal muscle fibers must then be trimmed away. The tibialis posterior is sutured to the tendon of the tibialis anterior and the flexor digitorum longus to the tendons of the extensor digitorum longus and extensor hallucis longus muscles. The attachment is of the loop type: the transferred tendon transfixes the paralyzed tendon and loops back to be sutured side to side to itself. Progressive upward splitting of the paralyzed tendon, resulting in loss of tension, is prevented by an arresting stitch in the recipient tendon. The tendon transfer should be attached as low as possible to allow tendons to pull in a straight line. Tendons should be sutured with maximum dorsiflexion of the foot and extension of the toes. When necessary, the Achilles tendon should be lengthened prior to tendon suture.

Postoperative Management A short-leg cast is applied with toes and foot maintained in dorsiflexion. Immobilization is discontinued after 3 weeks, when a drop-foot brace is applied and worn for 3 months.

The results of this procedure are quite satisfactory, especially in those patients whose foot drop resulted from trauma. In these instances, 15 degrees of dorsiflexion and more than 30 degrees of plantar flexion are obtained. A period of 3 to 6 months is necessary to obtain a full amplitude of motion, and fully automatic walking occurred after 6 months of active reeducation. Intrusion of the two tendons in the anterior compartment of the leg together with the two loops of tendon used to secure the transferred tendons prevents closure of the fascia in the leg; therefore, a hernia is visible.

Loss of Posterior Tibialis Muscle Function

Wrenn[116] described 12 patients with isolated injuries of the posterior tibial tendon in whom conventional end-to-end repair could not be done.

Since no functional deficit results from loss of flexor digitorum function, this tendon was used to restore the function of the posterior tibialis muscle. Subtalar or triple arthrodesis was not necessary, since the transferred tendon halted the progressive valgus deformity of the foot that occurs in this situation. Recently others[31,42,66] have described in more detail the technique of transfer of the flexor digitorum longus. These procedures have been described earlier in this chapter under Rupture of the Posterior Tibial Tendon.

Fried and Hendel [29] used the peroneus longus, flexor digitorum communis, the extensor hallucis longus, or the flexor hallucis longus to substitute for the tibialis posterior in children with polio. Many of these patients later required stabilization of the foot.[30]

When both the anterior and posterior tibialis muscles are paralyzed, as in poliomyelitis, the valgus deformity is severe. In addition to correction of the deformity and stabilization of the foot by triple arthrodesis, tendon transfer is required to restore dorsiflexion of the ankle. The tendon transfer chosen will depend on the deforming forces and available expendable musculature.

Other Conditions Requiring Tendon Transfers

Management of paralysis of the plantar flexors of the foot and ankle resulting in a calcaneus deformity is discussed in Section 9. The flail foot and ankle can be treated with a double upright AFO, which includes an ankle and foot lacer to provide medial and lateral stability or by pantalar arthrodesis. Before pantalar arthrodesis is done, the surgeon should be sure that the patient has the prerequisite musculature to stabilize the knee and hip. If the proximal portion of the limb is weak, preoperative casting or bracing in the proposed position of arthrodesis should be done to ensure that this position does not impair the patient's ability to ambulate.

Progressive Neuromuscular Atrophy

When symptoms of progressive neuromuscular atrophy (Charcot-Marie-Tooth disease) start in the second or third decade, these patients often present with a symmetric peroneal muscular atrophy that causes a bilateral varus deformity.[94] Later the atrophy spreads to the muscles of the anterior compartment. For this reason, transfer of the tibialis anterior tendon alone is not satisfactory, and anterior transfer of the posterior tibialis tendon should be considered.

Complete Sciatic Nerve Paralysis

Complete sciatic nerve paralysis seldom results in any gross muscular imbalance around the ankle, since the posterior tibial branch of the nerve often recovers when the peroneal portion does not. Therefore, although dorsiflexion of the foot may be lost, plantar flexion of the foot and ankle and sensation are preserved. This type of imbalance is usually adequately compensated for by a drop-foot brace. Attempting to restore dorsiflexion of the ankle by anterior transfer of the posterior tibialis muscle in this situation is frequently unsuccessful because the muscle has been weakened by the sciatic nerve injury.

Isolated injury to the posterior tibial branch of the sciatic nerve is exceedingly rare but could be expected to result in a calcaneus deformity due to the unopposed action of the dorsiflexors of the ankle. Bracing is not a satisfactory solution to this problem.[103] Recovery of plantar sensation of the foot would seem to be a prerequisite before any surgical procedure to correct the calcaneus deformity. If protective plantar sensation is recovered, stabilization of the foot by triple arthrodesis and posterior transfer of the peroneal and tibialis anterior tendons can be considered.[35,83,84,101] The extensors of the toes would be transferred to the metatarsals in a second procedure to improve dorsiflexion. The management of this problem is described in Section 9, Chapter 135.

Leprosy

Peroneal nerve paralysis is frequently seen in patients with leprosy and is often associated with anesthesia of the foot. Neurotrophic lesions, such as a varus deformity with ulceration along the outside of the foot, often develop in these unbalanced anesthetic feet.[37] The principles of tendon transfer, however, are much different from those for an ordinary peroneal nerve palsy due to trauma.[14,97,109] First, triple arthrodesis or any other type of bony stabilization should be avoided, if possible, since arthrodesis is difficult to obtain and delayed wound healing and chronic draining ulcers are frequent. Second, the tendon is transferred into tendon rather than into bone. Bone has a tendency to break down after surgery if a hole is made in it.

Anterior transfer of the tibialis posterior tendon to correct deformities seen in leprosy is possible, since posterior tibialis function if often affected in a later stage of the disease.[37] Several problems may arise after this transfer due to the unique pathologic process in leprosy. Inadequate elevation of the foot may develop due to inadequate tension in the transferred tendon. Varus and valgus deformities of the foot may develop and are related to the position of insertion of the transferred tendon. Talonavicular collapse is seen and may be caused by injury to the bone.[109] It may also be due to instability of the talonavicular joint due to removal of support to the joint by transfer of the tibialis posterior tendon. To maintain the muscular support to the talonavicular joint, Warren[109] suggested attaching the distal 5 cm of the tendon of the tibialis posterior to the flexor digitorum longus tendon. This enables the flexor digitorum longus to pull on the insertion of the tibialis posterior and thus maintain some muscular support to the arch of the foot. The tibialis posterior, now shorter because it was cut above the malleolus, is attached to the tendon of the tibialis anterior at the junction of the middle and lower thirds of the leg. Thus, the tibialis anterior tendon provides length to the transferred yet short tibialis posterior. To balance the foot, a slip of the peroneal tendon is woven through the tibialis anterior to form an inverted Y. When the transferred tibialis posterior muscle contracts, it dorsiflexes the foot without inverting it.

In an attempt to balance the foot without resorting to triple arthrodesis, Srinivasan et al.[98] split the posterior tibialis tendon into two tails. One is inserted into the extensor hallucis longus tendon and the other into the tendons of the extensor digitorum longus and peroneus tertius. Transfer of the flexor digitorum longus and tibialis posterior tendons as described by Carayon et al. obviates the need for triple arthrodesis, and is useful in patients with leprosy.

Stroke

Tendon transfer and release in the rehabilitation of a patient with stroke is covered in Section 9, Chapter 154.

Tendon Displacement

Displacement of the Peroneal Tendons

Eckert and Davis[24] studied the anatomy and mechanism of the peroneal tendon dislocation. They noted a dense aggregation of the collagen fibers that form a ridge along the lip of the posterior margin of the lateral malleolus. The ridge is most pronounced distally and tapers proximally. It is usually 3 to 4 cm long. The superior peroneal retinaculum, which is a thickened portion of the sheath of the peroneal tendons just above the tip of the fibula, lacks any strong connections with this dense strip of fibers and blends with the periosteum on the lateral aspect of the malleolus. For this reason, when the peroneal tendons dislocate, the ridge remains attached to the fibula while the retinaculum strips the periosteum from it. Also, the shallow depression on the posterior aspect of the distal fibula may sometimes be absent.

Displacement of the peroneal tendons from the posterior surface of the lateral malleolus most frequently occurs as a result of trauma. Most cases have been described in skiers who have fallen forward and sustained a severe dorsiflexion injury to the ankle.[24,25,72,75,100] The superior peroneal retinaculum elevates from the lateral surface of the lateral malleolus with the periosteum, enabling the tendons to move anteriorly. Occasionally a fragment of bone is avulsed from the lateral malleolus.[75] The injury is often misdiagnosed as a sprained ankle. However, the diagnosis can be made by palpating the displaced tendons over the lateral malleolus. This may require dorsiflexion of the ankle. A history of snapping over the lateral malleolus with ambulation is highly suggestive.

There are three patterns of injury.[24] In the first pattern, the retinaculum separates from the collagenous lip and the lateral malleolus. In the second, the distal 2 cm of the fibrous lip on the posterior edge of the lateral malleolus is elevated with the retinaculum. In the third pattern, a thin fragment of bone along with the collagenous ridge remains attached to the undersurface of the peroneal retinaculum.

Acute Dislocation

Treatment of the fresh injury is controversial. Stover and Bryan[100] advocated a short-leg cast with the foot in equinus after reduction of the dislocation. These workers stressed prohibiting weight bearing for 5 to 6 weeks and the use of a well-molded cast. Since closed methods of treatment are frequently unsuccessful, Eckert and Davis[24] and O'Donoghue,[81] recommended immediate exploration and repair of all acute injuries.

Treatment

Technique: Eckert and Davis

Local anesthesia is used and a J-shaped incision is made 1 cm behind the distal fibular shaft and extended 1 cm distal to the tip of the lateral malleolus.[24] If a fragment of bone or cartilage can be palpated operatively, the fascia and the periosteum are incised along the posterior margin of the fragment. Otherwise, the incision is extended proximally and distally just anterior to the skin incision along the posterior border of the fibula.

Grade I injuries are repaired by suturing the anterior edge of the incised fascia to the posterior margin of the intact collagenous ridge. The posterior edge of the incised deep fascia is then plicated over the repair and sutured to the surface of the collagenous ridge. In grade II injuries the distal 5 mm of the fibrous retinaculum is avulsed, and accurate replacement and firm suture fixation through the bone is adequate to hold the tendons in place. In grade III injuries, two small K-wires are inserted in a posterolateral to anteromedial direction through the fragment into the fibula. The wires resist subsequent pressure from the peroneal tendons against the fragment. It is often necessary to tack the fascia and periosteum proximally to the posterior border of the lateral malleolus. A posterior edge of the incised fascia is then sutured, as in grade I and II injuries.

Postoperative Management A short-leg cast is applied for 3 weeks without weight bearing and is followed with a short-leg walking cast for 2 to 3 weeks.

Recurrent Dislocation

The acute injury is often overlooked, and the patient later requires treatment for the feeling of instability, pain, and snapping of the tendons with dorsiflexion of the ankle. Various methods of treatment for recurrent dislocation of the peroneal tendons include retention of the displaced tendons by (1) formation of osteoperiosteal flaps fashioned from the lateral malleolus and looped posteriorly around the tendons; (2) deepening of the peroneal groove; (3) tenoplasty or tendon slings[99]; (4) bone block procedures; and (5) direct repair of the detached periosteum to the fibula. Several techniques of rerouting the peroneal tendons under the calcaneofibular ligament[85,93] have been described. These have two major drawbacks. Division of the peroneal tendons or the insertion of the calcaneo-

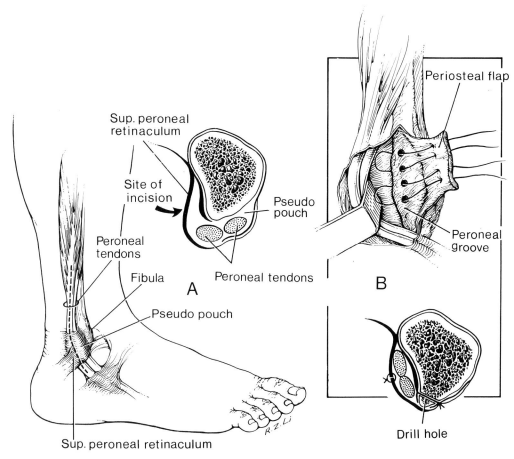

Fig. 130-20. Technique of direct repair of detached periosteum to the fibula for recurrent dislocation of the peroneal tendons. Diagrams include transverse sections of the lower end of the right fibula seen from above. **(A)** The false pouch formed by stripping of periosteum from the lateral malleolus incontinuity with the superior peroneal retinaculum. The arrow shows the site for incision of the retinaculum. **(B)** Normal anatomy restored by obliteration of the false pouch and closing the incision in the peroneal retinaculum. (Modified from Das De,[19] with permission.)

fibular ligament and repair are required and stenosis of the peroneal tendons when passed beneath the calcaneofibular ligaments seems to be a real possibility. Reattachment of the periosteum to the distal fibula,[19] the tenoplasty of Jones,[25,43] and the Thompson procedure to deepen the peroneal groove as described by Zoellner and Clancy[117] seem the most logical alternatives. Occasionally the peroneus quartus is present and may be used to reconstruct both the superior and inferior retinacula.[70] Das De and Balasubramaniam[19] advocate repair of the detached periosteum to drill holes in the distal fibula. We prefer this method of repair.

Treatment

Technique: Das De and Balasubramaniam

Using a tourniquet, a 10-cm skin incision is made posterior to the lateral malleolus.[19] Care is taken

not to injure the sural nerve. The superior peroneal retinaculum is divided 0.5 cm from its posterior margin (Fig. 130-20). Anterior retraction of the incised retinaculum reveals the pseudo pouch into which the peroneal tendons dislocate. Four drill holes, 1 cm apart, are made in the lateral edge of the peroneal groove. The superficial surface of the lateral malleolus is roughened with an osteotome, and #1 Dexon sutures are passed through the periosteal flap and drill holes and tied to obliterate the pouch. The incision in the superior peroneal retinaculum is then repaired. A below-the-knee cast with the foot in equinus is used for 6 weeks.

Jones, in 1932, described a procedure in which a portion of the Achilles tendon is transplanted through a hole in the fibula anterior to the peroneal tendons and sutured onto itself to substitute for the ruptured retinaculum. In performing this procedure, care should be taken to avoid damage to the sural nerve which lies between the lateral malleolus and the Achilles tendon.

Technique: Jones

The peroneal tendons are exposed by a straight incision 5 cm in length extending downward directly behind the lateral malleolus.[43] The Achilles tendon is exposed, and a tendon slip 6 to 7 cm long and 1 cm wide is freed from above downward and left attached at its calcaneal insertion. The pero-

neal tendons are retracted. A hole is drilled transversely through the fibula 2.5 cm above the tip of the malleolus. The tendon slip is passed from behind forward through the drill hole and looped posteriorly and sutured both to itself and the periosteum of the fibula (Fig. 130-21). The peroneal sheath is not opened. After the skin is closed and the wound is dressed, a short-leg plaster cast is applied with the foot at a right angle.

Postoperative Management The cast is changed after 2 weeks. A short-leg cast is reapplied to permit weight bearing. All fixation is removed at 6 weeks, when full activity is permitted. The long-term results reported by Escalas et al.[25] using this method recommend its continued use. Zoellner and Clancy described a procedure designed to deepen the peroneal groove without the use of metallic fixation or tendon transfer, which they ascribed to F. R. Thompson.

Technique: Zoellner and Clancy

A 5- to 7-cm J-shaped curvilinear incision is made posterior to the lateral malleolus along the course of the peroneal tendons.[117] The tendons are freed from their sheath and retracted anteriorly over the lateral malleolus. A cortical osteoperiosteal flap measuring 3 × 1 cm is raised along the posterior lateral aspect of the distal fibula and the lateral malleolus with the posterior medial border intact to act as a hinge. The flap is swung posteriorly; cancellous bone from the created fenestration in the fibula is removed to deepen the groove by 6 to 9 mm. The flap is then tamped back into position, creating a groove 3 to 4 cm in length. The floor continues to present a smooth gliding surface to the peroneal tendons. The tendons are replaced in the groove and the ankle is put through a full range of motion. The tendons should remain well seated and show no tendency to subluxate or dislocate. If the superior peroneal retinaculum is strong enough to use for repair, it is plicated over the tendons. If the retinaculum is tenuous, as in many ankles, an additional periosteal flap 1 cm² from the lateral surface of the malleolus is raised and hinged posteriorly and sutured to the medial part of the peroneal retinaculum (Fig. 130-22).

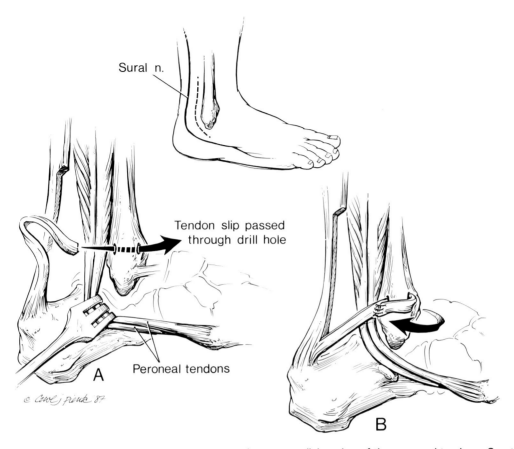

Fig. 130-21. (A,B) Jones technique for correction of recurrent dislocation of the peroneal tendons. See text. (Modified from Jones,[43] with permission.)

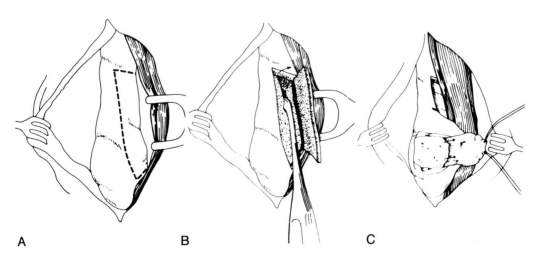

Fig. 130-22. Thompson technique of correction of recurrent dislocation of the peroneal tendons. **(A)** Outline of cortical flap. **(B)** Underlying cancellous bone is removed to permit impaction of the cortical flap. **(C)** Tendons are reduced in the deepened groove and covered with a periosteal flap. (From Zoellner,[117] with permission.)

Postoperative Management   The foot is immobilized in a short-leg cast for 3 weeks. A hinged short-leg cast is used for 3 more weeks, permitting dorsiflexion and plantar flexion exercises. Strenuous athletic activities are deferred until full range of motion and normal strength are regained.

In follow-up averaged 2 years in nine patients, all regained normal motion of the ankle and subtalar joint, and no recurrent dislocations, instability, or persistent pain were reported.

INFLAMMATORY CONDITIONS OF TENDONS

Tenosynovitis is an inflammation of the synovium of the tendon sheath.[58] Paratendonitis or peritendonitis, according to Lipscomb, refers to an inflammatory process around the tendon in areas lacking a tendon sheath. The inflammatory process is manifested by pain, tenderness, swelling, and, occasionally, a palpable crepitus. When the process is chronic, the tendon sheath may be thickened and the tendon substance weakened from thinning and fraying out of tendon. Bursitis refers to inflammation of the bursa. These inflammatory processes around the ankle result most commonly from overuse and usually respond to conservative measures when acute.

Processes requiring more specific treatment include: (1) inflammatory conditions such as Reiter's syndrome, ankylosing spondylitis, rheumatoid arthritis, and gout[31]; (2) pyogenic and granulomatous infections; (3) mechanical abnormalities; and (4) space-occupying lesions.

The major sites of tenosynovitis about the foot and ankle are the sheaths of the anterior tibial, posterior tibial, peroneal, and Achilles tendons.[13,58,107] Involvement of the anterior tibial and Achilles tendons most often results from problems with footwear. Tenosynovitis of the posterior tibial and peroneal tendons is likely to be stenosing since these tendons angle behind the malleoli in the tendon sheaths.[58]

McMaster,[69] using the experiments on loaded tendon muscle units, showed that normal tendon does not rupture but that rupture is at the insertion to bone, through the musculotendinous junction, or through the muscle, in decreasing order of frequency. For this reason in tenosynovitis unresponsive to rest, physical therapy, systemic anti-inflammatory medication, or local steroid injection, prophylactic surgical tenosynovectomy should be considered not only to relieve symptoms[51] but also to prevent weakening of the tendon.[2] When using steroids in these processes, injection into the substance of the tendon must be carefully avoided.

Surgery on or about the tendons in the distal portion of the leg is recommended for several conditions. In rheumatoid arthritis, synoviobursectomy has been advocated to prevent collagenolytic weakening of tendons.[47,87,89] Incision or excision and drainage of infectious tenosynovitis which fails to respond to antibiotics is also recommended. Tissue must be obtained for culture and histologic examination, since superinfection of granulomatous processes may result in misdirected antibiotic therapy. For nonspecific peritendonitis of the ankle and foot, when conservative measures have failed, surgical excision of inflamed tenosynovia with release of the constricting portion of the tendon sheath, if present, is indicated.[92,106] In the case of the peroneal and posterior tibial tendons, care must be taken to preserve a restraint to subsequent dislocation of these tendons.[76]

Calcaneal Paratenonitis

Pain in the posterior distal portion of the leg may result from calcaneal paratenonitis or partial rupture of the Achilles tendon. The symptoms are particularly apt to develop in runners, who complain of pain and tenderness above the heel. Pain is most severe at the onset of a particular sports activity or on rising in the morning. In acute calcaneal paratenonitis edema, crepitus and local tenderness are present. Treatment consists of oral anti-inflammatory medication, elevation of the heel, restriction of activity, and physical therapy.

In chronic paratenonitis, crepitus and edema have disappeared and a diffuse thickening of the soft tissues with tender nodules around the Achilles tendon is present. The fibrin in the tendon sheath becomes organized and adhesions develop between the tendon and paratenon and the surrounding soft tissues. Since nonoperative management of chronic calcaneal paratenonitis is usually unsuccessful, surgery is frequently indicated. Kvist and Kvist[49] reported remarkable success with lysis of adhesions and debridement of hypertrophied paratenon in Finnish runners. In this technique, the crural fascia on both sides of the tendon is incised and left open, adhesions around the tendon are trimmed away, the strongly hypertrophied portions of the paratenon are removed, and mobilization is immediately begun.

Technique: Kvist and Kvist

The surgery is performed with the patient prone using a general anesthetic.[49] A 7-cm incision is made along the lateral aspect of the calcaneal tendon. The sural nerve and saphenous vein are identified and carefully protected. The crural fascia is incised along the length of the tendon. All adhesions between the tendon and the ventral aspect of the crural fascia are excised. The peritenon externum and the crural fascia covering the dorsal part of the tendon are detached from the skin to which they have become adherent. The tendon is retracted and the procedure repeated on its medial aspect. The tendon is freed distally to within 1.5 cm of the calcaneus and proximally to the musculotendinous junction. Care must be taken to preserve the small vessels in front of the tendon. The attachment of the distal 2 cm of the tendon to the skin is left undisturbed. At this time, the freed tendon covered with its paratenon should be inspected, if the paratenon is considerably thickened dorsolaterally and constricting the tendon, it is removed. Hemostasis is obtained. The crural fascia and subcutaneous tissue are not sutured, but the skin is sutured. In instances in which degenerative nodules are found within the tendon substance the degenerative areas are excised.

Postoperative Management   The leg is not immobilized and the patient begins active dorsiflexion and plantar flexion of the ankle upon recovery from the anesthetic. Three to 4 weeks after the operation, gradual resumption of sports is allowed.

Kvist and Kvist reported 169 excellent results in 201 operations. There were recurrent symptoms in 26 patients. Further surgery was necessary on 20 occasions. There were seven poor results. Leach et al.[54] also found Achilles tenolysis an effective treatment for this problem.

Ossification may be seen in the Achilles tendon. If the patient has chronic pain, excision of the bone mass and repair of the tendon should be performed. A large ossification may weaken the tendon and lead to a tendon rupture.[62]

Painful prominences at the superior calcaneal tubercle in patients with a Achilles tendon or retrocalcaneal bursitis in whom conservative measures have failed occasionally require excision.[21,46] This is discussed elsewhere.

Lee and Weiss[55] and Fahey et al.[26] reported the operative resection of xanthomas in patients with type II hyperbetalipoproteinemia experiencing pain or poor appearance associated with lesions in the Achilles tendon. The lesion infiltrates the tendon and is therefore apt to recur if excised and often continues to grow if resection is incomplete. Substantial portions (one-half to four-fifths) of the Achilles tendon are removed and tendon reinforcement is usually required. Lee and Weiss[55] used total resection of the Achilles tendon and reconstruction with fascia lata. No ruptures of the Achilles tendon were found in the cases they reviewed. Early treatment with appropriate diet and drugs is essential in preventing further deposits in this and other areas.

Peroneal tendonitis may occur with widening of the calcaneus after calcaneal fractures and can be corrected by surgical decompression.[27,45,65] All the literature on peroneal tendonitis following calcaneal fractures stresses that subtalar or triple arthrodesis frequently does not relieve the symptoms. The simpler procedure of decompression the peroneal tendons where they are caught between the fracture callus and the lateral malleolus frequently will be corrective. These procedures are described elsewhere. Resistant peroneal tenosynovitis associated with stenosis or space-occupying lesions can be treated by opening the constricting retinacular enclosure and/or excising the lesion.[13,82,107,111]

REFERENCES

1. Abraham E, Pankovich A: Neglected rupture of the Achilles tendon. Treatment by V-Y tendinous flap. J Bone Joint Surg 57A:253, 1975

2. Anzel SH, Covey KW, Weiner AD, et al: Disruption of muscles and tendons. An analysis of 1,014 cases. Surgery 45:406, 1959

3. Arner O, Lindholm A: What is tennis leg? Acta Chir Scand 116:73, 1958

4. Arner O, Lindholm A: Subcutaneous rupture of the Achilles tendon. A study of 92 cases. Acta Chir Scand Suppl 239: 1959

5. Barfred T: Experimental rupture of the Achilles tendon. Comparison of experimental ruptures in rates of different ages and living under different conditions. Acta Orthop Scand 42:406, 1971

6. Barnes MJ, Hardy AE: Delayed reconstruction of the calcaneal tendon. J Bone Joint Surg 68B:121, 1986

7. Benum P, Berg V, Fretheim OJ: The strain on sutured Achilles tendons in walking cast. Eur Surg Res 16(suppl 2):14, 1984

8. Beskin JL, Sanders RA, Hunter SC, et al: Surgical repair of Achilles tendon ruptures. Am J Sports Med 15:1, 1987

9. Bock E, Colavita N, Cotroneo AR, et al: Xeroradiography of tenomuscular traumatic pathologic conditions of the limbs. Diagn Imag 50:235, 1981

10. Bosworth DM: Repair of defects in the tendo Achillis. J Bone Joint Surg 38A:111, 1956

11. Bredo L, Waddell JP, Hudson AR: Tendon transfer in the management of persistent foot drop. Presented at the Fifty-Fourth Annual Meeting of the American Academy of Orthopaedic Surgeons, January 1987

12. Bugg EI Jr, Boyd BM: Repair of neglected rupture or laceration of the Achilles tendon. Clin Orthop 56:73, 1968

13. Burman M: Stenosing tenovaginitis of the foot and ankle. Studies with special reference to the stenosing tendovaginitis of the peroneal tendons at the peroneal tubercle. Arch Surg 67:686, 1953

14. Carayon A, Bourrel P, Bourges M, et al: Dual transfer of the posterior tibial and flexor digitorum longus tendons for drop foot. Report of thirty-one cases. J Bone Joint Surg 49A:144, 1967

15. Cetti R, Christensen SE: Surgical treatment under local anesthesia of Achilles tendon rupture. Clin Orthop 173:204, 1983

16. Cole WH: The treatment of claw-foot. J Bone Joint Surg 22:895, 1940

17. Cozen L: Effect of lengthening the Achilles tendon on the strength of gastrocnemius-soleus musculature. Clin Orthop 49:179, 1966

18. Cummins EJ, Anson BJ, Carr BW, et al: The structure of the calcaneal tendon (of Achilles) in relation to orthopaedic surgery. Surg Gynecol Obstet 83:107, 1946

19. Das De S, Balasubramaniam P: A repair operation for recurrent dislocation of the peroneal tendons. J Bone Joint Surg 67B:585, 1985

20. Denstad TF, Roaas A: Surgical treatment of partial Achilles tendon rupture. Am J Sports Med 7:15, 1979

21. Dickinson PH, Coutts MB, Woodward EP, et al: Tendo Achillis bursitis. Report of 21 cases. J Bone Joint Surg 48A:77, 1966

22. Dooley BJ, Kudelka P, Menelaus MB: Subcutaneous rupture of the tendon of the tibialis anterior. J Bone Joint Surg 62B:471, 1980

23. Durig M, Schuppisser JP, Gauer EF, et al: Spontaneous rupture of the gastrocnemius muscle. Injury 9:143, (1977–1978)

24. Eckert WR, Davis Jr., EA: Acute rupture of the peroneal retinaculum. J Bone Joint Surg 58A:670, 1976

25. Escalas F, Figueras JM, Merino JA: Dislocation of the peroneal tendons. J Bone Joint Surg 62A:451, 1980

26. Fahey JJ, Stark HH, Donovan WF, et al: Xanthoma of the Achilles tendon. Seven cases with familial hyperbetalipoproteinemia. J Bone Joint Surg 55A:1197, 1973

27. Fitzgerald RH Jr, Gross RM, Johnson KA: Traumatic peroneal tendinitis. A complication of calcaneal fractures. Minn Med 58:787, 1975

28. Fox JM, Blazina ME, Jobe FW, et al: Degeneration and rupture of the Achilles tendon. Clin Orthop 107:221, 1975

29. Fried A, Hendel C: Paralytic valgus deformity of the ankle. Replacement of the paralyzed tibialis posterior by peroneus longus. J Bone Joint Surg 39A:921, 1957

30. Fried A, Moyseyev S: Paralytic valgus deformity of the foot. Treatment by replacement of paralyzed tibialis posterior muscle. A long term follow-up study. J Bone Joint Surg 52A:1674, 1970

31. Funk DA, Cass JR, Johnson KA: Acquired flat foot deformity secondary to posterior tibial tendon pathology. J Bone Joint Surg 68A:95, 1986

32. Gerster JC, Vischer TL, Bennani A, et al: The painful heel. Comparative study in rheumatoid arthritis, ankylosing spondylitis, Reiter's syndrome, and generalized osteoarthrosis. Ann Rheumatol Dis 36:343, 1977

33. Goldner JL, Keats PK, Bassett FH III, et al: Progressive talipes equinovalgus due to trauma or degeneration of the posterior tibial tendon and medial plantar ligaments. Orthop Clin North Am 5:39, 1974

34. Green WT: Tendon transplantation in rehabilitation. JAMA 163:1235, 1957

35. Green WT, Grice DS: The surgical correction of the paralytic foot. p. 343. In American Academy of Orthopaedic Surgery, Instructional Course Lectures. Vol. 10. JW Edwards, Ann Arbor, 1953

36. Griffiths JC: Tendon injuries around the ankle. J Bone Joint Surg 47B:686, 1965

37. Gunn DR, Molesworth BD: The use of tibialis posterior as a dorsiflexor. J Bone Joint Surg 39B:674, 1957

38. Haldeman KO, Soto-Hall R: Injuries to muscles and tendons. JAMA 104:2319, 1935

39. Hooker CH: Rupture of the tendo calcaneus. J Bone Joint Surg 45B:360, 1963

40. Inglis AE, Scott N, Sculco TP, et al: Ruptures of the tendo Achillis: Objective assessment of surgical and nonsurgical treatment. J Bone Joint Surg 58A:990, 1976

41. Inglis AE, Sculco TP: Surgical repair of ruptures of the tendo Achillis. Clin Orthop 156:160, 1981

42. Jahss MH: Spontaneous rupture of the posterior tibial tendon: clinical findings, tenographic studies and a new technique of repair. Foot Ankle 3:158, 1982

43. Jones E: Operative treatment of chronic dislocation of the peroneal tendons. J Bone Joint Surg 14:574, 1932

44. Kaplan SS: Burns following applications of plaster splint dressings. J Bone Joint Surg 63A:670, 1981

45. Kashiwagi D, Inamatsu N: Diagnosis and treatment of fractures of the os calcis. Kobe J Med Sci 11(suppl):21, 1965

46. Keck SW, Kelly PJ: Bursitis of the posterior part of the heel. Evaluation of surgical treatment of eighteen patients. J Bone Joint Surg 47A:267, 1965

47. Kelley WN, Harris ED Jr, Ruddy S, Sledge CB, et al (eds): Textbook of Rheumatology. WB Saunders, Philadelphia, 1981

48. Kettelkamp DB, Alexander HH: Spontaneous rupture of the posterior tibial tendon. J Bone Joint Surg 51A:759, 1969

49. Kvist H, Kvist M: The operative treatment of chronic calcaneal paratenonitis. J Bone Joint Surg 62B:353, 1980

50. Lagergren C, Lindholm A: Vascular distribution in the Achilles tendon. An angiographic and microangiographic study. Acta Chir Scand 116:491, 1958–1959

51. Lapidus PW, Seidenstein H: Chronic non-specific tenosynovitis with effusion about the ankle. Report of three cases. J Bone Joint Surg 32A:175, 1950

52. Lavallette R, Pope MH, Dickstein H: Setting temperatures of plaster casts. J Bone Joint Surg 64A:907, 1982

53. Lea RB, Smith L: Rupture of the Achilles tendon nonsurgical treatment. Clin Orthop 60:115, 1968

54. Leach RE, James S, Wasilewski S: Achilles tendonitis. Am J Sports Med 9:93, 1981

55. Lee CK, Weiss AB: Xanthomas of the Achilles tendons. J Bone Joint Surg 62A:666, 1980

56. Levy M, Velkes S, Goldstein J, et al: A method of repair for Achilles tendon ruptures without cast immobilization. Clin Orthop 187:99, 1984

57. Lindholm A: A new method of operation in subcutaneous rupture of the Achilles tendon. Acta Chir Scand 117:261, 1959

58. Lipscomb PR: Nonsuppurative tenosynovitis and paratendinitis. Tendons Symposium. p. 254. In American Academy of Orthopaedic Surgery Instructional Course Lectures. Vol. 7. JW Edwards, Ann Arbor, 1950

59. Lipscomb PR, Kelly PJ: Injuries of the extensor tendons in the distal part of the leg and in the ankle. J Bone Joint Surg 37A:1206, 1955

60. Lipscomb PR, Sanchez JJ: Anterior transplantation of the posterior tibial tendon for persistent palsy of the common peroneal nerve. J Bone Joint Surg 43A:60, 1961

61. Ljungqvist R: Subcutaneous partial rupture of the Achilles tendon. Acta Orthop Scand Suppl 113: 1968

62. Lotke PA: Ossification of the Achilles tendon. Report of seven cases. J Bone Joint Surg 52A:157, 1970

63. Lynn TA: Repair of the torn Achilles tendon, using the plantaris tendon as a reinforcing membrane. J Bone Joint Surg 48A:268, 1966

64. Ma GW, Griffith TG: Percutaneous repair of acute closed ruptured Achilles tendon. Clin Orthop 128:247, 1977

65. Magnuson PB: An operation for relief of disability in old fractures of os calcis. JAMA 80:1511, 1923

66. Mann RA, Thompson FM: Rupture of the posterior tibial tendon causing flat foot. J Bone Joint Surg 67A:556, 1985

67. Marti RK, van der Werken C, Schutte PR, et al: Operative repair of the ruptured Achilles tendon and functional after-treatment. I, II. Neth J Surg 35:61, 1983

68. Mayer L: The physiological method of tendon transplantation in the treatment of paralytic dropfoot. J Bone Joint Surg 19:389, 1937

69. McMaster PE: Tendon and muscle ruptures. Clinical and experimental studies on the causes and location of subcutaneous ruptures. J Bone Joint Surg 15:705, 1933

70. Mensor MC, Ordway GL: Traumatic subcutaneous

rupture of the tibialis anterior tendon. J Bone Joint Surg 35A:675, 1953

71. Mick CA, Lynch F: Reconstruction of the peroneal retinaculum using peroneus quartus. J Bone Joint Surg 59A:296, 1987

72. Moritz JR: Ski injuries. Am J Surg 98:493, 1959

73. Mubarek SJ, Hargens AR, Owen CA, et al: The Wick catheter technique for measurement of intramuscular pressure. J Bone Joint Surg 58A:1016, 1976

74. Mubarek SJ, Owen CA, Garfin S, et al: Acute exertional superficial posterior compartment syndrome. Am J Sports Med 6:287, 1978

75. Murr S: Dislocation of the peroneal tendons with marginal fracture of the lateral malleolus. J Bone Joint Surg 43B:563, 1961

76. Nava BE: Traumatic dislocation of the tibialis posterior tendon at the ankle. J Bone Joint Surg 50B:150, 1968

77. Nistor L: Surgical and nonsurgical treatment of Achilles tendon rupture. J Bone Joint Surg 63A:394, 1981

78. Norris SH, Mankin HJ: Chronic tenosynovitis of the posterior tibial tendon with new bone formation. J Bone Joint Surg 60B:523, 1978

79. Ober FR: Tendon transplantation in the lower extremity. N Engl J Med 209:52, 1933

80. O'Brien T: The needle test for complete rupture of the Achilles tendon. J Bone Joint Surg 66A:1099, 1984

81. O'Donoghue DH: Treatment of injuries to athletes. 3rd Ed. p. 704. WB Saunders, Philadelphia, 1976

82. Parvin RW, Ford LT: Stenosing tenosynovitis of the common peroneal tendon sheath. Report of two cases. J Bone Joint Surg 38A:1352, 1956

83. Peabody CW: Tendon transposition. An end-result study. J Bone Joint Surg 20:193, 1938

84. Peabody CW: Tendon transplantation in the lower extremity. Tendon transposition in the paralytic foot. p. 178. In American Academy of Orthopaedic Surgeons Instructional Course Lectures. Vol. 6. JW Edwards, Ann Arbor, 1949

85. Poll RG, Duijfjes F: The treatment of recurrent dislocation of the peroneal tendons. J Bone Joint Surg 66B:98, 1984

86. Pinzur MS, Kett N, Trilla M: Combined anterior/posterior tibial tendon transfer in traumatic paralytic peroneal foot-drop. Presented at the Fifty-fourth Annual Meeting of the American Academy of Orthopaedic Surgeons, January 1987

87. Potter TA, Kuhns JG: Rheumatoid tenosynovitis. Diagnosis and treatment. J Bone Joint Surg 40A:1230, 1958

88. Ralston EL, Schmidt E Jr: Repair of the ruptured Achilles tendon. J Trauma 11:15, 1971

89. Rask MR: Achilles tendon rupture owing to rheumatoid disease. Case report with a nine-year follow-up. JAMA 239:435, 1978

90. Rowley DI, Scotland TR: Rupture of the Achilles tendon treated by a simple operative procedure. Injury 14:252, 1982

91. Rubin BD, Wilson HJ Jr: Surgical repair of the interrupted Achilles tendon. J Trauma 20:248, 1980

92. Sammarco GT, Miller EH: Partial rupture of the flexor hallucis longus tendon in classical ballet dancers. J Bone Joint Surg 61A:149, 1979

93. Sarmiento A, Wolf M: Subluxation of the peroneal tendons. Case treated by rerouting tendons under calcaneofibular ligament. J Bone Joint Surg 57A:115, 1975

94. Shapiro F, Bresnon MJ: Orthopaedic management of childhood neuromuscular disease. II. Peripheral neuropathies, Friedreich's ataxia and arthrogryposis multiplex congenita. J Bone Joint Surg 64A:949, 1982

95. Sharrard WJW: Paralytic deformity in the lower limb. J Bone Joint Surg 49B:731, 1967

96. Shields CL, Kerlan RK, Jobe FW, et al: The Cybex II evaluation of surgically repaired Achilles tendon ruptures. Am J Sports Med 6:369, 1978

97. Shields CL, Redix L, Brewster MS: Acute tears of the medial head of the gastrocnemius. Foot Ankle, 5:186, 1985

98. Srinivasan H, Mukherjee SM, Subramaniam RA: Two tailed transfer of tibialis posterior for correction of drop foot in leprosy. J Bone Joint Surg 50B:623, 1968

99. Stein RE: Reconstruction of the superior peroneal retinaculum using a portion of the peroneus brevis tendon. J Bone Joint Surg 69A:298, 1987

100. Stover CN, Bryan DR: Traumatic dislocation of the peroneal tendons. Am J Surg 103:180, 1962

101. Straub LR, Harvey JP Jr, Fuerst CE: A clinical evaluation of tendon transplantation in the paralytic foot. J Bone Joint Surg 39A:1, 1957

102. Straehley D, Jones WW: Acute compartment syndrome (anterior, lateral, and superficial posterior) following tear of the medial head of the gastrocnemius muscle. Am J Sports Med 14:96, 1986

103. Sutherland DH, Cooper L, Daniel D: The role of the ankle plantar flexors in normal walking. J Bone Joint Surg 62A:354, 1980

104. Tachdjian MO: Pediatric Orthopedics. Vol. 2, p. 985. WB Saunders, Philadelphia, 1972

105. Teuffer AP: Traumatic rupture of the Achilles tendon reconstruction by transplant and graft using

the lateral peroneus brevis. Orthop Clin North Am 5:89, 1974

106. Thompson TC, Doherty JH: Spontaneous rupture of tendon of Achilles: A new clinical diagnostic test. J Trauma 2:126, 1962

107. Trevino S, Gould N, Korson R: Surgical treatment of stenosing tenosynovitis at the ankle. Foot Ankle, 2:37, 1981

108. Vazelle F, Rochcongar P, Masse M, et al: La pathologie du tendon d'Achille. Un emploi inattendu du mammographe. J Radiol 62:299, 1981

109. Warren AG: Correction of drop foot in leprosy. J Bone Joint Surg 50B:629, 1968

110. Watkins MB, Jones JB, Ryder CT Jr: Transplantation of the posterior tibial tendon. J Bone Joint Surg 36A:60, 1954

111. Webster FS: Peroneal tenosynovitis with pseudotumor. J Bone Joint Surg 50A:153, 1968

112. Westin GW: Tendon transfer about the foot, ankle, and hip in the paralyzed lower extremity. J Bone Joint Surg 47A:1430, 1965

113. White JW: Torsion of the Achilles tendon: Its surgical significance. Arch Surg 46:784, 1943

114. White RK, Kraynick BM: Surgical uses of the peroneus brevis tendon. Surg Gynecol Obstet 108:117, 1959

115. Williams R: Chronic non-specific tendovaginitis of tibialis posterior. J Bone Joint Surg 45B:542, 1963

116. Wrenn RN: Isolated injuries of posterior tibial tendon. J Bone Joint Surg 57A:1035, 1975

117. Zoellner G, Clancy W Jr: Recurrent dislocation of the peroneal tendons. J Bone Joint Surg 61A:292, 1979

Compartment Syndromes of the Lower Leg

131

Anthony A. Schepsis
Robert E. Leach

A compartment syndrome is one of the surgical emergencies that an orthopaedic surgeon must deal with. Failure to diagnose and treat this condition promptly will lead to devastating consequences. Our extremities contain multiple compartments, with muscles, arteries, veins, and nerves confined within a closed space. The boundaries are relatively noncompliant fascia and bone; thus any condition that causes either an increase of contents of the compartment, such as hemorrhage or edema, and/or external compression can lead to high pressures within the compartment. A compartment syndrome exists when the pressure within this closed space becomes high enough to impede capillary perfusion of the local tissue, leading to loss of tissue viability. Since permanent tissue damage may occur within a matter of hours, relief by decompression fasciotomy must be performed promptly. Otherwise, muscle necrosis as well as irreversible nerve damage may lead to permanent loss of function, limb contracture, and even amputation.

Commonly, a compartment syndrome is an acute phenomenon that occurs secondary to a fracture or soft tissue injury. A second form, the chronic or exertional compartment syndrome, occurs secondary to exercise-induced increase in the intracompartmental pressure. This temporary and reversible form commonly occurs in the lower leg, where exercise increases compartment pressure, causing pain and occasionally a temporary neurologic deficit that usually resolves with rest.

ANATOMY

The muscles within a given compartment tend to have a similar function; e.g., the muscles in the anterior tibial compartment dorsiflex the foot and toes. Each muscle has its own investing layer, the epimysium, which further subdivides the compartment into subcompartments. The arteries traversing through each individual compartment nourish these muscles. The nerve within the compartment usually innervates the muscles within that compartment but, like the arteries, may also have a distal destination and function. The investing fascia is strong, relatively noncompliant connective tissue. The fascia adds to the strength of the contained muscle as fascia removal reduces the force of the muscle contraction by almost 15 percent.[12]

This chapter deals primarily with the compartments of the lower leg. However, the general principles outlined are applicable to other body compartments. There are four anatomic compartments in the lower leg; the anterior, lateral, superficial posterior, and deep posterior (Fig. 131-1). The anterior tibial compartment is the most frequent site for the acute as well as the exertional compartment syndrome. It is bounded anteriorly by the crural fascia, laterally by the anterior intermuscular septum, posteriorly by the fibula and interosseous membrane, and medially by the tibia. The muscles within this compartment dorsiflex the foot and toes and consist of the tibialis anterior, extensor digitorum longus, extensor hallucis longus, and per-

oneus tertius. The nerve within the compartment is the deep peroneal nerve, which enters it after winding around the fibular neck and supplies all the muscles within the compartment before coursing distally into the foot to become the sensory nerve of the first dorsal web space. The major artery in the anterior compartment is the anterior tibial artery, which supplies the compartment muscles as it goes distally to become the dorsalis pedis artery.

The lateral compartment contains two muscles, the peroneus longus and peroneus brevis, which evert the ankle and foot. The major nerve within this compartment is the superficial peroneal nerve, which innervates these two muscles and divides into two sensory nerves that supply the remainder of the dorsum of the foot. There is no major vessel in this compartment, as the peroneal muscles are nourished by both the peroneal and anterior tibial arteries.

The superficial posterior compartment contains

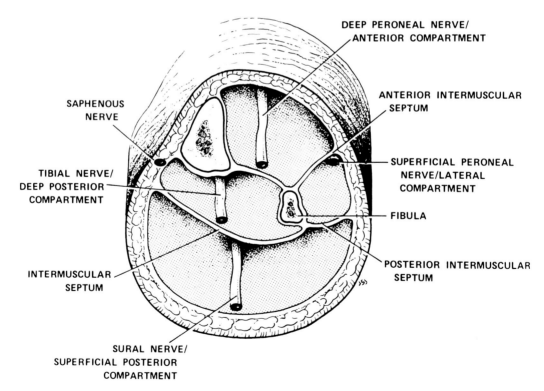

Fig. 131-1. The four compartments of the lower leg and their respective nerves. (From Mubarak,[33] with permission.)

the gastrocnemius, soleus, and plantaris muscles. There is no major vessel in this compartment, and the muscles are supplied by branches of the posterior tibial and peroneal arteries. Also, there is no major motor nerve in this compartment, with the muscles innervated by branches of the posterior tibial nerve. The only significant nerve that traverses this compartment in the proximal portion is the sural nerve, which exits from the compartment in its distal half and becomes subcutaneous, supplying sensation to the dorsolateral aspect of the foot and ankle.

The deep posterior compartment is separated from its superficial counterpart by a transverse intermuscular septum. In the proximal two-thirds of the leg, it is entirely deep, invested by the superficial compartment as well as the tibia and fibula. In the distal one-third of the leg, it has a superficial border behind the posteromedial aspect of the tibia, below the distal extent of the tibial origin of the soleus. This anatomic fact is important in the clinical examination as well as for pressure measurements of the deep compartment. The muscles in this group consist of the tibialis posterior, flexor hallucis longus, and flexor digitorum longus. They are innervated by the posterior tibial nerve, which goes distally to become the medial and lateral plantar nerves, which supply the intrinsic muscles of the foot as well as sensation on the sole of the foot. The major vessel in this compartment is the posterior tibial artery. Detailed knowledge of the anatomy of these compartments is essential in making the diagnosis of a compartment syndrome.

PATHOPHYSIOLOGY

The key to understanding a compartment syndrome lies at the microvascular level. Whether it be hemorrhage, edema, muscle fiber swelling, external constriction, or a combination of these factors that causes increased pressure within the compartment, it is the retardation of the capillary perfusion that leads to tissue ischemia[37] (Fig. 131-2). At rest, intracompartmental pressure is

close to 0 mmHg, allowing for normal blood flow. Hargens and Reneman's[16] study of capillary blood flow and pressures showed that a tissue pressure of 30 mmHg is sufficient to retard oxygenation to the muscles and nerves, leading to loss of tissue viability. At the same time, the large vessels remain patent unless the intracompartmental pressure rises above the arterial diastolic pressure, making the presence or absence of distal pulses an extremely unreliable sign in making the diagnosis of a compartment syndrome. Since the muscle capillary hydrostatic pressure has been measured at 25 mmHg pressure, exceeding this could conceivably prevent blood flow at the microvascular level.

Whitesides et al.[57] demonstrated a correlation between the critical intracompartmental pressure and the blood pressure and showed that someone with hypertension is "relatively protected" from a compartment syndrome, since higher pressures are required to cause critical closure. These workers suggested 45 mmHg as the critical level. However, most studies agree that 30 mmHg should be considered the critical level, above which irreversible damage may occur. The potential muscle and nerve tissue damage is a function of time as well as pressure. Lower pressures can be tolerated for longer periods of time. Rorabeck and Clarke[47] showed that muscle and nerve damage is progressively more severe with increasing time. Hargens et al.[15,18] demonstrated that irreversible injury within the anterior compartment of dog limbs is produced at 30 mmHg sustained for a period of 8 hours. They also showed that at an intracompartmental pressure of 30 mmHg, nerve conduction velocity is retarded after 6 to 8 hours.[16,17] It appears that a pressure of 30 mmHg sustained for 6 hours or longer may lead to permanent muscle and nerve damage, emphasizing that prompt treatment is necessary in a compartment syndrome.

ETIOLOGY

An acute compartment syndrome is often seen as the result of a fracture or soft tissue injury. Hemorrhage within the compartment causes an increase

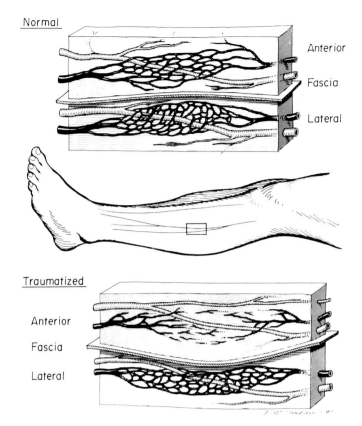

Fig. 131-2. Unifying principles of a compartment syndrome. In the enlarged figure above the leg, normal micro-circulation is viewed during rest in the anterior and lateral muscle compartments. These two compartments are separated by fascia. During rest, intracompartmental pressure in the anterior and lateral compartments is near zero, and blood flow in all capillaries (network of black vessels) and large arteries (shaded vessels entering figure from the right) is normal. If pressure in the anterior compartment reaches a threshold level close to 30 mmHg (enlarged figure below leg), capillary perfusion is inadequate to maintain tissue viability. If this high pressure in the anterior compartment is not relieved after approximately 8 hours, irreversible necrosis of muscle tissue and indwelling nerves may result in the anterior compartment. It is noteworthy that distal pulses are usually present in the foot primarily because intracompartmental pressure rarely rises above central artery diastolic pressure. (From Mubarak,[32] with permission.)

in pressure. This is further aggravated by an accumulation of interstitial edema fluid, which further increases the pressure. The most common injury causing an acute compartment syndrome is a fracture of the tibia, which occurs in open as well as closed fractures. The second leading cause of an acute compartment syndrome in the lower extremity results from a severe soft tissue injury. This is usually a crushing injury, with increased pressure resulting from hemorrhage as well as edema. The absence of a fracture should not make the clinician less suspicious of an acute compartment syndrome. Less common causes of an acute compartment syn-

drome result from bone bleeding after an osteotomy,[14] a Hauser or Maquet procedure,[51] and from hemophilia.[26]

The compartment syndrome may be the sequela of an arterial injury. If there is complete arterial occlusion, muscle and nerve damage will occur as the result of prolonged ischemia. Without restoration of the circulation, tissue necrosis will be the result rather than a compartment syndrome. Commonly, the compartment syndrome occurs after circulation is restored. This is secondary to postischemic swelling. Whitesides et al.[55] proved that in canines, 6 hours of tourniquet-induced ischemia produced markedly elevated intracompartmental pressures. Therefore, most authorities recommend fasciotomy as a routine procedure after arterial repair if ischemia has been present for 4 to 6 hours or more.[10,58]

A compartment syndrome may also result from a decrease in the size of the compartment, such as may occur from external constriction (e.g., a circular dressing or cast). Burns and frostbite may cause a compartment syndrome by forming a constricting eschar that decreases the size of the compartment. Thermal injuries are associated with increased edema fluid within the compartment, further increasing the pressure. It may be difficult to make the diagnosis of a compartment syndrome in these extensive thermal injuries, making compartment pressure measurements an important parameter on which to base the decision for decompression.

A less common but iatrogenic cause of a compartment syndrome is surgical closure of a fascial defect. A muscle hernia, secondary to a fascial defect may be seen in the anterior tibial compartment and has been associated by some with an increased incidence of the exertional compartment syndrome.[42] Leach et al.[23] as well as other investigators[3,8,31] have shown that closure of fascial defects may lead to an acute compartment syndrome on either an immediate or delayed basis. Closure of fascial defects should never be performed. A period of prolonged limb compression occur from drug overdose or a surgical procedure under general anesthesia,[41] particularly in a knee-chest position, may lead to a compartment syndrome.[25] More recently, the use of the pneumatic antishock trousers has been associated with increased intramuscular pressures inducing a compartment syndrome.[4,21,54]

CLINICAL DIAGNOSIS

Prompt recognition of either a fully developed or impending compartment syndrome is critical, since it has been shown that irreversible damage will occur within a matter of hours. Pain out of proportion relative to the primary injury should make the clinician immediately suspicious of a compartment syndrome. The pain is localized to the general area of the affected compartment and is constant and acute. In the presence of a neurologic deficit or with a multiply injured or comatose patient, pain becomes a less reliable sign. Otherwise, it is the most consistent and important clinical symptom. A tense and swollen compartment is the most important objective finding. The swelling is seen throughout the compartment and is not localized to just the area of injury. This is particularly true with the anterior tibial compartment. However, in the presence of a deep posterior compartment syndrome, this finding becomes less reliable.

Since a compartment syndrome produces ischemia to the muscles within the compartment as well as the nerve transversing the compartment, a careful neurologic examination is essential. One of the first signs of nerve ischemia is a sensory deficit, manifested by decreased sensation of the nerve passing through the compartment. For example, the first sign of nerve ischemia in the anterior tibial compartment would be decreased sensation in the first dorsal web space, indicating involvement of the deep peroneal nerve. Since the sensory deficit occurs earlier than muscle weakness, it is important to do a careful examination for light touch and pin prick. A motor deficit occurs later. This would be indicated by weakness of the muscles within the involved compartment. This finding alone might be hard to differentiate from proximal nerve injury as well as guarding due to pain at the site of injury. Another sign of muscle ischemia is pain with passive stretch of the muscles involved in the affected compartment. For example, in the presence of an anterior compartment syndrome, passive plantar flexion of the ankle and toes will cause pain in the anterior compartment muscles. This finding, while consistent, is not specific to a compartment syndrome and should be correlated with other findings. The presence of a distal pulse should not deter the clinician from making the diagnosis of a compartment syndrome. Unless the tissue pressure is extremely high, that is, higher than the mean blood pressure, there could still be a distal pulse in the presence of a fully developed compartment syndrome. Distal capillary filling is usually intact and is a poor physical sign upon which to base a diagnosis. An exception occurs in the presence of a major arterial injury.

MEASUREMENT OF INTRACOMPARTMENTAL PRESSURE

The clinical manifestations of a compartment syndrome and the signs described above should, in most cases, be what is needed for the diagnosis of a compartment syndrome. There are situations, however, in which quantitative measurement of compartment pressures become important in making the diagnosis. Patients who are unresponsive and comatose may present with only a swollen injured extremity and insufficient clinical data on which to base the presence or absence of a compartment syndrome. Some patients are uncooperative, unreliable, or emotionally distressed, making the clinical examination difficult. Finally, patients with nerve deficits, due to either injury or other factors, such as diabetes, make laboratory measurements imperative in making the diagnosis. Pressure measurements are helpful in making the diagnosis of an exertional compartment syndrome.

The most simple method with which to measure compartment pressure is that of the needle-injection technique described by Whitesides et al.[56] All the necessary equipment is usually available in the hospital. Its degree of reliability is not as good as other techniques, and it does not provide a method of continuous monitoring.[29] With practice, the results become more reproducible. Measurement by use of the wick catheter is a popular technique and has been well described by Mubarak et al.[34,36] This accurate reproducible method offers a means of constant monitoring of pressure. The slit catheter is another popular method for measuring intracompartmental pressure and is less susceptible to coagulation of blood around the tip, one of the problems with the wick catheter. Both the wick and slit catheters are commercially available and are relatively easy techniques to learn.

TREATMENT

Once the diagnosis of an acute compartment syndrome has been made by clinical and/or laboratory means, immediate surgical decompression by fasciotomy is imperative. If the clinician is presented with a traumatized limb in which massive swelling and the potential for a compartment syndrome exists, steps can be taken to minimize the chances that a compartment syndrome will develop. First, all external pressure in the forms of circular dressing and casts should be removed. Univalving a cast is not sufficient, and we believe that bivalving the cast and cutting all the underlying soft dressings is imperative. Garfin et al.[11] studied the compartment volume and pressure relationships in the casted extremities of dogs. These workers demonstrated that complete removal of the cast was necessary before all the external pressure was relieved. If there is no change in the injured and swollen extremity with these measures, immediate fasciotomy should be performed. Compartment pressure measurements may be helpful in selected cases.

Decompressive fasciotomy of the lower leg has been described by a variety of techniques, including fibulectomy/fasciotomy through a single lateral incision,[22] a single lateral incision or parafibular approach,[28] and the more popular and widely used double-incision technique.[35]

Authors' Preferred Technique

We consider the double-incision technique as described by Mubarak et al.[34] the preferred method for decompressive fasciotomy of the lower leg. Not only is the fibula left intact, but it is a simple and quick procedure that also permits exposure and debridement of any necrotic muscle or tissue. In cases in which only one compartment is involved, one of the incisions may be used rather than both. Two limited incisions are usually sufficient. In patients in whom there is massive swelling and in whom the skin is a restricting envelope, the incisions can be lengthened to the full length of the compartments. The longer the skin incisions, the more likely that later skin grafting rather than delayed primary closure will be necessary. If a limited incision is used, care must be taken to perform a complete fasciotomy; in some cases, it may be necessary to remeasure compartment pressures. If compartment pressure measurement techniques are not available or if there is massive swelling, full-length incisions should be used. The double-incision technique uses an anterolateral approach for the anterior and lateral compartments and a posteromedial incision for the superficial and deep posterior compartments.

Anterolateral Approach

A vertical incision is made halfway between the anterior tibial crest and the fibula shaft, in the vicinity of the anterior intermuscular septum that divides the anterior and lateral compartments. The skin incision for the limited-incision technique

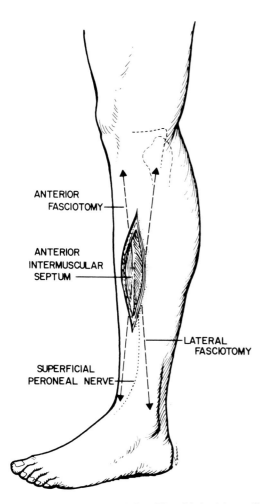

Fig. 131-3. Anterolateral incision. The skin incision utilized to approach the anterior and lateral compartments is placed halfway between the fibular shaft and the tibial crest. (From Mubarak,[33a] with permission.)

should be approximately 15 cm in length and may be extended to 25 cm or to the full length of the compartment when necessary. Sharp dissection is carried down to the fascia, and the skin is undermined proximally and distally as well as medially and laterally to permit full exposure of the fascia. The more limited the incision used, the more undermining should be performed. Large right-angle retractors are helpful when doing this. A small 2-cm transverse incision is then made through the fascia and the anterior intermuscular septum is then identified, separating the anterior and lateral compartments. The primary importance of identifying the septum that separates the compartments is to prevent damage to the superficial peroneal nerve, which travels in the lateral compartment just next to the anterior intermuscular septum. Vertical fasciotomy is then performed proximally and distally, using a 12-inch Metzenbaum scissors midway between the intermuscular septum and the tibial crest. The curved tip of the scissors should be pointed toward the patella proximally and the great toe distally, to prevent damage to the superficial peroneal nerve (Fig. 131-3). With skin retraction, verify that complete fasciotomy has been performed. If there is any doubt, the skin incisions should be lengthened.

The lateral compartment fasciotomy is made just anterior and parallel to the fibular shaft with the curved tip pointed toward the fibular head proximally and the lateral malleolus distally to again prevent damage to the superficial peroneal nerve. Debridement of necrotic muscle may be carried out as necessary.

Posteromedial Approach

Where the skin incision for the anterolateral approach is centered in the midportion of the lower leg, the posteromedial incision should be centered slightly distal to this, in order to identify the deep posterior compartment as it becomes superficial distally. A vertical incision is made 15 to 25 cm long, depending on the individual case, parallel and 2 cm posterior to the posteromedial tibial border. This approach avoids the saphenous nerve and vein, which travel just posterior to the tibial border. As in the anterolateral incision, extensive undermining of the skin incision is necessary to gain complete exposure of the fascia. The saphenous nerve and vein should be carefully dissected free of the fascia and retracted anteriorly. A transverse incision is made identifying the intermuscular septum separating the superficial and deep posterior compartments. The flexor digitorum longus muscle and tendon are usually visible in the deep compartment. The Achilles tendon and distal gastrocnemius and soleus muscles are visible posteriorly. The superficial posterior compartment is decompressed first using 12-inch Metzenbaum scissors and large right-angle retractors. The deep compartment fasciotomy is then extended distally behind the medial malleolus and proxi-

mally beneath the soleus bridge (Fig. 131-4). The distal end of the soleus bridge varies from case to case and, if it extends distally more than halfway down the tibia, it may be necessary to release the soleus bridge partially from its tibial attachment in order to complete the proximal portion of the deep compartment fasciotomy. In cases of massive swelling, complete detachment of the soleus bridge may be necessary. Intracompartmental pressure monitoring may be helpful in determining the extent of dissection necessary for full decompression.

POSTOPERATIVE MANAGEMENT

If the diagnosis is made early and there is relatively little swelling, primary skin closure may be possible. However, if there is any doubt, the wound should be left completely open. A delayed primary closure is often possible 5 to 7 days later, particularly if the initial incision had been small. In the case of a large open wound, split-thickness skin grafting is often necessary. Often, it is necessary to return the patient to the operating room in 48 to 72 hours, to determine the status of the muscle and the need for debridement of necrotic muscle tissue. Splinting may also be necessary to prevent contracture. Routinely, apply a posterior splint to hold the ankle in neutral to prevent any plantar flexion contracture. In the presence of a tibial fracture, external fixation has proved very useful not only in immobilizing and treating the fracture primarily but in facilitating wound management as well.

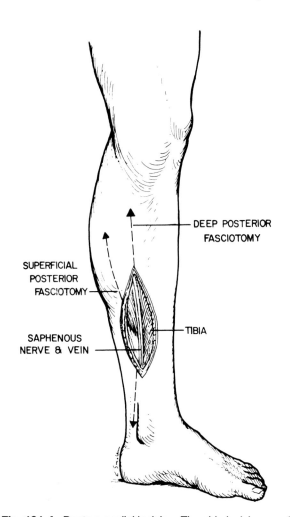

Fig. 131-4. Posteromedial incision. The skin incision used to decompress the superficial and deep posterior compartments is placed 2 cm posterior to the posterior tibial margin. (From Mubarak,[33a] with permission.)

EXERTIONAL COMPARTMENT SYNDROME

The exertional compartment syndrome has become an increasingly recognized cause of exercise-induced pain in the lower extremity. In this entity, exercise induces temporary increases in intracompartmental pressures sufficient to retard the blood flow to the tissue causing pain and occasionally a temporary neurologic deficit. With cessation of exercise, pressure is returned to normal. It most commonly involves the anterior tibial compartment and the deep posterior compartment.[50] On rare occasions, prolonged exercise may initiate an acute irreversible compartment syndrome requiring immediate treatment. However, the much more common chronic reversible syndrome is the topic of this discussion.

It has been well established that with exercise it is normal for intracompartmental pressures to increase. Logan et al.[24] studied the variations in compartment pressure with walking and jogging in normal individuals. This was performed with a slit catheter in the anterior tibial compartment. They found that with walking there was a mean pressure of 13 mmHg, which increased with walking speed. However, there were marked variations in pressure with peak to peak pressures up to 40 mmHg, which increased further with jogging. Also, during an acute muscle contraction, there is a temporary rise in intracompartmental pressure, probably as a result of tissue compression and temporary cessation of blood flow. Gershuni et al.[13] demonstrated by ultrasound techniques that there is an increased compartment width with exercise, up to 10 percent with running, secondary to an increase in the volume of the compartment contents. Furthermore, in a trained athlete with chronic muscle hypertrophy, there may be less room to accommodate for the acute swelling with exercise.

Many studies[30,36,39,40] have shown that in patients with exertional compartment syndrome, there is a statistically significant higher increase in pressure with exercise as compared with controls. Mubarak and Hargens[32] studied patients with symptoms of chronic compartment syndrome with the wick catheter before, during, and after exercise and compared it with normal controls. They found that the resting intracompartmental pressure in these patients was usually 15 mmHg or more, as compared with 0 to 5 mmHg in normal subjects. With exercise, they found that the mean pressure rose to above 75 mmHg and, at the completion of exercise, the pressure would usually remain at greater than 30 mmHg for 5 minutes or more (Fig. 131-5).

Using similar studies, Puranen and Alavaikko[39] also found that these patients had increased resting pressure as well as increased pressure after exercise compared with normal subjects. They performed muscle biopsies in these patients and demonstrated increased water content and muscle lactate content. They also demonstrated increased blood flow, using xenon-133 clearance techniques. In comparing symptomatic and asymptomatic controls, McDermott et al.[30] found that the only truly statistically significant difference was the mean pressure during exercise; they concluded that a mean pressure of more than 85 mmHg should be considered abnormal and diagnostic of a chronic compartment syndrome.

The clinical presentation is usually that of an athletic individual who complains of recurrent pain over the affected compartment with exercise.[27] Its symptoms are described as a recurrent tightness or aching in the general distribution of the compartment with activity. Sometimes this is described as a cramping or stabbing sensation. Symptoms slowly increase with exercise and often are reproducible for a specific speed and distance in a runner. It may reach the point where the athlete may have to stop the activity; usually, with a period of rest, the pain will gradually subside, only to recur with exercise. Occasionally, a temporary neurologic deficit may occur, including the feeling of numbness or paresthesias in the foot, as well as ankle weakness and the feeling of the ankle giving way. Rarely, an actual neurologic deficit may temporarily occur, usually in association with an anterior tibial compartment syndrome, causing a temporary foot drop.

There is usually a paucity of physical findings when examining the athlete in the office. Occasionally, muscle hypertrophy with the well-trained athlete will be noted; some of these patients are believed to have a thickened, less compliant fascia, although this is usually difficult to determine on physical examination. There appears to be an association with the presence of a muscle hernia with the chronic anterior tibial compartment syndrome. This herniation, which may be more evident after exercise, occurs in the lower third of the leg overlying the anterior intermuscular septum dividing the anterior and lateral compartments. It is possible that this fascial defect is in actuality an enlargement of the orifice through which the superficial

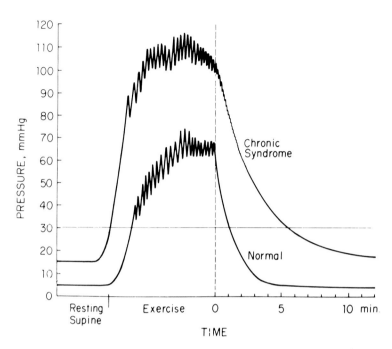

Fig. 131-5. Illustrative anterior compartmental pressures recorded with the wick catheter during exercise of a normal subject and a patient afflicted with a chronic anterior compartment syndrome. The resting pressure of the chronic syndrome is elevated over that of the normal control. During exercise, the pressure rises to greater than 75 mmHg and remains greater than 30 mmHg for more than 5 minutes in the patient with chronic syndrome. (From Mubarak and Hargens,[32] with permission.)

peroneal nerve exits the lateral compartment, to become superficial in the distal third of the leg.[20,23]

It is most helpful to have patients reproduce their symptoms with exercise. After exercise, the clinician may note a general increase in fullness over the affected compartment. A careful motor and sensory examination may indicate temporary deficits. This approach may also help differentiate this entity from other causes of exercise-induced lower leg pain, including stress fractures of the tibia or fibula, tenosynovitis, periostitis, or the medial tibial syndrome.[7,53]

Most of these patients will have had symptoms ranging from several months to years. Plain films and bone scan may be helpful to rule out stress fracture, periostitis, or other more unusual causes. When clinical findings warrant, the most conclusive way to make the diagnosis of an exertional compartment syndrome is by dynamic pressure measurements before, during, and after exercise. This is most commonly done with the wick or slit catheter, permitting clinical monitoring of the pa-

tient's symptoms and correlating them with the pressure measurements.[48] It is important to determine whether just one compartment is involved or, as in many cases, more than one, most commonly the anterior and deep posterior compartments. In one study of 100 patients with symptoms of compartment syndrome, the anterior compartment was involved 39 percent of the time and the deep posterior compartment 48 percent of the time.[9]

Treatment

Once a diagnosis has been made on the basis of history, physical examination, and pressure measurements, and other causes have been ruled out, nonoperative treatment options are few.[5] Many patients will prefer to limit their athletic activities once the problem has been outlined to them, in order to minimize their symptoms. However, if the patient wishes to continue the running or exercise program at the same level, fasciotomy is the only solution. The technique is similar to that described for the acute compartment syndrome, but the incisions used can be much smaller and the surgery can be performed on an outpatient basis.[49]

Anterior Tibial Compartment

For the anterior tibial compartment, a 5- to 6-cm vertical incision is made halfway between the anterior tibial crest and the fibula in the midportion of the leg. Dissection is carried right down to the fascia, and the anterior intermuscular septum is identified. Using large right-angle retractors, the edges are undermined proximally and distally and, using a 12-inch Metzenbaum scissors, fasciotomy of the anterior and then the lateral compartment is performed. We would recommend routine decompression of both compartments. If a muscle hernia is present, the skin incision should be centered over the defect so that the superficial peroneal nerve can be identified. Decompressive fasciotomy is then carried out proximally and distally from this defect. Under no circumstances should this defect be closed, for fear of precipitating an acute compartment syndrome. The decompression is performed exactly as described for the acute compartment syndrome. The skin is then closed and a compressive dressing is applied.

Deep Posterior Compartment

For the deep posterior compartment, a vertical 5-cm incision is made 2 cm posterior to the posteromedial edge of the tibia, centered at the junction of the mid- and distal third of the lower leg. Dissection is carried down to the fascia, and the saphenous nerve and vein are identified anteriorly and retracted. Decompression of both deep and superficial posterior compartments is performed using the 12-inch Metzenbaum scissors. The incision is closed, and a compressive dressing is applied.

Postoperatively, the patient is allowed immediate weight bearing. Crutches can usually be discarded within a couple of days after surgery and range-of-motion exercises are begun 1 week to 10 days after surgery. A gradual resumption of activities is allowed over the following 2 to 3 weeks, and full return to normal activities is usually possible

within 1 month after surgery. Numerous follow-up studies[1,9,46,52] have shown excellent results after a fasciotomy for exertional compartment syndrome. Our own experience parallels the experience of these investigators.

Rorabeck[45] suggested that the tibialis posterior is contained within its own osseofacial compartment and should be decompressed during the posterior compartment fasciotomy. Using pressure measurements on cadavers, he showed that the tibialis posterior is actually in its own separate compartment and that it is not decompressed by routine deep posterior compartment fasciotomy. He recommends decompression through a single lateral incision, which permits exposure of all the compartments, and releasing the fascial attachment of the tibialis posterior muscle to the fibula in order to decompress this muscle. We have not had experience with this technique.

Medial Tibial Syndrome

Medial tibial syndrome is a distinct clinical entity most often seen in runners, but it is also seen in athletes involved in jumping sports.[2] The pain is located along the medial border of the distal tibia. Pain is exacerbated by athletic activity and decreases with rest. It quite often becomes a chronic problem that is frequently bilateral. In more severe cases, the patient may also be symptomatic with the normal activities of daily living.

On physical examination, there is always palpable tenderness along the distal third of the posteromedial edge of the tibia. In some cases, there may be some soft tissue swelling or thickening in this area as well as a feeling of fullness. No neurovascular abnormalities will be noted, and the pain and tenderness will increase after athletic activity. Radiographs are usually negative, although in some chronic cases, cortical hypertrophy or periosteal bone formation may be seen along the distal medial third of the tibia. Bone scan frequently shows mildly increased uptake diffusely along the distal third of the medial tibia, but not always.[19] The localized intense uptake that one would see with stress fracture is not seen in these cases.

This entity was originally thought to represent a deep posterior compartment syndrome.[38] However, subsequently several studies using pressure measurements in these patients have refuted this theory. D'Ambrosia et al.[6] studied the pressures in the deep posterior compartment in patients with medial tibial syndrome and found all to be normal. Dynamic pressure measurements before, during, and after exercise have supported the fact that this does not represent a deep posterior compartment syndrome.[33,35] It appears that this entity most likely represents a periostitis or more appropriately a stress reaction in the periosteum as well as the fascia and bone at this location.

A very conservative approach appears to be the best way to manage these patients. The mainstay of treatment is a period of rest until signs and symptoms have disappeared. Running activities can usually be substituted for with biking and swimming. In the acute phase, ice application and nonsteroidal anti-inflammatory drugs (NSAIDs) have been used by some with limited success. Stretching and gentle strengthening exercises are often prescribed. Alteration of running shoes as well as the use of taping and orthotics have also proved helpful. Operative intervention has been proposed by some in recalcitrant cases. Interestingly, although evidence points to the fact that this is not a deep posterior compartment syndrome, some investigators reported satisfactory results after performing a deep posterior compartment fasciotomy in these patients.[38,52] Recently, Allen and Barnes[1] compared two groups of patients, one with a chronic anterior compartment syndrome and the other with a medial tibial syndrome. They found that although fasciotomy is the treatment of choice for the chronic anterior compartment syndrome, those patients with medial tibial syndrome did not show significant improvement with surgery. It is obvious that further well-controlled studies are necessary before it can be determined whether surgical intervention is ever indicated in these cases.

REFERENCES

1. Allen MJ, Barnes MR: Exercise pain in the lower leg. Chronic compartment syndrome and the medial tibial syndrome. J Bone Joint Surg 68B:815, 1986

2. Bates P: Shinsplints—a literature review. Br J Sports Med 19(3):132, 1985

3. Bleck SS, Brumback RJ, Poka A, et al: Compartment syndrome in open tibial fracture. J Bone Joint Surg 68A:1348, 1986

4. Chisholm CD, Clark DE: Effect of the pneumatic antishock garment on intramuscular pressure. Ann Emerg Med 13:581, 1984

5. Christensen JT, Eklof B, Wulff K: The chronic compartment syndrome and response to diuretic treatment. Acta Chir Scand 149:249, 1983

6. D'Ambrosia RD, Zelis RF, Chuinard RG, Wilmore J: Interstitial pressure measurements in the anterior and posterior compartments in athletes with shin splints. Am J Sports Med 5:127, 1977

7. Davey JR, Rorabeck CH, Fowler PJ: The tibialis posterior muscle compartment: an unrecognized cause of exertional compartment syndrome. Am J Sports Med 12:319, 1984

8. Delec J, Steihl JB: Open tibia fracture with compartment syndrome. Clin Orthop 160:175, 1981

9. Detmer DE, Sharpe K, Sufit RL, Firdley FM: Chronic compartment syndrome: diagnosis, management, and outcome. Am J Sports Med 13(3):162, 1985

10. Ernst CB, Kaufen H: Fibulectomy-fasciotomy: an important adjunct in the management of lower extremity arterial trauma. J Trauma 11:365, 1971

11. Garfin SR, Mubarak SJ, Evans KJ, et al: Quantification of intracompartmental pressure and volume under plaster casts. J Bone Joint Surg 63A:449, 1981

12. Garfin SR, Tipton CM, Mubarak SJ, et al: The role of fascia in the maintenance of muscle tension and pressure. J Appl Physiol 51:317, 1981

13. Gershuni DJ, Gosink BB, Hargens AR, et al: Ultrasound evaluation of the anterior musculofascial compartment of the leg following exercise. Clin Orthop 167:185, 1982

14. Gibson MJ, Barnes MR, Allen MJ, Chan RN: Weakness of foot dorsiflexion and changes in compartment pressures after tibial osteotomy. J Bone Joint Surg 68B:471, 1986

15. Hargens AR, Akenson WH, Mubarak SJ, et al: Fluid balance within the canine anterolateral compartment and its relationship to compartment syndromes. J Bone Joint Surg 60A:499, 1978

16. Hargens AR, Romine JS, Sipe JC, et al: Peripheral nerve-conduction block by high muscle-compartment pressure. J Bone Joint Surg 61A:192, 1979

17. Hargens AR, Mubarak SJ, Owen CA, et al: Interstitial fluid pressure in muscle and compartments syndromes in man. Microvasc Res 14:1, 1977

18. Hargens AR, Schmidt DA, Evans KL, et al: Quantitation of skeletal-muscle necrosis in a model compartment syndrome. J Bone Joint Surg 63A:631, 1981
19. Holder LE, Michael RH: The special scintigraphic pattern of "shin splints in the lower leg." Concise communication. J Nucl Med 25:865, 1984
20. Hoover JA: Exertional compartment syndrome with fascial hernias. J Foot Surg 22:271, 1983
21. Kabach KR, Sanders AB, Meislin HW: MAST suit update. JAMA 252:2598, 1984
22. Kelly RP, Whitesides TE Jr: Transfibular route for fasciotomy of the leg. J Bone Joint Surg 49A:1022, 1967
23. Leach RE, Hannomd G, Stryker WS: Anterior tibial compartment syndrome; acute and chronic. J Bone Joint Surg 49A:451, 1967
24. Logan JG, Rorabeck CH, Caste GSP: Measurement of dynamic compartment pressure during exercise. Am J Sports Med 11:220, 1983
25. Lydan JC, Spielman FJ: Bilateral compartment syndrome following prolonged surgery in the lithotomy position. Anesthesiology 60:236, 1984
26. Madigan RR: Acute compartment syndrome in hemophilia. A case report. J Bone Joint Surg 64A:313, 1982
27. Martens MA, Backaert M, Vermaut G, Mulier JC: Chronic leg pain in athletes due to a recurrent compartment syndrome. Am J Sports Med 12:148, 1984
28. Matsen FA, Kurgmire RB: Compartment syndromes. Surg Gynecol Obstet 147:143, 1978
29. McDermott AG, Marble AE, Yabsley RH: Monitoring acute compartment pressures with the STIC catheter. Clin Orthop 190:192, 1984
30. McDermott AG, Marble AE, Yabsley RH, Phillips MB: Monitoring dynamic anterior compartment pressures during exercise. A new technique using the STIC catheter. Am J Sports Med 10(2):83, 1982
31. Miniaci A, Rorabeck CH: Compartment syndrome as a complication of repair of a hernia of the tibialis anterior. A case report. J Bone Joint Surg 68A:1444, 1986
32. Mubarak SJ, Hargens AR: Compartment Syndromes and Volkmann's Contracture. Saunders Monographs in Clinical Orthopedics. Vol. III. WB Saunders, Philadelphia, 1981
33. Mubarak SJ, Gould RN, Leo YF, et al: The medial tibial stress syndrome. A cause of shin splints. Am J Sports Med 10(4):201, 1982
33a. Mubarak SJ, Hargens AR: Diagnosis and management of compartment syndromes. In AAOS: Symposium on Trauma to the Leg and Its Sequela. CV Mosby, St. Louis, 1981
34. Mubarak SJ, Hargens AR, Owen CA, et al: The wick technique for measurement of intramuscular pressure: a new research and clinical tool. J Bone Joint Surg 58A:1016, 1976
35. Mubarak SJ, Owen CA: Double incision fasciotomy of the leg for decompression in compartment syndromes. J Bone Joint Surg 59A:184, 1977
36. Mubarak SJ, Owen CA, Hargens AR, et al: Acute compartment syndromes: diagnosis and treatment with the aid of the wick catheter. J Bone Joint Surg 60A:1091, 1978
37. Owen CA, Mubarak SJ, Hargens AR, et al: Intramuscular pressures with limb compression; clarification of the pathology of the drug-induced muscular compartment syndrome. N Engl J Med 300:1169, 1979
38. Puranen J: The medial tibial syndrome. Exercise ischemia in the medial fascial compartment of the leg. J Bone Joint Surg 56B:712, 1974
39. Puranen J, Alavaikko A: Intracompartment pressure increase on exertion in patients with chronic compartment syndrome in the leg. J Bone Joint Surg 63A:1304, 1981
40. Quarfordt P, Christenson JJ, Edlaf B, et al: Intramuscular pressure, muscle blood flow, and skeletal muscle metabolism in chronic anterior tibial compartment syndrome. Clin Orthop 179:284, 1983
41. Reddy PK, Kaye KW: Deep posterior compartment syndrome; a serious complication of the lithotomy position. J Urol 132:144, 1984
42. Reneman RS: The anterior and the lateral compartment syndrome of the leg due to intensive use of muscles. Clin Orthop 113:69, 1975
43. Reneman RS, Slaaf DW, Lindbom L, et al: Muscle blood flow disturbances produced by simultaneously elevated venous and total muscle tissue pressure. Microvasc Res 20:307, 1980
44. Roberts RS, Csencsitz TA, Heard CW: Upper extremity compartment syndromes following pit Viper envenomation. Clin Orthop 193:154, 1985
45. Rorabeck CH: Exertional tibialis posterior compartment syndrome. Clin Orthop 208:61, 1986
46. Rorabeck CH, Bourde RB, Fowler PJ: The surgical treatment of exertional compartment syndrome in athletes. J Bone Joint Surg 65A:1245, 1983
47. Rorabeck CH, Clarke KM: The pathophysiology of the anterior tibial compartment syndrome: an experimental investigation. J Trauma 18:299, 1987
48. Russell WL, Apyan PM, Burns RP: Utilization and wide clinical implementation using the wick catheter for compartment pressure measurement. Surg Gynecol Obstet 160:207, 1985
49. Styf JR, Korner LM: Chronic anterior-compartment syndrome of the leg. Results of treatment by fasciotomy. J Bone Joint Surg 68A:1338, 1986

50. Veith RG, Matsen FA, Newell SG: Recurrent anterior compartment syndrome. Physician Sports Med 8:30, 1980

51. Wall JJ: Compartment syndrome as a complication of the Hauser procedure. J Bone Joint Surg 61A:185, 1979

52. Wallenstein R: Results of fasciotomy in patients with medial tibial syndrome or chronic anterior compartment syndrome. J Bone Joint Surg 65:1252, 1983

53. Wallenstein R, Eriksson E: Intramuscular pressures in exercise-induced lower leg pain. Int J Sports Med 5:31, 1984

54. Warbel GB, Shybut GT: Acute compartment syndrome caused by malfunctioning pneumatic compression boot. A case report. J Bone Joint Surg 68A:1445, 1986

55. Whitesides TE Jr: Compartment syndromes. Orthopedic Instruction Course. Am Acad Orthop Surg Dallas, TX, 1978

56. Whitesides TE Jr, Haney TC, Hirada H et al: A simple method for tissue pressure determination. Arch Surg 110:1311, 1975

57. Whitesides TE Jr, Haney TC, Morimoto K, Hirada H: Tissue pressure measurements as a determinant for the need of fasciotomy. Clin Orthop 113:43, 1975

58. Whitesides TE Jr, Hirada H, Morimoto K: Compartment syndromes and the role of fasciotomy, its parameters and techniques. Am Acad Orthop Surg Instruct Course Lect 26:179, 1977

Section 9

THE FOOT

Henry R. Cowell

Section Editor

Introduction

Henry R. Cowell

The orthopaedic surgeon with an interest in the foot will see many patients with painful foot deformities. This pain may be mild and only annoying or may be so severe as to be disabling at times. In either instance, the pain is usually secondary to deformity of one or more parts of the foot. This deformity may be flexible, and thus correctable in its early stages, or may progress to fixed deformity that cannot be corrected passively. When the deformity is flexible, soft tissue procedures such as tendon transfer may be performed to properly align the foot or toes into satisfactory position, thereby relieving the symptoms. However, once the deformity becomes fixed, bony reconstruction is frequently required to relieve the deformity and place the foot in a plantigrade position for weight bearing. When the foot is not plantigrade, one portion of the undersurface of the foot takes an excessive amount of weight, resulting in pain and callus formation. Most surgery on the foot is directed at realigning the foot in the plantigrade postion or aligning the toes, thus redistributing the pressure caused by weight bearing or shoes. Many deformities of the toes would not require surgery in a shoeless society.

This section is organized by anatomic location, by the position of the deformity, and by the etiology of the abnormalities. The first chapter covers the common disorders of the os calcis, including "pump bump." The next five chapters discuss positional deformities of the hind part of the foot and their conservative and surgical treatment. This is followed by a discussion of the treatment of the painful flatfoot and a chapter on the tarsal tunnel syndrome. Chapter 140, the final chapter in this subsection outlines the use of astragalectomy in treating problems in this anatomic area.

The next four chapters are devoted to abnormalities of the big toe, including hallux valgus, hallux rigidus, prosthetic arthroplasty of the hallux, and dorsal bunion. A discussion of bunionette deformity of the fifth toe (which is analogous to the common bunion) follows.

Four chapters are devoted to abnormalities of the lesser toes and splay foot. A discussion of surgical syndactyly follows. This subsection is concluded with a discussion of aseptic necrosis of the sesamoids and metatarsal heads.

Chapters on rheumatoid arthritis, the diabetic foot, and deformities secondary to cerebral vascular accidents follow. The next chapter discusses the management of skin and nail problems.

The final chapters cover the treatment of fractures of the talus and os calcis, and fractures and dislocations of the midpart and forepart of the foot.

The preoperative evaluation of the patient should include an examination of the foot in both the static and dynamic states. Pressure measurements under the foot may aid in planning realignment procedures. The patient should have good skin coverage, good circulation, and no infection. Skin incisions must be placed accurately and osteotomies must be preplanned. The radiograph may be traced and cutouts made to determine the appropriate location and extent of osteotomies. A duplicate of the radiograph may be cut to simulate the osteotomy and postoperative position.

The expected outcome and therapeutic goals should be agreed upon by the patient and the physician. Operations on the foot and ankle should involve meticulous care of the skin to avoid skin loss. The skin edges may be retracted with skin hooks rather than with rakes or other types of retractors; the skin should not be retracted with pickups or other instruments. Most surgical procedures on the foot should be carried out using a thigh tourniquet.[2] It should be noted that a tourniquet may be contraindicated in patients with certain problems such as diabetes, sickle cell disease, or circulatory abnormalities. If a thigh tourniquet is used, the leg can be exsanguinated and the tourniquet inflated prior to prepping the extremity when it is anticipated that the operation will last less than an hour. I prefer to do this, since it is difficult to adequately exsanguinate the leg once the drapes have been applied. The tourniquet is inflated to 150 mmHg above systolic pressure after exsanguination by elevation and an elastic bandage. The use of a tourniquet in this fashion does not increase the risk of venous thrombosis.[3] Many procedures may be done using regional blocks in association with an ankle tourniquet. The leg is prepped with Betadine soap and the skin painted with Betadine prior to the incision being made.

I prefer to deflate the tourniquet at the end of the procedure to be sure that all bleeding vessels are coagulated in order to prevent hematoma formation postoperatively. The only exception to deflating the tourniquet is in an individual who has undergone large bony resection where bone bleeding will be present. This may be seen in patients with triple arthrodeses. However, in most instances the tourniquet should be deflated and hemostasis obtained prior to closure. Following adequate hemostasis, deep tissue is generally closed with a 00 suture, subcutaneous tissue with a 000 suture, and the skin with either nylon or subcuticular wire.

When a postoperative cast is required polyurethane foam may be applied over the entire dorsum of the foot and leg. Polyurethane foam[1] is placed directly on the skin and a piece of foam approximately 3 inches wide is laid over the dorsal aspect of the foot, the anterior aspect of the leg, and the anterior aspect of the thigh. Webril is used over this, and a cast is applied. The polyurethane foam allows for some swelling; also, if it becomes necessary to split the cast during the postoperative period, this can be done through the plaster and sheetwadding (or Webril) down to the polyurethane foam, protecting the skin. Polyurethane foam is the only type of material that may be used for this; the use of sponge rubber or similar material causes skin maceration and should not be considered.

Most operative procedures involving tendon transfer require postoperative casting for 6 weeks, followed by protection in a brace. Operative procedures on bone, including osteotomies, involve at least 6 weeks in a cast. An above-knee cast may be required if the abnormality is in the hind part of the foot. The cast is removed at 6 weeks, radiographs are obtained, and the patient is allowed to ambulate (in a short-leg walking cast, if necessary). A few procedures will require weight bearing during the postoperative period, e.g., osteotomy of the second metatarsal, which is performed to relieve pressure from the second metatarsal head. Most operative procedures will require non-weight bearing at least in the immediate postoperative period. Also, elevation is recommended, since allowing the leg to be dependent causes increased swelling. However, the patient should be allowed to get out of bed and may ambulate with crutches even if weight bearing is restricted.

In summary, it must be emphasized that all surgery on the foot should be very carefully planned and may be facilitated by a preoperative radiograph cut-out to determine the optimum correction for placing the foot in a plantigrade position. The skin must be handled meticulously throughout the entire operative procedure. Attention to detail allows operative intervention without significant complications.

ACKNOWLEDGMENT

I would like to thank Mary Katherine O'Haire, Eileen Cunniffe, and Eda Flaxer for their assistance in the editing of this section.

REFERENCES

1. Cowell HR, Balecia T: Polyurethane foam in postoperative casts. Clin Orthop 131:259, 1978
2. Shaw JA, Murray DG: The relationship between tourniquet pressure and underlying soft-tissue pressure in the thigh. J Bone Joint Surg 64A:1148, 1982
3. Simon MA, Mass DP, Zarins CK, et al: The effect of a thigh tourniquet on the incidence of deep venous thrombosis after operations on the forepart of the foot. J Bone Joint Surg 64A:188, 1982

132

Henry R. Cowell

BONY RIDGES AND TUBEROSITIES OF THE OS CALCIS

Anatomically, the os calcis often has a superior tuberosity and a lateral bony ridge, either of which may become the source of irritation when tight shoes are worn. In addition, there are two bursae in this area. The subcutaneous bursa is found between the skin and the heel cord. The retrocalcaneal bursa is located at the point where the heel cord inserts, approximately 1.5 cm distal to the superior portion of the os calcis. Prolonged irritation from tight shoes gives a characteristic bony enlargement of the posterior lateral surface of the calcaneous in this area proximal to the insertion of the Achilles tendon. Because of its frequent occurrence in women, Dickinson, Coutts, Woodward, and Handler[6] have used the term "pump bump" to describe the syndrome of a painful enlargement of the os calcis, which is frequently associated with an overlying bursitis. They noted that these bumps are almost invariably found in women and are associated with wearing high-heeled shoes or shoes with a short vamp, both of which exert pressure on the posterior lateral surface of the os calcis.

By contrast, Heneghan and Pavlov[15] maintain that the symptoms seen with this condition are related to an increase in the pitch of the os calcis, noting that Fuglsang and Torup[9] found that retrocalcaneal bursitis was more common in patients with cavus feet. Apley[1] noted that there are developmental variations in the shape of the os calcis, and that there is frequently a prominence of the lateral calcaneal ridge. While this ridge is considered to be a normal variant, it may give rise to symptoms when pressure from shoes is present in the area, and Helfet and Lee[14] have used the name "winter heel syndrome" to describe this difficulty.

Individuals have no difficulty from pump bump or winter heel syndrome if they do not wear shoes, or if they wear sandals or other shoes which do not create pressure on this area. Moreover, it is generally noted that, while the os calcis may have a superior tuberosity or there may be a lateral ridge, these conditions in themselves do not cause difficulty, and tight shoes cause problems in only a small number of patients. The difficulty arising from the pump bump can generally be helped by changing shoes to eliminate pressure over the area or by inserting a felt pad inside the shoe to raise the heel away from the tender area. Operative intervention

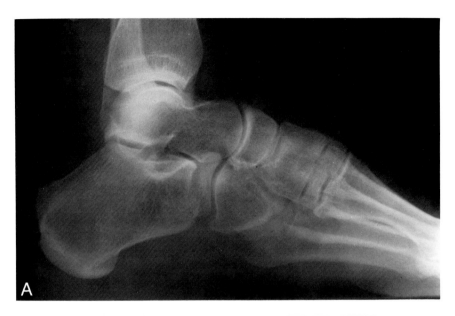

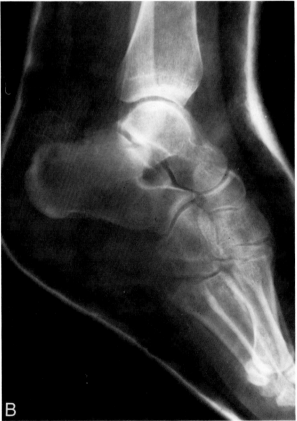

Fig. 132-1. (A) Preoperative radiograph of os calcis, illustrating a pump bump. There was redness of the skin and tenderness over the prominent portion of the os calcis. **(B)** Postoperative radiograph shows the amount of os calcis that must be excised to decompress the area under the skin.

is indicated only when symptoms have persisted and have not been relieved by the conservative measures outlined above. Heneghan and Pavlov[15] suggest that raising the heel, and thereby decreasing the calcaneal pitch, tilts the prominent portion of the os calcis away from the shoe, which relieves the symptoms.

Surgical Technique — Giannestras[11]

This procedure involves resection of a portion of the os calcis[11] and is carried out through a 4-cm incision on the medial aspect of the foot, equidistant between the posterior aspect of the medial malleolus and the posterior aspect of the heel cord. The incision is begun approximately 1 cm above the upper border of the os calcis and carried straight downward over the medial surface of the os calcis. The medial plantar branch of the posterior tibial nerve, located just forward of the incision, is retracted toward the medial malleolus. The os calcis is encountered, and the Achilles tendon is dissected from the portion of the os calcis proximal to the insertion of the Achilles tendon. This insertion is not violated. The soft tissue is dissected from the superior portion of the os calcis, and a bunion retractor may be slid around the os calcis to the lateral surface. A 1-inch osteotome is used to resect a triangular portion of the os calcis, measuring at least 1 cm at the base and approximately 2.5 cm on the hypotenuse of the triangle (Fig. 132-1). The osteotome is directed distally from medial to lateral to ensure removal of a satisfactory portion of the os calcis. I prefer this incision and resection both for the pump bump and to remove a piece of the lateral portion of the calcaneus, as described by Helfet for the winter heel syndrome. Following removal of the bone, the deep tissue is closed with interrupted sutures of 000 chromic catgut, the subcutaneous layer is closed with interrupted sutures of 000 plain catgut, and a subcuticular wire is used to approximate the skin. Giannestras recommends a below-knee weight-bearing plaster with the foot in mild plantar flexion for 4 weeks, followed by active weight bearing with crutches until full unsupported weight bearing is permitted, 6 weeks postoperatively.

Surgical Technique — Helfet[14]

Excision of the lateral calcaneal ridge is carried out through a vertical incision made over the os calcis,[14] lateral to the Achilles tendon. The sural nerve is identified and protected. The os calcis is identified, and the periosteum overlying the dome-shaped superior eminence of the os calcis beneath the Achilles tendon is incised vertically and stripped from the bone on the superficial and deep aspects to expose the calcaneal ridge. Helfet notes that this ridge is normally covered with a layer of articular cartilage. The lateral ridge is then excised by driving an osteotome obliquely through the full width of the bone. Helfet notes that extreme caution must be exercised not to strike the osteotome too hard, lest the instrument inadvertently penetrate the medial cortex of the os calcis with subsequent damage to the posterior tibial vessels. The skin edges are approximated and the os calcis is palpated to ensure that no ridge of bone is left; if any remains, it may be removed with a rongeur. Following this, the wound is closed with chromic catgut sutures in the deep fascia, and the skin is closed with subcuticular wire suture. Postoperatively, the foot is placed in a bulky dressing and is elevated. Weight bearing is allowed as soon as the patient can do so comfortably.

HEEL SPUR — PLANTAR FASCIITIS

While it has been suggested that the spur frequently seen on the inferior surface of the calcaneus is the cause of persistent heel pain, plantar fasciitis is the common cause of pain under the heel on weight bearing. The only physical finding is severe localized tenderness plantar to the spur of the os calcis, and thus the erroneous conclusion arises that the pain is secondary to the spurring and that excision of the spur will relieve the difficulty. In fact, the pain is secondary to a nonspecific inflammatory response in this area, and this difficulty frequently may be treated by conservative measures.

When operative intervention is required, removal of the heel spur or the prominence of the spur will relieve the symptoms in the weight-bearing surface of the foot. However, it should be emphasized that the main reason that removal of the spur relieves the difficulty is that it also excises the inflammatory tissue in the area; removal of the spur is specifically the cause of relief only when the spur is prominent and points down into the sole of the foot, causing an area of localized increased pressure on weight bearing. Numerous operative techniques have been suggested for the painful heel. These include excision of the spur, described by Du Vries[7]; plantar fasciotomy by Spitzy[23]; osteotomy by Steindler[24]; countersinking osteotomy by Michele and Krueger[20]; and drilling by Hassab and El-Sherif.[13]

There are many conservative treatment options for pain associated with plantar fasciitis. While custom inserts may be made with a depression in the insert below the prominence of the spur to relieve pressure from this area, the author has had excellent results with the use of a heel cup. This plastic heel cup, frequently referred to as a "high jumper's heel cup," will almost universally relieve the symptom of pain under the heel. This cup may be purchased at a sporting goods store and is worn under the heel, inside the shoe. Snook and Chrisman[22] have noted excellent results with this method of treatment. If the patient fails to respond, then a custom-fit insert may be made from a full insert of Plastizote, with the area underneath the heel spur depressed to prevent pressure. Full arch supports may also be made from leather, with a hollow in the area underneath the heel spur. Campbell and Inman[4] have suggested similar treatment with the use of a UC-BL shoe insert. If the individual fails to respond to a shoe insert, then Furey[10] suggests treatment with phenylbutazone, given 4 times a day for 7 days. He used this treatment in conjunction with a 2-cm foam rubber heel pad and high-heeled shoes, as well as arch supports. Lapidus and Guidotti[18] also suggest the use of phenylbutazone and, if this alone fails, the injection of local steroids. These investigators report satisfactory results in 323 patients with 364 painful heels. They state that no patient in their series required an operation. However, while an operation is seldom indicated, the following techniques are included for those patients who fail to respond to conservative measures.

Surgical Technique — DuVries[7]

A linear incision is made over the medial side of the os calcis, approximately 2 cm above the plantar border. This incision is begun at the posterior border of the os calcis and continued to the anterior third of the bone, approximately 5 to 6 cm in length. The incision is placed so that the spur is located immediately beneath and approximately in the midportion of the incision (Fig. 132-2). The incision is carried down through the skin and subcutaneous tissue until the medial border of the plantar fascia is exposed. The plantar fascia is separated from the inferior surface of the os calcis by blunt dissection, and the fascia is freed from the other subcutaneous tissue, also by blunt dissection. Following this, scissors are used to free the fascia over and around the spur until it is completely denuded on its superior and inferior surfaces across from the medial to the lateral side of the foot. A ⅜-inch osteotome is used to remove the spur from the os calcis. The surface is then smoothed with a rasp; the fascia is closed with interrupted sutures of 000 chromic, and the skin is closed with a subcuticular wire. A compression bandage is applied. The patient is allowed to ambulate with crutches in 4 days, and weight bearing may be resumed 4 weeks after surgery.

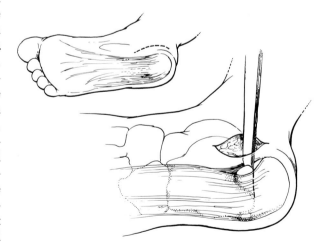

Fig. 132-2. Medial incision is made over the heel to excise the prominent portion of the os calcis and calcaneal spur (which in most instances is on the medial side of the os calcis). After stripping the periosteum from the area of the spur, the spur is excised, using a straight osteotome.

Surgical Technique — Bordelon[2]

A straight incision is made over the anterior three-fourths of the os calcis on the medial side of the foot. The distal portion of the medial calcaneal nerve is identified in the proximal portion of the incision, at the level of the proximal base of the spur, and decompressed. The nerve to the abductor digiti quinti is identified just distal to the spur, and is also decompressed. The plantar fascia is released, and the bone spur removed. After closure, a pressure dressing is applied. The patient is not allowed to bear weight on the foot for 3 weeks, following which a soft orthotic device is worn in the shoe.

Surgical Technique — Michele and Krueger[20]

Michele and Krueger[20] have described a procedure performed through a heel-flap incision to countersink the prominent portion of the os calcis while leaving the plantar fascia intact. A circumferential incision is made about the heel and the heel flap is raised, revealing the undersurface of the os calcis and the plantar fascia. A ¾-inch osteotome is driven into the os calcis medial, lateral, and posterior to the prominence of the os calcis. A small osteotome is used to divide the cortex anterior to the plantar fascia, thus freeing a block of bone with the plantar fascia attached. This block is countersunk into the os calcis, thus broadening the area for weight bearing and eliminating the bony prominence. No internal fixation is used. A below-knee cast is applied for 4 weeks and weight bearing is allowed. A longitudinal arch support is used following this. Because of the possibility that this procedure may injure the fat pad under the heel, I do not recommend its use.

Surgical Technique — Hassab and El-Sherif[13]

A small, curved incision approximately 3 cm in length is made on the lateral surface of the heel, extending below the lateral malleolus. The incision is carried down to the bone; the periosteum is stripped from the peroneal tendons anteriorly to the small muscles of the foot inferiorly. Retractors are then inserted between the bone and the Achilles tendon, and between the bone and the muscles of the sole. Approximately 7 to 10 small holes are drilled in the os calcis, traversing the bone from the lateral to the medial cortex. The deep tissue is closed with interrupted sutures of 000 chromic catgut, and the skin is closed with interrupted sutures of nylon. A soft dressing is applied. Postoperatively, the patient is allowed to walk on the third day, and the stitches are removed on the tenth day.

Complications

No investigators report any complications with these operative procedures. DuVries reports success in all 37 operative cases, and Hassab and El-Sherif report immediate and dramatic relief on the second postoperative day in 62 of 68 feet treated by their procedure. However, while these investigators have not reported complications, infection and neuropraxia of the posterior calcaneal nerve may occur, and the operation may fail to relieve the patient's symptoms. Hassab and El-Sherif note four failures: one in a patient with gout, one in a patient who had a postoperative infection, and two in patients with rigid flatfeet. They note that when the operation is used in patients who have recently developed symptoms the results are not so favorable. They therefore suggest the use of their procedure specifically in the chronic fasciitis/heel-spur syndrome.

REFERENCES

1. Apley AG: System of Orthopaedics and Fractures. 5th Ed. Butterworths, London, 1977
2. Bordelon RL: Adult forefoot. Subcalcaneal pain: present status, evaluation, and management. p. 283. American Academy of Orthopaedic Surgeons Instructional Course Lectures. Vol. 33. CV Mosby, St. Louis, 1984
3. Brahms MA: Common foot problems. J Bone Joint Surg 49A:1653, 1967

4. Campbell JW, Inman VT: Treatment of plantar fasciitis and calcaneal spurs with the UC-BL shoe insert. Clin Orthop 103:57, 1974

5. Chang CC, Miltner LJ: Periostitis of the os calcis. J Bone Joint Surg 16:355, 1934

6. Dickinson PH, Coutts MB, Woodward EP, et al: Tendo Achillis bursitis: report of twenty-one cases. J Bone Joint Surg 48A:77, 1966

7. DuVries HL: Heel spur (calcaneal spur). Arch Surg 74:536, 1957

8. Fowler A, Philip JF: Abnormality of the calcaneus as a cause of painful heel: its diagnosis and operative treatment. Br J Surg 32:494, 1945

9. Fuglsang F, Torup D: Bursitis retrocalcanearis. Acta Orthop Scanda 30:315, 1961

10. Furey JG: Plantar fasciitis: the painful heel syndrome. J Bone Joint Surg 57A:672, 1975

11. Giannestras NJ: Foot Disorders: Medical and Surgical Management. 2nd Ed. Lea & Febiger, Philadelphia, 1973

12. Griffith JD: Osteophytes of the os calcis. Am J Orthop Surg 8:501, 1910

13. Hassab HK, El-Sherif AS: Drilling of the os-calcis for painful heel with calcanean spur. Acta Orthop Scand 45:152, 1974

14. Helfet A, Lee DMG: Disorders of the Foot. JB Lippincott, Philadelphia, 1980

15. Heneghan MA, Pavlov H: The Haglund painful heel syndrome. Clin Orthop 187:228, 1984

16. Jones DC, James SL: Partial calcaneal ostectomy for retrocalcaneal bursitis. Am J Sports Med 12:72, 1984

17. Keck SW, Kelly PJ: Bursitis of the posterior part of the heel: evaluation of surgical treatment of eighteen patients. J Bone Joint Surg 47A:267, 1965

18. Lapidus PW, Guidotti FP: Painful heel: report of 323 patients with 364 painful heels. Clin Orthop 39:178, 1965

19. Martini M, Martini-Benkeddache Y, Bekhechi T, et al: Treatment of chronic osteomyelitis of the calcaneus by resetion of the calcaneus: a report of twenty cases. J Bone Joint Surg 56A:542, 1974

20. Michele AA, Krueger FJ: Plantar heel pain treated by countersinking osteotomy. Milit Surg 109:25, 1951

21. Porras ME, Hidalgo R, Quintana J: Partial excision of the os calcis in the treatment of lesions of the calcaneus. p. 176. In Bateman JE, Trott AW (eds): The Foot and Ankle. Thieme-Stratton, New York, 1980

22. Snook GA, Chrisman OD: The management of subcalcaneal pain. Clin Orthop 82:163, 1972

23. Spitzy H: Operation bei schmerzhaftem Kalkaneussporn. München Med Wehnschr 84:807, 1937

24. Steindler A, Smith AR: Spurs of the os calcis. Surg Gynecol Obstet 66:663, 1938

25. Wiltse LL, Bateman JG, Kase S: Resection of major portion of the calcaneus. Clin Orthop 13:271, 1959

Varus Foot

133

Henry R. Cowell

Varus of the foot may result from both paralytic and structural deformities in the adult. Paralytic varus deformities may be secondary to poliomyelitis, nerve injury, meningomyelocele, or the relative muscle imbalance seen in cerebral palsy. Varus deformities may also occur as a result of congenital problems, and may be seen in a patient who has an uncorrected club foot, or a partially corrected or a relapsed club foot. A foot may exhibit all components of the congenital club foot, with equinus, varus, and adduction deformities, or, in a partially corrected foot, only varus. The adult who has had a paralytic disorder since childhood generally has a structural as well as a paralytic deformity, but paralysis which has occurred at a later age, such as nerve injury, may lead to paralytic deformity without structural components.

INDICATIONS

Surgical correction of the varus foot is indicated in patients with structural deformities who are unable to place the foot plantigrade or who have diffi-culty with shoe wear because of the inverted position of the heel. When the deformity is dynamic, secondary to paralytic problems, and without structural components, bracing with a plastic orthosis may be considered to appropriately position the foot. However, if too much overpull is present in the posterior tibial muscle, bracing is not satisfactory, and operative correction is indicated to place the foot in the plantigrade position.

METHODS OF TREATMENT

The operative procedures available for correction of the varus foot include tendon transfer, bony stabilization with triple arthrodesis, or realignment of the os calcis by osteotomy. Tendon transfers are indicated in patients who have dynamic or paralytic deformities without structural instability. In patients who have mild imbalance, in whom the remaining active peroneal musculature is weak, lateral transfer of the anterior tibial muscle may be considered. If weakness is more profound and the peroneal muscles are only fair or poor, anterior transfer of the posterior tibial muscle may be considered. In patients with a relatively dynamic imbalance, such as those with cerebral palsy, a split transfer of the anterior tibial tendon may be performed. (The technique described by Hoffer[9] is included in Ch. 154.) When varus of the heel is the only component, with minimum or no muscle imbalance, then osteotomy of the os calcis, as described by Dwyer,[2,3] is the indicated procedure. When muscle imbalance and instability are present, or muscle imbalance and structural deformity, stabilization of the subtalar calcaneonavicular, talonavicular, and calcaneocuboid joints by triple arthrodesis should be considered. If the deformity is long standing, as seen in the uncorrected club foot of an adult, surgical release medially, followed by triple arthrodesis, as described by Herold and Torok,[8] may be considered. In patients who have long-standing deformity with structural varus and weakness of the peroneal muscles, who have had relative imbalance and have walked on the foot without support, laxity of the lateral ankle ligaments may be present. When the fibulotalar ligament has been elongated or stretched and ankle stability is present, triple arthrodesis may be combined with reconstruction of the ankle ligaments using the peroneal tendons, as described in Chapter 129.

Partial or total loss of sensation in the foot is a relative contraindication to stabilization of the foot by triple arthrodesis. When there is a lack of sensation on the sole of the foot, fusion of the joints of the foot may lead to pressure ulcers. This is particularly true if stabilization of the foot is not performed meticulously to ensure that weight bearing is distributed over the heel and the first and fifth metatarsals. When one of these points is prominent and insensitivity of the foot is present, excess pressure in the area that strikes the floor first will result in pressure sores; these may in turn lead to further skin breakdown. Healing is difficult when chronic osteomyelitis results, and amputation may be required. Therefore, while stabilization procedures may be considered in the insensitive foot, one must be certain that protective sensation is present, and that the foot is stabilized in such a position that no one weight-bearing area is prominent. In patients with insensitive feet, the postoperative use of Plastizote shoe inserts may help to obviate the prob-

lems caused by increased pressure in a concentrated area, but will not eliminate these problems completely.

Surgical Technique — Lateral Transfer of the Anterior Tibial Tendon

A 3-cm incision is made over the medial aspect of the foot, across the joint between the first metatarsal and the first cuneiform (Fig. 133-1). The anterior tibial tendon is located on the medial surface of the cuneiform as it runs under this bone. The tendon sheath is incised, and the tendon is freed from its distal attachment and tagged with a suture of 0 chromic catgut. Following this, the anterior tibial tendon is freed proximally and dissected sharply from the cuneiform and navicular.

A second incision is then made on the anterior surface of the leg, in the anterior medial aspect. This incision, approximately 5 cm in length, is made over the anterior tibial tendon, which can be palpated by pulling on the suture in the distal wound. The incision is carried down through the skin and subcutaneous tissue, the fascia is incised, and the anterior tibal tendon is identified by pulling on its distal aspect. A hemostat is placed under the anterior tibial tendon, which is pulled into the proximal incision. The distal incision is closed with subcutaneous sutures of 000 plain catgut, and the skin is closed with sutures of 000 nylon.

The bone chosen for the insertion of the tendon must be selected carefully. If the function of the posterior tibial tendon is normal, insertion into the cuboid should be considered. If the posterior tibial tendon is weak, insertion into the third cuneiform is appropriate. A 4-cm incision is made in the selected area through the skin and subcutaneous tissue; the extensor tendons are identified, and the incision is carried down to the appropriate bone. The periosteum is elevated and a hole is drilled in the bone for insertion of the tendon. The drill is carried through the proximal and distal cortices of the cuboid or cuneiform. The extensor tendon sheath is then split, and a tendon passer is inserted from the proximal incision to the distal lateral incision. The suture through the anterior tibial tendon is pulled into the distal wound. The anterior tibial

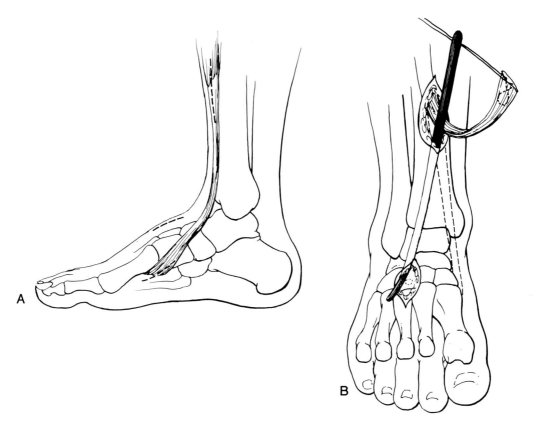

Fig. 133-1. **(A)** Incisions required for lateral transfer of the anterior tibial tendon are made over the medial side of the foot, over the anterior aspect of the leg, and on the dorsum of the foot. **(B)** After removing the anterior tibial tendon from its insertion and delivering the tendon into the proximal incision over the tibia, a tendon passer is used to thread the tendon to the lateral incision in the foot for insertion into bone.

tendon is delivered into the distal incision, and a wire pull-out suture is inserted into the anterior tibial tendon. Long, straight needles are used to pass the tendon into the bone. The wire exits through the sole of the foot, through a sponge, and is tied over a button, with the foot in the neutral position. This repair may be reinforced with sutures of 0 chromic catgut through the tendon and periosteum.

The incision is closed with interrupted sutures of 000 plain, and the skin is closed with interrupted 000 nylon. A below-knee cast is applied postoperatively and maintained for a 6-week period. At this time, the cast is split, and the posterior half is used as a splint until an ankle brace or an ankle-foot orthosis has been fitted to maintain the foot in the neutral position. This brace is worn full time for a

period of 4 to 6 months. The splint may be used at night, instead of the brace, if desired.

Surgical Technique — Anterior Transfer of the Posterior Tibial Tendon

The posterior tibial tendon may be transferred anteriorly around the tibia, or through the interosseous membrane.[14] Transfer through the interosseous membrane is the preferred approach. The surgical procedure is carried out through three incisions: one over the medial aspect of the foot; one over the posterior aspect of the leg; and one over the anterior aspect of the foot, for insertion (Fig. 133-2). The medial incision is placed on the inside

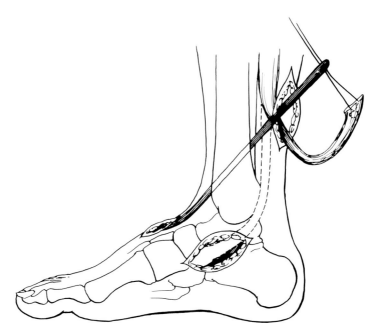

Fig. 133-2. Anterior transfer of the posterior tibial tendon, as carried out through three incisions. The tendon is removed from its insertion through the first incision, retracted into the second incision on the posterior aspect of the leg, and threaded to the dorsum of the foot through a window in the interosseous membrane.

of the foot, over the talus and the talonavicular joint. This incision is carried down through the skin and subcutaneous tissue, and the posterior tibial tendon is identified. The tendon sheath is then split, and the tendon itself is identified. The tendon is traced down to and split from the navicular, and the fibers coursing down under the arch of the foot are released as far distally as possible. The other attachments to this tendon, located over the navicular, are released, so that the tendon is free in the wound. The tendon is tagged with a suture of 0 chromic catgut.

A second incision is made in the posterior aspect of the leg, just behind the tibia. The tendon and muscle belly may be identified by pulling on the suture in the distal wound. This proximal incision should be 8 to 10 cm in length, and placed at least 6 to 8 cm proximal to the medial malleolus. The incision is carried down through the fascia, which is split, and the muscle belly and tendon of the posterior tibial muscle are identified. The muscle is dissected free, and a window is cut in the interosseous membrane. A tendon passer will usually fit through this window and should be directed distally underneath the extensor retinaculum to the lateral side of the foot. The area for insertion is selected and the tendon inserted, as described above for the anterior tibial tendon transfer laterally. The same postoperative regimen is used. If the tendon passer cannot be passed through the window easily, an incision is made over the anterior compartment to locate the tendon and subsequently pass it into the foot.

Surgical Technique — Triple Arthrodesis

Triple arthrodesis has been reported by Goldner and Irwin,[6] Hoke,[10] and Ryerson.[12] Goldner and Irwin report using triple arthrodesis in adults, followed 4 weeks later by transposition of the anterior tibial tendon to the lateral aspect of the tarsal bones. The posterior tibial tendon may be sectioned if overpulling is evident, or it may be transferred at the time of the second procedure. Triple arthrodesis is carried out through an anterolateral incision through the skin crease, which runs from the area of the talonavicular joint anteriorly, to the midportion of the talocalcaneal joint posteriorly. The incision, which is placed so that the calcaneo-cuboid joint can be excised as well, extends from the extensor tendons anteriorly to the peroneal tendons posteriorly. The extensor digitorum brevis is identified, dissected from its origin, and re-tracted distally. Once this has been done, the sinus tarsi is identified and all fatty material is debrided from the area. At this point, the talonavicular, cal-caneocuboid, and talocalcaneal joints should be identified and incised. Large osteotomes are used to remove two wedges, based on the lateral aspect of the foot, one from the talonavicular joint and the other from the calcaneocuboid joint. These wedges are removed to bring the foot into a position in which the metatarsals are aligned on the talus. For severe varus deformity, it may be necessary to re-move the entire portion of the head of the talus and place the navicular on the talar neck. Following excision of these two joints, a laterally based wedge is removed from the talocalcaneal joint. Removal of this wedge is facilitated by cutting the interosseous ligament between the talus and the calcaneus and using a lamina spreader to open the joint. The en-tire talocalcaneal joint can be visualized using this technique. The middle facet of the talocalcaneal joint is removed with a ⅜-inch osteotome by strip-ping the cartilage from both the talus and the cal-caneus. A laterally based wedge is then removed from the os calcis with a 1-inch osteotome. The entire posterior facet of the talocalcaneal joint is removed along with this wedge of bone. It should then be possible to bring the heel into the neutral position, aligning the forepart of the foot with the hindpart of the foot. Fixation may be obtained by stapling the calcaneocuboid and talocalcaneal joints, although this is not necessary in most in-stances. Once the foot has been placed in position, the previously removed bone is cut into small matchsticks, and the open areas in the sinus tarsi and joints are packed. A radiograph should be ob-tained in the operating room to ensure correction of the deformity. Following this, the extensor brevis is reattached with sutures of 000 chromic catgut, the subcutaneous tissue is closed with 000 plain catgut, and the skin with interrupted sutures of 000 nylon. Postoperatively, the patient is placed in an above-knee cast with the foot in neutral posi-tion, and the knee flexed at 90 degrees. The cast is maintained for 6 weeks, after which it is split, ra-diographs are obtained, and the patient is placed in a weight-bearing cast for another 4 to 6 weeks. If radiographs show satisfactory healing at this time, the patient is removed from the cast. If tendon transfers are indicated, these are performed at 6 weeks postoperatively. The patient is maintained in a below-knee cast for an additional 6 weeks, fol-lowed by the brace regimen outlined above.

Surgical Technique — Dwyer Osteotomy

When varus of the heel is the only component of the deformity and muscle function is intact, osteot-omy of the os calcis should be considered. Dwyer has described osteotomy of the os calcis through both medial and lateral incisions. The advantage of a medial incision is that an open-wedge osteotomy may be performed, thereby increasing the length of the os calcis and correcting the deformity. The disadvantages of a medial incision are delayed healing and skin slough. The procedure may also be performed through the lateral incision (this is my choice). This offers the advantage of easy skin clo-sure without subsequent difficulty, but it does have the disadvantage of shortening the os calcis.

The procedure is carried out through a 4- to 6-cm oblique incision over the lateral aspect of the foot, just distal to the peroneal tendons from the supe-rior to the inferior border of the os calcis (Fig. 133-3). The osteotomy is made at a 45-degree angle to the sole of the foot, in line with and approx-imately 1 cm distal to the peroneal tendons, so that a laterally based wedge may be removed. The os calcis is drilled and the bone is cut with an osteo-tome. Following removal of the laterally based wedge, the heel may be put into the corrected po-sition, in line with the forefoot. The osteotomy may be held with a staple, although this is not usually necessary, since the Achilles tendon will hold the osteotomy closed as the foot is dorsiflexed. The periosteum is closed with interrupted sutures of 000 chromic catgut, the subcutaneous tissue with interrupted sutures of 000 plain catgut, and the skin with interrupted sutures of nylon or subcu-ticular wire. A long-leg cast is applied with the foot

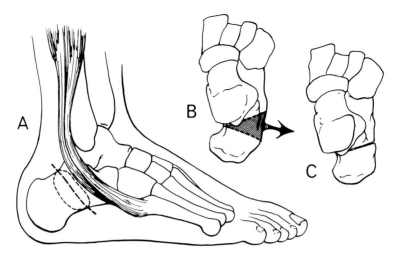

Fig. 133-3. (A) The skin incision for osteotomy of the os calcis, as described by Dwyer, is made over the lateral aspect of the foot, approximately one fingerbreadth below the peroneal tendons. The elliptical area shows the base of the wedge of bone to the removed through this lateral incision. **(B)** The amount of bone to be removed from the os calcis. **(C)** The position of the os calcis after removal of bone wedge and closure of the osteotomy.

dorsiflexed and the plaster molded to bring the heel out of varus. This cast is removed after 6 weeks and radiographs are obtained. Generally, sufficient healing has occurred by this time, and the patient is allowed to walk without protection. If healing has not been sufficient, a below-knee cast may be applied for an additional 6 weeks.

The results for correction of simple varus deformity with the Dwyer procedure are quite satisfactory. However, the procedure is not applicable to more serious conditions.

COMPLICATIONS

The results of triple arthrodesis for the varus foot are also satisfactory, although there are specific problems following this surgery. Complications include aseptic necrosis of the talus and lack of fusion of any of the joints involved. Marek and Schein[11] report on aseptic necrosis following arthrodesis procedures in the tarsal area. Their report includes two cases of aseptic necrosis in a series of 17 patients, and three cases in another series of 44 patients. Aseptic necrosis also followed a Lambrin-

udi-type triple arthrodesis in Marek and Schein's series.

Friedenberg[5] and Wilson et al.[15] reported on factors affecting fusion with triple arthrodeses. Friedenberg noted that the most common joint which failed to fuse was the talonavicular. Wilson et al. also noted problems with failure of fusion. In their report on 26 feet in which the Hoke technique was used, there was no pseudarthrosis and no avascular necrosis. However, when staples were used to maintain apposition of the bony surfaces, there were five pseudarthroses in 95 feet. These investigators also noted 26 feet in which early postoperative radiographs demonstrated the lack of bony contact in one or more joints. Fusion had not been obtained in 11 of these feet (42 percent) due to inappropriate bone removal. Wilson et al. also noted 11 feet with soft tissue infections, one of which demonstrated pseudarthrosis. Fifty other feet had superficial necrosis, maceration of the skin, separation of the wound edges, or hematoma. There were seven pseudarthroses among these patients. They had no evidence of osteomyelitis. However, with the high incidence of infection in this procedure in the foot, osteomyelitis is sometimes seen.

When pseudarthrosis occurs, it may not cause symptoms. If pain in the area and difficulty with walking persist, then refusion may be attempted by grafting the joint. This usually will produce satisfactory results.

REFERENCES

1. Dekel S, Weissman SL: Osteotomy of the calcaneus and concomitant plantar stripping in children with talipes cavo-varus. J Bone Joint Surg 55B:802, 1973
2. Dwyer FC: Osteotomy of the calcaneum for pes cavus. J Bone Joint Surg 41B:80, 1959
3. Dwyer FC: The treatment of relapsed club foot by the insertion of a wedge into the calcaneum. J Bone Joint Surg 45B:67, 1963
4. Fisher RL, Shaffer SR: An evaluation of calcaneal osteotomy in congenital club foot and other disorders. Clin Orthop 70:141, 1970
5. Friedenberg ZB: Arthrodesis of the tarsal bones: a study of failure of fusions. Arch Surg 57:162, 1948
6. Goldner JL, Irwin CE: Paralytic deformities of the foot. p. 190. In American Academy of Orthopaedic Surgeons. Instructional Course Lectures. Vol. 5. JW Edwards, Ann Arbor, 1948
7. Hart VL: Arthrodesis of the foot in infantile paralysis. Surg Gynecol Obstet 64:794, 1937
8. Herold HZ, Torok G: Surgical correction of neglected club foot in the older child and adult. J Bone Joint Surg 55A:1385, 1973
9. Hoffer MM, Reiswig JA, Garrett AM et al: The split spastic varus hindfoot of childhood. Orthop Clin North Am 5:31, 1974
10. Hoke M: An operation for stabilizing paralytic feet. Am J Orthop Surg 3:494, 1921
11. Marek FM, Schein AJ: Aseptic necrosis of the astragalus following arthrodesing procedures of the tarsus. J Bone Joint Surg 27:587, 1945
12. Ryerson EW: Arthrodesing operations on the feet. J Bone Joint Surg 5:453, 1923
13. Schwartz RP: Arthrodesis of subtalus and midtarsal joints of the foot: historical review, preoperative determinations, and operative procedure. Surgery 20:619, 1946
14. Turner JW, Cooper RR: Anterior transfer of the tibialis posterior through the interosseous membrane. Clin Orthop 83:241, 1972
15. Wilson FC Jr, Fay GF, Lamotte P, Williams JC: Triple arthrodesis: a study of the factors affecting fusion after three hundred and one procedures. J Bone Joint Surg 47A:340, 1965

Equinus Foot

134

John D. Hsu

The equinus foot (talipes equinus) is a condition in which the foot is in a plantar-flexed position. It is frequently referred to as a drop foot (Fig. 134-1) and can either be fixed or positional. Such a position is caused by one or a combination of the following conditions:

1. Weakness of the dorsiflexors of the ankle with inability to overcome the effects of gravity and the active plantar flexors
2. An overpull of the plantar flexors
3. A fixed contracture of the soft tissue and bony structures

Muscle imbalances usually lead to an equinovarus or an equinovalgus position, and thus a foot fixed in equinus without a varus or valgus component is seldom seen.

Talipes equinus may result from congenital conditions, such as hereditary Achilles tendon contracture, congenital hypoplasia of the leg, hypoplasia or absence of the tibia or fibula, congenital pseudarthrosis of the tibia, or congenital bowing of the tibia; or from leg length discrepancy secondary to growth or vascular abnormalities. Equinus deformity may be secondary to fracture of the lower extremity with subsequent leg-length discrepancy or to contracture of the injured gastrocnemius muscle. It may also result from peroneal nerve palsy, poliomyelitis, Guillain-Barré syndrome, cerebral palsy, head trauma, hereditary motor and sensory neuropathies, or muscular dystrophy.[32]

Because such a large number of conditions can produce a drop foot, a patient presenting with equinus, equinovarus, or equinovalgus of the foot should have a general clinical examination to determine the cause or the presence of associated conditions. A manual muscle test with grading of selective muscles in the lower extremity is crucial in assessing the residual effects of poliomyelitis and Guillain-Barré syndrome. A knowledge of the forces that create the deformity secondary to spasticity in cerebral palsy and head injury gives the examiner an idea of progress and possible recovery. Asymmetric joint weakness and contractures in neuromuscular disorders should be assessed, documented, and appropriately treated.

Diagnostic electromyography may be used to clarify certain neuromuscular conditions. Dynamic walking-gait electromyography (EMG) is used to show selective neuromuscular activity and may assist the surgeon in the selection of available treat-

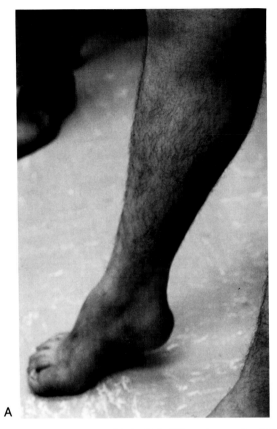 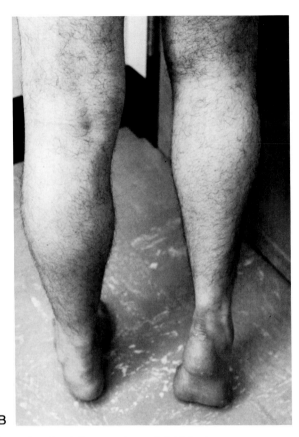

A   B

Fig. 134-1. Side **(A)** and posterior **(B)** views showing talipes equinus of right foot.

ment modalities.[25] Accurate leg-length measurements to confirm clinical discrepancies can only be made with use of the orthoradiograph (scanogram).[13]

NORMAL ANATOMY

A knowledge of the anatomic structure of the triceps surae and the Achilles tendon can assist the surgeon in selecting and accomplishing successful correction of talipes equinus.

Triceps Surae

The triceps surae consists of the two heads of the gastrocnemius and the soleus muscles, joining to form the Achilles tendon. The gastrocnemius mus-

cle originates from the condyles of the femur, whereas the soleus originates from the upper tibia and fibula. Therefore, the gastrocnemius crosses two joints and, in the growing child, three epiphyses.[22] Relaxation of this muscle can be effected by flexing the knee, which will relieve equinus if the gastrocnemius is the tight structure. If the soleus is tight or there are fixed contractures at the ankle, flexion of the knee will not relieve the equinus.

Achilles Tendon

The Achilles tendon in the adult is about 15 cm long and inserts into the posterior aspect of the os calcis. Anatomic studies by White[39] and by Cummins et al.[6] have shown a 90-degree twist of the fibers along the axis of the tendon before insertion (Fig. 134-2).

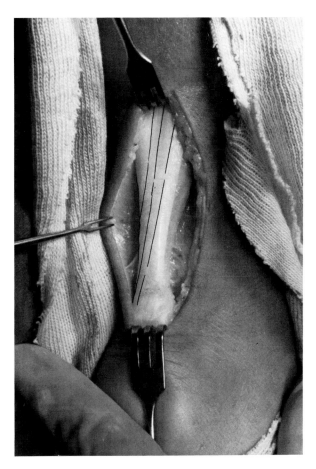

Fig. 134-2. Surgically exposed Achilles tendon showing fiber direction.

stand on the forefoot to maintain balance. Shoe wedges provide a better base of support and relief of metatarsalgia.

Procedures Directed to the Triceps Surae

Passive Stretching

Manual heel cord stretching is useful in correcting mild equinus. A daily regimen started as early as possible can effectively correct the deformity and maintain correction.

Night Splinting

Positioning in night splints can augment the passive stretching program.[8,16] In the growing child, frequent checking and padding of pressure areas eliminates discomfort and frequently enhances success.

Dynamic Splinting

The orthotic device to achieve active correction is shown in Figure 134-3.[8] Selective use is recommended, and proper fitting is extremely important, as the forces need to be properly distributed, especially in patients with sensory impairment.[38] Used improperly, pressure sores can develop at the heel.

Inhibitive Casts

This method can be used for selected cerebrospastic patients. The reflex-induced foot deformity and hypertonicity may be reduced.[7]

NONOPERATIVE TREATMENT

Shoe Correction

Shoe wedges and external shoe modifications may be used to compensate for mild equinus conditions. However, a leg weakened by muscle atrophy may not tolerate the added weight of a large and heavy buildup to the shoe.

Consideration of this type of support is most important in prolonging walking in the neuromuscular patient in whom the combined abdominal, gluteal, and quadriceps weakness can force a patient to

OPERATIVE TREATMENT

Surgical correction for the equinus foot is generally accomplished by release or lengthening of the triceps surae, the gastrocnemius and soleus muscles, or the Achilles tendon. Varus and valgus components should be corrected by appropriate releases or tendon transfers, which are generally done at the same time.

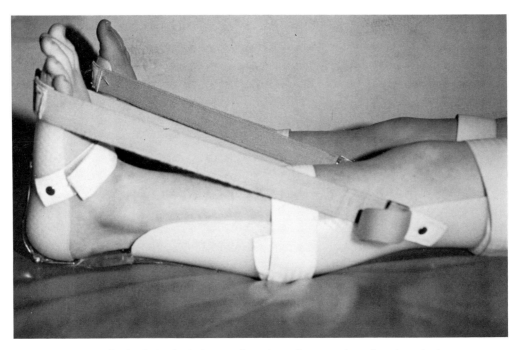

Fig. 134-3. Orthotic device to effect dynamic correction of equinus feet.

Achilles Tendon Lengthening

Lengthening can be accomplished either by the closed (percutaneous) or open methods.

Percutaneous Method

General anesthesia is used in this method of lengthening the Achilles tendon. The patient is placed in the prone position, although the supine position can be satisfactory to the experienced surgeon. With the foot held in maximum dorsiflexion, three percutaneous incisions are made—two on the medial side and one on the lateral side, between the two medial incisions.

Author's Preferred Method

The Achilles tendon, which is subcutaneous, is easily palpated. The medial and lateral borders are distinct, and, if desired, these margins can be outlined with a marking pen. A small #15 blade is introduced parallel and medial to the tendon and passed behind it (Fig. 134-4). After the knife enters the tissues behind the Achilles tendon to about

one-half the width of the tendon, the blade is turned 90 degrees toward the Achilles tendon. The foot is then grasped firmly with the other hand and dorsiflexed as much as possible, stretching the tendon. The selected half of the tendon is then cut from under the tendon to its subcutaneous surface, taking care to control the blade so that the skin is not button-holed. A second cut is made 2 inches distal to the first through the opposite half of the tendon. A third cut is made on the medial side of the tendon as close to the insertion of the tendon into the os calcis as possible. After all the cuts are made, the heel is grasped and the foot forcefully dorsiflexed in a smooth manner, applying a constant amount of pressure to the sole of the foot. An audible snap is heard. It is important to avoid jerking the foot, particularly in patients with neuromuscular disorders, since the distal tibia may become fractured by excessive sudden forces if it is osteoporotic as is commonly the case in these patients.

Care should be taken when the proximalmost cut is made, as muscle fibers may be present. Thus, this incision needs to be made as close to the palpable

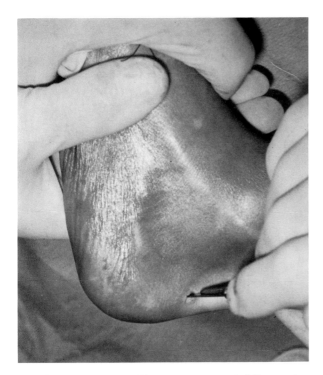

Fig. 134-4. Incision used for percutaneous Achilles tendon lengthening. Note (1) the knife blade is introduced at the medial border to make the distalmost cut, and (2) the foot is grasped firmly and held in maximum dorsiflexion before the incisions are made.

stretched tendon as possible. A #11 (lancet-tipped) blade should not be used for this procedure, as its large cutting surface cannot be well controlled.

This method of lengthening can be done in almost all instances, and 30 degrees of fixed contracture can be easily corrected (Fig. 134-4). Morbidity is minimal, and in more than 100 consecutive lengthenings, no complications have occurred.[17,18] Moreau and Lake[24] have also reported similar success in children with the percutaneous heel-cord lengthenings made on an outpatient basis. This method has also been successful in patients who have had a previous lengthening procedure, either open or closed.

Other Methods

Many techniques for percutaneous Achilles tendon lengthening exist. Hatt and Lamphier[14] described a similar type of procedure, except that the blade is introduced into the middle of the Achilles tendon and then turned to either the medial or lateral side for cutting. We have found that this method can lead to complications, as a force needs to be applied to cut through the tendinous portion of the Achilles tendon. If the force is too great, vital structures, including the posterior tibial artery, can be severed near the ankle.

The percutaneous methods of Frost[9] and of Conrad and Frost[5] are modifications of the procedure described by White.[39] Two cuts are made, the distal one being made medially, and both cuts are within the distal inch of the tendon.

Open Method

The tendinous portion of the Achilles tendon is exposed through an incision posterior to the ankle and medial to the tendon. The fibers are visualized, and a Z cut is made. The fibers are allowed to slide to achieve lengthening by dorsiflexion of the foot (Fig. 134-5). I use the method proposed by Gaines and Fort[10] for selected patients in whom there is a need to set the tension to counteract spasticity and to avoid overcorrection. After lengthening has been accomplished, the tendon is sutured together and continuity reestablished.

Heel-Cord Advancement

The heel-cord advancement operation, also known as the Murphy procedure, transplants the insertion of the Achilles tendon to the dorsum of the calcaneus. This technique alters the mechanical advantage of the gastrocnemius-soleus muscle and effectively weakens the pull of the Achilles tendon. Its main advantage is that it does not disturb the epiphyses and has been used successfully in the growing child.[26,35] I have not used this procedure in the adult.

Gastrocnemius Muscle Recession

This method was described by Vulpius in 1913 and was used successfully in cerebral palsy patients by Strayer.[19,34] The triceps surae is exposed and the musculotendinous junction identified. Lengthening is made by selectively cutting the junction in a

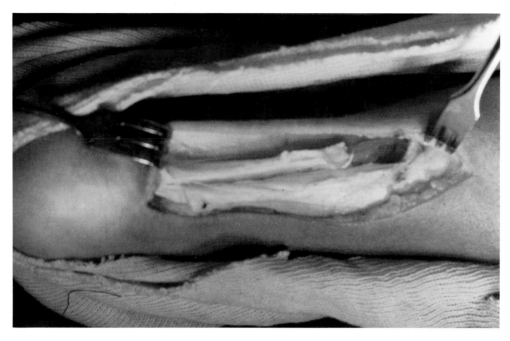

Fig. 134-5. Open Achilles tendon lengthening by the Z method. Note the sliding of the halves to accomplish correction.

V manner, following which the tendon is allowed to slide and the degree of lengthening may be controlled.[10] Variations of this procedure include the tongue-and-groove lengthening of Baker[1] and percutaneous intramuscular lengthenings as described by Majestro et al.[21]

Gastrocnemius Advancement

The Silfverskiold operation consists of releasing both heads of the gastrocnemius muscle at their origin and allowing them to slide distally, converting a two-joint gastrocnemius muscle to one spanning and influencing only the ankle joint. Silver and Simon[31] report a modification in which the motor nerve to only one of the gastrocnemius heads has been sectioned to prevent poor push-off during walking in spastic cerebral palsy children with equinus deformity. I have had no experience with these procedures in the adult.

Neurectomy

Selective motor neurectomy of one or more branches of the tibial nerve to the triceps surae was described by Stoffel[33] in 1913. It is no longer used today, except in combination with other procedures, such as gastrocnemius advancement.

Posterior Capsulotomy

Posterior capsulotomy is used in conjunction with procedures on the Achilles tendon in fixed contractures uncorrected by other methods. To accomplish the posterior capsulotomy satisfactorily, adequate exposure of the posterior ankle joint is needed. Generally, it is performed in conjunction with the open Z-type Achilles tendon lengthening. Before reapproximation of the tendon, the posterior capsule is identified and cut in a transverse manner. I wish to stress the need for identification and adequate protection of the medial and lateral structures of the ankle. Associated lengthenings and release of other tight structures can also be done to effect full correction.

Posterior Tibial Tendon Release or Transfer

Posterior tibial tendon release is indicated in instances in which its overpull is causing deformity and in which its transfer is impractical or will not

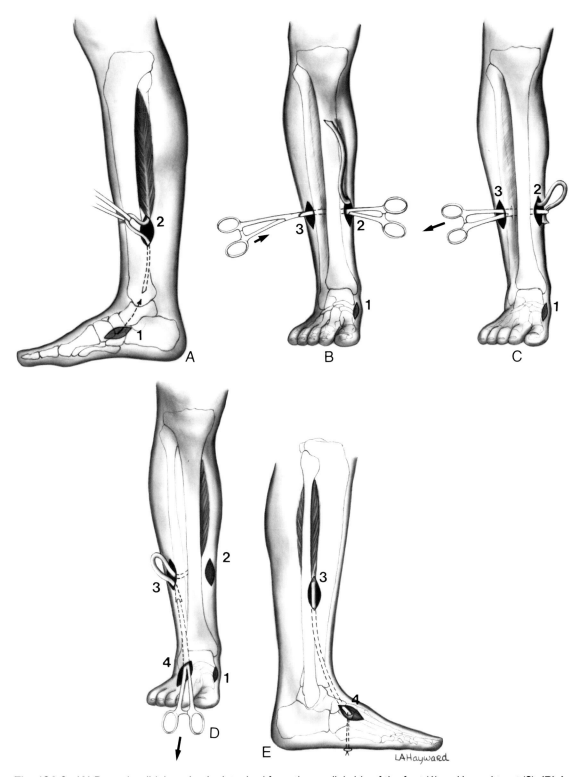

Fig. 134-6. **(A)** Posterior tibial tendon is detached from the medial side of the foot (1) and brought out (2). **(B)** A blunt instrument is pushed through the interosseous membrane following the contour of the tibia. The third incision (3) is made on the anterolateral side. **(C)** The clamp introduced from the lateral side (3) follows the pathway through the interosseous membrane and picks up the tendon bringing it anteriorly. **(D)** The posterior tibial tendon, now anterior to the interosseous membrane is brought down to the mid-lateral side of the foot (4) subcutaneously. **(E)** Anchoring of the tendon to the bottom of the foot is through a tunnel made in the tarsal bone.

contribute further to the balance of the foot.[16-20, 37,40] Otherwise, the preferred method is posterior tibial tendon transfer anteriorly through the interosseous membrane, as described in Chapter 133. This converts the deforming tendon into a dorsiflexor. This is especially useful in patients with polio, neuromuscular disorders[17,23,27] (Fig. 134-6) and traumatic drop foot.

Peroneus Brevis Release

Release of the peroneus brevis removes the deforming force in equinovalgus. Whenever possible, transfer to the second cuneiform through the interosseous membrane will assist in support of the ankle. Generally, in feet afflicted with paralysis, a triple arthrodesis may be required prior to this procedure so that the peroneal muscle becomes available for transfer.

Functional Electrical Stimulation and Implantable Peroneal Nerve Stimulation

These methods are discussed in Chapter 154.

Osteotomy and Fusion

Bone resection and fusion are indicated in conditions wherein the bony architecture of the distal tibia and/or proximal talus has been distorted and destroyed. Appropriate bone resections from the distal tibia and proximal talus are made. When there is need for correction of valgus or varus deformities, the bone removed is in the form of wedges. Although recently developed compression devices have resulted in a good fusion rate, use of the Charnley apparatus provides a simple and successful method to achieve bony union of the two surfaces.[4,5]

More extensive fusions, such as the pantalar fusion (fusion of the joints around the talus) or triple arthrodesis, may need to be considered in certain paralytic conditions. Selection of these procedures is dependent on the foot deformity. In cases in which there is a need to provide stability to the ankle and hindpart of the foot, triple arthrodesis may be indicated to make available tendons for transfer so that their pull could help modify or eliminate orthoses.

Bone Block

Construction of a bone block on the posterior aspect of the talus was initially described by Campbell.[11,12] Its success is limited, and residual pain and recurrence are frequently associated with this procedure. Tachdjian stated that the only indication for use of the posterior bone block today is in a female patient with fair strength of the triceps surae muscle and no dorsiflexors who desires to wear shoes with heels of varying height.[36]

POSTOPERATIVE MANAGEMENT

Wounds

When the skin and soft tissues have been stretched and placed under tension, an extra measure of care is needed after wound closure to ensure proper healing. The wounds should be closed in layers. In open Achilles tendon lengthening, Bands and Green[2] stress the importance of closing the sheath and including a small portion of the subcutaneous tissue over the newly lengthened tendon. We recommend dressing wounds carefully with a generous amount of soft dressings and padding. When there are multiple wounds, they should be treated individually. Windows should be made in the cast to inspect wounds at periodic intervals, and if the patient has the slightest complaint, or a sustained fever. Wound breakdown can result in painful and unsightly scars, which have frequently been associated with corrective surgeries (such as Achilles tendon lengthening) and other procedures around the foot and ankle in which correction is achieved by sudden stretching of the structures. With proper attention to wound closure and care, such problems are preventable.

Casts

Postoperatively, a short-leg cast should be applied with the ankle placed in a neutral position. The duration of immobilization averages 3 to 5 weeks, depending on the patient's age and the condition for which the surgery was done. Long-leg casts, however, should be used in spastic patients. In cases where walking in the cast after surgery is desired, the position of the ankle is important so that the patient can balance while standing. Difficulties may be encountered when the foot is placed in an overcorrected or undercorrected position. Patients with precarious balances (e.g., the neuromuscular patient) are apt to lose function if walking is not restored as soon as possible after surgery.

Undercorrection can lead to recurrence. Muscle readaptation at a later date may cause return of the patient's symptoms and further talipes equinus.

COMPLICATIONS

Skin breakdown with dehiscence, infection, and abnormal scar formation has been described. When this occurs it must be recognized and treated appropriately. Pressure ulceration can be prevented with a cast that is adequately padded, especially in areas where deforming forces may continue to exist or act unopposed.

Recurrence of the deformity with loss of correction can result in the need for additional surgery. Generally, the use of orthoses or night splints to support the foot and ankle minimizes recurrence and the need for reoperation.

Loss of function can occur, especially in the neuromuscular patient, as a result of limb immobilization in a cast or orthosis that may be too heavy for the patient to maneuver or lift.

Iatrogenic Complications

The timing, spacing, and sequencing of operative procedures and the recognition of certain primitive patterns are most important in the management of the spastic individual.[2] For instance, in the cerebral palsy patient, use of Achilles tendon lengthening to correct talipes equinus requires an understanding of the overall problem and of the relationship to other deformities; its correction requires detailed planning and precise timing. Unless special factors are involved, it is inappropriate to consider Achilles tendon lengthening in the first 3 to 4 years of life, as it is difficult to know exactly where the main problem will occur. A simple heelcord lengthening could affect the whole presenting pattern, leading to later confusion. In acquired childhood cerebrospasticity, Hoffer and Brink[15] advocate delaying reconstructive procedures until 1 year after onset of head injury. When multiple or combined procedures are carried out in the cerebral palsy patient, there is an increased incidence of calcaneus foot deformity.[29]

Sharrard and Bernstein[30] and Samilson and Hoffer[28] have pointed out other iatrogenic situations that can occur. For example, lengthening of the heel cord in a spastic patient with associated hip flexion, knee flexion, and equinus could result in the occasional iatrogenic calcaneus deformity.

REFERENCES

1. Baker LD: A rational approach to the surgical needs of the cerebral palsy patient. J Bone Joint Surg 38A:313, 1956
2. Banks HH, Green WT: The correction of equinus deformity in cerebral palsy. J Bone Joint Surg 40A:1359, 1958
3. Carney BT, Cracchiolo A III: Ankle arthrodesis by external fixation. Orthop Trans 10:495, 1986
4. Charnley J: Compression arthrodesis of the ankle and shoulder. J Bone Joint Surg 33B:180, 1951
5. Conrad JA, Frost HM: Evaluation of subcutaneous heel-cord lengthening. Clin Orthop 64:121, 1969
6. Cummins EJ, Anson BJ, Cann BW, et al: The structure of the calcaneal tendon (of Achilles) in relation to orthopedic surgery: with additional observations on the plantaris muscle. Surg Gynecol Obstet 83:107, 1946
7. Duncan WR, Mott DH: Foot reflexes and the use of the "inhibitive cast." Foot Ankle 4:145, 1983
8. Falewski de Leon G: Maintenance of mobility. Isr J Med Sci 13:177, 1977
9. Frost HM: Subcutaneous tendo Achilles lengthening. Am J Orthop 5:256, 1963
10. Gaines RW, Ford TB: A systematic approach to the amount of achilles tendon lengthening in cerebral palsy. J Pediatr Orthop 4:448, 1984
11. Gill AB: An operation to make a posterior bone

block at the ankle to limit foot-drop. J Bone Joint Surg 15:166, 1933

12. Girard PM: Ankle-joint stabilization with motion. J Bone Joint Surg 17:802, 1935

13. Green WT, Wyatt GM, Anderson M: Orthoroentgenography as a method of measuring the bones of the lower extremities. J Bone Joint Surg 28A:60, 1946

14. Hatt RN, Lamphier TA: Triple hemisection: a simplified procedure for lengthening the Achilles tendon. N Engl J Med 236:166, 1947

15. Hoffer MM, Brink J: Orthopedic management of acquired cerebrospasticity in childhood. Clin Orthop 110:244, 1975

16. Hsu JD: Management of foot deformity in Duchenne's pseudohypertrophic muscular dystrophy. Orthop Clin North Am 7:979, 1976

17. Hsu JD, Hoffer MM: Posterior tibial tendon transfer anteriorly through the interosseous membrane. Clin Orthop 131:202, 1978

18. Hsu JD, Jackson RB: Treatment of symptomatic foot and ankle deformities in the non-ambulatory neuromuscular patient. Foot Ankle 5:238, 1985

19. Javors JR, Klaaren HE: The Vulpius procedure for correction of equinus deformity in cerebral palsy. J Pediatr Orthop 7:191, 1987

20. Lipscomb PR, Sanchez JJ: Anterior transplantation of the posterior tibial tendon for persistent palsy of the common peroneal nerve. J Bone Joint Surg 43A:60, 1961

21. Majestro TC, Ruda R, Frost HM: Intramuscular lengthening of the posterior tibial muscle. Clin Orthop 79:59, 1971

22. Martz CD: Talipes equinus correction in cerebral palsy. J Bone Joint Surg 42A:769, 1960

23. Miller GM, Hsu JD, Hoffer MM, et al: Posterior tibial tendon transfer: a review of the literature and analysis of 74 procedures. J Pediatr Orthop 2:363, 1982

24. Moreau MJ, Lake DM: Outpatient percutaneous heel cord lengthening in children. J Pediatr Orthop 7:253, 1987

25. Perry J, Hoffer MM: Preoperative and postoperative dynamic electromyography as an aid in planning tendon transfers in children with cerebral palsy. J Bone Joint Surg 59A:531, 1977

26. Pierrot AH, Murphy OB: Heel cord advancement. A new approach to the spastic equinus deformity. Orthop Clin North Am 5:117, 1974

27. Pinzur MS, Kett N, Trilla M: Combined anterior/posterior tibial tendon transfer in traumatic paralytic peroneal footdrop. Orthop Trans 11:370, 1987

28. Samilson RL, Hoffer M: Problems and complications in orthopedic management of cerebral palsy. p. 258. In Samilson RL (ed): Orthopaedic Aspects of Cerebral Palsy. JB Lippincott, Philadelphia, 1975

29. Schwartz JR, Carr W, Bassett FH, et al: Lessons learned in the treatment of equinus deformity in ambulatory spastic cerebral palsy. Orthop Trans 1:84, 1977

30. Sharrard WJW, Bernstein S: Equinus deformity in cerebral palsy: a comparison between elongation of the tendo calcaneus and gastrocnemius recession. J Bone Joint Surg 54B:272, 1972

31. Silver CM, Simon SD: Gastrocnemius-muscle recession (Silfverskiold operation) for spastic equinus deformity in cerebral palsy. J Bone Joint Surg 41A:1021, 1959

32. Spencer GE Jr: Orthopaedic considerations in the management of muscular dystrophy. Curr Pract Orthop Surg 5:279, 1973

33. Stoffel A: The treatment of spastic contractures. Am J Orthop Surg 10:611, 1913

34. Strayer LM: Recession of the gastrocnemius: an operation to relieve spastic contracture of the calf muscles. J Bone Joint Surg 32A:671, 1950

35. Tachdjian MO: Pediatric Orthopedics. WB Saunders, Philadelphia, 1972

36. Throop FB, DeRosa GP, Reeck C, et al: Correction of equinus in cerebral palsy by the Murphy procedure of tendo calcaneus advancement: a preliminary communication. Dev Med Child Neurol 17:182, 1975

37. Watkins MB, Jones JB, Ryder CT, et al: Transplantation of the posterior tibial tendon. J Bone Joint Surg 36A;1181, 1954

38. Westin GW: Tendon transfers about the foot, ankle, and hip in the paralyzed lower extremity. J Bone Joint Surg 47A:143, 1965

39. White JW: Torsion of the Achilles tendon: its surgical significance. Arch Surg 46:784, 1943

40. Williams PF: Restoration of muscle balance of the foot by transfer of the tibialis posterior. J Bone Joint Surg 58B:217, 1976

Calcaneus Foot

135

Henry R. Cowell

The calcaneus foot, which has as its basic component a prominence of the posterior aspect of the os calcis in the weight-bearing surface of the foot, results from muscle weakness rather than structural deformity. This condition is particularly disabling because overpull of the anterior structures dorsiflexes the forepart of the foot so that it does not touch the floor during ambulation, and the absence of posterior muscle function eliminates the ability to push off with the toe while walking. Therefore, persons with calcaneus foot not only lack the stability of being able to place the foot on the ground but also ambulate as if the extremity ended in a peg.

Irwin[8] notes that the deformity is a result of muscle imbalance related to the loss of adequate function of the gastrocnemius-soleus muscle group. When the gastroc is absent or functionally inadequate, the metatarsal heads become the fixed area of muscle function in weight bearing. The structures on the undersurface of the foot, including the short flexors, decrease the distance between the metatarsal heads and the os calcis, since they are unopposed by the gastrocnemius action. Eventually, the plantar fascia contracts and maintains the deformed position of the foot. Since the relationship between the talus and os calcis is maintained,

the talus is dorsiflexed and the os calcis is forced into equinus. Thus, weight is borne on the anterior portion of the talar head and the neck of the talus (which articulates with the ankle mortise) and on the posterior aspect of the os calcis. When this occurs, weight is not borne on the sole of the foot but rather on the heel pad under the posterior aspect of the os calcis. Irwin[8] notes that this leads to a large callus under the heel and adaptive changes in the subtalar joint.

When this dorsiflexion position is created, the posterior tibial and peroneal muscles increase the cavus deformity by plantar-flexing the fore part of the foot. In addition, the anterior tibial muscle further elevates the fore part of the foot because it is unopposed by the gastrocnemius.

Once the cavus deformity has been established, the long plantar flexors of the foot have a shortened range for excursion, and the extensors have a relatively longer range because of the drop of the fore part of the foot. Therefore, the long toe extensors are not opposed adequately by the flexors, and clawing results. This produces flexion of the interphalangeal joints and hyperextension of the metatarsophalangeal joints, with depression of the metatarsal heads. In addition, the dorsal interosseous muscle increases the deformity, further depressing the metatarsal heads.

Relative weakness of the gastrocnemius-soleus group as compared with the anterior musculature and development of prominence of the heel are indications for treatment of a calcaneus deformity. When possible, consideration should be given to surgery at an early age to prevent progression of the deformity. When a patient develops an imbalance between the gastrocnemius-soleus and anterior tibial groups, either because of conditions such as poliomyelitis or spina bifida, or nerve injury, the foot should be placed in equinus during the early stages of management. This is an exception to the general rule that equinus should be avoided in the treatment of orthopaedic problems. Early treatment with bracing may also be attempted, but this, again, generally applies to the child rather than the adult. The prevention of calcaneus deformity is best handled with tendon transfers, as described by Banta, Sutherland and Wyatt,[1] Green and Grice,[6] Herndon et al.,[7] Irwin,[9] Peabody,[11] and Turner and Cooper.[13] While the majority of these procedures have been described for children, tendon transfer can be considered in the early treatment of older individuals with the potential to develop calcaneus deformity secondary to muscle imbalance.

METHODS OF TREATMENT

Treatment options for the condition include: tendon transfer, as outlined above; a combination of triple arthrodesis with tendon transfer, as reported by Cholmeley[2]; osteotomy of the os calcis accompanied by plantar release (see Ch. 137); a combination of triple arthrodesis tendon transfer and osteotomy, as reported by Lipscomb[10]; the addition of tenodesis of the Achilles tendon to the latter procedure; and, finally, if complete paralysis is present, pantalar arthrodesis. If the imbalance is mild, tendon transfer plus triple, arthrodesis is the procedure of choice. If severe muscle weakness is encountered and the deformity is fixed, then triple arthrodesis, osteotomy of the os calcis, tenodesis of the Achilles tendon, and tendon transfer are pre-

ferred, if sufficient muscles are available. Occasionally, a pantalar arthrodesis may be required due to a lack of sufficient musculature.

Surgical Technique — Herndon, Strong, and Heyman

This procedure involves transposition of the tibialis anterior and is carried out through three skin incisions (Fig. 135-1).[7] The first incision, which is approximately 4 cm in length, is made over the medial aspect of the navicular and the cuneiform. The anterior tibial tendon, which may be identified through this incision, is divided from its insertion underneath the first cuneiform bone. The second incision, approximately 4 to 6 cm in length, is made over the muscle belly of the anterior tibial tendon at its musculotendinous junction, approximately 6 to 10 cm above the medial malleolus. After dissecting the entire tendon free in the distal incision, the tendon and muscle belly may be delivered into the proximal incision; the distal incision is then closed with interrupted sutures of 000 plain catgut and skin sutures of 000 nylon. Herndon, Strong, and Heyman recommend making a window in the interosseous membrane by pushing a blunt instrument through the membrane and spreading the instrument to enlarge the opening.[7]

A third incision is then made over the medial aspect of the heel cord, running approximately 4 cm above the os calcis. A chromic suture is placed in the anterior tibial tendon, and a tunnel is made through the deep tissue, with a tendon passer bringing the tendon out at the level of the Achilles tendon. The Achilles tendon is split in half for a distance of 1 to 2 cm, and the anterior tibial tendon runs through this. A periosteal flap is raised in the os calcis, and the tendon is buried in a shallow gutter of bone under this flap. The repair is then reinforced by tautly suturing the Achilles tendon to the anterior tibial tendon, using 0 chromic catgut, with the foot in maximum plantar flexion. The patient is placed in a plaster cast for 6 weeks, and a brace with a dorsiflexion stop is used for 4 months postoperatively. The above authors report the use of this procedure in children, with excellent results in seven cases, good results in three, and fair results in two. While the oldest patient reported by the au-

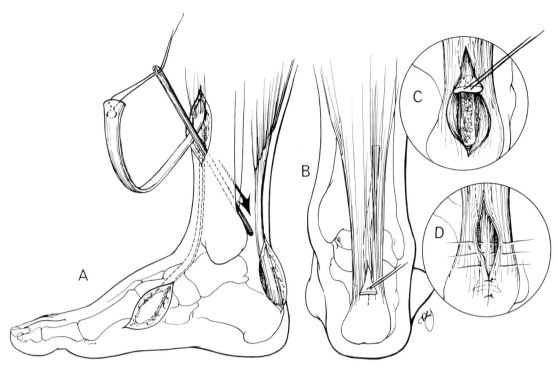

Fig. 135-1. **(A)** Posterior transfer of the anterior tibial tendon is carried out through three incisions. The tendon is passed through the interosseous membrane, and **(B)** directed through a split in the Achilles tendon. **(C)** After splitting the Achilles tendon and raising a subperiosteal window. **(D)** the anterior tibial tendon is sutured into its new location.

thors was 12 years of age, this technique may be used in the adult when combined with other procedures to correct any existing fixed cavus deformity.

Surgical Technique — Elmslie (Described by Cholmeley)

Elmslie's procedure is carried out in two stages (Fig. 135-2).[2] First, the plantar fascia is stripped from the undersurface of the os calcis through a medial incision, and the talonavicular joint is fused at the same time by resection of a dorsal wedge of bone through a medial incision. The foot is then placed in a position of maximum dorsiflexion for 6 weeks. At this time, a second operative procedure is performed through a vertical incision 4 to 5 inches in length along the inner border of the Achilles tendon. The tendons of the flexor hallucis longus, flexor digitorum longus, and peroneus longus and brevis are isolated, identified with su-

tures, and divided as far distally in the incision as possible. The talocalcaneal joint is identified and a wedge of bone is removed from its posterior aspect. The periosteum of the distal tibia is elevated, and a strip of the Achilles tendon is dissected free and sutured into the periosteum of the posterior aspect of the tibia, holding the foot in 20 degrees of plantar flexion. The tendons of the flexor hallucis longus, flexor digitorum longus, and peroneus longus and brevis are then sutured into the Achilles tendon at a point just above its insertion with 00 chromic catgut. The subcutaneous tissue is closed with interrupted sutures of 000 plain catgut and the skin with interrupted sutures of nylon or a subcuticular wire. The foot is placed in 20 degrees of plantar flexion and kept in this position for a total of 3 months. This technique has been described in children and is also applicable in the adult. However, I do not recommend the procedure, since it requires stabilization of the subtalar area at two different times.

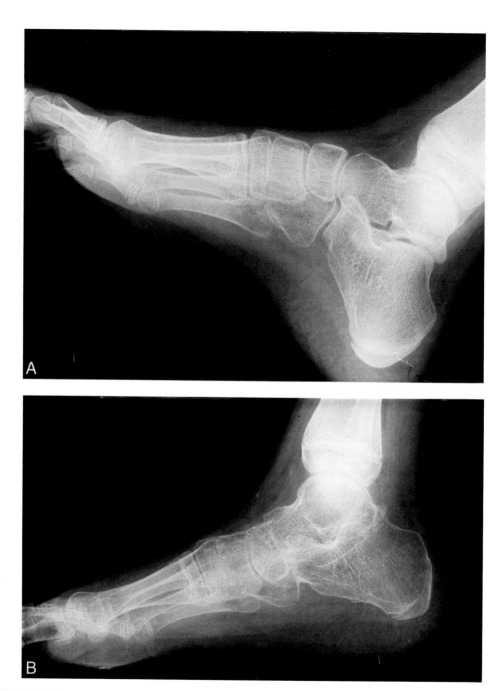

Fig. 135-2. **(A)** Preoperative radiograph of patient with calcaneus foot. **(B)** Nine months following correction with Elmslie's procedure. (From Cholmeley,[2] with permission.)

Surgical Technique — Lipscomb

Lipscomb reported the combined use of osteotomy, triple arthrodesis, and tendon transfer in one patient (Fig. 135-3).[10] He reported that all procedures were carried out at the same time, but that trouble was encountered in closing the skin. He suggested that the procedures be done separately in the future. A Steindler plantar fasciotomy was performed through a medial incision placed on the side of the heel.[12] A lateral incision was also used, extending distally to the subtalar joint and across the calcaneocuboid joint. A triple arthrodesis was performed through this incision, removing the calcaneocuboid joint, the talocalcaneal joint, and a portion of the head of the talus. Staples were placed through the calcaneus and cuboid and the calcaneus and talus to maintain correction. The os calcis was exposed through the medial and lateral incisions, and an osteotomy was carried out through the calcaneus, with an opening wedge based on the plantar surface of the os calcis. A Steinmann pin was then inserted through the heel into the posterior portion of the os calcis, creating an opening of approximately 30 degrees. The head of the talus was impacted into this space after the cartilage was removed. A third incision was made on the lateral aspect of the leg, and the peroneal tendons were identified and transferred to the posterior aspect of the os calcis. The skin edges were under tension when closed with interrupted sutures, and skin grafting was required postoperatively. The patient was maintained in a plaster cast for approximately 2½ months following surgery.

Lipscomb recommends a combination of the first two portions of the procedure, with tendon transfers being performed 6 weeks or more after the first procedure. He also notes that a skin graft should be considered if the wounds cannot be closed without tension. I have had no experience with this procedure.

Author's Preferred Technique

My preferred technique consists of triple arthrodesis, osteotomy of the os calcis, and tenodesis of the Achilles tendon, and is carried out in two

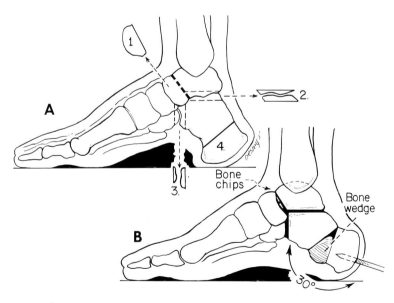

Fig. 135-3. (A) Correction of the calcaneus foot, as described by Lipscomb, involves triple arthrodesis. The talocalcaneal joint (2) and the calcaneocuboid joint (3) are excised. The talonavicular joint is excised, and a portion of the head of the talus is removed (1) and shaped into a wedge. **(B)** Following completion of the triple arthrodesis, the previously shaped wedge is inserted into an opening wedge osteotomy in the os calcis, thus obtaining realignment of the hindfoot area. (From Lipscomb,[10] with permission.)

stages (Fig. 135-4). A triple arthrodesis is performed through a lateral skin incision over the area of the sinus tarsi. Incision is made through the skin and subcutaneous tissue, and the origin of the extensor digitorum brevis muscle is removed to expose the sinus tarsi. After debriding all fatty tissue from the sinus tarsi, the calcaneocuboid, talonavicular, and talocalcaneal joints are identified. The calcaneocuboid joint is denuded of cartilage using a 1-inch osteotome. The joint between the talus and the navicular is cleared of all cartilage, using a ¾-inch osteotome, and a portion of the head and neck of the talus is removed to allow dorsiflexion of the foot. The area between the talus and the cal-

caneus is identified and the interosseous ligament is cut. The joint is opened with a lamina spreader, and a wedge is removed from the talocalcaneal joint. This wedge has it apex in the middle of the joint and is based posteriorly. Removal of the wedge with a broad osteotome allows approximation of the os calcis and talus posteriorly, thereby decreasing the cavus component. At this stage, plantar fasciotomy is performed with a tenotome placed in the sole of the foot just medial to the plantar fascia. The plantar fascia is transected by pushing it against the tenotome. Following this, the talonavicular joint is inspected, and, if necessary, further bone is removed to approximate the talus

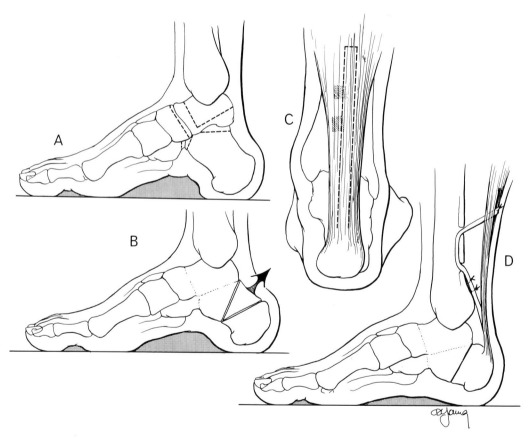

Fig. 135-4. **(A)** Triple arthrodesis is carried out by removal of wedges from the talocalcaneal and calcaneocuboid joint to align the os calcis with the talus and the cuboid. A rectangular piece of bone is removed from the area of the talonavicular joint. **(B)** At 6 weeks postoperatively, a wedge is removed from the os calcis. **(C)** Following this, the central portion of the Achilles tendon is dissected free after closure of the wedge, and threaded through two drill holes in the tibia. **(D)** Following suture of this portion of the Achilles tendon to the periosteum of the tibia, it is threaded back and reattached to the remainder of the Achilles tendon.

and the navicular. The area between the calcaneus and the talus is held by a staple, with the posterior aspect of the os calcis held against the talus; this decreases the cavus component and holds the forefoot in the corrected position. Subcutaneous tissue is closed with interrupted sutures of 000 plain, and the skin with interrupted sutures of nylon. An above-knee cast is applied, pushing up on the os calcis and the fore part of the foot to decrease the cavus component.

The second procedure is carried out 6 weeks later through a medial incision over the area of the Achilles tendon; this incision extends from the level of the os calcis, approximately 6 to 8 cm along the medial aspect of the tibia. The subcutaneous tissue is opened and the flexor hallucis longus muscle and the posterior tibial artery and nerve are identified. The artery and nerve are displaced medially. One-third of the Achilles tendon, from the center of the tendon, is dissected free from the area of insertion on the os calcis to the musculotendinous junction. This section is freed proximally and is left attached to os calcis. Drill holes are made in the posterior aspect of the tibia, approximately 3 and 5 cm above the ankle joint, and the freed section of the Achilles tendon is passed through the holes. The os calcis is identified and its dorsal aspect is stripped subperiosteally. A 1-inch osteotome is used to remove a wedge from the os calcis, based on the superior aspect. The slip of the Achilles tendon that was used for tenodesis is then made taut in the wound and resutured to the periosteum of the posterior aspect of the tibia. This is accomplished by pulling the talus into maximum plantar flexion. If the procedure is properly planned, it should leave the foot in approximately 10 degrees of equinus. Following transfer of the Achilles tendon into the periosteum with sutures of 0 chromic catgut, the deep tissue is closed with sutures of 000 chromic catgut, and the skin with a subcuticular wire. The patient is placed in a new above-knee cast, maintaining approximately 10 degrees of equinus. This should be the maximum amount of dorsiflexion possible after the Achilles tendon has been attached to the tibia. After 6 weeks, the triple should be sufficiently solid and the osteotomy adequately healed to change to a short-leg weight-bearing cast, which is worn for another 4 to 6 weeks. At this time the patient is placed in a brace with a dorsiflexion stop, which is maintained for at least 6 months. While this procedure has been used in a limited number of cases, I have been pleased with the results.

REFERENCES

1. Banta JV, Sutherland DH, Wyatt M: Anterior tibial transfer to the os calcis with Achilles tenodesis for calcaneal deformity in myelomeningocele. J Pediatr Orthop 1:125, 1981
2. Cholmeley JA: Elmslie's operation for the calcaneus foot. J Bone Joint Surg 35B:46, 1953
3. Dillin W, Samilson RL: Calcaneus deformity in cerebral palsy. Foot Ankle 4:167, 1983
4. Evans D: Calcaneo-valgus deformity. J Bone Joint Surg 57B:270, 1975
5. Goldner JL, Irwin CE: Paralytic deformities of the foot. p. 190. In American Academy of Orthopaedic Surgeons Instructional Course Lectures, Vol. 5. JW Edwards, Ann Arbor, 1948
6. Green WT, Grice DS: The management of calcaneus deformity. p. 135. In American Academy of Orthopaedic Surgeons. Instructional Course Lectures. Vol. 13. JW Edwards, Ann Arbor, 1956
7. Herndon CH, Strong JM, Heyman CH: Transposition of the tibialis anterior in the treatment of paralytic talipes calcaneus. J Bone Joint Surg 38A:751, 1956
8. Irwin CE: The calcaneus foot. South Med J 44:191, 1951
9. Irwin, CE: The calcaneus foot: a revision. p. 15. In American Academy of Orthopaedic Surgeons. Instructional Course Lectures. Vol. 15. JW Edwards, Ann Arbor, 1958
10. Lipscomb PR: Osteotomy of calcaneus, triple arthrodesis, and tendon transfer for severe paralytic calcaneocavus deformity: report of a case. J Bone Joint Surg 51A:548, 1969
11. Peabody CW: Tendon transposition in the paralytic foot. p. 178. In American Academy of Orthopaedic Surgeons. Instructional Course Lectures. Vol. 6. JW Edwards, Ann Arbor, 1949
12. Steindler A: Stripping of the os calcis. J Orthop Surg 2:8, 1920
13. Turner JW, Cooper RR: Posterior transposition of tibialis anterior through the interosseous membrane. Clin Orthop 79:71, 1971

Pes Cavus

136

Kamal Ibrahim

Pes cavus is a fixed equinus deformity of the forepart of the foot in relationship to the hindpart of the foot. It may occur as an isolated deformity or in conjunction with other deformities, such as claw toes or varus of the heel. Pes cavus is often seen in children but is most often treated in adults as a residual of childhood disease.

Many diseases can cause cavus deformity of the foot. It is most frequently associated with neurological disease.[4] Pes cavus may be the presenting complaint for a lesion of cauda equina.[27,48] The most common neuromuscular cause is Charcot-Marie-Tooth disease, followed by spinal dysraphism.[4,11,12,17,20,27] With the improved methods of diagnosis now available, idiopathic pes cavus seems to be an increasingly uncommon entity.[4,26,33] Table 136-1 lists its different etiologic groups.[4,20,26,27,31,36,45]

PATHOGENESIS

Pes cavus is produced by a poorly understood muscle imbalance. Many theories have been proposed to explain its pathogenesis, which can be classified as extrinsic muscle imbalance, intrinsic muscle imbalance, or combined extrinsic and intrinsic muscle imbalance. Some of the theories are outlined below.

Extrinsic Muscle Imbalance

One theory suggests that weak anterior tibial and strong peroneus longus muscles cause the first metatarsal and medial cuneiform to be pulled into equinus on the hindpart of the foot[1]; in fact, a strong peroneus longus will produce planovalgus foot.[12]

Weakness of the peroneus brevis may lead to peroneus longus hypertrophy, which will in turn overpower the anterior tibial muscle and pull the first metatarsal and medial cuneiform into equinus.[18]

Another theory holds that an overactive posterior tibial tendon functioning against a weak gastrocnemius will cause cavus foot.[30]

Intrinsic Muscle Imbalance

Duchenne proposed that claw foot is similar to claw hand—i.e., that paralysis or weakness of an intrinsic muscle will abolish the moderating effect

4015

Table 136-1. Etiologic Groups of Pes Cavus

Classification	Manifestations
Neuromuscular	
Muscle disease	Muscular dystrophy
Peripheral nerves and lumbosacral spinal nerve roots	Charcot-Marie-Tooth disease, spinal dysraphism, polyneuritis, traumatic peroneal palsy, intraspinal tumors
Anterior horn cell disease of the spinal cord	Poliomyelitis, spinal dysraphism, disatematomyelia, syringomyelia, spinal muscular atrophy, spinal cord tumors
Long tracts and central disease	Friedreich's ataxia, Roussy-Levy syndrome, primary cerebellar disease, cerebral palsy
Congenital	Isolated cavus foot, residual of clubfoot, arthrogryposis
Traumatic	Malunion of fractured foot bones, deep posterior compartment syndrome of the leg resulting in vascular damage and muscular fibrosis
Other	Infection of the foot, neoplasm of soft tissues or bones, debilitating disease, gravity and blanket weight on the feet of unconscious patients

on the long extensors and flexors of the toes, resulting in claw toes and cavus foot. However, the interossei of the foot are anatomically different from those of the hand.

Sabir et al.[37] proposed that the lumbricals and interossei may become denervated and weak, producing a "windlass" affect. Subsequently, the short plantar muscles of the foot undergo denervation, fibrosis, and shortening. They then act as a tie beam between the anterior and posterior pillars of the longitudinal plantar arch, drawing them closer, which produces a cavus foot.

Combined Extrinsic and Intrinsic Muscle Imbalance

Chuinard et al.[5] proposed that the muscles of the ankle and foot (extrinsic and intrinsic) form a right triangle. An imbalance in any portion of this triangle will result in pes cavus.

Coonrad et al.[8] observed that overactivity of intrinsics and short toe flexors in otherwise flail feet produced a cavus foot deformity.

In summary, pes cavus seems to be produced by different mechanisms involving imbalances in both intrinsic and extrinsic foot muscles.

Different investigators[23,24,35,37,38] propose that the primary deformity is the cavus component, which can be of three varieties. Either the first metatarsal bone is in rigid equinus and pronated position in relationship to the hindpart of the foot or the whole forepart of the foot is in a rigid equinus

position in relationship to the hindpart of the foot. The third less common deformity is a paralytic cavus foot, where the forepart of the foot is flail and in a flexible equinus position in relationship to the hindpart of the foot.

Claw toes and varus heel deformities are usually secondary to the drop of the forepart of the foot. The claw toes are initially mild and flexible, but

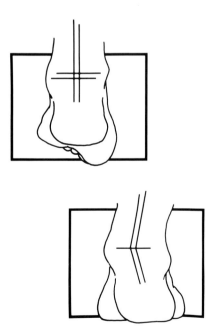

Fig. 136-1. Pathogenesis of varus of the heel. With the first metatarsal in cavus deformity, the whole heel will assume a varus position to balance the foot on the floor.

later become severe and rigid.[26] The heel will go into varus position in order to relieve the excessive weight that is placed on the first metatarsal.[35,45] This varus heel is also initially flexible but later develops into a fixed deformity (Fig. 136-1).

Calcaneal position of the hindpart of the foot may occur as a result of paralysis of the triceps surae muscle, as is seen in polymyositis and myelomeningocele.[3]

EVALUATION

Evaluation should be aimed at finding the etiology of pes cavus, and diagnosis of idiopathic pes cavus should be made only after all possible neuromuscular diseases have been investigated adequately. After a period of observation and a review of the patient's history, it should be determined whether the deformity is progressive or stationary. Finally, the deformity should be examined carefully in order to evaluate the severity and the rigidity of the three deformities—that is, cavus foot, claw toes, and varus of the heel.

An adequate history should be taken, including family history of any neuromuscular diseases, especially Charcot-Marie-Tooth disease. Thorough neurologic examination should be carried out. The foot should be examined relative to weight bearing. If cavus deformity is flexible, it should disappear with passive correction; if not, the obstructing structures need to be evaluated. These usually include the plantar fascia and short plantar muscles. The flexibility of claw toes can be examined by passive elevation of the metatarsal heads. If the toes are flexible, they will extend when the metatarsals are dorsiflexed by applying pressure under the metatarsal head of the affected toe. If the toe deformities are fixed by contracture, then this pressure will not correct the deformity. If the hindpart of the foot is in a varus position, its flexibility should be evaluated using the Coleman block test[7] (Figs. 136-2 A,B). The heel is placed on a block of wood at least 1 inch thick, and the patient stands with the lateral metatarsals on the wood and the first, second, and third metatarsal heads on the

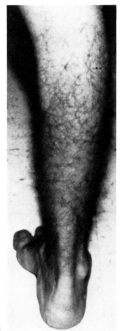
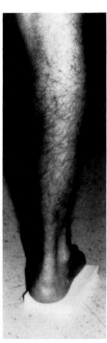
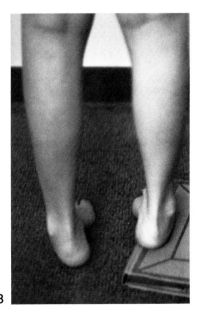

Fig. 136-2. (A) Flexible varus of the heel will correct with the block test. **(B)** Rigid varus of the heel does not correct with the block test.

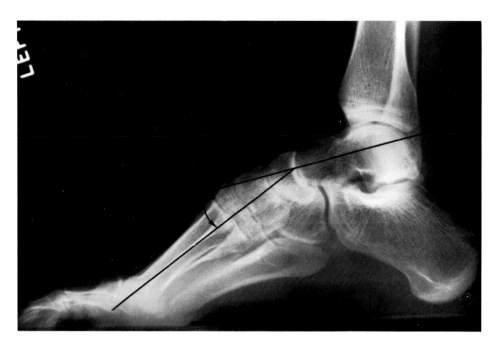

Fig. 136-3. The amount of cavus deformity may be determined on the lateral radiograph. Lines are drawn through the talus and the shaft of the first metatarsal. In a normal foot these lines should be continuous. The amount of cavus may be determined by the angle of intersection of the two lines.

floor. If the hindpart of the foot remains in varus, then the deformity is a fixed one; if the hindpart of the foot corrects to neutral with this test, then the deformity is flexible. The heel cord should be examined for tightness and contractures.

Radiographs of the foot should be done, including views in the lateral weight-bearing position. The angle of pes cavus may be measured from this view[45] (Fig. 136-3). Every patient with cavus foot should have electromyographic studies and radiographs taken of the entire spine. When spinal dysraphism is a possible etiology, magnetic resonance imaging or myelography should be done.

TREATMENT

Conservative measures should be taken while diagnosis is being established and the patient is being observed to decide if the deformity is progressive. These conservative measures should include stretching of the plantar fascia, short toe flexors, and heel cord (if tight). A metatarsal bar should be added to the shoes to distribute the weight and relieve some of the pressure on the metatarsal heads.

If the deformity is mild, flexible, and nonprogressive, conservative treatment is generally adequate in relieving the symptoms of pain and callosities under the metatarsal head. If the deformity is severe and progressive, or if conservative treatment has failed, surgery is indicated.

Release of soft tissue contractures alone or in combination with tendon transfers should be adequate for flexible deformities or in a patient who is skeletally immature. When the deformity is progressive, as in Charcot-Marie-Tooth disease, the soft tissue procedure should be considered as a temporary correction,[41] keeping in mind that bony procedures may be required later.[32] When muscle weakness or paralysis is demonstrated, appropriate tendon transfers should be done to balance the foot.

Bony procedures should be carried out when the deformity is rigid, fixed, or severe. When the deformity is isolated, a specific osteotomy should be carried out along with a release of tight soft tissue or a tendon transfer to decrease the effect of the deforming forces. Triple arthrodesis is indicated when the deformity is complex, severe, or rigid and includes many components (cavus, varus, and pronation).

Soft Tissue Procedures — Overview

When the cavus foot deformity is mild, flexible, and nonprogressive without claw toes, a Steindler procedure[44] should be adequate. In this procedure, the plantar fascia and origin of the short plantar muscles are stripped from the calcaneal attachment. A more extensive release may be carried out if this is not enough to correct the cavus deformity.[2,38,42] Such options include release of the posterior tibial muscle, long and short plantar ligaments, and the spring ligament. More radical plantar release, followed by serial casting, has recently been described by Paulos, Coleman, and Samuelson, with better than 85 percent acceptable results after more than 2 years of follow-up.[35]

Sherman and Westin[42] reported an 83 percent success rate using plantar release to correct cavus feet. They advised against plantar release in paralytic calcaneocavus deformity because it destabilizes the position of the os calcis.

When the cavus deformity is accompanied by flexible clawing of the toes or weakness of the anterior tibial muscles, transfer of the long extensor tendons to the neck of the metatarsal bones and fusion of the interphalangeal joints should be performed along with a Steindler procedure. In the Jones procedure,[29] the extensor hallucis longus is transferred to the neck of the first metatarsal, and the interphalangeal joint of the big toe is fused. In the second through fifth toes, the long extensor tendons are transferred by extensor shift operation,[15] the Hibbs operation,[6,21] or the method described by Chuinard and Baskin.[5] The purpose of these procedures is to eliminate the deforming force; the transferred tendon will actively elevate the metatarsal bones and may correct the cavus deformity. Fusion of interphalangeal joints will

give the long flexor tendons better leverage to flex the metatarsophalangeal joints and will eliminate hammer-toe deformity.

A moderate equinus deformity with pes cavus should be treated with heel cord lengthening and posterior ankle capsulotomy.

Other tendon transfer procedures are indicated to restore the foot balance when weakness of certain muscles is demonstrated. In the case of weakness or paralysis of the anterior tibial muscle, the peroneus longus is transferred to the base of the second metatarsal, and its distal stump is sutured to the peroneus brevis to avoid the development of dorsal bunions.[19]

When there is paralysis of peronei and anterior tibial and toe extensors, the overactive posterior tibial muscle produces cavus deformity as well as varus and equinus heel. Anterior transfers of the tibialis posterior to the third cuneiform through the interosseous membrane should be effective.[46]

All of these tendon transfers should be preceded by Steindler stripping and should be performed on nonrigid deformities before bony changes occur.

The transfer of posterior tibial tendon to the dor-

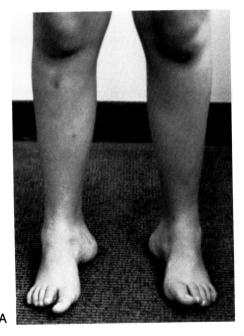

A

Fig. 136-4. (A) Cavus foot with first metatarsal equinus deformity as well as rigid varus heel. *(Figure continues.)*

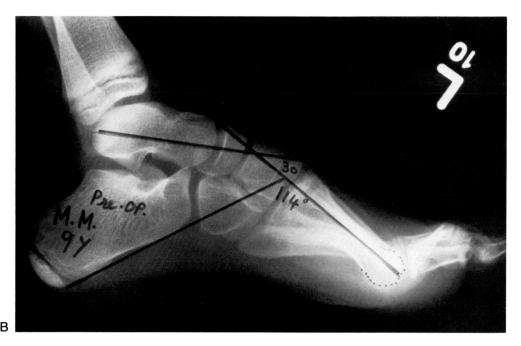

B

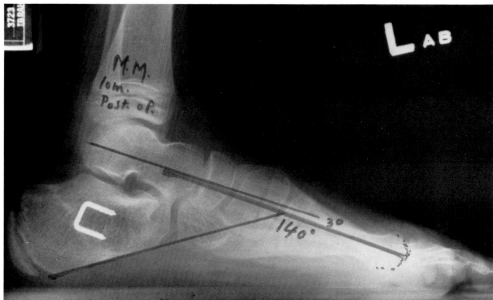

C

Fig. 136-4 *(Continued).* **(B)** Preoperative radiographs with Merry's angle of 30 degrees and Hibb's angle of 114 degrees. **(C)** Postoperative radiograph after first metatarsal dorsal wedge osteotomy and Dwyer's calcaneal osteotomy. *(Figure continues.)*

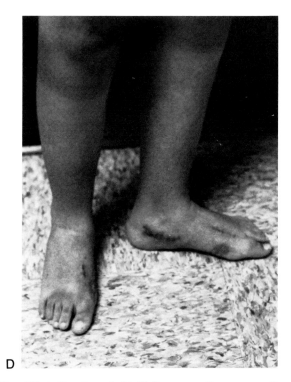
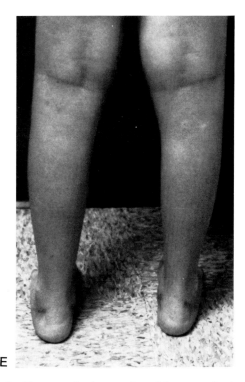

Fig. 136-4 *(Continued).* **(D,E)** One year after surgery, the patient has excellent correction of the cavus foot and varus heel.

sum of the foot, when the muscle is strong, has shown good results in correcting the paralytic flail cavus foot and the drop foot gait in these patients.[23,38]

At the Alfred I. duPont Institute, Steindler stripping and anterior transfer of the tibialis posterior were carried out on eight patients who had peronei and anterior tibial muscle weakness owing to Charcot-Marie-Tooth disease. The initial results were encouraging, but as the disease progressed the deformity recurred. All of these patients needed triple arthrodesis. These results support Levitt et al.,[32] who believe that soft tissue procedures in a progressive deformity such as Charcot-Marie-Tooth disease offer temporary relief of symptoms but often require subsequent surgery.

Garceau and Brahms[16] described a technique of selective denervation of short plantar muscles in cases in which the cavus deformity was a result of overactive intrinsic muscles in an otherwise flail foot. This procedure is indicated in children with poliomyelitis, but it has very limited use in adults.

Lateral transfer of the tibialis anterior to the cuneiform to correct the inversion component of cavovarus deformity has been described. However, it should not be used because it enhances the peroneus longus action as a flexor on the first metatarsal, making the cavus deformity worse. The Fowler procedure[14] of transferring the anterior tibial tendon to the head of the first metatarsal is an acceptable procedure in some cases.

Tendon transfer is performed in calcaneocavus deformity where the triceps surae muscle is paralyzed but should be preceded by a bony procedure such as calcaneal osteotomy or triple arthrodesis.[3,38]

Procedures on Bones — Overview

Bony procedures are more often indicated in adolescents and adults than soft tissue procedures. They are indicated when the cavus deformity is severe or rigid and when structural changes in the bones have taken place. Stripping and release of contracted soft tissue (Steindler operation) should take place prior to any bony procedure.

Specific osteotomies should be planned and implemented at the site of the deformity. Muscle weakness and imbalance should be corrected with appropriate tendon transfers, either in combination with the bony procedures or at a later stage.

Procedures on the first metatarsal are indicated when the first metatarsal is in equinus and the forepart of the foot is pronated (Fig. 136-4 A–E). The deformity must be confined to the forepart of the foot. The varus deformity of the heel should be flexible, as determined by the Coleman block test.[7] McElvenny and Caldwell[34] described elevation and supination of the first metatarsal by fusing the metatarsal cuneiform joint and, if necessary, the navicular cuneiform joint as well. Dorsal wedge osteotomy of the base of the first and second metatarsal bones[33] has been described for the same condition (Fig. 136-5). The Fowler procedure[14] may also be used when the equinus deformity is mainly

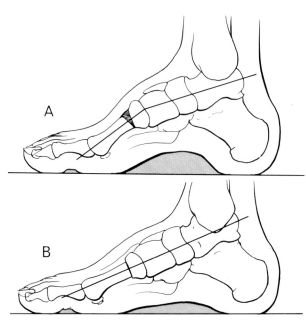

Fig. 136-5. (A) Osteotomy of the first metatarsal alone may be considered when the main deformity is a drop of the first ray. If the heel may be placed in neutral, with the lateral four metatarsals on a block and the first metatarsal resting on the floor, then osteotomy of the first metatarsal may be considered for a mild deformity. **(B)** Realignment of the first metatarsal with the talus can be seen following a proximal closing-wedge osteotomy of the first metatarsal.

confined to the first metatarsal. In this operation, medial cuneiform vertical osteotomy is carried out, and a wedge of autogenous bone graft is placed plantarward in the osteotomy site. Plantar fasciotomy is undertaken, and the anterior tibial tendon is transferred to the head of the first metatarsal.

A dorsal tarsal osteotomy is indicated if the cavus deformity involves the whole forepart of the foot (not only the first metatarsal bone) without rigid varus of the calcaneus. Different techniques have been described. In the anterior tarsal-wedge osteotomy described by Saunders[39] and popularized by Cole,[6] the wedge is removed from between the navicular-cuboid and cuneiform bones. This preserves the motion at midtarsal and subtalar joints, but it has the disadvantages of shortening the foot and risking vascular compromise of the toes.

The V-osteotomy of Japas[28] preserves the length and normal appearance of the foot. This procedure involves a V-wedge with its apex at the highest point of the cavus, usually within the navicular. One line of the V extends laterally through the cuboid to the lateral border of the foot, and the other extends medially through the first cuneiform to the medial border. No bone is excised, but the distal fragment of the osteotomy is depressed plantarward and the metatarsal bones are elevated, thereby correcting the deformity without shortening the foot.

Wilcox and Weiner[47] described a dome osteotomy in the mid tarsal bone to correct the deformity in different planes.

Jahss[26] described a technique of tarsometatarsal truncated-wedge arthrodesis, in which the osteotomy is carried out at the level of tarsometatarsal joints. This is indicated when the apex of the deformity is at that level—provided that the heel is not in fixed varus deformity, there is no muscle imbalance, and the foot has good circulation and normal skin. Jahss reported the results in 34 patients. Most had satisfactory correction of the deformity and relief of the symptoms without any major complications. He indicated that, if the procedure is carried out before hammer toes become rigid, spontaneous correction will occur and separate procedures will not be needed for the toes.

Dwyer[11,12] described a calcaneal-wedge osteotomy to correct varus of the heel as well as cavus deformities. In this procedure, the plantar fascia and the short muscles are released. A lateral closing-wedge osteotomy of the calcaneus is then carried out. Dwyer suggests that inversion of the heel is the primary deformity; thus, the gastrocsoleus group becomes a strong inverter, which is helped by the other plantar muscles that produce the cavus and varus deformities. Theoretically, this osteotomy should realign the heel cord and decrease its deforming force without attacking the main site of the deformity (the pes cavus). Many authors[9,33,43] believe that the Dwyer osteotomy is a good procedure for correcting the varus of the heel, but it has limited value in correcting cavus deformity.

If the foot is rigid and in a cavus and varus position, a dorsal tarsal osteotomy should be followed by a Dwyer osteotomy of the calcaneus. Preferably, this should be done in two stages to avoid vascular compromise of the foot.

I used the protocol mentioned above for 31 feet in 17 patients in whom the cavus deformity was treated with extensive plantar release, first metatarsal osteotomy or Japas osteotomy. Posterior tibial transfer was performed in patients who had a paralytic cavus foot. Dwyer osteotomy was performed only when the position varus was rigid and thus secondary to bony abnormality. Claw toes were corrected with Jones and extensor shift transfers. On follow-up of a minimum of 3 years, 16 patients had either good or excellent results in achieving pain relief and better gait. None of these patients required triple arthrodesis.[23,24]

Finally, if the deformity is complex, and rigid, and involves cavus of the forepart of the foot and varus of the heel, plantar fasciotomy and triple arthrodesis are indicated using the procedure of either Dunn,[10] Hoke,[22] or Siffert, Forster, and Nachamie.[40] If toe deformities still exist, they should be corrected 6 weeks later. Also, if the posterior tibial muscle is strong and acts as a deforming force, the tendon should be transferred to the dorsum of the foot.

Surgical Techniques

Surgical Technique — Steindler Stripping[13,44]

A longitudinal incision is made along the medial side of the calcaneus and carried distally to a point 4 cm anterior to the medial tubercle. Next, the superficial and deep surfaces of the plantar fascia are separated from the muscle and fat. The plantar fascia must be dissected from all other tissue from its medial to its lateral edge. The fascia is incised transversely, close to the point where it blends into the plantar surface of the calcaneus. With a blunt periosteal elevator, the muscles covered by the plantar fascia are stripped from the periosteum of the calcaneus, moving from the abductor of the great toe, to the short flexors of the second, third, and fourth toes, to the abductor of the fifth toe. It is important to avoid removing cortical bone with the fascia and muscle attachments; otherwise, new bone may form on the plantar surface of the calcaneus and cause pain on weight bearing. The dissection is continued distally to the calcaneocuboid joint. The long plantar ligament, which extends from the calcaneus to the cuboid, is released; this ligament is also contracted, and produces a convexity in the lateral border of the foot. By dissecting close to the bone, the plantar vessels are not injured. After all the structures have been released, the foot is forced into the corrected position.

When the deformity has been completely corrected by surgery, a below-knee cast is applied. Seven to ten days later, the sutures are removed and a new below-knee cast is applied, with padding beneath the metatarsal heads and over the dorsum of the foot to prevent pressure necrosis of the skin.

If the deformity is not completely corrected intraoperatively, the cast is gently wedged at intervals of 3 to 5 days until radiographs show the deformity to be corrected. Immobilization is continued for 3 weeks after complete correction has been obtained. The cast is removed, and a carefully molded weight-bearing boot cast is applied and worn for 2 or 3 weeks. Metatarsal bars are then applied to the shoes and plantar-stretching exercises are implemented.

Surgical Technique — Extensor Shift (Frank and Johnson[15])

The interphalangeal joint of the great toe is fused through a transverse incision made over the dorsum of the joint. The extensor hallucis longus tendon is isolated and divided ¼ inch proximal to the joint and reflected distally to expose the joint. After removal of all articular cartilage, a Kirschner wire is placed longitudinally through the phalanges and cut distally at the skin level for fixation. Further fixation is obtained by suturing the remaining distal portion of the extensor hallucis longus tendon to the periosteum of the proximal phalanx.

A second 1½-inch incision is made longitudinally over the dorsal aspect of the distal portion of the first metatarsal. The severed extensor tendon is delivered to this level, and at least 2 inches of the tendon sheath are carefully excised to prevent reestablishment of an insertion of the tendon on the phalanges. Each of the long extensor tendons of the lesser toes is exposed through two additional inci-

sions, each 1½ inches in length. These incisions are located in the distal portions of the second to third and fourth to fifth metatarsal interspaces. Each tendon is divided distally as far as possible, avoiding injury to the extensor digitorum brevis tendons. The distal portions of the severed tendons are allowed to retract. If necessary, capsulotomy of the metatarsophalangeal joints to relieve dorsal subluxation of the toes is performed. Transverse drill holes of sufficient size to accept the tendons are then made in the distal portion of the first metatarsal and the midportions of the third and fifth meta-

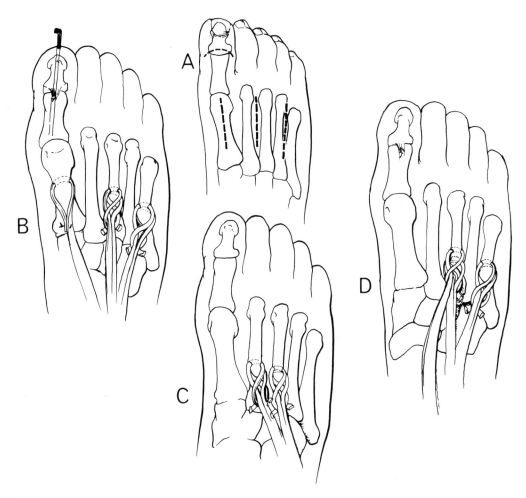

Fig. 136-6. (A) Incisions used for the extensor shift procedure are made over the interphalangeal joint of the first toe and over the metatarsals. **(B)** Standard procedure involves fusion of the interphalangeal joint of the great toe and shifting of the extensor tendons to the first, third, and fifth metatarsals. **(C)** Frank and Johnson also describe shift of the tendons to the second and third metatarsals to correct eversion, or **(D)** to the third and fifth metatarsals to correct inversion.

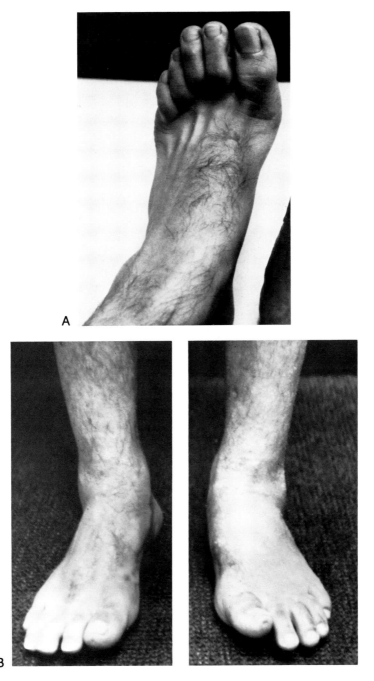

Fig. 136-7. (A) Preoperative rigid claw toes and first metatarsal cavus deformity. **(B)** Two years after standard extensor shift procedure and first metatarsal cuneiform fusion (McElvenny and Caldwell procedure).

tarsals. These holes may vary from ⅛ to ¼ inch in diameter. The tendons are then pulled through the holes with loops of silk.

In the standard shift (Fig. 136-6), the extensor hallucis longus is passed through a hole in the first metatarsal; the long extensor slips to the second and third toes through the third metatarsal, and the tendons slip to the fourth and fifth toes through the fifth metatarsal. The tendons are interwoven and sutured together over the dorsal aspects of the metatarsals with nonabsorbable sutures, under moderate tension, while the ankle is held in a neutral or slightly dorsiflexed position. This position is then maintained during closure of the subcutaneous tissue and skin and during the application of a below-knee cast.

An asymmetric shift is accomplished by the selection of other metatarsals for medial and lateral placement of the tendons in the correction of any element of forefoot inversion or eversion. The tendons are attached to the lateral metatarsal bones to correct inversion and to the medial metatarsal bones to correct eversion. Initially, other combined procedures are performed, such as plantar fasciotomy or lengthening of the Achilles tendon. A transverse or U-shaped skin incision may be used over the metatarsals to prevent reattachment of the extensor tendons to the phalanges through scar tissue.

Postoperative treatment consists of immobilization in a below-knee cast for 4 to 6 weeks, followed by physical therapy and ambulation. Under

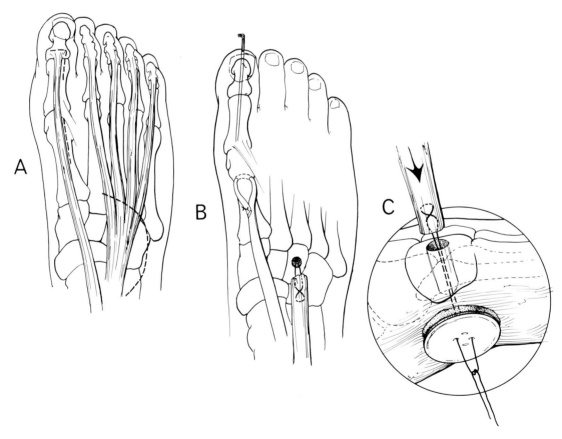

Fig. 136-8. (A) Hibbs technique for transfer of the long extensors carried out through three incisions on the dorsum of the foot, in combination with a plantar fasciotomy. **(B)** Interphalangeal fusion of the first toe is carried out, followed by recession of the extensor tendon to the neck of the metatarsal. **(C)** Extensor tendons are inserted into the third cuneiform with a pull-out-type suture, and tied over a button and sponge on the sole of the foot. A pull-out wire should be used, so that the suture may be removed after the tendon has attached to bone.

ordinary circumstances, the Kirschner wire is removed at 12 weeks or when bony fusion can be demonstrated by radiographic examination (Fig. 136-7A,B).

Surgical Technique — Transfer of Long Extensors (Hibbs[6,21])

The plantar structures are separated from the calcaneus as described in the Steindler operation. By forcibly elevating the forepart of the foot, the exaggerated arch is corrected and the position of the metatarsals is improved. Next, a curved incision 7.5 to 10 cm long is made on the dorsum of the foot proceeding laterally to the midline and exposing the common extensor tendons (Fig. 136-8). The tendons are divided as far distally as feasible. The proximal ends of the tendons are drawn through a tunnel in the third cuneiform and fixed with a silk suture or a pull-out wire. A Jones operation is performed for the big toe.

With the foot in the corrected position, a plaster boot cast is applied and worn for 6 weeks. Physical therapy is then started and continued for an additional 6 weeks.

Surgical Technique — Medial Cuneiform Metatarsal Fusion (McElvenny and Caldwell[34])

The first metatarsal and medial cuneiform are exposed through the medial longitudinal incision. The first metatarsocuneiform joint is opened and denuded of its cartilage. Sufficient joint capsule is excised so that the first metatarsal bone can be elevated and rotated (supinated). When this has been accomplished, gradual trimming of the cuneiform bone and the metatarsal base will allow full contact between these two bones (Fig. 136-9). The overcorrected position is maintained while two or three threaded wires are run through both bones and across the denuded joint to maintain position and contact. The wires should be long enough for incorporation into the plaster boot.

If the first metatarsal drop is marked, additional correction is easily obtained by fusing the naviculocuneiform joint, once full correction and stabilization of the metatarsocuneiform joint have been accomplished.

A plaster boot is applied with the forepart of the

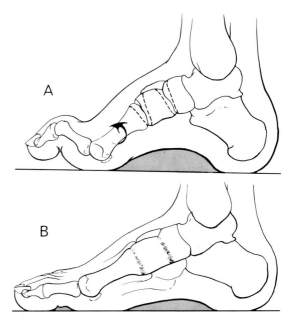

Fig. 136-9. **(A)** Medial cuneiform metatarsal fusion and navicular cuneiform fusion are carried out by removing wedges from the joints. The rotatory component of the first metatarsal may also be corrected by rotating the bone into the corrected position and holding this fixation with threaded wires or a staple. **(B)** Correction is shown.

foot supinated and the heel in valgus. Both positions of supination and valgus must be as extreme as possible without jeopardizing the soft tissue or the circulation.

At the end of 5 weeks, the wires are exposed in the plaster and spun out. A weight-bearing sole is provided. The boot is removed at the end of 9 weeks. If a radiograph shows union at the metatarsocuneiform joint, a self-adhering gauze stocking is provided, and the patient starts bearing weight on the foot.

Surgical Technique — Anterior Tarsal-Wedge Osteotomy (Cole[6])

A longitudinal incision is made on the dorsum of the foot and carried down between the tendons to the bone. The anterior tarsal region is exposed subperiosteally as far as possible. It is generally necessary to use a knife as well as a periosteal elevator to remove the periosteum by sharp dissection. When the bones have been identified, an almost vertical

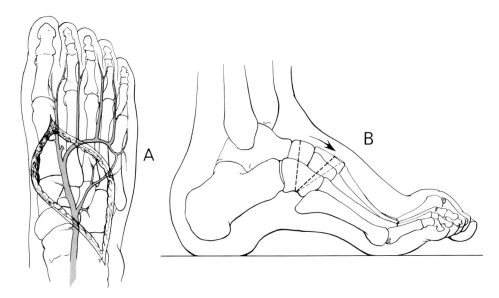

Fig. 136-10. **(A)** Anterior tarsal-wedge osteotomy may be carried out through a dorsal incision. It is important to identify the vascular structures to avoid injuring them. **(B)** A wedge is removed from the tarsal area.

osteotomy is made from approximately the center of the navicular and cuboid bones to the undersurface of the tarsus. A second osteotomy is then made, located anterior to the first osteotomy and connecting with it at its plantar edge (Fig. 136-10). The distance from the proximal cut depends on the width of the wedge required for a particular case. The forepart of the foot is brought up out of the dropped position, closing the gap left by removal of the wedge. A few interrupted sutures are used to close the periosteum and the skin.

A plaster-of-Paris dressing is applied from the toes to just below the knee. This dressing is maintained for about 8 weeks, at which time weight bearing without support can usually be implemented.

Surgical Technique — V-Osteotomy (Japas)

First, a plantar fasciotomy is performed through a medial incision on the heel, according to the Steindler technique (Fig. 136-11). Once the undersurface of the calcaneus has been denuded, the wound is packed with gauze, deferring the hemostasis and suture until the end of the operation.

The V-osteotomy is then made through a longitudinal incision, 6 to 8 cm long, on the dorsum of the foot. The incision runs along the extensor ten-

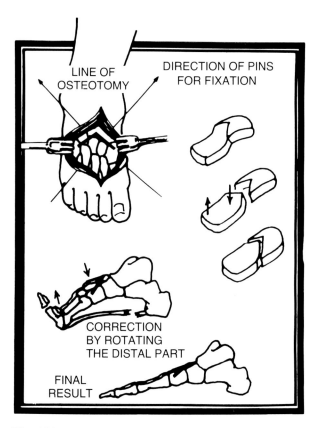

Fig. 136-11. Steps of the Japas osteotomy (see text for explanation).

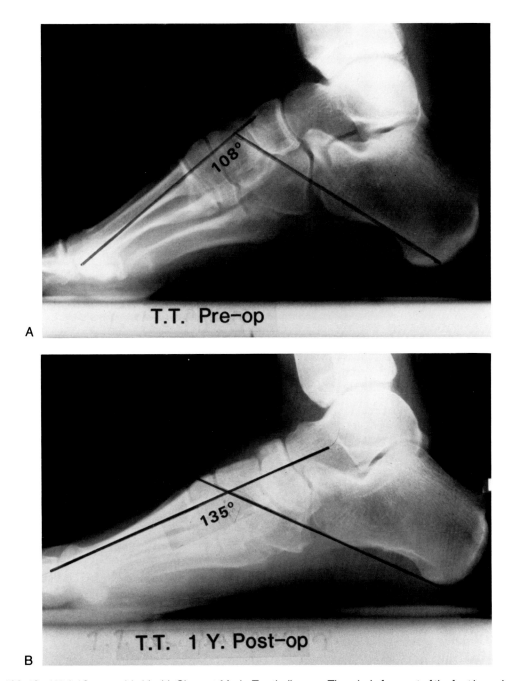

Fig. 136-12. (A) A 13-year-old girl with Charcot-Marie-Tooth disease. The whole forepart of the foot is equinus in relationship to the hindpart of the foot. The heel is in neutral position. **(B)** One year after a Japas osteotomy. The cavus deformity is corrected. Note the site of the osteotomy at the distal end of the navicular. *(Figure continues.)*

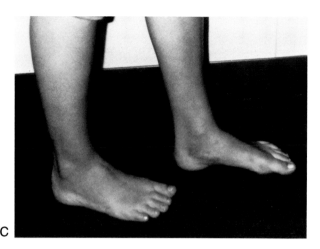

C

Fig. 136-12. *(Continued).* **(C)** Clinical results 1½ years after surgery.

don of the third toe and extends from the mid tarsal joint to the tarsometatarsal joints. The dissection passes between the extensor tendons of the second and third toes. The extensor digitorum brevis is retracted laterally. The site of the osteotomy is exposed extraperiosteally to avoid damage to the neurovascular bundle. The medial portion of the osteotomy should extend to the medial border of the foot, emerging proximal to the cuneiform-first metatarsal joint. The lateral portion of the osteotomy emerges on the lateral side of the foot through the cuboid, proximal to the cuboid-fifth metatarsal joint. Before making the osteotomies, the joint line of the talonavicular joint should be identified and avoided so that function of the mid tarsal joint will not be compromised. If a portion of the head of the talus is cut off by the osteotomy, avascular necrosis and traumatic arthritis may result.

With a Stryker saw or chisel, an osteotomy in the shape of a V is made with its apex in the midline of the foot and at the top of the arch of the cavus deformity. The osteotomy is extended distally, medially, and laterally toward both sides of the foot, keeping it proximal to the tarsometatarsal joints. By combining manual traction with leverage which is exerted by a curved periosteal elevator inserted into the osteotomy and used as a sliding surface (shoehorn or skid action), the distal segment of the foot is raised at its distal end and depressed at its proximal end to correct the cavus deformity.

If correction of abduction or adduction is necessary, it may be accomplished by simple manipulation of the forepart of the foot. It is not necessary to remove any bone to correct abduction or adduction.

The displacement of the distal segment to correct the cavus deformity must be done accurately to obtain satisfactory results; once the desired alignment is attained, the two segments are fixed by means of one or two Steinmann pins directed through the metatarsals toward the rear of the foot.

When correction has been effected, the tourniquet is removed, hemostasis is obtained, and the two wounds are closed in a routine fashion. A plaster cast is applied from the knee to the toes.

After surgery, the limb is elevated. Weight bearing is not permitted until the pin has been removed. At the end of 2 months, the cast is removed for clinical and radiographic examination and for removal of the Steinmann pins and stitches. A weight-bearing plaster boot is then applied and worn for 30 days. The cast is removed at this time and physical therapy is implemented (Fig. 136-12A–C).

Surgical Technique — Tarsometatarsal Truncated-Wedge Arthrodesis (Jahss[26])

No tourniquet is used. Using the tip of a finger, the slight indentation of the first metatarsal-medial cuneiform joint is palpated and a 3.8-cm vertical skin incision is made on the dorsum of the foot, 0.6-cm medial to the extensor hallucis longus. The incision is centered over the joint and, if necessary, may be extended slightly proximally and medially (Fig. 136-13). The underlying metatarsal-medial cuneiform joint is exposed. Using a thin, sharp, curved 4.8-mm chisel, the area to be resected is exposed subperiosteally after identifying and preserving the dorsalis pedis artery. Distal osteotomy through the base of the first metatarsal is done first using a thin, flat, sharp 2.5-cm osteotome. The proximal osteotomy of the medial cuneiform is then performed so that a dorsal truncated wedge may be removed. (If the proximal osteotomy is done first, it is difficult to cleanly osteotomize the now-movable distal fragment.) A medial wedge that will increase any adductus should be avoided. It is important to excise truncated rather than trian-

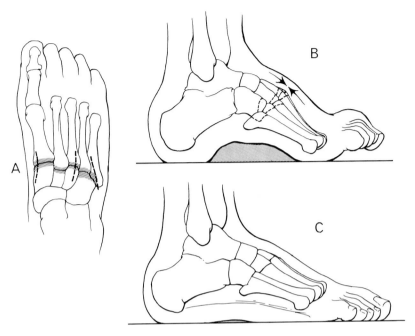

Fig. 136-13. (A) Tarsometatarsal truncated-wedge arthrodesis may be carried out through three incisions. **(B)** A wedge of bone is removed from each of the tarsometatarsal joints, and **(C)** correction is obtained by closing this wedge.

gular wedges of bone, or the plantar fascia will be too tight when the osteotomy is closed or may not even permit closure.

A second vertical skin incision of the same length is made between the bases of the second and third metatarsals (slightly closer to the third) and their cuneiforms. The base of the second metatarsal generally extends more proximally than the others. The second metatarsal-middle cuneiform joint is exposed by similar periosteal stripping to the first operative incision, which produces a medial longitudinal skin flap. This skin flap and the subsequently developed lateral skin flap must be handled very cautiously. They must not be retracted or subjected to pressure, except gently with a finger when inserting the osteotomes. A dorsal truncated wedge is removed from the second metatarsal-middle cuneiform joint. Working laterally through the same incision, the third metatarsal-lateral cuneiform joint is similarly exposed and resected.

A third vertical incision is made just medial to the base of the fifth metatarsal and, in a similar fashion, wedges are taken from the fourth and fifth metatarsal cuboid joints. There is a second lateral skin flap between the second and third incisions. If the third incision needs to be extended, the wound is lengthened proximally and laterally to permit a better blood supply to the second flap. However, the longer the skin incision, the less blood will be supplied to the flaps.

At this point, the forepart of the foot is dorsiflexed to close the dorsal wedges. A finger is used to palpate all of the wounds and under the flaps to see whether any small segments of bone remain that may block reduction. This should be confirmed by visual inspection. The osteotomy sites are closed again, palpating each metatarsal head on the plantar surface and feeling for residual depression while keeping the ankle in maximum dorsiflexion. When working under the two skin flaps, further bone may have to be removed proximally to permit the forepart of the foot to form a right angle with the tibia, while at the same time ensuring that all of the metatarsal heads remain absolutely level. Any rotation or adduction of the foot is also corrected in this manner. In more severe cases of pes cavus, the surgeon must guard against removal of too large a wedge when trying to bring up the forepart of the foot completely, as this will result in a lateral rocker-bottom when the wedge is closed. This is avoided by gradually increasing the size of the wedges and repeatedly checking while closing the osteotomy sites. If a prominence does occur at the base of the fifth metatarsal when the wedge is closed, it must be excised with a rongeur.

The wounds are irrigated and the skin is closed without subcutaneous sutures. The foot is held in its corrected position (at a right angle to the tibia) while a below-knee cast is applied. The metatarsals must be equally plantigrade and without excess abduction or rotation. The excellent stability obtained by closing the osteotomy site, while the forepart of the foot is held by the undisturbed plantar fascia, makes internal fixation unnecessary. The surgeon holding the foot should also make certain that the base of the fifth metatarsal has not slipped plantarward and caused a lateral rocker-bottom deformity.

The limb is elevated for 4 to 5 days. The cast is changed without anesthesia 14 days postoperatively, at which time the skin sutures are removed. Minor adjustment of the forepart of the foot may be made at this time, especially in regard to residual adductus angulation. Crutch walking without weight bearing is permitted about 10 days postoperatively, and full weight bearing is allowed 2 months postoperatively. The cast is removed 2½ months postoperatively, regardless of radiographic appearance, with immediate full weight bearing.

Surgical Technique — "Beak" Triple Arthrodesis (Siffert, Forster, and Nachamie[40])

The calcaneocuboid, talonavicular, and subtalar joints are exposed through the incision normally used for triple arthrodesis. Next, the calcaneocuboid and subtalar joints are denuded of cartilage. The dorsal cortex of the navicular is excised. The wedge of bone to be removed is planned prior to osteotomy of the anterior aspect of the calcaneus, the posterior aspect of the navicular, and the inferior aspect of the talar head and neck. The osteotomy is started inferiorly and carried superiorly to the inferior surface of the talus. The inferior part of the talar head and neck are resected to form a beak, leaving the soft tissue structures undisturbed on the superior aspect of the talus anterior to the ankle joint. The forepart of the foot is displaced plantarward, and the navicular is locked beneath the remaining part of the talar head and neck. When the bones fit together snugly, the position is maintained manually by applying slight pressure beneath the forepart of the foot while the cast is being applied. If the fit is not so snug, the navicular can be placed in proper relationship to the talus by a staple if desired; occasionally, it is advisable to fix the talus to the calcaneus.

At 10 to 14 days, the cast and sutures should be removed, the foot inspected, and radiographs taken. If the position is not satisfactory, the foot should be manipulated with the patient under general anesthesia. A new cast, snug but properly padded, is then applied and molded to the contour of the foot. This is maintained for 6 weeks without weight bearing.

REFERENCES

1. Bentzon PGK: Pes cavus and the medial peroneus longus. Acta Orthop Scand 4:50, 1933
2. Bost FC, Schottstaedt ER, Larsen LJ: Plantar dissection: an operation to release the soft tissues in recurrent or recalcitrant talipes equinovarus. J Bone Joint Surg 42A:151, 1960
3. Bradley GW, Coleman SS: Treatment of the calcaneocavus foot deformity. J Bone Joint Surg 63A:1159, 1981
4. Brewerton DA, Sandifer PH, Sweetnam DR: "Idiopathic" pes cavus: an investigation into its aetiology. Br Med J 2:659, 1963
5. Chuinard EG, Baskin M: Claw-foot deformity; treatment by transfer of the long extensors into the metatarsals and fusion of the interphalangeal joints. J Bone Joint Surg 55A:351, 1973
6. Cole WH: The treatment of claw-foot. J Bone Joint Surg 22:895, 1940
7. Coleman SS, Chestnut WJ: A simple test for hindfoot flexibility in the cavovarus foot. Clin Orthop 123:60, 1977
8. Coonrad RW, Irwin CE, Gucker T III, et al: The importance of plantar muscles in paralytic varus feet: the results of treatment by neurectomy and myotenotomy. J Bone Joint Surg 38A:563, 1956

9. Dekel S, Weissman SL: Osteotomy of the calcaneus and concomitant plantar stripping with talipes cavovarus. J Bone Joint Surg 55B:802, 1973

10. Dunn N: Stabilizing operations in the treatment of paralytic deformities of the foot. Proc R Soc Med 15:15, 1921

11. Dwyer FC: Osteotomy of the calcaneum for pes cavus. J Bone Joint Surg 41B:80, 1959

12. Dwyer FC: The present status of the problem of pes cavus. Clin Orthop 106:254, 1975

13. Edmonson AS, Crenshaw AH, Eds: Campbell's Operative Orthopaedics. 6th ed. CV Mosby Co, St. Louis, 1980

14. Fowler SB, Brooks AL, Parrish TF: The cavo-varus foot. J Bone Joint Surg 41A:757, 1959 (abst)

15. Frank GR, Johnson WM: The extensor shift procedure in the correction of clawtoe deformities in children. South Med J 59:889, 1966

16. Garceau GJ, Brahms MA: A preliminary study of selective plantar-muscle denervation for pes cavus. J Bone Joint Surg 38A:553, 1956

17. Giannestras NJ: Foot Disorders: Medical and Surgical Management. 2nd Ed. Lea & Febiger, Philadelphia, 1973

18. Hallgrimsson S: Studies on reconstructive and stabilizing operations on the skeleton of the foot with special reference to subastragalar arthrodesis in treatment of foot deformities following infantile paralysis. Acta Chir Scand 88 (Suppl 78):1, 1943

19. Herndon CH: Tendon transplantation at the knee and foot. p. 145. In American Academy of Orthopaedic Surgeons. Instructional Course Lectures. Vol. 18. JW Edwards, Ann Arbor, 1961

20. Heron JR: Neurological syndromes associated with pes cavus. Proc R Soc Med 62:270, 1969

21. Hibbs RA: An operation for "claw foot." JAMA 73:1583, 1919

22. Hoke M: An operation for stabilizing paralytic feet. J Orthop Surg 3:494, 1921

23. Ibrahim K: Cavus foot deformity in children: a comprehensive approach. Orthop Trans 9:417, 1985

24. Ibrahim K: Cavus foot deformity in children. Scientific Exhibit. American Academy of Orthopaedic Surgeons Meeting. Atlanta, February 1984

25. Irwin CE: The calcaneus foot. p. 135. In American Academy of Orthopaedic Surgeons. Instructional Course Lectures. Vol. 15. JW Edwards, Ann Arbor, 1958

26. Jahss MH: Tarsometatarsal truncated-wedge arthrodesis for pes cavus and equinovarus deformity of the fore part of the foot. J Bone Joint Surg 62A:713, 1980

27. James CCM, Lassman LP: Spinal dysraphism: the diagnosis and treatment of progressive lesions in spina bifida occulta. J Bone Joint Surg 44B:828, 1962

28. Japas LM: Surgical treatment of pes cavus by tarsal V-osteotomy: preliminary report. J Bone Joint Surg 50A:927, 1968

29. Jones R: The soldier's foot and the treatment of common deformities of the foot. Part II. Claw foot. Br Med J 1:749, 1916

30. Karlholm S, Nilsonne U: Operative treatment of the foot deformity in Charcot-Marie-Tooth disease. Acta Orthop Scand 39:101, 1968

31. Karlstrom B, Lonnerholm T, Olerud S: Cavus deformity of the foot after fracture of the tibial shaft. J Bone Joint Surg 57A:893, 1975

32. Levitt RL, Canale ST, Cooke AJ Jr, et al: The role of foot surgery in progressive neuromuscular disorders in children. J Bone Joint Surg 55A:1396, 1973

33. Lovell WW, Winter RB, Eds: Pediatric Orthopedics. JB Lippincott, Philadelphia, 1978

34. McElvenny RT, Caldwell GD: A new operation for correction of cavus foot: fusion of first metatarso-cuneiformnavicular joints. Clin Orthop 11:85, 1958

35. Paulos L, Coleman SS, Sanuelson KM: Pes cavovarus: review of a surgical approach using selective soft-tissue procedures. J Bone Joint Surg 62A:942, 1980

36. Rivera-Dominguez M, DiBenedetto M, Frisbie JH, et al: Pes cavus and claw toes deformity in patients with spinal cord injury and multiple sclerosis. Paraplegia 16:375, 1979

37. Sabir M, Lyttle D: Pathogenesis of Charcot-Marie-Tooth disease, gait analysis and electrophysiologic, genetic, histopathologic and enzyme studies in kinship. Clin Orthop 184:223, 1982

38. Samilson RL, Dillin W: Cavus canovarus and calcaneocavus. An update. Clin Orthop 177:125, 1983

39. Saunders JT: Etiology and treatment of clawfoot: report of the results in one hundred and two feet treated by anterior tarsal resection. Arch Surg 30:179, 1935

40. Siffert RS, Forster RI, & Nachamie B: "Beak" triple arthrodesis for correction of severe cavus deformity. Clin Orthop 45:101, 1966

41. Shanahan MDG, Douglas DL, Shanard WJW, et al: The long term results of the surgical management of paralytic pes cavus by soft tissue release and tendon transfer. Z Kinderchir 40(suppl 1):37, 1985

42. Sherman FC, Westin GW: Plantar release in the correction of the foot in children. J Bone Joint Surg 63A:1382, 1981

43. Stauffer RN, Nelson GE, Bianco AJ Jr: Calcaneal osteotomy in treatment of cavovarus foot. Mayo Clin Proc 45:624, 1970

44. Steindler A: Stripping of os calcis. J Orthop Surg 2:8, 1920

45. Tachdjian MO: Pediatric Orthopedics. WB Saunders, Philadelphia, 1972

46. Watkins MB, Jones JB, Ryder CT Jr, et al: Transplantation of the posterior tibial tendon. J Bone Joint Surg 36A:1181, 1954

47. Wilcox PG, Weiner DS: The Akron midtarsal dome osteotomy in the treatment of rigid pes cavus: a preliminary review. J Pediatr Orthop 5:333, 1985

48. Winter RB, Haven JJ, Mae JH, Lagaard SH: Diastematomyelia and congenital spine deformities. J Bone Joint Surg 56A:27, 1984

Osteotomy of the Os Calcis for the Calcaneocavus Foot

137

Robert L. Samilson

Osteotomy of the os calcis plays a role in the treatment of the calcaneocavus foot. In order to understand this role, it is necessary to classify cavus foot in general, and calcaneocavus foot specifically. Anterior cavus (cavus of the forepart of the foot), with the apex of deformity at Chopart's joint, may be subdivided into a global form, in which the entire transverse arch is involved, or the local form, in which only the first metatarsal is plantar flexed. When the first metatarsal is plantar flexed, the forepart of the foot is relatively pronated with respect to the hindpart of the foot. Posterior calcaneocavus is characterized by vertical orientation of the os calcis with increased calcaneal pitch. Calcaneal pitch is defined as the angle made with the horizontal by a plantar line drawn from the posterior to the anterior calcaneal tuberosity on a weight-bearing lateral radiograph. Angles greater than 30 degrees indicate a calcaneus position of the os calcis. Midtarsal cavus is characterized by the apex of the cavus deformity being at the talonavicular or calcaneocuboid joint. Combined cavus is one in which plantar flexion of the forepart of the foot coexists with increased vertical calcaneal orientation.

SURGICAL PROCEDURES

It is only in the posterior (calcaneocavus) type of cavus that calcaneal osteotomy is indicated. An integral part of the surgical procedure is an adequate plantar fasciotomy. Crescentic osteotomy of the os calcis for the calcaneocavus foot was first described in 1976.[2] It is indicated in ambulatory patients with symptomatic calcaneocavus feet where the calcaneal pitch is more than 30 degrees and the patient is over 10 years of age. It is best used in the fully established calcaneus deformity, since the developing calcaneus deformity associated with paralysis of the triceps surae can usually be prevented by early tendon transplantation. These tendon transplants are very well described in the preceding section.

Mitchell, in 1977, described posterior displacement osteotomy of the calcaneus, utilizing an oblique transverse osteotomy that permits upward and backward displacement of the posterior fragment.[1] It is to be noted that his operation was carried out in patients from 3 to 21 years of age. Although I have no personal experience with his procedure, I would suggest that the same age restrictions for crescentic osteotomy would apply to Mitchell's osteotomy as well.

Crescentic Osteotomy of the Os Calcis

Under tourniquet control, an obliquely placed lateral incision over the posterior tuberosity of the os calcis is made posterior to the subtalar joint. The peroneal tendons should be anterior to the posterior position of the incision. Dissection is carried down to the lateral aspect of the os calcis. The superior portion of the skin incision is about 4 cm posterior to the inferior end of the incision. The peroneal tendons are identified and are carefully protected. A complete plantar fasciotomy is performed. A crescentic osteotomy is then made in the os calcis, posterior to the subtalar joint. This may be done with a curved blade on a Stryker saw, or by joining multiple drill holes made in the os calcis with a large curved osteotome. The freed posterior tuberosity is shifted posterosuperiorly along the osteotomy line to correct the calcaneocavus (Fig. 137-1). The fragment may be secured with staples or with Kirschner wires left in place for 6 weeks, after which unprotected weight bearing is permitted.[2]

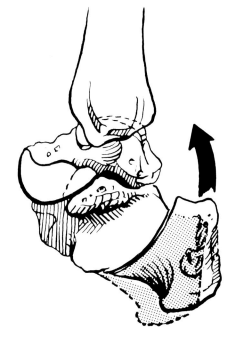

Fig. 137-1. Crescentic osteotomy of the os calcis with posterior fragment shifted superiorly along the osteotomy line. (From Samilson,[3] with permission.)

plied. A weight-bearing cast is retained for another month.[1]

Mitchell Osteotomy of the Calcaneus

A thorough plantar release is first carried out, including division of the long and short plantar ligaments. The calcaneocuboid and talonavicular joints are identified by sharp periosteal elevator, and the foot is manipulated to correct as much cavus as possible. The lateral aspect of the os calcis is exposed through a curved lateral incision. The osteotomy is carried out by oblique section of the bone, inclining the osteotomy forward and downward just posterior to the peroneal tendons. The posterior fragment is shifted upward and backward. The new position is fixed with a Steinmann pin. A below-knee cast is applied incorporating the Steinmann pin. The pin may be removed in 3 or 4 weeks, at which time a weight-bearing cast is ap-

RESULTS

Both the Mitchell and the crescentic osteotomy procedures are singularly free of complications. No nonunions or infections occurred in reported series.[1,2] In the crescentic osteotomies, there was no apparent alteration in triceps surae strength. Calcaneal pitch, which averaged 41 degrees preoperatively, was reduced to 19.5 degrees postoperatively with the crescentic osteotomy[2] (Fig. 137-2). Mitchell points out that, when some power of plantar flexion remains in the calcaneocavus foot, osteotomy of the os calcis (with adequate plantar release) may suffice. Otherwise, he regards it as a stage preparatory to further procedures such as tendon transplant or triple arthrodesis.[1]

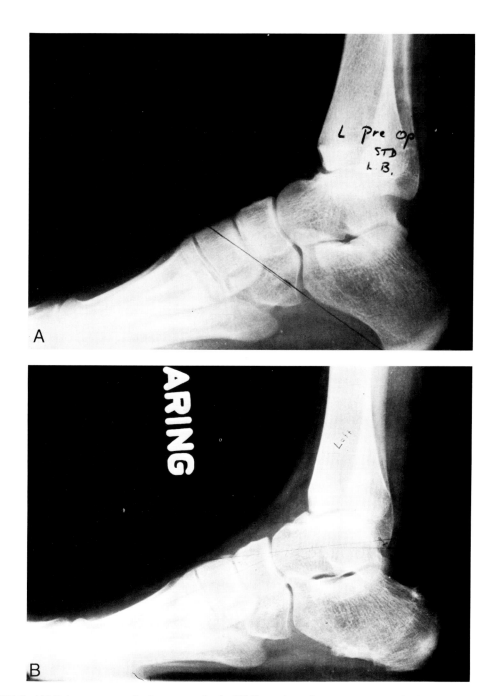

Fig. 137-2. (A) Calcaneocavus foot preoperatively. **(B)** Same foot, 5 years postoperatively, showing correction of increased calcaneal pitch. (From Samilson,[2] with permission.)

REFERENCES

1. Mitchell GP: Posterior displacement osteotomy of the calcaneus. J Bone Joint Surg 59B:233, 1977

2. Samilson RL: Crescentic osteotomy of the os calcis for calcaneocavus feet. p. 18. In Bateman JE (ed): Foot Science. WB Saunders, Philadelphia, 1976

3. Samilson RL, Specht EE: Neuromuscular disease affecting the foot. p. 271. In Inman VT (ed): DuVries' Surgery of the Foot. 3rd Ed. CV Mosby, St. Louis, 1973

Pes Planus

138

Henry R. Cowell

The term *pes planus* covers a wide range of foot abnormalities that require careful diagnosis and specific management. In the past, numerous operative procedures have been described for pes planus, but have frequently been applied indiscriminately to all forms of flatfoot. Radiographs enable the orthopaedic surgeon to differentiate among the varying anatomic manifestations of flatfoot and to implement the appropriate treatment regimen.

FLEXIBLE PES PLANUS

Flexible pes planus deformities may be divided into two types, according to whether an arch develops in the foot when the individual is not bearing weight. Children with flatfoot are often treated conservatively with corrective shoes and support devices. From the age of 2 to 5 years, a shoe with a medial cookie, medial heel wedge, and inner-heel advance may be used. Children may also have difficulties between the ages of 4 and 6, with pain over

the anterior tibial muscle belly and aching pain at night. This pain is dramatically relieved by a Thomas heel and medial cookie arch support. However, the use of shoe corrections in the child has not been shown to correct flattening of the foot, nor has it been shown to prevent difficulty in adulthood. In addition, children and adolescents with flexible flatfoot may demonstrate tightness of the heel cord. If detected during childhood, a tight heel cord may be improved by stretching exercises, or by serial casting with the foot in inversion to stretch the cord. While this tightness of the heel cord may be seen in the adult, it seldom causes symptoms or requires lengthening. It should be noted that, while several investigators have suggested heel cord lengthening for flexible flatfoot in the adolescent, in the adult it is a weakening procedure and should not be considered unless the foot is at least 15 degrees below neutral when the fore part of the foot is inverted. Anteroposterior (AP) and lateral radiographs in the standing position should be obtained for patients with this type of flatfoot.

There are two specific radiographic abnormalities which may appear in these films, leading to specific diagnoses of navicular cuneiform sag or talonavicular sag. Talonavicular sag is usually associated with abduction and pronation of the fore-part of the foot. In the normal foot, a line drawn on the lateral radiograph through the talus should be continuous with a line drawn through the plane of the first metatarsal. In navicular cuneiform sag, a line drawn through the talus creates an angle with a line drawn through the metatarsal which has its apex at the navicular cuneiform joint. In talonavicular sag, a line drawn through the talus will intersect with a line drawn through the metatarsal and navicular at the talonavicular joint, and the apex of the angle formed by these two lines will be at the talonavicular joint (Fig. 138-1). On the standing AP film, a line drawn through the talus should run

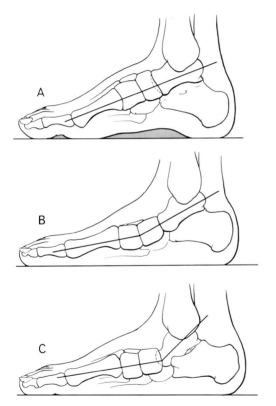

Fig. 138-1. **(A)** In the normal foot, a line drawn through the talus will continue through the shaft of the first metatarsal. **(B)** In a foot with navicular cuneiform sag, the line through the talus will form an angle with the line through the metatarsal. The apex of this angle will be at the navicular cuneiform joint in a patient with navicular cuneiform sag. **(C)** In a patient with talonavicular sag, a line drawn through the long axis of the talus will form an angle with a line through the metatarsal in the area of the talonavicular joint.

through the first metatarsal. In a foot with talonavicular sag, when abduction of the fore part of the foot is present, a line drawn through the talus will project medial to the first metatarsal. The operative procedures appropriate for navicular cuneiform sag are those reported by Butte,[1] Caldwell,[2] Giannestras,[6] Hoke,[12] and Miller.[22] Procedures appropriate for talonavicular sag have been reported by Harris and Beath,[10] Lowman,[19] and Young.[33]

A second variety of pes planus is the foot that is flat with or without weight bearing. This foot may be flexible and have subtalar motion; however, it cannot be treated with an arch support in the child, since placing a correction under the foot will not create an arch but will increase pressure under the medial aspect of the foot. Any use of wedges or corrections in this foot will result in pain. In the adolescent and adult, this type of flatfoot is best managed conservatively by a Plastizote insert. If severe symptoms warrant surgery, the appropriate operative procedure for this type of foot is triple arthrodesis.[16] Subastragalar arthrodesis, as described by LeLièvre,[17] may also be considered. When the deformity occurs along with minimal deviation of the forefoot and clinically detectable valgus of the os calcis, but without subluxation of the talonavicular joint, it may be well to consider one of the procedures for osteotomy of the os calcis, as described by Gleich,[7] Koutsogiannis,[15] or Lord.[18]

A third variation of the flexible flatfoot occurs in conjunction with an accessory navicular bone. An individual with an accessory navicular may have difficulty because the prominence on the medial side of the foot makes finding comfortable shoes difficult. This condition normally does not cause problems if shoes are not worn. The only individuals who are likely to have trouble without shoe wear are those who have a cornual navicular, which is much more prominent than a typical accessory navicular (Fig. 138-2).

Generally, the use of a proper shoe with adequate room will relieve the symptoms. If this is not effective, a felt pad may be placed inside the shoe with a hollowed out area in the region of the prominence. A moleskin donut may also be applied to the skin to hold the shoe away from the prominence and thereby decrease the irritation to the skin in this area. Occasionally, the use of a below-knee

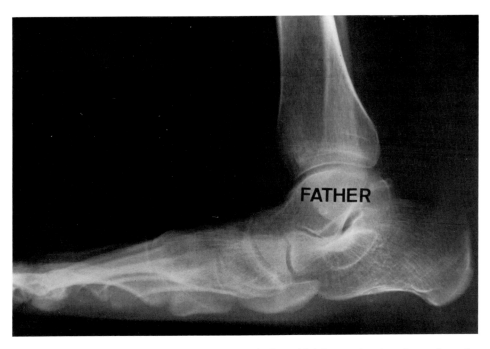

Fig. 138-2. This radiograph shows a large accessory navicular, which is prominent on the undersurface of the foot. Weight bearing causes pressure on this prominent area, and pain develops. This patient's son had a similar abnormality. Removal of the accessory navicular will relieve pain but will not improve the pes planus.

cast with a felt donut placed over the prominence may be required. One or more of these conservative methods is often effective in relieving the symptoms; once these modalities are discontinued, the symptoms may not recur. Excision of the accessory navicular, along with the medial prominence of the navicular, is indicated only when the patient does not respond to an adequate trial of conservative therapy.

Since the accessory navicular is associated with pes planus, Kidner[13] suggested that the accessory bone displaced the posterior tibial tendon medially, thereby compromising its function. He therefore suggested that, in addition to excision of the accessory navicular, the main portion of the posterior tibial tendon be rerouted under the navicular in an attempt to restore the normal direction or pull of the tendon. However, Macnicol and Voutsinas[20] report that pes planus did not improve following the Kidner procedure, except as a function of growth and time. Those of their patients who had the Kidner procedure had no better results than did those who had only an excision of the

accessory navicular, provided the navicular was contoured as well.

Finally, Mann and Thompson[21] reported progressive painful pes planus secondary to rupture of the posterior tibial tendon. Thirteen of seventeen patients that they saw with this condition had a history of injury, and while these patients never required emergency care, most of them sought medical care within several weeks of the injury. The patients had a flatfoot deformity that was unilateral in all but five patients. In those five who previously had had pes planus, the deformity was much more severe in one foot than the other. The diagnosis was apparent in all patients because of the poor function of the posterior tibial tendon. At operation, three patients had an intact but scarred adhesed tendon; three a rupture in situ with proliferative synovitis, thickening, and adhesions; and 11 a complete rupture.

In three patients in whom the rupture was close to the navicular, treatment consisted of advancing the tendon and reinserting it into the navicular. In eight patients, the flexor digitorum longus was identified, sutured to the flexor hallucis longus distally, transected just proximal to the site of the suture, and then inserted into the navicular after passing the tendon through the sheath of the posterior tibial tendon. In six patients in whom scarring of the sheath of the posterior tibial tendon was excessive, the flexor digitorum longus tendon was left in its own tendon sheath. Following transection, the distal end was tenodesed to the flexor hallucis longus and the proximal end anchored to the navicular. In four patients, three of the eight, and one of the six, the transfer was augumented by tenodesing the proximal stump of the posterior tibial tendon to the flexor digitorum longus. Postoperatively, a non-weight-bearing cast with the foot placed in equinus and inversion was used for 4 weeks. The cast was then changed, the foot placed in the plantigrade position, and a weight-bearing cast used for 6 weeks.

RIGID PES PLANUS

The other major type of flatfoot is the rigid deformity seen in conjunction with either congenital vertical talus or tarsal coalition. When found in conjunction with congenital vertical talus, rigid flatfoot is normally treated in the child. If it remains untreated until adulthood, the only satisfactory procedure is triple arthrodesis with excision of a major portion of the talus. The peroneal spastic flatfoot seen in tarsal coalition requires anatomic diagnosis. An oblique radiograph will demonstrate a calcaneonavicular bar that may be treated by resection and extensor digitorum brevis interposition, as I have described.[5] Talocalcaneal coalition may be resected in certain instances but generally will not give satisfactory results. In individuals with persistent symptoms of talocalcaneal coalition, triple arthrodesis is the recommended procedure.

The indication for operation in all adolescents and adults with pes planus is intractable pain which has failed to respond to conservative measures. The use of a Thomas heel and medial heel wedge should be considered first in those individuals with flexible flatfoot.[3] The use of Plastizote inserts is the appropriate treatment for patients with rigid flatfoot. When this deformity is accompanied by tightness of the peroneal musculature, a below-knee weight-bearing cast worn for three weeks may relieve the difficulty. The operative procedure for a calcaneonavicular coalition restores subtalar motion and may be considered for a patient with mild symptoms. However, I have not performed this procedure unless pain was present. The operative procedure for talocalcaneal coalition, triple arthrodesis, is a more disabling procedure in the adolescent or young adult, and should be reserved for the painful foot which has failed to respond to a regimen of Plastizote inserts and the use of a series of plaster casts.

NAVICULAR CUNEIFORM SAG

All operative procedures aimed at the correction of navicular cuneiform sag include fusion of the navicular cuneiform joint. Various investigators combine this fusion with tendon transfer, and some recommend heel cord lengthening.[2,6,12,22] Most of these workers suggest that the treatment of navicular cuneiform sag is more effective when carried out before the age of 14, although each has reported using the procedure in a number of selected adults. Most authorities note, however, that the same good results should not be anticipated in adults as in adolescents. The indication for these procedures in the adult is severe disabling pain. Before performing a procedure for navicular cuneiform sag, a plantar-flexion lateral radiograph of the foot should show that the cuneiform can be placed in proper position in relation to the navicular. The following investigators have described their procedures as being appropriate at least occasionally in the adult.

Surgical Techniques

Giannestras' Technique

A slightly curved medial incision is made from approximately 1 cm posterior and inferior to the medial malleolus, extending forward across the midportion of the navicular, and then curving plantarward to the midshaft of the first metatarsal (Fig. 138-3).[6] The abductor hallucis muscle is identified and reflected from the medial and plantar surfaces of the cuneiform bone, navicular bone, and spring ligament. The flexor digitorum longus tendon is identified in the posterior tibial nerve. The posterior tibial tendon is located and its sheath is split from the medial malleolus to its insertion on the navicular. The tendon is then detached from the navicular, preserving as much length as possible. A 00 chromic suture is used to tag the tendon for future reinsertion and retraction. The anterior tib-

ial tendon is dissected free of its sheath, proceeding from the inferior border of the extensor retinaculum to the insertion at the first tarsometatarsal joint. It is divided from the bone at this point. A suture of 00 chromic catgut is passed through this tendon, to be used for reattachment and retraction.

A proximal flap is planned, approximately 1.5 cm in width and having its base over the talus, extending down across the navicular and the cuneiform. Two parallel incisions are made on the dorsal and plantar aspects of the talus, navicular, and cuneiform. These incisions are connected to create a

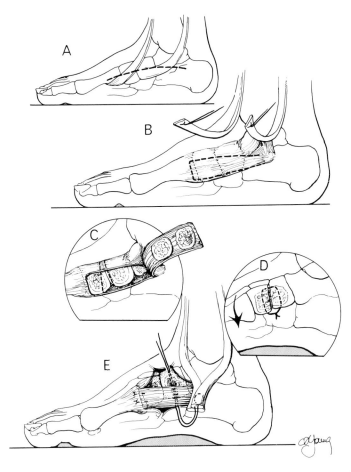

Fig. 138-3. **(A)** The Giannestras procedure is performed through a medial skin incision. **(B)** After the anterior and posterior tibial tendons have been free from their insertions, an osteoperiosteal flap is raised. **(C)** After raising this flap, the navicular cuneiform joint is identified, and a wedge of bone removed. **(D)** Following removal of this wedge, the forefoot is plantar flexed to oppose the navicular and the cuneiform, and the area is fixed with a suture. **(E)** The anterior and posterior tibial tendons are threaded through the navicular from its undersurface, the osteoperiosteal flap is reattached, and the tendon sutured to the flap.

flap that has its distal portion at the level of the joint between the first metatarsal and the cuneiform. Following incision of the capsule of the first metatarsal cuneiform joint, a sharp osteotome is used to raise the flap, shaving off a portion of the cartilage and a small fragment of bone from the cuneiform and the navicular. The spring ligament is then identified and dissected free to the level of the sustentaculum tali, revealing the medial surface of the head and neck of the talus as well as the medial edge of the talocalcaneal joint. The cortex of the plantar surface of the navicular is roughened to form a bed for the tibialis anterior and posterior tendons, which will later be inserted here.

Next, a thin wedge of bone is removed from the navicular cuneiform joint with a thin osteotome, its base directed toward the plantar surface of the foot. Giannestras recommends that this wedge be no more than 2 to 3 mm wide, since removal of a larger wedge will cause overcorrection. The articular surfaces of the navicular and cuneiform are cleared of cartilage to expose the underlying bone. The forepart of the foot is placed in pronation and plantar flexion to assure that the bony deformity of the navicular cuneiform sag has been corrected. Following this, a $\frac{5}{16}$-inch drill hole is made in the cuneiform, from the plantar surface toward the area of the osteotomy, exiting just below the dorsal cortex. A second drill hole is made in the navicular, extending dorsally and distally from the plantar surface so that it exists approximately at the midpoint of the osteotomy surface of the navicular. A double suture of 2 chromic catgut is passed from the plantar surface of the navicular, through the drill hole, across into the cuneiform, and out through the plantar surface of the cuneiform. The foot is placed in the corrected position and the suture is tied to maintain this correction. The previously created flap is now sutured to the periosteum at the base of the first metatarsal, producing a bolstering effect across the arch. The flap is sutured under tension with 0 chromic catgut while the foot is held in the corrected position. Additional sutures are then used to hold the flap in place.

A $\frac{7}{64}$-inch drill hole is then made through the navicular, for insertion of the posterior and anterior tibial tendons. The previously placed sutures are threaded through the navicular from the plantar surface, pulling the tendons into the navicular.

The sutures are tied on the dorsal surface of the navicular, bringing the foot into a slight varus. Additional sutures are then applied through the tendons and underlying spring ligament to hold them in place. The tendon sheath of the posterior tibial tendon is repaired. A Hemovac drain that exits through the calf is used. The subcutaneous tissue is closed with interrupted sutures of 000 plain catgut, and the skin is closed with subcuticular wire.

Lengthening of the Achilles tendon, if necessary, may be carried out through a separate lateral incision. The decision to lengthen this tendon should be made prior to surgery; the procedure is indicated only if the foot does not come within 5 degrees of the neutral position when the fore part of the foot is held in the corrected position. Giannestras recommends that the cast be applied with the foot in its corrected position (not overcorrected). The cast is applied in sections, with the first portion covering the leg and ankle, beginning at the mid-metatarsal level; the foot is held in the neutral position with the knee in 90 degrees of flexion for this part of the casting. Next, the arch is molded and the tourniquet released. When this has set, the foot is placed in full pronation and the remainder of the cast is applied. The foot is elevated for 24 hours and the Hemovac unit is removed after 72 hours. Postoperative radiographs are taken to ensure that correction has been maintained in the cast. The patient is allowed to walk and bear weight 5 to 7 days following surgery. Mobilization is continued for a minimum of 8 weeks. If no union is present after this period, a second weight-bearing cast should be applied and maintained for 4 weeks. Giannestras recommends that the casting be discontinued at 12 weeks postoperatively, even if union does not appear to be firm.

After removal of the cast, a rigid-shank shoe is worn for 3 months. No athletic activities are allowed for 6 months postoperatively. Giannestras noted excellent to good results in 127 of 146 postoperative feet. Three adults who underwent this procedure had satisfactory results and were able to perform a full day's activity without difficulty, although pain sometimes returned. Complications in this procedure include nonunion of the navicular cuneiform joint and metatarsalgia and callus formation under the second and third metatarsal heads. A two-team approach is not recommended, since one patient complained that the feet were not symmetrically corrected.

Durham's Technique

Caldwell[2] reported the results of the Durham procedure for navicular cuneiform sag, which involves fusion of the navicular cuneiform joint. He reported that the oldest patient treated with this procedure was 15 years of age. The Durham procedure is comparable to that of Giannestras and is carried out through an identical incision. However, Caldwell described fusion of the navicular cuneiform joint with a bone peg, with the flap raised on a distal base at the area of the first metatarsal. This flap is sutured into the tissue at the sustentaculum tali to obtain a bowstring effect, and only the posterior tibial tendon is routed underneath the navicular. Caldwell reported that, in a series of 76 feet, 58 feet had results classified as excellent, 14 as good, and 4 as poor. It should be noted again that these results were obtained in patients under 15 years of age.

Hoke's Technique

The technique of Hoke[12] involves fusion of the navicular cuneiform joint combined with sliding-lengthening of the Achilles tendon. Here again, the procedure was performed in children, and a piece of the tibia was used as an inlay graft in the navicular cuneiform area. The Achilles tendon was lengthened in all cases. The Hoke technique is mentioned for the sake of completeness, since a modification of the procedure is a routine part of the Giannestras operation. Butte[1] reported on end results of the Hoke procedure, stating that in a series of 138 feet results were excellent in 30, good in 40, fair in 34, and poor in 34. The data strongly suggest that the Hoke operation produces a number of unsatisfactory results. Butte noted that this procedure should be used only in the early adolescent patient, and only if no other deformity of the tarsal bones and no arthritis are present in the foot.

Miller's Technique

The Miller procedure[22] is carried out through the same incision and in the same fashion as the procedure outlined by Giannestras. The Miller procedure, however, involves only the steps in which a proximally based flap is combined with navicular cuneiform fusion, and reinsertion of the flap occurs underneath the periosteum at the base of the first metatarsal. No other tendon transfers are performed.

TALONAVICULAR SAG

Operative correction of talonavicular sag has been described by Harris and Beath,[11] and by Lowman[19] with fusion of the talonavicular joint. Young[33] suggested elevation of this joint with a rerouting of the anterior tibial tendon.

Surgical Techniques

Harris and Beath's Technique

A medial incision is made approximately 1 cm distal to the medial malleolus, extending approximately 4 cm beyond the midpoint of the talonavicular joint. The talonavicular joint is incised transversely, and the cartilage is removed from the talus and the navicular; sufficient cartilage is removed from the head of the talus to allow the forepart of the foot to swing around into the neutral position. The forepart of the foot is aligned with the hindpart of the foot to create an arch, and the navicular is aligned with the talus. The joint between the talus and the os calcis is approached through an incision on the dorsal border of the sustentaculum tali, and the middle facet of the talocalcaneal joint is removed and packed with bone. An intraoperative AP radiograph is obtained to ensure that the fore part of the foot has been corrected in relationship to the hindpart of the foot and the talus. Following this, subcutaneous closure is effected with interrupted sutures of 000 plain catgut, and the skin is closed with 000 Dermalon. An above-knee cast is applied with the foot in the corrected position and maintained for 6 to 8 weeks, at which time the cast is removed and fusion of the joint is checked radiographically. If fusion has not occurred, another 4 weeks of immobilization in plaster are indicated.

Lowman's Technique

A curved incision is begun approximately 1 cm below the medial malleolus and extended forward over the middle surface of the navicular to the base of the first metatarsal (Fig. 138-4). The skin flap is retracted, and a separate incision is made through the fascia in a straight line from just below the medial malleolus down to the base of the first metatarsal. The talonavicular ligament is incised in the line of the joint, and a periosteal elevator is used to strip the fibrous tissue from the navicular along with all ligamentous attachments.

At this point, the Achilles tendon is tenotomized and the foot is dorsiflexed to neutral. A wedge is excised from the talonavicular joint, with a major

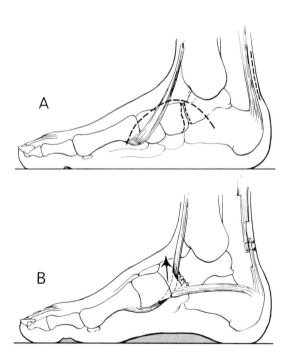

Fig. 138-4. (A) The Lowman procedure is carried out through medial and posterior incisions. The talonavicular joint is identified and excised, and the anterior tibial tendon is rerouted around the edge of the navicular and through the joint. **(B)** Following this, the remainder of the joint is packed with bone chips and the heel cord is lengthened. A second slip of the heel cord is directed forward and used as a suspensory ligament to maintain the arch and hold the plantar surface of the navicular and talus approximated.

portion being removed from the navicular. Adequate bone must also be removed from the head of the talus so that the forepart of the foot can be reduced on the hindpart of the foot; therefore, a plantar and medially based wedge should be excised. Lowman noted that the Achilles tendon may be tenotomized if only a few degrees of dorsiflexion are needed, but recommended that an open procedure be used if more than a mild amount of tendon lengthening is required. (While Lowman also included tenotomy of the peroneal muscles in his procedures, this is generally not indicated in the case of a flexible flatfoot.) Next, the anterior tibial tendon is dissected free without damaging the insertion. The anterior tibial tendon is displaced around the navicular, so that it lies on the plantar surface of the navicular and is routed through the talonavicular joint. With the tendon held in this position and with the fore part of the foot plantar flexed and adducted, sutures are placed in the undersurface of the talonavicular joint to maintain correction. Number 1 chromic sutures are used for this placement. The fascia and periosteum over the navicular and in the talonavicular area are closed with interrupted sutures of 000 chromic catgut, the subcutaneous tissue with interrupted sutures of 000 plain catgut, and the skin with Dermalon. Postoperatively the foot is placed in an above-knee cast with the knee flexed and maintained in this position for 4 weeks. At the end of this period, the plaster is changed to a weight-bearing cast. Lowman suggested that weight bearing be initiated at 10 weeks in a shoe with an arch support and brace.

Young's Technique

Young modified the procedure described by Lowman by rerouting the anterior tibial tendon without fusion of the joint (Fig. 138-5). Through a similar incision, the area of the navicular and talonavicular joint are approached, but the talonavicular joint is not opened. Young's incision passes superior to the medial aspect of the navicular bone. The posterior tibial tendon is temporarily separated subperiosteally from its attachment to the inferior surface of the navicular tuberosity. A drill hole approximately 6 mm in diameter is made through the navicular and located approximately 1

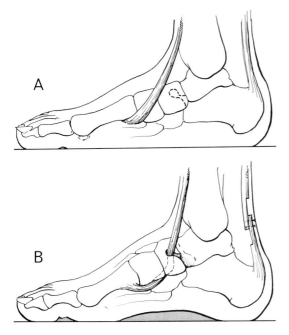

Fig. 138-5. The Young procedure is carried out through lateral and posterior incisions. **(A)** A channel is made in the navicular, and **(B)** the anterior tibial tendon is routed around the navicular and run through this channel, thus providing a mechanical advantage in creating an arch in the foot. The heel cord is usually lengthened also.

cm from the medial aspect of the bone. Once this hole has been drilled, a Gigli saw is used to remove the section between the hole and the portion of the navicular medial to the talus. A gouge is used to make a groove on the inferior surfaces of the first cuneiform and the navicular bones. The anterior tibial tendon is then identified, and the tendon sheath is incised in its distal 6 cm. Once the tendon has been freed, it is pulled posteriorly and passed through the slot in the navicular and into the drill hole. The previously removed bone chips are placed in the slot and 00 chromic catgut sutures are used to close the periosteum, returning the posterior tibial tendon to its original position. A below-knee cast is applied postoperatively and maintained for 8 weeks. Young noted that this procedure had been used in adolescents with satisfactory raising of the arch and the correction of the forefoot. One adult patient was also treated this way and was relieved of his symptoms.

PES PLANUS WHEN NON-WEIGHT BEARING

The foot that is flat when standing and remains flat with non-weight bearing is frequently asymptomatic. However, this condition may give pain in the midtarsal area; this pain is generally secondary to degenerative changes occurring in the subtalar joint, since the os calcis is shifted into valgus and the head of the talus is frequently depressed. This type of flatfoot cannot be managed with arch supports since there is no arch, even without weight bearing. However, the flatfoot with no arch can frequently be managed with a Plastizote insert, which serves both as a shock absorber and as a mechanism for redistributing weight to all aspects of the foot. Since the only applicable surgery for this type of foot involves fusion of joints, it should be delayed until a conservative regimen with Plastizote inserts has been tried. An operation is indicated only in individuals who have severe, painful flatfeet with degenerative changes of such magnitude that activity is limited.

Surgical Techniques

Triple Arthrodesis

The operative procedure used for this type of flatfoot is triple arthrodesis. A lateral incision is made over the talonavicular joint from the level of the extensor tendons, curving backward underneath the lateral malleolus, to the level of the peroneal tendons over the lateral talocalcaneal joint. Following incision through the skin and subcutaneous tissue, the extensor digitorum brevis muscle is encountered. The insertion of this muscle is separated from the os calcis by sharp dissection and is reflected distally. The sinus tarsi is cleaned of fat and all other fibrous tissue, and the joints between the talus and the navicular, the talus and the os calcis, and the os calcis and the cuboid are identified and incised in the direction of the joint lines. Since the heel is in valgus and the fore part of the foot is abducted, wedges must be removed from the medial side of the talonavicular joint and the medial side of the talocalcaneal joint. These wedges must be removed in such a fashion that the foot is brought back to the neutral position and an arch is created. The talonavicular is approached first and a ¾-inch osteotome is used to remove a biplane wedge from the talus and the navicular, with the apices based laterally and dorsally.

Since the osteotomes are directed so that they diverge from each other from the lateral side of the foot, it may be necessary to make a second skin incision over the medial side of the foot. If this is required, a Freer periosteal elevator is inserted into the talonavicular joint and advanced until the skin is tented medially to identify the level of skin incision on the medial side of the foot. A straight skin incision is made on the medial side of the foot, running from the area just anterior to the navicular, posteriorly along the joint between the talus and the os calcis. The wedge that is removed should be 2 to 3 mm wider at the plantar surface of the joint than at the dorsal surface, and approximately ½ cm should be removed from the medial side of the foot to allow the fore part of the foot to come into a neutral position. More bone is removed from the talus if necessary.

The cartilage is then cleared from the calcaneocuboid joint, and two minimal wedges are removed: one with a dorsal apex and one with a lateral apex. The talocalcaneal joint is approached, and a lamina spreader is placed between the talus and the calcaneus to gently open the joint. The interosseous ligament is cut, allowing the joint to open even further. Once proper visualization is possible, the cartilage is removed from the talus and the os calcis, taking care to extract a wedge that is based medially in the foot. The posterior and middle facets are carefully removed through this incision. Special effort must be made not to disturb the neurovascular bundle and the extensor hallucis longus, which are visible in the posterior medial aspect of the wound. If the middle facet cannot be removed through the lateral incision, the medial incision is extended.

Following removal of all excess bone, the foot is placed in the corrected position with the surfaces in contact. Staples may be used to maintain this position, and if used are placed medially to hold the correction obtained between the talus and the navicular. The talus and the calcaneus should be in contact as well. Following this, the bone which has been removed is denuded of all cartilage and used to pack the area between the talus and the calcaneus laterally, and any other open areas.

The extensor digitorum brevis muscle is reattached, and the subcutaneous tissue is closed with interrupted sutures of 000 plain catgut. The skin is closed with interrupted sutures of Dermalon. An above-knee cast is applied with polyurethane foam padding over the dorsum of the foot, the anterior surface of the tibia, and the anterior surface of the femur. The cast may be changed at 5 to 7 days postoperatively to improve position, if necessary. This may be done in the castroom without anesthesia, unless a marked change in position is required. The above-knee cast is maintained for 6 to 8 weeks, at which time it is removed and radiographs are obtained. Generally, a below-knee weight-bearing cast is applied for an additional 4 to 6 weeks, at which time radiographs should show consolidation of the fusion.

A major complication of this procedure is nonunion, usually in the talonavicular joint. Aseptic necrosis of the talus has not been a problem in my series of adolescent patients. Other authors have reported an increased incidence of degenerative arthritis in the ankle joint; however, in a recent review of patients 10 to 30 years after triple arthrodesis (for various conditions including flatfoot), I found a very low incidence of degenerative arthritis in the ankle joint. The most common complication of triple arthrodesis for flatfoot is fusion in an incorrect position. Frequently, the foot is fused with the heel in valgus and the forefoot abducted. When this happens, the individual may have continued pain when weight bearing because of bony prominences on the undersurface of the foot, and the inability to compensate for these bony prominences through subtalar motion.

Complications of Triple Arthrodesis in Pes Planus

As noted, the most common complication of arthrodesis in pes planus is a prominence on the undersurface of the foot due to failure of the surgery to reconstruct the arch. When a triple arthrodesis is done with the foot in an uncorrected position, the undersurface of the os calcis may remain prominent on the sole of the foot. When this occurs, two subsequent operative procedures are available to the surgeon: either the area which is prominent may be resected, or the triple arthrodesis must be osteotomized and redone. If there is a single tender area on the undersurface of the foot, resection is advisable; if the triple is not solid, or if the foot remains in valgus and there are multiple problems, a repetition of the procedure should be considered.

Resection of Prominence of Os Calcis When there is an area of tenderness and pain or a prominence of the undersurface of the foot, resection is required (Fig. 138-6). Prior to resection, a radiograph is taken with a marker over the tender area to be sure that prominence of the os calcis is, indeed, the cause of the pain. When indicated, resection is accomplished through an incision on the lateral aspect of the foot. The incision is carried down through the skin and subcutaneous tissue, and the plantar lateral border of the os calcis is identified. The periosteum is stripped subperiosteally. A

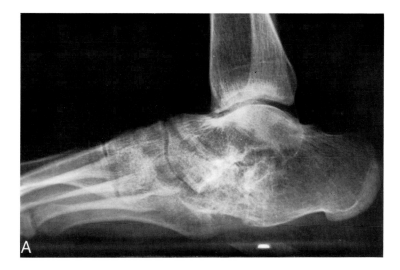

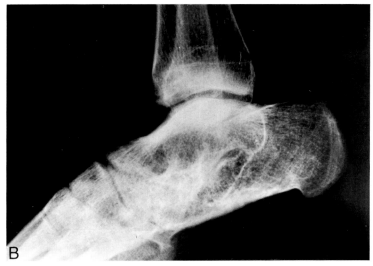

Fig. 138-6. (A) Radiograph of a patient who previously underwent triple arthrodesis for pes planus without satisfactory reconstruction of the arch. The undersurface of the os calcis is prominent in the weight-bearing surface of the foot. A metal marker has been placed over the area of the patient's pain to identify the prominence. **(B)** Postoperative radiograph of the same patient following removal of the undersurface of the os calcis.

broad osteotome is used to excise all areas of prominence from the undersurface of the foot. Once this has been done, a radiograph should be obtained in the operating room to confirm that a sufficient portion of the os calcis has been removed. The periosteum is closed with interrupted sutures of 000 chromic catgut, the subcutaneous tissue with 000 plain, and the skin with interrupted sutures of Dermalon. A below-knee weight-bearing cast is applied with a polyurethane foam support under the foot. Weight bearing is allowed. The cast may be

changed at 10 to 14 days, and a new cast is applied with a sole cutout of polyurethane foam. Sutures are removed at 3 weeks, and ambulation is then allowed.

Reconstruction of Previous Triple Arthrodesis If there is more than one area of tenderness, if the heel is in valgus, or if there is incomplete healing of any joint in the triple arthrodesis, the triple should be osteotomized and redone with the foot in proper position (Fig. 138-7). A straight incision is

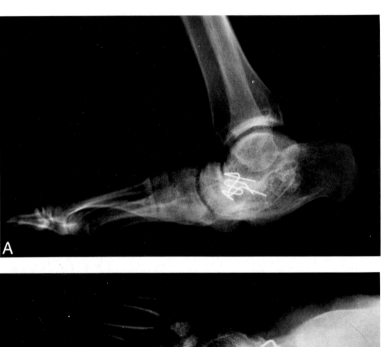

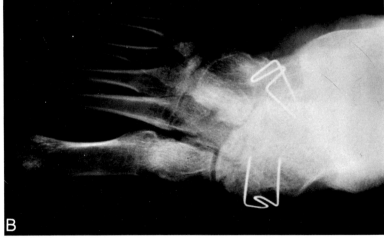

Fig. 138-7. (A) Radiograph of a patient who previously underwent triple arthrodesis for pes planus without reconstruction of the arch. The patient was weight bearing on the undersurface of the cuboid and anterior portion of the os calcis. **(B)** AP radiograph shows the marked abduction of the forepart of the foot, demonstrating that the triple arthrodesis had been performed without reconstituting the arch, and with the forepart of the foot left in the valgus position. *(Figure continues.)*

made on the medial aspect of the foot, approximately 1 cm below the medial malleolus. This incision extends from just anterior to the heel cord, directly across the talonavicular joint on its plantar surface. After incision through the skin and subcutaneous tissue is completed, the neurovascular bundle, the posterior tibial tendon, and the flexor digitorum longus and flexor hallucis longus tendons are identified in the middle of the wound; a rubber drain is placed around the neurovascular bundle to protect it for further dissection. The area

of the talonavicular joint is approached from the medial aspect, and the periosteum is freed by subperiosteal dissection. At this point, the incision described previously for triple arthrodesis is made on the lateral side of the foot, beginning over the lateral area of the talonavicular joint and curving backward approximately 2 cm below the lateral malleolus. This incision runs from the level of the extensor tendons anteriorly to the peroneal tendons posteriorly.

The original area of the calcaneocuboid, talocal-

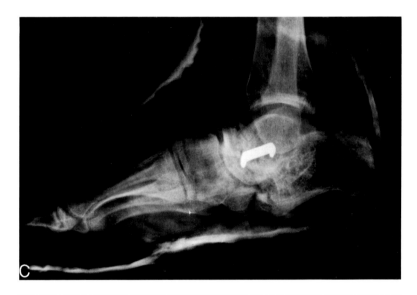

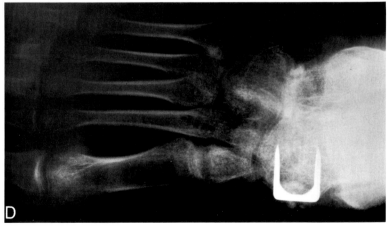

Fig. 138-7 *(Continued).* **(C)** Postoperative radiograph of same patient following wedge resection and realignment with reconstruction of a plantigrade foot. Notice that the forepart of the foot has been plantar flexed more than 20 degrees from the previous radiograph. **(D)** AP radiograph shows the alignment of the forepart of the foot on the hindpart of the foot after removal of a large, medially based wedge to correct the abduction of the forepart of the foot.

caneal, and talonavicular joints is identified. Attention is redirected to the medial incision, where any prominence of the talus is excised. A wedge is planned through the area, having its base on the plantar surface of the foot and its apex on the dorsal surface. Sufficient bone is removed from this wedge to permit reconstruction of the arch. Another wedge is planned on the medial side of the foot, between the talus and the calcaneus with the base medially and the apex laterally. This wedge is planned to bring the heel out of valgus. After removal of the two wedges, the foot is positioned and evaluated. If further bone needs to be removed, it is done at this time. A staple is placed on the medial aspect of the talonavicular area with the foot held in the corrected position. This staple maintains correction of the talus and the navicular. If necessary, a second staple may be placed between the talus and the calcaneus to hold these bones in position. This staple is removed 6 months postoperatively.

While this procedure is occasionally carried out through the medial incision, it is usually necessary to use a lateral incision to remove the wedge and to allow for full correction. Following removal of the bone and placement of the staples, the subcutaneous tissue is closed with 000 sutures of plain catgut and the skin with interrupted sutures of nylon. An above-knee cast is applied with the foot in the corrected position. This cast is removed at 6 to 8 weeks postoperatively and radiographs are obtained. Generally, a below-knee weight-bearing cast is applied at this time and maintained until radiographs show consolidation of healing. I have been pleased with results of this procedure, although it has been used in only a few cases. No complications have occurred in these patients.

LeLièvre's Technique

LeLièvre[17] described a procedure that he calls arthroereisis, involving the use of a piece of bone in the lateral tarsal area to hold the foot in the corrected position and prevent valgus of the os calcis. LeLièvre stated that the advantage to this procedure is that abnormal motion of the os calcis into valgus is blocked but motion is not totally limited, as in an arthrodesis performed between the talus and the calcaneus. LeLièvre reported using arthroereisis in adults up to 69 years of age and

states that he has had no complications as a result of this technique.

The sinus tarsi is exposed through a curvolinear lateral skin incision, similar to that described for triple arthrodesis. The extensor digitorum brevis muscle is identified and its origin is removed from the talus and calcaneus. The ligament between the talus and the calcaneus is identified and resected. The calcaneus is then aligned with the astragalus by displacing it medially. If the os calcis is not mobile, this maneuver may be facilitated by the use of a periosteal elevator. A small cone-shaped bone graft is cut and inserted into the sinus tarsi, with the foot held in the corrected position. (LeLièvre reported the use of homologous bone for this procedure.) A graft that fits firmly into the sinus tarsi with the os calcis held in neutral position should be selected. A staple may be inserted between the talus and the calcaneus if the graft is not stable. If used, this staple should be removed after 4 months. The origin of the extensor digitorum brevis is reattached. The subcutaneous tissue is then closed with interrupted sutures of 000 plain catgut, and the skin is closed with interrupted sutures of nylon.

LeLièvre reported that a plaster cast need not be applied, and the patient may ambulate with support at the end of 2 weeks. He also noted that, in the adult, heel cord lengthening is necessary and should be carried out in such a way as to leave the medial portion of the heel cord attached to the os calcis, thereby pulling the heel into varus. This procedure was used in 80 patients, 21 of whom were over the age of 20. LeLièvre reported satisfactory results in a majority of patients. While he did not break down the statistics as to the benefits in adults, he did note that the results were excellent in 73 of 80 cases. He reported no complications from this procedure.

PES PLANUS WITH VALGUS HEEL

When valgus of the os calcis is the main component of pes planus, osteotomy of the os calcis may be considered. Medial displacement of the portion of the os calcis which is attached to the heel cord was originally described by Gleich[7] in 1893 and discussed by Lord[18] in 1923. This procedure was originally reported for children, but has more recently been used in adults. It is carried out through a lateral incision over the os calcis. Koutsogiannis[15] reported on this technique; while it was primarily intended for use in children, that author has employed it in at least two adults.

Surgical Techniques

Os Calcis Osteotomy

A lateral incision is made over the os calcis in line with and approximately 1 cm below the peroneal tendons. This incision is carried from anterior to the Achilles tendon to the undersurface of the os calcis. Following incision of the skin and subcutaneous tissue, the os calcis is identified and the periosteum is incised in a line running parallel and inferior to the peroneal tendons. A narrow strip of periosteum is stripped from the dorsal and plantar surfaces of the os calcis. The os calcis osteotomy is planned and marked with an osteotome at an angle of 45 degrees with the undersurface of the os calcis. Following this, multiple holes are drilled along this line in both the medial and lateral cortices of the os calcis. A broad osteotome is used to complete this osteotomy through the medial and lateral surfaces of the os calcis. The superior and inferior cortices are cut with a ⅜-inch osteotome. Once the osteotomy has been completed, the entire os calcis may be shifted medially by a distance approximately one-half the width of the os calcis. In most instances, the osteotomy is stable in this position with the foot brought into maximum dorsiflexion. If not, a single Kirschner wire may be used to maintain fixation. This wire is inserted through the posterior aspect of the os calcis and run anteriorly toward the toes into the second portion of the os calcis. The wire exits through the skin and, thus, may easily be removed 3 weeks postoperatively when the cast is changed. Following displacement of the os calcis, the subcutaneous tissue is closed with interrupted sutures of 000 chromic catgut and the skin with interrupted sutures of 000 nylon.

A below-knee cast is applied and maintained for 3 weeks, at which time it is changed and the sutures and wire are removed. A second below-knee weight-bearing cast is applied for 3 weeks. I have used this procedure in children and adolescents and have been pleased with it. The only complication has been the displacement of the pin in one young patient who kicked the cast against the ground. Koutsogiannis noted some difficulty with his patients, with complications in two patients with tight heel cords. Both patients were unable to dorsiflex the foot to a right angle. This operative procedure should not be considered for individuals who have tight heel cords.

PES PLANUS WITH ACCESSORY NAVICULAR

Occasionally an individual will present with a flatfoot with symptoms related to the marked prominence of an accessory navicular on the medial side of the foot. This is caused by pressure from the medial counter of the shoe on the accessory navicular, and excision of this bone may be considered for relief. This procedure, originally described by Kidner for flatfoot, is intended to excise the prominence, and treat the flatfoot itself. The procedure will relieve symptoms but may not reconstitute a normal arch, and the patient should be made aware of this prior to the surgery.

Surgical Technique — Kidner's Technique

Incision is carried out on the dorsomedial aspect of the foot. A curvolinear incision is placed over the navicular and runs approximately 3 to 4 cm from the talus over the dorsal surface of the navicular to the area of the first cuneiform. This incision should be placed sufficiently dorsal that it will not be rubbed by the shoe. The incision is carried down through the skin and subcutaneous tissue, and the prominence of the navicular and the posterior tibial tendon are identified. The posterior tibial tendon is freed by sharp subperiosteal dissection from the navicular. A wafer of the accessory bone is left attached to the tendon. A broad osteotome is used to remove both the accessory navicular and the prominent portion of the medial aspect of the navicular at the same time. All of the navicular bone, which projects medial to the first cuneiform, should be excised. This may require removal of 0.75 cm from the lateral aspect of the navicular. A sufficient amount should be taken from the lateral aspect of the navicular so that there will no longer be a prominence on the medial side of the foot. Following this, two drill holes are placed through the navicular distally from the dorsal to the ventral surface. The foot is held in an inverted and supinated position. A suture of 0 chromic catgut is then placed through the posterior tibial tendon, and the suture is threaded up through the navicular using straight needles. The suture is tied over the dorsum of the navicular and has the effect of pulling the posterior tibial tendon underneath the plantar surface of the navicular, creating an arch. The subcutaneous tissue is closed with interrupted sutures of 000 chromic catgut, and the skin with interrupted sutures of nylon. A subcuticular wire may be used. A below-knee cast is applied, which is changed 7 to 10 days postoperatively, and a new below-knee weight-bearing cast is applied for 4 more weeks. The specific use of this procedure for resection of the medial portion of the navicular has given satisfactory results in most instances.

Complications of the procedure include incomplete removal of the accessory navicular and incomplete removal of a sufficient amount of the navicular. Rerouting of the posterior tibial tendon may result in severance of the tendon if care is not taken to dissect the posterior tibial tendon free at the time of resection. I have not observed recurrence of the deformity, but I have seen patients with painful scars caused by injudicious placement of the incision.

PERONEAL SPASTIC FLATFOOT

Patients who present with a rigid flatfoot, showing limited subtalar motion and contraction of the peroneal tendons and going into valgus when the foot is inverted, should be reviewed systematically to ascertain the anatomic cause. Rigid flatfoot may occur secondary to systemic causes such as rheumatoid arthritis, or may be seen secondary to trauma or to coalitions in the area of the talocalcaneal and calcaneonavicular joints.[8,14,27] Coalition between the calcaneus and the navicular is a common finding in younger individuals, with symptoms often appearing between the ages of 8 and 12. Coalition between the talus and the calcaneus frequently causes symptoms during the adolescent period.

Identification of coalitions should be carried out by means of a systematic radiographic approach. Lateral radiographs may indicate coalition in the talocalcaneal joint if beaking of the head of the talus, broadening of the lateral process of the talus, or narrowing of the talocalcaneal joint is seen. An oblique film of the area will show the presence or absence of a calcaneonavicular bar. Next, a second special film, an axial view of the talocalcaneal joint, should be obtained. (The axial view, originally described by Korvin,[14] was popularized by Harris and Beath[10] as the axial or skijump view of the talocalcaneal area.) Computed tomography (CT) of the talocalcaneal joint may also be used to determine coalitions between the talus and the calcaneus in any of the three facets between these bones. Scintigraphy using technetium 99m-methylene diphosphonate may also be of value.[25]

Treatment varies according to the type of coalition. In a younger individual, resection of the calcaneonavicular coalition should be considered. However, resection of a calcaneonavicular coalition cannot be considered in the older individual if any degenerative changes, such as beaking of the talonavicular joint, have occurred. A regimen of conservative therapy should be undertaken when beaking of the talonavicular joint is present in a patient with calcaneonavicular coalition, or when the coalition occurs between the talus and the calcaneus. Frequently a Plastizote insert in the shoe will relieve the symptoms seen with tarsal coalition. When this fails, a below-knee weight-bearing cast is applied for 3 to 4 weeks to rest the foot and allow the symptoms to subside; the cast is then followed by a Plastizote insert. If the individual still fails to respond to conservative therapy, excision of the calcaneonavicular bar is indicated, as long as the patient is young and has not undergone degenerative changes. Resection of the bar is particularly likely to be effective when the bar is cartilaginous but may also be considered with an osseous bar for a calcaneonavicular coalition.

Recent studies[23,26] have also reported good results with resection of talocalcaneal coalitions in the middle facet. Prior to resection of any coalition, the presence of other coalition in the same foot should be ruled out, since talocalcaneal and calcaneonavicular coalitions have been reported in the same foot.[31]

Author's Preferred Technique

The calcaneonavicular coalition is approached through a lateral Ollier-type incision, placed approximately 2 cm inferior and anterior to the lateral malleolus.[5] This curvolinear incision, located over a skin crease, is made through the skin and subcutaneous tissue from the extensor tendons anteriorly to the peroneal tendons posteriorly. The coalition can usually be palpated under the skin as a fullness below the extensor digitorum brevis muscle belly. After incision of the skin and subcutaneous tissue, the origin of the extensor digitorum brevis muscle is identified, and the entire extensor digitorum brevis muscle belly is dissected free of the os calcis. The fascia is incised dorsally to free it from any attachment to the talus. This incision extends as far as the level of the nerve supply to the extensor digitorum brevis, which is identified and protected. Following this, the muscle belly is retracted distally to identify the calcaneonavicular coalition. The calcaneocuboid joint is also identified, but care is taken not to cut the ligament between the calcaneus and the cuboid. The talonavicular joint is identified, as well as the area between the navicular and the third cuneiform. Osteotomes are driven perpendicular to the calcaneonavicular coalition and on either side of the cartilaginous portion of the coalition directly through to the medial side of the foot. A section of the coalition at least 1 cm in length must be excised. Care must be taken not to damage the cartilage of the joint between the talus and the navicular, between the navicular and the cuneiform, and between the os calcis and the cuboid. The joint surfaces may be protected by using Freer periosteal elevators. An oblong of bone is removed. Care must be taken to ensure that all cartilaginous portions are removed from both the navicular and the os calcis sides of the coalition; if this cartilage remains, reformation of the bar may occur. Care must also be taken not to disturb the middle or anterior facets of the talocalcaneal joint. Once the bar has been removed, a suture of 1 chromic is threaded through the muscle belly of the extensor digitorum brevis and passed through the arch of the foot using two Keith needles. This pulls the muscle belly of the extensor digitorum brevis down into the resected defect. It is tied on the medial surface of the foot over a sponge and button. Range of motion of the subtalar joint is noted prior to insertion of the extensor digitorum brevis and is recorded in the operating room. Following this, the subcutaneous tissue is closed with interrupted sutures of 000 plain and the skin with interrupted sutures of nylon.

Postoperatively the patient is placed in a below-knee cast with polyurethane foam padding over the area of the incision. This cast is maintained for 5 to 7 days, at which time it is split and subtalar motion is initiated three times daily. The posterior half of the cast is used as a splint. The sutures are removed at 3 weeks, at which time the chromic suture through the extensor digitorum brevis will usually break and may be pulled out. If it does not break, it should be cut and removed. No weight bearing is allowed until subtalar motion reaches the level measured in the operating room. This is accomplished with daily physical therapy and reinforcement of range of motion by the patient.

The results of this procedure show that 90 percent of adolescent patients have a satisfactory range of motion, no recurrent symptoms, and the ability to participate in sports. In an older age group, approximately three-fourths of patients operated on without signs of degenerative changes have had satisfactory subtalar motion, no pain, and have been able to participate in all activities including sports (Fig. 138-8).

The only complication seen from this procedure occurred in two patients who had limited extension of the toes. If care is not directed toward protecting the extensor digitorum brevis nerve, the muscle will not function and extension of the toes may be limited. In addition, care must be taken not to cut the sensory nerves on the dorsum of the foot, or an area of decreased sensation will result.

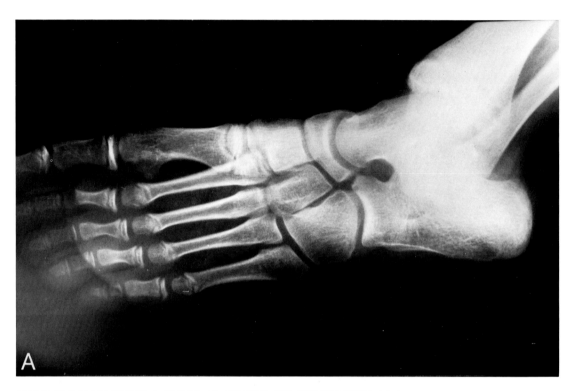

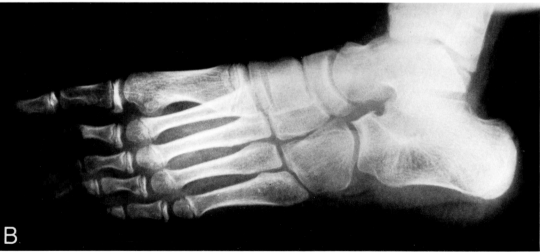

Fig. 138-8. (A) Calcaneonavicular coalition preoperatively. **(B)** Calcaneonavicular coalition postoperatively, showing resection of the midportion of the osseous and cartilaginous coalition.

Resection may also be considered for talocalcaneal coalition. Prior to resection, a CT scan should be used to identify the extent of the coalition. A 4-cm oblique incision is made on the medial aspect of the hindpart of the foot distal to the medial malleolus. The posterior tibial tendon is palpated before the incision is made, and the incision is made along a line tangent to the posterior tibial tendon and just distal to it. The neurovascular bundle is identified and preserved. The flexor digitorum longus and flexor hallucis tendons are located where they pass below the medial malleolus and the sustentaculum tali identified. The periosteum is incised between the two tendons and the flexor digitorum longus and its sheath are reflected toward the ankle, and the flexor hallucis tendon and its sheath toward the sole of the foot. The posterior facet of the talocalcaneal joint is located and the anterior portion of the middle facet or the anterior facet identified. A truncated wedge of bone, the medial base measuring 1 cm, and the lateral portion measuring 4 mm is removed from the bridge between the talus and os calcis. Once this truncated wedge has been removed, 10 to 15 degrees of subtalar motion should be present. This motion may be confirmed by observing the motion in the area of the posterior facet, which should be easily visualized in the proximal portion of the incision. While some authors suggest placing fat in the defect, I do not consider this necessary. The periosteum is tacked down to the bone with two or three sutures of 000 chromic, the subcutaneous tissue closed with sutures of 000 plain, and the skin with 000 nylon. The postoperative care is generally the same as that following excision of calcaneonavicular coalition.

If degenerative changes are present in the talonavicular joint, if the symptoms are severe, and if the patient has failed to respond to conservative measures, triple arthrodesis may be considered. If the heel is in valgus, the coalition should be resected prior to completing the triple arthrodesis. This may be done through the lateral incision for triple arthrodesis described above. A sufficient amount of the coalition is resected through the lateral incision to allow the os calcis to be placed underneath the talus and to produce proper positioning of the foot.

If the talocalcaneal fusion is bony and the symptoms are secondary to the valgus position of the heel, medial displacement osteotomy of the os calcis may be considered.

REFERENCES

1. Butte FL: Navicular-cuneiform arthrodesis for flatfoot: an end-result study. J Bone Joint Surg 19:496, 1937
2. Caldwell GD: Surgical correction of relaxed flatfoot by the Durham flatfoot plasty. Clin Orthop 2:221, 1953
3. Chambers EFS: An operation for the correction of flexible flat feet of adolescents. West J Surg Obstet Gynecol 54:77, 1946
4. Clark WA: A rebalancing operation for pronated feet. J Bone Joint Surg 13:867, 1931
5. Cowell HR: Diagnosis and management of peroneal spastic flatfoot. p. 94. In American Academy of Orthopaedic Surgeons. Instructional Course Lectures. Vol. 24. JW Edwards, Ann Arbor, 1975
6. Giannestras NJ: Flexible valgus flatfoot resulting from naviculocuneiform and talonavicular sag: surgical correction in the adolescent. p. 67. In Bateman JE (ed): Foot Science. WB Saunders, Philadelphia, 1976
7. Gleich A: Bietrag zur operativen Plattfussbehandlung. Arch Klin Chir 46:358, 1893
8. Harris RI: Rigid valgus foot due to talocalcaneal bridge. J Bone Joint Surg 37A:169, 1955
9. Harris RI: Retrospect: peroneal spastic flatfoot (rigid valgus foot). J Bone Joint Surg 47A:1657, 1965
10. Harris RI, Beath T: Etiology of peroneal spastic flat foot. J Bone Joint Surg 30B:624,1948
11. Harris RI, Beath T: Hypermobile flatfoot with short tendo Achillis. J Bone Joint Surg 30A:116, 1948
12. Hoke M: An operation for the correction of extremely relaxed flat feet. J Bone Joint Surg 13:773, 1931
13. Kidner FC: The prehallux (accessory scaphoid) in its relation to flat-foot. J Bone Joint Surg 11:831, 1929
14. Korvin H: Coalitio talocalcanea. Z Orthop Chir 60:105, 1934
15. Koutsogiannis E: Treatment of mobile flat foot by displacement osteotomy of the calcaneus. J Bone Joint Surg 53B:96, 1971
16. Leavitt DG: Subastragaloid arthrodesis for the os calcis type of flat foot. Am J Surg 59:501, 1943

17. LeLièvre J: Current concepts and correction in the valgus foot. Clin Orthop 70:43, 1970
18. Lord JP: Correction of extreme flatfoot: value of osteotomy of os calcis and inward displacement of posterior fragment (Gleich operation). JAMA 81:1502, 1923
19. Lowman CL: An operative method for correction of certain forms of flatfoot. JAMA 81:1500, 1923
20. Macnicol MF, Voutsinas S: Surgical treatment of the symptomatic accessory navicular. J Bone Joint Surg 66B:218, 1984
21. Mann RA, Thompson FM: Rupture of the posterior tibial tendon causing flat foot. J Bone Joint Surg 67A:556, 1985
22. Miller OL: A plastic flat foot operation. J Bone Joint Surg 9:84, 1927
23. Olney BW, Asher MA: Excision of symptomatic coalition of the middle facet of the talocalcaneal joint. J Bone Joint Surg 69A:539, 1987
24. Purvis GD: Surgery of the relaxed flat-foot. Clin Orthop 57:221, 1968
25. Sartoris DJ, Resnick DL: Tarsal coalition. Arthritis Rheum 28:331, 1985
26. Scranton PE Jr: Treatment of symptomatic talocalcaneal coalition. J Bone Joint Surg 69A:533, 1987
27. Slomann HC: On coalitio calcaneo-navicularis. J Orthop Surg 3:586, 1921
28. Slomann HC: On the demonstration and analysis of calcaneo-navicular coalition by roentgen examination. Acta Radiol 5:304, 1926
29. Stewart SF: Human gait and the human foot: an ethnological study of flatfoot. Clin Orthop 70:111, 1970
30. Stewart SF: Human gait and the human foot: an ethnological study of flatfoot. II. Clin Orthop 70:124, 1970
31. Wheeler R, Guevera A, Bleck EE: Tarsal Coalitions: review of the literature and case report of bilateral dual calcaneonavicular and talocalcaneal coalitions. Clin Orthop 156:175, 1981
32. Wright DG, Desai SM, Henderson WH: Action of the subtalar and ankle-joint complex during the stance phase of walking. J Bone Joint Surg 46A:361, 1964
33. Young CS: Operative treatment of pes planus. Surg Gynecol Obstet 68:1099, 1939
34. Zadek I: Transverse-wedge arthrodesis for the relief of pain in rigid flat-foot. J Bone Joint Surg 17:453, 1935

Tarsal Tunnel Syndrome

139

Roger A. Mann

The tarsal tunnel syndrome results from an entrapment of the posterior tibial nerve or one of its branches, which results in a clinical syndrome that can be extremely disabling for the patient. In most patients, the condition, which was named by Keck and Lam in separate articles in 1962,[1,2] is characterized by burning pain on the plantar aspect of the foot, usually aggravated by activity and diminished by rest. Some patients will complain of similar pain that is worse at night and relieved by activity. The burning, tingling, numb feeling cannot be well localized on the foot. Occasionally, it will be distributed along one of the three terminal branches of the posterior tibial nerve. In about one-third of patients, the pain will radiate along the medial aspect of the leg to the midcalf.

The condition is idiopathic in approximately 50 to 60 percent of patients. Others will identify the gradual onset of symptoms following an injury, such as an ankle sprain, crush injury, severe fracture of the distal tibia, fracture dislocation of the ankle, or fracture of the calcaneus. Local causes I have observed include:

1. A ganglion of one of the tendon sheaths that pass next to the tarsal canal or next to the branches of the posterior tibial nerve
2. A lipoma involving the fat surrounding the posterior tibial nerve or one of its terminal branches
3. An exostosis from the distal tibia or one of the tarsal bones
4. A tarsal coalition with a medial talocalcaneal bar that produces a large area of bony proliferation and presses on the medial plantar nerve
5. An enlarged venous plexus surrounding the posterior tibial nerve within the tarsal canal

OR

6. Severe pronation of the hindpart of the foot that results in stretching of the posterior tibial nerve

The diagnosis of the tarsal tunnel syndrome is made by the correlation of the patient's history, physical findings, and electrodiagnostic studies. If any of these three criteria does not point toward a tarsal tunnel syndrome, one should be very cautious about making the diagnosis. Although the diagnosis is often not recognized, the other end of the spectrum is also true: the condition at times is overdiagnosed and overtreated.

CLINICAL EVALUATION OF THE PATIENT

Subjective Complaints

The most frequent complaint elicited from a patient with a tarsal tunnel syndrome is a burning pain on the plantar aspect of the foot, which is usually aggravated by activities and diminished by rest. There are, however, a certain group of patients whose main complaint will consist of a burning, aching pain in the plantar aspect of the foot that is worse at nighttime while in bed and relieved somewhat by being on the feet.

The pain is characterized as a burning tingling numbness that cannot be well localized on the plantar aspect of the foot. On occasion, the pain will be distributed along one of the three terminal branches of the posterior tibial nerve — namely, the medial plantar, lateral plantar, or medial calcaneal branch. The patient will often seek relief of this pain by rubbing the foot, moving about, and at times soaking the feet in either hot or cold water.

Initially the symptoms are quite mild, but over a period of time they usually become progressively bothersome to the patient. In approximately 30 percent of patients the pain will be noted to radiate up along the medial aspect of the leg to the level of the midcalf. It is most unusual for the pain to go any farther than midcalf, and I have never seen the pain radiate up past the knee.

Physical Examination

The main physical finding is that of a positive Tinel's sign along the posterior tibial nerve over the tarsal canal. If a positive Tinel's sign is not elicited in this area, one should carefully percuss along the terminal branches of the posterior tibial nerve, in an attempt to elicit a Tinel's sign. I have never

seen a tarsal tunnel syndrome in which there has not been a positive Tinel's sign over the posterior tibial nerve or one of its terminal branches. At times, the positive Tinel's sign will extend proximally up the medial side of the leg, along the course of the posterior tibial nerve. The etiology of the Tinel's sign proximal to the tarsal tunnel canal cannot be explained.

In a few patients with a tarsal tunnel syndrome, the gait is abnormal because of tethering of the nerve within the tarsal canal. These patients will usually take a short step with the involved leg in order to prevent stretching of the posterior tibial nerve by striding to a normal step length.

The neurologic examination at times is confusing in that although the patient clinically complains of pain and numbness, in only 50 percent of the patients will the clinician be able to demonstrate actual numbness or loss of two-point discrimination. Weakness of the intrinsic muscles has been a very infrequent finding in my experience.

Although a tarsal tunnel syndrome can be caused by severe valgus of the hindpart of the foot, I have not been able to reproduce the patient's symptoms by forcing the foot into marked valgus.

In the patient who has a local cause for the tarsal tunnel syndrome, such as a ganglion, lipoma, or exostosis, the diagnosis is readily made in that the area in which the pressure is being applied to the nerve will be the point at which the positive Tinel's sign can be elicited.

Electrodiagnostic Studies

The third criterion for the establishment of the diagnosis of a tarsal tunnel syndrome is a decrease of the conduction velocity of the posterior tibial nerve or one of its terminal branches.

It is important to determine the conduction velocity of the posterior tibial nerve before the tarsal tunnel, which will help rule out an abnormality of the posterior tibial nerve before it enters the area of the tarsal tunnel — e.g., peripheral neuritis. The terminal latency of the medial plantar nerve to the abductor hallucis and of the lateral plantar nerve to the abductor digiti quinti should be obtained. One should not obtain the nerve conduction to only one of the terminal branches.

The terminal latency of the medial plantar nerve to the abductor hallucis should be less than 6.2 msec, and of the lateral plantar nerve to the abductor digiti quinti should be less than 7 msec.

The abductor hallucis and the abductor digiti quinti should be sampled in order to determine whether any fibrillation potentials are present in either of these muscles. The sensory examination of the posterior tibial nerve can be useful; however, accurate determination of the sensory delay is technically somewhat difficult and is not as readily obtained as the previously mentioned studies.

DIFFERENTIAL DIAGNOSIS

If the criteria previously put forth are carefully adhered to in obtaining the history, the physical findings, and the electrodiagnostic studies, there

Table 139-1. Differential Diagnosis of Tarsal Tunnel Syndrome

Remote causes
    Interdigital neuroma
    Intervertebral disc lesion
    Plantar fasciitis
    Plantar fibromatosis

Intraneural causes
    Peripheral neuritis
    Peripheral vascular disease
    Diabetic neuropathy
    Leprosy
    Neurilemoma
    Neuroma

Extraneural causes
    Ganglion
    Nerve tethering
    Fracture (callous, malunion, nonunion, displaced fragment)
    Blunt trauma
    Valgus hindfoot
    Rheumatoid arthritis
    Venous varicosities
    Tenosynovitis
    Ligament constriction
    Abductor hallucis origin constriction
    Metatarsal arch strain
    Longitudinal arch strain
    Lipoma

(From Wilemon,[3] with permission.)

should be little doubt as to whether a true tarsal tunnel syndrome exists. If all three criteria are not present, one should strongly consider a diagnosis other than that of a tarsal tunnel syndrome (Table 139-1).

TREATMENT

Once the three criteria for the diagnosis of a tarsal tunnel syndrome have been met, one should take steps to correct the etiology, if possible. If the etiology is valgus of the hindpart of the foot, some type of orthotic device may alter the clinical course of tenosynovitis or rheumatoid arthritis. Antiinflammatory medications may be used either systemically or locally. Following blunt trauma or a fracture in the area with resulting edema, the use of an elastic stocking may be beneficial in reducing the edema and then controlling it. On occasion, one may be justified in placing the patient into a below-knee weight-bearing cast, just to immobilize the ankle joint and the posterior tibial nerve to see whether this in itself would be sufficient to permit the symptom complex to subside.

In attempting to decide whether a surgical release should be carried out in the treatment of a tarsal tunnel syndrome, one should be guided by the fact that even after the tarsal tunnel has been released, the clinical symptoms may persist and on rare occasions may even worsen. It is crucial to explain to the patient the fact that even after the successful release of a tarsal tunnel syndrome, complete relief of symptoms may not occur; even if the patient does initially experience complete relief, there is sometimes a recurrence of the symptom complex several years later.

Surgical Approach

The surgical approach to the tarsal tunnel syndrome is carried out under thigh tourniquet hemostasis. The skin incision is made, starting about 5 cm proximal to the tip of the medial malleolus and 1 cm posterior to the posterior border of the tibia (Fig.

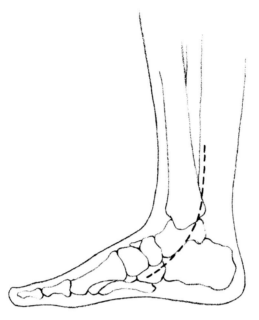

Fig. 139-1. Skin incision.

139-1). The skin incision then passes behind the medial melleolus, proceeding approximately 1 cm plantar to the course of the posterior tibial tendon and ending at the area of the talonavicular joint. The incision is deepened through subcutaneous tissue and fat in order to expose the deep fascial layers. Then, in the proximal portion of the wound, the fascia is opened posterior to the posterior tibial tendon sheath in order to expose the posterior tibial nerve before it actually enters the tarsal canal. By so doing, the nerve is still rather mobile and the possibility of inadvertently traumatizing the nerve is minimized. Once the nerve has been identified, the remainder of the deep fascia that forms the roof over the tarsal canal is opened throughout the length of the skin incision. As one proceeds past the level of the malleolus, the dorsal aspect of the abductor hallucis muscle is identified and is retracted plantarward (Fig. 139-2) in order to continue to expose the nerve in this area. Returning now to the proximal portion of the wound, the posterior tibial

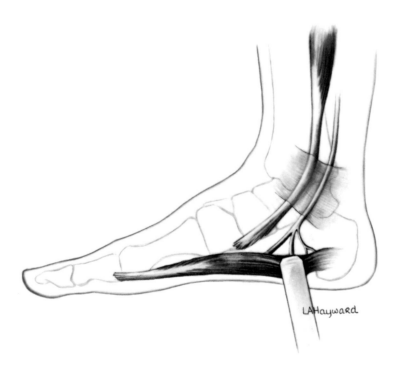

Fig. 139-2. The posterior tibial nerve as it branches into the medial and lateral plantar nerves. Following removal of the fascia of the tarsal tunnel, the plantar nerves can be seen clearly. The medial plantar nerve is seen along the dorsal aspect of the abductor hallucis muscle.

nerve, which is usually present as a single trunk (on rare occasions two trunks are noted in this area), is then traced distally by careful blunt dissection. The bifurcation into the medial and lateral plantar nerve is identified in the midportion of the tarsal canal. Next, the medial plantar nerve is traced distally along or just beneath the dorsal border of the abductor hallucis muscle until it starts to cross the foot, at about the level of the talonavicular joint. A hemostat should be placed into the fibro-osseous tunnel in the abductor hallucis, through which the medial plantar nerve passes as it begins to move across the foot (Fig. 139-3). This maneuver is carried out to look for any type of constriction of the nerve in this area. As one traces the medial plantar nerve beneath the numerous veins and arteries that cross it, the dissection at times becomes tedious and time consuming, particularly if there is a moderate amount of fibrosis present. Other than generally separating the nerve from the vessels, no effort is made to ligate the venous plexus, which may be accompanying the posterior tibial nerve through the tarsal canal. Next, the lateral plantar nerve is identified proximally. It is located posterior to the medial plantar nerve, proceeding distally, almost

in a straight line, deep to the vascular leash, passing beneath the abductor hallucis muscle and then proceeding laterally across the foot. Again, the fibroosseous tunnel through which the nerve passes should be carefully identified so as to rule out any constriction of the nerve in this area.

In the dissection of the lateral plantar nerve, care should be taken to identify the medial calcaneal branches. There may be one or more medial calcaneal branches coming off the posterior aspect of the lateral plantar nerve. These branches vary in size from 1 to 2 mm. It is important, therefore, to always initially dissect the lateral plantar nerve along its anterior border so as not to inadvertently disrupt one of the medial calcaneal branches.

Once the posterior tibial nerve and its terminal branches have been carefully dissected free, it is important to inspect the nerve carefully for evidence of constriction. We use the same criteria in evaluating the posterior tibial nerve as we use for the median nerve as it passes through the carpal tunnel—namely, a change in the color of the nerve, the presence or absence of a fine capillary tree, and the presence or absence of fat along the course of the nerve.

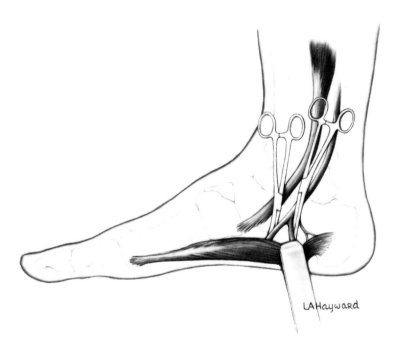

Fig. 139-3. The lateral plantar nerve is located posterior to the medial plantar nerve. Both nerves should be freed where they pierce the abductor hallucis muscle, to ensure decompression.

Once the dissection has been completed and all structures constricting the nerve have been released, pressure should be applied to the wound, the tourniquet released, and careful hemostasis obtained. The wound is then closed in a routine manner and a sterile compression dressing is applied. Postoperatively the patient is kept non-weight bearing for a period of 3 weeks and encouraged to keep the extremity elevated as much as possible in order to relieve edema and promote healing of the surrounding soft tissues. Progressive ambulation is then begun with the use of an elastic stocking for support; following this, activities are permitted to increase as tolerated.

Clinical Results

Generally speaking, patients who feel that the pain they had previously experienced is relieved immediately after surgery tend to have the best prognosis for a successful tarsal tunnel release. The outlook is not as favorable if, immediately following surgery, the patient does not feel that there has been any significant relief of the preoperative symptoms.

Occasionally, a great deal of scarring is present about the posterior tibial nerve or one of its terminal branches, which will require both an external and internal neurolysis. Occasionally, one may carry out microdissection of the posterior tibial nerve or its terminal branches. In following this group of patients postoperatively, the Tinel's sign has usually persisted in the area of the tarsal tunnel and, roughly speaking, less than 25 percent of the patients will lose this sign. In some patients the Tinel's sign will progress down along the terminal branches, following the release of the tarsal tunnel. This is an indication that true compression of the nerve was present. Even when this occurs, it is unusual for the patient to lose the Tinel's sign completely.

Approximately 70 percent of patients who have a release of the tarsal canal will experience relief of symptoms. The patient will often still note mild dysesthesias, but generally speaking most are quite satisfied with the surgical outcome. Approximately 30 percent of patients will demonstrate little or no improvement from the surgical procedure. I have noted that patients who have symptoms and a positive Tinel's sign proximal to the tarsal tunnel generally tend to do worse than those whose symptom complex is entirely located distal to the tarsal canal.

CONCLUSION

The diagnosis of tarsal tunnel syndrome is dependent on three specific criteria. It must be carefully brought out by the history, elicited in the physical examination, and confirmed by electrodiagnostic studies. If all three of these criteria are present and the patient's clinical symptoms warrant it, release of the tarsal tunnel is justified if conservative measures have failed. Even following a successful release of a tarsal tunnel syndrome, approximately 30 percent of patients will report that they have had minimal or no improvement from the surgical procedure. A small group of patients will have relief of the symptoms following the surgical procedure, only to have symptoms recur months or years later. It is for these reasons that the surgical release of the tarsal canal should be undertaken only when all other forms of treatment have failed.

REFERENCES

1. Keck C: The tarsal-tunnel syndrome. J Bone Joint Surg 44A:180, 1962
2. Lam SJS: A tarsal-tunnel syndrome. Lancet 2:1354, 1962
3. Wilemon WK: Tarsal tunnel syndrome: a 50-year survey of the world literature and a report of 2 new cases. Orthop Rev 8(11):111, 1979

Astragalectomy

140

Eugene R. Mindell

Astragalectomy was originally performed on rare occasions for trauma.[14] In 1872 Edward Lund of Manchester described talectomy for congenital talipes equinovarus and devised a special knife for the operation.[7] Royal Whitman initiated enthusiasm for this operation in 1901 by publishing a report of 13 cases of talectomy performed for paralytic talipes calcaneus.[19] It then became a common operation in some centers but was never universally practiced. Overenthusiasm led to its misapplication, and it became unpopular. In many centers talectomy was almost completely replaced by bracing, tendon transfer procedures, and selected foot stabilization techniques such as triple arthrodesis.[5]

However, today astragalectomy remains a useful procedure in carefully selected cases of calcaneus or calcaneovalgus deformity in poliomyelitis, of equinovarus deformity in patients with meningomyelocele, or of arthrogrypotic clubfoot in children, as well as occasionally in talar injury[11] or disease.

INDICATIONS

Calcaneus and calcaneovalgus foot deformities were common problems in the past in postpoliomyelitis paralysis patients. In such deformities the talus is perched on an os calcis that is vertical rather than horizontal. The mechanics of weight bearing are poor, with the entire body weight thrown upon the tuberosity of the os calcis. The forepart of the foot serves little useful function. Many methods of treatment are available for such foot deformities, including bracing, surgical correction of fixed deformities, tendon transfers, selected foot stabilization procedures, and astragalectomy.[5,13] Each procedure has its indications and contraindications. Astragalectomy, as the preferred treatment for paralytic calcaneus and calcaneovalgus deformity, was designed[17,19] to correct deformity, displace the foot backward, produce good contact between the foot and the ground, eliminate lateral instability, and bring the lower end of the tibia over the center of the weight-bearing area of the foot. Astragalec-

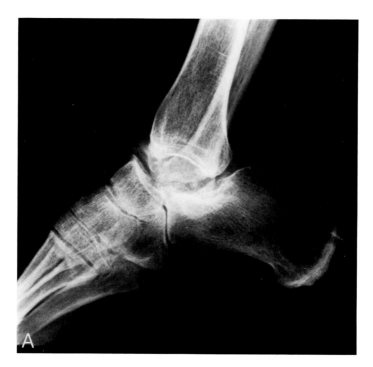

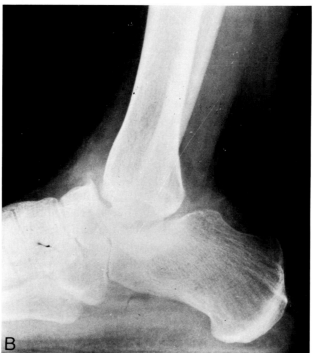

Fig. 140-1. (A) This lateral radiograph shows the ankle of a 45-year-old woman 12 years after talectomy was performed for a severe open comminuted fracture-dislocation of the entire talus. **(B)** The tibia is balanced nicely on the os calcis, as can be seen in the standing weight-bearing lateral radiograph. She has little discomfort and can walk all day.

tomy may be performed in poliomyelitis patients under the age of 10 years, for whom arthrodesing operations on the foot are usually not advisable.[2]

Children with rigid equinovarus deformities secondary to meningomyelocele may develop adaptive changes in the bones of the feet that prevent adequate correction by soft tissue surgical release alone. Astragalectomy should be considered for the younger child with meningomyelocele in whom soft tissue releases are inappropriate and who are too young for triple arthrodesis.[15]

Children with clubfoot deformity secondary to arthrogryposis not infrequently have persistent rigid equinovarus deformity despite having had manipulation prior to cast application and soft tissue releases. These children can be improved significantly by astragalectomy.[3,4,7,8,10] According to Drummond and Cruess,[4] talectomy is the procedure of choice in the young child with a very severe or recurrent clubfoot secondary to arthrogryposis.

In certain fracture-dislocations of the talus, particularly when the proximal fragment is comminuted, markedly displaced, and obviously necrotic, excision of the talar head and fusion of the tibia to the distal talar fragment, as described by Blair,[1] should be considered. Total talectomy may be considered as treatment for a markedly comminuted or infected open fracture-dislocation of the talus but should be performed rarely, as the results are unpredictable. Proper alignment and maintenance of the tibia on the calcaneus in a stable position are necessary for a satisfactory result (Fig. 140-1).

Slowly growing neoplasms, such as giant cell tumors, or chronic low-grade infections are occasionally encountered in the talus. Astragalectomy may be considered as a surgical option.

SURGICAL TECHNIQUE

Although the specific technique for astragalectomy and the postoperative management required vary with the underlying disease, certain common principles apply. A generous anterolateral skin incision should be made. The ligaments are stripped off both the malleoli and the os calcis, so that the foot can easily be displaced posteriorly. A meticulous resection of the talus from the tibiotalar, sub-

talar, and talonavicular joints must be done cleanly, leaving no fragments behind. Following talectomy, the foot is displaced posteriorly. The calcaneus is then positioned so that its anterior aspect is between the malleoli with good opposition of the superior surface of the calcaneus under the tibia. With the calcaneus in this position, the lateral malleolus rests opposite the calcaneocuboid joint, while the medial malleolus lies just above and behind the navicular bone. For this to be accomplished the foot must be externally rotated beneath the leg. The foot must be aligned not with the patella but with the malleoli. After the foot has been correctly placed, a Kirschner wire or Steinmann pin is driven through its plantar surface into the tibia to prevent posterior drift of the foot.

When the deformity is secondary to neuromuscular disease, as in meningomyelocele, Trumble et al.[15] state that following the lateral skin incision, the dissection is directed to the interval between the extensor digitorum longus and the peroneus tertius tendons in order to locate the prominent lateral articular margin of the navicular bone. The forepart of the foot is inverted and plantar-flexed. A towel clip placed around the neck of the talus delivers the talus into the wound, and this facilitates deep dissection of its ligaments. The talus must be excised intact, as retained cartilage remnants from it may interfere with the proper positioning of the foot at surgery. Moreover, cartilage remnants may grow and cause late deformity and loss of correction.

Next, the forepart of the foot is derotated. After removal of the talus, the calcaneus is displaced posteriorly into the ankle mortise until the navicular bone abuts the anterior edge of the tibial plafond. The exposed articular surface of the tibial plafond should be opposite the middle articular facet of the calcaneus. Excision of the tarsal navicular may be required to obtain the necessary amount of posterior displacement of the foot. Both the deltoid and the lateral collateral ligament of the ankle require sectioning. In older patients with extreme deformity, the articular surface of one or both malleoli may require shaping or resection to obtain alignment of the calcaneus. Equinus deformity of the hind part of the foot is corrected by sectioning the Achilles tendon, allowing its proximal end to retract. In a foot with uncorrected severe equinovarus deformity, the dome of the talus may be extruded anterior to its normal relationship in the ankle mortise. In such feet the adaptive narrowing of the mortise may require release of the anterior and posterior tibiofibular ligaments of the syndesmosis to allow proper posterior positioning of the calcaneus within the ankle mortise.

When the plantigrade position of the foot is obtained, the calcaneus should be aligned with its long axis at a right angle to the bimalleolar axis of the ankle. This usually requires 20 to 30 degrees of external rotation of the foot. The calcaneus is held in its new position by two Steinmann pins introduced from the heel into the distal end of the tibia. An above-knee cast is then applied with the knee flexed to 60 degrees. The Steinmann pins are removed 6 weeks postoperatively and a below-knee weight-bearing cast is applied and worn for an additional 18 weeks. Bracing, to maintain the foot in the corrected position together with the use of well-molded night splints, should be maintained until the patient's growth is completed.

The deformity seen in a clubfoot secondary to arthrogryposis may recur after talectomy.[4,7,15] To prevent this Drummond and Cruess[4] recommend that a large incision be made through which a meticulous resection of the talus can be done without cutting into its substance. After tenotomy of the Achilles tendon, partial excision of the tendon allows good positioning of the calcaneus below the tibia. When total talectomy seems inadequate or when an earlier incomplete talectomy is being revised, the navicular bone can also be excised to achieve correction.[7] Partial excision of the calcaneus should be avoided, as this leads to a small, deformed heel. When correctly placed, the calcaneus can be held with a Kirschner wire driven from the sole of the foot into the tibia, preventing posterior drift. Although the Kirschner wire may be removed at 3 weeks, the limb should be immobilized in plaster for a minimum of 3 months.

BLAIR FUSION

The fusion described in 1943 by Blair[1] for certain fracture-dislocations of the talar neck with aseptic necrosis of the talar body has since been modified and popularized by Morris et al.[12] This procedure may be considered for a severe closed injury to the talus but is more commonly applied to open fracture-dislocations. The proximal talar body may be removed at the time of initial wound debridement. Subsequent fusion of the tibia to the distal talar fragment may be carried out once soft tissue healing has occurred.

The Blair procedure utilizes a standard anterior approach to the ankle joint. The neurovascular bundle is retracted medially, and the joint is widely exposed. The entire body of the talus is removed if this has not been done previously. Neither the talar neck nor head should be disturbed since these are usually not damaged. The talonavicular joint and the anterior and medial portions of the talocalcaneal joint should also be avoided. A 2.0 cm by 6.0 cm cortical bone graft is cut from the distal anterior portion of the tibia. No cartilage needs to be removed from the articular surface of the tibia where it contacts the superior border of talar neck or from the distal end of the sliding cortical graft.

With the ankle in 10 degrees of plantar flexion, a quadrilateral slot is created in the talar neck. This slot must be deep enough to receive 2.0 cm of the graft. The graft is then slid into place, and its proximal portion is secured to the posterior cortex of the distal end of the tibia with a screw. A Steinmann pin is placed through the plantar surface of the heel, traversing the calcaneus and extending into the tibia to provide some stability postoperatively. Bony contact must be attained between the superior border of the talar neck and the inferior border of the distal anterior tibia. Cancellous bone is packed around the tibial graft and into the remaining space between the talar neck and the tibia (Fig. 140-2).

An above-knee plaster cast is maintained for 6 weeks, after which the Steinmann pin is removed and a below-knee weight-bearing plaster cast applied.

The Blair fusion avoids shortening between the tibia and os calcis and allows a few degrees of both eversion and inversion of the forepart of the foot. Little if any pain or limp occurs in patients who undergo this procedure, and excellent function can usually be expected.

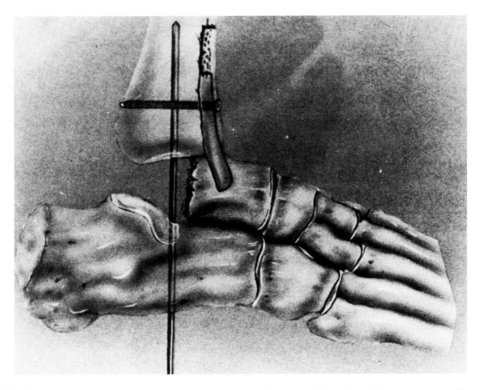

Fig. 140-2. Diagram of the Blair procedure. Following open fracture-dislocation of the talar neck with complete extrusion and necrosis of the proximal fragment, the head may be removed and the tibia fused to the remaining distal talar fragment. The clinical result is often quite good. (From Morris,[12] with permission.)

RESULTS

The results of astragalectomy depend on many factors, including the severity of the underlying disease, the nature of the foot deformity, the type of muscle imbalance, and the technical excellence of the surgical procedure and follow-up care. Cooper and Capello[3] reported on 26 talectomy patients with long-term average follow-up of 20 years. The preoperative diagnoses included 10 poliomyelitis, 6 meningocele, 4 arthrogryposis, 4 congenital clubfoot, 1 cerebral palsy, and 1 Marfan's syndrome. The average age at surgery was 10 years, and the results seemed equally good regardless of preoperative deformity—the procedure produced stable, painless plantigrade feet. These authors also found that posterior displacement of the foot did not appear to influence the result. The time of immobilization averaged 8 weeks. Their results were satisfactory in 24 of 26 patients (92 percent).

Trumble et al.[15] reported their results in nine patients with myelomeningocele (17 involved feet) who had talectomy for the correction of equinovarus deformity, with an average follow-up of 7 years 4 months. Their average age was 3 years 6 months, with a range of 1 year 9 months to 7 years 4 months, and the mean follow-up was 7 years 4 months. Fifteen feet had a good and two had a poor correction of the deformity of the hindpart of the foot, the result being directly related to the intraoperative correction of the equinovarus deformity. The correction of the deformity in the forepart of the foot was rated good in eight, fair in one, and poor in eight. Residual deformity of the forepart of the foot did compromise the functional result in six feet that had an acceptable correction of the deformity of the hind part of the foot. The authors feel that the chief cause of a compromised result is residual deformity of the forepart of the foot. They state that residual muscle imbalance must be corrected either by tenotomy or by tendon transfer prior to talectomy and that postoperative casts for 6 months and adequate bracing and night splints until the patient has reached skeletal maturity are necessary. In these patients the best age for talectomy was between 1 and 5 years.

When performed on arthrogrypotic patients with clubfoot, the result of talectomy is considered satisfactory if a stiff, deformed foot in poor weight-bearing position is corrected to a stiff plantigrade foot. Long-term follow-up studies show that feet usually remain in the plantigrade position and that gait is significantly improved.[3,5,6] Green et al.[7] reported in 1984 on 18 patients with arthrogryposis, in whom 34 feet were treated by talectomy for rigid equinovarus deformity with an average follow-up of 11 years. In 71 percent the results were considered satisfactory, and the remainder were improved. Seven feet required further operations to correct recurrence of deformity. All patients could be fitted with boots and shoes, and all patients could walk.

Drummond and Cruess[4] found lasting and permanent correction of the hindpart of the foot in their primary talectomies performed for arthrogrypotic clubfoot deformity. Failure of this procedure was the result of poor technique.

Patients who undergo total astragalectomy for local disease or severe injury sometimes have an excellent result, with little pain and a good gait, which endures for years. The loss of height in the foot, which averages ½ inch, is not a problem. However, the results in such patients remain somewhat unpredictable, with approximately half obtaining satisfactory long-term results. Patients who have had a successful Blair fusion for severe talar injury uniformly do well.

In conclusion, astragalectomy remains a surgical alternative worthy of consideration in selected patients.

REFERENCES

1. Blair HC: Comminuted fractures and fracture dislocations of the body of the astragalus: operative treatment. Am J Surg 59:37, 1943

2. Carmack JC, Hallock H: Tibiotarsal arthrodesis after astragalectomy: a report of eight cases. J Bone Joint Surg 29:476, 1947

3. Cooper RR, Capello W: Talectomy. A long term follow-up evaluation. Clin Orthop 201:32, 1985

4. Drummond DS, Cruess RL: The management of the foot and ankle in arthrogryposis multiplex congenita. J Bone Joint Surg 60B:96, 1978

5. Edmonson AS, Crenshaw AH: Campbell's Operative Orthopaedics. 6th Ed. CV Mosby, St. Louis, 1980

6. Gibson DA, Urs NDK: Arthrogryposis multiplex congenita. J Bone Joint Surg 52B:483, 1970

7. Green ADL, Fixsen JA, Lloyd-Roberts GC: Talectomy for arthrogryposis multiplex congenita. J Bone Joint Surg 66B:697, 1984

8. Hsu LCS, Jaffray D, Leong JCY: Talectomy for club foot in arthrogryposis. J Bone Joint Surg 66B:694, 1984

9. Lloyd-Roberts GC, Lettin AWF: Arthrogryposis multiplex congenita. J Bone Joint Surg 52B:494, 1970

10. Mead NG, Lithgow WC, Sweeney HJ: Arthrogryposis multiplex congenita. J Bone Joint Surg 40A:1285, 1958

11. Mindell ER, Cisek EE, Kartalian G, Dziob JM: Late results of injuries to the talus. J Bone Joint Surg 45A:221, 1963

12. Morris HD, Hand WL, Dunn AW: The modified Blair fusion for fractures of the talus. J Bone Joint Surg 53A:1289, 1971

13. Tachdjian MO: Pediatric Orthopaedics. WB Saunders, Philadelphia, 1972

14. Thompson TC: Astragalectomy and the treatment of calcaneovalgus. J Bone Joint Surg 21:627, 1939

15. Trumble T, Banta JV, Raycroft MD, Curtis BH: Talectomy for equinovarus deformity is myelodysplasia. J Bone Joint Surg 67A:21, 1985

16. Whitman AJ: The Whitman operation as applied to various types of paralytic deformities of the foot: results in the average case. Med Rec 99:304, 1921

17. Whitman AJ: Astragalectomy and backward displacement of foot: an investigation of its practical results. J Bone Joint Surg 4:266, 1922

18. Whitman AJ: Astragalectomy: ultimate result. Am J Surg 11:357, 1931

19. Whitman R: The operative treatment of paralytic talipes of the calcaneus type. Am J Med Sci 122:593, 1901

Hallux Valgus

141

Ray J. Haddad, Jr.

Hallux valgus or the less descriptive term *bunion,* is a technical classification which basically denotes the lateral deviation of the great toe and medial displacement of the first metatarsal and metatarsal head associated with changes at the metatarsophalangeal and internal cuneiform first metatarsal joint (Fig. 141-1).

Much debate can be undertaken regarding the primary and secondary causes for this deformity. Which develops first — the primus varus or the lateral deviation of the great toe? Metatarsus primus varus is probably a manifestation of splaying of the forefoot; this splaying leads to lateral deviation of the great toe at the metatarsophalangeal joint (Fig. 141-2).

NORMAL ANATOMY

In order to understand the descriptive anatomy and pathophysiology of hallux valgus, the normal anatomy of the medial metatarsophalangeal joint should be reviewed. Differing from other joints of the other toes, the metatarsophalangeal joint of the great toe contains two plantar sesamoids. The plantar surface of the first metatarsal is grooved to articulate with each sesamoid; it is separated by a small ridge and by a fibrous groove that receives the ridge of the metatarsal head (Fig. 141-3). The dense fibrous plantar pad embeds the sesamoids and anchors each to the base of the proximal phalanx. Its medial and lateral margins fix ligaments and muscles. The proximal aspect receives the flexor hallucis brevis before the sesamoid ligaments attach to the distal end of the first metatarsal. Covered with articular cartilage, the sesamoids protrude through the dorsal surface of the pads, each longitudinally and dorsally concave to fit the plantar articulating surface of the metatarsal head[13] (Fig. 141-4).

The sesamoid bones may both lie at the same level, or the lateral one may lie just proximal to the medial one. If the sesamoids are small, the flexor hallucis longus may pass in the interval between them and actually groove the metatarsal head plantarly; otherwise, the flexor hallucis longus tendon lies in the groove plantar to, but formed by, the

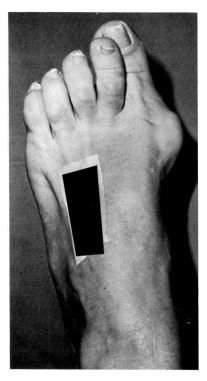

Fig. 141-1. Typical appearance of hallux valgus, demonstrating lateral deviation of the great toe and medial eminence, or bunion.

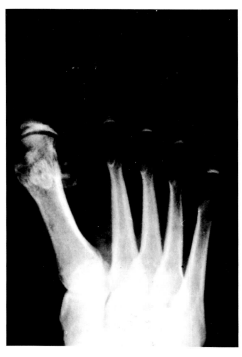

Fig. 141-2. Splaying of the forepart of the foot, which leads to lateral deviation of the great toe at the metatarsophalangeal joint.

sesamoids and the intervening fibrous tissue of the plantar pad (Fig. 141-5).

To consider the sesamoids as developing in two heads of the flexor hallucis brevis may well be erroneous; the flexor hallucis brevis inserts not only into the sesamoids, but also into some of the fibers of the abductor and adductor of the great toe, as well as into a strong band of the plantar aponeurosis. Matzen[27] regards the sesamoids as ossifications in the substance of the fibrous plantar pad.

Ligaments of the lateral and medial sesamoids and the collateral ligaments arise from the epicondyle of the metatarsal head both medially and laterally, forming the ligamentous complex at the metatarsophalangeal joint. The collateral ligaments, which are more anterior, fan out distally and plantarad to anchor into the base of the proximal phalanx. The more proximal sesamoid ligaments insert into the margin of the fibrous plantar pad and the sesamoids. The intermediate fibers unite the collat-

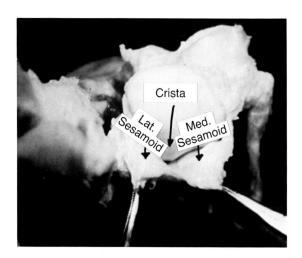

Fig. 141-3. The plantar surface of the first metatarsal is grooved to articulate with each sesamoid and is separated by a small ridge, the crista, and by fibrous grooves that receive the ridge of the metatarsal head.

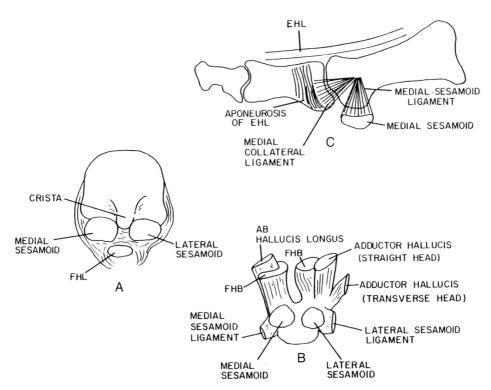

Fig. 141-4. (A) Drawing showing the relationships between the medial and lateral sesamoids, the crista, and the fibrous osseous tunnel of the flexor hallucis longus. **(B)** The tendinous and ligamentous insertions about the sesamoids of the first metatarsal head. **(C)** The medial sesamoid ligament, its relationship to the medial collateral ligament of the metatarsophalangeal joint, and the aponeurosis of the extensor hallucis longus.

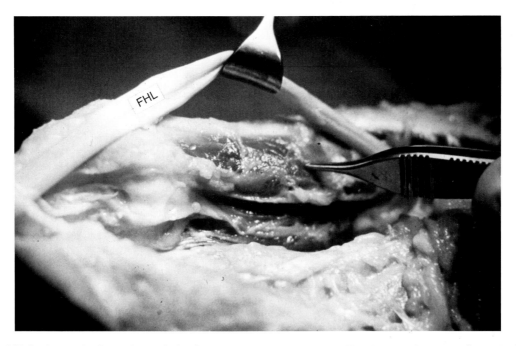

Fig. 141-5. Anatomic dissection with the flexor hallucis longus tendon *(FHL)* lying in the grove plantar to, but formed by, the sesamoids in the intervening fibrous tissue of the plantar pad.

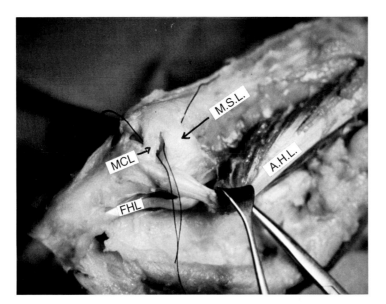

Fig. 141-6. Medial sesamoid ligament is demonstrated in its relationship to the medial collateral ligament of the metatarsophalangeal joint.

eral ligaments with the ligaments of the sesamoids. The collateral ligaments provide the metatarsophalangeal joint stability. The ligaments of the medial and lateral sesamoids hold the sesamoids in their respective grooves[12] (Figs. 141-6, 141-7).

Obviously, these ligaments of the medial and lateral sesamoid are altered in the pathologic anatomy of hallux valgus deformity.

PATHOPHYSIOLOGY

Hallux valgus is a technical classification for lateral deviation of the great toe with medial displacement of the first metatarsal. The first metatarsophalangeal joint is dislocated or subluxed laterally

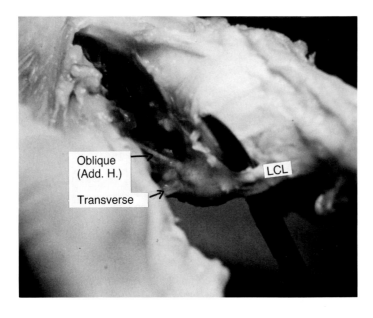

Fig. 141-7. Relationship between the adductor hallucis, oblique and transverse heads, their insertion and relationship to the lateral collateral ligament of the metatarsophalangeal joint.

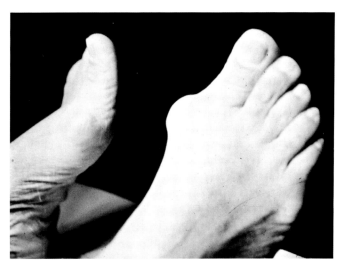

Fig. 141-8. External pressure on the medially displaced metatarsal head causes thickening over the medial capsule and a resultant bunion deformity.

and may occur in conjunction with a bunion, the painful soft tissue swelling over the medial prominence of the metatarsal head. In addition to the great toe being deviated laterally and the first metatarsal being in varus, there is often pronation of the great toe. Once displacement of the great toe occurs, other deforming factors come into play.[25]

Medial Deviation and Migration of the Metatarsal Head

As the subluxation at the metatarsophalangeal joint occurs with lateral deviation of the proximal phalanx of the great toe, medial migration occurs at the metatarsal head. This causes displacement of the metatarsal head, occasionally in conjunction with a congenitally wide metatarsal head, which is affected by external pressures (e.g., shoe pressure). This thickening over the medial capsule produces a so-called bunion (Fig. 141-8). This pressure is also associated with periosteal reaction at the metatarsal head on the medial side of the first metatarsal. As the first metatarsal head migrates medially, it assumes a dorsally displaced position, as seen occasionally with migration of the fifth metatarsal head in a splay foot. The three central metatarsal heads remain fixed at their immobile tarsometatarsal joints.

The deformities occur at the medially displaced metatarsal head. The medial articular surface of the metatarsal head is exposed to the overlying capsule and is subjected to soft tissue and extrinsic pressure, thus causing degenerative changes. Centrally, the opposing proximal phalangeal base, despite its valgus attitude, undergoes sparse articular surface degenerative changes. The so-called sagittal groove[4] (Fig. 141-9), which may be due to capsular distraction, evolves and will determine the level of osteotomy for the removal of the exostosis on the medially displaced metatarsal head.

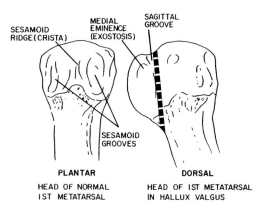

Fig. 141-9. Diagrammatic illustration of the sagittal groove and its relationship to the medial eminence.

The etiology of the sagittal groove has been discussed by several authors. Jordan and Brodsky[20] conclude that it might be due to pressure of the margins of the phalanx. Clark[4] stated that the sagittal groove evolved from the erosion of the articular cartilage and degeneration of the medial metatarsal head. Haines and McDougall[13] suggested that it was formed by degeneration of the articular cartilage and weakness of the bony trabeculae deep to the groove. This is considered an area of minimal pressure due to the lack of stimulation rather than erosion secondary to external pressure. Anatomic studies show that the sagittal groove incorporates the old groove of the medial sesamoid. Similar degenerative changes can be seen on the plantar aspect of the first metatarsal head at the crista. A degenerative state on the articular surface of the metatarsal head ensues secondary to loss of the congruent articular surfaces of the medially displaced metatarsal head and the laterally migrated medial sesamoid.

Two theories can be advanced for the development of the medial protuberance or medial eminence seen in hallux valgus on the first metatarsal head (Fig. 141-10). One is that a true exostosis is caused primarily by deviation of the great toe. As a result of lateral subluxation of the great toe, the first metatarsophalangeal joint capsule lies on the medial articulating surface of the metatarsal head. The stretch in the medial ligaments causes inflammation of the medial aspect of the metatarsal head.

By a traction phenomenon, this causes a fibrocartilaginous outgrowth that ossifies.[9] The other theory considers the eminence not to be a new growth, but a part of the metatarsal head that was originally articulated with the proximal phalanx. It suggests that the new bone, if it forms, appears on the lateral side in relation to the displaced phalanx and sesamoids. The medial prominence is therefore part of the normal head, which was originally supported proximally by the medial ligaments and distally by the proximal phalanx. After displacement of the phalanx, the medial aspect of the metatarsal head articulates only with the stretched capsule and ligaments.[13]

Pronation of the Great Toe

With lateral deviation of the great toe and varus of the first metatarsal head, pronation of the great toe often occurs. This is a further deforming force generally attributed to the dorsal displacement of the metatarsal heads. The muscle imbalance between the proximal phalangeal insertion of the abductor hallucis longus and adductor hallucis causes the pronation. Pronation of the great toe is also seen in many patients in whom pes planus or pes valgus is present, particularly in young patients in whom pronation of the first metatarsal occurs. This pronation of the great toe is also a manifestation of a pronated first metatarsal, as seen in pes valgus. Concomitant callosity on the pronated interphalangeal joint of the great toe is due to pressure from weight bearing associated with friction.

Lateral Displacement of the Sesamoids

In hallux valgus deformity, the two sesamoids sublux laterally in their relationship to the metatarsophalangeal joint. Generally, these sesamoids appear to migrate in relation to the lateral deviation of the proximal phalanx of the great toe. As a metatarsal head migrates medially, the sesamoids remain with the proximal phalanx; thus, the sesamoids are held in position laterally by the tendinous insertion of the tendons of the abductor hallucis longus and adductor hallucis, as well as by the

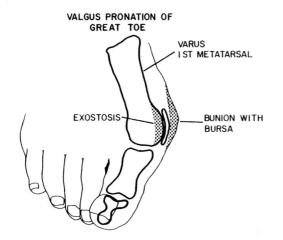

Fig. 141-10. Lateral subluxation of the great toe with resultant exostosis.

tenacious fibrous pad. Abnormal stress and weight bearing are placed on the sesamoids in their new location beneath the metatarsal head (Fig. 141-11).

The new location of the sesamoids facilitates erosion and chondromalacia secondary to incongruity of the metatarsal sesamoid joints. The amount of displacement of the fibular or lateral sesamoids may vary from mild subluxation in varus to severe displacement, so that the lateral sesamoid will lie almost between the first and second metatarsal heads. The amount of displacement must be demonstrated by radiographic views of the metatarsophalangeal joints in the sagittal plane. These sagittal radiographs must be done prior to any surgical procedure, particularly when contemplating excision of the lateral sesamoid.

Structures involved in the displacement include muscle, ligament, capsule, tendons, and bone. These changes and the relationships of the first metatarsophalangeal joint and sesamoids all differ from the normal anatomy to varying degrees. With mild hallux valgus, the major deformity is lateral deviation of the great toe and, as the severity increases, pronation of the great toe and the fibular displacement of the sesamoids occur. If the plantar fibrous pads and sesamoids become laterally displaced, the medial joint and sesamoid ligaments are stretched.[36] The groove for the lateral sesamoid remains normal but the groove for the medial sesamoid is eroded and encroaches on the bony ridge (crista) that separates the sesamoid facets. Eventually, the crista will be flattened and no resistance

will remain for lateral subluxation of the plantar pads along with the sesamoids. The ligaments of the lateral sesamoid will shorten, thus resisting replacement of the sesamoids into their original position. As the deformity becomes more severe, the lateral sesamoid will appear to turn onto the lateral surface of the metatarsal head. The medial sesamoid will shift to the flat surface of the crista, and a new intermediate groove of the long flexor of the toe will form on the metatarsal head between the sesamoids. It should be noted that the sesamoids move laterally only after destruction of the crista.

On anterior and posterior radiographs, the lateral sesamoid may be seen lying lateral to the metatarsal head and protruding into the first intermetatarsal space. When a shoe is worn, the first metatarsal is supported medially and is not displaced as far into varus, but the great toe and sesamoids are displaced more laterally. In a severely affected toe, the sesamoids are larger than normal.[13]

Tendinous Deformities

As lateral displacement of the great toe progresses, tendinous deformities and forces come into play, causing the bowstring effect of the plantar-displaced abductor hallucis longus. The dorsal extensor aponeurosis of the extensor hallucis longus becomes attenuated and migrates laterally with loosening of the medial capsule structure, and the extensor hallucis longus is displaced laterally. The flexor hallucis longus, along with the displaced

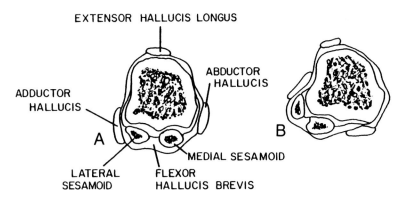

Fig. 141-11. (A) Normal relationship of the medial and lateral sesamoids to the peritendinous structures. **(B)** Lateral shift of the sesamoids and the concomitant shift of the peritendinous structures.

sesamoids, is then bowstrung to a more lateral position.

The binding mechanism of the metatarsal heads cannot be discussed without mention of the long extensor tendon's medial fibers, or medial hood ligaments. These square–shaped fibers attach the extensor hallucis longus to the plantar fibrous bed, proximal phalanx, periosteum, and the fibrous tunnel to the flexor hallucis longus. On the dorsum of the proximal phalanx, the medial hood ligaments cover the insertion of the extensor hallucis brevis but pass deep to the conjoined tendon (the abductor hallucis longus and the medial head of the flexor hallucis brevis) and the plantar aponeurosis to insert into the proximal phalanx. All the above-mentioned structures blend together medial to the metatarsophalangeal joint. They attach to the proximal phalanx and not to the metatarsal.[12] When the great toe is adducted, it carries with it all these attachments and exposes the medial metatarsal articular surface. The collateral ligaments and ligament of the medial sesamoid are the only structures that originate from the metatarsal.

During the 1930s, Lapidus[24] and McMurray[31] popularized the theory that when the metatarsals are spread, the transverse ligaments are stretched. However, Haines and McDougall[13] later demonstrated quite the contrary: as the first metatarsal head moves medially, the deep transverse ligaments remain intact, as does the fibrous plantar pad with its sesamoid. What attenuates is the ligament of the medial sesamoid. Thus, upon radiographic evaluation, the sesamoids look as if they are moving laterally when, in fact, they remain embedded in the fibrous pad and are held snugly in place laterally by the deep transverse ligament.[13] The same type of attenuation at the fifth metatarsal (the lateral ligament of the fifth pad) would constitute the pathology of the splay foot.

In the normal foot, the flexor hallucis longus and the extensor hallucis longus and brevis are placed such that, in addition to their main function of flexion-extension, they also adduct the great toe toward the second toe. Thus, this adductive force becomes greater as the ligament of the medial sesamoid stretches. The medial ligament of the extensor hood is attenuated, displacing the extensor apparatus laterally. The abductor hallucis moves to a plantar relationship as the metatarsal head dis-

places medially, thereby losing the direction of pull necessary to abduct. The long flexor that is embedded plantar and slightly between the two sesamoids is effectively lateral to the medially displaced metatarsophalangeal joint, providing a valgus force to the great toe. The two heads of the flexor hallucis brevis have a similar relationship, adding to the valgus deformity.

Metatarsus Primus Varus

A frequent association of hallux valgus is that of metatarsus primus varus.[24] The hallux of the human embryo has simian features that are lost with growth. Varus of the first metatarsal (as measured by the angle of the long axis of the first and second metatarsals) is more marked in the fetus at eight weeks (32 degrees) but decreases to 6 to 10 degrees in the normal adult foot[37] (Fig. 141-12). Varus deviation can be associated with obliquity of the articular surface of the first cuneiform or obliquity of the base of the first metatarsal, as one sees in

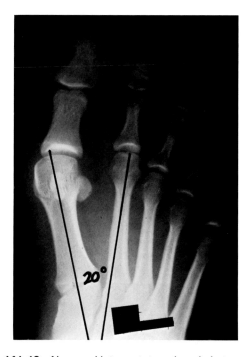

Fig. 141-12. Abnormal intermetatarsal angle between the first and second metatarsal heads in metatarsus primus varus.

Blount's disease of the tibia.[24] The normal cuneiformfirst metatarsal joint is set transversely and occasionally obliquely, without hallux valgus.[33]

In summary, the pathologic anatomy of hallux valgus involves many structures, making the term *simple bunion* a gross simplification. The essential pathology rests with the ligaments of the medial sesamoid and the base of the proximal phalanx, with gradual disintegration of the bony ridge (crista) that separates the sesamoid groove, thus leaving no resistance to medial splaying of the first metatarsal. The deep transverse metatarsal ligaments remain intact, holding the position of the two great toe sesamoids. The medial eminence probably is a combination of preexisting bone, as well as exostosis.

ETIOLOGY

Shoes

Many factors predispose to hallux valgus; certainly, there is a higher incidence in people who wear shoes than those who do not.[10] Most statistical data show a higher frequency in females because footwear with higher heels and more pointed toes forces the toes toward the midline.[1,19] Higher heels also add to adduction and equinus, which further accentuate the valgus of the great toe and varus of the lesser toes, particularly in a splay foot (Fig. 141-13).

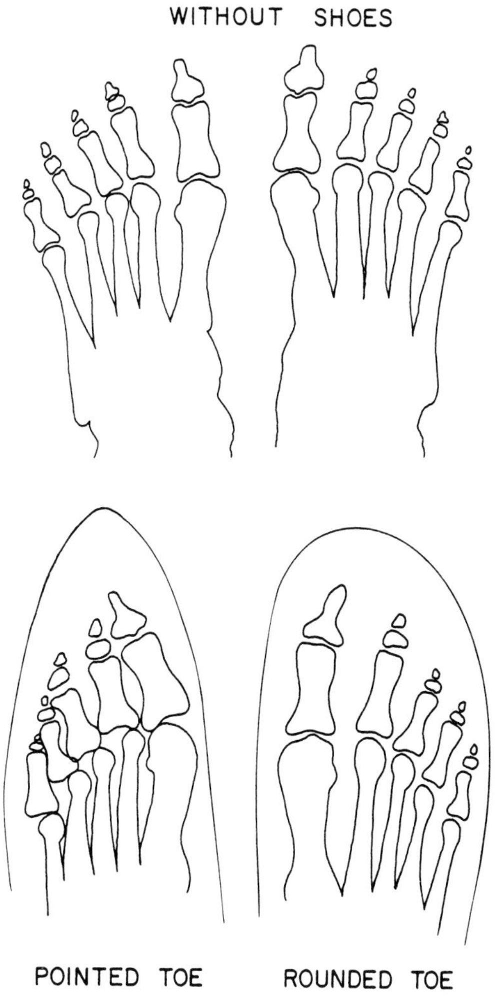

Metatarsus Varus

Metatarsus primus varus with a short first metatarsal, which may well be hypermobile, often predisposes to lateral deviation of the great toe.[1,7,8,10,14,34] This also may be a congenital variant, as is more commonly seen in association with adolescent hallux valgus. Many investigators dispute this fact, but others associate the syndrome with a short, hypermobile first metatarsal with hallux valgus. First and second metatarsal lengths, in my opinion, are instrumental in determining the

WITHOUT SHOES

POINTED TOE   ROUNDED TOE

Fig. 141-13. The phenomenon that occurs at the metatarsophalangeal joint with and without shoes, and the difference between pointed and roundtoed shoes.

type of correction of the primus metatarsus varus. The short first metatarsal should be lengthened by opening wedge and bone grafting. The long first metatarsal should be shortened by a closing laterally based wedge.

Pes Planus and Pes Valgus

In the pronated valgus foot, pronation of the first metatarsal forces the first metatarsal head into a more plantarward position, causing the sesamoids to migrate laterally through the sesamoid ligaments.[8,10] Shifting the great toe laterally at the metatarsal joint can cause more pressure in the hallux, increasing the valgus deformity. With the cuneiform-metatarsal joint in pronation and valgus, the obliquity of the plane of this joint increases, making it less resistive to forces such as weight bearing, and to extrinsic pressure, such as that caused by shoes.

SURGICAL TREATMENT

The bunion deformity is the principal problem of the forefoot. Many surgical procedures have been described for hallux valgus. Kelikian listed at least 80 references to various types of metatarsal osteotomies and soft tissue procedures for correction, with 75 percent of these being modifications of basic operations.[21,22.] Several of the most frequently used procedures are described. With each, successful hallux valgus surgery depends on preoperative planning, meticulous technique, and meticulous dissection.

Preoperative Evaluation

Consideration of any surgery for hallux valgus must take into account the patient as a whole. All bony operations and plastic procedures must conform with the patient's age, circulatory status, and goal expectation and should be included in patient selection. For example, in a patient with metatarsalgia and hallux valgus, it must be considered that the metatarsalgia may not be related to the hallux valgus deformity and may even be made worse as a result of a surgical procedure. The cause(s) of concomitant metatarsalgia must be considered before any bunion operation is undertaken.

Many surgical procedures are available to correct hallux valgus and proper selection will help obtain a satisfactory result and correction. In selecting the best procedure, one must always study weight-bearing radiographs done in the anteroposterior and lateral views, and if any symptoms suggest a problem of the forefoot, multiple views should be performed.

In evaluating the radiographs, the length of the first metatarsal is of the utmost importance in its relationship to the second metatarsal length. The hallux valgus angle, the metatarsus primus varus angle, the degree of splaying of the forefoot, the shape of the first metatarsophalangeal joint, and the presence of degenerative changes in the first metatarsophalangeal joint and the interphalangeal joint of the great and small toes must be considered. Concomitant associated disease, such as rheumatoid arthritis, may affect selection of the surgical procedure.

Surgery should never be done on a patient who has evidence of peripheral vascular disease; a decrease in pulses, abnormal Doppler studies, and calcification in the area of the small arteries about the foot and ankle are all contraindications to surgery.

In younger patients (under 50 years of age) with good circulation, most plastic procedures and bony correctional operations can be done without any significant problem. In elderly patients, surgery is almost never indicated. Each patient must be assessed as an individual. Generally, in the patient with diabetes or other diseases which affect the peripheral blood supply and/or the peripheral nerves, surgery must be undertaken with great caution. With this in mind, the following surgical procedures will be discussed.

McBride Procedure

This procedure, described by McBride[28] in 1928, is based on the soft tissue procedures as described by Silver[35] in 1923. One of Silver's procedures describes resection of the medial eminence, release of the adductor tendon and lateral capsule, and a tightening capsulorrhaphy of the medial capsule of the first metatarsophalangeal joint. McBride modified this procedure by combining it with excision of the lateral sesamoid and reattaching the adductor tendon to the head of the first metatarsal in an attempt to correct the metatarsus varus deformity[29,30] (Fig. 141-14).

The indications for the McBride procedure are:

1. A young patient who has a congruous metatarsophalangeal joint and who does not have signif-

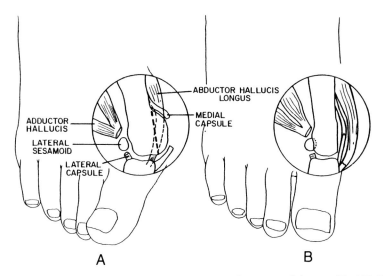

Fig. 141-14. **(A)** Exostosis and **(B)** subsequent tendinous realignment of the modified McBride procedure.

icant metatarsus primus varus or marked lateral migration of the sesamoid (Fig. 141-15).
2. The more moderate valgus deformities
3. Patients seeking relief from joint pain
4. Patients who want to alter their type of footwear by creating a narrow forefoot

The McBride procedure is made more complicated because it depends on the tendon and capsule to rebalance the foot and, as has been reported in the past, overcorrection may lead to a varus deformity; undercorrection will lead to recurrence of valgus deformity.

Author's Preferred Technique

A medial incision is made over the metatarsophalangeal joint. The tendon of the abductor hallucis longus is dissected and detached from its insertion into the volar base of the proximal phalanx. The medial capsule and bursa over the eminence of the metatarsal head are opened in a V-Y incision, with the V-flap left attached distally to the proximal phalanx (Fig. 141-16). Usually, a separate skin incision is made between the first and second metatarsal heads (Fig. 141-17). The dissection can then be carried down easily to the conjoined tendon of the adductor. The tendon is tenotomized; it is not reattached to the metatarsal head, as we have found that this attachment really does not give any

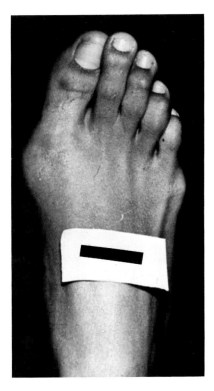

Fig. 141-15. Hallux valgus deformity prior to McBride procedure in a young patient.

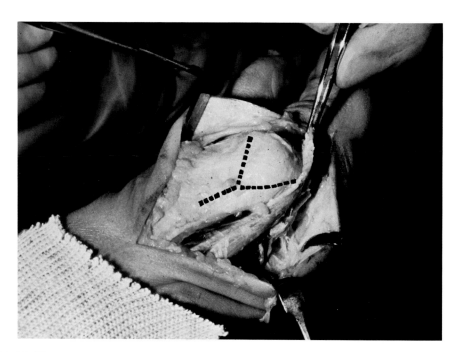

Fig. 141-16. The VY incision in the medial capsule and bursa over the eminence of the metatarsal head.

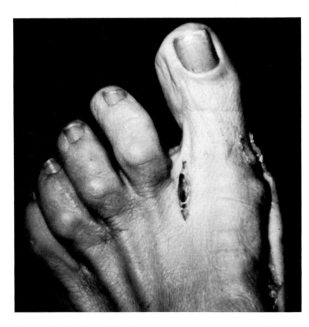

Fig. 141-17. Medial incision over the metatarsophalangeal joint and the secondary incision in the web between the great and second toes for lateral capsule release and adductor tenotomy.

additional correction to the valgus position of the metatarsal head and shaft. The adductor will reattach itself. Excision of the lateral sesamoid is not done unless there is marked migration of the lateral sesamoid between the first and second metatarsal heads, or there is actually a bony ankylosis of the displaced sesamoid to the first metatarsal head, as is occasionally seen in rheumatoid patients with severe deformity.

When the tenotomy of the adductor is completed, the lateral capsule is also tenotomized. The medial eminence is then osteotomized along the line of the sagittal groove. Following osteotomy of the medial eminence, bone wax has been found to decrease the amount of bleeding from the osteotomized metatarsal head and also will prevent calcification.

The great toe is then placed into the corrected position (Fig. 141-18). Further correction is carried out by imbricating the medial capsule. The abductor hallucis is then resutured to the base of the proximal phalanx to further hold the toe straight. It is important that the toe be placed in a degree of extension, not flexion (Figs. 141-19,

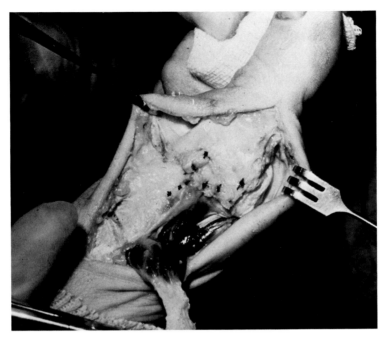

Fig. 14-18. Closure of the medial capsule and bursa over the first metatarsal head, further correcting the hallux valgus.

141-20). Postoperatively, the patient is treated with soft tissue dressings, which are first changed at least four to five days after surgery. It is very important that dressings be changed weekly thereafter, in an attempt to maintain the correction while soft tissue healing occurs. The patient may walk in a cast-shoe as soon as tolerated. If too much

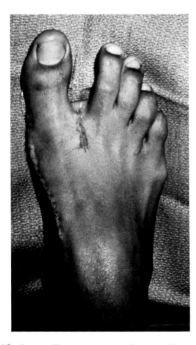

Fig. 141-19. Immediate postoperative position of the great toe after the modified McBride procedure.

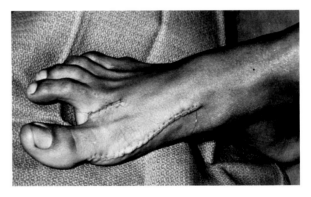

Fig. 141-20. Lateral view of the great toe after the modified McBride procedure. Note that the toe is placed in extension.

varus is present, this can be corrected with soft tissue dressings. If too much valgus of the great toe persists, this can also be corrected with soft tissue dressings during the immediate postoperative period (Fig. 141-21). Generally, the dressings can be removed at three weeks, at which time the patient is started on motion and can be protected with a toe spreader between the great and second toes (Fig. 141-22). This protective pad should be worn full time for 3 weeks, then used at night for an additional 6 weeks.

Keller Procedure

It is believed that the Keller procedure is basically indicated in older patients, particularly those with an associated hallux rigidus (Figs. 141-23, 141-24). It is effective in correcting severe valgus deformity but frequently results in a foreshortened great toe (occasionally flail), which leads to poor great toe function and toe-off in weight bearing, particularly if the great toe drifts into extension.

The Keller procedure, however, is an excellent salvage procedure, one that can be tolerated in the older patient. It is a less tedious operation and has less morbidity than other bunion procedures.

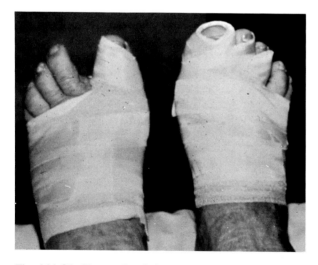

Fig. 141-21. Types of soft dressings that can be used immediately postoperatively to correct varus (left) or valgus (right) deformity of the great toe after the modified McBride procedure.

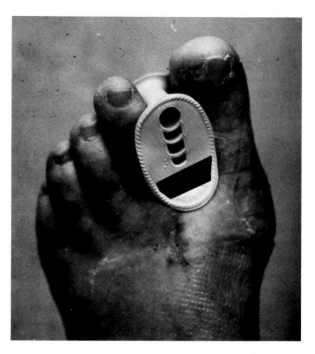

Fig. 141-22. Commercial toe spreader used postoperatively.

Author's Preferred Technique

In the classic Keller procedure,[23] the first metatarsophalangeal joint is exposed by a medial incision through a medial approach. It is important that the incision in the medial capsule be made in a linear manner — *not* in a V-Y incision, which would leave a distally based flap unattached once the base of the proximal phalanx is excised (Fig. 141-25). After excision of the medial eminence along the sagittal groove, the proximal one-third of the proximal phalanx is resected (Fig. 141-26). The lateral capsule is sutured into the remaining medial capsule in an attempt to interpose capsule between the metatarsal head and the remaining proximal phalanx; however, I have found this procedure generally not to be indicated. If one wishes to form an interposition, the method described by Kelikian, in which he uses a flap of the adductor longus tendon sutured over the head of the first metatarsal to the tendon of the adductor, is preferable to the capsular interposition; however, the great toe can be balanced extremely well simply with imbrication of the medial capsular structure if it has been excised

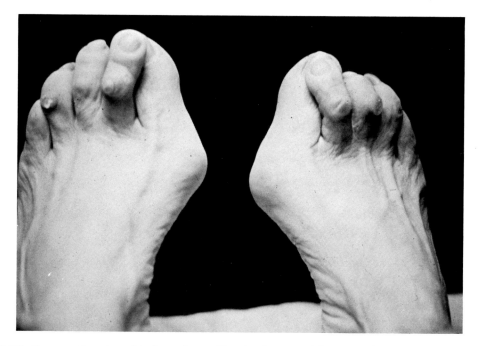

Fig. 141-23. Preoperative view of hallux valgus with splay feet overriding second toes, and degenerative joint disease of the metatarsophalangeal joints.

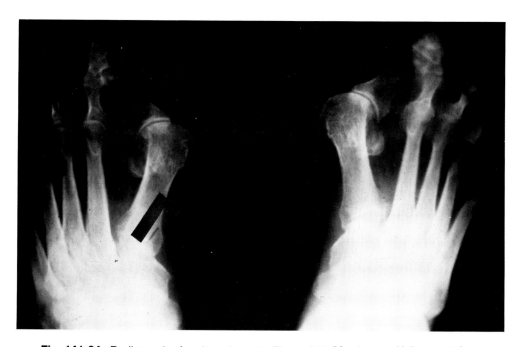

Fig. 141-24. Radiograph of patient shown in Figure 141-23 prior to a Keller procedure.

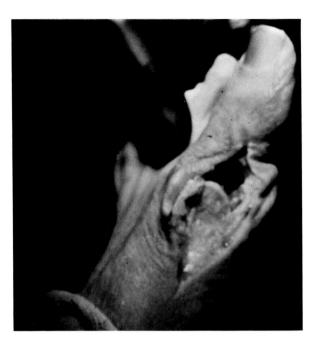

Fig. 141-25. Opening of the medial capsule of the metatarsophalangeal joint and partial resection of the proximal phalanx of the great toe and excision of the medial eminence.

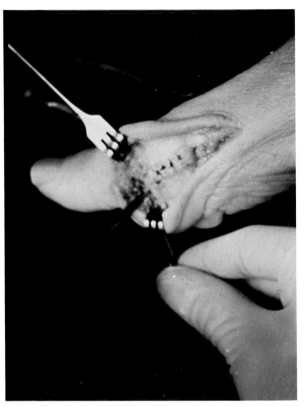

Fig. 141-26. Linear closure of the capsule in the Keller procedure after medial tenorrhaphy.

in a linear manner. The great toe is then pinned with an intramedullary smooth Steinmann pin that exits through the tip of the great toe (Figs. 141-27 to 141-30). In a patient with hallux rigidus and/or marked degenerative arthritis with an incongruity at the metatarsophalangeal joint and a significant metatarsus primus varus, an opening- or closing-wedge osteotomy (depending on the lengths of the metatarsals) can be done at the base of the metatarsals to correct the valgus; the same intramedullary pin can then be driven across this osteotomy site (Figs. 141-31, 141-32). The intramedullary pin can be removed 3 weeks postoperatively without osteotomy and in a period of 4 to 6 weeks with osteotomy of the proximal metatarsal.

Mitchell Osteotomy

The Mitchell procedure involves an osteotomy of the distal metatarsal shaft. Varus of the toe is corrected at the level of the osteotomy.[16,33] The details of this operation must be carefully adhered

to, since this is basically an extracapsular osteotomy. The lateral capsular attachments of the first metatarsal head must not be sectioned, or the blood supply to the metatarsal head will be in jeopardy. Adequate correction of the metatarsus primus varus is dependent on sufficient lateral displacement of the metatarsal head and slight medial angulation of the fragments at the site of the osteotomy. Plantar angulation of the distal fragment must be avoided to prevent first metatarsal head metatarsalgia.

Indications for this procedure include the younger patient with a congruent joint and an angle of more than 10 degrees between the first and second metatarsals, as demonstrated on weight-bearing radiographs. Mitchell considered it better to correct the metatarsus primus varus close to its point of origin. He found the distal osteotomy to be a simple and sure method of correcting the metatarsus primus varus at the metatarsopha-

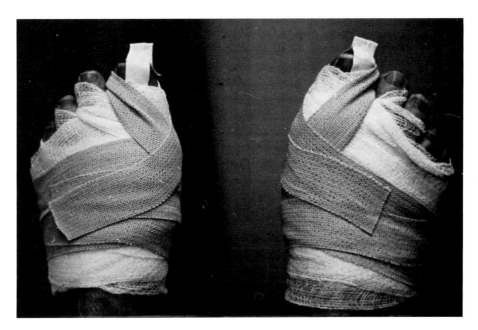

Fig. 141-27. Immediate postoperative dressings for the Keller procedure, with pins extruding through the tips of the great toes.

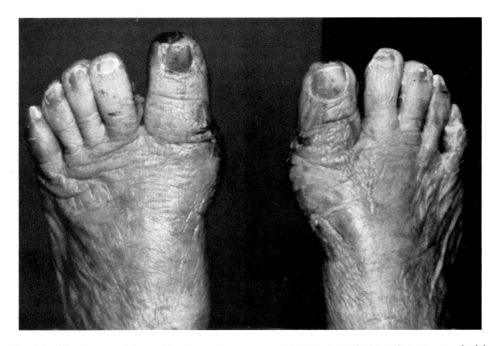

Fig. 141-28. The great toes after the Keller procedure (approximately 1 week postoperatively).

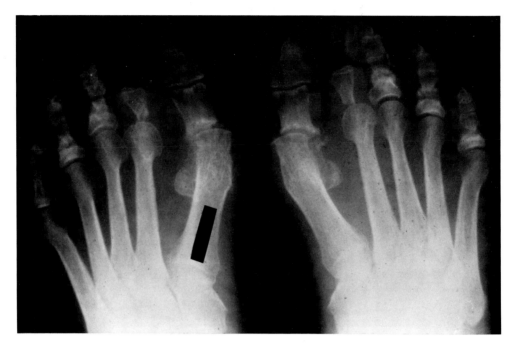

Fig. 141-29. Radiographic result of the Keller procedure 1 year postoperatively.

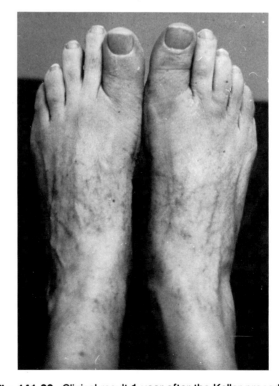

Fig. 141-30. Clinical result 1 year after the Keller procedure.

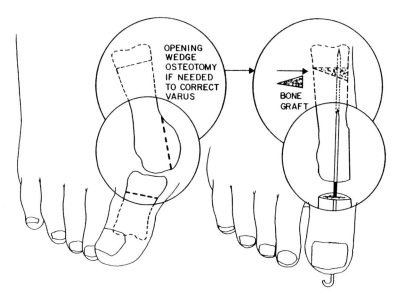

Fig. 141-31. Keller procedure for marked metatarsus varus. Varus can be corrected by an opening or closing basal wedge. The metatarsal is internally fixed with the same intermedullary pin that is used for great toe fixation.

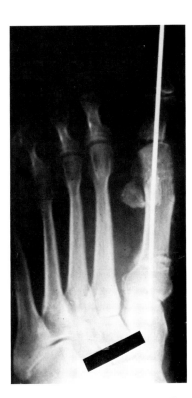

Fig. 141-32. Postoperative radiograph illustrating the Keller procedure combined with an opening-wedge corrective osteotomy for metatarsus varus.

langeal joint. The slight shortening that recurs as a result of a resection osteotomy allows relaxation of the lateral capsule and adductor hallucis muscles so that lateral release of the metatarsophalangeal joint is usually not required. A significant narrowing of the foot is obtained by a combination of exostectomy and lateral shifting of the metatarsal head. This narrowing will often allow the patient to wear high-heeled shoes. It is felt that the results of this operation are somewhat superior cosmetically and functionally even to a good result from the Keller operation or other excision arthroplasties (Figs. 141-33 to 141-36).

Author's Preferred Technique

A dorsomedial incision is made over the metatarsophalangeal joint. A V-Y incision is made through the medial capsule down to the medial eminence. The neck and shaft of the metatarsal are then stripped subperiosteally. One of the complications with this type of distal osteotomy is avascular necrosis of the first metatarsal head. This can occur because lateral capsular attachments are not released, and these are the structures that will provide blood to the metatarsal heads. In performing this procedure, one must be aware of the impor-

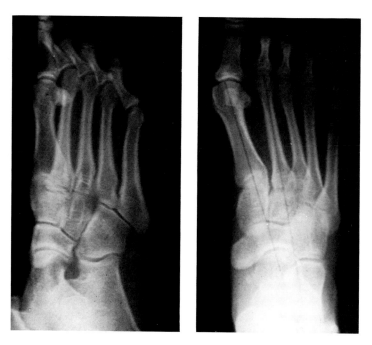

Fig. 141-33. Radiograph prior to the Mitchell procedure.

tance of not disturbing the insertion of the adductor tendon or lateral capsule of the metatarsophalangeal joint. Kelikian[21] emphasized that stripping of the medial and lateral capsules should not be combined with removal of the exostosis, release of the adductor tendon, and osteotomy of the meta-tarsal head from the shaft, since this combination of procedures will destroy the blood supply to the head.

After the V-Y incision has been made in the medial capsule, an osteotomy is then carried out along the sagittal groove of the medial eminence and the

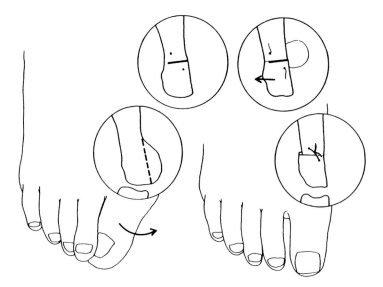

Fig. 141-34. Distal osteotomy of the first metatarsal head as described by Mitchell.

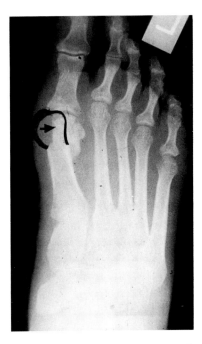 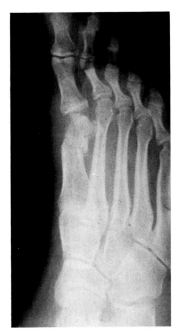

Fig. 141-35. Anteroposterior and oblique views of results of the Mitchell procedure 1 year after surgery.

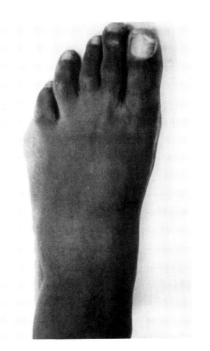

Fig. 141-36. Standing view of the results of the Mitchell procedure 1 year after surgery.

exostosis is removed flush with the shaft of the metatarsal. Two drill holes are then placed, one ⅓ inch and the other 1 inch from the articular surface. The distal drill hole is slightly medial so that the holes will be in line when the lateral shift of the head is accomplished. Care is taken to place these drill holes perpendicular to the metatarsal shaft. A #1 chromic catgut suture is then placed through the holes by means of a ligature carrier or straight needle.

A double incomplete osteotomy is then done ¾ inch from the articular surface between the drill holes and perpendicular to the shaft. The thickness of the bone between the two cuts depends on the amount of shortening of the metatarsal that will be necessary to relax the contracted lateral structures. Usually, about ⅛ inch of bone is removed. The size of the lateral spur depends on the amount of metatarsus primus varus to be neutralized by the lateral shift of the metatarsal head. Generally, ⅙ of the width of the shaft is left to form the lateral spur. The osteotomy is completed proximally with a thin saw blade.

The metatarsal head is then shifted laterally until the lateral spur locks over the proximal shaft. The head is angulated slightly lateral so that its articular surface parallels the axis of the second metatarsal head. Slight plantar displacement or angulation is desired to prevent first metatarsal head metatarsalgia. The suture is then tied, giving stability to the osteotomy site.

Tightening medial capsule imbrication and capsulorrhaphy are then carried out with the hallux held in slight overcorrection. After this capsulorrhaphy is completed, the wounds are closed in a routine manner and a pressure dressing is applied. Mitchell recommends that splints of padded tongue depressors be applied with the toe in slight overcorrection and 5 degrees of plantar flexion to avoid dorsal displacement or angulation at the osteotomy site. This splint is worn for 10 days. Following suture removal, a below-knee cast is applied to the leg, incorporating the great toe. Again, care is taken not to displace or angulate the osteotomy site dorsally.

Complications

Technical failures that may occur with this operation are as follows:

1. If the osteotomy is done too far proximally and is done more in the compact bone than the cancellous bone, the fragments will take longer to heal and will be more difficult to maintain in the desired position.
2. Displacement of the osteotomy may occur if the sutures break because of rough handling or incorrect application of the splint or cast. An unstable osteotomy will result because of loose suturing or overlapping of the drill holes with the osteotomy site.
3. Incomplete correction of the metatarsus primus varus may occur due to failure to laterally angulate the head of the metatarsal. The head of the first metatarsal must be lined up with the second metatarsal so that the metatarsus primus varus is corrected at the metatarsophalangeal joint.
4. Dorsal angulation and displacement of the metatarsal head may occur, causing metatarsalgia from increased weight on the second metatarsal head.
5. Avascular necrosis of the metatarsal head may occur as a result of stripping of the lateral capsule and adductor tendon.

Chevron Osteotomy*

The chevron osteotomy, first described by Corless[6] in 1976, is an osteotomy of the distal first metatarsal used for the correction of valgus deformity of the great toe and alleviation of discomfort due to a prominent medial eminence. The chevron osteotomy is recommended for the patient with an intermetatarsal of 1 to 2 angles of less than 15 degrees and a metatarsophalangeal of 1 angle of less than 30 degrees on anteroposterior standing radiographs of the feet. According to Meier and Kenzora,[32] patients of all ages are suitable candidates for this procedure, as they found similar subjective results in patients both under and over 40 years of age. This was not the finding of Hattrup and Johnson,[15] however, who reported a marked decrease in patient satisfaction for patients more than 50 years of age. Adolescents with hallux valgus deformity are also appropriate candidates for the chevron osteotomy.

Patients with advanced degenerative changes in the first metatarsophalangeal joint or reduced first metatarsophalangeal motion should not be considered for this procedure.

Treatment Options

The operative procedure chosen should be tailored to the severity of the deformity and the patient's needs. Distal metatarsal osteotomies are most effective when the deformity is mild. When the intermetatarsal angle exceeds 15 degrees and there is a passively correctable hallux valgus deformity, a proximal crescentic first metatarsal osteotomy with a distal soft tissue resection and realignment (modified McBride) is a good way of achieving correction. Fixed valgus deformity of the hallux with pronounced lateral subluxation of the proximal phalanx probably cannot be corrected by a metatarsal osteotomy, and first metatarsophalangeal arthrodesis or a Keller resection arthroplasty should be considered. Of these latter two options, the arthrodesis, which retains the weight-bearing function of the great toe and is not subject to recur-

---

* This section was prepared by Dr. Ian J. Alexander and Dr. Kenneth A. Johnson.

rent angulation or other displacement of the hallux, probably is preferable, except in the most sedentary patients.

Multiple distal metatarsal osteotomies have been described. The most widely used of these are the chevron, Mitchell, Wilson, and biplanar osteotomies.[17] Each of these procedures has certain advantages and disadvantages. The major advantages of the chevron osteotomy include relatively simple surgical technique with a minimum of soft tissue dissection, excellent stability, usually without the need for internal fixation, and minimal shortening. The major disadvantage, compared with the other distal osteotomies, is the more limited correction possible with this technique.

Authors' Preferred Technique

The chevron procedure for hallux valgus deformity involves resection of the medial eminence, lateral displacement of the metatarsal head by osteotomy, and tightening of the medial capsular structures.[18]

A dorsomedial incision provides access to the medial capsular area of the first metatarsophalangeal joint. The medial capsule is incised longitudinally at a level plantarad from the skin incision, and an ellipse of capsule is removed. The medial prominence is removed by the use of a microsagittal saw (Fig. 141-37A). Care is taken to keep the cut medial to a sagittal groove and to make the cut parallel

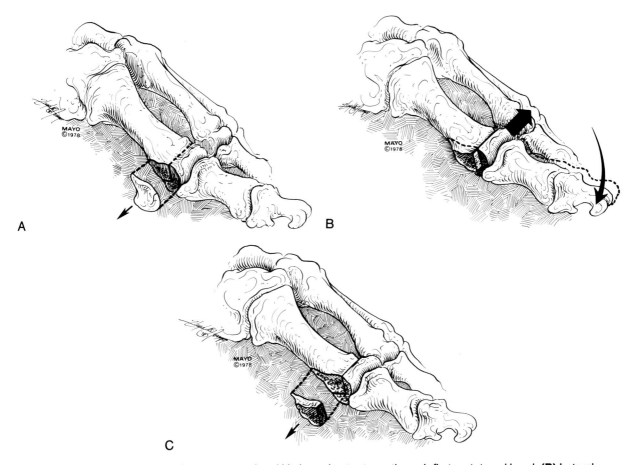

Fig. 141-37. (A) Medial eminence removal and V-shaped osteotomy through first metatarsal head. **(B)** Lateral displacement of first metatarsal head. **(C)** Removal of the protruding first metatarsal shaft parallel to medial border of foot. (From Johnson et al.[19] By permission of Mayo Foundation.)

to the medial border of the foot, not the shaft of the first metatarsal joint. Only the medial third of the capsule around the metatarsal head is elevated, so as to preserve the blood supply to the head; the retained blood supply to the head after osteotomy enters through the lateral capsular attachments. The transverse V-osteotomy in the metatarsal head is made using the microsagittal saw with a narrow sharp blade. The blade is 5 mm wide and has an in-line tooth configuration. The osteotomy is placed such that maximal width of the metatarsal head is available for displacement and stability. The distal apex of the osteotomy is approximately 3 to 5 mm from the subchondral bone of the metatarsal head, and the acute angle formed by the V is approximately 50 degrees. The metatarsal head is laterally displaced by grasping the distal metatarsal shaft with a towel clip and applying thumb pressure over the metatarsal head. The head is moved approximately 4 mm laterally (Fig. 141-37B). The medial projection of the metatarsal shaft is then resected (Fig. 141-37C); again, the cut remains parallel to the medial border of the foot. If there is a question about stability, a single smooth Kirschner wire is used to prevent potential displacement. The wire is removed 3 to 4 weeks after operation. Special attention is given to provide a tight capsular closure by holding the great toe in an overcorrected position. When released, the toe should assume a position of about 10 degrees of valgus angulation.

A plaster-reinforced soft compressive dressing is used to splint the great toe in the corrected position; 2 to 3 days after the operation, a below-knee weight-bearing cast is applied. Three weeks after surgery, the cast is removed, and the patient is instructed to use a postoperative shoe until a conventional shoe can be worn comfortably. Key technical points in the procedure are to avoid excessive (1) medial eminence resection, (2) soft tissue stripping from the metatarsal head, and (3) lateral displacement of the metatarsal head.

Complications

Most complications of chevron osteotomy can be avoided by careful patient selection and adherence to correct surgical technique. The most frequently documented postoperative problems are persist-

ent valgus deformity (due to either inadequate initial correction or gradual recurrence of the deformity),[15] displacement of the metatarsal head,[15] and injury to the dorsomedial digital nerve of the hallux.[32] Avascular necrosis of the metatarsal head has been described, but the incidence is extremely low if soft tissue mobilization from the metatarsal head is minimized. A lateral soft tissue release should not be used in conjunction with any type of distal metatarsal osteotomy because of the high risk of devascularizing the metatarsal head.[32] The practice of combined distal metatarsal and proximal phalangeal osteotomy also is not recommended. Other described but less frequent complications of the procedure are included in Table 141-1.

Results

In most series, overall patient satisfaction with the chevron osteotomy has been good, ranging between 80 percent and 90 percent. Persistent or recurrent deformity, with or without pain, is the most common reason for failure. Objective correction of both the angle between the first and second metatarsal and the metatarsophalangeal angle of the first toe is variably reported and depends somewhat on the method of measurement employed. An early series of patients treated at the Mayo Clinic showed an average correction of 5 degrees in the intermetatarsal angle between the first and second toe and an average correction of 12 degrees in the metatarsophalangeal angle of the first toe.[19] Although this degree of correction has not been achieved in all published series, the patient satisfaction rate is consistently between 80 percent and 90 percent.[32]

Table 141-1. Reported Complications of First Metatarsal Chevron Osteotomy

Recurrent hallux valgus
Neuromas of dorsal medial and plantar medial digital nerves
Displacement of distal metatarsal fragment
Avascular necrosis
Joint stiffness
Shortening
Hallux varus
Malunion
Fracture of metatarsal head at apex of osteotomy
Septic arthritis
Superficial wound infection
Marginal skin necrosis
Reflex sympathetic dystrophy

Chevron osteotomy of the distal first metatarsal is a relatively simple procedure that can effectively realign the hallux and eliminate a painful medial prominence in patients with mild metatarsus primus varus and no degenerative changes in the metatarsophalangeal joint. The stable configuration of the osteotomy permits early ambulation, reducing patient morbidity. With proper patient selection and adherence to the described surgical technique, excellent patient satisfaction can be achieved with a minimal complication rate.

Metatarsal Osteotomy°

The hallux valgus deformity consists of a soft tissue component and an osseous component. The soft tissue component results from the proximal phalanx drifting laterally on the metatarsal head, which results in a contracture of the tissues on the lateral side of the metatarsophalangeal joint and an elongation of the soft tissues on the medial aspect. In order to correct the hallux valgus deformity, the soft tissues on the lateral aspect need to be released and those on the medial aspect need to be plicated. Once this is accomplished, the first metatarsophalangeal joint can be realigned in relation to the long axis of the metatarsal, providing the distal articular surface of the metarsal is perpendicular or nearly so to the long axis of the metatarsal. If the articular surface of the metatarsal head slopes laterally, then more than a simple soft tissue procedure is needed in order to realign the metatarsophalangeal joint. The treatment of this latter type of hallux valgus problem has been covered elsewhere in this section.

The following discussion regarding the use of a metatarsal osteotomy is predicated on the fact that the articular surface of the metatarsal head is perpendicular to the long axis of the metatarsal. Once the metatarsophalangeal joint has been realigned to form a congruent joint, the soft tissue portion of the procedure is completed. The next decision that needs to be made is whether the first metatarsal can be realigned to the second metatarsal. The upper limit of the intermetatarsal angle is about 9 de-

grees, and if a soft tissue type of repair about the first metatarsophalangeal joint is to succeed, the intermetatarsal angle must be corrected. The correction of the intermetatarsal angle after a soft tissue repair is dependent on the mobility at the tarsometatarsal joint. Obviously, if there is to be any correction of the intermetatarsal angle without an osteotomy, it has to occur at that joint. In a study of 100 patients who underwent a soft tissue repair of their hallux valgus deformity, using a DuVries modification of the McBride procedure, the average correction of the intermetatarsal angle was 5.2 degrees.[26] Those patients whose intermetatarsal angle failed to correct usually had a recurrence of their deformity of a varying degree. The recurrence of the hallux valgus in these patients results from the fact that a soft tissue procedure, namely the repair of the hallux valgus deformity, will not be successful if there is a fixed bony deformity present, that is, a fixed metatarsus primus varus. As the proximal phalanx moves lateralward (i.e., subluxes) on the metatarsal head, the intermetatarsal angle increases. Therefore, once the lateral soft tissue contractures are released the first metatarsal can then move back into better alignment. The degree of the correction is dependent on the mobility of the tarsometatarsal joint. If, however, a fixed bony deformity is present such that there is little or no correction at the metatarsocuneiform joint or there is increased medial deviation of the articular surface of the first metatarsocuneiform joint, creating a metatarsus primus varus, some type of osteotomy needs to be carried out in order to realign the first and second metatarsals. Once this is achieved, a satisfactory long-term result should occur. If, however, the bony deformity is not corrected, the hallux valgus deformity will usually recur, since the same anatomic alignment of the first and second metatarsals is still present after the operation as was present prior to the operation.

Many types of metatarsal osteotomies have been advocated in the past. Careful examination of the principles involved when performing an osteotomy of the first metatarsal brings into question the wisdom of some of these methods.

The ideal metatarsal osteotomy should be stable and relatively easy to complete and stabilize and should not produce shortening of the metatarsal. If a lateral closing wedge osteotomy is used to correct

---

° This section was prepared by Dr. Roger A. Mann.

the intermetatarsal angle, shortening of the metatarsal occurs to a varying degree, since a lateral wedge is being removed from the bone. If the first metatarsal is short in relationship to the second to begin with, this may result in metatarsalgia because of the decreased weight bearing of the first metatarsal. If the first metatarsal is longer than the second, then a closing wedge osteotomy may produce a satisfactory result. A second problem with a lateral closing wedge osteotomy involves the operative technique. More bone is usually removed from the dorsal aspect of the metatarsal than from the plantar aspect. This results in dorsiflexion of the first metatarsal of varying degrees when the osteotomy site is closed. It is therefore imperative, when doing a lateral closing wedge osteotomy, to make the dorsal and plantar cuts parallel in order to prevent this technical error.

The use of an opening wedge osteotomy has also been advocated in order to correct the intermetatarsal angle. The osteotomy that is produced at the base of the first metatarsal is held open, either by using the medial eminence of bone removed from the distal aspect of the first metarsal (which may or may not be of the correct size) or by placing a bone graft into the site. However, since the tissues across the metatarsophalangeal joint are somewhat tight in a patient with severe deformity, lengthening the metatarsal by 3 or 4 mm increases the tension across the joint, and this may prevent the phalanx from maintaining a balanced position on the metatarsal. Another problem is that this type of osteotomy is somewhat unstable, and if weight bearing occurs prior to bony union, the metatarsal head may be displaced dorsally, which results in increased weight bearing on the second metatarsal, with possible metatarsalgia.

The osteotomy type that I prefer is the crescentic or curved osteotomy, which is made with a fine-toothed curved saw blade and an oscillating saw. This produces a thin osteotomy site, which is located about 5 to 7 mm distal to the metatarsocuneiform joint. Once this osteotomy site is created, more than 2 cm of cancellous bone oppose each other, creating a very stable osteotomy site. This neither lengthens nor shortens the first metatarsal in relation to the second. If the first metatarsal is markedly shorter than the second, the entire metatarsal shaft can be displaced plantarward 2 to 4 mm

to increase weight bearing and still leave a stable osteotomy site once it has been fixed.

Author's Preferred Technique

First, the skin incision is made on the dorsal aspect of the first metatarsal, beginning at the metatarsocuneiform joint and proceeding distally for a distance of about 2 to 2.5 cm. The incision is carried down to the extensor tendon, which is retracted either medially or laterally.

The periosteum over the metatarsal is then cut and stripped from the dorsal, medial, and lateral aspects of the metatarsal base. The metatarsocuneiform joint is identified for orientation, and a mark is made about 7 mm distally on the metatarsal, where the osteotomy site is to be created.

Using an oscillating saw and curved blade, the osteotomy site is then cut. The plane of the osteotomy should be perpendicular neither to the long axis of the metatarsal nor to the bottom of the foot, but rather in a plane bisecting these two planes. In order to cut the osteotomy the saw is firmly held against the bone in order to produce a scar on the bone, following which the saw is gently rocked medially and laterally along its arc in order to produce the osteotomy site. It is imperative to avoid torquing the blade, as it is thin and can be fractured.

Once the osteotomy site has been completed, the soft tissues are freed up from around the site, so that the distal metatarsal can be displaced in order to correct the abnormal intermetatarsal angle. If the osteotomy site has been cut so that the concavity of the cut is proximally based, the base of the osteotomy is displaced medially about 1 to 1.5 mm as the first metatarsal head is shifted laterally, adjacent to the second metatarsal, so the intermetatarsal angle is corrected. If the base of the osteotomy is displaced any further medially, excessive correction of the intermetatarsal angle occurs, which should be avoided. If the osteotomy is cut so that the concavity of the distal fragment faced proximally, the osteotomy site locks on itself as the first metatarsal head is moved laterally. As the distal portion of the metatarsal is shifted laterally, a Freer elevator is used to push the proximal metatarsal fragment medially. The distal portion of the metatarsal is literally rolled laterally around the osteotomy site as the metatarsal head is deviated laterally against the second metatarsal. When using the osteotomy in this configuration, overcorrection of the metatarsal rarely occurs.

Finally, the osteotomy site is fixed with an oblique pin, a series of pins, or a screw. I prefer an oblique ⁵⁄₆₄-inch smooth Steinmann pin, which holds the osteotomy site rather firmly. The only problem associated with the use of the pin is that it sticks out through the skin and requires careful observation. The pin is left in place for approximately 4 weeks. Other surgeons have used multiple small pins to stabilize the osteotomy site and buried them beneath the skin, while others have used a screw in order to compress the osteotomy site, bringing it either from the dorsal or the medial aspect. This is technically somewhat more difficult and, at times, if the bone is too osteoporotic, gaining rigid fixation is difficult.

Following the operation all patients are treated with a firm gauze and adhesive tape dressing that binds the metatarsal heads together and maintains the great toe in proper alignment. This dressing is changed on a weekly basis for 8 weeks. The pin is removed at approximately 4 weeks.

Following this osteotomy, the patient is allowed to walk in a wooden shoe and no cast immobilization is used. Union of the osteotomy site usually occurs after 8 weeks of immobilization. If delayed union occurs, cast immobilization will allow healing in an additional 4 to 6 weeks.

Proximal Phalangeal Osteotomy in Hallux Valgus

In 1929, OP Aiken of Portland, Oregon, reported a procedure for hallux valgus in which he described the condition as the deflexion of the great toe toward the others, accompanied by varying amount of exostosis at the terminal end of the metatarsal and the proximal end of the first phalanx. As the great toe goes into valgus, the portion of the first metatarsal head which originally was covered with thick articular cartilage degenerates, leaving only a thin eroded cartilaginous surface. However, the part in contact with the base of the proximal phalanx continues to have good cartilage.[3,5]

Aiken described an excision of the exostosis of the first metatarsal head and excision of the overgrown bone on the medial aspect of the base of the proximal phalanx accompanied by a medially based osteotomy of the proximal phalanx of the great toe with the toe being rotated slightly inward to alter the direction of the pull of the extensor tendon.

This operation is one in which there is easier realignment of the long extensors and flexors to the great toe. Since they deviate to the lateral side, they act as a bowstring and continue to pull the great toe further into valgus. Placing the base of the phalanx in the position in which it has been functional for many years leads to fewer arthritic changes postoperatively; this is done simply by osteotomizing the base of the proximal phalanx to correct the alignment of the great toe (Fig. 141-38).

A dorsomedial approach is made. The skin and subcutaneous tissues are reflected toward the plantar surface of the foot. A U-shaped flap is cut, with its base proximally, going down through the soft tissue to the cortex of the metatarsal area superiorly and inferiorly. A separate small intermetatarsal incision is made between the first and second metatarsal heads. This exposes the adductor hallucis and the lateral capsule. Tenotomy and lateral capsulotomy are then performed under direct vision. The medial eminence of the metatarsal head is resected in line with the medial border of the proximal phalanx to avoid a step or overhang. This same incision is then extended distally to expose the basal portion of the proximal phalanx. The osteotomy is performed in the metaphyseal region of the proximal phalanx within ¼ inch of the joint. The medial wedge is removed and the wedge is closed to allow correction of the deviated toe. An abnormal degree of rotation (pronation) may also be corrected at the osteotomy site. The site of osteotomy is transfixed with a small simple staple fashioned from a conventional Kirschner-wire. Reapproximation of the capsule and bursal incision are done without tension and without altering the opposing joint surface. A compression dressing is applied. Immediate motion is encouraged postoperatively. Ambulation is encouraged early, within 5 to 7 days, with a cutout cast shoe. Through early joint mobilization, almost every patient is able to maintain free postoperative motion at the metatarsophalangeal joint of the great toe.

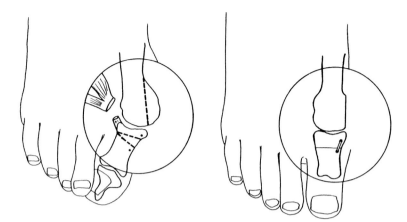

Fig. 141-38. Method for proximal phalangeal osteotomy.

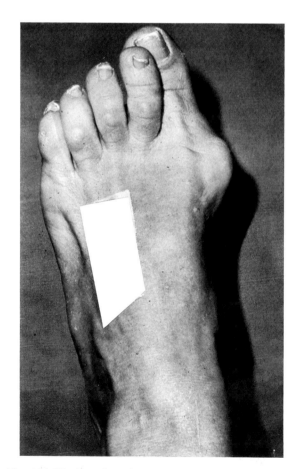

Fig. 141-39. Standing photograph prior to realignment of the great toe by proximal metatarsal osteotomy and soft tissue reconstruction.

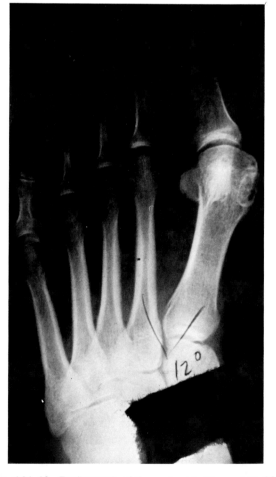

Fig. 141-40. Radiograph of the patient in Figure 141-39.

If metatarsus primus varus is severe (more than 10 degrees), this procedure can be combined with a proximal metatarsal osteotomy. This may be indicated especially in patients who have congenital interphalangeal hallux valgus. A metatarsal osteotomy, either distal or proximal, will not correct this type of hallux valgus and a basal proximal phalangeal osteotomy is more appropriate. The proximal phalangeal osteotomy is generally not recommended in severe cases of metatarsus primus varus, hallux rigidus, or rheumatoid arthritis.

AUTHOR'S PREFERRED TECHNIQUE FOR HALLUX VALGUS

Many proponents of osteotomy to correct the primus metatarsus varus favor the proximal osteotomy for the following reasons:

1. It does not encroach upon the blood supply to the metatarsal head.
2. The correction is easier to maintain.
3. Fewer technical failures occur.

Rapid healing will occur if the osteotomy is done promixally through the metaphyseal area of the first metatarsal.

This procedure is a combination of the modified McBride procedure and the proximal metatarsal osteotomy.[8,11] Again, this is indicated in those patients who have congruent joint surface, who do not have hallux rigidus, and who are generally in a younger age group with good blood supply.

The skin incision is made to the level of the callus of the first metatarsal exostosis. Sharp dissection is then carried out to avoid injury to the medial digital nerve of the great toe. The callus and medial capsule of the first metatarsophalangeal joint are then opened in a V-Y incision, leaving a triangular, distally based fascia and capsule flap attached to

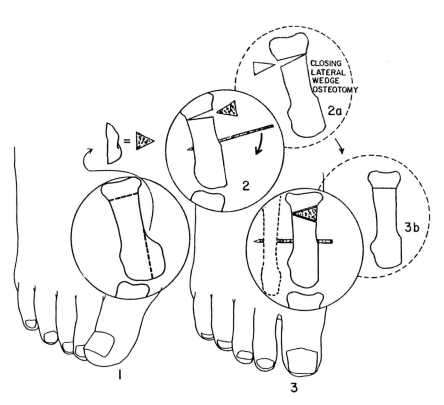

Fig. 141-41. The author's preferred method for proximal metatarsal osteotomy. Basal osteotomy is done either by opening or closing wedge with pin fixation.

the proximal phalangeal base. The capsule and synovial attachments provide material for strong resuturing of the distally based triangular flap and medial capsulorrhaphy; therefore, they are not stripped to the first metatarsal neck. The tendon of the abductor hallucis longus is then dissected from its flexed position and from the proximal phalangeal base. The tendon is not detached from the proximal phalangeal base; it is left attached, as this will correct in closure the pronation of the great toe. The long head of the abductor hallucis longus is dissected free. The muscular motor branch at the proximal muscle belly of the adductor is avoided. The oblique head of the abductor, which inserts into the medial sesamoid and medial pad, is not disturbed.

Next, a separate straight incision is made in the web space between the great and second toes. The tenotomy of the adductor hallucis is done, but the tendon is not resutured. Resection of the lateral sesamoid generally is not done unless a severe lateral and dorsal migration of the lateral sesamoid has occurred between the first and second metatarsal heads. A sharp incision of the contracted lateral capsule and part of the metatarsophalangeal joint of the great toe is made in attempt to bring the

great toe out of its valgus position. This release of soft tissue allows good repositioning of the proximal phalanx on the first metatarsal head.

Using the standard method of resection at the sagittal groove, the medial eminence is removed from the first metatarsal head. Care is taken in this resection so that a solid piece of bone will be available to fashion a bone graft.

The bone graft is then denuded of callus and articular surface, if any remains. Dissection is then carried out over the dorsomedial aspect of the first metatarsal base. Care is taken in identifying the metaphyseal base of the first metatarsal for the site of the osteotomy. At this point, with prior planning, one has decided whether an opening, lengthening wedge, or a closing, laterally based wedge is indicated. If an opening wedge is to be done, a simple straight osteotomy is then carried out using a sagit-

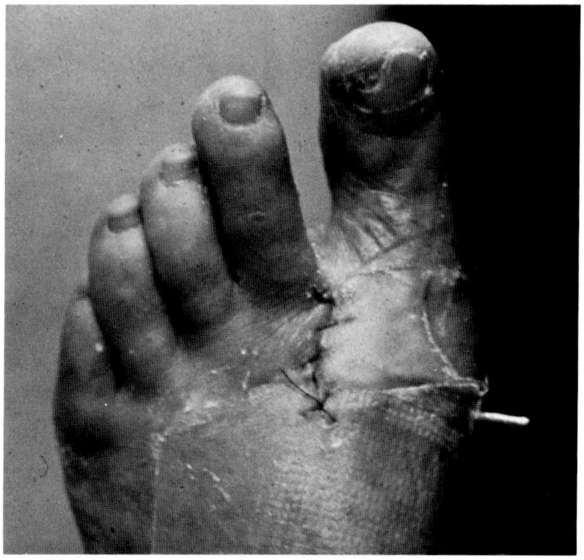

Fig. 141-42. Patient 1 week following our method of proximal metatarsal osteotomy.

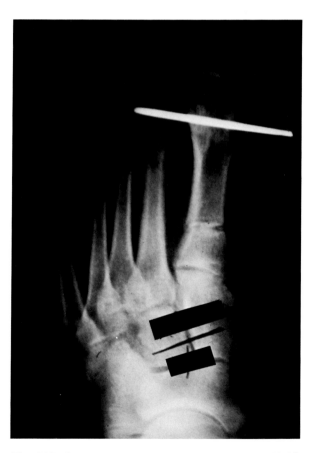

Fig. 141-43. Radiograph of the patient in Figure 141-42.

tal power saw. At this point a ³/₃₂-inch Steinmann pin is inserted at the very base of the medial eminence osteotomy site in the cortical part of the medial metatarsal shaft. The pin is then drilled through the lateral cortex of the metatarsal shaft. This ³/₃₂-inch threaded Steinmann pin allows a good levering force to place the varus first metatarsal into valgus. This also allows very easy opening or closure of the basal metatarsal osteotomy, as planned. If the opening wedge is to be done, then a wedge-shaped piece of bone obtained from the resected medial exostosis is driven into the osteotomy site. After the varus deformity has been corrected, the ³/₃₂-inch Steinmann pin is drilled into the second metatarsal neck. This affords stability

and maintains correction of the first metatarsal. The pin is then cut so that it will protrude through the wound and suture line on the medial aspect of the great toe. Closure of the medial capsule flaps of the first metatarsal joint is then carried out, and shortening of the distally based flap can be accomplished at this time to allow straight positioning of the great toe. Once this has been accomplished, the abductor hallucis longus—which has been dissected free, particularly the long head, and left attached to the base of the proximal phalanx—is brought back to its more normal position in the center of the medial aspect of the metatarsophalangeal joint. If the extensor is laterally displaced, it can be corrected at this time by suturing the abductor hallucis longus to the capsule and to the extensor conjoined tendon. Subcutaneous tissue is then closed. A gauze divider is placed between the great and second toes. Generally, only a well-padded pressure dressing is applied. The patient is kept on partial weight bearing for a period of 3 weeks, at which time the pin is removed; the patient can then be placed into a hardsole shoe or below-knee weight-bearing cast. The osteotomy generally heals in about 6 weeks (Figs. 141-39 to 141-44).

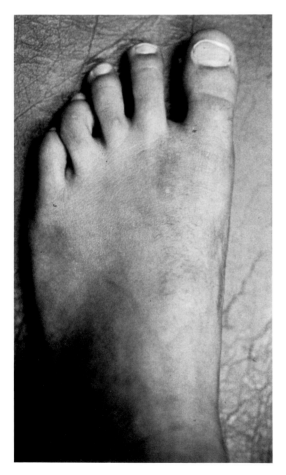

Fig. 141-44. Correction maintained by realignment and proximal metatarsal osteotomy. Same patient as illustrated in Figure 141-42 at 2 years postoperatively.

REFERENCES

1. Bargman J, Corless J, Gross AE, Langer F: A review of surgical procedures for hallux valgus. Foot Ankle 1:39, 1980
2. Bonney G, Macnab I: Hallux valgus and hallux rigidus: a critical survey of operative results. J Bone Joint Surg 34B:366, 1952
3. Butterworth RD, Clary BB: A bunion operation. Va Med Monthly 90:11, 1963
4. Clarke JJ: Hallux valgus and hallux varus, Lancet 1:609, 1900
5. Colloff B, Weitz EM: Proximal phalangeal osteotomy in hallux valgus. Clin Orthop 54:105, 1967
6. Corless JR: A modification of the Mitchell procedure. (abstr) J Bone Joint Surg 58B:138, 1976
7. Durman DC: Metatarsus primus varus and hallux valgus. Arch Surg 74:128, 1957
8. Edgar MA: Hallux valgus and associated conditions.

p. 83 In Klenerman L (ed): The Foot and Its Disorders. Blackwell Scientific, London, 1976

9. Froriep R: De ossis metatarsi primi exostosi. Landes, Industrie, Comptoir 1, 1834

10. Giannestras NJ: Problems of the forepart of the foot. p. 218. In American Academy of Orthopaedic Surgeons. Instructional Course Lectures. Vol. 22. CV Mosby, St. Louis, 1973

11. Haddad RJ Jr: Hallux valgus and metatarsus primus varus treated by bunionectomy and proximal metatarsal osteotomy. South Med J 68:684, 1975

12. Haines RW: The mechanism of the metatarsals and spread foot. Chiropodist 2:197, 1947

13. Haines RW, McDougall A: The anatomy of hallux valgus. J Bone Joint Surg 36B:272, 1954

14. Hardy RH, Clapham JCR: Observations on hallux valgus; based on a controlled series. J Bone Joint Surg 33B:376, 1951

15. Hattrup SJ, Johnson KA: Chevron osteotomy: analysis of factors in patients' dissatisfaction. Foot Ankle 5:327, 1985

16. Hawkins FB, Mitchell CL, Hedrick DW: Correction of hallux valgus by metatarsal osteotomy. J Bone Joint Surg 27:387, 1945

17. Jahss MH, Troy AI, Kummer F: Roentgenographic and mathematical analysis of first metatarsal osteotomies for metatarsus primus varus: a comparative study. Foot Ankle 5:280, 1985

18. Johnson KA: Chevron osteotomy of the first metatarsal: patient selection and technique. Contemp Orthop 3:707, 1981

19. Johnson K, Cofield RH, Morrey BF: Chevron osteotomy for hallux valgus. Clin Orthop 142:44, 1979

20. Jordan HH, Brodsky AE: Keller operation for hallux valgus rigidus; an end result study. Arch Surg 62:586, 1951

21. Kelikian H: Hallux Valgus, Allied Deformities of the Forefoot and Metatarsalgia. WB Saunders, Philadelphia, 1965

22. Kelikian H: The surgical management of hallux valgus complex. Orthop Dig 11, 1979

23. Keller WL: The surgical treatment of bunions and hallux valgus. NY Med J 80:741, 1904

24. Lapidus PW: The author's bunion operation from 1931 to 1959. Clin Orthop 16:119, 1960

25. Mann RA (ed): DuVries' Surgery of the Foot. 4th Ed. CV Mosby, St. Louis, 1978

26. Mann RA, Coughlin MJ: Hallux valgus—etiology, treatment, and surgical considerations. Clin Orthop 157:31, 1981

27. Matzen PF: Beitrag zur operativen Behandlung extremer Foremen von Hallux valgus. Zentralbl Chir 74:828, 1949

28. McBride ED: A conservative operation for bunions. J Bone Joint Surg 10:735, 1928

29. McBride ED: The conservative operation for "bunions": end results and refinements of technique. JAMA 105:1164, 1935

30. McBride ED: Hallux valgus bunion deformity. p. 334. In American Academy of Orthopaedic Surgeons. Instructional Course Lectures. Vol. 9. CV Mosby, St. Louis, 1952

31. McMurray TP: Treatment of hallux valgus and rigidus. Br Med J 2:218, 1936

32. Meier PJ, Kenzora JE: The risks and benefits of distal first metatarsal osteotomies. Foot Ankle 6:7, 1985

33. Mitchell CL, Fleming JL, Allen R et al: Osteotomy-bunionectomy for hallux valgus. J Bone Joint Surg 40A:41, 1958

34. Piggot H: The natural history of hallux valgus in adolescence and early adult life. J Bone Joint Surg 42B:749, 1960

35. Silver D: The operative treatment of hallux valgus. J Bone Joint Surg 5:225, 1923

36. Stein HC: Hallux valgus. Surg Gynecol Obstet 66:889, 1938

37. Straus WL Jr: Growth of human foot and its evolutionary significance. Contrib Embryol 19:93, 1927

Hallux Rigidus

Andrea Cracchiolo III

Hallux rigidus is a condition of the hallux metatarsophalangeal joint characterized by pain and limitation of motion. This entity has been known for 100 years and is probably second only to hallux valgus as a cause of hallux symptoms. The original description of this condition was probably by Davies-Colley in 1887, which he called hallux flexus. Many other names have been used to characterize the pathology, such as hallux dolorous, dorsal bunion, and hallux limitus. However, the name proposed by Cotterill—hallux rigidus—remains in use today.

Almost all patients present with symptoms of pain and restriction of motion in the hallux metatarsophalangeal joint. These usually are of gradual onset, and the patient may give a completely negative history for any possible etiology. One characteristic of pain in hallux rigidus is that it is present with any walking, whereas patients with hallux valgus usually complain of pain when walking in shoes.[11] The motion initially most severely restricted is dorsiflexion; plantar flexion may be un-affected. However, patients may also present with some restriction of almost all motion. Various degrees of inflammation can be seen within the joint. However, the foot often appears completely normal (Fig. 142-1), with no detectable swelling or erythema and with only some degree of spasm of the extensor hallucis longus. There is usually considerable tenderness when the joint is palpated, and any forceful motion, especially dorsiflexion, causes pain. The visible signs of deformity are usually very mild. Angular deformities such as hallux valgus are rarely seen. Patients with rigidus have a particularly difficult time finding any shoe which will allow more comfortable walking. Whenever a shoe with any significant elevation of the heel is worn, pain increases and walking is more limited. Patients with this condition usually show no sign of arthritis in any other joints.

Hallux rigidus is found in both men and women, being somewhat more common in women.[7,10] However, since restriction of dorsiflexion is more disabling in women, they may more often seek

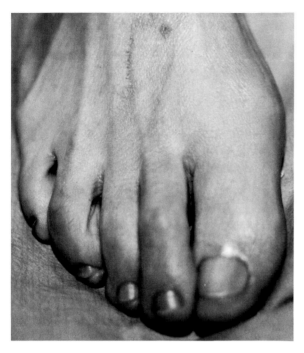

Fig. 142-1. Hallux rigidus in a 54-year-old man. The absence of grossly observable deformities is common.

care. The condition may be present in any age group from adolescents through older adults. Unilateral cases are the most common.

ETIOLOGY

Many factors have been implicated as possibly causing or contributing to the development of hallux rigidus. A partial list of etiologic factors would include the following:

1. Abnormalities of anatomy, such as a long narrow foot, pronated foot, a long first metatarsal, and abnormalities of the hallux metatarsophalangeal joint
2. Improper shoes, especially those causing hyperextension of the joint
3. Abnormalities of gait
4. Osteochondritis dissecans
5. Miscellaneous factors such as obesity and occupation

6. Trauma to the joint
7. Chip fractures of the dorsal lip of the proximal phalanx as well as small subchondral defects in the metatarsal head[10]

Patients occasionally report a specific history of injury that seems consistent with the degree of pathology seen clinically, radiographically, and at the time of surgical exploration of the joint.

PATHOLOGY AND RADIOGRAPHIC FEATURES

Patients are usually seen initially with advanced changes that resemble the pathology of degenerative joint disease (Fig. 142-2). Extensive osteophytes are present, usually on the dorsum of the metatarsal head and phalanx and along the tibial and fibular borders of the head, which is usually flattened (Figs. 142-3, 142-4). The joint space is greatly narrowed and almost obliterated at times. Subchondral sclerosis is seen, and cysts may be present in the head and may also occur in the phalanx. However, patients seen early in their disease

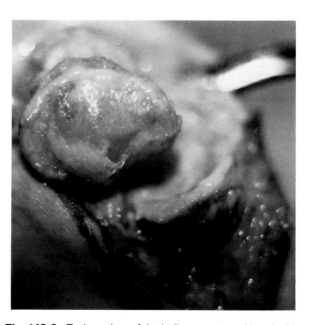

Fig. 142-2. End-on view of the hallux metatarsal head with complete loss of articular cartilage.

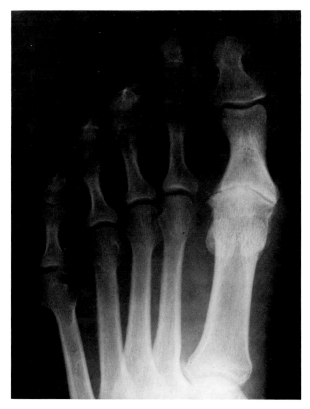

Fig. 142-3. AP radiograph of hallux rigidus. Note the distortion of both the base of the proximal phalanx and the metatarsal head. Some subchondral sclerosis is present.

may have minimal radiographic changes showing only some narrowing of the joint and slight flattening of the head. A loose body has been described within a joint, as well as a traumatic flap of cartilage that was found between the apex of the dome of the head and its dorsal border.[10] Therefore, it does appear that direct trauma or indirect trauma such as stubbing the hallux can produce lesions that result in hallux rigidus.

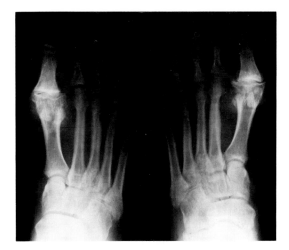

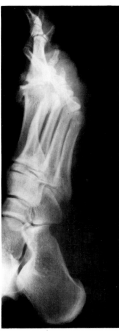

Fig. 142-4. AP and lateral radiographs of a 48-year-old man with bilateral hallux rigidus. The pathology is more advanced than that shown in Figures 142-2 and 142-3. Note the dorsal osteophyte of the metatarsal head.

METHODS OF TREATMENT

Nonoperative Procedures

Treatment should be indicated by the severity of the patient's symptoms. Some individuals have little discomfort or restriction of activities and initially may only require reassurance. Pressure about the hallux should be relieved, if possible, by having the patient wear a shoe with an adequate last and toe box. Shoe modifications may be helpful, including a full shank for the sole to restrict motion at the metatarsophalangeal joint, use of a rocker-bottom sole to allow a smoother toe-off, or a SACH-type heel. Nonsteroidal anti-inflammatory drugs (NSAIDs) can provide relief, since the pathology of hallux rigidus, regardless of etiology, is that of degenerative joint disease. Injections of corticosteroids may give only temporary relief. Such injections carry some well-known risks, including atrophy of subcutaneous tissues.

Operative Procedures

Patients with significant symptoms, especially those who are active, usually cannot find sufficient relief with nonoperative measures and require more definitive treatment. A routine preoperative evaluation usually suffices, as most patients with hallux rigidus are not elderly. If pulses cannot be palpated at the ankle and foot or if there are any signs or symptoms of vascular insufficiency, Doppler evaluations and vascular consultation should be obtained.

A variety of operations have been performed to correct painful hallux rigidus. These procedures include the following:

1. Arthrodesis of the hallux metatarsophalangeal joint
2. A Keller procedure to resect the base of the proximal phalanx
3. Cheilectomy, which is a debridement of the joint with special emphasis on removing the osteophytes about the metatarsal head
4. Implant arthroplasty, either with a single stem to replace the base of the proximal phalanx or with a double-stem implant so that both arthritic surfaces may be removed.

Indications

Choosing the correct procedure depends on two factors: first, the surgeon's familiarity with the available procedures, and second, the patient's age, sex, severity of the disease, and postoperative activity expectations.

Age and Activity Level

It would indeed be a rare patient who required an operation prior to completion of skeletal

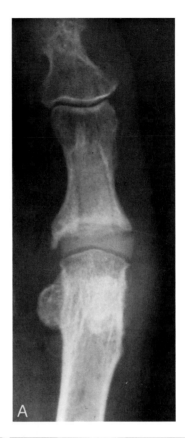

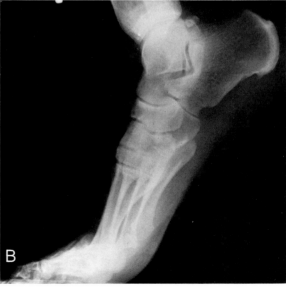

Fig. 142-5. (A) Single-stem implant with 2 years of follow-up. The position is excellent and the patient is pain free. **(B)** Weight-bearing lateral radiograph with the patient on tiptoes shows the degree of passive motion in the hallux.

growth. Patients with chip fractures or osteochondritis would be best treated by removal of the fragments. A young active patient might not appreciate so definitive a procedure as an arthrodesis and would be a candidate for cheilectomy. Implant arthroplasty might be more advisable in the middle-aged active patient (Fig. 142-5). Elderly patients could be candidates for implants or arthrodesis. However, age itself cannot completely determine the type of operation; many older patients jog or play tennis, and these activities may be restricted by an arthrodesis.

Sex

Women usually require mobility of the metatarsophalangeal joint, especially if they wish to wear any type of fashionable shoe. Such patients should be considered for cheilectomy or implant arthroplasty.

Contraindications

Aside from the absolute contraindications for surgery (insufficient symptoms, poor general health, peripheral vascular disease, poor skin coverage, local infection), each of the following procedures has specific drawbacks.

Keller Procedure

It is difficult to recommend the Keller procedure because its main disadvantage is that it frequently results in a loss of hallux function. In addition, malalignment of the hallux may develop. Since so many other good operations are available, this procedure should not often be considered (Fig. 142-6).

Cheilectomy

Debridement of a severely arthritic joint may be unwarranted if significant motion and function are the goals. While these joints may show significant motion in the face of cartilage deterioration, long-term improvements in function are seldom seen.

Arthrodesis

Successful arthrodesis will certainly relieve pain. However, the disadvantages of this operation are

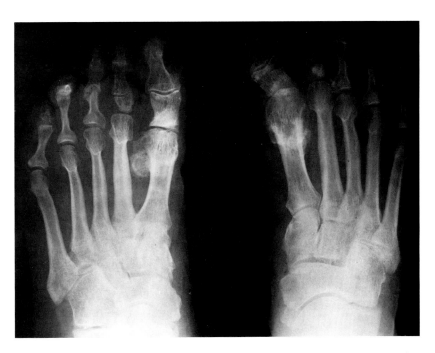

Fig. 142-6. Radiograph of patient in Figure 142-4, 5 years following bilateral Keller procedures. Both hallux metatarsophalangeal joints are now painful. Severe malalignment of the right hallux has resulted in symptoms along the entire hallux.

many. Interphalangeal motion should be normal preoperatively and must not be damaged by the procedure. Should the interphalangeal joint deteriorate later, the patient's gait will be further impaired. The technique of arthrodesis must be precise, and the angle of arthrodesis is critical. Time required for fusion as well as cast immobilization is lengthy and may produce difficulties, especially for the older patient. Joint fusion is a definitive procedure; if the result is unsatisfactory, little can be done for the patient.

Operative Techniques

Several steps are common to all operations involving the hallux metatarsophalangeal joint. Most surgeons prefer to use a tourniquet so that the procedure is performed in a bloodless field. Instruments should be similar to those used for surgery of the hand. The incisions are almost always longitudinal and are placed on the dorsomedial side of the joint. For arthrodesis, however, a direct dorsal longitudinal incision may be preferable.

Other steps in the operative technique depend on the individual bias and experience of the surgeon. These include such factors as

1. Whether to release the tourniquet and achieve hemostasis prior to closure
2. The use of drains
3. The type of postoperative dressing (most surgeons prefer a soft compression dressing; however, following arthrodesis, most advocate use of a cast)

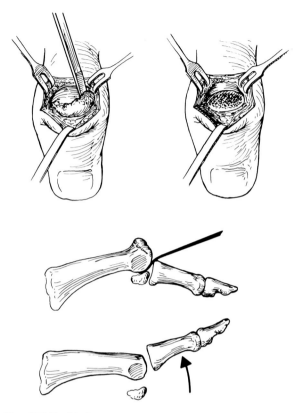

Fig. 142-7. Cheilectomy, or debridement of the hallux metatarsophalangeal joint, is frequently indicated in early hallux rigidus. A sharp osteotome or rongeur is used to remove the osteophytes, particularly those on the dorsum of the metatarsal head. An elevator is inserted to make certain that there are no adhesions or tightness of the plantar structures, particularly between the sesamoid and the plantar aspect of the metatarsal head. It is necessary to establish free passive dorsiflexion during this procedure.

Cheilectomy — Mann[7]

The hallux metatarsophalangeal joint is exposed through a dorsal longitudinal incision. (Fig. 142-7) The extensor hallucis longus is retracted either medially or laterally depending on the size and location of the dorsal bone spurs. The capsule is incised in a similar longitudinal line. Bony spurs can be removed by using rongeurs and the metatarsal head further trimmed using either a sharp osteotome or a power oscillating saw with a new blade. Approximately the dorsal 25 to 35 percent of the metatarsal head should be obliquely excised, with the cut made from distal in a proximal and dorsal

direction. This also avoids fracture to the head if an osteotome is used. A small amount of bone wax can be used to decrease the posttourniquet bleeding. The medial and lateral osteophytes should be removed in a similar fashion. Any significant osteophytes on the dorsum of the base of the proximal phalanx should also be removed. At this point, at least 70 to 90 degrees of passive dorsiflexion must be obtained. Since approximately one-half of that motion will be lost postoperatively, it is important to obtain the maximum degree of motion at the operation. If this proves difficult, insufficient bone may have been removed or there may be adhesions between the sesamoids and the metatarsal head on the plantar surface. This area should be inspected routinely and can be easily done by plantar-flexing the hallux. The area can be probed with a smooth elevator. Blunt dissection is usually sufficient to clear these restrictive adhesions. The dorsal capsule is closed loosely with an absorbable suture and the skin is closed routinely. A compressive dressing is placed and changed at approximately 18 to 24 hours.

Postoperatively, the patients can walk on the second or third day and remain in wooden-soled shoe for about 10 to 14 days. However active and passive motion of the toes should be instituted as soon as possible. Thus, patients can come out of their wooden shoe and walk either barefoot or in sandals. The postoperative dressing is further changed at about the tenth day; the sutures can be removed if wound healing is satisfactory. A smaller dressing is placed to hold the hallux in a corrected position, permitting more potential motion. Pain and swelling usually subside after 2 to 3 months, and maximum results are usually seen by 6 months. It must be stressed that the patients must actively participate in a vigorous rehabilitation program if they are to regain motion.

Arthrodesis — Lipscomb

The surgeon must decide what type of internal fixation will be used to immobilize the metatarsophalangeal joint. The types of internal fixation are (1) a screw,[6] (2) Steinmann pins driven across both the interphalangeal and metatarsophalangeal joints,[8] and (3) a circumferential wire.[4,5]

One of these techniques must be selected prior to the removal of any remnants of the articular surfaces.

A second critical decision is what position to place the joint in for the fusion. Basically, the plantar skin of the calcaneus, the metatarsal head, and the distal phalanx of the hallux should touch a flat surface simultaneously when the foot is at a right angle to the leg.[6] Most studies state that the angle between the proximal phalanx and the metatarsal should be between 20 and 30 degrees in the horizontal plane (Fig. 142-8).[6,12] If a screw is selected for internal fixation, a drill hole of 2 to 3 mm is placed through the distal medioplantar surface of

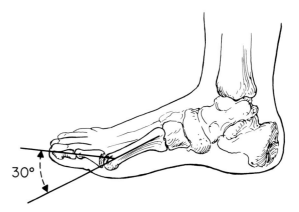

Fig. 142-8. Arthrodesis must be performed using an angle that will allow either a plantigrade position or slight dorsiflexion of the hallux in relationship to the remainder of the foot. It is important that the hallux is not hampered in toe-off. Many toes have little extension at the interphalangeal joint. This should be considered in positioning the hallux for arthrodesis.

the base of the proximal phalanx. Then, with the toe reduced in proper position, the drill is passed into the metatarsal shaft. Usually a 5-cm screw is selected, and the hole in the phalanx is slightly overdrilled to produce some compression. The screw is placed tightly enough to hold both surfaces firmly together.[6]

The use of threaded Steinmann pins across the entire phalanx to hold the hallux firmly to the metatarsal gives solid fixation. Usually two pins are placed in a retrograde fashion; it is important that they have trochar points at both ends. The pins are placed after first properly preparing the bone ends with whatever method one is accustomed for arthrodesis. Parallel cuts through good cancellous bone of the metatarsal head and base of proximal phalanx probably give the best stability.

If a firm surface is available on the operating table, the knee flexion is normal, the knee can be fully flexed and the foot placed in a plantigrade weight-bearing position. An assistant must then hold the phalanx tightly to the metatarsal, while the surgeon drives the pins across the arthrodesis site. This must be done using a large power drill.

The diameter of pins selected can vary between $\frac{9}{64}$ inch (3.6 mm), $\frac{1}{8}$ inch (3.2 mm), or $\frac{3}{32}$ inch (2.4 mm) and may vary, depending on the size of the patient and the bone available for fusion. The pins are cut long enough distally to permit subsequent removal. Well-fitting plastic caps are helpful to avoid anything from impinging on the cut end of the pin.

One theoretical disadvantage of this fixation is that it passes through the interphalangeal joint. Although radiographic deterioration of this joint may be seen in as many as 60 percent of feet, a painful interphalangeal joint occurs infrequently. Degenerative changes of the interphalangeal joint can also be seen following arthrodesis techniques that do not involve placing a pin across the joint. The interphalangeal joint normally only flexes, but with a solid arthrodesis of the MTP joint the interphalangeal joint is exposed to the stresses of extension forces, which are also increased by the greater length of the fused proximal phalanx and metatarsal. Despite early evidence of fusion, which may occur as early as 8 weeks, the average time to fusion is 13 to 14 weeks postoperatively.[8,9] Therefore, the external fixation device should not be removed prematurely.

Cerclage wire fixation provides stable fixation when performing a cone arthrodesis.[4,5] The surfaces must be carefully prepared, and minimal length is sacrificed. Holes for the wires must be accurately drilled in the metatarsal and phalanx. The latter must pass distal to the point at which the prepared metatarsal head will rest. Thus, when the wire is tightened, full axial compression occurs. Usually, the ends of the wire exit on the lateral side of the joint, where they are twisted and buried in soft tissue.

Postoperative immobilization is provided by a below-knee cast or by a compression dressing and a wooden-soled shoe.[6] Depending on the type of fixation, it may be difficult to determine when arthrodesis has been achieved. Despite early evidence of fusion, which may occur at about 8 weeks postoperatively, the internal fixation device should not be removed prematurely. In many cases, the screw or wire need not ever be removed unless it causes irritation.

Results

The best possible result in treating a painful hallux rigidus would be to provide the patient with painless functional motion which would allow return to full activities. Cheilectomy has been reported to provide substantial relief of symptoms in 17 of 20 patients, with the remaining three patients having minimal discomfort.[7] Despite the small number of patients reported, these results appear promising, especially since little progression of the degenerative joint changes were seen in the follow-up evaluation. Moreover, no complications were reported.[7]

Arthrodesis has also been reported to satisfy most patients.[5,6] This is obviously a technically more demanding procedure, and good results will occur only if fusion is achieved in the proper position.

Implant arthroplasty has also shown favorable results. Patients with either single- or double-stem implants have had almost complete relief of pain.[2,13,15] The single-stem implant appears to give a significantly increased range of motion, and to date only one implant failure has been reported.[13] The use of high performance silicones should assure future implant integrity. Stokes has studied the distribution of load on the forefoot pre- and postoperatively in six patients with hallux rigidus following silicone arthroplasty.[14] As compared to patients having a Keller procedure, patients with implants were found to have more normal foot function. Although favorable results have also been reported when Swanson finger implants have been used to treat hallux rigidus,[16] the specially designed toe implants should be used.

Thus, it appears that the surgeon may select one of three possible operations to treat patients with symptomatic hallux rigidus nonresponsive to conservative measures. No single operation is satisfactory for every patient. Should the patient require a movable joint and no need exists to use an implant, then cheilectomy appears the procedure of choice. The same patient with more advanced pathology should be considered for implant arthroplasty. Arthrodesis appears suitable for selected patients, but it must be done correctly to avoid unsatisfactory results.

REFERENCES

1. Cotterill JM: Condition of stiff great toe in adolescence. Edinb Med J 33:459, 1887

2. Cracchiolo A, Swanson AB, Swanson G: The arthritic great toe metatarsophalangeal joint. A review of flexible silicone implant arthroplasty from two medical centers. Clin Orthop 157:64, 1981

3. Davies-Colley JNC: Contraction of the metatarsophalangeal joint of the great toe. Br Med J 1:728, 1827

4. Fitzgerald JAW: A review of long-term results of arthrodesis of the first metatarsophalangeal joint. J Bone Joint Surg 51B:488, 1969

5. Fitzgerald JAW, Wilkinson JM: Arthrodesis of the metatarsophalangeal joint of the great toe. Clin Orthop 157:70, 1981

6. Lipscomb PR: Arthrodesis of the first metatarsophalangeal joint for severe bunions and hallux rigidus: a review of the literature and a method of treatment. Clin Orthop 142:48, 1979

7. Mann RA, Coughlin MJ, DuVries HL: Hallux rigidus. Clin Orthop 142:57, 1979

8. Mann RA, Oates JC: Arthrodesis of the first metatarsophalangeal joint. Foot Ankle 1:159, 1980

9. Mann RA, Thompson FM: Arthrodesis of the first metatarsophalangeal joint for hallux valgus in rheumatoid arthritis. J Bone Joint Surg 66A:687, 1984

10. McMaster MJ: The pathogenesis of hallux rigidus. J Bone Joint Surg 60B:82, 1978

11. Möberg E: A simple operation for hallux rigidus. Clin Orthop 142:55, 1979

12. Moynihan FJ: Arthrodesis of the metatarsophalangeal joint of the great toe. J Bone Joint Surg 49B:544, 1967

13. Sethu A, D'Netto D, Ramakrishna B: Swanson's silastic implants in great toes. J Bone Joint Surg 62B:83, 1980

14. Stokes IAF, Hutton WC, Mech MI, et al: Forces under the hallux valgus foot before and after surgery. Clin Orthop 142:64, 1979

15. Swanson AB, Lumsden RM, Swanson G: Silicone implant arthroplasty of the great toe: a review of single stem and flexible hinge implants. Clin Orthop 142:30, 1979

16. Wenger RJJ, Whalley RC: Total replacement of the first metatarsophalangeal joint. J Bone Joint Surg 60B:88, 1978

Prosthetic Arthroplasty of the Hallux

143

Andrea Cracchiolo III

Deformities of the forepart of the foot occur frequently and may vary in severity. The causes of such pathology are multiple and vary from congenital deformities to local degenerative and systemic arthritic diseases. Treatment should be based on the etiologies of these deformities and the severity of symptoms they produce. In most cases, conservative care will suffice; however, should this fail or should the deformity be severe, operative correction must be considered.

Since many deformities of the forepart of the foot may involve multiple joints, the integrity of all joints must be evaluated closely when planning to treat the pathology. Joints that are normal on physical or radiographic examination usually are not painful. They move freely and show no evidence of inflammation. Areas directly adjacent to joints may produce significant symptoms, such as seen in the painful bunion or callus. Such conditions are usually treated surgically by excision of a bony prominence or by an osteotomy. However, a joint that is not significantly damaged should be preserved.

THE ARTHRITIC JOINT

Symptoms produced by joint pathology usually have several common features. Pain usually occurs with any type of joint motion. Therefore, a patient will complain of pain with any walking, whether bare-footed or in shoes. Tight-fitting high-heeled shoes will usually cause more severe pain.

Swelling of a metatarsophalangeal joint other than the hallux may not be obvious. The lateral joints of the forepart of the foot are covered by extensive subcutaneous tissues, especially on the plantar side. However, careful inspection and palpation as well as soft tissue shadows on radiographs can demonstrate such pathology. Bursal formation may also indicate joint pathology. This is most commonly seen in rheumatoid arthritis, where a bursa forms over the plantar dislocated metatarsal head, or on the medial side of the hallux when a bunion is present.[1]

Malalignment may be further evidence of joint pathology. This may precede joint deterioration, as

4113

in the long-standing hallux valgus that results in a degenerative metatarsophalangeal joint.

Areas of skin pressure may also point to an abnormal joint. Plantar calluses may be evidence of malalignment with no significant joint deformity or they may be evidence of a dislocated joint. Corns on the dorsum of the toes are similar landmarks of joint pathology.

SURGICAL TREATMENT

A joint with satisfactory articular integrity should be maintained. Deformities about such a joint should be treated by such procedures as excision of an exostosis, osteotomy, or soft tissue repositioning. There is no current operative procedure that can replace a normal functioning joint.

Joints with insufficient articular integrity have usually been treated by either (1) excising part or all of the joint, or (2) fusion of the joint. These procedures are designed to give only pain relief, and both have the disadvantage of sacrificing function. In addition, excising a joint may lead to recurrence of the deformity, and arthrodesis is a procedure in which the angle of fusion must be absolutely correct.

Prosthetic Arthroplasty

An alternative treatment for the painful arthritic joint is to excise all or part of the articular surfaces and replace them with an implant. Such implants have been made of silicone rubber and initially were only for the replacement of the resected base of the proximal phalanx (single-stemmed implant).[3] (See Ch. 142, Fig. 142-5.) Subsequently, a double-stemmed silicone implant was developed that could be placed across the resected surfaces of an arthritic joint with one stem fitting into the proximal phalanx and the other into the metatarsal intramedullary canal. These implants are now made of a newer, high-performance silicone rubber, which should provide great durability to the implant.

Advantages and Disadvantages

Successful implant arthroplasty provides a movable, pain-free joint with good stability. This does increase or maintain function of the toe and prevents secondary deformities that can occur from resection of all or part of a joint. At times, implants are the only method of salvaging a previously failed operation or of avoiding an arthrodesis. However, should the implant fail, it can easily be removed, and an excisional arthroplasty or an arthrodesis can be performed.

The major disadvantage of the procedure is that of possible implant failure. Thus, the same uncertainties common to all joint arthroplasties apply to foot implants. These procedures also require precise surgical technique. The operation requires careful handling of tissues and precise reconstruction of the soft tissues. Moreover, the use of these implants in patients with a very high activity level should be avoided. It is usually possible to select alternative operative procedures as the first attempt to relieve pain and correct deformity in a patient who has a high activity level. Thus, careful patient selection is also necessary to avoid fatigue of the silicone implant with subsequent fragmentation and fracture.[2]

Indications

Implant arthroplasty should be used only in painful joints that have completely destroyed or severely deteriorated articular surfaces without evidence of sepsis. Conditions that could produce such joint pathology are:

1. Local factors, such as hallux valgus, hallux rigidus, or traumatic arthritis
2. Systemic arthritic diseases, the most characteristic being rheumatoid arthritis
3. Failed previous operations, such as a failed Keller procedure, where fusion or resection of bone are the only other alternatives

Preoperative Patient Evaluation

In addition to the general history-taking and physical evaluation, patients who are to undergo implant arthroplasty should have some additional evaluation. This should reveal:

1. No evidence or history of sepsis in the joints or bones subjected to this operation
2. Good skin coverage
3. Adequate peripheral vascular circulation
4. Absence of diseases such as diabetes that could complicate the result

Therefore, evaluation should include:

1. Routine laboratory studies, including specific studies for the various arthritic or metabolic diseases when indicated
2. Evaluation of pulses by physical examination and evidence of adequate perfusion seen by an examination of the skin, hair, and nail growth, and, occasionally, special studies, such as Doppler evaluation
3. Medical evaluation of the entire patient; an inquiry into the past history to determine the presence of recent cardiorespiratory diseases; a careful analysis of all medications being taken, as well as allergies to antibiotics
4. Weight-bearing radiographs, including anteroposterior (for viewing the forepart of the foot), lateral (for viewing the midpart and hindpart of the foot), and when indicated, views of the os calcis and ankle

Operative Procedure

Most operations are performed under tourniquet control, taking care to limit the pressure and length of time the tourniquet is inflated.

Implant arthroplasty for the hallux metatarsophalangeal joint requires precise surgical technique. As is true with any other prosthetic implant, antibiotics should be utilized in the preoperative period. Intravenous dose of antibiotics can be given approximately 30 minutes prior to inflation of the tourniquet, and it is safest to do this in the preoperative room. Postoperatively antibiotics can be continued intravenously and orally for 48 hours. Obviously if there are serious problems with wound healing the postoperative use of antibiotics may need to be extended, but this is most unusual.

The joint is approached through a longitudinal incision on the dorsomedial aspect of the joint. The incision extends from the middle of the proximal phalanx to the distal metatarsal shaft (Fig. 143-1). Care is taken not to injure the superficial dorsal

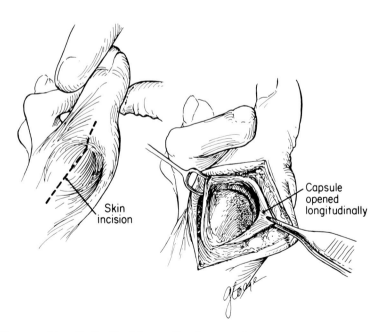

Fig. 143-1. Slightly curved longitudinal incision on the dorsomedial aspect of the hallux metatarsophalangeal joint is recommended. The capsule is again opened longitudinally, taking care not to strip the base of the proximal phalanx of its capsular and muscle attachments.

sensory nerves, and the capsule is exposed from the long extensor tendon to the medial sesamoid. The capsular incision is quite important; it should also be longitudinal and slightly offset from the skin incision. The metatarsal head should be exposed by sharply dividing the soft tissue attachments on its medial and dorsal sides. The articular surfaces can be visualized by distracting the joint. A few millimeters of the capsule and soft tissues surrounding the base of the phalanx can also be sharply released. However, care should be taken not to completely release the insertion of the tendons that attach to the base. Occasionally a more extensive release of the base of the proximal phalanx is necessary. In addition, it is sometimes necessary to excise more of the bony base of the proximal phalanx; in so doing, the insertion of the short toe flexors and the medial capsule are completely released. Following preparation of the intramedullary canal, it is important to reattach these structures. At this point a final decision can be made about whether to perform a single-stemmed implant that replaces the base of the proximal phalanx or a double-stemmed implant with resection of both joint surfaces.[1]

Bone Preparation

Single-Stemmed Implant

This type of implant usually requires more exposure of the base of the proximal phalanx. However, one should stop short of removing all soft tissue insertions. Using one of the trial components as a guide, several millimeters of bone are resected using a small power saw or a side-cutting burr. It is critical that the insertion of the short flexor tendons not be damaged or cut. Should this occur, the tendons and the medial capsule must be resutured to the bone. Before placing the implant a 1- or 1.5-mm drill is used to make holes through the proximal phalanx through which a 3-0 or 4-0 absorbable suture is passed for reattaching the tendons and the medial capsule. The intramedullary canal is opened with an awl or a small straight curette. The

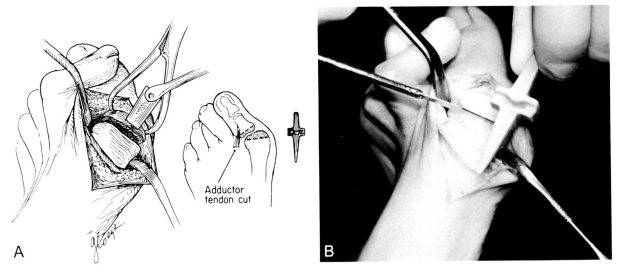

Adductor tendon cut

A   B

Fig. 143-2. (A) Since double-stemmed implants come in a variety of sizes, excessive bone resection is not necessary. A small, thin-bladed oscillating saw removed the damaged articular surface of the metatarsal head. Only a partial resection of the head is necessary. The base of the proximal phalanx must be preserved as much as possible. Frequently, the concave base can simply be flattened using a saw or a very high-speed power burr. A trial implant is helpful in judging the amount of bone to be resected. Usually a number 1 or 2 trial implant is used. **(B)** Trial double-stemmed silicone implant used to determine the amount of bone requiring excision. This is a size 0 trial, one of the smaller implants for use in the hallux. The special retractors are helpful in delivering the head into the wound.

pilot burrs are most helpful in widening and shaping the canal to accept the implant. The implant should fit snugly — that is, neither tight nor loose. All bone edges should be smoothed. The medial exostosis of the metatarsal head should be excised.

Double-Stemmed Implant

A trial implant, approximately the size of the intramedullary canals, should be used as a guide (Fig. 143-2). Usually, this is a number 1-3 trial implant. The metatarsal head is resected first with a small power saw or side-cutting burr using the width of the hinge portion of the implant as a guide (Fig. 143-3). It is important not to resect an excessive amount of the metatarsal head. Usually it is possible to retain that portion of the head which articulates with the sesamoids when the toe is in neutral alignment. The intramedullary canals of the metatarsal and proximal phalanx are then opened. If there is significant osteoporosis, a hand broach will suffice. If the bone is sclerotic, then graduated sizes of pilot burrs are available. It is not necessary to try and place the largest possible implant across this joint;

however, an implant of suitable size that will maintain the normal alignment is desirable. The mouth of each of the intramedullary cavities must be carefully shaped to accept the rectangular silicone stem. Titanium grommets in various sizes are now available, which serve to protect the silicone stem from the surrounding bone. This will require removing slightly more bone. A trial fit using the grommet that can be placed on the silicone stem should than be made. A full trial reduction of the double-stemmed silicone implant is essential. This will check the extent of the very important soft tissue releases that may be necessary or have already been done. It will also check the overall alignment of the ray, and if the appropriate soft tissue releases have been accomplished then this will point to the need for doing a proximal osteotomy of the metatarsal base (Fig. 143-4).

Soft Tissue Procedures

Once the trial implant is placed within the prepared bones, an estimate of the soft tissue procedures that must be performed can be made (Fig.

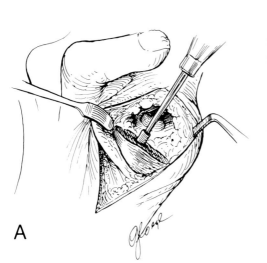
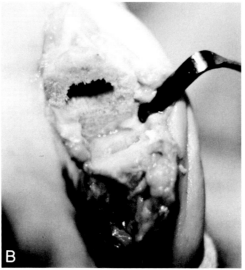

Fig. 143-3. (A) The intramedullary canals of the proximal phalanx and the metatarsal must be prepared using a special high-speed pilot burr to accept the double-stemmed implant. If only a single-stemmed implant is being used to replace the base of the proximal phalanx, then only the proximal phalanx requires this procedure. Care must be taken to remove all sharp edges either on the cut surface or in the intramedullary canals to avoid injury to the patient. **(B)** The intramedullary canals of both the metatarsal and the phalanx have been prepared using the pilot burr to accept the double-stemmed implant. All surfaces should be smooth to avoid injury to the implant.

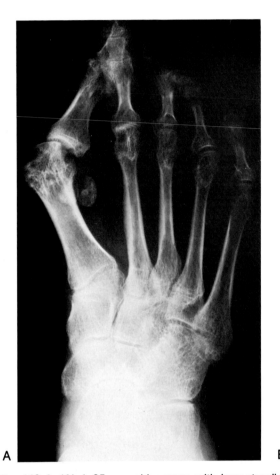 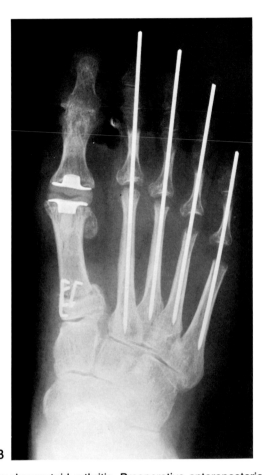

A   B

Fig. 143-4. (A) A 35-year-old woman with long-standing rheumatoid arthritis. Preoperative anteroposterior weight-bearing views show extensive destruction of the rheumatoid forefoot. The patient had severe metatarsalgia and had failed conservative care. **(B)** Postoperative anteroposterior view 7 days following reconstruction of the forepart of the foot. A #1 double-stemmed silicone implant with proximal and distal titanium grommets has been placed across the hallux metatarsophalangeal joint. The sesamoids are properly repositioned. A curved proximal osteotomy of the hallux metatarsal using pneumatic-powered titanium staples was also necessary to gain correction of the hallux ray. The obliquity of the metatarsocuneiform joint made an osteotomy desirable since passive correction of the metatarsal would be limited and the intermetatarsal 1-2 angle could not be reduced. The metatarsal heads were excised and a volar plate arthroplasty was performed. The volar plate was dissected from the base of the proximal phalanx, the flexor tendons were inspected and centralized and then a 0.062-inch Kirschner-wire was placed in a retrograde fashion first through the toe and then back across the volar plate into position between the base of the proximal phalanx and the metatarsal. The Kirschner-wire extends to the base but not through the base of the metatarsal, so that the toe is not impaled and stretched out. This will minimize any neurovascular complication that might require removal of the pin.

143-5). The goal of these procedures is to restore the hallux to as near normal a position as possible before the wound is closed. Occasionally, nothing more is needed than to close the capsular incision. However, if significant deformity exists, the following should be considered:

1. A careful capsular release, especially if a severe hallux valgus exists: The release may be performed in one of three ways: a separate longitudinal incision between the first and second metatarsal heads easily exposes the adductor tendon and the lateral sesamoid; this area can also be reached through the original incision by continuing the dissection of the capsule dorsal and lateral to the long extensor tendon; however, it may suffice to find the lateral sesamoid through the excised joint and perform a longitudinal lateral release of the adductor and capsule.

2. The sesamoids should be freed from the undersurface of the metatarsal if adhesions exist.

3. Closure of the capsule: This is the final step in properly positioning the hallux (Fig. 143-6). If a single-stemmed implant has been placed, it may

be necessary to reattach some of the capsule to the phalanx. This is done using two 1- or 1.5-mm drill holes through which is passed a 0 or 00 absorbable suture. The capsule must be sutured securely to the bone. With the hallux held in slight supination, the remainder of the capsule is attached to the metatarsal in a similar fashion. The position of the sesamoids should be checked before finally reattaching the capsule. If they have been properly released, their position should be under the metatarsal head. Usually, some redundant capsule remains and may be excised. The capsular incision is closed using the same suture material with interrupted buried sutures. These soft tissue procedures also aid in reducing the metatarsus primus varus that is frequently present.

4. The abductor hallucis may also be advanced, which is most helpful in cases of severe hallux valgus deformity. The abductor tendon is not fully detached but is freed from the capsule, leaving its distal insertion intact and sutured more dorsally and distally (Fig. 143-7). This should be done carefully, especially if a wide

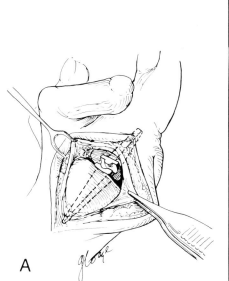
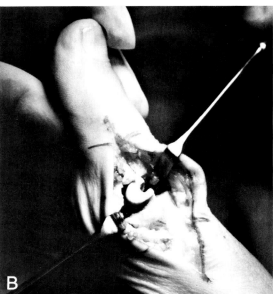

Fig. 143-5. **(A)** Trial reduction should always be done with one of the trial prostheses. It is important to see not only that sufficient bone has been resected but also that enough soft tissue releases have been performed so that the hallux aligns itself normally. **(B)** With the trial implant in place, soft tissue abnormalities can now be assessed.

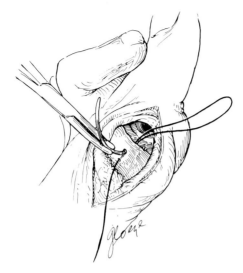

Fig. 143-6. Before placing the actual silicone implant, it is necessary to use a small (1-mm) high-speed burr to place two holes at the distal edge of the metatarsal shaft. Through these holes are woven an absorbable suture, usually size 0. Since such sutures usually come with very large needles it is important to obtain a suture with an appropriate small needle to facilitate passing through the holes. Once the suture is in place, the implant is placed and closure of the important lateral capsule to the bone can be accomplished. Advancement of the lateral capsule dorsally and proximally controls the amount of valgus and rotation of the hallux. Care should be taken to avoid any residual pronation.

lateral release has been performed, because an unopposed tight abductor can lead to subsequent varus deformity of the hallux.

5. It may be necessary to release the extensor hallucis brevis tendon. However, it is rarely necessary to lengthen the extensor hallucis longus. Such a lengthening can produce a weakness in extension and may be bothersome to the patient.

A few 4-0 absorbable sutures may be placed subcutaneously, and the skin is closed with interrupted 5-0 Prolene sutures, care being taken to handle the skin gently. One or two silicone drains are inserted into the wound, and a sterile compression dressing is used to hold the hallux and lateral toes in proper alignment. At this point, the tourniquet is released and removed from the upper thigh.

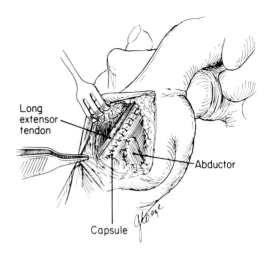

Fig. 143-7. The remainder of the capsule is closed with either 0 or 00 interrupted sutures. In addition, it may be necessary during the procedure to lengthen the long extensor tendon. In toes that have severe hallux valgus or that are excessively pronated, the abductor tendon can be advanced more dorsally and distally into the capsule to provide more stability. If an excessive lateral release has been performed, including release of the adductor, care must be taken not to over-balance the hallux and incur a resultant varus deformity.

Proximal Metatarsal Osteotomy

Following a full soft tissue release and placement of the trial component, it is essential to check whether normal alignment will be possible. The medial capsule should be held with a tissue forceps in the appropriate position. If there is still malalignment, it will be necessary to perform a proximal metatarsal osteotomy. A curved osteotomy is preferable, and this can be performed using a special curved crescentic blade on an oscillating saw. The plane of the osteotomies should be at right angles to the foot and not at right angles to the metatarsal shaft. Some type of internal fixation should be used to hold the osteotomy securely. A 4.0-mm cancellous bone screw does a very effective job and can be placed with the metatarsal held in a corrected alignment. The distal hole should be drilled prior to completing the osteotomy as this will make placement of the screw easier. When some osteoporosis is present it is possible to obtain good internal fixation using titanium staples placed via a pneumatic-powered gun. However, even a Steinmann pin or multiple 0.062-inch Kirschner wires can be used for fixation. Should fixation be questionable, it might be necessary to place the patient in a short-leg or slipper cast; this is rarely needed. The osteotomy should be performed approximately 1.5 cm distal to the metatarsocuneiform articulation. It is best not to cross that joint with any of the internal fixation devices. One should not hesitate in performing the osteotomy if that step is necessary to achieve the final goal of normal alignment of the hallux ray. Once it has been determined that an osteotomy is necessary, it is best to perform the osteotomy after the implant, with the grommets both proximally and distally firmly in place within the intramedullary cavity so as to avoid unnecessary stress on the metatarsal after the osteotomy has been performed and internally fixed. Before placing the actual implant and the grommet, the drill holes for subsequent reattachment of the medial capsule and the suture through the drill holes must be placed. After the skin is closed, flat silicone drains are placed in all the wounds, and a compression dressing is placed over the foot to hold the hallux in the corrected position.

POSTOPERATIVE MANAGEMENT

The foot is elevated and a cradle keeps the bed covers from resting on the foot. The patient is allowed to stand the first postoperative day, using support and a postoperative wooden-soled shoe. Ambulation is restricted, allowing only bathroom privileges. On the second postoperative day, the drains are removed and the wound is carefully redressed by the surgeon, using strict aseptic technique. An identical dressing is reapplied. The patient's discharge from the hospital depends on many factors but usually occurs on the second or third postoperative day. Home activities are strictly limited to allow the wound to heal uneventfully. Sutures are removed between 10 and 14 days after the operation.

Early motion should be initiated; however, the wound must first appear to be healing well. The postoperative wooden-soled shoe should be modi-

fied by placing a 2.5-cm lift within the shoe that extends from the heel to just proximal to the implant. A commercial orthosis is available that keeps the hallux in position and permits flexion and extension. However, the therapist can easily attach such a device to the shoe. Similarly, the therapist can construct a night splint to hold the toe in the corrected position; this is especially important in patients with severe hallux valgus. Such devices should be used for about 4 weeks. However, if stiffness is noted early, the night splint may be discontinued. During this time, the patient is instructed to move the hallux actively and passively. Hydrotherapy may be helpful when the wound is healed. Wide shoes should be worn until swelling has subsided. Shoes with a narrow toe box and heels higher than 3 to 4 cm should be avoided. Most of these adjunctive measures are needed, especially when operating on markedly abnormal joints, so that a well-aligned implant is the result (Fig. 143-8).

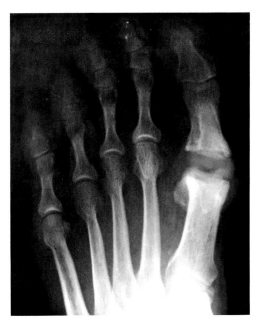

Fig. 143-8. Radiographic view of a properly positioned double-stemmed implant. The hallux metatarsal was significantly shorter than the second metatarsal in this patient. However, the sesamoids retain their normal position and the length of the hallux has been maintained. Excisional arthroplasty or arthrodesis might have further shortened this toe.

CURRENT STATUS

Implant arthroplasty offers the surgeon another option in treating abnormalities of the hallux metatarsophalangeal joint. Traditionally, osteotomy or a soft tissue procedure has been the initial treatment for most correctable bunion deformities. However, when the joint is beyond saving, the procedures available are excisional arthroplasty and arthrodesis. Both procedures sacrifice function and may result in malalignment of the hallux. Therefore, it is useful to have a procedure such as implant arthroplasty, which offers the possibility of some postoperative function while controlling alignment of the toe. Moreover, arthrodesis may be difficult when dealing with a previously failed operation in which a portion of the joint has been removed or has resorbed, and a double-stemmed implant may be an alternative solution.

Therefore, implant arthroplasty is certainly not a procedure that should replace any operation to salvage a normal metatarsophalangeal joint. However, the use of implants now adds yet another good operation that can be used in treating painful and deformed toe joints.

REFERENCES

1. Cracchiolo A, Swanson AB, Swanson GD: The arthritic great toe metatarsophalangeal joint: a review of flexible silicone implant arthroplasty from two medical centers. Clin Orthop 157:64, 1981
2. Shiel WC, Jason M: Granulomatous, inguinal lymphadenopathy after bilateral metatarsophalangeal joint silicone arthroplasty. Foot Ankle 6:216, 1986
3. Swanson AB, Lumsden RM, Swanson GD: Silicone implant arthroplasty of the great toe: a review of single stem and flexible hinge implants. Clin Orthop 142:30, 1979

Dorsal Bunion

144

Craig E. Blum

The dorsal bunion is a pathologic deformity of the great toe characterized by dorsiflexion of the first metatarsal and plantar flexion of the first metatarsophalangeal joint (Fig. 144-1). With regular footwear, prominence of the first metatarsal head produces a painful dorsal exostosis. In addition, symptoms develop in the forefoot lateral to the first ray, due to the loss of the prime weight-bearing function of the distal first metatarsal (Fig. 144-2). An abnormal painful gait ensues.

The etiology of this condition is usually one of two types of muscular imbalance, although other causes have also been noted (Table 144-1). In the first, and more frequent, of the types, there is over-pull of the anterior tibial muscle relative to a weak, paralyzed, or transferred peroneus longus (Fig. 144-3). Dorsiflexion of the first metatarsal is compensated for by plantar flexion at the metatarsophalangeal joint; contractures of the joint capsules and the flexor hallucis brevis ensue.

In the second type of imbalance, overpull of the flexors to the great toe leads to a primary plantar-flexion contracture of the first metatarsophalangeal joint with dorsiflexion of the first metatarsal occurring secondarily. In cases of hallux rigidus associated with a dorsal bunion, a "voluntary" muscle imbalance occurs when dorsiflexion of the first metatarsophalangeal joint is painful due to articular cartilage degeneration. The patient maintains the joint in flexion to avoid pain, and the plantar capsule contracts. The first metatarsal dorsiflexes secondarily, and degenerative spur formation spreads dorsally.

Evaluation of the patient with a dorsal bunion requires a careful history and a detailed physical examination in order to fully understand the etiologic factors involved and to plan a treatment program. Anteroposterior and lateral radiographs should be obtained with the patient standing before surgical correction is attempted (Fig. 144-4).

4123

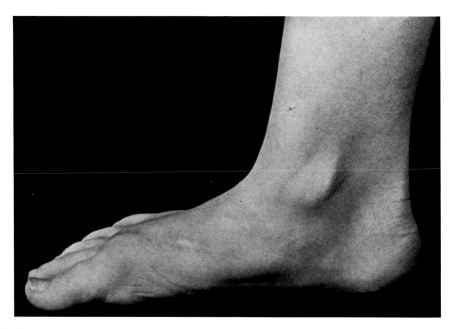

Fig. 144-1. Clinical appearance of dorsal bunion deformity resulting from malunion of metatarsal osteotomy.

Only after the sites of pain have been located, and the magnitude of deformity, the gait, degree of contracture, neurologic balance, and osteology have been assessed for a particular patient can a logical management program be formulated.

MANAGEMENT

The indications for orthopaedic treatment of the dorsal bunion include persistent pain, gait deterioration, difficulty in fitting with footwear, and cosmesis.

Nonoperative Treatment

Nonoperative treatment is generally ineffective except in patients with mild deformities, or it is unacceptable because of cost or for cosmetic reasons. It consists of the use of analgesics, anti-inflammatory agents, customized shoe wear, and curtailment of activity level. It is best not to tarry with

these therapies except in patients with mild deformity, or when an operation is not feasible, since well-planned and executed operative correction is generally gratifying and permanent. Contraindications to operative correction include the nonambulatory patient, continuing progression of the neurologic deficit causing muscular imbalance, or poor local conditions for wound healing.

Operative Treatment

In all attempts at operative correction, one must address the muscular imbalance as well as the fixed deformity for optimal results. Those patients in whom the deformity is not related to an imbalance can be treated in a more straightforward fashion. Thus, the dorsal bunion associated with hallux rigidus is best corrected by the standard methods of fusion or arthroplasty preferred for primary treatment of hallux rigidus. Similarly, malunion at the first metatarsal, secondary to trauma or poorly controlled osteotomy, is rather easily treated by corrective osteotomy with appropriate repositioning and fixation.[2] The dorsal bunion associated with another primary or secondary foot deformity must

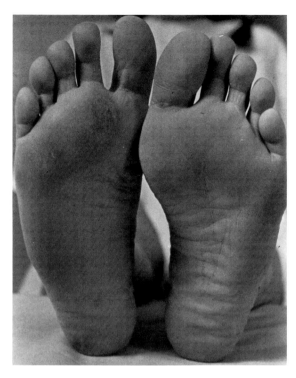

Fig. 144-2. Plantar view of same patient with dorsal bunion on the right foot, revealing abnormal callus pattern under metatarsal heads. No weight is being borne by the first metatarsal head, while the lateral rays are subjected to abnormally high stresses with resultant pain and reactive callus formation.

Table 144-1. Dorsal Bunion Etiologic Classification

Etiology	Underlying Condition
Muscle imbalance	
Overpull of the tibialis anterior vs. the peroneus longus	Neurologic disease (flaccid and spastic
	Posttraumatic
Overpull of the great toe plantar flexors	Iatrogenic (i.e., injudicious tendon transfers)
Associated with hallux rigidus	Arthritis
Associated with congenital and/or paralytic foot deformity	Clubfoot Rocker-bottom foot Cavus foot
Secondary to malunion of the first metatarsal	Posttraumatic Following osteotomy for metatarsus primus varus
Sequelae of a local disease	Infection Tumor Inflammation

have its correction integrated into the overall management of the entire problem.

For a dorsal bunion resulting from muscle imbalance, the following surgical corrections are available.

Surgical Technique — Hammond

Preoperatively, the underlying muscular imbalance must be identified. Most commonly, this imbalance is related to the anterior tibial tendon or a

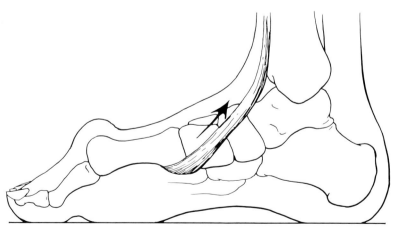

Fig. 144-3. Dorsiflexion of the first metatarsal caused by unbalanced pull of the tibialis anterior. The first metatarsophalangeal joint flexes and the dorsal aspect of the metatarsal head becomes prominent.

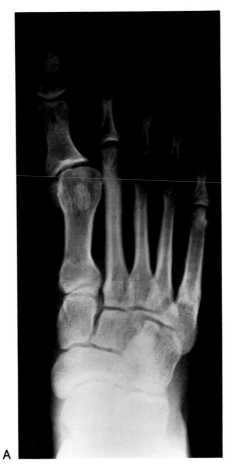

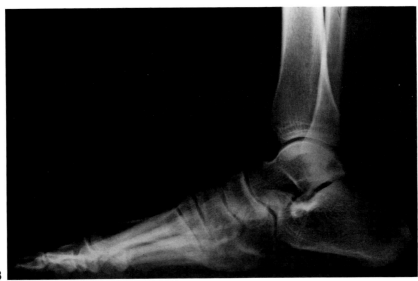

Fig. 144-4. Standing anteroposterior **(A)** and lateral **(B)** radiographs.

muscle that has been transferred to it.[1] The dorsal aspect of the foot is exposed medially from the navicular to the proximal shaft of the first metatarsal through a longitudinal skin incision. Next, the attachment of the anterior tibial tendon is freed at the first cuneiform and the first metatarsal base; in doing so, as much length as possible should be preserved. Next, the capsule of the first metatarsal-cuneiform joint is incised dorsally. If the deformity is severe, the first cuneiform-navicular joint should also be exposed. The articular cartilage is then removed. The first metatarsal is manipulated back into its normal position. Next, the wedge-shaped defect that has been created is filled with a cortico-cancellous graft obtained from the ilium (Fig. 144-5). Proper trimming of the graft can provide stable realignment. If the repositioning is not stable, fixation may be effected with Kirschner wires.

Following realignment of the first metatarsal with the arthrodesis, fixed plantar-flexion deformity at the metatarsophalangeal joint usually responds to manipulation. Occasionally, plantar capsulotomy and sectioning of the flexor hallucis brevis may be required through a separate plantar incision. With the deformity thus corrected, the anterior tibial tendon is reattached to the midpart of the foot in the midline dorsally. A separate skin incision is usually necessary. The third cuneiform is then exposed, and the tendon is passed subcutaneously to this incision. The tendon is then reinserted so that the dorsiflexion pull is neutral — that is, neither eversion nor inversion is produced. Reattachment can be made in one of two ways: through a tunnel drilled in the bone with the use of a pull-out wire; or, if the tendon is long enough, it can be sutured to itself after being routed through an osseous tunnel. The wounds are then closed in a routine fashion and a below-knee cast is applied.

Postoperative Care

The patient is allowed to stand non-weight bearing when comfortable, and discharged when proficient in ambulating with crutches. If a pull-out wire or Kirschner wires were used, they are removed after 6 weeks. Weight bearing in a below-knee cast is then allowed, and this cast is removed following

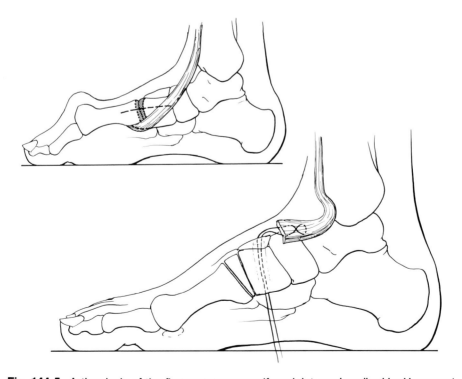

Fig. 144-5. Arthrodesis of the first metatarsocuneiform joint, as described by Hammond.

healing of the arthrodesis, normally at 8 to 10 weeks. Regular footwear is allowed thereafter.

Surgical Technique — Lapidus

For this procedure the dorsal capsule of the first metatarsophalangeal joint is exposed through a dorsomedial longitudinal incision.[3] The capsule is raised as a tongue-shaped flap based distally on the phalanx. The dorsal exostosis of the metatarsal head is excised. Next, the first cuneiform-metatarsal joint (and, if necessary, the first cuneiform-navicular joint) is exposed through a separate longitudinal incision. If there is an overactive tibialis anterior, this should be detached and translocated posteriorly into the tendon of the tibialis posterior. A wedge-shaped resection with a plantar base is performed at the first cuneiform-metatarsal joint and, if necessary, at the first cuneiform-navicular joint. Preoperative calculation of the width of the base with radiograph and cut-outs will allow for close approximation of the resected bone surfaces. At this step, simultaneous correction of a metatarsus primus varus deformity can be accomplished if necessary. Next, the flexor hallucis longus tendon is detached at its insertion and pulled into the proximal wound. An oblique tunnel is drilled into the shaft of the first metatarsal, running from distal and dorsal to proximal and plantar. The flexor hallucis longus is then passed through this tunnel and into the distal wound (Fig. 144-6). Next, the flexor hallucis brevis and the plantar capsule are subcutaneously incised at the metatarsophalangeal joint just

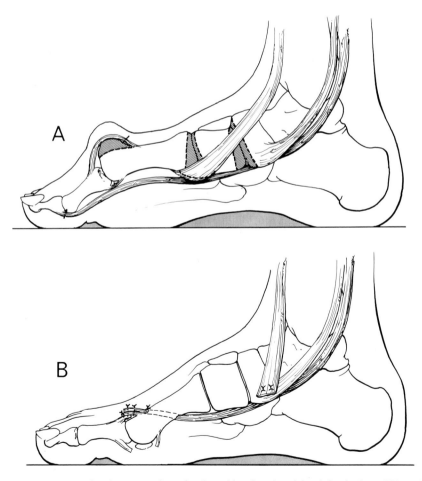

Fig. 144-6. Lapidus technique for the correction of a dorsal bunion, involving joint fusions **(A)** and relocation of the tibialis anterior **(B).**

distal to the sesamoids. Closure is begun by repairing the dorsal capsule of the first metatarsophalangeal joint in an overlapping "vest-over-pants" manner, with the joint held in a few degrees of dorsiflexion. The distal end of the transplanted flexor hallucis longus tendon is anchored into the repaired capsule, thereby reinforcing it. Also, the tendon is sutured to the periosteum where it exits the tunnel dorsally. The skin is closed in standard fashion and a well-molded, well-padded below-knee cast is applied with the foot in the corrected position.

Postoperative Care

When comfortable, the patient is allowed to stand on crutches, non-weight bearing, and is discharged when proficient with crutches. After 2 weeks, the cast is removed and the wound is inspected. The sutures are removed and a below-knee weight-bearing cast that allows dorsiflexion of the great toe is applied. Full weight bearing is allowed in this cast, which is continued until the arthrodesis sites have united at about 8 to 10 weeks. The cast is removed to allow regular shoe wear and gradual reconditioning thereafter.

Surgical Technique — LeLièvre

For mild deformity, the base of the first metatarsal is exposed through a medial incision.[4] A triangular wedge of bone based plantarly is excised and the osteotomy site coapted with a suture or Kirschner wire. When there is significant contracture at the metatarsophalangeal joint, it is exposed through a

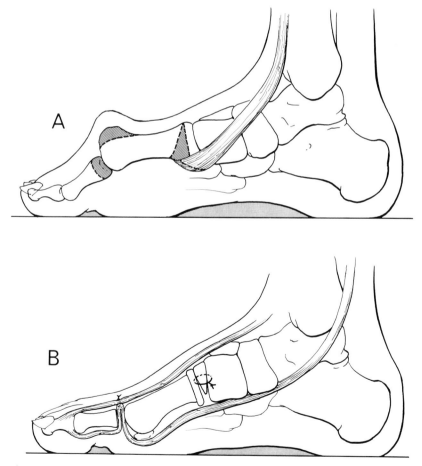

Fig. 144-7. LeLièvre's options for correction of a dorsal bunion, involving metatarsal osteotomy **(A)** and tendon transfer **(B).**

longitudinal dorsomedial incision. The dorsal exostosis as well as the base of the proximal phalanx is excised. If greater correction is required to realign the first metatarsal, the bone removed from the proximal phalanx may be used as a graft, substituting arthrodesis at the first metatarsal-cuneiform joint for metatarsal osteotomy (Fig. 144-7A). The realignment this produces may again be held with a suture or Kirschner wire. Following this, muscular imbalance is restored as follows: for relative overpull of the anterior tibial tendon, the tendon is transferred laterally to the midline; for relative overpull of the flexor hallucis longus, the muscle is sutured to the extensor hallucis longus as a combined great toe dorsiflexion force and interpositional arthroplasty at the first metatarsophalangeal joint level (Fig. 144-7B). Routine capsular and skin closures are performed, and a well-molded, below-knee cast is applied with the foot in the corrected position.

Postoperative Care

The skin sutures are removed after 2 weeks, and the Kirschner wires, if used, are taken out after 6 weeks. Weight bearing in the cast is permitted after 6 weeks and all immobilization is discontinued after osseous union occurs 8 to 10 weeks postoperatively.

placed in the midline anteriorly when using it to substitute for the tibialis anterior. Due to these more refined procedures and the decline in patients with poliomyelitis around the world, the dorsal bunion is an infrequently seen deformity. The preferred treatment is corrective osteotomy of the base of the first metatarsal. The procedure is relatively simple and does not sacrifice joint motion. Muscular balance must be restored, most often by lateral transfer of the anterior tibial tendon to the midline. Contracture of the first metatarsophalangeal joint is treated by plantar capsulotomy and release of the flexor hallucis brevis. Contracture of the flexor hallucis longus usually responds to stretching; however, fractional lengthening at the musculotendinous junction can be performed in conjunction with metatarsal osteotomy when necessary. If severe contractures exist at the metatarsal-cuneiform-navicular level, these will need to be released; if the contractures are particularly severe, wedge resection and arthrodesis may be required instead of metatarsal osteotomy. If no fixed contractures are present, osteotomy is not needed and operative restoration of muscle imbalance alone will correct an early deformity.

DISCUSSION

In the past, many cases of dorsal bunion have been the result of injudicious transfer of the peroneus longus tendon. This complication can be avoided by transferring the anterior tibial tendon to the midline when transferring the peroneus longus posteriorly. The peroneus longus should be

REFERENCES

1. Hammond G: Elevation of the fist metatarsal bone with hallux equinus. Surgery 13:240, 1943
2. Lambrinudi C: Metatarsus primus elevatus. Proc R Soc Med 31:1273, 1938
3. Lapidus PW: "Dorsal bunion": its mechanics and operative correction. J Bone Joint Surg 22:627, 1940
4. LeLièvre J: Pathologie du pied. 4th Ed. Masson, Paris, 1971

Bunionette

145

Henry R. Cowell

The term *bunionette* has been used to refer to a prominence of the fifth metatarsal head on the lateral side of the foot.[8] This prominence occurs in most individuals but seldom causes symptoms. The normal fifth metatarsal deviates from the fourth metatarsal by approximately 5 degrees. In addition, the fifth metatarsal head is generally broader than the shaft of the metatarsal itself and therefore causes a prominence on the lateral side of the foot. In a normal infant, the phalanges of the fifth toe are aligned on the metatarsal shaft. However, in most adults a medial deviation of the phalanges is seen on the metatarsals, thus making the metatarsal head even more prominent.

Davies[2] noted that the outer border of the foot is seldom prolonged straightforward along the little toe, but rather that the head of the fifth metatarsal interrupts this line by protruding outward, and that the axis of the little toe protrudes inward. He also noted that most feet have a bunionette, but that the degree of symptoms varies greatly. When the lateral portion of the metatarsal head is irritated by chronic pressure from shoes, a soft tissue bursa develops over the fifth metatarsal head and thick callusing of the skin results. This area becomes painful, is markedly tender, and is called a bunionette

or tailor's bunion. (The term *tailor's bunion* results from the assumption that tailors sit with their legs crossed, putting pressure on the outer borders of their feet,[4] causing hypertrophy of the callus over the fifth metatarsal head.[5]) Symptoms from this normal prominence of the fifth metatarsal head are commonly seen in conjunction with pes planus, hallux valgus, and splaying of the forepart of the foot.

INDICATIONS

While the condition is seen frequently, surgical treatment is seldom indicated. A bunionette usually can be treated by wearing an adequate shoe that has sufficient room over the area of the prominence. A leather shoe may be stretched in this area with an instrument called a swan to relieve the pressure. A mole-skin donut may also be placed over the callus to absorb pressure from the shoe and thus relieve stress on the tender callous area.

The indications for operation are limited. The only patients who should be considered for an operation are those who have painful tender calluses over the fifth metatarsal head that have been unrelieved by conservative methods. Surgical treatment of bunionettes is seldom required when there are no other problems in the foot, but is occasionally indicated in conjunction with repair of a bunion deformity of the first toe.

METHODS OF TREATMENT

Operative options include simple removal of the exostosis, removal of a portion of the metatarsal head combined with excision of a portion of the proximal phalanx, osteotomy of the metatarsal head, osteotomy of the metatarsal base,[7] resection of a portion of the fifth metatarsal, or complete ray resection. The method of treatment I prefer is removal of the prominent portion of the fifth metatarsal head, along with removal of a portion of the proximal phalanx (Fig. 145-1). This is a simple operative procedure which may be performed by itself or as a part of the repair of a hallux valgus. I have been pleased with the results of this procedure and, while other investigators have reported only temporary relief, I have not found it necessary to perform more extensive procedures. If the patient fails to respond to simple removal of the exostosis, then resection of a portion of the fifth meta-

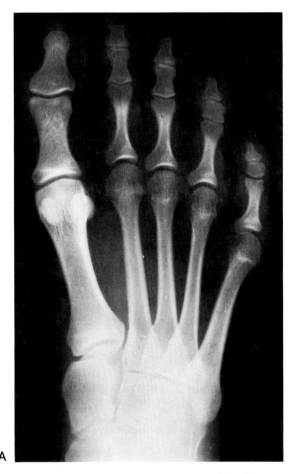
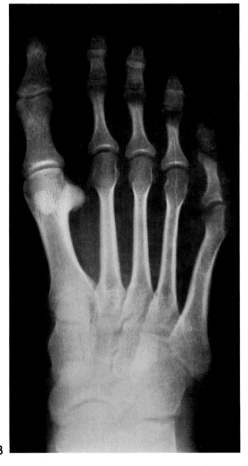

A   B

Fig. 145-1. (A) Preoperative radiograph of a patient with bunionette. Note the prominence of the metatarsal head and proximal phalanx. Soft tissue swelling may be seen. **(B)** Postoperative radiograph showing removal of a portion of the metatarsal head and the prominent portion of the condyle of the proximal phalanx.

tarsal may be considered. Osteotomy at the base of the fifth metatarsal head has also been reported to have good results by Leach and Igou.[6] Diebold and Bejjani[3] reported good early results at 1 year with basal osteotomy of the fifth metatarsal. Sponsel[10] reported satisfactory results in 27 patients treated with a distal oblique osteotomy of the metatarsal neck, but 11 patients had a delayed union that although mostly asymptomatic, persisted for as long as 2 years. Removal of the fifth digit, as described by Brown,[1] is mentioned for the sake of completeness, but I do not recommend this procedure.

Surgical Technique — McKeever

A straight dorsal incision is made over the metatarsal shaft from the midshaft of the metatarsal to the base of the proximal phalanx.[9] This incision is carried down through the subcutaneous tissue, lateral to the extensor tendon. The fifth metatarsal is approached and the periosteum split on the dorsal surface. A periosteal elevator is used to shell out the fifth metatarsal from the midpoint of the metatarsal shaft down to and including the metatarsal head. Sharp dissection may be necessary to release the collateral ligaments of the metatarsal phalangeal joint. After the fifth metatarsal has been dissected, an osteotome is driven across the metatarsal in an oblique fashion to resect the distal two-thirds of the metatarsal. The bone is cut at approximately a 45-degree angle from proximal to distal, laterally to medially. The periosteum and soft tissue are closed with sutures of 000 chromic catgut, and the skin is closed with 000 nylon. A pressure dressing is applied. The patient may ambulate in a below-knee weight-bearing cast or a postoperative shoe 10 days following the procedure.

McKeever noted that the operation was successful in 38 patients who had the procedure performed on 60 feet (22 bilateral). He stated that the only patients who had difficulty were ones in whom a sufficient amount of the metatarsal was not removed. During the early part of his series, he noted that he removed less of the metatarsal and that he had more satisfactory results when he removed at least half of the metatarsal. He also noted that the fifth toe retracted from 0.5 to 0.75 cm but that this caused no difficulty.

Surgical Technique — Leach and Igou

A dorsal-curvolinear incision is made from the metatarsal phalangeal joint, over the metatarsal head to the midpoint of the metatarsal shaft. The bone is encountered and the dorsal periosteum incised. Following this, a periosteal elevator is used to dissect subperiosteally around the neck of the metatarsal. Two small holes are drilled approximately 5 mm proximal and distal to the proposed osteotomy site, which should be located approximately 1.5 cm from the metatarsal phalangeal joint (Fig. 145-2). Two parallel osteotomy cuts are planned perpendicular to the long axis of the metatarsal shaft, and located midway between the two drill holes. The distal cut is made ¾ of the way across the bone from the lateral side. A 3-mm (⅛-inch) osteotome is used to make a second cut in a proximal direction at 90 degrees from the distal cut at its medial end. The bone is then divided by an osteotomy across the entire shaft 3 mm proximal to the first cut. Thus, a small edge of bone is left on the

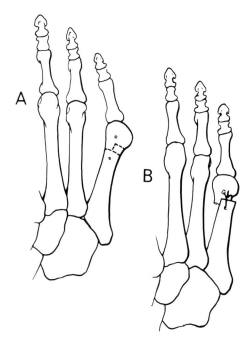

Fig. 145-2. (A) Mitchell-type osteotomy as described by Leach and Igou[6] for bunionette deformity. **(B)** Corrected position.

medial side of the metatarsal head fragment. These cuts are made in a fashion similar to Hammond's[5] description of the Mitchell osteotomy for the first toe. The head is displaced medially, and a 00 chromic catgut suture is inserted through the drill holes and used to secure the osteotomy once it has been displaced medially. Care must be taken to ensure that the metatarsal head does not tilt dorsally. Forward displacement will result in increased pressure on weight bearing. Leach and Igou report that it is seldom necessary to remove any of the lateral aspect of the fifth metatarsal or the bursum. Following displacement, any bone prominent on the lateral aspect of the proximal shaft should be removed with a rongeur or rasp.

Postoperatively, the patient is placed in a below-knee cast and allowed gradual weight bearing with a walking boot and crutches. The cast remains in place for 6 weeks. Leach and Igou reported good results in eight patients who underwent eleven operative procedures (three bilateral). They reported no complications in their series. The authors suggest that the operation is particularly valuable in patients who have an angulation of greater than 9 degrees between the fourth and fifth metatarsals.

Surgical Technique — Diebold and Bejjani

Two 0.8-mm smooth Kirschner wires, placed one centimeter apart, are inserted into the midshaft of the metatarsal, perpendicular to the shaft. The tip of the wire is placed just through the medial cortex and the tips of the wires are cut 5 cm from the skin. A 4-cm skin incision is made on the dorsolateral surface of the foot, beginning 1 cm distal to the styloid process of the fifth metatarsal and proceeding distally just lateral to the shaft of the metatarsal. The sural nerve is visualized and retracted dorsally. The lateral metaphysis of the metatarsal is exposed 1 cm distal to the insertion of the peroneal brevis tendon. A chevron cut is then marked on the lateral surface of the metatarsal, the apex of the cut directed toward the base of the metatarsal with a distal angle of 60 degrees. The lateral cortex is cut, and the osteotomy is completed in the transverse plane through the medial cortex. Correction is obtained by pivoting the shaft in this plane, and fixation maintained by advancing the wires through the shaft of the fourth metatarsal. If a prominent edge projects laterally from the distal fragment, it is resected and used as a bone graft in the osteotomy site. The metatarsal head may be shifted dorsally, or plantarward, by inserting the graft in the plantar, or dorsal aspect of the chevron osteotomy. The subcutaneous tissue is closed with sutures of 000 plain catgut and the skin closed with sutures of 000 nylon. A below-knee cast is applied and maintained for 4 weeks, at which time radiographs are obtained. The wires are removed if bony union has occurred, or left in place for an additional 2 weeks if it has not. Partial weight bearing, as tolerated, is permitted after the wires have been removed. The patient can usually resume normal activities within 3 months.

Author's Preferred Technique

The procedure involves excision of the lateral portion of the metatarsal head and the lateral portion of the proximal phalanx. A 2-cm skin incision is made on the dorsal aspect of the foot over the fifth metatarsal head and the base of the proximal phalanx. Care must be taken to place this incision so that the side of the shoe will not press on the incision postoperatively. Following incision through the skin and subcutaneous tissue, the bone is approached and the dorsal lateral periosteum is incised over the metatarsal head and the base of the proximal phalanx. A Freer periosteal elevator is used to dissect the periosteum from the metatarsal head and the base of the proximal phalanx. A ½-inch Hoke osteotome is driven from proximally to distally parallel to the shaft of the metatarsal. That portion of the metatarsal head which is lateral to the metatarsal shaft is then removed in one piece. The prominent portion of the phalanx is also removed with a Hoke osteotome. Following irrigation of the wound, the periosteum is approximated with sutures of 4-0 chromic catgut, the subcutaneous tissue closed with 000 plain catgut, and the skin with sutures of 000 interrupted nylon. A soft dressing is applied.

The patient may ambulate in a cast shoe or a weight-bearing cast on the third postoperative day. The only complication noted from simple removal of a portion of the fifth metatarsal head has been recurrence of the deformity. This is not common in the author's experience. McKeever[9] has also reported subluxation of the metatarsal phalangeal joint following resection of a large portion of the metatarsal head. He suggests that the procedure which he describes is preferable to this, particularly if there is also a callus present under the base of the fifth metatarsal.

REFERENCES

1. Brown JE: Functional and cosmetic correction of metatarsus latus (splay foot). Clin Orthop 14:166, 1959
2. Davies H: Metatarsus quintus valgus. Br Med J 1:664, 1949
3. Diebold PF, Bejjani FJ: Basal osteotomy of the fifth metatarsal with intermetatarsal pinning: a new approach to tailor's bunion. Foot Ankle 8:40, 1987
4. Giannestras NJ: Foot Disorders: Medical and Surgical Management. 2nd. Ed. Lea & Febiger, Philadelphia, 1973
5. Hammond G: Mitchell osteotomy-bunion-ectomy for hallux valgus and metatarsus primus varus. p. 246. In American Academy of Orthopaedic Surgeons. Instructional Course Lectures. Vol. 21. CV Mosby, St. Louis, 1972
6. Leach RE, Igou R: Metatarsal osteotomy for bunionette deformity. Clin Orthop 100:171, 1974
7. LeLièvre J: Pathologie du Pied. 4th Ed. Masson & Cie, Paris, 1971
8. Margo MK: Surgical treatment of conditions of the fore part of the foot. J Bone Joint Surg 49A:1665, 1967
9. McKeever DC: Excision of the fifth metatarsal head. Clin Orthop 13:321, 1959
10. Sponsel KH: Bunionette correction by metatarsal osteotomy. Preliminary report. Orthop Clin North Am 7:809, 1976

Claw Toes

146

Bruce K. Foster

Claw toe deformities are characterized by hyperextension of the metatarsophalangeal joints and flexion of the interphalangeal joints. In relationship to new pressure areas, painful callosities develop under the heads of the metatarsals, the tips of the toes, and over the dorsum of the proximal interphalangeal joints, causing symptoms. All the toes are usually affected, although great toe claw deformity is often the most severe.

Claw toes occur commonly in association with neuropathic conditions such as Friedreich's ataxia, polio, and spinal cord injury. There is also an association with myopathic conditions such as peroneal muscle atrophy. There is often a positive family history for the deformity. The initiating mechanism of deformity remains unknown.

The position of the proximal phalanx at the metatarsophalangeal joint is subject to the antagonistic action of the extensors and intrinsic flexors—the lumbricals and the interosseous muscles. The common explanation for claw toes is paralysis of the intrinsic muscles of the foot with subsequent muscle imbalance. In 1951, Taylor[15] observed in surgery that the intrinsic muscles appeared normal and reacted normally to physical stimulation, and that biopsy showed no evidence of degeneration.

Ineffectiveness of the intrinsic flexors has been attributed to a shift of the line of action dorsal to the transverse axis of the movement of the metatarsophalangeal joints.[8] Scheck,[12] in 1977, was unable to demonstrate this shift in cadaver dissections despite extensive dorsiflexion of the toes. The etiology, therefore, remains unknown, but association of this deformity with other conditions should be considered in patient assessment and management.

METHODS OF TREATMENT

Operative treatment for claw toe deformity should not be undertaken unless conservative measures have failed to give relief from symptoms due to the pressure of shoes on painful callosities. Such conservative measures include passive stretching, faradic stimulation of the intrinsic muscles, active exercises, adequate trimming of callosities, and appropriate shoe modification.

Metatarsal bars and reverse heel pads may be particularly beneficial. Haines and McDougall[6] described the continuous band of the plantar aponeurosis that extends from the calcaneus to the proximal phalanges and transmits a pull when under tension. In weight bearing, the toes are plantar-flexed by the tensing of the plantar aponeurosis. Some of the benefits derived from metatarsal bars and reverse heel pads may be due to the fact that these mechanical aids increase the tension of the plantar aponeurosis.[12]

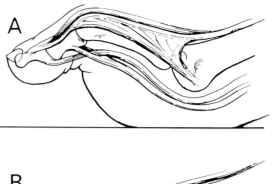

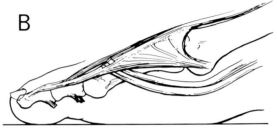

Fig. 146-1. Girdlestone-Taylor tendon transfer for correction of claw toes. **(A)** Preoperative deformity. **(B)** The tendons of both long and short toe flexors after being transferred to the extensor expansions.

SURGICAL PROCEDURES

In 1922, Stiles and Forrester-Brown[14] described the transfer of the sublimis flexor tendons into the extensor of the fingers to counteract intrinsic paralysis. Forrester-Brown,[3] in 1938, applied the same principle to the claw deformity of the great toe. Taylor,[15] in 1951, reported that Girdlestone first suggested transfer of the long flexors into the dorsal expansion of the extensor tendons to assume the function of the intrinsics in producing active plantar flexion of the metatarsophalangeal joint. In this operative method, both long and short flexors are transferred (Fig. 146-1).

Taylor's report indicated that in 38 patients with associated cavus, 27 obtained good results, 5 had some difficulty because of one or more toes with residual deformity, and 6 showed poor results. Of 23 patients with valgus foot, 21 had good results, 1 fair, and 1 poor. Of 7 patients with claw toes, only 2 were good, 4 fair, and 1 poor. Pyper,[11] in 1958, was not as encouraging, with an overall finding of 60 percent stiffness (Figs. 146-1, 146-2) of toes and 20 percent regeneration of the extensor tendons and recurrence of deformity. Newman and Fitton,[10] in 1979, recommend the procedure only in children.

Clawing of the Lateral Toes

Surgical Technique — Girdlestone-Taylor[15]

The first step is to correct fixed deformity by manual stretching. Using tourniquet control, a 2.5-cm mid-lateral incision is made on the lateral side of the toe from the metatarsal neck to the distal interphalangeal joint. The neurovascular bundle is protected plantarward. The extensor expansion is defined and the long and short flexors caught with a small, blunt hook and divided at their insertions. These are then brought around the lateral side of the proximal phalanx and sutured to the extensor expansion over the interphalangeal joint. For the little toe a medial incision prevents a painful scar. In modifying this technique I have found that the same result may be obtained by transfer of the long flexor only. This enables less bulk to the dorsal transfer position in the extensor.

When dorsal capsulotomy of the metatarsophalangeal joints or interphalangeal plantar capsulotomy is necessary, the capules should be divided prior to suturing the rerouted tendons. Z-plasty elongation of the extensor tendon may also be necessary if the tendon proves too tight.

A modified Lambrinudi splint and stay suture around the proximal phalanx have been recommended by Taylor to immobilize the toes in this corrected position, but a well-padded plaster boot cast carefully molded over the toes will maintain position without use of the splint; this cast is applied while holding the foot in dorsiflexion by pressure and elevation of the transverse metatarsal arch. A felt pad is placed over the gauze dressing on the dorsal surface of the toes. Toe tips are left uncovered to observe circulation.

The operative intention is to correct all fixed deformities. Elongation of extensor tendons, dorsal capsulotomy of the metatarsophalangeal joints, and plantar capsulotomy of the interphalangeal joints should be done without hesitation.

Postoperatively, elevation is very important and must be maintained until the patient can comfortably hold the feet in a dependent position. This is usually within the first 2 to 3 days. Mobilization and full weight bearing are encouraged as soon as possible. After 6 weeks, the casts and sutures are removed. Metatarsal bars, inner soles, or specific exercises are usually not necessary.

Alternative Surgical Techniques (for Nonfixed Deformity)

The long flexor tendon can be tenotomized through a short incision on the plantar surface of the toe and the proximal phalanx. This reinforces the active flexion of the metatarsophalangeal joint and distal alignment. To protect the neurovascular bundle and ensure complete tendon division I prefer to openly divide the flexor tendons through the midlateral toe incision as previously described.

Alternatively, beginning distally at the level of the metatarsal joints, a 4- to 5-cm skin incision is made dorsally between both the second and third, and the fourth and fifth metatarsals. The medial edges of these incisions are retracted and by a long Z-plasty incision, and the long extensor tendons divided. The dorsal capsule of the second and fourth metatarsophalangeal joints are exposed and completely resected. The joint positions are then forcibly overcorrected. The lateral skin edges are retracted and the procedure repeated on the third and fifth rays. The tendons should not be sutured. The deformity will recur if percutaneous tenotomy is performed without attention to the metatarsophalangeal joint capsule.

Postoperatively, the corrected position is maintained with a bulky cotton and gauze bandage with individual cotton wool strips separating the toes, and a dorsal dressing over the proximal phalanx held by a 1-inch noncompressive ribbon gauze bandage over the toes and forefoot. The patient is mobilized fully, permitted to bear weight as pain allows, and reviewed in 3 weeks for change of dressing and removal of sutures. A similar dressing with toes held in corrected position is maintained for a total of 6 weeks. The total time before normal shoe wear is permitted averages 3 months.

Fixed Claw Toe Deformity

As the patient becomes older, joint deformities may be increasingly difficult to overcome, placing the claw toes in the same treatment classification as the degenerative hammer toe deformity. Shortening of the toe must be undertaken to allow adequate relaxation of contracted tendon and ligament structures. The technique of DuVries is described for this condition, since it has the advantage of simplicity and is atraumatic.

DuVries Technique

A 0.5-cm-wide eye-shaped transverse incision is made over the proximal joint prominence (Fig. 146-2). The skin and subcutaneous tissue are excised, and the tendon and joint capsule are exposed by sharp dissection. A section of tendon and capsule are removed along the outline of the original incision. The head of the proximal phalanx is exposed by division of the collateral ligaments of the joint. If the distal joint is involved, then the head of the middle phalanx is exposed. The head of the proximal phalanx (or middle phalanx in the case of the distal joint) is freed by superiosteal elevation with sharp dissection, incising the capsule on both sides of the joint. Using a small pair of bone-cutting forceps, the head of the bone is amputated across the sulci, which are present on each side of the head. The cut surface is smoothed with a rasp. The margins are sutured with a mattress suture so that the base of the stitch includes the capsule and tendon and the apex includes only the skin. Occasionally, a tenotomy and capsulotomy at the metatarso-

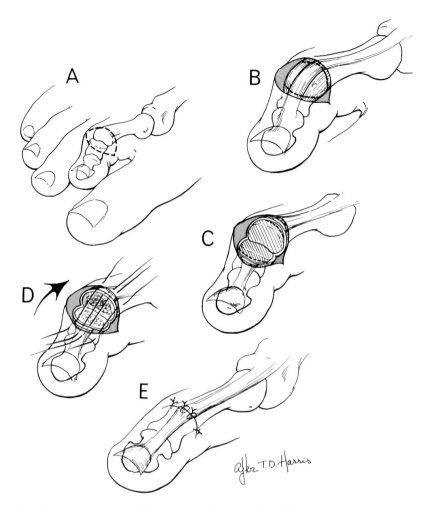

after T.D.Harris

Fig. 146-2. (A–E) DuVries' recommended procedure for correction of hammered second, third, and fourth toes involves removal of sections of the tendon and capsule and amputation of the head of the proximal phalanx and the base of the middle phalanx. (Redrawn from Mann.[9])

phalangeal joint are necessary so that the toe will lie flat.

The postoperative technique is as described in the previous section. DuVries recommended a cradle-gauze bandage, but this has a potential tourniquet effect on the toes and is difficult to apply.

Many other procedures have also been offered for the correction of the rigid claw or the C hammer toe deformity. Figure 146-3 shows the surgical options outlined by DuVries. Glassman et al.[5] advised total phalangectomy, and Newman and Fitton[10] reaffirm that suggestion.

Clawing of the Great Toe

Surgical Technique — DuVries

When the deformity is not fixed and can be reduced passively, this procedure involves tenodesis and shortening of the extensors and dorsal capsule of the interphalangeal joint. The tendon and capsule are sectioned on the plantar surface of the phalangeal joint through a medioplantar incision, to permit immediate reduction of deformity. To maintain reduction, a longitudinal incision is made over the dorsum of the phalangeal joint; a trans-

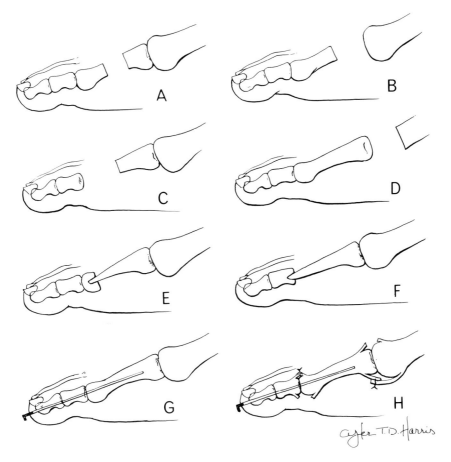

Fig. 146-3. Surgical options outlined by DuVries. **(A–E)** Excision techniques. **(F, G)** Arthrodesis. **(H)** Soft tissue release using a Kirschner wire. (Redrawn from Mann.[9])

verse oval section about 0.5 cm in width is removed from the dorsophalangeal capsule and tendon of the extensor hallucis longus. The dorsal capsule and tendon of the extensor hallucis longus are sutured in the shortened position, and then the skin is sutured. The toe is partly immobilized by adhesive splinting for 2 to 3 weeks. This splinting is achieved by bandaging the great toe to the three adjacent toes and carrying the bandage over all the metatarsophalangeal joints.

Surgical Technique — Dickson-Diveley

The Dickson-Diveley technique is recommended when fixed clawing of the great toe persists after appropriate foot stabilization and tendon transfer for insufficiency of the plantar flexors of the ankle.[1]

To proceed, the flexor hallucis longus tendon is exposed through a medioplantar incision at the level of the metatarsophalangeal joint (Fig. 146-4). The tendon is grasped with forceps proximally and placed under tension, and the metatarsophalangeal and interphalangeal joints flexed acutely. Through a second direct dorsal incision from the base of the first metatarsal to the first phalanx along the extensor hallucis longus, the extensor hallicus longus is divided just proximal to the interphalangeal joint. A subcutaneous tunnel is made medially between these incisions and the proximal end of the extensor tendon rerouted to the plantar aspect of the joint.

Under tension, the extensor is attached to the

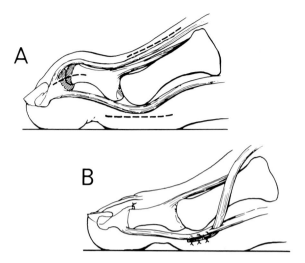

Fig. 146-4. (A, B) Dickson-Diveley procedure for clawing of the great toe involves tendon transfer and arthrodesis. (Redrawn from Dickson and Dively.[1])

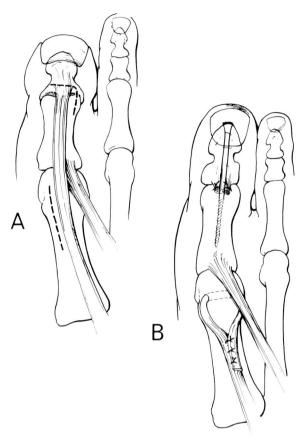

Fig. 146-5. (A, B) Jones transfer of the extensor hallucis longus to the first metatarsal, showing immobilization of the distal interphalangeal joint with an AO cancellous lag screw to secure arthrodesis.

taunt flexor tendon with 4-0 nylon sutures. Finally, arthrodesis of the interphalangeal joint is done with resection of the surfaces of the joint to permit arthrodesis with the joint in a neutral position. The approach to arthrodesis can be through a separate incision medially, although this will cause discomfort with shoe wear. A separate L-shaped dorsomedial incision will prevent contracture over the metatarsophalangeal joint that continuation of the second dorsal incision could involve. After arthrodesis, the short part of the extensor tendon should be sutured to the soft tissues on the dorsum of the proximal phalanx to assist in maintaining apposition of the right joint surfaces.

Kirschner wire fixation, cut off just under the skin, has been recommended to supplement the maintenance of joint position.

Surgical Technique — Jones

When clawing of the great toe is caused by insufficiency of the dorsiflexor of the ankle and contracture of the Achilles tendon, where there is a fixed rigid deformity, Jones[2,7] technique for transference of the extensor hallucis longus to the first metatarsal and interphalangeal arthrodesis offers the best results (Fig. 146-5).

Arthrodesis of the interphalangeal joint is performed as described above, dividing the extensor

hallucis longus at the joint level. A second longitudinal incision is made dorsomedially along the extensor hallucis longus tendon for 2.5 cm, extending distally to the level of the proximal extensor skin crease. The extensor hallucis longus tendon is dissected free to limit possible regrowth of the extensor hallucis longus. The neck of the first metatarsal is then exposed. Initially, a 2- to 3-mm hole is drilled from the inferomedial aspect transversely to the long axis of the bone to emerge on the dorsolateral aspect. According to tendon size, this hole may need to be widened. A stainless steel wire is threaded through the end of the previously freed tendon with a straight needle. The needle is passed through the drill hole and the tendon guided through it. The end of the tendon is sutured to itself with interrupted sutures on the dorsum of the first metatarsal shaft. Judgment of the correct tension for suture is critical to the success of the procedure and is measured as the amount of tension required to hold the first metatarsal in a neutral position at 90 degrees of ankle dorsiflexion. The skin is closed and a below-knee plaster splint applied, holding the first metatarsal and great toe in the corrected position.

After wound healing is assured, physical therapy and exercises are begun to strengthen the transferred muscle. Weight immobilization is maintained for 6 weeks. In the case of Kirschner wire fixation, internal fixation should be removed when arthrodesis is solid.

Author's Preferred Technique for Interphalangeal Arthrodesis

A 4-mm AO cancellous screw with lag effect provides for a more rigid fication and will increase the achievement of successful arthrodesis by providing interfragmentary compression.[13]

First, the interphalangeal joint is exposed, the cartilage excised, and the joint surfaces fitted together. Through the L-shaped dorsal incision, a 2-mm drill bit is inserted through the distal phalanx in line with its long axis from proximally to distally. A second 10- to 15-mm-long fish-mouth incision is made through the pulp, down onto the pointing drill bit. The 2-mm drill bit is removed and, without using the drill, the bit is inserted through the tip of the toe into the predrilled distal phalanx. The joint is reduced and the position checked. The drill is advanced into the proximal phalanx and then removed, and the screw length measured. Then the fragments are fixed with a 4.0-mm lag cancellous screw that provides interfragmentary compression. It is not necessary to pretap the screw.

It should be noted that arthrodesis of the interphalangeal joint may be difficult in a child because the epiphysis is largely cartilage prior to skeletal maturity. On one occasion with a good result I had to replace a broken 4.0-mm cancellous screw with a large-fragment 6.5-mm screw. Use of a malleolar screw would be an alternative method of fixation (Sutherland AD: Personal communication).

REFERENCES

1. Dickson FD, Diveley RL: Operation for correction of mild claw-foot, the result of infantile paralysis. JAMA 87:1275, 1926
2. Edmonson AS, Crenshaw AH (eds): Campbell's Operative Orthopaedics. Vol. 2. 6th Ed. CV Mosby, St. Louis, 1980
3. Forrester-Brown MF: Tendon transplantation for clawing of the great toe. J Bone Joint Surg 20:57, 1938
4. Frank GR, Johnson WM: The extensor shift procedure in the correction of clawtoe deformities in children. South Med J 59:889, 1966
5. Glassman F, Wolin I, Sideman S: Phalangectomy for toe deformities. Surg Clin North Am 29:275, 1949
6. Haines RW, McDougall A: The Anatomy of hallux valgus. J Bone Joint Surg 36B:272, 1954
7. Jones R: Notes on Military Orthopaedics. Cassell & Co., London, 1917
8. Kelikian H: Hallux Valgus, Allied Deformities of the Forefoot and Metatarsalgia. WB Saunders, Philadelphia, 1965
9. Mann RA (ed): DuVries' Surgery of the Foot. 4th Ed. CV Mosby, St. Louis, 1978
10. Newman RJ, Fitton JM: An evaluation of operative procedures in the treatment of hammer toe. Acta Orthop Scand 50:709, 1979
11. Pyper JB: The flexor-extensor transplant operation for claw toes. J Bone Joint Surg 40B:528, 1958
12. Scheck M: Etiology of acquired hammertoe deformity. Clin Orthop 123:63, 1977
13. Shives TC, Johnson KA: Arthrodesis of the interphalangeal joint of the great toe—an improved technique. Foot & Ankle 1:26, 1980
14. Stiles HJ, Forrester-Brown MF: Treatment of Injuries of the Peripheral Spiral Nerve. Oxford University Press, New York, 1922
15. Taylor RG: The treatment of claw toes by multiple transfers of flexor into extensor tendons. J Bone Joint Surg 33B:539, 1951

Interdigital Neuroma

147

Roger A. Mann

Interdigital neuroma is a frequent cause of metatarsalgia. The condition was first described by Lewis Durlacher in 1845[3] and was given the eponym Morton's neuroma following a report by Thomas G. Morton in 1876.[10] In 1892, Thomas S. K. Morton[11] confirmed the findings of Thomas G. Morton. An unrelated form of metatarsalgia was described in 1935 by Dudley J. Morton.[9] Because of this confusion of eponyms, the term *interdigital neuroma* is used here.

Patients with an interdigital neuroma will complain of a burning pain that is localized in the plantar aspect of the foot and that often radiates out to the tips of the toes of the involved interspace. Some patients will report tingling, numbness, or cramping on the plantar aspect of the foot; an occasional patient will have pain radiating to the dorsal aspect of the foot. The onset of symptoms is rarely acute. The pain is usually aggravated by activity and by tightly fitting, high-heeled shoes. It is relieved by rest and massage and returns after resumption of activity.

The causes of this condition include trauma, mechanical pressure against the transverse metatarsal ligament, enlargement of the intermetatarsal bursa, the anatomic arrangement of the nerve sup-

ply to the third interspace, mobility of the fourth metatarsal head, impingement by a synovial cyst, and vascular changes. Trauma to the plantar aspect of the foot can be localized to an interspace, producing a contusion of the common digital nerve. Thickening of the digital nerve or surrounding tissues may be aggravated by the wearing of high-heeled shoes. A synovial cyst, frequently arising from the second metatarsophalangeal joint, can push the nerve against the firm edge of the transverse metatarsal ligament and cause neuritic symptoms.

The anatomic arrangement of the nerve in the plantar aspect of the foot is such that the common digital nerve to the third interspace receives a communicating branch from the lateral plantar nerve; Winkler et al.[13] believe that this predisposes the patient to an interdigital neuroma (Fig. 147-1). The biomechanical arrangement of the foot is such that the fourth metatarsal is the most mobile, and this is readily noted upon clinical examination of the foot. T. G. Morton[10] and DuVries[4] both believed that this type of mobility may play a role in the irritation of the digital nerve to the third interspace. This increased motion of the fourth and fifth rays against the more firmly fixed third ray may

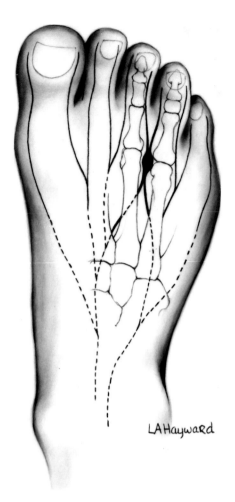

Fig. 147-1. A neuroma of the interdigital nerve may be seen between the third and fourth toes in the location of the metatarsal heads.

produce sufficient friction or irritation against the nerve to cause thickening of the tissues surrounding the nerve. This in turn could lead to irritation of the common digital nerve. Betts said in 1940[2] that the anatomic difference from other digital nerves, along with contraction of the flexor digitorum brevis, would set into motion a series of circumstances that would result in thickening of the tissues surrounding the nerve. The concept that the changes about the nerve were degenerative in nature was put forth by McElvenny in 1943[8] and by Baker and Kuhn in 1944.[1] The possibility of this

being a vascular type of degeneration was put forth by Nissen in 1948.[12]

CLINICAL EVALUATION

The most frequent complaint noted by patients with an interdigital neuroma is pain localized in the plantar aspect of the foot. The patient can usually place a finger close to the spot from which the pain emanates. The pain frequently radiates toward the tips of the toes on either side of the involved interspace. The pain is characterized as a burning type of pain by the vast majority of patients. Occasionally the patient will complain of a tingling or numb feeling on the plantar aspect of the foot. Only on rare occasions does this pain radiate proximally in the foot. Occasionally the patient will state that the pain seems to radiate to the dorsal aspect of the involved interspace. A few patients complain of a cramping feeling in the plantar aspect of the foot.

In general, the pain is aggravated by activities and by wearing shoes. The patient will often state that the looser the shoe and the lower the heel, the more comfortable the foot. Conversely, the tighter the shoe and the higher the heel, the more bothersome the symptom complex. Usually the pain is relieved by sitting down, removing the shoe, and rubbing the foot. In a few minutes, the patient can resume activities, only to have the pain recur. It is unusual for a patient with an interdigital neuroma to have significant night pain.

The onset of symptoms is gradual and may be intermittent. A few patients state they have no symptoms in the foot but will periodically step on a "lump" on the bottom of the foot, following which they feel a sharp pain on the plantar aspect of the foot that radiates toward the toes. Rarely is the onset of an interdigital neuroma acute.

The incidence of interdigital neuroma is much higher in females than in males, by a ratio of about 10 to 1. The third interspace is involved about 55 percent of the time and the second interspace about 45 percent. An interdigital neuroma of either the first or fourth interspace is rare. Two interdigital neuromas occurring simultaneously in the same foot are very uncommon. Although an interdigital neuroma can occur in almost any decade of adult life, it occurs most frequently in the fifth and sixth decades.

Some patients will have a synovial cyst associated with an interdigital neuroma. They will often initially manifest symptoms secondary to the cyst and only later on, as the cyst enlarges, will neuritic symptoms begin. The patients with a synovial cyst will complain of a squishing feeling on the plantar aspect of the foot, which may be associated with pain radiating out toward the tip of the toes.

Physical examination should permit precise localization of the neuroma and simultaneously rule out other conditions that may mimic an interdigital neuroma. By having the patient stand when examining the foot, one may determine the presence of any thickening within the involved interspace. This thickening may bulge into the interspace dorsally or may cause the toes to diverge with weight bearing, which may not be manifest when there is no pressure on the plantar aspect of the foot. The patient should then sit while the examiner carefully palpates the interspaces, beginning away from the area of the pain. Once the involved interspace is identified by reproducing the patient's pain by palpation, the metatarsal heads should be carefully palpated. In most cases, the metatarsal heads will not be sensitive, even though they are adjacent to the involved neuroma. Synovitis of the metatarsophalangeal joint or degeneration of the plantar capsule of the metatarsophalangeal joint may mimic an interdigital neuroma. For this reason, utmost care should be exercised in differentiating whether one is palpating the interspace or the metatarsal head. At times a thickening can be noted in the interspace on the plantar aspect of the foot; if a synovial cyst is present, the cyst can be rolled beneath the examiner's fingers, reproducing the squishy feeling with relative ease. Occasionally more than one interspace will be sensitive and the examiner should make every effort to ascertain which interspace is the most sensitive. If more than one interspace is sensitive, it is important to percuss over the area of the tarsal tunnel and the medial and lateral plantar nerves in order to rule out the possibility of a tarsal tunnel syndrome or a le-

sion involving the medial or lateral plantar nerve; either may mimic an interdigital neuroma. It has been my experience that significant sensory loss in the involved interspace is rare in patients with a neuroma.

A weight-bearing radiograph of the foot should be obtained to rule out bone or joint pathology.

DIFFERENTIAL DIAGNOSIS

The following conditions should be considered when evaluating a patient for an interdigital neuroma:

1. Other neuritic causes of pain
   a. Degenerative disc disease
   b. Tarsal tunnel syndrome
   c. Lesion of the medial or lateral plantar nerve
   d. Peripheral neuritis
2. Metatarsophalangeal joint pathology
   a. Synovitis of the joint, secondary to rheumatoid arthritis, nonspecific synovitis, gout, trauma, etc.
   b. Impending subluxation or dislocation of the metatarsophalangeal joint
   c. Freiberg's infraction
   d. Degenerative lesion of the plantar capsule
3. Lesions on the plantar aspect of the foot
   a. Synovial cyst
   b. Lesions not involving the metatarsophalangeal joint, such as ganglion, lipoma, or other soft tissue tumor
   c. Tumor involving a metatarsal bone

TREATMENT

The treatment of an interdigital neuroma should be directed toward relieving the pressure over the symptomatic interspace. This is best accomplished by having the patient wear a low-heeled shoe with a soft sole material. The shoe should have a round toe box to allow the foot to spread. A metatarsal support is placed in the shoe proximal to the metatarsal head to relieve pressure on the affected interspace. Occasionally, the use of an anti-inflammatory medication or even local steroids may be of benefit, although in my experience the success rate has been low.

Twenty to 30 percent of patients treated conservatively will be satisfied with this mode of treatment and their pain will subside. Most patients, however, will not be sufficiently relieved to accept this as definitive treatment and will require surgical excision of the neuroma.

Surgical Treatment

An interdigital neuroma should be excised through a dorsal approach made in the webspace which contains the neuroma. The incision is made directly in the midline so as to avoid the small superficial dorsal cutaneous nerves present on either side of the webspace (Fig. 147-2). The incision is deepened directly in the midline, following which a Weitlander retractor is placed into the wound between the metatarsal heads in order to stretch the transverse metatarsal ligament to its full length. Once this is accomplished, the transverse metatarsal ligament is cut, thereby exposing the structures beneath it, which consist of the neurovascular bundle and plantar fat. Working longitudinally in the webspace, using a neurologic freer, the nerve is readily identified just beneath the area of the transverse metatarsal ligament and traced distally and proximally. The common digital nerve should be traced proximally to the level of the neck of the metatarsal and distally past the bifurcation into its terminal branches. Once this has been accomplished, the nerve is cut sharply proximally (Fig. 147-3) and then resected distally just past its bifurcation.

If a synovial cyst coexists with the interdigital neuroma, this too can be excised through the dorsal approach. After the nerve has been removed, a search is carried out for the synovial cyst. The synovial cyst almost invariably seems to arise from the plantar aspect of the metatarsophalangeal joint. This cyst is usually poorly defined and the walls can

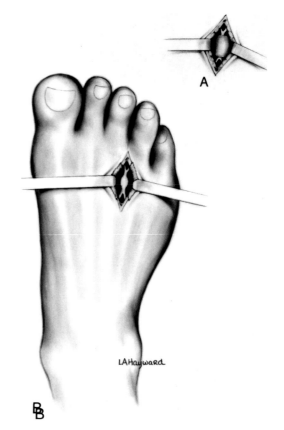

Fig. 147-2. (A) Incision showing transverse metatarsal ligament. **(B)** Incision showing exposure of neuroma.

be extremely thin and friable. An effort should be made to excise as much of the cyst as possible, but this must be tempered by the fact that we do not wish to excise too much of the plantar fat pad for fear of creating scar tissue sufficient to cause metatarsalgia.

It is interesting to note that there is occasionally a communicating branch to the common nerve trunk, which may come from either the medial or lateral side of the interspace. This more than likely represents an accessory nerve trunk. I believe that these small aberrant trunks probably cause the occasional symptomatic postoperative foot. Once the nerve has been excised, the wound is closed only at the level of the skin, a compression dressing is applied, and the patient is ambulated in a wooden-sole shoe.

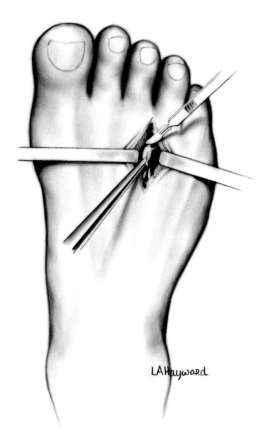

Fig. 147-3. Excision of neuroma.

Postoperative Management

The patient's foot is bandaged for a period of 3 weeks in order to permit adequate reconstitution of the transverse metatarsal ligament. Following removal of the dressing, the patient is encouraged to regain foot function as tolerated. The patient should not wear a high-heeled narrow shoe for another month if feasible.

Complications

I do not favor the plantar approach for the excision of an interdigital neuroma because it is possible to develop scar tissue beneath a metatarsal head if the incision is not accurately placed between the metatarsal heads. Thus, not only is there scar tissue on a weight-bearing area but, if the scar tissue becomes hyperkeratotic or is otherwise symptomatic, it is a significant problem for the patient. I believe

that the approach from the dorsal webspace is the preferred approach because it is so simple and because the possibility of any type of significant scarring along the incision is so insignificant.

RESULTS

In a review[7] of 62 of my patients with 81 interdigital neuromas that were excised, 80 percent of the patients stated that they were substantially improved and 6 percent felt that they were made better by the surgery but still noted some tenderness on the plantar aspect of the foot. Fourteen percent of the patients felt that the surgery did not significantly change the preoperative symptom complex.

The reason that some of these patients did not improve following their surgery is somewhat difficult to explain. The technique of excising the neuroma is essentially the same in all cases, yet there is a group of 14 percent of the patients who continue to have the same postoperative complaint. These patients were all carefully reevaluated; the diagnosis was thought to be correct, and no other etiology for the persistence of the postoperative pain could be found.

I have seen a number of patients in whom a neuroma has been excised through a small dorsal incision, in whom I did not believe an adequate amount of nerve tissue had been removed. These patients, if symptomatic, were subsequently reexplored and at surgery it was noted that indeed most of the common digital nerve was still intact. Reexcision of the nerve in these patients will often bring about a satisfactory result. There is, however, still a small group within this subgroup who will continue to have pain in the foot despite surgical excision of the neuroma.

Following excision of a neuroma, approximately 60 percent of patients will note numbness in the webspace and in a small localized area on the plantar aspect of the foot. This numbness is occasionally bothersome to the patient immediately following the surgery but gradually seems to fade away and become minimally symptomatic in time.

The concept of just releasing the transverse metatarsal ligament, as reported by Gauthier,[5] will not give lasting relief for this condition, since the transverse metatarsal ligament will reconstitute itself and can once again cause irritation of the nerve.

Patients who have had excision of a neuroma and who continue to have discomfort should be treated conservatively initially, once again using the proper shoe, metatarsal support, possible steroid injections, and a course of physical therapy involving ultrasound. If all these measures fail to produce significant relief, reexploration of the interspace would be indicated.

REFERENCES

1. Baker LD, Kuhn HH: Morton's metatarsalgia: localized degenerative fibrosis with neuromatous proliferation of the fourth plantar nerve. South Med J 37:123, 1944
2. Betts LO: Morton's metatarsalgia: neuritis of the fourth digital nerve. Med J Aust 1:514, 1940
3. Durlacher L: A treatise on Corns, Bunions, the Disease of Nails and the General Management of the Feet. Simpkin, Marshall, London, 1845, p. 52
4. DuVries, HL: Surgery of the Foot. 2nd Ed. CV Mosby, St. Louis, 1965
5. Gauthier G: Thomas Morton's disease: A nerve entrapment syndrome. Clin Orthop 142:90, 1979
6. Lassmann G: Morton's toe: clinical, light, and electron microscopic investigations in 133 cases. Clin Orthop 142:73, 1979
7. Mann RA, Reynolds JD: Interdigital neuroma: a critical clinical analysis. Foot Ankle 3:238, 1983
8. McElvenny RT: Etiology and surgical treatment of intractable pain about the fourth metatarsophalangeal joint (Morton's toe), J Bone Joint Surg 25:675, 1943
9. Morton DJ: The Human Foot: Its Evolution, Physiology and Functional Disorders. Columbia University Press, New York, 1935, pp. 184 and 211
10. Morton TG: A peculiar and painful affection of the fourth metatarsophalangeal articulation, Am J Med Sci 71:37, 1876
11. Morton TSK: Metatarsalgia (Morton's painful affection of the foot). Ann Surg 17:680, 1893
12. Nissen KI: Plantar digital neuritis, J Bone Joint Surg 30B:84, 1948
13. Winkler H, Feltner JB, Kimmelstiel P: Morton's metatarsalgia, J Bone Joint Surg 30A:496, 1948

Overlapping Toes

148

Henry R. Cowell

Overlapping of the second toe on the first, as reported by Branch,[1] may occur (1) following trauma to the metatarsophalangeal joint; (2) in patients with inflammatory joint disease in this area[13]; (3) secondary to chronic hyperextension of the metatarsophalangeal joint, as may be caused by wearing a shoe with an extremely high heel[4]; or (4) as a result of extrinsic pressure on the toe secondary to hallux valgus. Patients with this condition may report the acute onset of pain in the second metatarsal interspace, or the onset may be insidious, leading to increasing discomfort.[4] Over time, the second toe migrates up and over the first toe with hyperextension of the proximal phalanx. The patient may eventually complain of pain in both in the second intermetatarsal space, where the symptoms may be difficult to differentiate from an interdigital neuroma, and on the dorsal aspect of the toe, where the pain is secondary to pressure from the shoe.

Overlapping of the second, third, fourth, and fifth toes on the other small toes is a common congenital deformity. However, this condition is generally mild and seldom requires treatment. The condition may frequently be corrected passively when it occurs in the second, third, and fourth toes,

and may also improve with weight bearing. Occasionally, overlapping of the toes due to congenital angulation or a delta phalanx may cause symptoms that call for surgical correction.[6,10]

Overlapping of the fifth toe on the fourth with dorsal displacement and angulation may cause shoe-fitting problems and sometimes requires treatment (Fig. 148-1). Fixsen[5] notes that when the overlapping occurs in the second or third toe it is frequently associated with minor degrees of syndactyly or hypoplasia. Sweetnam[17] notes that strapping of the toes is seldom indicated and seldom effective. Overlapping deformities are often cosmetic and of little functional consequence.

INDICATIONS

The presence of the deformity alone is seldom an indication for surgery; indications for surgery relate to symptoms caused by the condition. When overlapping of the second, third, and fourth toes is so severe that one toe sits atop another, a callus will

4151

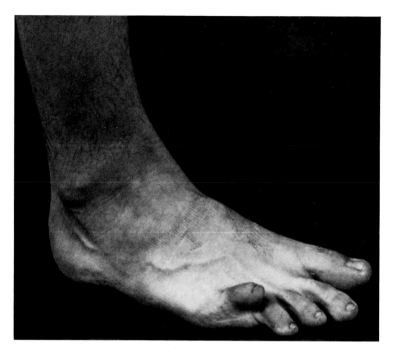

Fig. 148-1. Photograph of patient with severe overriding of the fifth toe.

develop on the dorsal or lateral aspect of the toe, becoming tender and creating pain secondary to pressure from the shoe. This is also true when the fifth toe overrides the fourth; here again, the indication for surgery is a painful, tender callus over the dorsum of the fifth toe.

While the operative procedures described for the second, third, and fourth toes may be carried out in the young individual, surgery for the fifth toe should be delayed until adolescence, and all the procedures described may be carried out in the adult. The contraindications for operative correction are related to the adequacy of circulation to the foot. If circulation is impaired in the older patient because of cardiovascular problems, or in the presence of diabetes, conservative methods consisting of extra-depth shoes and Plastizote inserts should be considered, since the corrective procedures for the fifth toe require extensive exposure for this otherwise minor procedure. Correction of the second, third, and fourth toes is usually a less extensive procedure, but, again, adequate circulation should be present prior to surgery.

METHODS OF TREATMENT

When the second toe overlaps the first toe treatment alternatives depend on the severity of the deformity.[4] For acute deformities that are mild, Coughlin[4] suggests pulling the toe into the correct position using a piece of tape placed over the dorsal aspect of the toe with the ends of the tape applied to the sole of the foot. Coughlin suggests metatarsophalangeal capsulotomy, extensor tenotomy, or extensor tendon lengthening, followed by Kirschner wire fixation for mild deformities. In five of 15 patients, Coughlin repaired the lateral capsule of the metatarsophalangeal joint when it was found to be ruptured at the time of the operation. In more severe deformities, the procedures described for claw toes (Ch. 146) may be used.

When dealing with the second, third, and fourth toes, treatment includes osteotomy of the phalanx, which may or may not be combined with excision of a portion of the phalanx, and fusion of the interphalangeal joint or joints.

Operative correction of the fifth toe may be performed by soft tissue procedures such as tendon transfer of the extensor tendon of the fifth toe, or by bony procedures which involve excision of the bone with rotation of skin flaps,[19] or rotation of the entire toe. My preferred method of treatment is a modification of the method described by Lapidus. The principal difference between the methods described by Lapidus and my modification is the placement of the skin incision so that a Z-plasty may be used to release the tight band of skin running between the fourth and fifth toes that is frequently seen as an accompaniment of this lesion.

Surgical Technique for the Middle Toes (Author's Preferred Technique)

A dorsal longitudinal incision is made from the base of the proximal phalanx to the proximal interphalangeal joint. Following incision through the skin, the extensor tendon is displaced medially, and the periosteum is incised on the dorsal aspect and stripped from the midshaft of the proximal phalanx. If the toe is the correct length and no shortening is indicated, the proximal phalanx is divided with a Hoke osteotome. If the toe is long (as is frequently the case) and shortening is desired, a rongeur may be used to excise a section of the midshaft of the phalanx. A Steinmann pin may be threaded distally through the middle phalanx and out the distal tuft of the toe and then threaded proximally to hold the toe in the corrected position. The subcutaneous tissue is closed with interrupted sutures of 000 chromic catgut and the skin with 4-0 nylon. If a delta phalanx is present, the proximal interphalangeal joint can be excised through the same incision by extending the incision distally and removing the proximal portion of the middle phalanx with an osteotome. An alternative method of fixation that may be used in the third and fourth toes is temporary suture of the third toe to the second and fourth or, in the case of the fourth toe, to the third and fifth with two sutures of 0 nylon. If this method is chosen, one suture is placed through the distal tuft of the third and fourth toes to pull the toe into the corrected position, and a second suture is placed through the tuft of the second and third toes to maintain the alignment of all three. In either case, a soft dressing is applied postoperatively. The patient may ambulate on the second or third postoperative day with a wooden-soled shoe. If a Kirschner wire or Steinmann pin has been used for internal fixation, this is maintained for a 4-week period. The wooden-soled shoe must be worn during this time. If the toe is positioned by suturing it to the adjacent toes, then the patient may wear a regular shoe as soon as the swelling has subsided and comfort permits. In any event, the stay sutures are left in place for 4 to 6 weeks.

Surgical Technique — Lapidus

The technique described by Lapidus[11] involves the rerouting of the extensor digitorum longus to the fifth toe, with reinsertion into the abductor and short flexor of the fifth toe. Lapidus performs his procedure through a dorsal longitudinal incision that starts over the dorsal medial aspect of the fifth toe at the level of the distal interphalangeal joint. The incision is carried back over the dorsal medial aspect of the toe to the webspace, then laterally over the dorsum of the toe to the dorsolateral aspect of the toe and proximally past the head of the fifth metatarsal. A second dorsal transverse incision is made over the extensor tendon in the midportion of the metatarsal so that the extensor tendon may be released and drawn out through the distal incision (Fig. 148-2). The tendon is pulled out through this incision and dissected free of its insertion on the distal phalanx. Following this, the capsule of the metatarsal phalangeal joint of the fifth toe is incised on the dorsal and medial aspects to correct the deformity of the phalanx in relationship to the metatarsal. A hemostat is used to make a tunnel from the medial aspect of the middle phalanx under the plantar surface of the proximal phalanx, passing laterally to the proximal phalanx at its base. The free end of the long extensor tendon is then passed through this tunnel and inserted into the abductor and short flexor of the fifth toe with sufficient tension to align the phalanx of the fifth toe on the metatarsals. This may be accomplished with 000 chromic sutures. The subcutaneous tissue is closed with 000 plain catgut sutures, the skin

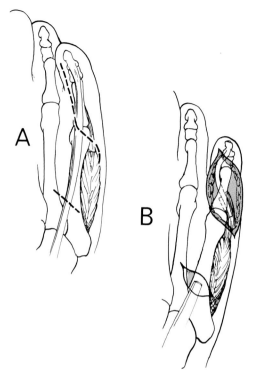

Fig. 148-2. (A) Lapidus procedure for repair of overriding fifth toe is carried out through two incisions. **(B)** Following proximal release of the extensor tendon, the tendon is routed underneath the middle phalanx and sutured to the abductor digiti quinti muscle.

with nylon. Lapidus recommends the use of an aluminum splint for a 4-week period, during which time walking may be allowed in a cutout shoe. A wooden-soled shoe with an open top is also satisfactory for the postoperative regimen.

Alternative Surgical Techniques

Various techniques have been described involving the resection of a portion of the phalanx with various skin incisions and closures.[3,9,12,16] Janecki and Wilde[8] have reported the technique ascribed to Ruiz-Mora, in which an elliptical segment of skin is removed from the plantar aspect of the fifth toe; the incision begins in the midplantar aspect of the fifth toe distal to the proximal phalanx, runs back over the proximal phalanx, and deviates medially in the proximal one-third of the phalanx. An elliptical

section of skin is removed with the proximal tip of the ellipse pointing medially. The flexor tendons are isolated and cut and allowed to retract into the foot. The proximal phalanx is exposed by subperiosteal dissection, and the collateral ligaments and joint capsule are freed by sharp dissection proximally and distally. Janecki and Wilde[8] recommend osteotomy of the phalanx to facilitate distal and proximal dissection for removal of the entire phalanx. Following this removal, the wound is closed by bringing the long ends of the ellipse together with one suture and closing each side of the ellipse to itself with a second suture of absorbable material. Postoperatively the patient is placed in a pressure dressing. Once the swelling has subsided, the patient is allowed to walk as soon as tolerated.

Morris et al.[15] suggest that the procedure described by Hulman[7] is simple and effective. They note that passive separation of the fourth and fifth toes makes an abnormal skin crease obvious, which runs from the dorsal aspect of the fourth toe at the webspace to the plantar aspect of the fifth toe. After an ellipse is marked on the skin, this ellipse is excised being careful not to injure the neurovascular bundle. The extensor tendon and the dorsal joint capsule of the metatarsophalangeal joint of the fifth toe are then divided. The defect in the skin is then closed with sutures of 000 nylon, the sutures being placed obliquely to pull the tissues into line. More skin is removed if necessary during closure to ensure accurate alignment. A soft dressing is applied.

Thompson[18] has described the removal of the proximal phalanx through a dorsal Z-plasty incision (Fig. 148-3). The skin incision is begun on the lateral aspect of the middle phalanx, carried down to the midportion of the proximal phalanx, and then carried down medially and proximally on the medial aspect of the fifth toe to the level of the metatarsal phalangeal joint. The extensor tendons are retracted medially and the phalanx is exposed by subperiosteal dissection. The capsule and collateral ligaments are released by sharp dissection and the phalanx excised. Next, 000 chromic sutures are used to approximate the capsule of the interphalangeal joint to the capsule of the metatarsal phalangeal joint. The skin is closed with interrupted sutures, reversing the Zs and thereby pulling the fifth toe into a corrected position.

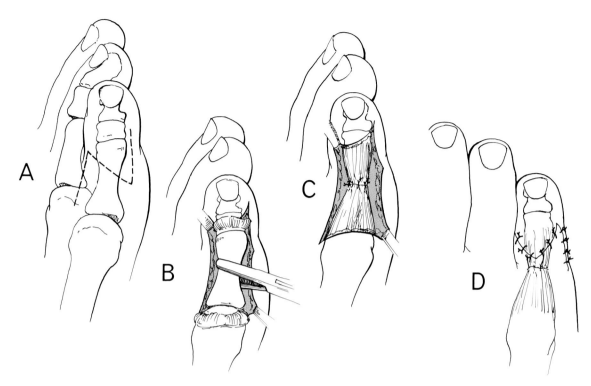

Fig. 148-3. **(A)** Thompson procedure for repair of overriding fifth toe is carried out through a Z-plasty incision. **(B)** After incising the skin and subcutaneous tissue and displacing the extensor tendon, the proximal phalanx is identified and excised. **(C)** The periosteum around the phalanx is closed, and closure of the skin is effected by reversing the limbs of the Z-plasty. **(D)** Thus, the skin is lengthened and the toe realigned.

McFarland[14] described a technique for resecting the proximal phalanx and subsequently syndactylizing the proximal portion of the fourth and fifth toes. I have not used this technique.

Cockin[2] described an operative procedure, ascribed to Butler, carried out through a racquet incision of the fifth toe with extensions of the incision on both the dorsal and plantar surfaces (Fig. 148-4). The circumferential incision is made around the toe at the level of the distal portion of the proximal phalanx. The dorsal incision is made to extend 1 cm proximally from the location of the extensor tendon. The plantar incision is made to extend laterally, about 2 cm in length, under the proximal phalanx of the toe.

Once the skin has been incised, the extensor tendon is located and cut, taking care to preserve the neurovascular bundles. The dorsal capsule of the metatarsophalangeal joint is incised, and the plantar capsule is dislodged from the metatarsal head by blunt dissection. The toe should then align satisfactorily, rotating externally to assume a more neutral position by displacing itself proximally in the plantar skin incision. After this repositioning, the plantar skin incision is less than 1 cm long, while the dorsal incision is at least 2 cm in length. In effect, the head of the racquet has been displaced plantarward, filling in the plantar extension of the racquet and increasing the length of the dorsal extension. Closure of the incision is effected with interrupted sutures and the remaining skin is closed while holding the toe in its corrected position, thereby eliminating the need for postoperative fixation.

Complications

When the Lapidus or my own described procedure is used, the major postoperative complication is recurrence of the deformity, caused by scar and

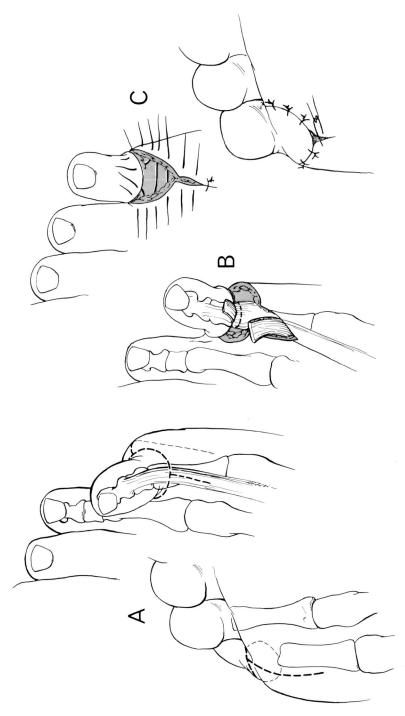

Fig. 148-4. **(A)** Butler procedure, described by Cockin, carried out through a double racquet incision. **(B)** The purpose of this incision is to free the fifth toe totally and displace it plantarward and laterally in the racquet incision. Following release of the extensor tendon and lateral and plantar displacement of the toe, the toe is rotated into the correct position. **(C)** The dorsal incision is closed, and one or two sutures are placed in the plantar aspect of the incision.

keloid formation from the Y-V or Z-plasty. Janecki and Wilde report that 10 of 28 patients who underwent the Ruiz-Mora procedure developed corns over the proximal interphalangeal joint of the fourth toe. Seven patients also developed painful bunionettes. Five of the seven had a combination of a bunionette and a corn on the fourth toe. The corn on the fourth toe was associated with underlying hammertoe deformity. None of these patients had preoperative hammertoe deformities in the fourth toe. Cockin reports that 64 of 70 feet that underwent the Butler procedure were satisfactory to both patient and surgeon. Four patients had partial correction of the deformity with a residual rotation. Two patients had a rapid recurrence of the deformity, and amputation of the toe was performed in these cases. It should be mentioned that, while amputation of the toe has been suggested by some, I do not recommend the procedure.

REFERENCES

1. Branch HE: Pathological dislocation of the second toe. J Bone Joint Surg 19:978, 1937
2. Cockin J: Butler's operation for an overriding fifth toe. J Bone Joint Surg 50B:78, 1968
3. Colonna PC: Regional Orthopedic Surgery. WB Saunders, Philadelphia, 1950
4. Coughlin MJ: Crossover second toe deformity. Foot Ankle 8:29, 1987
5. Fixsen JA: The foot in childhood. p. 73. In Klenerman L (ed): The Foot and Its Disorders. Blackwell Scientific Publications, Oxford, 1976
6. Goodwin FC, Swisher FM: The treatment of congenital hyperextension of the fifth toe. J Bone Joint Surg 25:193, 1943
7. Hulman S: Simple operation for the overlapping fifth toe. Br Med J 2:1506, 1964
8. Janecki CJ, Wilde AH: Results of phalangectomy of the fifth toe for hammertoe: the Ruiz-Mora procedure. J Bone Joint Surg 58A:1005, 1976
9. Kelikian H, Clayton L, Loseff H: Surgical syndactylia of the toes. Clin Orthop 19:208, 1961
10. Lantzounis LA: Congenital subluxation of the fifth toe and its correction by a periosteocapsuloplasty and tendon transplantation. J Bone Joint Surg 22:147, 1940
11. Lapidus PW: Transplantation of the extensor tendon for correction of the overlapping fifth toe. J Bone Joint Surg 24:555, 1942
12. Leonard MH, Rising EE: Syndactylization to maintain correction of overlapping 5th toe. Clin Orthop 43:241, 1965
13. Mann RA, Mizel MS: Monoarticular nontraumatic synovitis of the metatarsophalangeal joint: a new diagnosis? Foot Ankle 6:18, 1985
14. McFarland B: Congenital deformities of the spine and limbs. p. 107. In Platt Sir H (ed): Modern Trends in Orthopaedics. Hoeber, New York, 1950
15. Morris EW, Scullion JE, Mann TS: Varus fifth toe. J Bone Joint Surg 64B:99, 1982
16. Scrase WH: The treatment of dorsal adduction deformities of the fifth toe. J Bone Joint Surg 36B:146, 1954 (abst)
17. Sweetnam R: Congenital curly toes: an investigation into the value of treatment. Lancet 2:398, 1958
18. Thompson TC: Surgical treatment of disorders of the fore part of the foot. J Bone Joint Surg 46A:1117, 1964
19. Wilson NJ: V-Y correction for varus deformity of the fifth toe. Br J Surg 41:133, 1953

Splayfoot

149

Henry R. Cowell

Splayfoot has been defined by Giannestras as a spreading of the metatarsals such that the first metatarsal deviates from the second metatarsal by more than 10 degrees, and the fifth metatarsal deviates from the fourth metatarsal by more than 5 degrees. While this deviation results in a wide forepart of the foot, it is of little clinical consequence in most instances. When the splayfoot is associated with a hallux valgus deformity and a bunionette, symptoms may result from attempts to place the foot into a tight shoe. While the problem can frequently be overcome by wearing adequately sized shoes, occasionally the foot splays so much that standard size shoes will not fit comfortably. This, in my experience, is particularly common in patients with Ehlers-Danlos syndrome.

OPERATIVE PROCEDURES

Although certain of the procedures described for splayfoot are designed to allow the individual to wear a stylish shoe, I do not believe that surgery should be used in every case. Rather, operative procedures should be employed only when a patient's foot is splayed so severely that there is an associated bunion and bunionette deformity, which makes it impossible to wear any shoe without painful pressure over the first and fifth toes.

Giannestras[3] described an osteotomy of the bases of the first and fifth metatarsals, along with correction of the bunion deformity for the splayfoot. I have modified this technique to include fusion of the first metatarsal to the second metatarsal in patients with Ehlers-Danlos syndrome.

Joplin[4-6] and Bateman and Colwill[1] described soft tissue techniques combined with removal of the exostosis of the great toe for the correction of splayfoot. Brown[2] has suggested amputation of the fifth toe for this problem. I have had no experience with this last procedure and therefore cannot recommend it.

Surgical Technique — Giannestras

The procedure is carried out through two incisions on the dorsum of the foot (Fig. 149-1). The first incision extends along the medial aspect of the

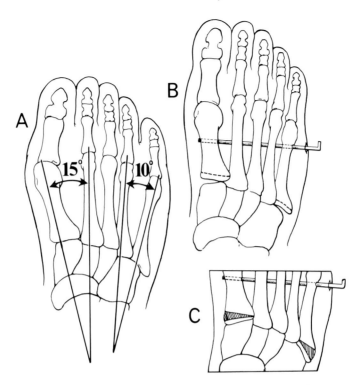

Fig. 149-1. (A) The Giannestras procedure is indicated for deviation between the first and second metatarsals of more than 15 degrees, and between the fourth and fifth metatarsals of more than 10 degrees. **(B)** Following exposure of the first and fifth metatarsals and removal of the exostosis from the first metatarsal, the first and fifth metatarsals are compressed and held in this position with a pin. **(C)** Osteotomies are then carried out at the base of the first and fifth metatarsals. The bone removed from the first metatarsal head is placed into the opening-wedge osteotomies created in the first and fifth metatarsals.

first metatarsal shaft, from the base of the metatarsal to just past the metatarsal phalangeal joint; this incision may curve laterally around the head of the first metatarsal. The second incision extends over the dorsal lateral aspect of the fifth metatarsal, from its base to the proximal phalanx of the fifth metatarsal. Each incision is carried down through the skin and subcutaneous tissue, and the dorso medial periosteum of the first toe is incised over the metatarsal head. The periosteum is elevated, and a distally based flap is developed on the proximal phalanx. This flap is approximately 1 to 1.5 cm in width. The flap is dissected from the metatarsal head. An osteotome is used to remove the prominent portion of the metatarsal head medially to allow correction of the hallux valgus deformity.

If the toe cannot be aligned by pulling the flap attached to the phalanx proximally, then a second incision may be made in the space between the first and second toes. The incision is carried down

through the subcutaneous tissue to the adductor, which is released to allow the phalanx to be placed in the corrected position.

The lateral incision is carried down through the skin and subcutaneous tissue; the fifth metatarsal is identified and the exostosis or bunionette prominence is removed from the fifth metatarsal head. A piece of sterile gauze is then wrapped around the metatarsal level of the foot to oppose the metatarsals.

Following this, a threaded Kirschner wire is driven carefully across the neck of the fifth metatarsal, then plantar to the fourth, third, and second, into the neck of the first metatarsal, exiting through the medial cortex of the first metatarsal (Fig. 149-1B). The wire is cut just medial to the first metatarsal, and sufficient wire is left to protrude laterally, for removal at 6 weeks postoperatively. This wire holds the metatarsals in a corrected position so that the bones may be osteotomized. (If osteotomy is performed before insertion of the wire, the first and fifth metatarsals may drift dorsally or plantarly, altering the weight-bearing mechanics of the foot.) Also prior to performing the osteotomies, a radiograph is obtained to ensure that correction has been effected. Next, an osteotomy is performed through the base of the first metatarsal, approximately 0.75 cm from the metatarsal joint, and a similar osteotomy is performed on the lateral side of the foot at the base of the fifth metatarsal, approximately 1 cm from the metatarsal base (Fig. 149-1C).

Once these osteotomies have been performed, the first and fifth metatarsals will spring open, since the wire holds the metatarsals in their corrected positions. The osteotomy may be opened slightly with an osteotome or with a laminar spreader. The osteotomy of the first metatarsal is opened medially, leaving the lateral cortex intact, and the osteotomy of the fifth metatarsal is opened laterally, leaving the medial cortex intact if possible. The bone previously removed from the exostosis is then placed into the first and fifth metatarsal osteotomies. The subcutaneous tissue is then closed with sutures of 000 plain catgut, and the skin is closed with interrupted sutures of nylon or subcuticular wire. A pressure dressing is applied.

On the seventh postoperative day the dressing is changed; if the incisions are healing satisfactorily, a below-knee weight-bearing cast is applied snugly about the forefoot. The author, unlike Giannestras, does not allow the patient to ambulate until the wire has been removed. The wire is removed at 6 weeks and, if the osteotomies do not show satisfactory healing at that time, the patient is placed in another short-leg walking cast for 4 weeks. Giannestras notes that the feet may be edematous following the procedure and that an elastic stocking may be indicated during the postoperative regimen.

Author's Preferred Technique

I have used the Giannestras technique but modified it by fusing the first and second metatarsals at their bases in patients with Ehlers-Danlos syndrome. The operative technique is carried out as above; however, the first incision is curved over the dorsal aspect of the first metatarsal and carried back to the first cuneiform. Prior to placing a wire

across the foot, the area between the first and second metatarsals is freed by blunt dissection, and, after removal of the periosteum in this area, the area of the first and second metatarsals is roughened by fishscaling the first and second metatarsal bases. A threaded wire is then inserted, as described by Giannestras. The first metatarsal is osteomized by drilling the bone from the dorsal surface, and the osteotomy is opened medially. Correction is maintained by inserting a wedge of bone into the osteotomy site. Next, fragments of bone from the exostosis are placed in the area between the first and second metatarsals. Following packing of the bone in this area, the procedure is carried out as described by Giannestras. The patient is maintained in a below-knee cast for 6 weeks. No weight bearing is allowed. The wire is removed at 6 weeks and radiographs are obtained. If sufficient healing has occurred, the patient is allowed to bear weight at this time; if not, a below-knee weight-bearing cast is applied until sufficient healing has occurred to allow weight bearing without the cast.

Surgical Technique — Joplin

Joplin has used this technique on patients between the ages of 10 and 20 years.[4-6] While it may be considered for the young adult, it is basically a procedure to be used on the adolescent patient. Joplin has noted that there are many patients who have unsightly bunion deformities associated with splayfoot and metatarsus primus varus deformity without pain. He notes that surgery is indicated only when splayfoot and the associated hallux valgus are causing pain. He also notes that the rheumatoid foot is better treated by other methods, and that this procedure is not advised for diabetics or patients with circulatory problems.

The first incision is a 5-cm-long incision over the dorsal medial aspect of the foot, curving slightly to the plantar side of the bony overgrowth of the bunion (Fig. 149-2A). Dissection is carried down to the capsule, and the bunion and abductor hallucis tendon are exposed. The capsule is opened through a linear incision on the medial aspect of the bony overgrowth, and this bony overgrowth is removed with a sharp osteotome. Joplin recommends closing the incision temporarily with a towel clip; however, I use one subcutaneous suture to approximate the incision, which I find preferable to placing a towel clip through the skin. A second incision is made in the web space between the first and second toes, extending proximally between the first and second metatarsal shafts for a distance of approximately 5 cm. The interosseous muscle to the second toe is identified and retracted. The adductor hallucis is identified by blunt dissection, and the lateral sesamoid bone is encountered. The adductor hallucis tendon is detached from the lateral lip of the proximal phalanx. It is lifted up and separated from the sesamoid and the flexor hallucis brevis tendon to which it is joined. After separation, excess capsular tissue should be trimmed from the abductor hallucis tendon with scissors. The skin incision is closed temporarily with a suture. A third incision is made 5 cm in length, curved dorsally over the fifth toe, exposing the capsule, bunionette, and lateral half of the proximal phalanx. The capsule is divided longitudinally and retracted to permit excision of the bony overgrowth on the lateral aspect of the fifth metatarsal head and the projecting lateral lip of the proximal phalanx. The ex-

tensor tendon is exposed by opening its sheath, and a tendon stripper is placed around the tendon and passed upward along the tendon until its end can be palpated beneath the skin at the level of the ankle. A short, 1-cm, transverse incision is made in this area to expose the tendon. The tendon is divided and withdrawn through the distal incision. The proximal incision may be closed with interrupted sutures of 000 plain catgut, and the skin is closed with interrupted sutures of nylon. The tendon is retracted through the distal wound and threaded with a tendon passer beneath the neck of the fifth metatarsal and across the foot beneath the necks of the four lateral metatarsals, but over the neck of the first metatarsal. The free end of the tendon is thus delivered into the first incision (Fig. 149-2B).

A bone perforator is used to form a small hole in the cancellous bone of the head of the fifth metatarsal. A number 2 chromic catgut suture is passed and tied over the transplanted fifth extensor tendon, securing it against the raw bony surface of the fifth metatarsal, where the bunionette was previously excised (Fig. 149-2C). Joplin notes that certain feet have flexion and external rotation of

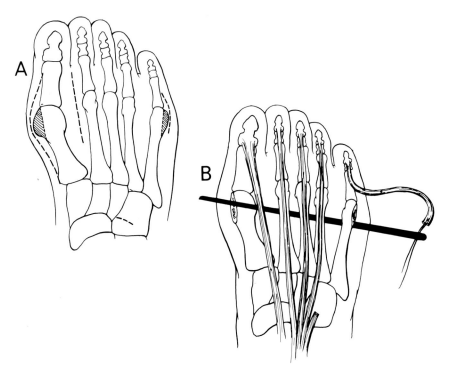

Fig. 149-2. **(A)** Joplin procedure carried out through four incisions. **(B)** The long extensor of the fifth toe is routed underneath the second, third, and fourth metatarsals and over the neck of the first metatarsal. *(Figure continues.)*

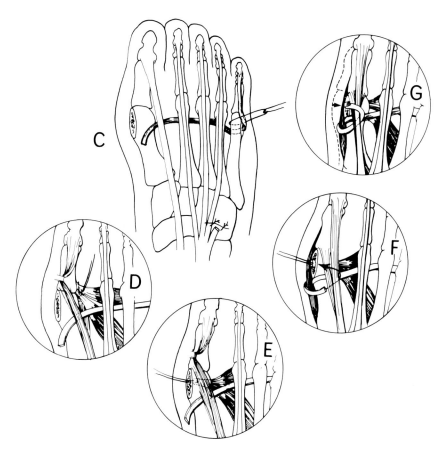

Fig. 149-2 *(Continued).* **(C)** The tendon is then fixed to the area of the fifth metatarsal where the bunionette was. **(D)** The adductor muscle is released, and **(E)** reinserted into the metatarsal head. **(F)** The tendon from the extensor of the fifth toe is threaded under the extensor tendons to the first toe, under the abductor of the first toe, routed around the extensor tendons to the first toe, and **(G)** sutured into the area of the adductor transfer through the metatarsal head.

the fifth toe secondary to this procedure, and he recommends that the extensor brevis tendon to the fourth toe be detached at its distal end and transplanted into the fifth extensor tendon distal to the site of the tenodesis. The capsule of the metatarsal phalangeal joint of the fifth toe is sutured to prevent dislocation of this joint. A drill hole is then made through the head of the first metatarsal, and the severed adductor tendon is pulled into this drill hole with a 00 chromic catgut suture. (Fig. 149-2D,E). One end of the suture is passed through the dorsal portion of the capsule and the other end through the ventral portion of the capsule. The fifth extensor tendon is passed over the shaft of the first metatarsal, down and under the abductor hallucis muscle, brought back up on top

of the first metatarsal, and sutured to itself in this position. This fifth extensor tendon is sutured while maintaining tension on the tendon in order to correct the deformity (Fig. 149-2F). Once this tendon has been sutured, the sutures from the adductor hallucis, previously placed in the dorsal and plantar edges of the capsule, are tied easily without undue tension. The remaining 2 to 3 cm of the fifth extensor tendon are used to form a wide loop around the extensor hallucis longus and brevis tendons. In order to form a pulley to reroute these tendons in the correct position, the final end of the extensor tendon from the fifth toe is sutured into the capsule to create this loop. Subcutaneous tissue is closed with interrupted sutures of 000 plain catgut and the skin is closed with 5-0 nylon. The patient is then placed in a compression dressing, which is changed on the fourth postoperative day. At this time, plaster of Paris slippers with a walking heel are applied and weight bearing is begun with crutches. Increased weight bearing is allowed as the patient tolerates it. The slippers are left on for 4 weeks, at which time they are discarded and the sutures removed. A 2-inch gauze bandage is worn circumferentially just proximal to the heads of the first and fifth metatarsals for 6 months postoperatively.

Joplin notes that deformity may recur in the older patient because of the malalignment of the first cuneiform metatarsal joint. This may be prevented by an opening-wedge osteotomy of the cuneiform. A medial incision is made in the perios-

teum of the cuneiform after extending the original incision proximally. A medial opening-wedge osteotomy is performed. A wedge of bone from the exostosis is inserted into the medial side of the cuneiform to maintain the opening of the osteotomy. The remainder of the sling procedure is then carried out as described.

Surgical Technique — Bateman and Colwill

Bateman and Colwill[1] used this same basic technique employing the peroneus tertius tendon. The first incision is placed dorsomedially over the metatarsal phalangeal joint of the great toe (Fig.

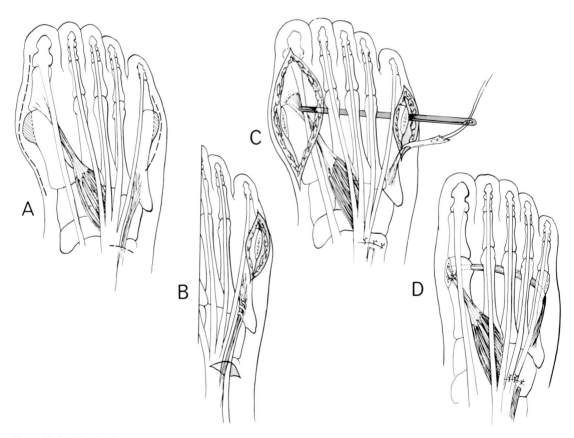

Fig. 149-3. The Joplin procedure has been modified by Bateman and Colwill, using the peroneus tertius muscle. This muscle is identified in the foot and released proximally. **(A)** Repair of the bunion and bunionette is carried out, and **(B)** a special corkscrew tendon stripper is used to free the peroneus tertius to its insertion on the metatarsal. **(C)** Following this, the peroneus tertius is routed underneath the second, third, fourth, and fifth metatarsals into the area of the first metatarsal. **(D)** After release of the adductors, the peroneus tertius tendon is threaded through the metatarsal head and sutured to the extensor hallucis brevis of the first toe.

149-3A). The capsule is incised longitudinally, and the prominent portion of the first metatarsal is excised using a reciprocating saw. The metatarsal is then retracted dorsally and laterally, the sesamoids medially. By sharp dissection, the lateral sesamoid is identified and removed, taking care to shell it from its bed to avoid injury to the flexor hallucis longus tendon. A lateral incision is made, similar to that described by Joplin. The bunionette of the fifth metatarsal is removed with a reciprocating saw. An area approximately 1 cm in length is dissected on the lateral aspect of the metatarsal to receive the peroneus tertius tendon, which will be used as a wraparound sling in this area.

The peroneus tertius tendon is identified just lateral to the extensor tendon of the fifth toe. Bateman and Colwill use a special corkscrew stripper to dissect the peroneus tertius tendon proximally and free it from the muscle belly. The peroneus tertius tendon is then subcutaneously routed out through the lateral incision at the fifth toe, and the tendon is passed underneath the fifth metatarsal head, around the lateral side of the metatarsal, and brought out between the first and second metatarsals through the medial incision (Fig. 149-3B).

Attention is then directed to the medial incision, where the extensor hallucis brevis is identified and severed at its insertion. This tendon is then used as the medial portion of the sling. A hole is drilled through the first metatarsal head and the peroneus tertius tendon is passed through the first metatarsal, pulling it out on the medial side of the bone (Fig. 149-3C). Following compression of the metatarsals, the peroneus tertius tendon is sutured to the extensor hallucis brevis tendon (Fig. 149-3D). Bateman and Colwill note that, if the malalignment of the phalanx has not been completely corrected, it may be corrected at this time by passing the peroneus tertius through the abductor hallucis and tying it in this position under tension so that it pulls the phalanx into proper alignment. They caution that care must be taken at this time not to overcorrect the phalanx. They note that, if the sesamoid has been removed carefully without severing the adductor, a portion of it will still be attached and firm resistance will be met in attempting to bring the toe into varus. They conclude that it is safe to tie the suture under tension. They report that the peroneus tertius was present and utilizable in 78 percent of their patients. If the peroneus tertius is not encountered, then the Joplin procedure may be carried out as originally described.

Postoperatively, Bateman and Colwill recommend application of a plaster cast that covers the toes completely and extends to above the incision in the region of the extensor retinaculum. The plaster permits ankle motion, and care is taken to fix the toes in plantar flexion and to mold the transverse arch to retain the correction obtained by the tendon sling. Weight bearing with a cut-out shoe is allowed 48 hours after surgery. Plaster is removed after 3 weeks, at which time the patient may ambulate. Bateman and Colwill note the complication of stiffness of the great toe in varus and dorsiflexion and note that this can be avoided by careful shelling out of the lateral sesamoid, leaving a portion of the abductor intact. Bateman and Colwill also note delayed healing in certain instances when bony reconstruction is a part of the procedure, particularly in the elderly patient.

REFERENCES

1. Bateman JE, Colwill JC: Modified Joplin sling procedure for splayfoot using peroneus tertius. p. 288. In American Academy of Orthopaedic Surgeons. Instructional Course Lectures. Vol. 21. CV Mosby, St. Louis, 1972
2. Brown JE: Functional and cosmetic correction of metatarsus latus (splay foot). Clin Orthop 14:166, 1959
3. Giannestras NJ: Foot Disorders: Medical and Surgical Management. 2nd Ed. Lea & Febiger, Philadelphia, 1973
4. Joplin RJ: Sling procedure for correction of splayfoot, metatarsus primus varus, and hallux valgus. J Bone Joint Surg 32A:779, 1950
5. Joplin RJ: Some common foot disorders amenable to surgery. p. 144. In American Academy of Orthopaedic Surgeons. Instructional Course Lectures. Vol. 15. Edwards, Ann Arbor, 1958
6. Joplin RJ: Sling procedure in the teen-ager. p. 269. In American Academy of Orthopaedic Surgeons. Instructional Course Lectures. Vol. 21. CV Mosby, St. Louis, 1972

Surgical Syndactyly

150

Paul Dubravcik

A search of the relevant literature on the subject of surgical syndactyly reveals A.M. Phelps[4] to be the first investigator credited with performing this procedure. More recently, H. Kelikian et al[3] perfected the procedure and described it in further detail, advocating its use in the surgical treatment of numerous lesser-toe deformities.

This chapter in the previous edition of this book dealt with my personal experience using this procedure and was based on 200 surgical syndactylizations performed on 130 patients over a period of 10 years (1970 to 1980). My aim in revising this chapter has been to take account and evaluate surgical syndactyly as the procedure of choice in an additional 100 syndactylizations performed between 1981 and 1985. These were reviewed as to indications, surgical technique, and complications, where applicable.

The indications for surgery employed in the first group of 200 surgical syndactylizations were only slightly altered for the latter group of surgeries performed. Those recommended are as follows:

1. Multiple rigid hammertoe deformities with contractures or subluxation of the metatarsophalangeal or proximal interphalangeal joints

2. Overlapping fifth toe
3. Clawing of the lesser toes
4. Iatrogenic hallux varus deformity, or recurrent hammertoe deformities after unsuccessful soft tissue surgery
5. Freiberg's infraction

As compared with the original group, in which two-thirds of patients required concomitant surgery for other deformities of the forepart of the foot (e.g., hallux valgus), only one-third of the latter group required correction of other forefoot deformities. This may be attributed to the fact that, as the success of well-indicated surgical syndactylization became more evident, the number of patients referred who required a revision of recurrent lesser-toe deformities increased (10 patients combined with four patients with unsuccessful primary syndactylization surgery).

Surgical treatment of hammertoe deformities depends to a great extent on the degree of flexibility involved. The rigidity of the metatarsophalangeal joints in the lesser-toe deformities, with or without subluxation or dislocation of the proximal phalanx, may easily be assessed by Kelikian's "push-up test."[2] This is done in conjunction with preoperative evaluation of the degree of flexibility of the metatarsal rays involved. A flexible hammertoe condition, which occurs as a part of a cavus or equinus foot deformity, may disappear spontaneously after successful correction of the basic deformity.

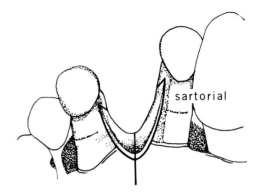

Fig. 150-1. Webspace bisected by the interdigital incision (Redrawn from Kelikian,[3] with permission.)

METHODS OF TREATMENT

Surgical procedures, such as those employing the transplant or lengthening of the tendons, metatarsophalangeal capsulotomies, proximal interphalangeal arthrodesis, partial excision of the proximal phalanx, and diaphysectomy, are indicated in the treatment of hammering of lesser toes. Conversely, soft tissue release alone is notoriously inadequate in the correction of fixed hammertoe contractures.

SURGICAL TECHNIQUE

The surgical procedure is carried out under tourniquet control with general anesthesia used in most patients. Two holding silk sutures are placed in the pulp of the terminal phalanges of the toes for retraction to facilitate exposure. The midline of the adjacent medial and lateral toe surfaces is outlined by a methylene blue marker, to facilitate visualization of a reference point for the placement of the interdigital incisions. This small addition to our technique proved to be of great assistance, particularly when attempting to correct a rotational deformity of the involved toes. Five skin incisions are made:

1. An interdigital incision bisecting the web space (Fig. 150-1)
2. Paradigital skin incisions (Fig. 150-2)
3. Two connecting sartorial incisions (Fig. 150-3)

One or both proximal phalanges are exposed and a proximal one-third to one-half of the phalangeal length is resected. A triangular skin flap between the paradigital and sartorial skin incisions is then excised to facilitate the syndactylia. The skin edges are slightly undermined with digital blood vessels and nerves thus exposed, protected or ligated.

In syndactylizations of the second and third toes, and as was suggested by Giannestras, about one-half (both series combined) of procedures resulted in the partial resection of one phalanx.[1] The syndactylizations of the fourth and fifth toes required only a resection of the fifth proximal phalanx in 60 percent of the 25 patients from our first group, and in 71 percent of the last 38 patients (Fig. 150-4).

The primary criteria for this modification, however, remains as cited earlier. The nonresected syndactylized toe must be either free of any deformity or have only a mild flexible hammering with

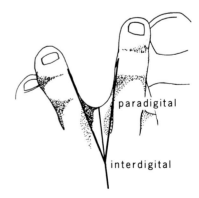

Fig. 150-2. Paradigital skin incision. (Redrawn from Kelikian,[3] with permission.)

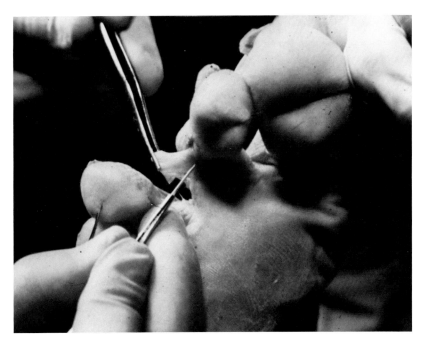

Fig. 150-3. A triangular piece of skin is removed between the connecting sartorial and paradigital incision.

no subluxation or dislocation of the metatarsophalangeal joint. The paradigital incision of the resected toe must extend beyond the distal interphalangeal joint to avoid malalignment. It is also recommended that the incision on the toe in which the phalynx is not resected extend slightly distal

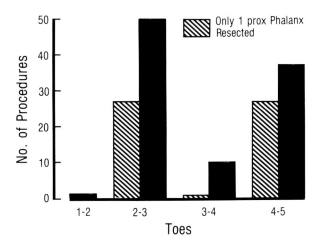

Fig. 150-4. Location of 100 syndactylizations performed during 1981 to 1985.

to the distal interphalangeal joint. The excision of the proximal phalanx should, in this instance, include only the proximal one-third to avert excessive toe shortening.

Holding sutures of 000 Vicryl are placed in the distal corners of the two paradigital incisions in order to evaluate the degree of alignment. When only one proximal phalanx is resected, manual pressure is exerted beneath the metatarsal head of the unresected toe in order to simulate weight-bearing conditions and to further test toe alignment.

At this stage, any required corrections in the skin incisions may be effected. For further enhancement of the esthetic appearance of the syndactylized toes, the skin and subcutaneous tissue is sutured in the following manner. Interrupted sutures of 000 Vicryl are placed on the dorsal aspect proximally and extended to the level of the interdigital web space. At the most distal part of the incision, inverted sutures — knots tied and embedded in the incision — are used. The remainder of the incision (approximately 2 cm into the plantar aspect of the interdigital space) is closed by interrupted sutures with knots tied exteriorly. This maneuver simulates

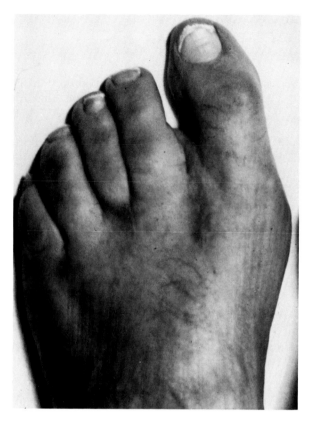

Fig. 150-5. Postsyndactylization of the second and third toes and of the fourth and fifth toes.

a dorsal interdigital skin crease and serves to improve the cosmetic result (Fig. 150-5). Fixed flexion contractures of the proximal interphalangeal joints are corrected manually, followed by only a slight compressive dressing.

POSTOPERATIVE MANAGEMENT

By the second postoperative day the patient usually may be fitted with an oversized running shoe, toe box removed, and laces loosely tied to secure a snug fit. Crutches may be of assistance during early ambulation. If surgical syndactylization alone was performed, the patient may be discharged as early as 3 days postoperatively. The dressing is removed between the tenth and fourteenth postoperative day. Healing is usually complete by that time, and the patient is permitted mild foot bathing, with application of a dry dressing if necessary. The running shoes are usually worn for a period of 3 to 4 weeks.

COMPLICATIONS

The only major complication I have encountered with this procedure in the initial 66 patients was a recurrence of the deformity in two cases and a gross malalignment of the toes due to incomplete syndactyly in three instances. In the latter 100 syndactylizations, a subsequent malalignment (three patients with gross malalignment, and five with lesser malalignment) was the principal complication.

Only one of five patients with minor malalignment, however, was significantly concerned with his results. Two patients, judged as having a gross malalignment due to a shortness and retraction of the resected toe, were so improved in their symptoms that they felt adequately compensated, particularly when wearing comfortable shoes. Three superficial infections occurred and were resolved with appropriate antibiotic therapy. Similarly, as witnessed in our first group, a mild spreading of the adjacent toes, although clinically asymptomatic, occurred in four patients. The formation of two hypertrophic scars were noted, both in patients of black extraction.

DISCUSSION AND RESULTS

In my experience, surgical syndactylization done for the indications noted, and precisely executed, yields satisfactory results in 90 percent of patients. Multiple lesser toe syndactylizations done on the same foot, present slightly more complex problems, and necessitate an even more rigid adherence to the technique. A pitfall to avoid in this group is the excessive shortening of the medial couple of toes, since even a minimal malalignment will then become more noticeable and progressively worse. This is possibly due to the removal of the supporting structures, which is unavoidable during the surgical resection. If metatarsalgia is present, in conjunction with rigid hammertoe deformities, a surgical correction such as osteotomy of the involved metatarsal is indicated and may be performed at the time of syndactylization surgery.

REFERENCES

1. Giannestras NJ: Other problems of the forepart of the foot. p. 410. Giannestras NJ (ed): In Foot Disorders. Medical and Surgical Management. 2nd ed. Lea & Febiger, Philadelphia, 1973
2. Kelikian H: Hallux Valgus, Allied Deformities of the Forefoot and Metatarsalgia. WB Saunders, Philadelphia, 1965
3. Kelikian H, Clayton L, Loseff H: Surgical syndactylia of the toes. Clin Orthop 19:208, 1961
4. Phelps AM: A new method of curing inveterate soft corns between the toes. Trans Am Orthop Assoc 6:237, 1894

Osteochondritis of the Forepart of the Foot

151

Henry R. Cowell

OSTEOCHONDRITIS OF THE SESAMOIDS OF THE GREAT TOE

Giannestras[6] reports that Ilfeld in 1971 described osteochondritis of the sesamoids of the great toe. Apley[1] also noted that this condition shows changes similar to those associated with osteochondritis dissecans in other bones and may lead to transverse rupture of the bone. In addition, Inge and Ferguson[10] note that these changes in the sesamoids may cause persistent metatarsalgia. While trauma to the sesamoids is rare, I have noted osteochondritic changes in the sesamoids secondary to trauma, with subsequent splitting of the bone (Fig. 151-1). By contrast, bipartite sesamoid bones may occur without trauma and do not cause symptoms. The diagnosis of osteochondritis should be made only when serial radiographs over a period of time show changes in a sesamoid bone.

Pain caused by pressure over the sesamoids may be secondary to osteochondritis, but in many instances the true cause of the pain cannot be ascertained. When this symptom complex presents, treatment should be directed at pain relief by conservative methods. The use of a below-knee weight-bearing cast for a 3-week period will frequently relieve tenderness over the sesamoids. The use of a full-sole Plastizote insert with hollowing in the area under the sesamoids may also relieve pain, as will a metatarsal bar applied to relieve weight bearing from the area of the sesamoid.

The rare indications for surgery are persistent pain on weight bearing with tenderness over the sesamoids and associated changes suggestive of necrosis. As noted above, an absolute diagnosis of osteochondritis cannot be made unless serial films are obtained. However, in some instances, the patient will not present until long after the onset of the condition, when the lesion may be so advanced that serial films will not show further changes.

Most investigators note that excision of the sesamoid frequently results in persistent pain during the postoperative period and disability that may last many months. I feel that the procedure is an appropriate one in selected feet when a specific diagnosis of osteochondritis with associated pain has been made. This diagnosis should be confirmed by injecting 1.5 cc of procaine into the affected sesamoid; this should relieve the symptoms if osteochondritis is, in fact, the cause of the difficulty. The surgeon should be aware of other possible

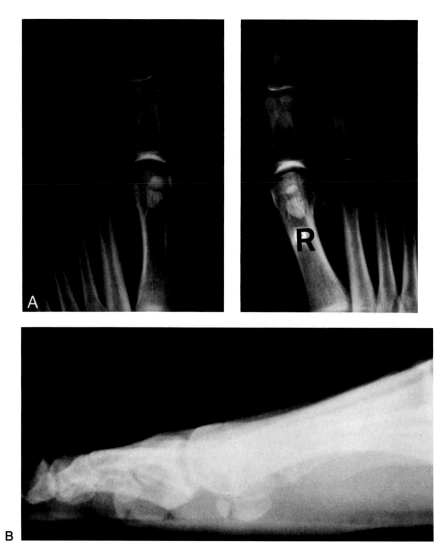

Fig. 151-1. (A) Radiograph of patient with aseptic necrosis of the sesamoid on the right side. Note the separation of the bone and the dense distal fragment, which may be compared with the normal bipartite sesamoid on the left. **(B)** Lateral view of the sesamoid showing the separation and displacement of the distal fragment, as compared with the proximal fragment. *(Figure continues.)*

causes of pain in this area, such as infection[7,14] and tumor.

Surgical Technique for Removal of the Sesamoid

A 2- to 3-cm incision is made on the inferomedial aspect of the great toe. This longitudinal incision runs in the direction of the flexor tendons, and should be placed away from the weight-bearing surface and below the area in which the shoe will press against the medial border of the foot. The incision is carried down through the skin and subcutaneous tissue, and the sesamoid is identified. The long toe flexor is split on the medial aspect, and the sesamoid is enucleated by subperiosteal dissection from the tendon sheath. Following complete excision and curettage of the remaining portions of

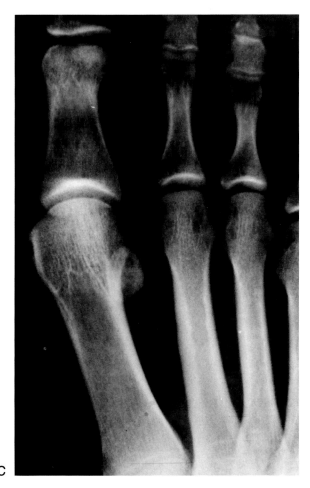

C

Fig. 151-1 *(Continued).* **(C)** Complete relief of symptoms was obtained after removal of the sesamoid.

the sesamoid, the tendon is closed with interrupted sutures of 4-0 plain catgut. Following this, the subcutaneous tissue is approximated and the skin is closed with interrupted sutures of 000 nylon.

Postoperatively, the patient is placed in a below-knee weight-bearing cast and allowed to walk as soon as comfort allows. After partial weight bearing with crutches, the patient is advanced to full weight bearing on the cast as tolerated. After 3 weeks, both plaster and sutures are removed, and the patient is allowed to advance from partial to full weight bearing as tolerated.

Complications noted from this procedure include tenderness in the area of the incision and division of the flexor brevis tendons. Inge and Fer-

guson[10] note that 41 percent of their patients obtained complete relief with restoration or maintenance of normal function. Twenty-nine percent of their patients showed improvement but continued to have minor difficulties postoperatively; these included tender keloid scars and impaired motion at the metatatarsophalangeal joint, as well as persistence of mild pain under the metatarsal head. In their series, 17 percent of the patients whose symptoms were relieved also had inadvertent division of the flexor hallucis brevis tendon. This occurred in six patients in whom both sesamoids had been removed, but in only one patient where a single sesamoid was removed. Another 12 percent (five patients) had persistent pain with inflammation in the area of the sesamoid.

OSTEOCHONDRITIS OF THE HEAD OF THE SECOND METATARSAL

Osteochondritis of the head of the second metatarsal was described by Freiberg[4] in 1914 as an infraction of the second metatarsal bone. Kohler also described the lesion in 1915, and both authors reported on it a second time: Kohler[12] in 1923 and Freiberg[5] in 1926.

Smillie[17] described five stages in the development of this condition. In stage I, a fissure develops in the ischemic epiphysis. In stage II, the contour of the articular surface is altered as the central portion of the joint surface subsides into the metatarsal head. In stage III, the central portion of the joint surface subsides further leaving lateral projections on both sides of the head. In stage IV, loose bodies occur as the plantar attachment of the cartilaginous surface of the joint breaks and the lateral projections of the remaining head fracture. In stage V, flattening of the head occurs with resultant degenerative arthritis.

This condition is generally found in the adolescent with an open epiphysis and was reported by Giannestras[6] in patients between the ages of 12 and 19. However, while the condition may be active during this period, its residuals occasionally cause difficulty in the adult. When the metatarsal head has undergone degenerative changes, there is often a flattening and irregularity of the head, resulting in prominence and lateral enlargement. The same condition may occur in the other metatarsals (Fig. 151-2). In addition, there may be some enlargement on the plantar surface of the foot. While pain may be secondary to this lipping and degeneration, it is more likely that the symptom complex results from enlargement of the metatarsal head and pressure underneath the foot. Therefore, a patient with radiographic findings that suggest Freiberg disease should be evaluated carefully

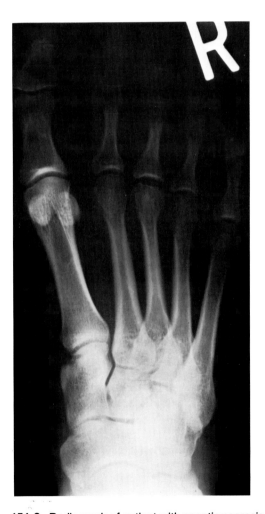

Fig. 151-2. Radiograph of patient with aseptic necrosis of the third metatarsal head with residual pain on weight bearing. This pain was relieved with a full-sole Plastizote insert, which shifted the weight to the shaft of the metatarsal.

to be sure that the symptoms are not a result of pressure underneath the head of the second metatarsal.

As with osteochondritis of the sesamoids, conservative treatment is indicated in all patients; this may consist of a Plastizote insert to relieve the pressure underneath the metatarsal head, or a metatarsal bar applied to the shoe. I have found that the Plastizote insert relieves the difficulty in most patients. An operation is indicated only when conservative measures have failed to give relief.

If the main symptoms relate to tenderness underneath the head of the second metatarsal the condition may be treated by oblique osteotomy of the metatarsal shaft to allow the metatarsal to ride up, thus relieving the pressure on the undersurface of the foot. Helal and Gibb[8] suggest an osteotomy and bone graft as described by Smillie[18] in the early stages (I and II) of this condition. In the later stages (III to V), these investigators suggest osteotomy,[9] if there is no pain on forced movement of the joint and the symptoms are secondary to pressure metatarsalgia. If arthritis has occurred, replacement arthroplasty is suggested. However, if the metatarsal head is enlarged both dorsally and on the plantar surface, this procedure will not be effective and other options must be considered. Freiberg[5] originally described removal of the loose pieces of bone. Campbell[2] described resection of the metatarsal head. Kelikian[11] suggests resection of the head with syndactylization of the second and third toes.

Surgical Technique — Smillie

The Smillie procedure is performed through a dorsal incision placed over the distal shaft and head of the metatarsal.[15] The incision is continued down through the skin and subcutaneous tissue, the extensor tendon is identified and retracted medially, and the periosteum over the distal shaft and proximal portion of the head incised. A slot approximately 1.5 by 0.5 cm is made in the dorsal aspect. The necrotic bone is removed with a curette and the epiphyseal plate drilled. The articular surface and subchondral plate are wedged into the correct position and held in this position by a graft of cancellous bone. Helal and Gibb[8] recommend holding the distal fragment in place by inserting a pin through the metatarsal head into the shaft of the bone. The periosteum is closed with interrupted sutures of 000 chromic catgut, the subcutaneous tissue with interrupted sutures of 000 plain catgut, and the skin with interrupted sutures of 000 nylon. A below-knee cast is applied and maintained for 6 weeks. Helal and Gibb suggest that the patient may bear weight on the cast during this period.

Surgical Technique — Campbell

The Campbell procedure for resection of the metatarsal head is carried out through a dorsal incision over the lateral portion of the distal shaft of the second metatarsal, which runs from approximately 1 cm proximal to the metatarsal head to just distal to the metatarsophalangeal joint. This incision is continued down through the skin and subcutaneous tissue. The extensor tendon is identified and shifted medially; the periosteum is incised with a knife, and subperiosteal dissection is carried out approximately 0.5 cm proximal to the metatarsal head. The bone is then osteotomized with a sharp osteotome or power saw, and the metatarsal head is grasped in a Kocher clamp. The metatarsal head is freed by subperiosteal dissection and delivered. The periosteum is reclosed with interrupted sutures of 000 chromic catgut, the subcutaneous tissue with interrupted sutures of 000 plain catgut, and the skin with interrupted sutures of 000 nylon. A pressure dressing is applied and a below-knee weight-bearing cast or walking shoe is used for 3 weeks, after which full weight bearing is allowed. The major complications of simple excision of the metatarsal head are shortening of the second toe with subsequent retraction and the shift of weight bearing to the lesser metatarsal head, with resultant metatarsalgia.

Surgical Technique — Kelikian

A dorsal incision is made between the second and third metatarsals, running from the midshaft of the second metatarsal distally to the web space between the second and third toes. The incision is carried down through the skin and subcutaneous tissue, and the second metatarsal is approached from the dorsal lateral aspect. The periosteum is incised and a periosteal elevator is used to dissect the periosteum from the metatarsal, approximately 0.5 cm proximal to the metatarsal head. The metatarsal head is grasped and removed, cutting the collateral ligaments around the joint capsule by sharp dissection. All fragments of bone present in the area should be excised as well. An ellipse of skin is excised from both the medial portion of the third toe and the lateral portion of the second toe, and the toes are syndactylized. The periosteum is closed with interrupted sutures of 000 chromic and the subcutaneous tissue with 000 plain catgut. The toes are syndactylized with interrupted sutures of 000 nylon.

Postoperatively the patient is managed in a below-knee weight-bearing cast or wooden-soled shoe for 3 weeks, at which time the sutures are removed and ambulation is begun. One complication reported from this procedure is shortening the second toe, if it has not been syndactylized. Kelikian reports good results with his procedure without significant complications when syndactylization accompanies resection of the metatarsal head. Care must be taken to ensure that the skin flaps are not traumatized, as this could lead to postoperative necrosis.

REFERENCES

1. Apley AG: System of Orthopaedics and Fractures. 5th Ed. Butterworths, London, 1977
2. Campbell WC: Infraction of the head of the second and third metatarsal bones: report of cases. Am J Orthop Surg 15:721, 1917
3. Colwill M: Osteomyelitis of the metatarsal sesamoids. J Bone Joint Surg 51B:464, 1969
4. Freiberg AH: Infraction of the second metatarsal bone: a typical injury. Surg Gynecol Obstet 19:191, 1914
5. Freiberg AH: The so-called infraction of the second metatarsal bone. J Bone Joint Surg 8:257, 1926
6. Giannestras NJ: Foot Disorders: Medical and Surgical Management. 2nd Ed. Lea & Febiger, Philadelphia, 1973
7. Gordon SL, Evans C, Green RB: Pseudomonas osteomyelitis of metatarsal sesamoid of the great toe. Clin Orthop 99:188, 1974

8. Helal B, Gibb P: Freiberg's disease: a suggested pattern of management. Foot Ankle, 8:94, 1987

9. Helal B, Greiss M: Telescoping osteotomy for pressure metatarsalgia. J Bone Joint Surg 66B:213, 1984

10. Inge GAL, Ferguson AB: Surgery of the sesamoid bones of the great toe: an anatomic and clinical study, with a report of forty-one cases. Arch Surg 27:466, 1933

11. Kelikian H: Hallux Valgus, Allied Deformities of the Forefoot, and Metatarsalgia. WB Saunders, Philadelphia, 1965

12. Kohler A: Typical disease of the second metatarsophalangeal joint. Am J Roentgenol 10:705, 1923

13. Mann RA (ed): DuVries' Surgery of the Foot. 4th Ed. CV Mosby, St. Louis 1978

14. Nuber GW, Anderson PR: Acute osteomyelitis of the metatarsal sesamoid. Clin Orthop 167:212, 1982

15. Painter CF: Infraction of the second metatarsal head. Boston Med Soc J 184:533, 1921

16. Panner HJ: A peculiar characteristic metatarsal disease. Acta Radiol 1:319, 1921–1922

17. Smillie IS: Freiberg's infraction. J Bone Joint Surg 39B:580, 1957

18. Smillie IS: Treatment of Freiberg's infraction. Proc Soc Med 60:29, 1967

Management of the Rheumatoid Foot and Ankle

152

Alan H. Wilde
Ian J. Alexander

Rheumatoid arthritis commonly involves the foot. Vainio[24] reported that 89 percent of adult patients with rheumatoid arthritis had arthritis in the foot. In 16 percent of patients, the initial manifestation of the disease was in the foot, particularly in the fourth or fifth metatarsophalangeal joints.[19]

PROBLEMS IN THE FOREPART OF THE FOOT

Initially, there is synovitis of the metatarsophalangeal joints. With persistent synovitis, distention of the joint capsule occurs, permitting dorsal subluxation and/or dislocation of the metatarsophalangeal joints. Clawing of the lesser toes occurs due to inability of the intrinsic muscles to flex the metatarsophalangeal joints and extend the proximal interphalangeal and distal interphalangeal joints. Dorsal subluxation of the metatarsophalangeal joint and loss of intrinsic function reduces weight bearing by the toes, and loads normally taken by the toes are transferred to the metatarsal heads, leading to metatarsalgia caused by this increased pressure. Hallux valgus commonly develops and, as the metatarsal heads spread apart due to relaxation of the intermetatarsal ligaments, a splay foot may develop. Rarely, hallux varus, with medial drift of the toes, is seen. This has been attributed to a rupture of the adductor hallucis, but this is not invariably the case. In addition to clawing of the toes, hammer toes and overlapping toes are commonly seen (Fig. 152-1). Divergent toes may occur as a result of the development of a large bursa between the metatarsal heads. As deformities become more pronounced, bursae may develop on the sole of the foot beneath the protruding metatarsal heads (Fig. 152-2). Keratoses may occur over the prominent metatarsal heads or over the dorsal aspects of the proximal interphalangeal joints in the clawed toes or hammer toes or on the ends of the toes if they are weight bearing. The keratoses and bursae may become secondarily infected, and draining sinuses may appear. Subcutaneous rheumatoid nodules are seen in the weight-bearing areas over bony promi-

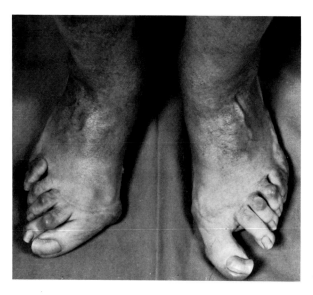

Fig. 152-1. Photograph of dorsum of the foot in a patient with rheumatoid arthritis, bilateral hallux valgus, and clawing of the lesser toe with keratoses on the proximal interphalangeal joints.

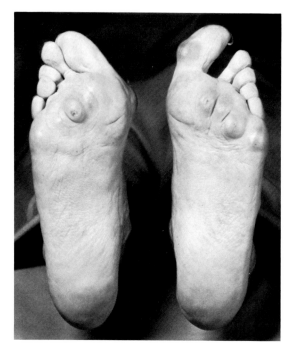

Fig. 152-2. Photograph of the plantar aspect of the feet shown in Figure 152-1 exhibiting bursae beneath protruding metatarsal heads and a keratosis on the plantar aspect of the distal joint of the left great toe.

nences or on the Achilles tendon. The clinical syndrome of Morton's neuroma is also seen in rheumatoid arthritis, most commonly between the third and fourth metatarsal heads. The intermetatarsal bursa may be the site of an inflammatory bursitis and may be responsible for symptoms.[2] Vasculitis can occur on the foot as it does in the hand. The lesions are small macules or papules and may have a necrotic center.

Conservative Treatment of Problems of the Forepart of the Foot

Initially, keratoses can be trimmed and protected by pads over the proximal interphalangeal joints or by applying metatarsal pads proximal to the painful metatarsal heads. As the deformities become more pronounced, the use of custom orthotics to unload the metatarsal heads may become necessary. In order to accommodate the deformed toes and the orthotics, a shoe with an extra-depth toe box may be necessary. Custom-molded shoes may be required if the depth inlay shoe cannot accommodate the deformed forefoot. Many patients will use athletic shoes for everyday use. Some patients resort to the use of sandals and/or slippers or to cut-out portions of their shoes in order to accommodate their forefoot deformities.

Surgical Treatment of Problems of the Forepart of the Foot in Rheumatoid Arthritis

Isolated hallux valgus, hammer toes, curled toes, or Morton's neuromas can be treated in a conventional manner as discussed in Chapters 141, 146, 147, and 148. When there are multiple subluxations and/or dislocations of the metatarsophalangeal joints associated with hallux valgus, reconstruction of the forepart of the foot is indicated. We agree with Clayton, who has stated that "if more than two metatarsal heads require surgery, it is preferable to perform the entire forefoot resection so that one may achieve a new weight-bearing alignment across the entire metatarsophalangeal region."[5] Using this as a guide for reconstruction of the forepart of the foot, one will occasionally have to resect one or more normal metatarsal heads. This is preferable to leaving a few normal metatarsal heads that may later cause pain requiring further surgery.

There are a number of ways to perform reconstruction of the forepart of the foot. These include implant arthroplasty of the first metatarsophalangeal joint and the lesser metatarsophalangeal joints, implant arthroplasty of the great toe metatarsophalangeal joint and resection of metatarsal heads 2 through 5, Keller arthroplasty and resection of metatarsal heads 2 through 5, arthrodesis of the first metatarsophalangeal joint and resection of metatarsal heads 2 through 5, the Hoffman procedure, the Clayton procedure, and transmetatarsal amputation. The results of each of these procedures are discussed below.

Implant Arthroplasty

Cracchiolo et al.[6] reported their results with double stem silicone rubber implants in the first metatarsophalangeal joint in 159 feet, followed between 18 months and 6 years. Pain relief was obtained in all patients. The amount of hallux valgus was reduced by 50 to 70 percent of the preoperative deformity. The lateral four metatarsal heads were excised. Thirty-nine percent of patients stated that they were able to wear stylish shoes postoperatively.

Keller Arthroplasty and Resection of Metatarsal Heads 2 Through 5

McGarvey and Johnson reported their results in 49 feet with an average follow-up of 4.9 years. There was recurrent hallux valgus in 53 percent, instability of the forepart of the foot in 27 percent, and continuing metatarsalgia in 20 percent of patients.[15] These results indicate a high number of unsatisfactory results when the first metatarsal head is retained with the use of the Keller arthroplasty.

Arthrodesis of Metatarsophalangeal Joint of the First Toe and Resection of Metatarsal Heads 2 Through 5

Results of this procedure in 18 feet in 11 women were reported by Mann and Thompson.[13] They had an average follow-up of 4.1 years, the longest being 7.25 years. Fusion of the first metatarsophalangeal joint was achieved in 94 percent of patients. This procedure effectively eliminated hallux valgus, and all patients were able to wear ordinary shoes. Reoperation was necessary in 11 percent for additional metatarsal head resection. Degeneration of the interphalangeal joint of the great toe was commonly seen radiographically, but was not symptomatic. These workers reported that the results of this procedure did not deteriorate with time.[13] Care must be taken to shorten the great toe so that it is not greatly longer than the lesser toes; otherwise, shoe fitting may be difficult. A great toe that is significantly longer than the remaining toes is also cosmetically unacceptable.

The Hoffman Procedure

The Hoffman procedure consists of resection of all metatarsal heads 1 through 5. Robson and Taylor[17] reported the results of 115 forefoot arthroplasties with an average follow-up of 4 years. At follow-up, 65 percent had no pain, in 30 percent pain had improved, in 4 percent it was unchanged, and in 1 percent it was worse. The cosmetic appearance of the foot improved in 89 percent of patients. Most patients had doubled their preoperative walking distance. Only 16 percent of patients used their toes normally when walking. Seventy-six percent of patients were able to wear normal shoes postoperatively. Spurs on the resected metatarsals were present in 70 percent of patients but were seldom symptomatic. All operations were performed from the dorsal approach.[17]

Amuso and Wissinger and co-workers[1] reported their results in 179 operations followed up for an average of 28 months. These investigators reported good or satisfactory results in 88 percent of cases and poor or unsatisfactory results in 12 percent of cases. The usual cause of an unsatisfactory result was insufficient bone resection or an irregular bone resection. The rate of wound infection was 1.4 percent. Supplemental surgery was required in eight percent of patients, usually to resect one metatarsal head.[1]

The Clayton Procedure

The Clayton procedure is performed through a dorsal approach and removes all five metatarsal heads through the necks and a portion of each of the proximal phalanges. Clayton[5] reported good results in 85 percent of patients with a minimum follow-up of 3 years. Reoperation was required in 10 percent of patients.

Transmetatarsal Amputation

In some patients, the deformities have been so severe as to require transmetatarsal amputation. A candidate for this operation would likely have dislocation of the proximal interphalangeal joints as well as the metatarsophalangeal joints with the presence of infection and vasculitis. This procedure has been performed mainly in Europe. The results have been good without an effect on balance from the loss of the toes. Gait is usually unchanged. The indications for this procedure are few in the United States, as most patients would rather retain their toes, even though some deformities remain (Savill DL, Wilde AH: unpublished data, 1966).

Authors' Preferred Technique

The technique for the Hoffman procedure of arthroplasty of the forepart of the foot is discussed, as it is the senior author's (AHW) preferred method of correction of problems of the forepart of the foot in rheumatoid arthritis. The senior author has had experience with more than 265 Hoffman operations.

Intravenous antibiotics are given at the start of anesthesia. We have been using cefazolin, 1 g q6h, IV for 24 hours. The operation is usually performed through a dorsal transverse incision at the level of the metatarsophalangeal joints (Fig. 152-3). A plantar approach may also be used; however, due to occasional incisional pain, the senior author (AHW) prefers the dorsal approach. The dorsal veins are carefully preserved. Longitudinal incisions are made over the shafts of the metatarsals through the extensor retinaculum, preserving the extensor tendons. A subperiosteal dissection is made over the metatarsals and the collateral ligaments of the metatarsophalangeal joints are released. The metatarsal heads are osteotomized with a power saw in a gentle curve (Fig. 152-4). No

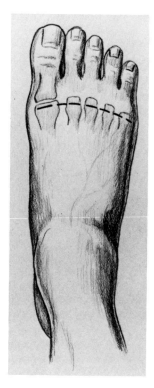

Fig. 152-3. Incision for the Hoffman procedure illustrated as a dotted line at the level of the metatarsophalangeal joints on the dorsum of the foot.

one metatarsal shaft is allowed to remain longer than another. The line of resection is made such that more bone is removed from the plantar surface than the dorsal surface to avoid having a residual condylar spike directed toward the plantar surface of the foot. The resected ends of the metatarsals are treated with bone wax to aid in hemostasis and perhaps limit spur formation. The medial and lateral sesamoids of the flexor hallucis are also removed in order to eliminate all bony prominences from the sole of the foot. The wound is irrigated. Hemostasis of any incised vessel should be obtained with the electric cautery. If the toes are contracted, they are gently manipulated into a straightened position. A portion of the redundant medial capsule of the first metatarsophalangeal joint can be resected or imbricated such that the great toe is not in valgus. Capsule repair is performed with 2-0 suture. The subcutaneous tissues are repaired with 3-0 suture. The sutures are placed at the junction of the dermis

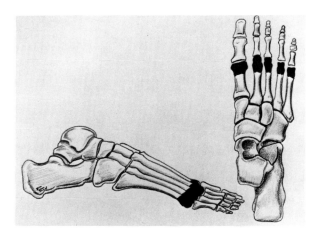

Fig. 152-4. AP and lateral drawings of the skeleton of the foot show the line of resection in a Hoffman procedure. Note that more bone is removed on the plantar aspect of the foot than the dorsal. The level of resection will vary depending on the deformity. More bone should be removed when the deformity is severe. The metatarsal heads are osteotomized in a gentle curve so that no one head is longer than another.

and the subcuticular fat. Drains are placed at the medial, central, and lateral portions of the wound. The skin is approximated loosely with 4-0 sutures. The dressing should be applied as carefully as with hand surgery. After applying a sterile dressing to the incision, a compression dressing of sterile Dacron is applied. The toes are carefully positioned with a small wisp of Dacron between the lesser toes and more Dacron between the first and second toes to prevent hallux valgus. After release of the tourniquet, all the toes should be inspected for ischemia. If the circulation of any toe is impaired, the dressing should be loosened.

Postoperative Management

Postoperatively, ice is applied to the foot, which is elevated. Active exercise of the ankle is encouraged. When comfortable enough, usually 48 hours, the patient may begin walking using a wooden-soled postoperative shoe. The dressing is changed prior to discharge. The sutures are removed 21 days after surgery, and Jacoby splints are applied to the great toes for an additional three to four weeks. The patient may begin wearing a shoe with a wide toe box, such as an athletic shoe, at 3 to 4 weeks.

Regular shoes may be able to be worn at 8 to 10 weeks postoperatively.

PROBLEMS IN THE MIDPART OF THE FOOT

While erosive changes can be seen in the joints of the midpart of the foot, they usually do not produce enough symptoms to require treatment other than the use of arch supports.

PROBLEMS IN THE HINDPART OF THE FOOT

Rheumatoid arthritis has been found in the subtalar joint, talonavicular joint, and calcaneocuboid joint. It can occur solely in the subtalar joint and in the talonavicular joint.[8] Commonly, the deformity seen is valgus of the hindpart of the foot. In advanced cases, the deformity may be so extreme that the head of the talus may subluxate from the navicular and become weight bearing on the medial side of the foot. In these cases, a rupture of the posterior tibial tendon may also be present. In the early stages of the disease in the hindpart of the foot, rheumatoid arthritis of the subtalar or talonavicular joint can be treated by the use of the combination of longitudinal and transverse arch supports and an extra-depth shoe. If this should not be sufficient to relieve the patient's symptoms, arthrodesis of the involved joints can be performed. If two of the three joints of the subtalar joint complex (subtalar, talonavicular, and calcaneocuboid) show erosive changes, all three joints should be fused. The valgus deformity should be corrected as much as possible. Bone grafts can be wedged in the subtalar joint laterally to aid in correcting the valgus deformity. We prefer to use two incisions: one oblique incision over the sinus tarsi and a dorsal medial incision over the talonavicular joint. Internal fixation is advisable, and bone staples are usually effective. Weight bearing should not be allowed before 6 weeks, particularly if bone graft has been used in the subtalar joint. A below-knee non-weight-bearing cast is used for the first 6 weeks postoperatively, followed by a below-knee weight-bearing cast for the duration of immobilization.

In the case of severe valgus deformity due to subluxation of the talonavicular joint, it is wise to resect the talonavicular joint surfaces first. The ball-and-socket nature of the talonavicular joint should be preserved to facilitate correction of the deformity. After resection of the subtalar and calcaneocuboid joints, the head of the talus is pushed dorsally and laterally while the forefoot is moved medially and plantarward. The correction can be held with a bone staple across the talonavicular joint. If severe valgus of the hindpart of the foot has been corrected, careful attention to rotation of the forepart of the foot is necessary before definitive fixation to ensure a plantigrade forepart of the foot. Failure to derotate fixed supination of the forepart

of the foot will invariably lead to lateral metatarsalgia. Associated ruptures of the posterior tibial tendon require no additional treatment.

Occasionally, an equinovarus deformity may be seen in a patient with limited tarsal motion. A closing-wedge supramalleolar osteotomy of the distal tibia and fibula has been described by Heywood.[11] The distal fragment including the ankle joint is displaced medially, slightly, in order to avoid a zigzag appearance. Ankle-joint motion decreased postoperatively, and five of eight ankles went on to bony ankylosis. However, tarsal motion was preserved, deformity corrected, and pain relieved, no nonunion occurred.

Bursal cysts of the subtalar joint and ankle joint are encountered rarely (Fig. 152-5). They are similar to Baker's cysts of the knee. The site of origin of the cysts can be confirmed by the injection of radiopaque material into the cyst and the use of roentgenograms. In the case of the subtalar joint, if the articular surfaces are intact, the cyst alone can be excised. Cysts of the ankle joint can present anteromedially or anterolaterally.

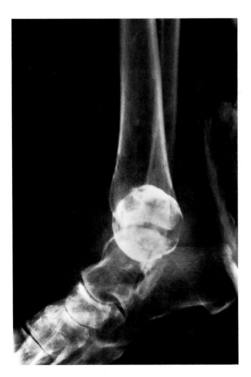

Fig. 152-5. Lateral radiograph of a foot and ankle showing that radiopaque dye has been injected into a bursal cyst communicating with the subtalar joint.

TENOSYNOVITIS OF THE ANKLE

Inflammation of the tendon sheaths around the ankle has been estimated to occur in 6 percent of patients with rheumatoid arthritis.[19] The tendons involved are the peroneus longus and brevis, anterior tibial, posterior tibial, and extensor digitorum longus. The peroneal tendons and the subtalar joint are frequently the site of combined inflammation. Tendon ruptures do occur, particularly the posterior tibial tendon and the Achilles tendon. Repair of a ruptured posterior tibial tendon is usually not indicated as there is frequently associated articular disease in the talonavicular joint or subtalar joint requiring fusion of one or both of these joints. Repair of a ruptured Achilles tendon is necessary. If much tendon substance is lost, a tendon graft may be necessary to bridge the gap.[18] Occasionally, tenosynovitis occurs without radiographic evidence of disease of the ankle joint. Tenosynovectomy is indicated when conservative measures consisting of medications, local steroid injections, or a period of rest in a cast or a splint have not relieved symptoms. In performing tenosynovectomy of the tendons on the anterior aspect of the ankle, care must be taken to avoid incising the extensor retinaculum directly over the anterior tibial tendon. This very powerful muscle tendon unit can easily disrupt the repair of the extensor retinaculum and skin closure and bow string through the wound. Following tenosynovectomy, the extensor retinaculum is repaired to prevent bowstringing of the tendons. In performing tenosynovectomy of the peroneal tendons, a portion of the peroneal retinaculum is also preserved in order to prevent subluxation of the peroneal tendons.

Subcutaneous nodules may also be excised if they are troublesome. Recurrence of the nodules is common unless the offending bony prominence has also been removed.

The tarsal tunnel syndrome has been reported in patients with rheumatoid arthritis. The posterior tibial nerve can be compressed by tenosynovitis of the posterior tibial tendon as it passes between the medial malleolus and calcaneus. The presence of burning pain and paresthesia on the sole of the foot in the medial plantar nerve distribution should not be attributed to the tarsal tunnel syndrome without considering other causes, such as peripheral neuropathy. Electromyograms and nerve conduction time should be performed. Conservative treatment consists of local steroid injections in the tarsal tunnel and weight reduction. Surgical decompression of the posterior tibial nerve may be considered if conservative treatment fails and electrophysiologic tests strongly indicate nerve compression as the cause of the symptoms.[13]

THE ANKLE JOINT

The ankle joint is not as frequently involved as other joints in rheumatoid arthritis. The disease can present in the ankle joint alone or in combination with disease in the articulations of the hindpart of the foot as well.

In the early stages of the disease, synovitis may be present without erosions or joint space narrowing. If the synovitis should persist in spite of conservative treatment of antirheumatic medications and local steroid injection, synovectomy can be considered. There are limited indications for synovectomy as not many patients will be seen at an early stage of the disease without erosions or joint space narrowing.

Once radiographs show joint destruction in the form of erosions and joint space narrowing, it is more appropriate to consider ankle fusion. Arthrodesis is now the treatment of choice rather than arthroplasty of the ankle. In an editorial entitled "Can the Ankle Joint be Replaced?," Hamblen[9] concluded the answer to be a resounding "No." A review of several series of ankle replacements reveals a significant rate of complications. Wound complications, including skin slough, may occur in as many as 40 percent of patients and skin grafting may be required. Infection rates vary between 2 and 5 percent. Loosening of the implant may occur in up to 25 percent of cases. Malleolar impingement and fractures are also frequent.[7,10,12,16,20] Bolton-Maggs et al.[4] reported satisfactory results in only 25 percent of cases. Until the current design and means of fixation of ankle prostheses are improved, arthrodesis of the ankle remains the treatment of choice for the arthritic ankle.

Operative Technique — Ankle Arthrodesis

The preferred position for ankle fusion is neutral, or at most, 5 degrees of equinus. Gait is considered the best in that position.[14,21] A variety of techniques are available for arthrodesis of the ankle. The senior author (AHW) prefers the technique described by Stewart et al.[21] The ankle is approached through anteromedial and anterolateral incisions. The medial and lateral malleoli are osteotomized. The articular surfaces of the distal tibia and talus can be completely removed. By removing wedges of bone from the medial side of the talus, medial side of the tibia, and the inner one-third of the medial malleolus, the lateral side of the body of the talus, lateral side of the distal tibia, and the medial two-thirds of the fibula, the ankle can be narrowed, which is cosmetically pleasing to the patient. This approach also completely removes the articular surfaces and allows maximum surface area for fusion. The malleoli are fixed to the distal tibia with screws. A Charnley clamp is applied for compression. One Steinmann pin is passed through the distal tibia, the other through the body of the talus. Any gaps between the osteotomized surfaces are packed with cancellous bone graft. The compression clamp is removed after 6 to 8 weeks. A below-knee weight-bearing can then be applied for an additional 6 to 8 weeks. Stewart reported successful arthrodeses in 92.8 percent of cases using this method.[21]

Pantalar Arthrodesis

In the event that the subtalar, calcaneocuboid, and talonavicular joints need to be fused as well as the ankle joint, pantalar arthrodesis will need to be performed.[22,23] The ankle joint and foot need to be placed in neutral with respect to dorsiflexion and plantar flexion and pronation and supination. The senior author (AHW) prefers to perform pantalar arthrodesis in one stage unless there is a major deformity in the hindpart of the foot that requires a correction. In the latter instance, a triple arthrodesis should be performed first. For a one-stage pantalar fusion, anteromedial and anterolateral approaches are made. The subtalar, calcaneocuboid, and talonavicular joints can be fixed with bone staples. The ankle joint can be fixed with AO screws. The position of the ankle joint should be confirmed radiographically in the operating room. Postoperatively, patients walk with a stiff gait and lack take-off. The use of a solid ankle, cushion heel (SACH) heel and rocker bottom sole may aid in gait and help to relieve any pain that is present.

REFERENCES

1. Amuso SJ, Wissinger HA, Margolis HM, et al: Metatarsal head resection in the treatment of rheumatoid arthritis. Clin Orthop 74:94, 1971
2. Awerbuch MS, Shephard E, Vernon-Roberts B: Morton's metatarsalgia due to intermetatarsophalangeal bursitis as an early manifestation of rheumatoid arthritis. Clin Orthop 167:214, 1982
3. Baylan SP, Paik SW, Barnert AL, et al: Prevalence of the tarsal tunnel syndrome in rheumatoid arthritis. Rheumatol Rehabil 20:148, 1981
4. Bolton-Maggs BG, Sudlow RA, Freeman MAR: Total ankle arthroplasty. A long-term review of the London hospital experience. J Bone Joint Surg 67B:785, 1985
5. Clayton ML: Correction of arthritic deformities of the foot and ankle. p. 785. In McCarty NJ (ed): Arthritis and Allied Conditions. 10th Ed. Lea & Febiger, Philadelphia, 1985
6. Cracchiolo A, Swanson A, Swanson GN: The arthritic great toe metatarsophalangeal joint. A review of flexible silicone implant arthroplasty from two medical centers. Clin Orthop 157:64, 1981
7. Demottaz JD, Mazur JM, Thomas WH, et al: Clinical study of total ankle replacement with gait analysis. A preliminary report. J Bone Joint Surg 61A:976, 1979
8. Elbaor JE, Thomas WH, Weinfeld MS, et al: Talonavicular arthrodesis for rheumatoid arthritis of the hindfoot. Orthop Clin North Am 7:821, 1976
9. Hamblen DL: Can the ankle joint be replaced? J Bone Joint Surg 67B:689, 1985
10. Herberts P, Goldie IF, Korner L, et al: Endoprosthetic arthroplasty of the ankle joint. Acta Orthop Scand 53:687, 1982
11. Heywood AWB: Supramalleolar osteotomy in the management of the rheumatoid hindfoot. Clin Orthop 177:76, 1983
12. Lachiewicz PF, Inglis AE, Ranawat CS: Total ankle replacement in rheumatoid arthritis. J Bone Joint Surg 66A:340 1984
13. Mann RA, Thompson RM: Arthrodesis of the first metatarsophalangeal joint for hallux valgus in rheumatoid arthritis. J Bone Joint Surg 66A:687, 1984
14. Mazur JM, Schwartz E, Simon SR: Ankle arthrodesis. Long term follow up with gait analysis. J Bone Joint Surg 61A:964, 1979
15. McGarvey SR, Johnson KA: Keller arthroplasty in combination with resection arthroplasty of the lesser metatarsophalangeal joint. Orthop Trans 10:624, 1986
16. Newton SE: Total ankle arthroplasty. J Bone Joint Surg 64A:104, 1982
17. Robson MF, Taylor AR: Excision arthroplasty of the forefoot in rheumatoid arthritis. J Bone Joint Surg 61B:519, 1979
18. Sbarbaro JL Jr: Surgery of the rheumatoid foot and ankle. 4:Sect. 9:191. In Evarts CM (ed): Surgery of the Musculoskeletal System. Churchill Livingstone, New York, 1983

19. Short CL, Bauer W, Reynolds WF: Rheumatoid Arthritis. Harvard University Press, Cambridge, 1957

20. Stauffer RN, Segal NM: Total ankle arthroplasty: four years' experience. Clin Orthop 160:217, 1981

21. Stewart MJ, Beeler TC, McConnell JC: Compression arthrodesis of the ankle. Evaluation of a cosmetic modification. J Bone Joint Surg 65A:219, 1983

22. Vahvanen V: Rheumatoid arthritis in the pantalar joints. Acta Orthop Scand 107(Suppl):9, 1967

23. Vahvanen V: Arthrodesis of the TC or pantalar joints in rheumatoid arthritis. Acta Orthop Scand 40:642, 1969

24. Vainio K: The rheumatoid foot: a clinical study with pathologic and roentgenological comment. A Chir Gynaecol 50(Suppl):1, 1956

Surgery of the Diabetic Foot   153

F. William Wagner, Jr.

Sir Frederick Grant Banting, an orthopaedic surgeon, and Charles Herbert Best, a medical student, isolated the pancreatic hormone insulin in 1921. The subsequent injectable animal extracts were heralded as a cure for diabetes mellitus. Unfortunately, the use of insulin has not lived up to this bright prediction and only a relatively small part of its promise has come true. Prior to the use of insulin, the typical downhill course of the diabetic patient was through emaciation, ketoacidosis, coma, and death.[27] Now, injectable insulin aids in promoting the entry of glucose into the cells of the body's systems and saves most patients from the typical pathway to coma. However, the later complications leading to morbidity and mortality have not been prevented. The most notable vascular problems are coronary heart disease, peripheral vascular disease, and small vessel disease of the eyes and kidneys. There appears to be an increased incidence of hypertension and cerebral vascular accident. Life expectancy is reduced to 70 percent of normal, occlusive disease in the lower extremities is 35 times more common, gangrene is more than 150 times more common in the fifth decade of life, and, despite advances in all areas of treatment, the death rate for juvenile-onset diabetes has not changed for the past 37 years.[25,27] The most common septic problem leading to hospitalization of a diabetic patient is an infected foot.[31]

As of this writing, it is estimated that there are between 11 million and 12 million diabetics in the United States. Of these 2 million are over 60 years of age. Diabetes is the twelfth leading cause of loss of years of potential life. This relatively small group accounts for at least 50 percent of major lower-extremity amputations.[12]

Since the pathophysiology of diabetes mellitus cannot be reversed, treatment is directed at symptoms, laboratory findings, and secondary manifestations. This leads to a multifaceted approach with many specialties involved. The team approach appears to be superior.[5,13,17,19] Medical members of the team include a diabetologist, orthopaedist, vascular surgeon, radiologist, general surgeon, infectious disease consultant, pathologist, psychiatrist, and anesthetist. Others are consulted as necessary. Paramedical personnel include nurses, medical social worker, psychologist, orthotist, prosthetist, cast technician, vascular technician, pedorthist, occupational therapist and physical therapist. The makeup of the team obviously will vary at different institutions.

Table 153-1. 277 Consecutive Dysvascular Surgical Cases, with Ischemic Index Over 0.45 in Diabetics and Over 0.35 in Nondiabetics

Level of Surgery	Cases	Healing Rates (%)		
		Diabetic	Nondiabetic	Combined
Above-knee	29	88	100	93
Through-knee	25	100	100	100
Below-knee	49	95	88	92
Syme's	79	82	95	91
Transmetatarsal	21	100	100	100
Ray and partial ray	33	81	100	91
Toe	30	100	100	100
Incision and drainage	11	100	100	100
Total	277	93	98	96

Care of the diabetic foot has changed markedly in the past 37 years. At one time, many patients with a gangrenous toe underwent an above-knee amputation. On a nationwide average, 80 percent of all lower limb amputations were done above the knee. Now 80 percent are below the knee, and at our institution the greatest percentages are at or below the ankle (Table 153-1). Surgery of the diabetic foot is ablative, reconstructive, and prophylactic. The progression of pathological changes is caused by deformity, peripheral neuropathy, infection, ischemia, or combinations of the four.

Peripheral neuropathy is present in most diabetics[23] and has been found in all who have had the disease for more than 20 years. There is no known treatment for neuropathy except palliation. Biochemical or metabolic changes and vascular changes are implicated in different theories.[9-11] Dysesthesias may be quite disturbing during the early stages. Motor changes are seen in the intrinsic muscles of the foot and are part of the pathogenesis of clawing of the toes (Fig. 153-1). Common peroneal involvement may lead to foot drop. Neurogenic bone changes can range from mild osteopenia to serve arthropathy (Charcot's joints).[16,18] Joints of the foot are involved more frequently than those of the ankle or knee (see Fig. 153-5). De-

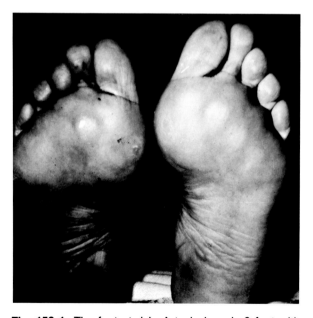

Fig. 153-1. The foot at risk. A typical grade 0 foot with hallux valgus, claw, toes, depressed metatarsal heads, and plantar keratoses. There are no open areas.

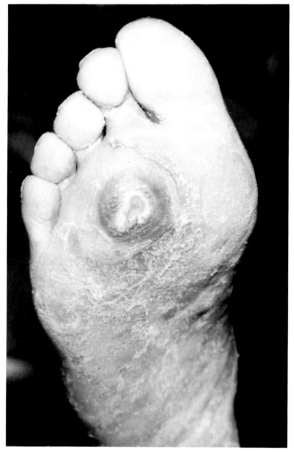

Fig. 153-2. Grade 2 lesion that extended to joint capsule. The open area is now closing after 2 weeks in a weight-bearing cast. Note thickened callus around ulcer.

struction of the midtarsal joints leads to bony deformity which, in turn, can lead to ulcer formation. The midtarsal joints are involved in approximately 80 percent of cases. During acute joint breakdown, the symptoms and findings may mimic an acute phlebitis or soft tissue infection. Bed rest and non-weight-bearing casts are used until the involved area has returned to normal skin temperature. Then weight-bearing casts are applied until healing is evidenced by radiographic examination (Fig. 153-2). If ulcers are present, weight-bearing casts aid in healing. As in major nerve injuries of the lower extremities, most ulceration occurs only after bony deformity has developed.[6] Any remain-

ing bony deformities are protected with polypropylene ankle-foot orthoses until healing is complete. If ulcers do not heal, underlying bone is removed through separate incisions; this procedure has resulted in virtually 100 percent healing. If deformity progresses, a triple arthrodesis is usually indicated (see Fig. 153-7).

Infection of the diabetic foot appears to be more frequent than in the normal population. Many factors appear to affect the outcome. The function of diabetic white cells has been shown to be impaired.[26] Basement membrane thickening may interfere with vessel wall transfer of nutrients and humoral factors.[36] Increased glucose content of

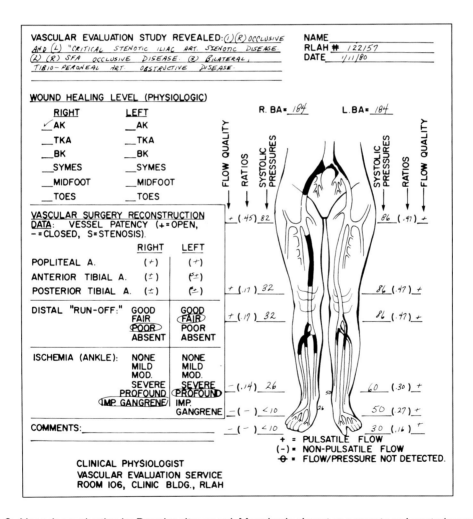

Fig. 153-3. Vascular evaluation by Doppler ultrasound. Mapping is almost as accurate as by arteriography. The ischemic index shows amputation level only at the hip on the right. Patient admitted for gangrene of toes on the right foot. Patient was referred for revascularization treatment.

blood and tissues may offer better culture media for bacteria. The autosympathectomy of diabetic neuropathy may decrease the normal vascular response to infections. Bacteriologic studies show a mixture of organisms present in most open lesions. Many times there is little concordance between organisms found in surface cultures and those found in the deep tissue after debridement or amputation.[35] Appearance of gas in the tissues is almost never due to clostridia but more likely to anaerobic streptococci, *Proteus* species, and *Escherichia coli.*[5,38] Surgical procedures appear to heal in a higher percentage of cases when the temperature is dropping and the white blood count is decreasing at the time of surgery.[13] If the temperature is in-

creasing and the white count is rising despite intensive medical care, this usually indicates deep infection that will require immediate evacuation or amputation above the level of infection.

The ischemic lesion in the diabetic foot is due partly to large and medium atherosclerosis[3,21] and partly to the microangiopathy of the skin and muscle capillaries.[1,29,36] Purely arteriosclerotic lesions usually occur after the age of 45 and are most often seen in the vessels distal to the knee. Although aortoiliac lesions are less frequent, they are more often amenable to endarterectomy, profundaplasty, and bypass grafts.[24,39] Symptoms of decreased vascularity are much the same in the diabetic as in the general population. However, in the diabetic they may

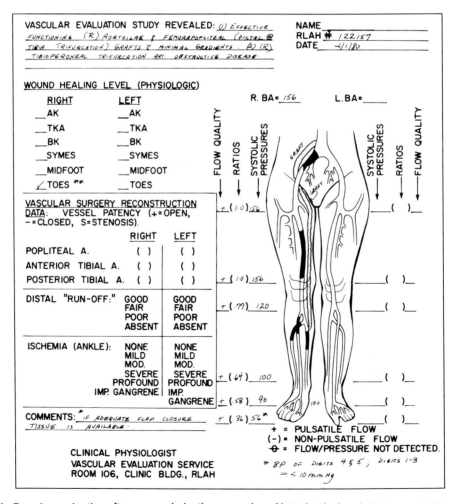

Fig. 153-4. Doppler evaluation after revascularization procedure. Note that ischemic index now indicates healing to toe level. The skin was not viable at toes, and a transmetatarsal amputation was done successfully.

be confused with neuritic symptoms, or they may be masked by hypoesthesia or frank anesthesia. Patients with intermittent claudication, rest pain, absence of distal pulses, nonhealing ulcers, and dependent rubor should be assessed by the vascular service for possible revascularization procedures.

An excellent example of the value of revascularization is the case of a 75-year-old diabetic presenting with infected gangrene of several toes. The initial Doppler evaluation showed a low ischemic index in the whole lower limb and the only possible area of amputation just below the hip. After arteriograms confirmed the areas of blockage, the patient underwent an aortoiliac and femoropopliteal bypass. Reevaluation by Doppler ultrasound showed healing potential at the transmetatarsal level. The patient underwent a successful transmetatarsal amputation and is now ambulatory (Figs. 153-3, 153-4).

With these multiple factors in mind, a system of grading the diabetic lesion and evaluating the blood supply by Doppler ultrasound has been developed. The accompanying treatment system has had a success rate of over 90 percent[43,44] (see Table 153-1). Lesions of the diabetic foot are divided into six grades, depending on the depth of the wound, presence of abscess or osteomyelitis, and the extent of gangrene.

Grade 0. The skin is intact. There may be multiple callosities and multiple deformities such as claw toes, depressed metatarsal heads, depressed longitudinal arch, and bony prominences resulting from Charcot arthropathy (Fig. 153-1).

Grade 1. The skin is open with a lesion that extends through skin only. The base may be clean or purulent.

Grade 2. The skin is open and the ulcer extends to bone, tendon, or joint. The base may be clean or purulent (Fig. 153-2).

Grade 3. The lesion extends to a deep abscess or osteomyelitis. Drainage may be absent, minimal, or profuse.

Grade 4. There is gangrene of a toe, toes, or part of the forefoot (see Fig. 153-11).

Grade 5. There is gangrene of such an extent that no foot salvage is possible and at least a below-knee amputation is required.

VASCULAR EVALUATION

Although neuropathy and infection appear to be interrelated with ischemia in the progression of lesions from simple to severe, the patient's ability to heal is most closely correlated with the blood supply to the area.[47] It seems evident that it takes more blood to heal a lesion than it does to keep the same area at a steady state in ordinary daily use. Patients are seen in the clinic with no symptoms and no open lesions but with an ischemic index well below 0.35. Methods of assessment of blood supply include oscillometry, skin temperature measurements, fluorescein tests, histamine wheals, plethysmography, ergometry, radionuclide scans, transcutaneous oximetry, radioactive xenon,[30] and similar procedures. Despite the use of these tests, the selection of amputation level has often been difficult and prediction of healing of lesions of the foot has not been easy.[32]

In recent years, the transcutaneous Doppler ultrasound flowmeter has been used as a sensitive stethoscope to map the arterial tree, to assess the quality of flow, and to measure the systolic blood pressure at various levels in the lower extremity[2,42,48] (see Figs. 153-3, 153-4). The American Heart Association has recommended that the width of the blood pressure cuff be 120 percent of the diameter of the limb being measured (e.g., a 6-inch cuff for a 5-inch diameter limb segment).[20] The systolic pressures obtained are used to calculate the ischemic index. The ischemic index is the ratio between the systolic pressure in the leg divided by the systolic pressure of the brachial artery, measured at the antecubital fossa. For example, if the brachial artery pressure is 120 mmHg and the pressure at the ankle is 60 mmHg, the ischemic index is 0.5. Healing can be predicted with over 90 percent success wherever the index is above 0.45 in the diabetic lower limb (see Table 153-1).

In order to plan a surgical treatment program, the presenting lesion is graded, the vascularity is assessed by Doppler ultrasound, and the medical treatment is begun. This includes vigorous control of the blood sugar, intravenous antibiotics, and local wound treatment.[15,19,43,44]

It is important that the ischemic index be measured at the level of healing desired. This may be for an ulcer or for a proposed surgical procedure. Midfoot or toe indices are measured to determine healing potential at those specific sites. The calf or ankle index is of no predictive value for toe or midfoot procedures.

TREATMENT PROGRAM FOR EACH GRADE

Grade 0

The intact skin is the greatest protection for the foot. All efforts are directed toward prevention of hyperkeratotic areas by pressure relief in shoewear. However, there may be deformities such as claw toes, hammer toes, depressed metatarsal heads, plantar keratoses, hallux valgus with bunions or bunionettes, Charcot arthropathy with bony deformities, and similar lesions. Protective shoe wear and patient instruction in the care of the feet are the most important starting points. If the deformities progress, prophylactic surgery may be performed before open lesions occur, or after healing if they do occur. Standard orthopaedic procedures, as described elsewhere in this text, can be done in the diabetic foot if the vascularity is sufficient. Bunionectomy, claw toe procedures, metatarsal osteotomies, resection of bony prominences, and even arthrodesis of Charcot joints can heal successfully (Figs. 153-5 through 153-7).

Grade 1

With ulceration present in the skin only, treatment is planned to produce a viable base that will heal by epithelialization or skin graft. Debride-

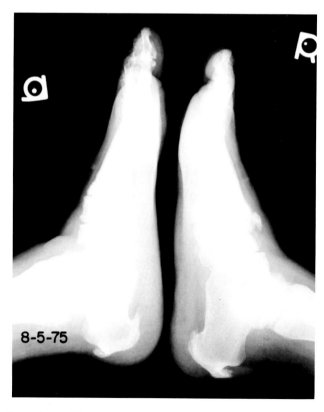

Fig. 153-5. Diabetic arthropathy in 52-year-old woman. Left foot developing ulcer under depressed head of talus. Right foot has been treated in cast and progression of deformity has stopped.

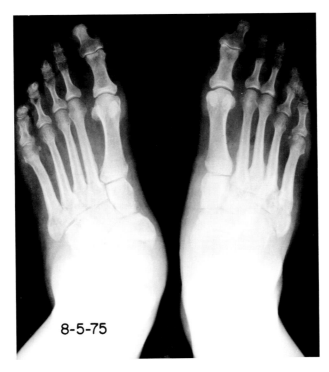

Fig. 153-6. Standing view of left foot shows marked lateral deviation of navicular and forepart of the foot from the head of talus, which has allowed the arch to collapse.

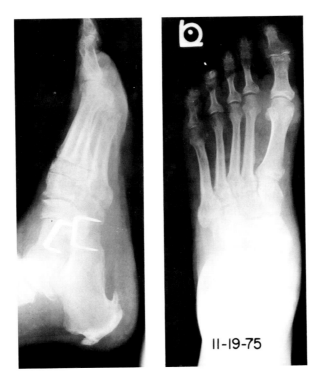

Fig. 153-7. Triple arthrodesis has been performed with inset grafts across the joints and staple fixation. The position of the longitudinal arch has been restored to that of the opposite side. Eighteen months of casting and bracing were required to obtain union. In December 1987 the patient had intact feet 12 years following triple arthrodesis on the left and cast treatment on the right.

ment can be surgical, enzymatic, or through wet-to-dry dressings. Weight-bearing casts aid greatly in the reduction of edema, healing of open lesions, and treatment of Charcot changes. Iodine in the form of Collen's solution,[7] povidone-iodine, or Iodoform packs aids in bacterial control. If there is surrounding cellulitis, antibiotics are used as indicated by cultures and sensitivities. After healing is complete, the residual deformities must be protected with suitable shoewear [29] (see Fig. 153-9). If there is any sign of recurrence, or if protection is not readily provided with shoes, surgical correction by standard orthopaedic procedures is indicated.

Grade 2

Since this lesion is deeper and penetrates to tendon, bone, or joint, debridement is usually surgical. An absolute must is the removal of all devitalized and infected tissue, especially fascia, tendon, and ligament. Ulcers less than 2 cm in diameter usually do not require skin grafts. Some ulcers require removal of underlying bone to allow closure. Walking casts are used for open ulcers and after operative procedures. Remaining bony deformities may be corrected following healing.

Grade 3

The lesion has progressed to deep infection, abscess, or osteomyelitis. Infected tissue of this type does not respond to small incision and drainage openings. An increased white blood cell count, increased fever, and difficulty in controlling the diabetic state all indicate the need for emergent surgery.[13] All infected tissue must be removed. Toe and ray amputations are usually quite successful for infections in the plantar space of the central toes. Removal of the lateral rays and toes through an oblique incision is successful and leaves a functioning foot (see Fig. 153-9). For surgery of this type, Kritter described an irrigation system that has worked well in our hands[22] (see Fig. 153-18). A small plastic tube is drawn into the wound through a separate stab incision. The irrigation fluid, usually containing an antibiotic, laves the wound and exits between the sutures, removing minor bits of debris and diluting the hematoma and residual bac-

teria. After the tube is removed, a cast is applied. Weight bearing is allowed at 10 to 14 days.

Grade 4

There is gangrene of some portion of the foot (see Fig. 153-14). It may be at the toes, metatarsal heads, beneath a Charcot deformity, or in the heel. Surgical level is determined by the ischemic index and the condition of the skin at the level of the proposed surgery. Multiple toe involvement usually requires a transmetatarsal amputation. Heel gangrene can be treated with excision of the os calcis if sufficient skin is available to close the wound. If the heel pad is intact, a two-stage Syme amputation is indicated. If the Doppler pressure and ischemic index are not high enough for a foot procedure, major amputation is carried out at the level indicated by the ischemic index. Consultation with the vascular service is obtained to be sure that revascularization is not possible before a higher amputation is performed.

Grade 5

In this grade, gangrene involves the major portion of the foot and no local procedures are possible. Amputation is performed at the level determined by the ischemic index. All efforts should be made to save the knee.[46]

SURGERY

The surgeon is usually not responsible for control of the blood sugar. However, an emergency may arise when some decision must be made before medical consultation can be obtained. Bessman[4] and Rossini and Hare[34] have excellent articles that will aid in the management of the diabetic surgical patient.

Specific Surgical Techniques

Toe Amputation

Gangrene or infection of a toe or toes can be removed through amputation or disarticulation. The flaps must be long enough to close without

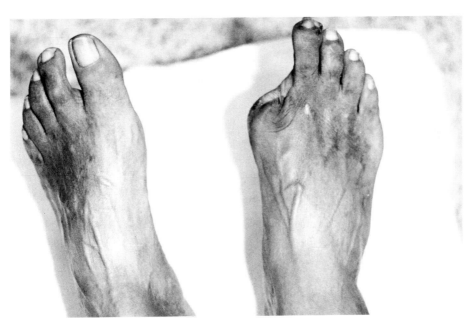

Fig. 153-8. Disarticulation of the great toe. A racquet incision was used on the medial side. A rocker-bottom shoe aids in roll-off during walking.

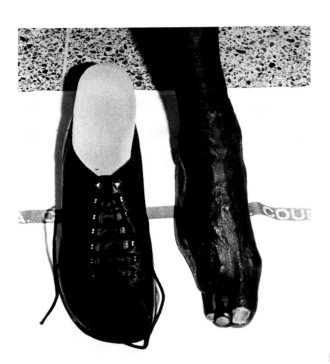

Fig. 153-9. Oblique removal of the fourth and fifth metatarsal rays and toes. A shoe filler of Plastizote keeps the foot secure in the shoe. Gait is normal.

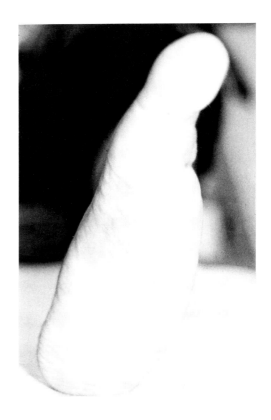

Fig. 153-10. The foot of an 80-year-old diabetic man 4 years after resection of lateral toes and rays. He has a below-knee amputation on right side. The patient is fully ambulatory.

tension. Disarticulation at the metatarsophalangeal joint is quite satisfactory (Fig. 153-8). If not enough skin is available to close readily, the metatarsal head may be removed. We have found that open wounds do not heal rapidly and skin grafts do not stand up well. It has been our experience that removal of bone with primary closure has left a far more functional foot than attempts at skin grafting. The period of hospitalization is also much shorter.

Toe and Ray Resection

Any combination of toes and rays can be removed (Fig. 153-9). Resection of the lateral rays, leaving the first ray and great toe, leaves a remarkably functional foot (Fig. 153-10). Gait after removal of the first toe and ray can be well compensated in a rocker-bottom shoe.

Metatarsal Head Resection

Persistent plantar ulcerations (mal perforans ulcers) respond well to removal of the overlying metatarsal head through a dorsal incision. The foot must be protected by a cast and then a polypropylene ankle-foot orthosis for several months to prevent midtarsal breakdown from altered foot mechanics. Disruption of the metatarsophalangeal joints may be severe enough to require a complete resection of the metatarsal heads. Again, the wounds are protected postoperatively with weight-bearing casts. Following this, protective

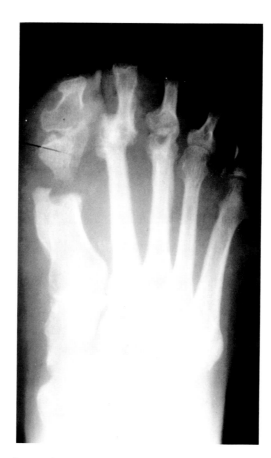

Fig. 153-11. Infection of the plantar ulcer led to osteomyelitis of the first metatarsal and proximal phalanx. All infected bone was removed. One year later, the patient has developed a pressure lesion under the dislocated second metatarsal head. The third metatarsophalangeal joint is subluxed.

shoe wear is prescribed (Figs. 153-11 through 153-13).

Transmetatarsal Amputation

McKittrick et al.[28] first performed this procedure for the diabetic patient in 1945, for gangrene of a single toe. Their satisfactory results in 67 percent of patients were excellent for the type of diagnostic procedures available at that time. Quoting from his article of 1949, "Careful review of the available data does not indicate how a more accurate decision might have been reached."[28] Now, at Rancho Los Amigos Hospital, with Doppler ultrasound for preoperative evaluation, our healing rate is well over 90 percent (see Table 153-1). The reoperation rate and late failure rate are both less than 5 percent. Most articles in the literature relate 25 to 35 percent rates of late reoperation.[45]

Indications

This procedure is indicated when a single or multiple toe amputation cannot be performed. The ischemic index should be 0.45 or higher in the midfoot. The ulceration or gangrene should not extend far enough into the midfoot that the flap will not be viable.

Surgical Technique

The incision starts medially and laterally at the midthickness of the foot at the level of the necks of the metatarsals. It then goes across the dorsum, neither undermining nor dissecting the dorsal flap. The incision is carried straight down to the bone (Fig. 153-14). The metatarsals are cut at the level of the incision with a motorized saw on an oblique line from medial to lateral. The outer edges of the first and fifth metatarsals as well as the inferior

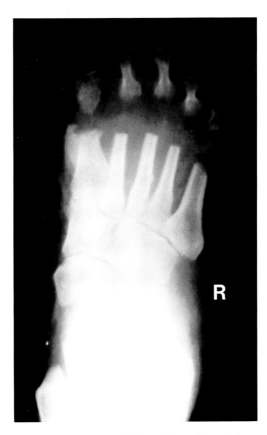

Fig. 153-12. Foot of patient described in Figure 153-11. Resection of the metatarsal heads and proximal portions of the phalanges relieved all plantar pressure points. The patient walks without difficulty.

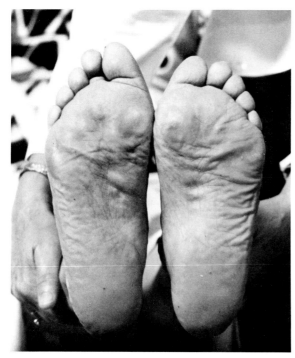

Fig. 153-13. Photograph of the patient described in Figure 153-1, 3 weeks after removal of metatarsal heads. This was done 2 years after Figure 153-1. In the interim, the patient had two episodes of plantar ulcers that were severely infected. She had a satisfactory gait for the 2 years she lived after her last foot surgery.

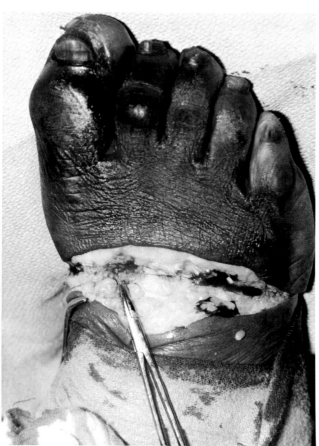

Fig. 153-14. Transmetatarsal amputation for grade 4 lesions of toes. Clamp is on first dorsal metatarsal artery. Incision is to bone.

edges of all the shafts are beveled to reduce soft tissue pressure concentrations (Fig. 153-15). The distal foot is then raised and the plantar flap dissected from the metatarsals on a bevel to the distal skin incision which is 1 cm proximal to the toe cleft. The tendons are pulled down, divided, and allowed to retract (Fig. 153-16). Hemostasis is secured with fine ligatures and pinpoint electrocoagulation. A Kritter drain is introduced[22] (Fig. 153-17). Closure is in one layer with nonabsorbable sutures (Fig. 153-18). When there is insufficient skin to close a transmetatarsal amputation at its usual length, enough bone is removed to allow the wound to be closed without tension. If the second and third metatarsals are left longer, pressure areas can develop when weight bearing is resumed (Fig. 153-19).

Postoperative Care

Irrigation is continued for 48 to 72 hours. The irrigation tube is removed aseptically and the tip is sent for cultures and sensitivities. A non-weight-bearing cast is applied. The wound is inspected at 2 weeks and walking is started in a weight-bearing cast. At 6 to 8 weeks, the incision is healed (Fig. 153-20) and the patient is able to wear protective shoes. Stiffened soles and rocker bottoms have aided markedly in walking.

Midtarsal Amputation

Lisfranc, Chopart, Boyd, Piragoff, and Vasconcellos procedures are rarely done, since most amputations in the diabetic foot are performed for infection or infected gangrene. In general, the most successful amputations from a healing and functional standpoint are distal to the tarsometatarsal joints.[14,15] Much of the postoperative equinus of the Lisfranc and Chopart levels can be prevented with transfer of the extensor tendons to the middorsum. However, this is rarely indicated in the face of infection. Dr. Richard Jacobs of Albany,

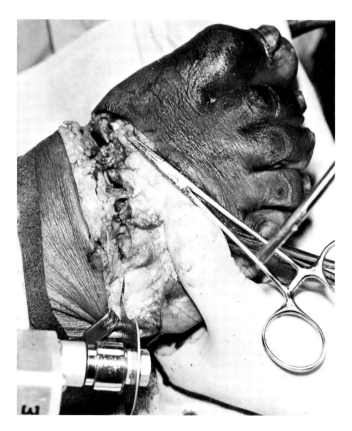

Fig. 153-15. Transmetatarsal amputation. Beveling of fifth metatarsal laterally to reduce pressure in shoe wear.

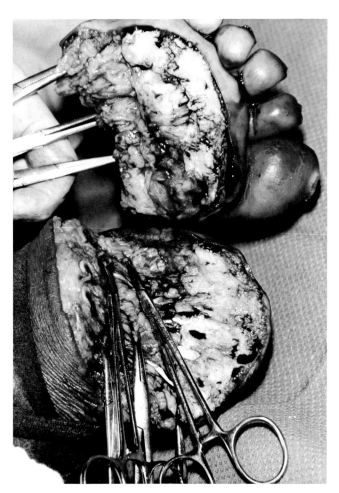

Fig. 153-16. Transmetatarsal amputation. Beveling of plantar flap and removal of distal foot. The plantar incision is made 1 cm proximal to toe clefts. Note tendons which are pulled down and divided.

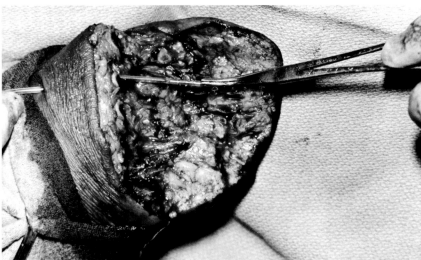

Fig. 153-17. Transmetatarsal amputation. A Kritter irrigating tube is brought in through a separate incision. Note that inferior edges of metatarsal shafts are beveled.

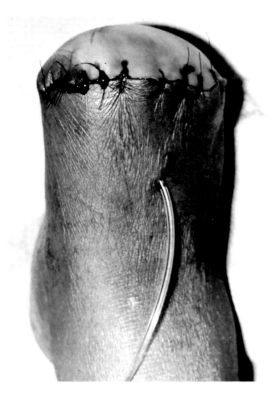

Fig. 153-18. Kritter irrigation system dilutes the postoperative hematoma aids in evacuation of debris and bacteria. Fluid exits between sutures.

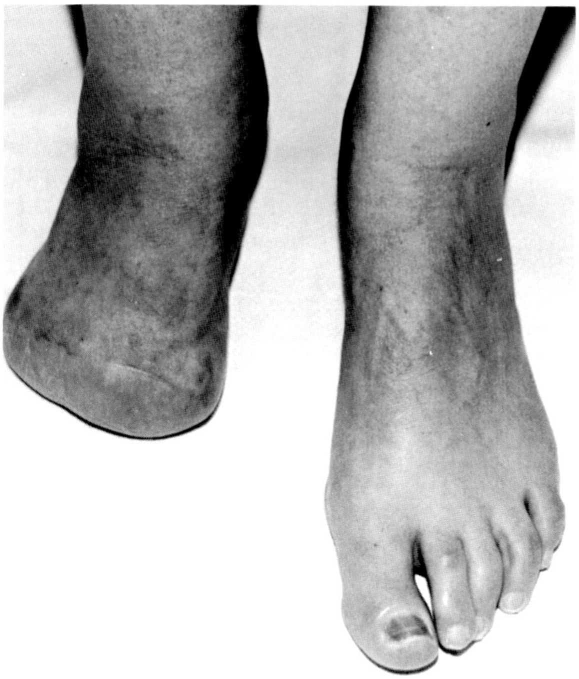

Fig. 153-20. Postoperative result of short transmetatarsal amputation.

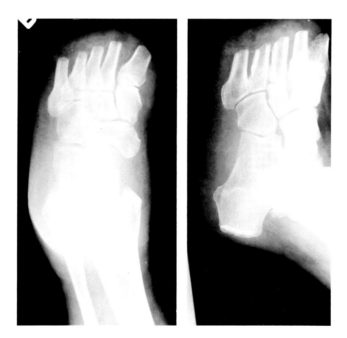

Fig. 153-19. Radiographic examination of residual foot in Figure 153-16. Note that second ray is slightly longer. An ulcer can be seen at the end of the second metatarsal. This occurred despite inferior rounding because of the slightly increased length of the second metatarsal.

New York, has reported satisfactory results with intraoperative percutaneous Achilles tendon lengthening for these two levels and postoperative support in a plastic ankle-foot orthosis.[17]

The fusion between calcaneus and tibia in the Boyd, Piragoff, and Vasconcellos amputations does not add any additional function to that obtained with a Syme amputation. The major disadvantages are the time required for fusion and the painful stump that can result from nonunion or fibrous union.

Syme Amputation

Although no movable ankle or foot is present, the residual limb is actually a partial foot because the heel pad remains. This pad, plus the length of the leg, provides function closer to that of the foot than that of the below-knee amputation.[41,46] Bilateral amputees with a Syme and below-knee combination favor the Syme side. They generally feel that the Syme stump acts more like their previous foot, is more stable, gives them better function, and is more of an annoyance than a disability. Despite this increased function, few centers have reported success with the Syme amputation in diabetic and dysvascular patients.[8,33,40]

Indications

This amputation is performed most often for infection and/or gangrene of the forefoot when no level of transmetatarsal or tarsal amputation is possible. The Doppler ischemic index should be 0.45 or greater at the ankle. If the posterior tibial artery is completely blocked, the amputation probably will fail and is not indicated. The skin of the heel pad should be free of open lesions. A two-stage method is indicated because of the residual bacteria present whenever infection of the forepart of the foot is present. Experience in the military with draining wounds of the forepart of the foot was disappointing with the single-stage Syme.[37] There was a high secondary infection rate in the distal tibia; this dropped to virtually zero with the two-stage method. The first stage consists of ankle disarticulation to remove the infected forepart of the foot. Removal of the malleoli and final shaping of the stump are carried out in the second stage.

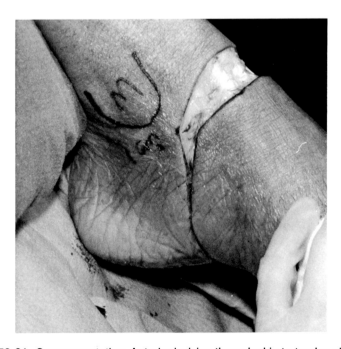

Fig. 153-21. Syme amputation. Anterior incision through skin to tendon sheaths.

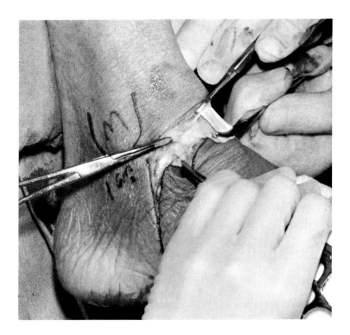

Fig. 153-22. Syme amputation. Incision carried through tendons.

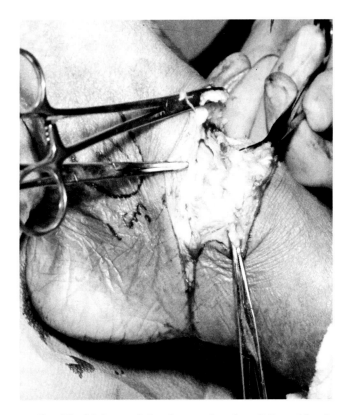

Fig. 153-23. Syme amputation. The joint capsule has been entered medially and the dome of the talus is visible.

Surgical Technique

The incision starts 1 to 1.5 cm more distal and more anterior than the classical Syme, which starts at the tips of the malleoli[41] (Fig. 153-21). From here, it goes across the dorsum of the ankle joint and plantarward just proximal to the base of the fifth metatarsal. No planes are dissected. The incision goes directly to bone. Tendons are drawn down, divided, and allowed to retract (Fig. 153-22). After entering the joint capsule (Fig. 153-23), the collateral ligaments are divided from side to side, allowing the talus to dislocate forward (Fig. 153-24). A bone hook driven into the dome aids in control of the foot and provides distal trac-

tion to tauten the ligaments as they are dissected (Fig. 153-25). Subperiosteal dissection of the os calcis is begun laterally and is carried medially until the flexor hallucis longus tendon is encountered, and dissected free from its tunnel under the sustentaculum tali. The tendon then acts as a protection for the posterior tibial artery and nerve while the medial surface of the calcaneus is dissected subperiosteally (Fig. 153-26). The Achilles tendon is severed sharply from the posterior base of the os calcis. Care must be taken, as there is almost always a ridge of bone at the inferior edge. Deflection of the scalpel on this ridge can sometimes result in button-holing of the thin skin posteriorly. Dissection along the plantar aponeurosis frees the foot.

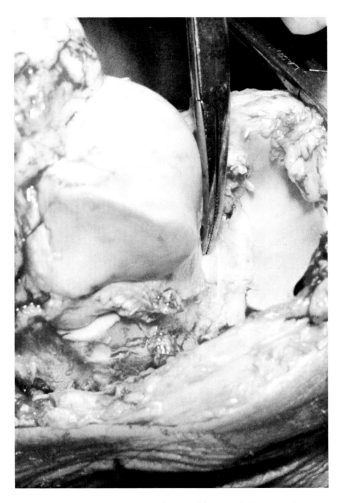

Fig. 153-24. Syme amputation. The talus has been dislocated forward. Flexor hallucis longus tendon is at the tip of the clamp. The tendon lies lateral to the posterior tibial nerve and artery.

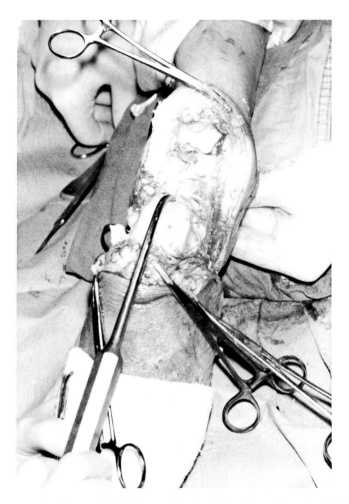

Fig. 153-25. Syme amputation. Flexor hallucis longus tendon is just above bone hook in talus. Neurovascular bundle lies just to the left of the tendon.

The wound is checked for devitalized bits of fascia and tendon and other minor bits of debris, which are removed. Hemostasis is secured with ligatures to the major vessels and electrocoagulation to the minor ones. The flaps are closed over a Shirley abdominal sump drain, which is modified for irrigation by perfusing through the air tube (Fig. 153-27). The perforated exit tube is connected to a collecting bag. Pressure and flow are regulated by the height of the irrigating bottle. The outlet tube is clamped off for approximately 5 minutes every 3 to 4 hours to provide lavage to all areas of the cavity. A soft compressive dressing is applied. The irrigation system is removed aseptically at 48 to 72 hours. The tip is cut off and sent to the laboratory for cultures and sensitivities.

Postoperative Care

After removal of the irrigation system, the limb is placed in a cast. At 14 days, the wound is checked; if the wound is secure, the patient is allowed to walk in a weight-bearing cast. Holes are cut into inch-thick felt to protect the dog ears. The patient is discharged and followed as an outpatient.

Second Stage

At 6 to 8 weeks, the second stage is performed. The malleoli are removed because they act as pressure points in the prosthesis in older patients. On occasion, if the pad is especially thick, a younger patient may have a prosthesis applied without a second stage. The malleoli are removed through

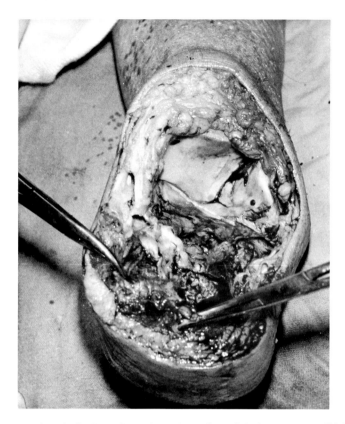

Fig. 153-26. Syme amputation. Left clamp is on branches of medial plantar nerve. Right clamp is on lateral plantar artery.

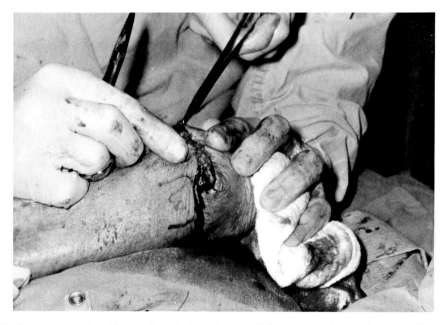

Fig. 153-27. Syme amputation. Testing flaps before closure. If closure is under tension, two slits may be cut in the fascia of the pad, which will permit nesting of the malleoli with relief of the tension.

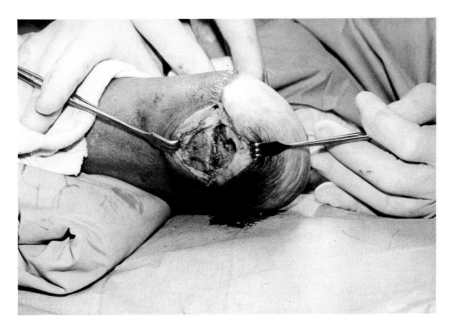

Fig. 153-28. Syme amputation—second stage. The lateral malleolus has been removed through an elliptical incision. The slight flare remaining is smoothed down.

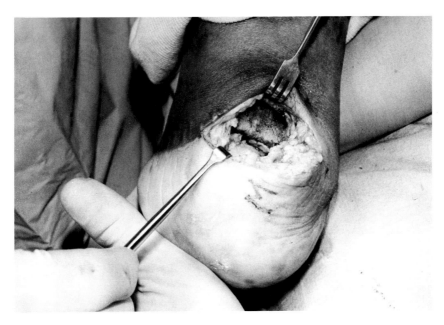

Fig. 153-29. Syme amputation—second stage. The medial malleolus has been removed and the flare of the tibia smoothed flat.

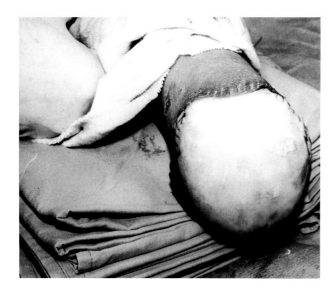

Fig. 153-30. Syme amputation—second stage. Completed closure of elliptical incision. Removal of wedge of tissue has tightened the pad against the tibia and fibula.

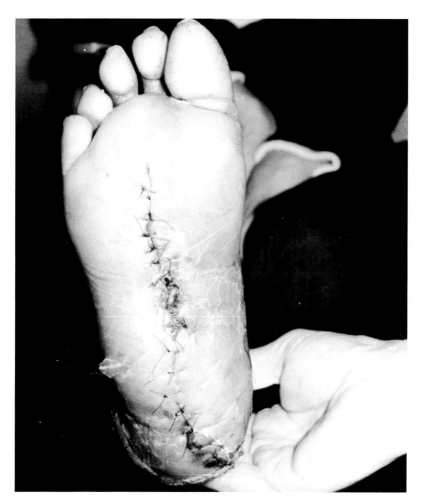

Fig. 153-31. Excision of os calcis. A heel ulcer and plantar abscess were removed. Sufficient os calcis was removed to close the skin.

elliptical incisions which outline the dog ears (Fig. 153-28). A wedge of soft tissue is removed to tighten the pad against the raw bone The sharp edge of the tibia and fibula are smoothed to alleviate any pressure points (Fig. 153-29). Deep fascia of the pad is sutured to the periosteum. If this is not sufficient to hold tightly, drill holes are made in the tibia and/or fibula for suturing of the pads (Fig. 153-30). Soft dressings are applied in surgery.

Postoperative Care

The patient begins weight bearing in a cast at 7 to 10 days and is discharged from the hospital in a few more days. The first prosthesis is fitted in about 6 to 8 weeks.

Excision of Os Calcis — Partial or Total

The heel is frequently involved with pressure lesions, especially in older diabetics who have had a hospital stay that required prolonged bed rest. It does not take long for pressure against the bony prominences of the os calcis to produce a gangrenous area. This can also occur from pressure and/or blisters from new or ill-fitting shoes. Because of the lack of supporting subcutaneous tissue, the healing process is slow and infection frequently supervenes. We have had excellent results in excising the ulcer and a sufficient amount of the os calcis to allow closure (Figs. 153-31 and 153-32). A Kritter or Shirley drain is used, depending on the size of the cavity. After removing the drain at 72 to 96 hours, the foot is placed in a cast. Weight bearing is not allowed for 3 weeks. In several cases, the wound has not healed per primum, and a small additional open area and more bone had to be removed. If the wound still does not heal, a below-knee amputation is necessary.

After complete healing and maturation of the wound in a weight-bearing cast, the patient is fitted with a polypropylene ankle-foot orthosis. There is excellent patient acceptance of this procedure, and the gait in this orthosis is obviously superior to that of a below-knee amputee in a prosthesis, the next possible level of treatment.

Surgical Mortality

Cooperation between the medical and surgical departments can provide optimum care for the surgical diabetic patient. Many of our procedures are performed under spinal, regional, or local block in medically unstable patients. For all surgical procedures from the through-knee level to toe procedures, the surgical mortality is less than 1 percent.[19]

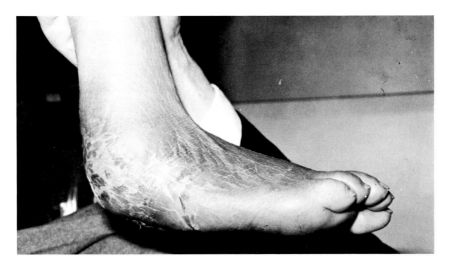

Fig. 153-32. Excision of os calcis. After healing of the wound, the patient walks with a polypropylene ankle-foot orthosis.

SUMMARY

The increase in numbers of diabetic patients has created a large segment of the population that requires highly specialized treatment for the feet, in addition to the treatment for the basic disease. The complications of atherosclerosis, microangiopathy, neuropathy, and infection produce problems in the feet in a high percentage of patients. Revascularization procedures increase blood supply to the lower extremity, aid in healing of local lesions, and allow surgical procedures and lower amputations to be performed. Because both lower extremities are frequently involved, it is most important to preserve as much of the foot as possible.[12] Although many of the surgical procedures are ablative, reconstructive and prophylactic surgeries can be performed to relieve pressure points and prevent further breakdown. The ischemic index obtained by measurement of the systolic pressure by Doppler ultrasound has aided in prediction of healing and selection of amputation levels with a success rate of over 90 percent in treatment of diabetic foot lesions.

REFERENCES

1. Banson BB, Lacy PE: Diabetic microangiopathy in human toes. Am J Pathol 45:41, 1964
2. Barnes RW, Shanik GD, Slaymaker EE: An index of healing in below-knee amputation: leg blood pressure by Doppler ultrasound. Surgery 79:13, 1976
3. Bell ET: Atherosclerotic gangrene of the lower extremities in diabetic and nondiabetic persons. Am J Clin Pathol 28:27, 1957
4. Bessman AN: Management of the diabetic surgical patient. Compr Ther 5:57, 1979
5. Bessman AN, Wagner W: Nonclostridial gas gangrene report of 48 cases and review of the literature. JAMA 233:958, 1975
6. Clawson DK, Seddon HJ: The late consequences of sciatic nerve injury. J Bone Joint Surg 42B:213, 1960
7. Collens WS, Vlahos E, Dobkin GB, et al: Conservative management of gangrene in the diabetic patient. JAMA 181:692, 1962
8. Dale GM: Syme's amputation for gangrene from peripheral vascular disease. Artif Limbs 6:44, 1961
9. Dry TJ, Hines EA: The role of diabetes in the development of degenerative vascular disease: with special reference to the incidence of retinitis and peripheral neuritis. Ann Intern Med 14:1893, 1941
10. Fagerberg SE: Diabetic neuropathy: a clinical and histological study on the significance of vascular affections. Acta Med Scand 164(suppl 345):1, 1959
11. Gabbay KH: The sorbitol pathway and diabetic complications: prospects for therapy. p. 594. In James VHT (ed): Endocrinology. Vol. 2. Excerpta Medica, New York, 1977
12. Goldner MG: The fate of the second leg in the diabetic amputee. Diabetes 9:100, 1960
13. Goodman J, Bessman AN, Teget B, Wagner W: Risk factors in local surgical procedures for diabetic gangrene. Surg Gynecol Obstet 143:587, 1976
14. Harris WR, Silverstein EA: Partial amputations of the foot: a follow-up study. Can J Surg 7:6, 1964
15. Hunter GA: Results of minor foot amputations of ischemia of the lower extremity in diabetics and nondiabetics. Can J Surg 18:273, 1975
16. Jacobs JE: Observations of neuropathic (Charcot) joints occurring in diabetes mellitus. J Bone Joint Surg 40A:1043, 1958
17. Jacobs RL, Karmody AM, Wirth C, Vedder D: The team approach in the salvage of the diabetic foot. Surg Annu 9:231, 1977
18. Jordan WR: Neuritic manifestations in diabetes mellitus. Arch Intern Med 57, 307, 1936
19. Kahn O, Wagner W, Bessman AN: Mortality of diabetic patients treated surgically for lower limb infection and/or gangrene. Diabetes 23:287, 1974
20. Kirkendall WM, Burton AC, Epstein FH, Freis ED: Recommendations for human blood pressure determination by sphygmomanometers. Circulation 36:980, 1967
21. Kramer DW, Perilstein PK: Peripheral vascular complications in diabetes mellitus. A survey of 3,600 cases. Diabetes 7:384, 1958
22. Kritter AE: A technique for salvage of the infected diabetic gangrenous foot. Orthop Clin North Am 4:21, 1973
23. Lamontagne A, Buchtal F: Electrophysiological studies in diabetic neuropathy. J Neurol Neurosurg Psychiatry 33:442, 1970
24. LoGerfo FW, Corson JD, Mannick JA: Improved results with femoropopliteal vein grafts for limb salvage. Arch Surg 112:567, 1977
25. Malone JI: Newer aspects of diabetes. Adv Pediatr 24:1, 1977

26. Martin SP, McKinney GR, Green R, Becker C: The influence of glucose, fructose, and insulin on the metabolism of leukocytes of healthy and diabetic subjects. J Clin Invest 32:1171, 1953

27. Maurer AC: The therapy of diabetes. Am Sci 67:422, 1979

28. McKittrick LS, McKittrick JB, Risley TS: Transmetatarsal amputation for infection or gangrene in patients with diabetes mellitus. Ann Surg 130:826, 1949

29. Mooney V, Wagner FW Jr: Neurocirculatory disorders of the foot. Clin Orthop 122:53, 1977

30. Moore WS: Determination of amputation level: measurement of skin blood flow with Xenon Xe_{133}. Arch Surg 107:798, 1973

31. Pratt TC: Gangrene and infection in the diabetic. Med Clin North Am 49:987, 1965

32. Romano RL, Burgess EM: Level selection in lower extremity amputations. Clin Orthop 74:177, 1971

33. Rosenman LD: Syme amputation for ischemic disease in the foot. Am J Surg 118:194, 1969

34. Rossini AA, Hare JW: How to control the blood glucose level in the surgical diabetic patient. Arch Surg 111:945, 1976

35. Sapico FL, Canawti HN, Witte JL, et al: Quantitative aerobic and anaerobic bacteriology of infected diabetic feet. J Clin Microbiol 12:413, 1980

36. Siperstein MD, Norton W, Unger RH, Madison LL: Muscle capillary basement membrane width in normal, diabetic and prediabetic patients. Trans Ass Am Physicians 79:330, 1966

37. Spittler AW, Brennan JJ, Payne JW: Syme amputation performed in two stages. J Bone Joint Surg 36A:37, 1954

38. Spring M, Kahn S: Nonclostridial gas infection in the diabetic: review of literature and report of 3 cases. Arch Intern Med 88:373, 1951

39. Stabile BE, Wilson SE: The profunda-femoris-popliteal artery bypass. Arch Surg 112:913, 1977

40. Srinivasan H: Syme's amputation in insensitive feet. A review of twenty cases. J Bone Joint Surg 55A:558, 1973

41. Wagner FW Jr: Amputations of the foot and ankle. Current status. Clin Orthop 122:62, 1977

42. Wagner FW Jr: Orthopedic rehabilitation of the dysvascular lower limb. Orthop Clin North Am 9:325, 1978

43. Wagner FW Jr: The diabetic foot and amputations of the foot. In p. 341. Mann RA (ed): DuVries Surgery of the foot. 4th Ed. CV Mosby, St. Louis, 1978

44. Wagner FW Jr: A classification and treatment program for diabetic, neuropathic, and dysvascular foot problems. p. 143. In American Academy of Orthopaedic Surgeons. Instructional Course Lectures. Vol. 28. CV Mosby, St. Louis, 1979

45. Wheelock FC Jr, McKittrick JB, Root HF: Evaluation of the transmetatarsal amputation in patients with diabetes mellitus. Surgery 41:184, 1957

46. Waters RL, Perry J, Antonelli D, Hislop H: Energy cost of walking of amputees: the influence of level of amputation. J Bone Joint Surg 58A:42, 1976

47. Williams HTG, Hutchinson KJ, Brown GD: Gangrene of the feet in diabetics. Arch Surg 108:609, 1974

48. Yao ST, Hobbs JT, Irvine WT: Ankle systolic pressure measurements in arterial disease affecting the lower extremities. Br J Surg 56:676, 1969

Management of the Foot Following Cerebrovascular Accident

154

John D. Hsu

Damage to the motor and sensory centers of the brain as a result of a cerebrovascular accident (CVA) causes loss of the ability to effect smooth selective muscle control for coordinated activities. A list of possible causes is included in Table 154-1. Most patients over the age of 40 who sustain a CVA have it as a result of either cerebral thrombosis or intracranial hemorrhage, whereas in younger patients the main cause is accidental head injury.

PATIENT ASSESSMENT

The patient's early clinical presentation may be expected to improve over time. This is because secondary control centers in the brain become active, leading in many instances to spontaneous recovery.[13] Most neurologic recovery occurs within the first 6 months after the CVA. The normal sequence of events may consist of a period of initial flaccidity followed by hypertonicity and hyperreflexia.[17] Factors that negatively affect a patient's chances of functional recovery were discussed by Bloch and Bayer.[1] These include persistent incontinence, decreased cognition, inability to move in bed, obesity, prior CVA, diabetes mellitus, hemianopia, aphasia, and increasing age.

The use of a knowledgeable interdisciplinary team for the treatment of a patient with cerebrovascular injury is crucial in restoring useful function. Treatment goals include maximizing the following abilities: physical, cognitive, communicative, and self-care.[4,14,18]

Gait Observation

An analysis of the walking cycle with specific attention paid to the ability of the patient for selective muscular control, and the assessment of patterns, deformities, and velocity can assist the examiner in the overall evaluation of the needs of the

Table 154-1. Possible Causes of Cerebrovascular Accident

Occlusive	Hemorrhagic
Cerebral thrombosis	Subarachnoid hemorrhage
Arteriosclerotic vascular disease (associated with diabetes)	Ruptured aneurysm
Vessel wall inflammation	Head trauma
Syphilis	Spontaneous
Acute or chronic meningitis	Neoplasm
Encephalitis	Hemorrhagic disease
Polyarteritis	Syphilis
Lupus erythematosus	Angiopathy
Thromboangitis obliterans	
Drug-induced (i.e., oral contraceptives)	Intracranial hemorrhage
	Rupture of arteriosclerotic vessel associated with
Cerebral embolus	hypertension
Cardiac disease	Arteriovenous malformation
Rheumatic heart disease	Aneurysm
Bacterial endocarditis	Trauma
Atrial fibrillation	Acute infection
Mural thrombi from aortocranial arterial tree	Vessel damage as a result of
Pulmonary thrombus	Syphilis
Fatty embolus from long bone fracture	Blood dyscrasias
	Collagen disease
Extracranial occlusive vascular disease (internal carotid,	Diabetes
vertebral)	Toxins
Arteriosclerotic vascular disease	Anticoagulants
Trauma	Neoplasm
Compression	
Embolism	
Syphilis	
Angiitis	

(From Montgomery,[11] with permission.)

hemiplegic patient following a cerebrovascular accident. The recording of these parameters of gait via motion pictures and videotapes allows for more detailed analysis, including pre- and posttreatment comparison.

Electromyographic Analysis

Walking gait electromyograms (EMGs) are done to determine the pattern of muscle activity in the leg muscles sampled in relationship to the deformity under consideration for correction. A report by Perry et al.[16] in 40 preoperative patients (6 of whom required surgery for equinus, 22 for equinovarus, and 12 for varus) was summarized as follows:

Although the exact pattern of muscle activity varied with each patient, premature firing of the triceps surae due to release of primitive locomotor control mechanisms and a hyperactive stretch response during limb loading are important causes of equinus. Prolonged firing of the tibialis anterior

during stance and inactivity of the peroneus brevis are the principal factors responsible for varus.

EARLY MANAGEMENT

Supportive medical care, proper management of the causative factors, and the support of bulbar weakness are of primary importance. The prevention of the patient's physical deterioration should be a part of the overall early management program. Special care must be given to the lower extremities:

1. Range of motion should be maintained; the residual range should be sufficient to permit standing, thus, a plantigrade foot is necessary.
2. Positioning of the patient in bed if important.
3. Splints should be used if proper positioning in bed is not possible.

PREOPERATIVE TREATMENT

Anesthetic Block

Local anesthesia, 0.5 to 1 percent lidocaine (Xylocaine), injected to block the posterior tibial nerve at the popliteal fossa assists the examiner in determining whether a persistent ankle deformity may be secondary to spasticity or to tissue contracture. Examination by this method provides information to help plan definitive treatment.

Phenol Nerve Block

One method for achieving temporary relief of spasticity prior to definitive surgical treatment involves the use of 3 percent phenol in glycerine injected to the motor branches of the posterior tibial nerve under direct vision.[8,12] A temporary reduction of spasticity is obtained and is useful while ambulation trials are being carried out. Specific indications for the use of phenol block are brought out by Garland et al.[3] as follows:

1. Equinus position not responsive to therapy or serial casting
2. Elevation of the heel in an orthosis while ambulating
3. Excessive ankle clonus

The effects of phenol block usually last about 6 to 9 months. After this period, there is a gradual return of spasticity with restoration of the deforming forces and abnormal clinical findings.

ORTHOTIC MANAGEMENT

Use of the ankle-foot orthosis is extremely important as a support to the leg in which there is (1) weakness of the anterior tibial muscle causing footdrop, (2) plantar flexion weakness with an unstable knee, or (3) proprioceptive loss. All are seen as early foot problems and can change with motor recovery.

The use of orthoses is important in the early treatment program, since the ability to walk may mean the difference between nursing home placement and living at home with the assistance of family members.[9,15,21]

Although many types of orthoses have been developed and are commercially available, the preferred brace is one that is as lightweight as possible with a rigid but adjustable ankle joint. The bichannel adjustable ankle lock (BiCAAL) was developed for this purpose and is illustrated in Figure 154-1. This ankle lock is incorporated into braces used in ambulation trials because it allows for fine adjustments in the angle of the brace at the ankle joint. Each component has an anterior and posterior channel, allowing the ankle joint to be set at any position either in dorsiflexion or plantar flexion. When the desired position is obtained, the channels are blocked with a steel rod and fixed with a screw. When changes become necessary, the ankle position can be readjusted.[13]

Therefore, in addition to the corrective value, use of such a brace is also important to the patient with proprioceptive loss; the presence or absence of pressure of the orthosis on the calf provides the afflicted patient with important sensory input. In cerebrospastic patients, especially those with hemiplegia secondary to head injury, the dynamic forces of spastic muscles and the development of static soft tissue contractures may render bracing difficult or impossible.[6]

Electronic Peroneal Orthosis

Functional electrical stimulation (FES) may be used for the hemiplegic patient with footdrop. FES is described by Vodovnik et al.[19] as follows:

> The brace was proposed by Liberson and various versions are presently manufactured in Europe and in the United States. The Ljublijana electronic peroneal brace functions as follows: An inner sole with a tape-switch at the heel is inserted in the shoe of the affected foot. Wires from the switch lead to a small stimulator which is usually worn at the belt of the patient. The output impulses of the stimulator are applied to cutaneous electrodes which are attached within a kneestocking. Cutaneous elec-

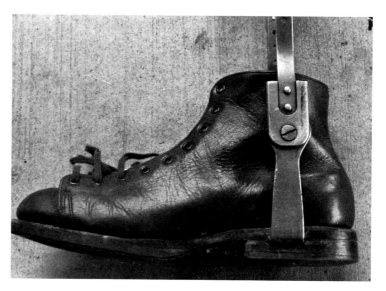

Fig. 154-1. Bichannel adjustable ankle lock (BiCAAL).

trodes are placed over the peroneal nerve. The exact location of the electrodes is determined experimentally so that good dorsiflexion and slight eversion of the foot is obtained. Generally the electrodes are applied over the peroneal nerve, behind the knee in the popliteal fossa. When the system is operational, the heel switch triggers the stimulator each time the patient lifts his affected heel to start a new stride. The triggered stimulator sends a train of pulses to the electrodes causing swing phase dorsiflexion. The patient is able to walk easier, safer, and faster. The stimulation of dorsiflexors normally contributes, also, to reduction of circumduction.

Modifications and refinements to this "brace" have been made. As an example, stimulation may be effected directly on the peroneal nerve by a surgically placed electrode operated and controlled using radio frequency. This eliminates potential interface problems between the skin and the stimulating electrode.[10]

SURGICAL TREATMENT

Surgical treatment of foot deformities should be considered as a part of the overall aggressive rehabilitative program. Because of the possible neuro-logic recovery of the associated changes, definitive treatment should not be performed until 6 months after the CVA. Preoperative planning is important. EMG gait analyses before and after operative treatment for hemiplegic foot deformities have shown that the abnormal pattern of muscle activity does not change significantly with the surgical procedure(s).[23] An appropriate surgical plan should be devised such that maximum benefit can be gained through operative intervention.

Once the patient has recovered cognition and sufficient motor control to permit walking, the situation can be improved in several foot and ankle deformities. These deformities include (1) flexion deformities of the toes (toe curling); (2) equinus, inadequate dorsiflexion and/or plantar-flexion weakness; (3) varus or equinovarus; and (4) plano-valgus. These deformities generally occur in combination and in most cases are greatly affected by the position of the limb and by the attitude, muscle tone, and strength throughout the body, especially the hip and knee.

Flexion Deformities of the Toes

Curling of the toes is a very common deformity; in most instances, it is a part of the overall foot problem. The toe extensors are usually inactive in this condition; thus, it can be differentiated from clawing of the toes.[22]

Surgical release should be done when pain occurs. Selective tenotomy is the treatment of choice when one or two toes are involved. If all the toes show curling, a tenotomy should be performed on the flexor hallucis longus and flexor digitorum longus in the sole of the foot distal to the insertion of the quadratus plantaris muscle. This procedure (Fig. 154-2) is described by Waters et al.[22]:

> An incision is made in the medial aspect of the foot along the upper border of the abductor hallucis. . . . The abductor is reflected plantarward and access to the flexor hallucis longus and flexor digitorum longus is obtained between the intervals of the first and third layers of plantar muscles. . . .

A more recent study by Keenan et al.[7] recommends considering additional releases at the base of each toe, which include the flexor digitorum brevis and intrinsic tendons.

Equinus Deformity

The treatment of choice for equinus deformity is lengthening of the Achilles tendon using percutaneous triple hemisection. The proximal and distal cuts should be placed medially. This procedure is described in detail in Chapter 134 and illustrated in Figure 134-4.

In the patient who has had a stroke, special attention should be given to the position of the foot after correction, as overcorrection causes plantar-flexor weakness. Postoperative casting in the neutral position or in 5 degrees of plantar flexion is desirable.

Curling of the toes may occur because of the relative shortening of the toe flexors after correction of the equinus deformity. This problem can be treated by lengthening or release of the toe flexors as described above.

Varus or Equinovarus Deformity

The varus and equinovarus deformities represent the most commonly seen foot problems.[2] The muscle that contributes to exert the most deforming varus force is the anterior tibial muscle. Although pure varus deformities can exist, equinovarus with curling of the toes is the most frequent condition. This deformity is best seen in Figure 154-3, in which the spastic anterior tibial muscle

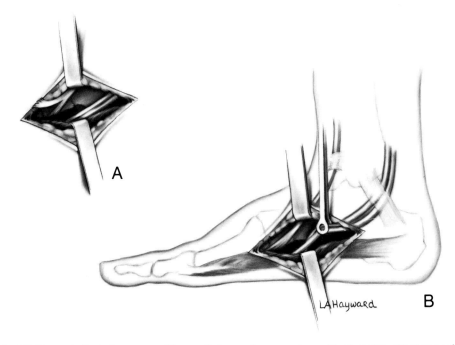

Fig. 154-2. **(A)** Flexor hallucis longus and flexor digitorum longus released in the interval between the first and third layers of plantar muscles. **(B)** Abductor hallucis reflected plantarward. (From Waters,[22] with permission.)

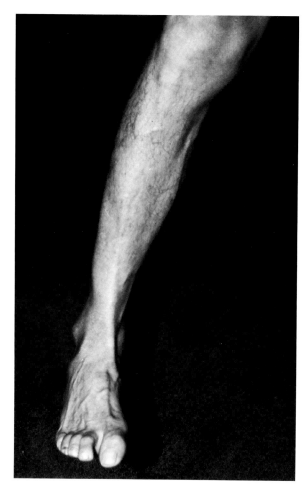

Fig. 154-3. Equinovarus deformity, post-CVA foot.

and tendon stand out. The surgical treatment of choice may be a combination of the following maneuvers:

1. Achilles tendon lengthening, by the percutaneous method
2. Split anterior tibial tendon transfer (SPLATT)
3. Long toe flexor release

SPLATT Operation

The SPLATT procedure is described by Hoffer et al.[5] (Fig. 154-4A):

> First incision is dorsomedial over the medial cuneiform. The anterior tibial tendon is identified and split with an umbilical tape. A second longitudinal

incision is made over the anterolateral aspect of the ankle. The anterior tibial tendon is identified. The umbilical tape is drawn into the second incision. The lateral half of the anterior tibial tendon is released, tagged, and brought up to the second incision. A third incision is made in a longitudinal direction on the dorsum of the cuboid. The lateral half of the anterior tibial tendon is passed subcutaneously into the third incision. By use of a 7/64-inch drill, two holes are placed in the cuboid at converging angles. A small curette is then used to join the depths of the hold, making a tunnel. Care should be taken to preserve a roof of bone. The lateral slip of the anterior tibial tendon is passed through the tunnel and sutured to itself with the ankle in slight dorsiflexion.

To prevent recurrence of equinus and stretching out of the SPLATT, reinforcement of the SPLATT by using the flexor hallucis longus and/or the flexor digitorum longus is recommended by Waters et al.[19] The required tendons are detached and passed through the interosseous membrane and then attached to the lateral transferred portion of the anterior tibial tendon (Fig. 154-4B).

Planovalgus

In the planovalgus deformity, the peroneal muscles are overactive and pull the ankle and heel into valgus. Planovalgus is seen only in patients who have pes planus and in whom the heel is in a valgus position prior to the CVA.

The surgical treatment of choice after failed use of an orthosis is percutaneous Achilles tendon lengthening. However, the uppermost and lowermost cuts should be based laterally. In addition, as indicated, release of the peroneal tendons or peroneal transfer to the dorsum of the foot may be used.[20]

POSTOPERATIVE CARE

Generally, 6 weeks immobilization in a below-knee weight-bearing cast is sufficient following tendon transfer or Achilles tendon lengthening in

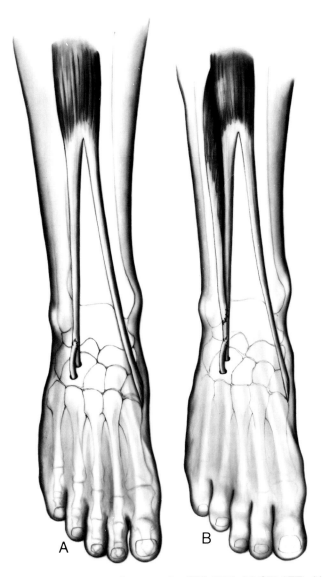

Fig. 154-4. (A) Split anterior tibial tendon-transfer operation (SPLATT). **(B)** SPLATT with toe flexor(s) reinforcement. Toe flexor(s) transferred through the interosseous membrane. (From Hoffer,[5] with permission.)

an adult patient. Ambulation the day after surgery is encouraged if possible.

After cast removal, the patient should use a locked-ankle orthosis when walking and night splints while resting; this is important for a period of up to 6 months. A range-of-motion, stretching, and exercise program can be started as soon as the cast is removed.

COMPLICATIONS

In the properly selected patient, complications generally are few and mild in nature. The chief problems encountered are skin necrosis and recurrence.

Skin Necrosis

Attention to hemostasis and meticulous closure of skin wounds are necessary to minimize skin necrosis and slough after correction has been effected. Skin problems occur mostly on the deformed side of the foot.

Recurrence

1. *Residual footdrop.* This problem can occur with increasing spasticity of the plantar flexors or further weakness of the anterior structures.
2. *Loss of correction.* In equinovarus, whenever possible, the SPLATT procedure should be reinforced by using the flexor hallucis longus and/or the flexor digitorum longus to minimize this problem.
3. *Triceps surae weakness.* Triceps surae weakness can affect knee stability. It occurs when the heel cord is overlengthened; thus, overcorrection should be avoided and positioning at neutral or 5 degrees of plantar flexion is desirable when casting after surgery.

REFERENCES

1. Bloch R, Bayer N: Prognosis in stroke. Clin Orthop 131:10, 1978
2. Capen DA, Garland D, Waters R: Orthopaedic surgery in patients with neurological dysfunction. Orthop Rev 8:125, 1979
3. Garland DE, Lucie RS, Waters RL: Current uses of phenol nerve block for adult acquired spasticity. Unpublished manuscript
4. Hoffer MM, Garrett A, Brink J, et al: The orthopaedic management of brain-injured children. J Bone Joint Surg 53A:567, 1971
5. Hoffer MM, Reiswig JA, Garrett AM, et al: The split anterior tibial tendon transfer in the treatment of spastic varus hindfoot of childhood. Orthop Clin North Am 5:31, 1974
6. Keenan MA, Creighton J, Garland DE, et al: Surgical correction of spastic equinovarus deformity in the adult head trauma patient. Foot Ankle 5:35, 1984
7. Keenan MA, Gorai P, Smith CW, et al: Intrinsic toe flexion deformity following correction of spastic equinovarus deformity in adults. Foot Ankle 7:333, 1987
8. Khalili AA, Betts HB: Peripheral nerve block with phenol in the management of spasticity. JAMA 200:1155, 1967
9. McCollough NC III: Orthotic management in adult hemiplegia. Clin Orthop 131:38, 1978
10. McNeal DR, Reswick JB: Control of skeletal muscle by electrical stimulation. Adv Biomed Eng 6:209, 1976
11. Montgomery J, Gillis MK, Winstein C: Physical Therapy Management of Patients with Hemiplegia Secondary to Cerebrovascular Accident. Professional Staff Association of Rancho Los Amigos Hospital, Inc., Downey, CA, 1979
12. Mooney V, Frykman G, McLamb J: Current status of intraneural phenol injections. Clin Orthop 63:122, 1969
13. Mooney V, Perry J, Nickel VL: Surgical and non-surgical orthopaedic care of stroke. J Bone Joint Surg 49A:989, 1967
14. Nickel VL, Hsu JD: Current treatment techniques and rehabilitation for neurological disorders. p. 45–53. In Arnold L, Billingsley JB (eds): Technology and the Neurologically Handicapped. National Aeronautics and Space Administration, Washington, DC, 1974
15. Perry J: Lower-extremity bracing in hemiplegia. Clin Orthop 63:32, 1969
16. Perry J, Waters R, Perrin T: Electromyographic analysis of equinovarus following stroke. Clin Orthop 131:47, 1978
17. Roper BA: Orthopedic management of the stroke patient. Clin Orthop 219:78, 1987
18. Treanor WJ: The role of physical medicine treatment in stroke rehabilitation. Clin Orthop 63:14, 1969
19. Vodovnik L, Kralj A, Stanic V, et al: Recent applications of functional electrical stimulation to stroke patients in Ljubljana. Clin Orthop 131:64, 1978
20. Waters RL: A surgical and orthotic management of limb deformities following stroke. Lecture presented at San Francisco Orthopaedic Review Course, June, 1980
21. Waters R, Montgomery J: Lower extremity management of hemiparesis. Clin Orthop 102:133, 1974
22. Waters RL, Perry J, Garland D: Surgical correction of gait abnormalities following stroke. Clin Orthop 131:54, 1978
23. Waters RL, Frazier J, Garland DE, et al: Electromyographic gait analysis before and after operative treatment for hemiplegic equinus and equinovarus deformity. J Bone Joint Surg 64A:284, 1982

Management of Skin and Nail Problems

155

Malcolm A. Brahms

CORNS

A corn is a hyperkeratotic lesion of skin that commonly occurs on the toes. It is usually found on the dorsum of the toes.

Corns are readily identified by the characteristic appearance of a thickened epidermis with a conical center. Corns are the result of irritation to the skin when it is compressed between an internal and an external source of pressure, such as a shoe. The pressure supplied from the inside is usually that of an enlarged phalangeal condyle, a bony prominence, an unreduced dislocation of the interphalangeal joint, or an exostosis.

Irritation from a shoe or any unyielding surface results in an inflammatory reaction with increased cellular production and a cone-shaped thickening of the skin. Corns may occur even in children if there is irritation from friction. Pronated feet with elevation of the lateral border of the foot and resultant pressure of the toe against the side of the shoe produce an irritative phenomenon and may result in the formation of a corn.

A corn may occur on any of the lesser toes, most frequently on the fifth toe[1] (Fig. 155-1). It is not an uncommon finding over a flexed proximal or distal interphalangeal joint,[2] as commonly seen in deformities such as hammertoes (Fig. 155-2). When there is a flexion deformity such as a mallet toe, a corn may form at the tip of the toe; this is known as an end corn (Fig. 155-3).

TREATMENT

The treatment of corns is as follows: conservative treatment involves shaving or paring of the hyperkeratotic areas with special knife blades. The central portion of the corn is called the apex. This should be enucleated without cutting into the dermal layers. The source of toe pain can be relieved by this management. The technique can be learned easily, and the razor-sharp blades are disposable.

The palliative treatment of a corn may be conservative, involving removal of the hyperkeratotic conical layers followed by the application of protective padding. Such padding may be made of thin

4223

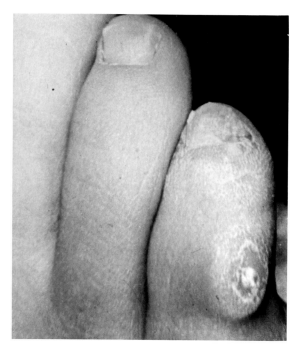

Fig. 155-1. Hyperkeratotic lesion (corn) on outer side of fifth toe. (From Brahms,[1] with permission.)

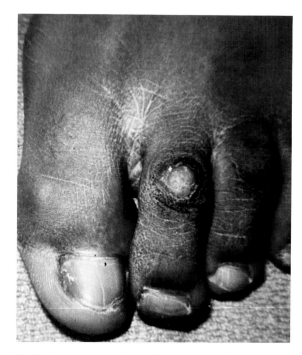

Fig. 155-2. Corn on second toe. (From Brahms,[2] with permission.)

Fig. 155-3. End corn. (From Brahms,[2] with permission.)

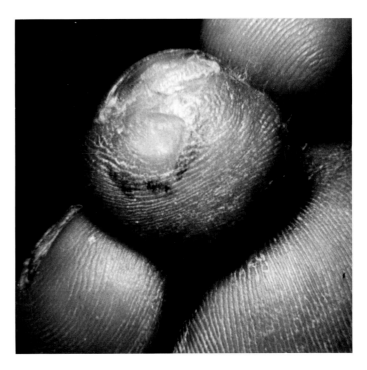

moleskin, felt, rubber, Plastizote, or a similar product (Fig. 155-4). This may be supplied commercially, with adhesive backing. It is applied to remove the pressure from the area of the corn and redistribute it to the toe. Latex pads (Fig. 155-5) are available in different sizes, and fit like a rubber glove over the toe to distribute the pressure from the area of pain to the noninvolved areas of the toe. Such pads are easily removed, washed, and reapplied.

Surgical Treatment

If the corn fails to respond to conservative therapy, surgical treatment may be considered, but only after careful evaluation of the patient is made. The vascular status of the foot should be intact, and the patient should have no metabolic problems.

When surgical treatment is indicated, the offending (prominent) portion of the condyle is removed, or a hemiphalangectomy can be performed.

An incision is made on the dorsum of the toe, either directly in line with the toe or obliquely across the involved joint. The incision should be carried through the skin directly to the bone. The prominent portion of the condyle should be removed. It is advisable to use sharp, small instruments similar to those used in hand surgery: a small rongeur, thin osteotome, rasp, and power equipment.

Technique

A 2-cm incision is made on the dorsum of the toe across the proximal interphalangeal joint. This incision may be oblique or straight and should be made boldly through the skin to the bone, avoiding the extensor tendon. Small nasal elevators or Freer elevators are used to retract the extensor tendon and/or the capsule on either side of the phalanx (Fig. 155-6). The proximal interphalangeal joint is flexed to help clear the soft tissues. The protruding portion of the bone is removed with a small bone-cutting forceps, a rongeur, or power equipment (Fig. 155-7). If the extensor tendon has not been transected, closure may be made through the skin edges. If the extensor tendon has been transected, it should be repaired in order to avoid the development of a flail toe (Fig. 155-8). Sutures can be removed in 7 to 10 days.

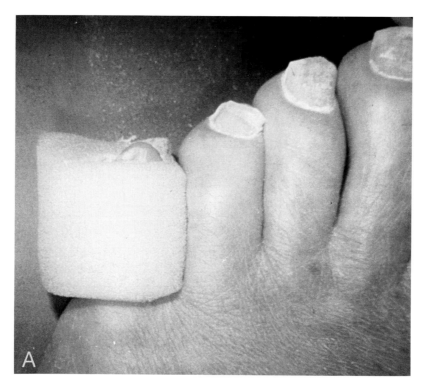

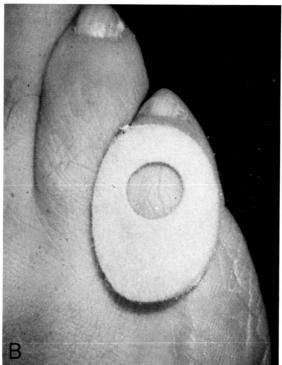

Fig. 155-4. **(A)** Moleskin (felt) pad applied to toe after removal of hyperkeratotic tissue. **(B)** Foam pad. (From Brahms,[2] with permission.)

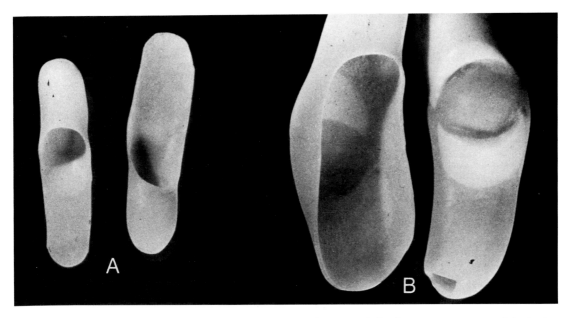

Fig. 155-5. Custom-made or commercial pads that fit over the toe and distribute pressure around the lesion. (From Brahms,[2] with permission.)

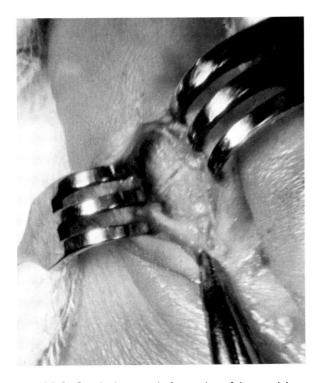

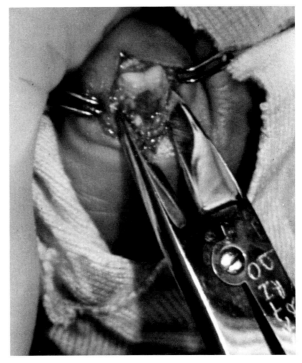

Fig. 155-6. Surgical removal of a portion of the condyle or condyles, following which the remaining bone is rasped smooth. (From Brahms,[2] with permission.)

Fig. 155-7. Bone-cutting forceps are used to remove the distal end of the proximal phalanx. (From Brahms,[2] with permission.)

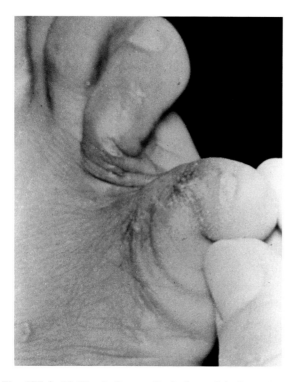

Fig. 155-8. Flail toe is the result of a loss of the integrity of the extensor tendon. (From Brahms,[2] with permission.)

SOFT CORNS

A soft corn is a painful hyperkeratotic lesion found between the toes. It represents pressure of one condyle against a contiguous condyle of the opposing toe (Fig. 155-9). Soft corns may be located in the web space or opposite any of the interphalangeal joint areas.

Treatment

The palliative treatment for soft corns — which involves relieving the lesions by shaving them with a small, sharp instrument, followed by the use of pads and/or lamb's wool between the toes — usually does not produce lasting relief because effective padding between the toes is difficult. Unless there are serious medical contraindications, surgery should be performed.

Surgical management of soft corns necessitates the removal of the protruding condyle of either one or both toes. The approach to the bony prominence

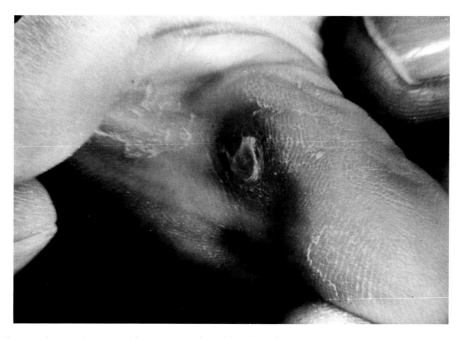

Fig. 155-9. A soft corn between the toes produced by chronic irritation of contiguous bony ridges. (From Brahms,[2] with permission.)

should be made through the dorsum of the toes. Incisions into web spaces should be avoided in order to prevent scars and sinus tract infections.

The incision is made through the skin to the bone. The condyle of the phalanx is cleared of all soft tissues with a nasal elevator. The condyle should be removed with a sharp, small instrument and smoothed with a rasp (Fig. 155-10).

Soft corns may also result from an unreduced interphalangeal joint dislocation (Fig. 155-11). Removal of the projecting condyle is recommended in such cases.

Soft corns may be confused with fungus infections when the corn is located near the web space and maceration occurs (Fig. 155-12). Frequently, surgical treatment as outlined will result in the

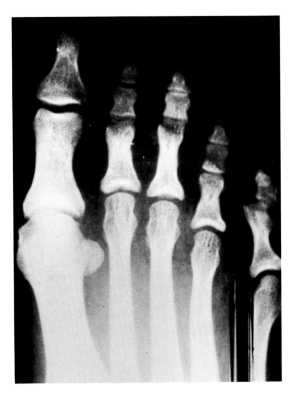

Fig. 155-11. Dislocation of interphalangeal joint may cause interdigital soft corn formation. (From Brahms,[2] with permission.)

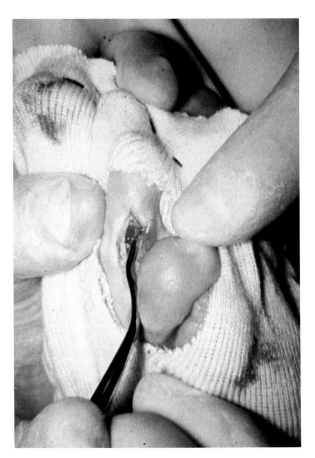

Fig. 155-10. Following surgical removal of a soft corn, the bone is rasped smooth. (From Brahms,[2] with permission.)

elimination of the maceration as well as of the irritation.

Not infrequently, excisions of soft corns in the interdigital space result in a painful scar or a draining sinus (Fig. 155-13). The basic reason for these complications is that the bone producing the lesion will continue to promote irritation unless the bony prominences are treated as described. The scar produced by the surgery or a sinus tract infection may necessitate excision of the sinus tract and the bony prominences beneath it and syndactyly of the toes.

Following shaving, pain is relieved by applying pads to the foot or the shoe to distribute the pressure away from the metatarsal head. The pad is placed under the metatarsal shaft, just proximal to the metatarsal head. The pad may be made of lamb's wool, rubber, moleskin, or one of the new materials such as Plastizote.

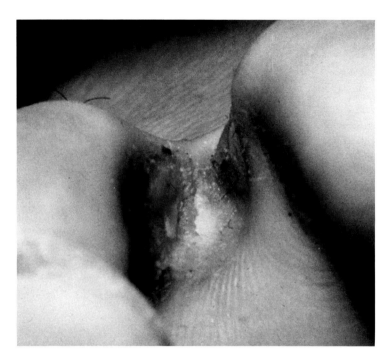

Fig. 155-12. Soft corn in the web space. Maceration occurs and lesion may be confused with a fungal infection. (From Brahms,[2] with permission.)

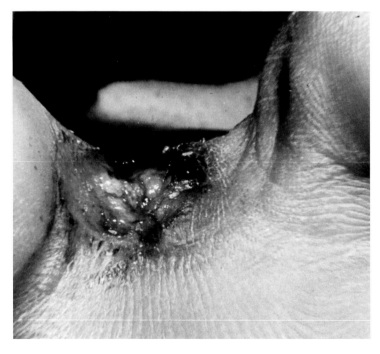

Fig. 155-13. Interdigital sinus tract infection following interdigital space surgery. (From Brahms,[2] with permission.)

PLANTAR HYPERKERATOSIS
(CALLUSES)

Plantar hyperkeratosis may be the result of abnormal localized pressure on the plantar surface of the foot caused by improper footwear, muscle imbalance, arthritis, cavus deformity, or trauma. The callus may occur under one or more metatarsal heads. Loss of the integrity of the metatarsophalangeal joint results in the malalignment of the joint and the protective soft tissues beneath it.

In the normal alignment of the foot, there is a balance between the extrinsic and the intrinsic musculature and the proximal phalanx is directed in front of the metatarsal head. Dorsal displacement of the proximal phalanx results in shortening of the extrinsic tendon, increased pressure on the metatarsal head, and a subsequent increase in the pressure of the metatarsal head on the plantar surfaces of the foot. Displacement of the soft tissues — namely, the plantar pad, the protective fat pad, and the flexor mass — produces increased pressure against the projecting articular metatarsal heads on the plantar surface of the metatarsal bone. Soft tissue hyperkeratosis (Fig. 155-14), either localized or generalized, may develop across the ball of the foot. Each metatarsal head has bifid condyles on the plantar surface (Fig. 155-15). With increasing

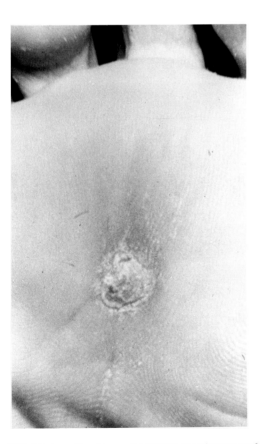

Fig. 155-14. Localized hyperkeratosis on plantar surface caused by isolated pressure of a metatarsal head. (From Brahms,[1] with permission.)

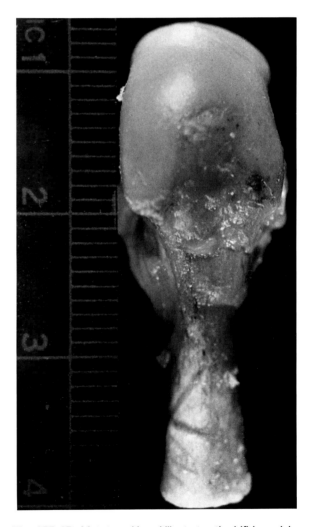

Fig. 155-15. Metatarsal head illustrates the bifid condyles on the plantar aspect of the bone.

irritation, these condyles become enlarged, producing further pressure on the underlying skin. The use of keratylitic agents, radiation therapy, or similar insult may result in permanent damage to the plantar skin in this region, adding to the discomfort. Such agents may cause atrophy of the normal skin, producing chronicity to the lesion.

Treatment

Palliative measures — involving use of pads, arch supports, or special shoes — frequently are helpful in relieving plantar hyperkeratotic lesions.[6]

Conservative treatment includes removal of the layer of hyperkeratotic tissue by shaving it off with a sharp, razorlike instrument. Removal of the callus results in relief of localized areas of pressure under the metatarsal heads.

The use of metatarsal pads is often sufficient to make a patient comfortable. A felt pad is useful for the acute care of a painful metatarsal problem (Fig. 155-16). A more permanent arch support may be the appropriate method of treatment. Insoles fitted with pads are used as a temporary measure to determine if an arch support will provide the long-term relief desired. Metatarsal bars properly placed on the shoes are advantageous in some pa-

tients. One or any of these measures may avert the need for surgical treatment. The preparation of a pad or a prescription-type arch support is recommended for ongoing management. Felt pads may be applied to the plantar surface of the foot or the shoe. The thickness need not be greater than 3/16 to 1/4 inch. To provide maximum comfort, the thickest portion of a felt pad should be placed behind the metatarsal heads and not directly on them.

The type of surgical treatment indicated for plantar hyperkeratosis depends on whether the lesion is localized or generalized. In general, if there is a diffuse plantar callus, conservative management with the use of supports or special shoes is the treatment of choice. Osteotomies of the neck are not recommended.

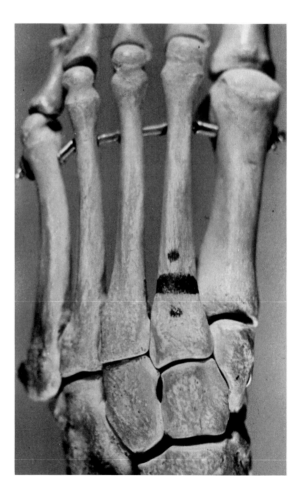

Fig. 155-17. Dorsal wedge osteotomy performed at the base of the metatarsal.

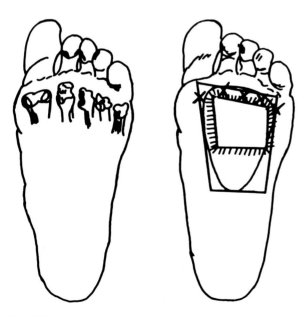

Fig. 155-16. The proper preparation and positioning for a metatarsal pad. (From Brahms,[1] with permission.)

DuVries[3] popularized the method of removal of a portion of the plantar aspect of the metatarsal head. A dorsal incision is made over the metatarsophalangeal joint of the foot. The extensor tendon is identified and retracted. The metatarsophalangeal joint is opened through a capsulotomy and is hyperflexed. The plantar aspect of the metatarsal, after being delivered into the wound, is removed obliquely with an osteotome and smoothed with a rasp. Early walking is encouraged.

Surgical Technique — Brahms

Shortening of the metatarsal as described by Brahms is another method of treatment.[4] This is achieved through an osteotomy at the base of the metatarsal. A wedge of bone is removed from the dorsum of the metatarsal at its base (Fig. 155-17). This has proven to be highly effective for patients in whom the hyperkeratosis is limited to one or two metatarsal heads.

A longitudinal incision is made at the base of the metatarsal. The extensor tendon is identified and

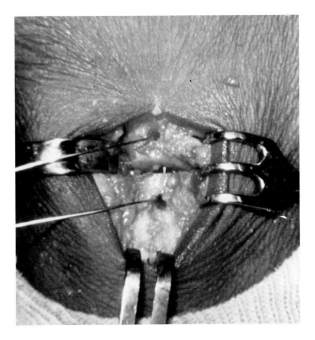

Fig. 155-18. Osteotomy at the base of the metatarsal, using a wire to close the wedge and approximate the bone.

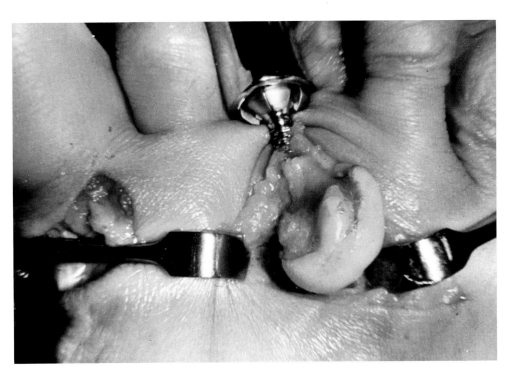

Fig. 155-19. Removal of a metatarsal head may be facilitated by inserting a screw into the neck of the bone and flipping it 180 degrees.

retracted. The periosteum is incised using a nasal elevator and is then stripped toward either side. Drill holes are made through the dorsal cortical surface of the metatarsal. Between the drill holes, a V-shaped osteotomy is performed, with the apex dorsally. It is recommended that the wedge removed be no greater than ³⁄₁₆ inch. The osteotomy is closed and held with a wire suture placed through the dorsal drill holes (Fig. 155-18). After the osteotomy is closed, the subcutaneous tissue and skin are closed. A plaster cast is applied. A weight-bearing cast is recommended for 4 weeks. Walking is permitted as soon as tolerated.

All the methods recommended are designed to relieve the pressure on the plantar surface of the foot or to shift weight bearing from the involved metatarsal head.

Localized plantar hyperkeratosis in the diabetic foot is best treated by resection of the involved metatarsal head through a dorsal incision.[7] Surgical removal of the metatarsal head is facilitated by the introduction of a screw into the osteotomized neck and head of the metatarsal (Fig. 155-19). By rotating the screw 180 degrees toward the toes, the metatarsal head is delivered and removed, usually cutting only one ligamentous attachment. This eliminates the need for blind surgical excursions into the depths of the wound to remove the metatarsal head. In the rheumatoid foot, however, this technique is not as easily applied because of the softness of the bone.

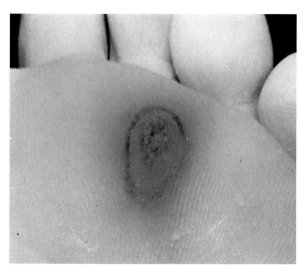

Fig. 155-20. Plantar verruca situated distal to the metatarsal head, painful to pinch, and containing vascular papillae.

PLANTAR VERRUCA

A verruca is a common lesion that may be found on the plantar surface of the foot (Fig. 155-20). It is necessary to differentiate a verruca from a callus. This may be difficult. Verrucae do not commonly occur directly under metatarsal heads. They are more frequently found proximal or distal to the metatarsal head.

A verruca is painful to compression, that is, to lateral pressure. A callus is not painful when pinched. This may help in differentiating one from the other. The verruca has small, visible, black papillae that bleed easily. A callus that is pared does not bleed, but is characterized by a hard, cone-shaped hyperkeratosis. It is not uncommon for a callus to be diagnosed improperly and receive the treatment commonly used for warts—for example, radiation therapy, keratolytic drugs, or caustic agents. Such treatments usually produce a plantar lesion that is more painful than a verruca and is resistant to treatment. The verruca and the callus differ microscopically as well. Verruca may be treated dermatologically by the use of keratolytic agents and/or caustic agents. The use of cautery has also been used. A method popularized by Dr. William Wagner is injection of an anesthetic agent between the lesion of the verruca and the dermal layer. Pressure necrosis seemingly destroys the verruca. The more recent advent of laser surgery is also a method of successful treatment of plantar verruca. A plantar verruca may be surgically enucleated without a resultant scar.

The Enucleation Procedure

The foot is cleansed in the usual preoperative manner. The area of the verruca is infiltrated with a local anesthetic. A #11 knife blade is used to make a small keyhole window at the junction of the verruca and the normal skin (Fig. 155-21). Direct incision into the verruca must be avoided to prevent

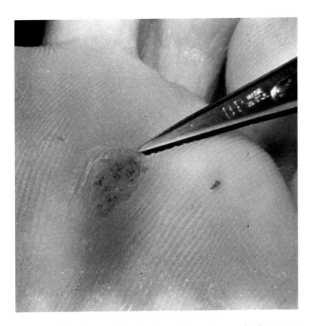

Fig. 155-21. A small keyhole window is made between normal and abnormal skin.

bleeding. The keyhole is not extended into the dermal layer. A small curette is inserted into the keyhole and manipulated to find a proper plane between the verruca and the normal tissue (Fig. 155-22). The verruca is enucleated. A large portion of the verruca will be below the level of the skin. When the verruca has been enucleated, the base of the lesion appears white. The overhanging edges are removed with an iris scissors. Next, the base of the lesion should be gently curetted. The lesion is packed with sterile gauze that has been soaked in ointment, and a dressing is applied. The surgical defect will promptly fill without scarring if the dermal layer has not been traumatized. After the second day, the foot is soaked in warm, soapy water. A Band-Aid may be used to cover the area.

INGROWN TOENAIL

Ingrown toenails are less likely to occur when there is proper care of the nails (Fig. 155-23). The penetration of a nail edge into the skin fold results

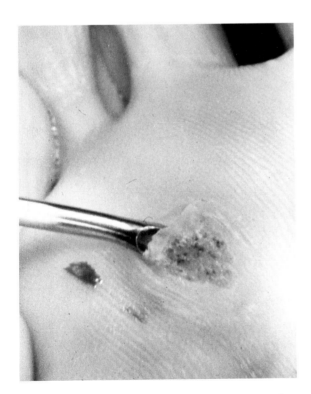

Fig. 155-22. Introduction of a small curette to enucleate the verruca.

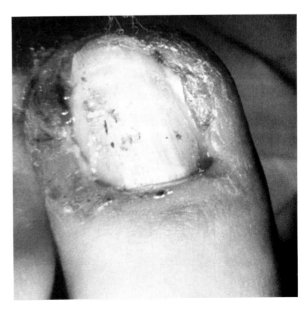

Fig. 155-23. Acute infected toenail caused by penetration of the nail into the nailfold. (From Brahms,[1] with permission.)

in infection. Improper nail cutting, trauma, or the development of incurving, thickened nails may interrupt the integrity of the skin and cause acute infection. Treatment of such acute infection involves the removal of the cause of the local abscess. This may mean the removal of a portion of the nail or the avulsion of the nail. Elective surgery should not be performed when there is an acute paronychia, but should be postponed until the acute process subsides.

Concentrated antiseptic solutions *should not* be used to soak the foot. Dilute solutions, in warm rather than hot water, are recommended.

Nail Edge Removal

After an acute infection has been treated, unilateral or bilateral nail edge removal may be indicated. The skin is prepared in the usual surgical manner. Local block anesthesia is recommended. A tourniquet can be used at the base of the toe. A nail-splitting instrument such as the Beaver #62 knife blade will provide a clean-cut nail border (Fig. 155-24). The nail is split throughout its length, extending the incision under the eponych-

ium. The nail fragment is then grasped with a hemostat and rolled out (Fig. 155-25). The granulation tissue or the nailfold is surgically excised. The tissue under the eponychium should be thoroughly curetted to remove the underlying germinal cells completely (Fig. 155-26). A gauze wick soaked in ointment is inserted and the wound is packed lightly. The tourniquet is then removed. A pressure dressing is applied.

The drain should be removed in 24 to 36 hours. Warm soaks are recommended until healing is complete.

Radical treatment is required for nails with chronic, recurrent infection, fungus infection, or psoriasis, or nails disturbed by a subungual exostosis. One of two methods may be chosen.

Surgical Procedure — Radical Removal of Nail

Radial incisions are made at the base of the nail from the eponychium in a proximal direction (Fig. 155-27). The edge of the skin-fold is labeled with a suture, separated from the top of the nail, and folded backward. The nail is avulsed with an eleva-

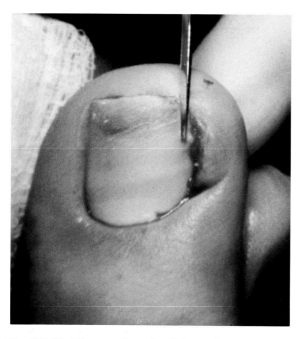

Fig. 155-24. The use of a nail-splitting knife blade to facilitate the removal of a segment of the nail.

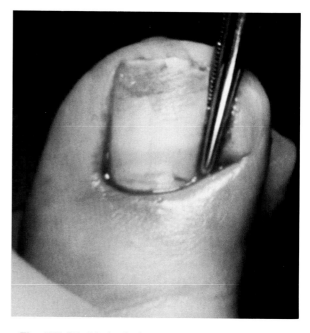

Fig. 155-25. Method of removal of the cut nail edge.

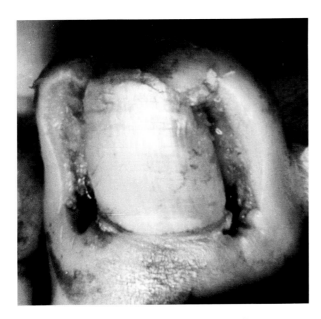

Fig. 155-26. Excision of granulation tissue.

tor or a hemostat. At the site where the eponychium was removed from its normal position, a transverse incision is made through the matrix of the toenail to the periosteum. The nail base and all the soft tissues are completely excised to the phalanx. The corners under the eponychium are curetted. The eponychium is permitted to fall back into place, and sutures are placed on either side to approximate the skin edges. A gauze dressing soaked in ointment is inserted under the eponychium for 24 to 36 hours. A pressure dressing is applied. The sutures may be removed in 7 to 10 days.

Surgical Procedure — Terminal Syme Operation

The terminal Syme operation is performed with tourniquet control at the base of the nail. An incision is made approximately ¼ inch proximal to the nailfold, circling the toe around the nail borders (Fig. 155-28). The nail is completely excised from the proximal to the distal end, removing the nail, the nail bed, and all the soft tissues down to the proximal phalanx (Fig. 155-29). The soft tissues at the end of the toe are then separated from the phalanx with a periosteal elevator and stripped back-

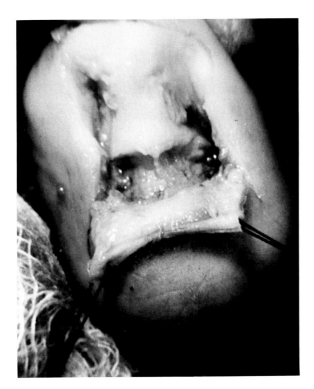

Fig. 155-27. Radial incision at base of nail and removal of all tissue down to the phalanx under the eponychium flap.

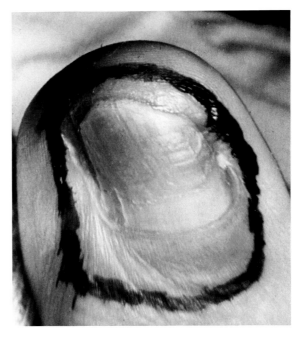

Fig. 155-28. Skin incision for terminal Syme procedure.

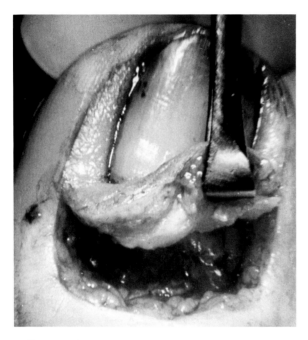

Fig. 155-29. Radical excision of nail and nail bed.

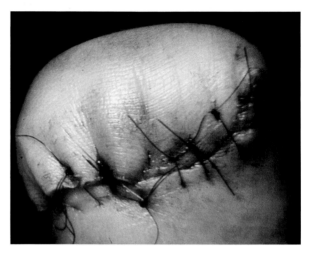

Fig. 155-31. Closure of the skin edges.

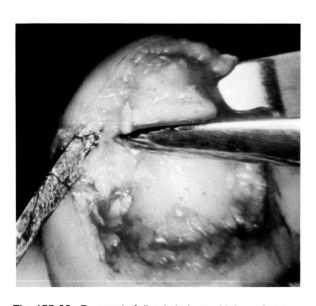

Fig. 155-30. Removal of distal phalanx with bone forceps. Note that enough bone is removed to permit skin approximation.

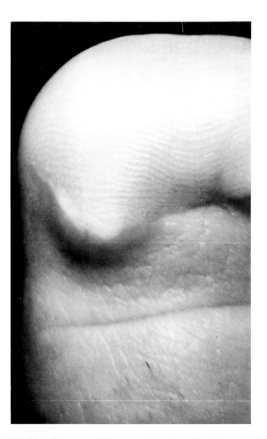

Fig. 155-32. One possible complication of nail surgery is an inclusion cyst.

ward. The distal portion of the phalanx, or as much as is necessary, is removed with a bone-cutting forceps (Fig. 155-30). Enough bone is removed to permit approximation of the skin edges without tension. The plantar aspect of the skinfold is folded over the end of the osteotomized phalanx and is approximated to the dorsal skin with fine interrupted sutures (Fig. 155-31). The skin incision on the top of the toe is slightly curved in the same contour as the distal end of the toe. The plantar skin is folded over the bone and is tailored such that no "dog ears" result. Drains are not necessary. Postoperative management is similar to that for any other procedure in which primary healing is anticipated. The patient must be advised that the procedure will result in shortening of the distal end of the toe, but this is of no functional importance.

A frequent complication of any nail surgery is the formation of an inclusion cyst[5] (Fig. 155-32). If this occurs, the cyst is removed in a manner similar to that described for nail surgery.

REFERENCES

1. Brahms MA: Common foot problems. J Bone Joint Surg 49A:1653, 1967
2. Brahms MA: The small toes. p. 622. In Jahss MH (ed): Disorders of the Foot. Vol. 1. WB Saunders, Philadelphia, 1982
3. DuVries HL: New approach to the treatment of intractable verruca plantaris (plantar wart). JAMA 152:1202, 1953
4. Giannestras NJ: Other problems of the fore part of the foot. In Giannestras NJ (ed): Foot Disorders. Lea & Febiger, Philadelphia, 1973
5. Kelikian H, Clayton LL, Loseff H: Surgical syndactylia of the toes. Clin Orthop 19:208, 1961
6. Milgram JE: Office measures for the relief of the painful foot. J Bone Joint Surg 46A:1095, 1964
7. Thompson TC: Surgical treatment of disorders of the fore part of the foot. J Bone Joint Surg 48A:1117, 1964

Fractures of the Talus

156

William M. Deyerle
Thomas Comfort

Barry W. Burkhardt
William Giles

Displaced fractures of the neck and body of the talus present the orthopaedic surgeon with a most difficult challenge. No one surgeon sees many of these complicated fractures. The literature suggests that avascular necrosis will occur in 40 to 50 percent of type II fractures of the talar neck.[1,6,14,17,21] While the operative approach should include osteotomizing the medial malleolus, some authors suggest surgical release of the deltoid ligament as an alternative. This is not acceptable, as it does not give adequate exposure and causes additional trauma to the blood supply, which enters the talus through the lower portion of the deltoid ligament.[7]

Hawkins' classification of vertical fractures of the neck of the talus, which has become the standard, is as follows:

Type I: Undisplaced. The fracture enters the subtalar joint between the middle and posterior facets. Frequently a portion of the fracture line will enter the talar body and involve the posterior facet of the subtalar joint or the most anterior portion of the articular cartilage of the talus. The body of the talus retains its normal position in relation to the ankle and subtalar joint.

Type II: Displaced. The subtalar joint is subluxated or dislocated, and the ankle joint is normal. The fracture line frequently enters a portion of the talar body and the posterior facet of the talus.

Type III The subtalar joint is displaced as in type II fractures, and the body of the talus is dislocated from both the ankle and the subtalar joint.

Undisplaced, Hawkins' type I fractures require immobilization only and not internal fixation. Talar dome and osteochondral fractures can be treated by open arthrotomies or arthroscopic debridement. If the fragment is small enough, non-weight-bearing but continual motion of the joint is indicated for this type of fracture.

We advocate a more aggressive approach to the treatment of all type II and type III fractures and for those in a fourth group, which includes displaced fractures of the body. Immediate open reduction, with an osteotomy of the medial malleolus, and internal fixation are indicated. In patients with multiple injuries, treatment of talar fractures in these categories should be given a high priority and should not be postponed until after treatment of other fractures.

Coltart[2] was one of the first to recognize that in talar neck type III fractures, in which the talar body is dislocated medially, the deltoid ligament is often the only ligamentous structure left intact. Hawkins[6] further stressed the importance of the medial blood supply and made the observation that revascularization usually takes place in a medial to lateral direction. To minimize avascular necrosis and increase the chances of revascularization, the medial blood supply should be preserved. This can be accomplished by medial malleolar osteotomy with preservation of the deltoid ligament.

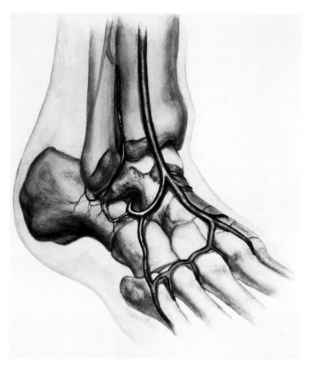

Fig. 156-1. The dorsalis pedis and the perforating peroneal arteries primarily supply the talar neck and send a branch to the sinus tarsi to anastomose with the vessels approaching from the medial side through the tarsal canal.

BLOOD SUPPLY TO THE TALUS

Mulfinger and Trueta[16] in 1970 gave the classic description of the blood supply to the talus. This blood supply has been correlated with various fracture types by several investigators.[1,5,6,9,10,21,22] In a Hawkins talar neck type I fracture, only the dorsalis pedis branches coming into the talar neck may be disrupted. In type II, with subtalar dislocations, the dorsalis pedis branches as well as the artery of the tarsal canal may be disrupted. In type III fractures all three of the major arterial supplies to the body of the talus (dorsalis pedis, tarsal canal artery, and tarsal sinus artery) may be disrupted. We believe that the deltoid artery is the last to be ruptured and may be preserved in many type II and type III talar neck and displaced body fractures. The tarsal canal artery arises from the posterior tibial artery (Fig. 156-1), usually 1 cm proximal to the origin of the medial and lateral plantar arteries. The deltoid branch is given off ½ cm distal to the origin of the artery and supplies the medial talar wall (Fig. 156-2). It anastomoses with the dorsalis pedis artery. The deltoid artery lies within the substance of the deltoid ligament, between the talocalcaneal and talotibial ligaments (Fig. 156-3). Preservation of this ligament usually means that the deltoid artery, and thus the medial blood supply, are intact.

Osteotomy of the medial malleolus and reflection with the attached deltoid ligament accomplishes two major goals: (1) it preserves the medial blood supply that enters the distal edge of the medial talar wall and (2) it gives excellent exposure for the anatomic reduction and internal fixation of the fractured talus. Three-fifths of the talus is covered by articular cartilage, and the functional results are dependent upon the accuracy with which the surgeon can restore the anatomic continuity of the joint surfaces and bony opposition. Exact anatomic impacted reduction and adequate internal fixation are essential in obtaining primary bone healing, good functional results, and the preservation of the medial blood supply to avoid avascular necrosis.

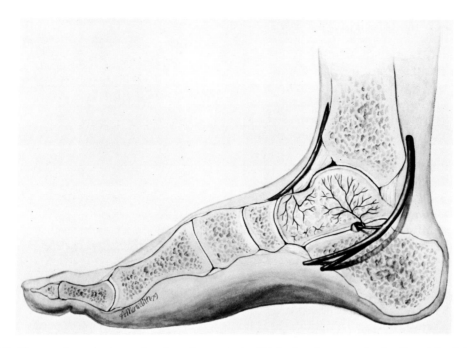

Fig. 156-2. The tarsal canal artery arises from the posterior tibial artery 1 cm proximal to the origin of the medial and lateral plantar arteries. The deltoid branch, supplying the medial wall, is given off ½ cm distal to the origin of this tarsal canal artery. The anastomoses inside of the talus, with the branches from the dorsalis pedis, are shown.

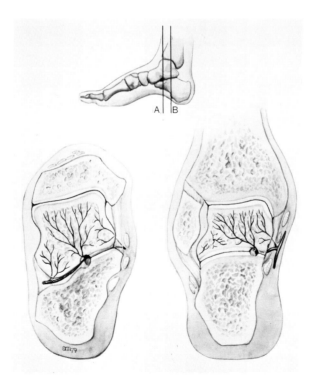

Fig. 156-3. The tarsal canal artery is shown as it passes between the os calcis and the talus to the point at which it anastomoses with the branch from the dorsalis pedis and peroneals.

RESULTS OF TREATMENT

We reviewed the results of 45 fractures treated at three locations: the Medical College of Virginia, the Ramsey Hospital in St. Paul, Minnesota, and Hattiesburg, Mississippi. Twenty-seven patients had open reduction and internal fixation and had a follow-up of over 2 years. Of these 27 fractures 5 were compound; no avascular necrosis occurred in these. There were no infections or wound sloughs. Only three patients had the screws removed from the medial malleolus or any internal fixation removed (Tables 156-1, 156-2).

Of 23 patients who underwent open reduction and internal fixation, 12 had an osteotomy of the medial malleolus so that the reduction and fixation could be accomplished with protection of the deltoid ligaments and the vital blood supply. These 12 comprise group I. Of the 12 patients 7 had Hawkins type III fractures; one developed avascular necrosis. Five patients had Hawkins type II fractures, with no avascular necrosis. Group II consisted of 11 patients who underwent open reduction and internal fixation without medial malleolar osteotomy. Three of these were Hawkins type III, of whom one developed avascular necrosis; the other eight had Hawkins type II fractures; and one of these developed avascular necrosis. Thus the avascular necrosis rate in the group with medial malleolar osteotomies was 1 in 12; and in those without osteotomy it was 2 in 11. These figures are not statistically significant. In the Hawkins type III fractures in which the medial malleolus was removed for reduction, and avascular necrosis rate was 1 in 7; the rate in the group without release of the medial malleolus was 1 in 3 (Tables 156-2, 156-3). The four patients (group III) who did not undergo open reduction and internal fixation all suffered avascular necrosis (Fig. 156-4).

The 18 fractures not included in either of the above three groups were treated by varying types of procedures or had no follow-up, and had to be excluded from our evaluation. Although these cases are not included in our statistics, inappropriate treatment led to problems in a number of these patients. For example, one operative note describing a type III fracture stated that it was "impossible to reduce the fracture without releasing the deltoid ligament, and while reducing the fracture the deltoid ligament was in such bad condition that it was completely excised" (Fig. 156-5). This completely removed the major blood supply to the talus with resulting avascular necrosis.

Table 156-1. Classification of 45 Talar Fractures Studied

Talar neck type I	8
Talar neck type II	22
Talar neck type III	8
Body	7
	45
Talar neck type I not included	8
Lost to follow-up	10
	27

Table 156-2. Method of Treatment

Group	No. of Patients	Treatment
Group I	12	ORIF[a] with reflected medial malleolus 7 talar neck type III 5 talar neck type II
Group II[b]	11	ORIF[a] — poor modification of proper treatment 1 talar neck type III 10 talar neck type II
Group III	4	Poor treatment

[a] ORIF, open reduction and internal fixation.

[b] Note that Group II has the larger number of Type II fractures as compared to Group I and should show a higher percentage of good results because Type II fractures are less severe fractures.

Table 156-3. Incidence of Avascular Necrosis

Group	No. of Patients	Treatment	AVN[a] Incidence
I	12	ORIF[a] with reflected medial malleolus	10% (1/12)
II	11	ORIF[a] without reflected medial malleolus	18% (2/11)
III	4	Poor treatment	100% (4/4)

[a] AVN, avascular necrosis; ORIF, open reduction and internal fixation.

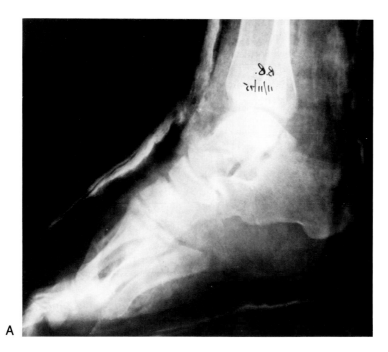

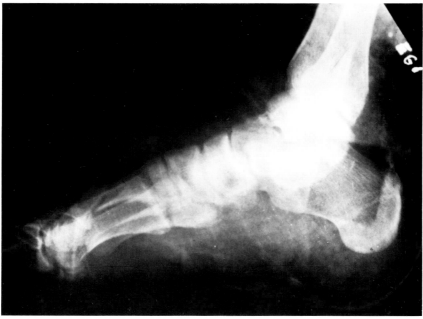

Fig. 156-4. **(A)** This patient with a type II fracture had a closed reduction, which is not adequate treatment for this fracture. **(B)** Three days later the reduction has not been maintained. *(Figure continues.)*

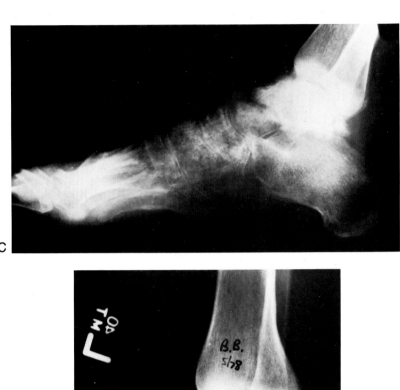

C

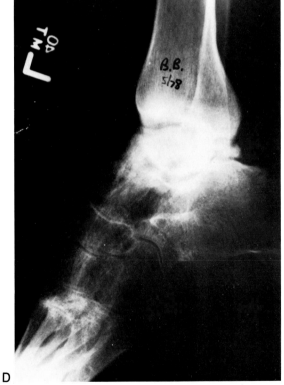

D

Fig. 156-4 *(Continued).* **(C)** Avascular necrosis and nonunion have occurred at 6 months postinjury. **(D)** At 29 months postinjury the ankle is painful, and fixed equinus has occurred. Walking tolerance is three blocks. Early open reduction and internal fixation through a medial malleolar osteotomy could have prevented this poor result.

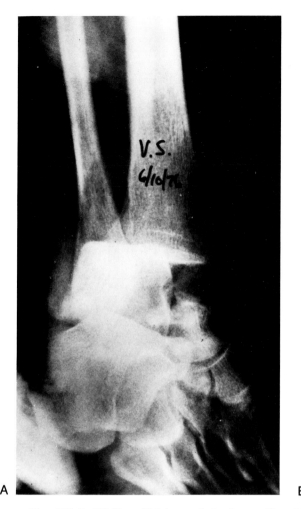
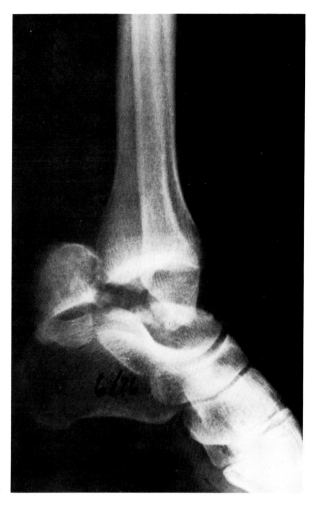

Fig. 156-5. (A) Type III talar neck fracture, with subtalar dislocation and total posterior dislocation of body. **(B)** Medial malleolus fracture from severe initial trauma. *(Figure continues.)*

ANATOMY

A surgical approach employing osteotomy of the medial malleolus, which reflects it with the deltoid ligament distally and thus preserves the medial blood supply, is recommended for adequate exposure of the talar neck and body. This approach has never been fully described in the English-language literature. It was first reported by Koenig in Germany in 1921.[11] Others have recommended lateral malleolar osteotomy in order to preserve the me-

dial blood supply.[5] This does not give as adequate an exposure as the medial osteotomy. Other investigators have mentioned osteotomy of the medial malleolus as a possible aid in exposure.[6,17]

SURGICAL TECHNIQUE

It is absolutely essential to make a 4-inch incision, starting 2 inches proximal to the medial malleolus and extending distally across the medial mal-

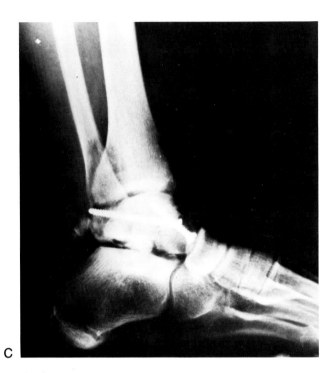

C

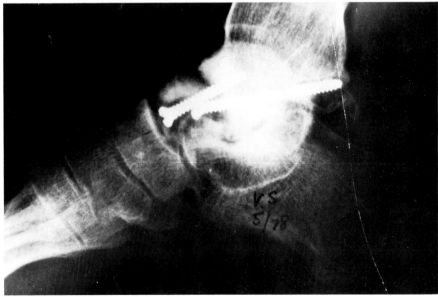

D

Fig. 156-5 *(Continued).* **(C)** Open reduction and internal fixation were difficult to perform. The surgeon removed the fragment of the medial malleolus with the deltoid ligament attached; this destroyed the blood supply. **(D)** Two years later avascular necrosis, collapse, and nonunion are noted.

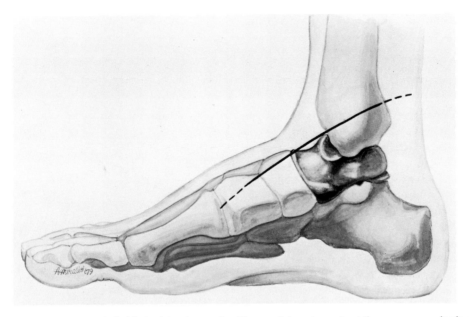

Fig. 156-6. The extended skin incision is used, with care taken to protect the neurovascular bundle.

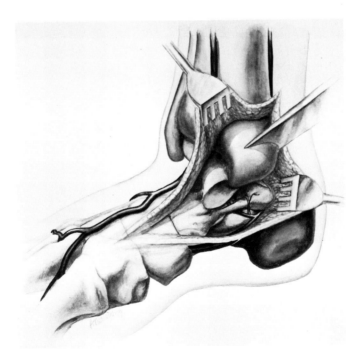

Fig. 156-7. With the osteotome in place, all the soft tissues are shown dissected away from the medial malleolus (for illustration only; this is not done in the actual approach). The deltoid ligament and its blood supply are illustrated.

leolus for 2 inches, with the convex portion of the incision placed posteriorly (Figs. 156-6, 156-7). An oblique osteotomy is made so as to enter the ankle mortise at its anterior medial corner. The attachment of the deltoid ligament is carefully preserved, as well as the small branches of the deltoid artery entering the medial talar cortex inferiorly (Figs. 156-8, 156-9). This osteotomy allows for adequate exposure for easy reduction rather than using retraction and leverage on already-traumatized soft tissue. This exposure makes the necessity of reinsertion of Kirschner wires or screws less likely. Before wound closure, good radiographs must be made to see that there is, in fact, anatomic reduction and compression of the fracture surface, and to ensure that the talus fits properly within the ankle mortise. The medial malleolus is then reattached, and one or two screws are inserted. To complete the procedure, the periosteum is sutured.

If the osteotomy is performed with the oscillating saw it is essential to cool the oscillating blade to

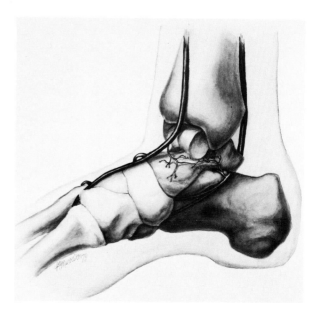

Fig. 156-9. The relationship of the deltoid branch and tarsal canal artery to the medial side of the talus is shown, revealing the bony skeleton, with the arterial tree to the tarsal canal and the branch through the deltoid.

avoid causing necrosis, which results in delayed union of the osteotomy.

POSTOPERATIVE CARE

Postoperative care consists of immobilization in an above-knee cast without weight bearing until the fracture is healed. The patient is given a regimen of isometric exercises for the muscles of the calf, which include dorsiflexion, plantar flexion, inversion, and eversion. These exercises are continued during cast wear and after the cast is removed, at which time they are supplemented with range-of-motion therapy. This usually takes from 10 to 12 weeks.

After this, the modality and duration of treatment depends on whether any evidence of avascular necrosis exists. Whether or not avascular necrosis is evident, the total stress on the talus should be limited for an additional 3 months. This is ac-

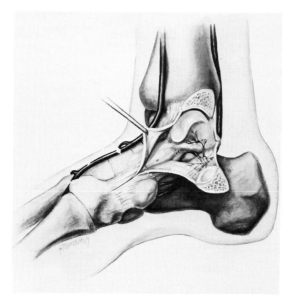

Fig. 156-8. The completed osteotomy is reflected carefully while protecting the deltoid ligament and its blood supply to the medial wall of the talus and the tarsal canal artery, shown entering between the os calcis and the talus. This provides excellent visualization for open reduction and internal fixation, as well as protecting the remaining blood supply.

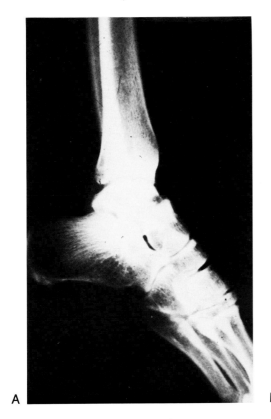

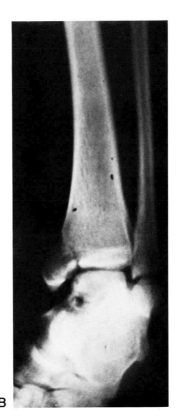

Fig. 156-10. (A) Talar body fracture with subtalar dislocation. **(B)** Reflected medial malleolus fracture at the time of open reduction and internal fixation prevents additional damage to the blood supply. **(C)** Reflected medial malleolus allows direct visualization for anatomic reduction and internal fixation. *(Figure continues.)*

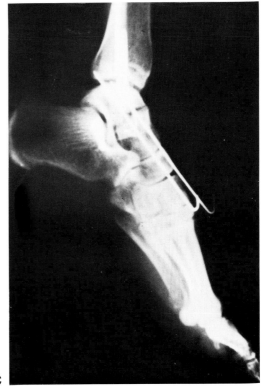

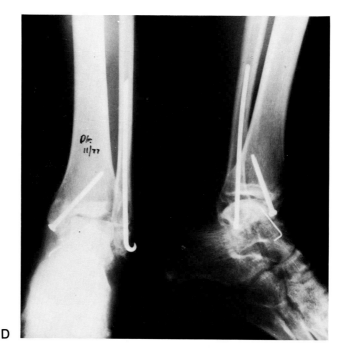

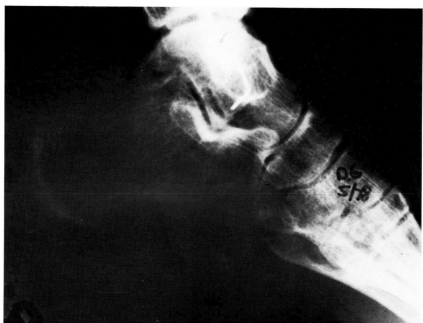

Fig. 156-10 *(Continued).* **(D)** Fracture healed at 3 months; note Hawkins revascularization sign. **(E)** Further revascularization is evident at 19 months. *(Figure continues.)*

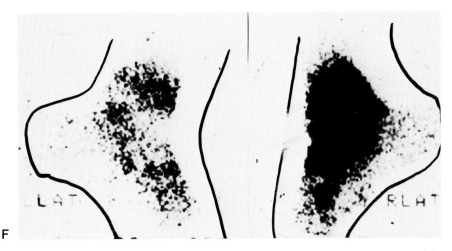

F

Fig. 156-10 *(Continued).* **(F)** Bone scan: normal left side compared with revascularization at right side at 19 months.

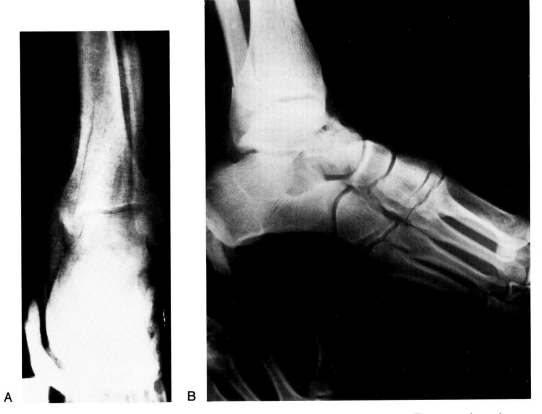

A   B

Fig. 156-11. Type II talar neck fracture: **(A)** AP view and **(B)** lateral view. *(Figure continues.)*

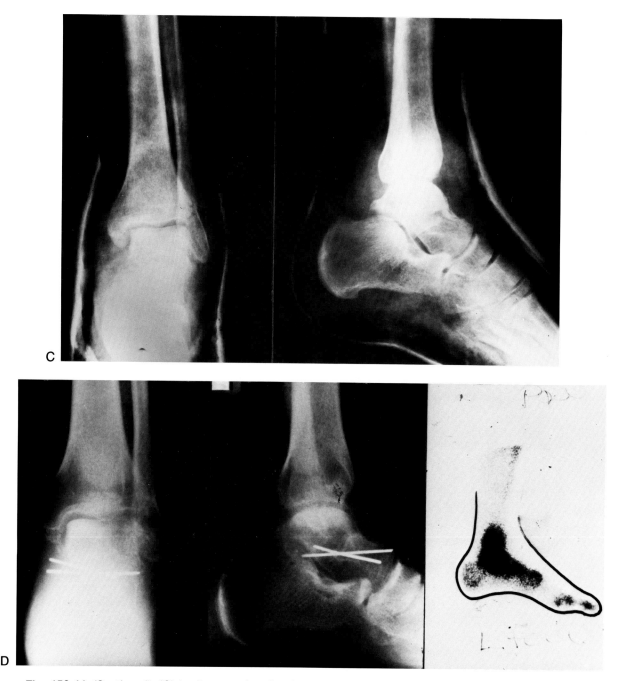

Fig. 156-11 *(Continued).* **(C)** Inadequate closed reduction. **(D)** The surgeon performed an open reduction without a malleolar osteotomy. This procedure violates the medial blood supply of the talus. *(Figure continues.)*

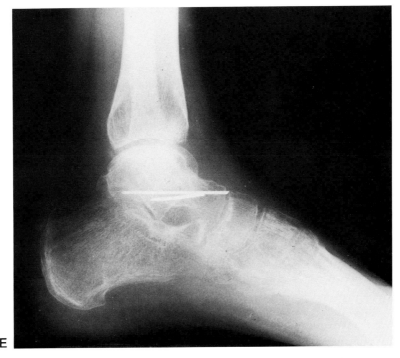

E

Fig. 156-11 *(Continued)*. **(E)** Further revascularization is seen at 6 months.

complished by one of three methods, which are individualized for each patient. One choice is to allow the patient to walk non-weight bearing with crutches. A second choice is to use a patellar tendon bearing brace on the affected side, which is better tolerated by the patient than non-weight bearing. This brace decreases the stress on the talus and transmits considerable stress beyond the talus through the brace to the shoe.

Finally, the third option is a 2-inch, elevated heel, which is easily tolerated by the patient. The talus is the apex of a 2:1 lever from the area of heel strike to the metatarsal heads.[27] If the heel is elevated by 2 inches, this represents 2 inches through which that the calf muscles do not have to elevate the weight of the body with each stride. The heel cord must exert twice the body weight in order to raise the foot by 2 inches. This stress is taken out of each step. Considering that the average person walks 1 to 4 miles a day at 2,000 steps per mile, the stress removed from the talus is considerable. V. Frankel (personal communication) estimated that this lift decreases stress on the talus by 25 percent with each stride.

AVASCULAR NECROSIS

A radiographic aid in diagnosing avascular necrosis is the Hawkins revascularization sign. The subchondral radiolucency seen in the body of the talus as early as 6 weeks postinjury indicates disuse osteopenia and suggests that some vascularity to the talar body is intact. The presence of this sign suggests that the talus has not undergone complete avascular necrosis (Figs. 156-10, 156-11), but its absence has no prognostic value.

Canale and Kelly[1] referred to the use of the technetium 99m bone scan, with pinhole technique, in monitoring revascularization of the talus with avascular necrosis. We believe that the early scan (6 to 10 weeks) is positive because of either fracture healing and/or early revascularization; however, it is helpful to have these early scans during the latter period of convalescence for following the revascularization process. The early scan makes it possible to compare and evaluate these subtle later changes. Continued protective treatment, designed to decrease the stresses on the talus until the bone scan shows a decrease in activity, is recommended by Canale and Kelly.[1] The end point for treatment of avascular necrosis is difficult to define and must be individualized for each patient.[15]

SUMMARY

In summary, we believe that displaced fractures of the talus require an operative approach, which should include osteotomy of the medial malleolus, with immediate open reduction and internal fixation of all type II and type III fractures of the neck of the talus and displaced fractures of the body of the talus. Medial malleolar osteotomy preserves the medial blood supply, gives atraumatic exposure, and permits accurate reduction. After the fracture is healed, continued protective treatment to decrease the stresses on the talus is indicated for a prolonged period of time. Finally, the technetium 99m bone scan may be a helpful technique to determine the type and length of care for prevention and treatment of avascular necrosis. The reader is also referred to the many studies of talar neck fractures that are available in the literature.[1,3–6,8,9,12,13,17–21,23,24]

REFERENCES

1. Canale ST, Kelly FB: Fractures of the neck of the talus. Long-term evaluation of seventy-one cases. J Bone Joint Surg 60A:143, 1978
2. Coltart WD: Aviator's astragalus. J Bone Joint Surg 34B:545, 1952
3. Detenbeck LC, Kelly PJ: Total dislocation of the talus. J Bone Joint Surg 51A:283, 1969
4. Deyerle W: Long term follow-up of fractures of os calcis. Diagnostic peroneal synoviagram. Orthop Clin North Am 4:213, 1973
5. Dunn AR, Jacobs B, Campbell RD: Fractures of the talus. J Trauma 6:443, 1966
6. Hawkins L: Fractures of the neck of the talus. J Bone Joint Surg 52A:991, 1970
7. Kelly PJ, Sullivan CR: Blood supply of the talus. Clin Orthop 30:37, 1963
8. Kenwright J, Taylor RG: Major injuries of the talus. J Bone Joint Surg 52B:36, 1970
9. Kleiger B: Fractures of the talus. J Bone Joint Surg 30A:735, 1948
10. Kleiger B: Injuries of the talus and its joints. Clin Orthop 121:243, 1976
11. Koenig F, Schaefer P: Osteoplastic surgical exposure of the ankle joint. Forty-First Report of Progress in Orthopedic Surgery. (Abstr) Z Chir 215:196, 1929
12. McKeever FM: Fracture of the neck of the astragalus. Arch Surg 46:720, 1943
13. McKeever FM: Treatment of complications of fractures and dislocations of the talus. Clin Orthop 30:45, 1963
14. Mindell ER, Cisek EE, Kartalian G, et al: Late results of injuries to the talus, analysis of forty cases. J Bone Joint Surg 45A:221, 1963
15. Morris HD: Aseptic necrosis of the talus following injury. Orthop Clin North Am 5:177, 1974
16. Mulfinger GL, Trueta J: The blood supply of the talus. J Bone Joint Surg 52B:160, 1970
17. Pantazopoulos PG, Galanos P, Vayanos E, et al: Fractures of the neck of the talus. Acta Orthop Scand 45:296, 1974
18. Pennal GF: Fractures of the talus. Clin Orthop 30:53, 1963
19. Peterson L: Fracture of the neck of the talus. Publication of the Department of Orthopaedic Surgery II. Univ of Goteberg, Goteberg, Sweden, 1974, p. 17
20. Peterson L: Romanus B, Dahlberg E: Fracture of the collum tali—an experimental study. J Biomechan 9:277, 1976
21. Peterson L, Goldie IF, Irstram L: Fractures of the neck of the talus, a clinical study. Acta Orthop Scand 48:696, 1977
22. Peterson L, Goldie I, Lindell D: The arterial supply of the talus. Acta Orthop Scand 45:260, 1974
23. Schrock RD: Fractures and dislocations of the astragalus p. 361. In American Academy of Orthopaedic Surgeons. Instructional Course Lectures. Vol. 9. JW Edwards, Ann Arbor, 1952
24. Sneppen O, Buhl O: Fractures of the talus. Acta Orthop Scand 45:307, 1974
25. Williams M, Lissner I, LeVeau B: Biomechanics of Human Motion, 2nd Ed. WB Saunders, Philadelphia, 1977

Fractures of the Os Calcis 157

Wallace E. Miller

A fracture of the os calcis is quite common in relation to fractures in other tarsal bones and seldom a disastrous occurrence, even if it is bilateral. Indeed, if the subtalar joint is not involved, the care of the injury can usually consist of a closed reduction and application of a below-knee cast. There are variations in how this is accomplished. Little or no manipulative effort may be indicated to try to reshape the bone. Attempts at manual molding can be tried to a greater extent under anesthesia. Frequently an early gradual resumption of weight bearing in a cast or in a bulky dressing is possible. External support, to assist in weight bearing, is usually discarded by the patient as pain decreases, sometimes in a few days, more often in several weeks, or after a few months.

By using closed techniques, approximately 60 to 65 percent of all fractures of the os calcis, those with minimal subtalar joint involvement, are adequately treated. With subtalar joint involvement, an acceptable and satisfactory plan of treatment may still be a closed reduction in an additional 12 to 15 percent. A minimal treatment plan for disruptive subtalar fractures has also been used successfully in another 5 to 8 percent. These figures total up to 77 to 88 percent and are derived from my

experience and interpretation of published reports.

As closed treatment is extended in its use for the more severe fractures, there is less predictability of gaining a good result. Once the decision of the type of care is made, neither the patient nor the physician expects a bad or poor result. Yet it is well known that often there will be residual complaints, whether simple or complicated treatment is used. Lessening the degree of residual pain, improving the time and ability to stay on the injured foot, and improving the gait with better joint mobility are the three major goals. In my experience in choosing treatment to obtain these goals, 87 percent of all patients with fractures of the os calcis were able to be treated with closed reduction as the final choice. Initially all (100 percent) of the fractures were treated closed, but eventually 13 percent were treated with an open reduction.[15]

Most authorities concede, as do I, that some form of permanent functional disability can be expected in one of five patients with a fracture of the os calcis, whether treatment is closed or open.[25] It is interesting to note that in the 6th edition of Campbell's Operative Orthopaedics, the statement was made, "We have probably favored non-operative

4257

treatment too much in the past. . . ."[22] Disenchantment with closed treatment (or nontreatment) has encouraged a renewed interest in open reduction. The late expectation that after 1 to 2 years the patient with a fracture of the os calcis would recover to tolerate weight bearing and gain an increase in mobility of the hind part of the foot did not always occur. However, there were other complaints following closed reduction or no treatment at all. The findings were poor shoe fitting, poor cosmesis associated with a widened flat heel, a more valgus malaligned foot, and a persistently swollen foot that had limited motion.

The implication in noting residual complaints is that more than 20 percent (or more than 13 percent in my series) might have been changed from a fair result to a good or excellent result if the reduction had been more accurate. In nearly all instances, the disruptive fractures os calcis are those that caused most concern. These will be the focus of attention in this chapter, with emphasis placed on the indications for surgical intervention.

INDICATIONS

Classification of Fractures of the Os Calcis

The classifications of fractures of the os calcis most frequently referred to are attributed to either Rowe or Essex-Lopresti. Both classifications have been helpful in sorting out the different mechanisms of injury and comparing results of reported series. Other authors tend to develop their own variations. All classifications are based on the radiographic interpretation. It would seem in retrospect that whether the original injury was viewed on radiograph (or a scan) or whether a clinical study was made after a closed reduction, the larger concern should have been the restoration of functional anatomy, rather than the fitting of a treatment plan to a classification type. For most purposes it seems useful to remember that fractures of the os calcis that do not involve a disruption of the subtalar joint, fit into the I, II, or III type. (Rowe)[21] or an A, B, C type (Essex-Lopresti).[2] The fractures that result from a greater force, as in Types IV, V (Rowe) or D, E, F,

(Essex-Lopresti), involve more distorted anatomy and disruptive articular surfaces. Classifications are helpful, and not to be ignored, but one must take care that the treatment plan is not dictated by a preordained recipe for a certain type.

Radiographs and Scans

In the radiographic interpretation of fractures of the os calcis, four views are essential: anteroposterior (AP), lateral, oblique, and axial. It has been helpful in the extremely distorted fractures to have the same views of the opposite uninjured os calcis for comparison. It is not necessary to add scans to the basic radiographs, although there may be additional information, such as the degree of rotation of fragments and soft tissue involvement that may be obtained from computed tomographic (CT) scans. CT studies recently suggested a means of determining the best surgical approach, whether lateral or medial. When indicated, both approaches are used to restore both the lateral wall and the medial cortex.[3]

Anatomic Guidelines

The os calcis has a unique double function. The structure, both in extrinsic configuration and in the intrinsic stress lines is primarily to support the body weight.[6] The height of the intact os calcis accommodates the function of unimpeded action of the tendons as they glide on both the medial and lateral aspects of the bone. The height of the os calcis must allow for the use of traditional shoewear. If the os calcis is not sufficiently high to accommodate a normal shoe counter, special shoes have to be used. Taking these considerations into account, the choice of treatment must accomplish the following:

Guideline 1. Restoration and maintenance of maximal os calcis height
Guideline 2. Elimination of bone expansion both laterally and medially by the restoration of the normal size and shape of the os calcis

Closed reduction as the treatment of choice may satisfy both of the above guidelines. As a corollary the presence of extreme comminution or distortion of the os calcis may be a contraindication to open reduction.

A second role of function beyond that of structural integrity and height is the need to accommodate the articulations with the talus and midtarsal bones. The superior surface of the os calcis has three talar facets. The dome-shaped posterior articular facet supports the major amount of weight, since it is the largest facet. It also must function in approximately 45 degrees of forward inclination. The axis of motion of the subtalar joint runs obliquely from the medial dorsal position of the talar neck in a plantar, posterior, and somewhat lateral direction.[8] As motion occurs the middle articular facet, supported by the sustentaculum tali, allows a forward guided action. The anterior articular facet directs the line of action to accommodate for the axis of midtarsal joint motion. This is determined by a horizontal and downward inclination of the calcaneo-cuboid articulation. An alteration of any one of these three facets will affect the other two, primarily in gait or in accommodative motion for the ankle and the forefoot. The result is a universal joint action that allows movement in two planes perpendicular to each other. The calcaneo-cuboid joint permits a gliding motion of inversion, adduction, and plantar flexion. The subtalar joint action, dorsiflexion, and plantar flexion complements the dorsiflexion and plantar flexion motion that occurs at the ankle joint.

Further considerations, then, in the decision of the type of treatment are:

Guideline 3. Anatomically restoring the posterior facet by reducing the os calcis to a sufficient height to allow for subtalar joint motion to a 45-degree inclination obliquely forward to further accommodate this motion

Guideline 4. Anatomically restoring the middle and anterior facets to further facilitate this motion and to allow motion in the midtarsal area

All the above four guidelines lead to secondary benefits when the structures are restored as close as possible to their previous anatomical positions. For example, a loss of height of the lateral side of the os calcis causes bulging of the os calcis, which can impinge on the peroneal tendons. A loss of height of the os calcis also lowers the position of the distal fibula, causing direct contact with the upper edge of the shoe. A bulging heel and prominent

lowered lateral malleolus is both disfiguring and functionally compromising, the result being foreshortened gait both with and without shoes.

A distorted medial wall may result in compromise to the tarsal tunnel through which plantar vessels, nerves, and long tendons pass. The flexor hallucis longus glides through a groove along the inferior surface of the sustentaculum tali.

The attachments of ligaments may be altered by comminution of the fracture. Involvement of the anterior margin of the eminence on the medial surface where the plantar calcaneonavicular and deltoid ligaments attach[1] or involvement of the sites of attachment of the flexor digitorum brevis, plantar aponeurosis, the long plantar ligament, and quadratus plantae may lead to structural changes in these areas.[9]

Posteriorly, elevation of the calcaneal tuberosity, the attachment of the Achilles tendon, may result in weakening of plantar flexion on weight bearing.

The final decision regarding management of the fracture must take into account the four major guidelines. Failure to do so will result in unacceptable results, whether the treatment is nonoperative, surgical, or simply an acceptance of the position of the fracture without reduction. The eventual long-term clinical functional result, whether good or bad, will be directly proportional to the acceptance and fulfillment of all four of the main guidelines.

Loss of height of the os calcis, loss[6] of the Bohler or Gissane angles of 25 to 40 degrees, subtalar joint involvement, loss of substance, the degree of comminution, the type of fracture, and all other structural features of the bone are determined radiographically.

There is another feature of the anatomy that is unique and sometimes overlooked, namely, the heelpad directly under the bone.[13] The heelpad has a structure of vertical columns made up of large fat globules, strategically placed, on top of each other and contained in septae, which allow for a pistonlike action. When this system is disrupted, there is atrophy of the fat pad and a loss of protective resiliency. In the injured heelpad, the fat columns are dispersed, disorganized, and as a result their shock absorber function is lost. Furthermore, once the heel is damaged, it can never be restored to its original condition and remains a flattened painful heelpad.[16] Residual pain following severe os calcis fractures may be attributed to the exposed unprotected nerve endings in the damaged heelpad.[14] Taking this into account, an additional anatomic feature must be considered. It is crucial, when taking the history, to find out how high a fall caused the injury as well as the kind of surface of impact. Ignoring this aspect of the injury may lead to the wrong choice of care. For example, if the decision should be to do a primary arthrodesis, and the heelpad has been severely injured, the final outcome will still be a painful heel, whether the arthrodesis is successful or not. A similar faulty decision may be made in choosing an arthrodesis as a salvage procedure since the damaged heelpad will still be the source of pain.[16,19]

Although consideration of the injury to the heelpad is not listed with the other four guidelines, it is a feature of the injury that must be taken into account. Therefore, one additional anatomical guideline is:

Guideline 5. Any os calcis fracture sustained by a fall of 40 feet or more or by a force from below (as an injury from a land mine or an acoustic mine injury in water)[27] may result in persistent pain even though the other four anatomical components have been corrected. The damage is intensified in a fall on a concrete surface and lessened when the fall is on grass or a yielding ground surface.

TREATMENT OPTIONS

Open versus Closed

The basis for the following observations is 40 years of first-hand experience in surgery of the musculoskeletal system culminating in a well-delineated study on when to use closed or open reduction for the treatment of os calcis fractures.[12] A consecutive series of 125 disruptive os calcis fractures was treated from 1975 through 1980 using the previously mentioned five guidelines. Closed treatment was used in 108 instances (87 percent).

In this group, 93 underwent reduction and 15 did not. In this group, six (5 percent) fractures were treated with the insertion of a pin but were still considered closed reductions. An average followup of 3.4 years of 109 patients provided data on all patients. Seventeen patients (13 percent) were treated by open reduction. Only one complication occurred in the patients treated by open reduction: an infection with drainage and sequestration of bone graft that responded to treatment and resolved after 18 months. When open reduction was indicated, the Palmer technique was used. However, since the greater number of decisions were for nonoperative care, I obviously favor closed treatment. An unexpected finding in the closed reduction results has caused renewed efforts to select open reduction more often: the large number of fair (as opposed to good) results in the patients who underwent closed treatment. A comparison showed that the results of closed reduction were excellent in 12 (13 percent), good in 54 (58 percent), and fair in 27 (29 percent); there were no poor results. Results of open reduction were excellent in 4 (23 percent), good in 10 (63 percent), fair in 1 (7 percent), and poor in 1 (7 percent). The criteria for an excellent result were no pain and return to work, full activity within 4 months, good if this activity range was 4 to 8 months. In addition, the fair results were identified with residual soreness and aching, an inability to walk long distances, lack of endurance, and an inability to tolerate activity beyond normal activity hours. Furthermore, the total of excellent and good results was 86 percent in the open reduction cases compared with 71 percent in the closed reductions.

CONSIDERATIONS REGARDING THE DECISION FOR OPEN REDUCTION TREATMENT OF OS CALCIS FRACTURES

Age

Open reduction of os calcis fractures is not advised and is probably contraindicated in children and elderly patients. While an exact cutoff age is unknown, the presence of mature bone, perhaps close to 14 years of age in the young, is the lower age limit for open reduction. In the elderly, the presence of good bone structure in an active alert patient is the determining factor. Overall, age may not be a major factor in the decision to perform an open reduction.

Activity

Surgical intervention is contraindicated in a wheelchair-bound or nonactive patient. Similarly, there is a lessened indication in a relatively inactive person or in someone who has been unemployed for a long period. By contrast, an employed person, particularly one who needs to be on the injured foot the entire day, is a candidate for open reduction. Patients with compensable injuries need more detailed surgical attention in spite of the greater risks that seem to be present in such patients. The reason for operation is to ensure a better chance of retaining gainful employment (usually as a laborer).

GENERAL MEDICAL CONDITION

Open reduction of fractures of the os calcis is contraindicated in a patient who is irrational, mentally disturbed, or suicidal or who has serious medical problems and is in poor general health. The operation is not contraindicated in a moderately overweight person but should be considered a less appropriate choice in anyone classified as obese. Surgery is contraindicated in a patient who has had severe trauma involving other areas of the body such as severe head injury, organ ruptures, ipsilateral multiple fractures, at least in the early days or weeks of care, for individuals with multiple life threatening injuries. Frequently, the decision for surgical intervention comes at a much later time in these individuals when the prognosis is good for returning such a person to an active weight-bearing life. By the time the definitive procedure is considered in such instances, it has become a salvage procedure. The difficulty of restoring the anatomy of the os calcis after injury increases after 3 or 4 weeks and becomes almost impossible after 6 or 8 weeks.

BILATERAL OS CALCIS FRACTURES

The presence of bilateral fractures may increase the need for consideration for surgical intervention. Frequently these injuries are job related. Each foot has to be considered separately before establishing the plan of care. If open reduction appears appropriate in both feet, it may be best to do one foot at a time, and on separate days spaced 1 week apart. The force of the injury varies. Sometimes the injured person has fallen from his own roof or is a housewife who has fallen off a ladder. More often the bilateral injury involves a gainfully employed individual who is working at a height (i.e., a telephone lineman, roofer, or a construction worker). If the landing is "soft" and from a medium height, both os calci will show a split caused by the wedge action of the lateral process at the talus as it pushes downward into the neutral triangular zone at the os calcis, which is devoid of strong supporting trabeculae. If the person is obese or the height of the fall is great or on a hard surface, the result is usually a joint depression fracture with the posterior articular facet rotated and forced within the substance of the comminuted bone.

Waiting 1 week between the open reduction of bilateral fractures helps avoid the possibility of a complication such as infection, which may be related to performing an operation on both feet simultaneously. In addition, there is a better chance of assessing the need for surgical intervention on the second procedure, usually the least injured of the two bones. However, the decision to operate on one foot and not the other does not ensure a better result on either one. Residual pain may be the result in either foot. If the greater pain is found on the nonoperated side, the supposition would be that the surgery should have been done on both. If residual pain is present in both feet that have been operated on, the conclusion may be that a wrong decision was made in both instances and nonoperative treatment should have been the choice.

THE CONDITION OF ADJACENT TISSUES

A contraindication to proceeding with an open reduction of fractures of the os calcis is the presence of compromised skin and subcutaneous tissues with blistering, abrasions, or lacerations. The skin must be healed before proceeding, which in most instances requires weeks rather than days. The swelling, which may be prolonged, even after 5 to 7 days of 24-hour elevation, should usually subside sufficiently within 10 days to allow surgical intervention. Even at this time, there is always some inflammatory reaction secondary to the increased fluid and blood associated with impeded lymphatic and venous drainage. Operative trauma, imposed on the tissues that are already compromised, usually produces more scar tissue, which results in a stiff, painful foot as the result of poor soft tissue healing. Another reason to delay the operation is the possibility of wound breakdown or dehiscence if the condition of the skin is impaired. Consistent elevation of the foot above the heart level may be a key factor prior to performing an open reduction in order to ensure an uncomplicated result.

SURGICAL PROCEDURES

Primary Arthrodesis

Performing a primary arthrodesis in the treatment of fresh fractures of the os calcis has never gained popularity, although reports continue to indicate predictable success.[17,23,24] There have been more negative reports or reserved observations than favorable comments, as Essex-Lopresti noted in his review of this procedure.[2] Palmer[18] tried the procedure and stopped using it. My early difficult experiences lead me to concur with this position, and I have now completely discarded arthrodesis in the acute phase and, instead, now use it as a salvage procedure, as the comminution of the fresh frac-

ture fragments makes the procedure technically difficult. Moreover, it is rarely possible to maintain good bone stock and, with the removal of articular surfaces, the heel height is reduced and the foot is shortened. Swelling is more of a problem following arthrodesis than after open reduction. Postoperative skin and wound breakdown is more frequent, since excessive retraction may be used to obtain more extensive exposure. Once the procedure has been done, there is no salvage procedure left for the patient if the fusion does not succeed. Either subtalar fusion or triple arthrodesis are excellent procedures when used for late arthritic changes, but their use for early treatment of os calcis fractures is questionable and should seldom be the acceptable mode of surgical intervention. Now that CT scanning has made surgical planning for joint alignment and replacement of fracture pieces more accurate, more consideration should be more directed toward open reduction.

Open Reduction

The French have been credited for their aggressiveness in first advocating open reduction. Essex-Lopresti notes that, in 1902, Morestin was one of the earliest individuals to document open reduction as a method to restore fracture fragments.[2] Gissane[4] introduced open reduction aided by insertion of a large pin, and Palmer recommended placing a cancellous bone graft in the cavity left beneath the depressed fragment after the open reduction.

Open Reduction — Essex-Lopresti

A variation of this technique is sometimes considered a closed procedure and is called axial fixation, since the insertion of a pin in the posterior portion of the os calcis is the only open part of the procedure. The reduction is accomplished by manipulative efforts using the pin or spike. A Gissane spike is preferred and inserted a short distance through the tuberosity. This pin is used for levering the depressed fragment into place. Good results have been reported by King.[7] The author's experience has not been as good.

Essex-Lopresti[2] describes the pin technique as

an assistive part of an open reduction. A lateral incision is made with the patient on their side. The incision is 5 to 6 cm in length and parallel to the superior border of the os calcis, below the tip of the lateral malleolus. The depressed superior border of the os calcis is approached through the sinus tarsi, which allows for identification of the rotated, displaced, and depressed posterior subtalar facet. The calcaneal fibular ligament and lateral capsule may need to be partially incised to aid in reduction, but the soft tissue attachments should not be widely dissected. An additional instrument is used as a lever under the lateral displaced fragment to elevate this fragment and bring it as far as necessary to hold the corrected and elevated position. The bone is compressed to restore the normal width of the bone. Essex-Lopresti does not suggest the use of a bone graft if the operation is done in the first few days after injury, the implication being that cancellous bone later fills the cavity below the depressed area. One modification is to use a bone graft and metallic fixation to maintain the elevated position. The procedure always requires the use of a pin which protrudes posteriorly. The pin or spike is incorporated in a padded slipper cast, which is left on for 6 weeks (if the procedure is done without an open incision, the time period is 4 weeks). A second cast is then used from tibial tubercle to toe. Weight bearing is not allowed until 8 to 10 weeks after reduction, regardless of whether closed or open reduction was performed.

Open Reduction — Palmer

This technique is described in great detail, since I have followed it and preferred it with no variation. Palmer[18] believes that there are three steps to follow and it is his contention that all three steps must be completed for a successful result. These steps are (1) reduction of the entire lateral block, (2) reduction of the secondary compressed articular surfaces, and (3) filling of the bony defect.

A shallow curved incision is made, 6 cm in length, beneath the lateral malleolus. Proximally, the incision can be deepened, if necessary, to divide the middle part of the fibulocalcaneal ligament. The sheath of the peroneal tendons is incised and the tendons are displaced forward. A wide

moist Penrose drain can be used to protect the tendons during the necessary retraction. The cutaneous nerve is identified and protected by placing the self-retaining retractors without tension. The lateral border of the os calcis is identified and the periosteum opened with sharp dissection (Fig 157-1). A dull but wide periosteal elevator is used to separate the fragments and elevate the compressed bone to obtain an accurate alignment of the talocalcaneal joint (Fig. 157-2). When the elevator is withdrawn, there may be a loss of position and displacement of the subtalar joint may recur. Without bony support, Palmer believes that there will be a loss of position and a resultant valgus foot. Palmer places a piece of autologous bone from the iliac crest, the "size of the end of one's thumb" in the defect to maintain the correction. In my experience, the hole left is too large to leave unfilled.

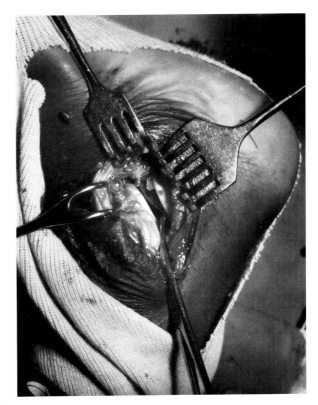

Fig. 157-1. View showing the unreduced state of the comminuted os calcis with the gap between the articular surfaces caused by the impaction of the dome-shaped posterior articular facet.

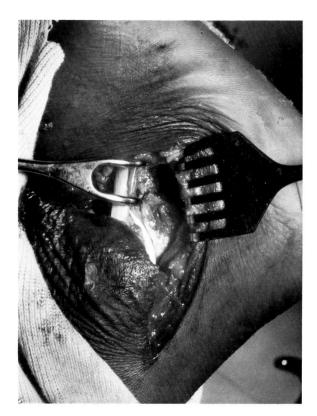

Fig. 157-2. The articular facet has now been elevated and the reduction is being maintained by position alone without the pressure of the periosteal elevator to hold the reduction. The large cavity that remains will be filled with iliac cortical cancellous bone.

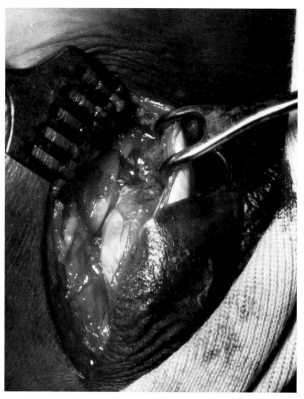

Fig. 157-3. The bone graft has now been inserted. The cavity has been completely filled. Joint articular surfaces are now in juxtaposition. Joint motion is tested for stability before the wound is closed.

Layered pieces of the iliac crest may be used as an alternative to fill the gap, as long as these pieces are not forced into position and do not crowd the medial side of the bone (Fig.157-3). The iliac bone is hammered into the cavity with a tamp. No pins or metallic fixation are used, since grafts are inserted until stability is maintained and motion is possible, as tested while the wound is open (Fig. 157-4). Although no mention is made by Palmer of two additional features, I believe that the procedure is best done under tourniquet control and an antibiotic solution is used to irrigate the wound before closure to protect against infection. The tourniquet is left inflated until a compressive cast has been applied. The cast padding is applied loosely. Tightly woven padding should be avoided.

The postoperative program of Palmer is followed. A below-knee cast is used. The patient is allowed up in 2 to 4 days with crutches and no weight bearing allowed for 12 weeks. It is anticipated the patient will be back to work or full activity in 4 to 5 months.

Open Reduction — McReynolds

McReynolds has not published details of his procedure, but others have done so.[22] The distinguishing characteristic of this procedure is the medial approach, in contradistinction to the more popular lateral approach. It is McReynolds' contention that the medial approach is preferable because displacement and overriding of the medial cortex is common, and this reduction can be best accom-

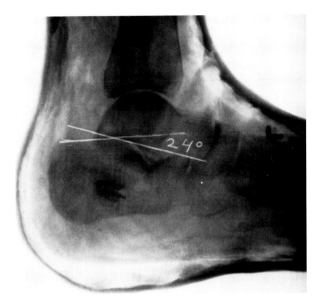

Fig. 157-4. Postoperative radiographs show a reduced os calcis fracture, as evidenced by the restored height of the bone and an acceptable Böhler angle of 24 degrees.

plished from the medial side. I do not agree that the problem is more common on the medial side, but I do agree that excellent exposure can be obtained with this approach. While I have used the medial approach in the treatment of fractures of the talus with osteotomy of the distal tip of the medial malleolus and later replacement and fixation with a screw. I still prefer the lateral approach for fractures of the os calcis because of the need to correct the lateral bulging and impingement which is a more common problem than is overriding on the medial side. The lateral side cannot be evaluated with a medial approach. Thus, it would require two incisions to reconstruct the os calcis if the problem must be corrected both medially and laterally. This may be something to consider as suggested by Gilmer et al.[3] Although the greater number of residual complaints of patients in long-term studies are those of the lateral side,[9] McReynolds still maintains that he prefers the medial approach because of the common displacement and overriding of the medial cortex which can be reduced only from the medial side.[10,11]

A straight horizontal incision of 5 to 7.5 cm is made on the medial side of the calcaneus and the neurovascular bundle identified and retracted.

Bone fragments are reduced under direct vision and stabilized by one or more metal staples. McReynolds has paid attention to detail and has evidentally mastered his technique well, but it is difficult to duplicate his efforts. The fracture fragments are reduced with extreme care since as McReynolds admits, the field of vision near the fracture site is very limited. Cautious leverage must be used to avoid breaking part of the superomedial fragment, since the elevation of the depressed or impacted areas is done blindly. The accuracy of reduction is checked by radiographs during the procedure. Placing the staples may require the prior placement of a drill hole to avoid splitting the thin cortical margin of the medial wall. Two-point or special three-point staples are used. The tabletop Stone staple, or staples with tapered tines, are not satisfactory for this operation. After the depressed fragments of the articular surfaces are corrected and the talar angle has been restored, radiologic confirmation of the reduction and staple positions is required before closure of the wound. A bulky dressing and a light cast is used, and the leg is elevated postoperatively. A plaster cast is applied and walking allowed at 2 weeks, with full weight bearing by 4 weeks. The cast is removed at 7 weeks, or shortly thereafter, depending on the amount of walking done by the patient. The patient is encouraged to walk 4 to 5 miles/day.

McReynolds reports 29 fractures in 25 patients, with 50 percent regaining subtalar motion and 76 percent with good or excellent results. His patients returned to work in 3 months and, if the fractures were bilateral, returned to work in 4½ months.

COMPLICATIONS

Residual Persistent Pain

A persistent painful stiff foot may occur regardless of the method of treatment. Rowe et al.[21] and Lindsay and Dewar[9] reported that this complication is more common with open reduction, but these findings seem more related to diffuse pain. Localized pain has been noted by these authors as well as others in addition to the diffuse pain. The lateral pain is secondary to the displaced fragments impinging on the peroneal tendons. The medial pain is associated with excessive fragmentation or poor reduction. All pain is brought on by weight bearing. Some additional pain is brought on by motion or by a gait involving midtarsal joint motion. Pain at rest is not a common feature.

Altered Heel Height and Shape

When reduction is not maintained, there is a gradual loss of bone stock. Various factors cause this complication, but the most common reason is too much compressive force caused by full weight bearing without external support too soon after reduction. The change in the size and shape of the heel causes problems with shoewear. In my study series,[12] 17 percent had difficulty with shoewear after open reduction, but an even higher number, 41 percent, had shoewear problems after closed reduction.

Swelling

Persistent swelling on standing or walking continues for a prolonged time and may never completely resolve. The exact reason is unknown. The swelling is aggravated by the dependent position and it is likely that altered lymphatic and venous drainage are the major causes. Since the swelling does not always subside overnight, or with elevation of the foot, there may be an additional factor of prolonged low-grade inflammatory changes that are unresolved with time.

Loss of Motion

If this complication is not associated with pain and instead is related to stiffness, there is less complaint. The presence of normal ankle or forefoot range of motion allows accommodation for the loss of subtalar or middorsal motion. Pain accentuates this complication when it is an accompanying feature. If the loss of motion alters the gait, this complication becomes more of a handicap at work or in daily activity. One must recall that stiffness and loss

of motion are an acceptable solution when arthrodesis is done to eliminate pain.

Infection

The choice of open reduction may bring on this complication, although there is the possibility of a pintract infection in the closed reduction technique. Infection in the os calcis is a devastating occurrence. The bone is a flat bone and therefore does not have the protective mechanism of a tubular bone with a strong periosteal envelope to help form an involucrum. Antibiotics cannot penetrate the substance of the os calcis when the infection becomes chronic. If bone grafts have been used, then sequestra will result and need to be removed. These will also need to be removed if metallic devices have been used.

Osteomyelitis

Not all infections of the os calcis will progress to the condition of osteomyelitis, but when this occurs the solution is drastic and drainage must be established. This can best be done with the split-heel incision of Gaenslen. It is possible that there will even need to be a complete excision of the os calcis as first advocated by Leriche and later by Pridie.[20] The final and most serious step to deal with this complication is amputation. The choice of open reduction means that both the patient and the physician will have to accept the complication of osteomyelitis as a possibility.

RESULTS

McReynolds reports 76 percent good or excellent results.[10] Palmer does not record his results, although the impression gained is that it is very high in the 80 to 90 percent range. The author used Palmer's technique and had 86 percent good or excellent results.[12] Pennel and Yadov[19] had 92 percent good or excellent results. Hammesfahr and Fleming report 80 percent good or excellent results.[5] The lowest quoted is 65 percent, reported by Vestad.[26] All these figures reflect reports of open reduction. Those investigators who profess to use only closed reduction report similar or better results and suggest that open reduction is less reliable and to less likely ensure a good or excellent result.

Striving for the best result possible, whether by a closed or open reduction, may be aided by the analysis of the fracture by better means. Often much helpful information may be gained with 30-degree coronal CT scan or a transverse CT scan. These techniques can be used in the presence of cast immobilization as suggested by the most recent study by Gilmer et al.[3]

In the future, additional sophisticated techniques may need to be considered following the initial closed reduction to determine whether open reduction is warranted. Eighty-seven percent of patients in my series were treated with closed reduction, and there were no poor results. The other 13 percent underwent open reduction. Eighty-six percent of patients who had an open reduction had results that were beneficial to them. Open reduction is a procedure with risks, but these risks may be justified by the better results that may be obtained in patients in whom this approach is indicated.

REFERENCES

1. Acton RK: Surgical anatomy of the foot. J Bone Joint Surg 49A:555, 1967
2. Essex-Lopresti P: The mechanism, reduction technique, and results in fractures of the os calcis. Br J Surg 39:395, 1952
3. Gilmer PW, Herzenberg J, Frank JL, et al: Computerized tomographic analysis of acute calcaneal fractures. Foot Ankle 6:184, 1986
4. Gissane W: Fractures of the os calcis. J Bone Joint Surg 29:255, 1947
5. Hammesfahr R, Fleming LL: Calcaneal fractures: a good prognosis. Foot Ankle 2:161, 1981
6. Harty M: Anatomic considerations in injuries of the calcaneus. Orthop Clin North Am 4:179, 1973
7. King RE: Axial pin fixation of fractures of the os calcis (method of Essex-Lopresti). Orthop Clin North Am 4:185, 1973
8. Lapidus PW: Spastic flat-foot. J Bone Joint Surg 28:126, 1946
9. Lindsay WRN, Dewar FP: Fractures of the os calcis. Am J Surg 95:555, 1958
10. McReynolds IS: Open reduction and internal fixation of calcaneal fractures. J Bone Joint Surg 54B:176, 1972
11. McReynolds IS: The case for operative treatment of fractures of the os calcis. p. 232. In Leach RE, Hoaglund PT, (eds): Controversies in Orthopaedic Surgery. WB Saunders, Philadelphia, 1982
12. Miller WE: Fractures of the calcaneus-open reductions vs. closed treatment. Orthop Trans 4:145, 1980
13. Miller WE: The heel pad. Am J Sports Med 10:19, 1982
14. Miller WE: The heel pad. (Letters to the editor.) Am J Sports Med 11:48, 1983
15. Miller WE: Pain and impairment considerations following treatment of disruptive os calcis fractures. Clin Orthop 177:82, 1983
16. Miller WE, Lichtblau PO: The smashed heel. South Med J 58:1229, 1965
17. Noble J, McQuillan WM: Early posterior subtalar fusion in the treatment of fracture of the os calcis. J Bone Joint Surg 61A:90, 1979
18. Palmer I: The mechanism and treatment of fractures of the calcaneus. Open reduction with the use of cancellous grafts. J Bone Joint Surg 30A:2, 1948
19. Pennel GF, Yadov MP: Operative treatment of comminuted fractures of the os calcis. Orthop Clin North Am 4:197, 1973
20. Pridie KH: A new method of treatment for severe fractures of the os calcis, a preliminary report. Surg Gynecol Obstet 82:671, 1946
21. Rowe CR, Sakellarides HT, Freeman PA, et al: Fractures of the os calcis: a long-term follow-up study of 146 patients. JAMA 184:920, 1963
22. Sisk TD: Fractures. p. 547. In Edmonson AS, Crenshaw AH: Campbell's Operative Orthopaedics. 6th Ed. CV Mosby, St. Louis, 1980
23. Thompson KR: Treatment of comminuted fractures of the calcaneus by triple arthrodesis. Orthop Clin North Am 4:189, 1973
24. Thompson KR, Friesen CM: Treatment of comminuted fractures of the calcaneus by primary triple arthrodesis. J Bone Joint Surg 41A:1423, 1959
25. Trickey EL: Treatment of fractures of the calcaneus. J Bone Joint Surg 57B:411, 1975
26. Vestad E: Fractures of the calcaneum open reduction and bone grafting. Acta Chir Scand 134:617, 1968
27. Weiland AH: Lest we forget. South Med J 53:175, 1960

Fractures and Dislocations of the Midpart and Forepart of the Foot

158

James D. Heckman

INJURIES OF THE MIDPART OF THE FOOT

Injury to the Midtarsal Joint

The midtarsal (Chopart's) joint is a confluent articulation composed of the talonavicular and the calcaneocuboid joints. These two joints work in unison to provide modest but critical motion of the midfoot. This motion is linked to subtalar joint motion during normal walking. At heel strike, the subtalar joint everts, creating a parallel alignment of the axes of the talonavicular and the calcaneocuboid joints. This parallel alignment allows the midtarsal joint to move and absorb much of the energy of impact at heel strike. By contrast, during toe-off the subtalar joint inverts and the axes of the two component articulations of the midtarsal joint are no longer parallel. This configuration produces stability of the midtarsal joint, creating an efficient lever arm for push-off.[9] Thus, injury to the midtarsal joint has the potential to disturb the normal mechanics of gait. Fortunately, the joint complex is not particularly vulnerable to injury, and reports of significant injury are rare.

Complete isolated dislocation of the midtarsal joint is rare and is often associated with avulsion fractures of the navicular tuberosity or the corner of the head of the talus. In Kenwright and Taylor's series[7] of 10 such injuries, dislocation occurred medially in five, dorsally in three and plantarly in two, due to severe rotational forces applied to the fixed foot in falls from a height.

Reduction of a complete midtarsal dislocation can usually be achieved by closed means, although open reduction is occasionally necessary for severely displaced injuries. Good long-term results have been reported following simple closed reduction and immobilization in a below-knee non-weight-bearing cast for 4 to 5 weeks (Fig. 158-1). Care must be taken, however, to assure an anatomic, stable reduction. Residual subluxation of either individual joint or the entire joint complex may lead to persistent joint pain as described below. In the severely swollen foot, plaster immobilization may be insufficient to assure the maintenance of an adequate reduction. If there is any doubt about the stability of the joint once reduced, reduction should be maintained for 4 to 6 weeks with one large Kirschner wire driven axially across each joint.

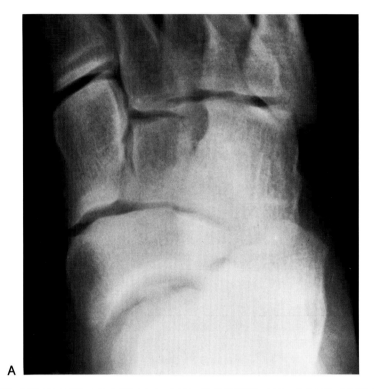

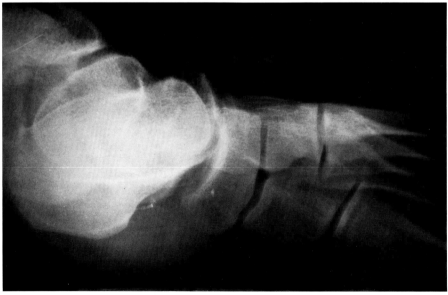

Fig. 158-1. (A,B) Oblique views of plantar lateral dislocation of the talonavicular and calcaneocuboid joints. A stable closed reduction was achieved and maintained with plaster immobilization. These injuries are often overlooked on initial routine radiographs taken to evaluate foot injuries.

Recently, subluxation of the midtarsal joint was identified as a sometimes overlooked injury that when untreated leads to symptomatic posttraumatic arthritis of this joint complex.[6] As with complete midtarsal dislocation, subluxation is often associated with avulsion fractures of the bones that comprise this joint; in particular, avulsion fracture of the navicular tuberosity. The posterior tibial tendon spans this joint and has its primary insertion on the navicular tuberosity. Thus, subluxation or dislocation of the midtarsal joint, particularly laterally, may result in avulsion of the tendon's insertion. Because these avulsion fractures are only minimally displaced, they are assumed to be isolated insignificant injuries, and the subluxation of the midtarsal joint is overlooked. Howie et al.[6] reviewed 14 patients who were initially diagnosed as having an isolated navicular tuberosity fracture and found that seven had, in addition, an avulsion fracture of the anterior process of the calcaneus, indicative of injury of the entire midtarsal joint complex. While the seven patients with isolated navicular avulsion fractures had no long-tem residual symptoms after 4 weeks of cast treatment, the seven patients with occult subluxation of the midtarsal joint all had a prolonged recovery, and three had persistent symptoms at long-term follow-up.

Dewar and Evans[2] and Stark[14] similarly have reported a total of six patients with occult fracture-subluxation of the midtarsal joint. Four of these injuries were initially misdiagnosed as an ankle sprain and, upon resumption of weight bearing, persistent pain and deformity (depression of the midtarsal joint with forefoot abduction) were noted. Of these four, two had persistent long-term symptoms without further treatment, and two underwent reduction and calcaneocuboid arthrodesis with restoration of alignment and resolution of their symptoms.

In an extensive review of 71 injuries in the midtarsal region, Main and Jowett[8] identified two patterns of subtalar subluxation: medial and lateral. In the medial subluxation, the forefoot is displaced medially; with the lateral subluxation, it is displaced laterally and a crushing fracture of the calcaneocuboid articulation occurs. These investigators also describe medial and lateral swivel dislocations, which are variants of the respective types of subtalar dislocations; however, with the swivel dislocation, axial rotation of the calcaneus occurs on the talus around the axis of the intact talocalcaneal ligament. In both types of swivel dislocations, the talonavicular joint dislocates, while the calcaneocuboid joint remains intact, and the calcaneus rotates about the talocalcaneal ligament axis, either medially or laterally. Closed reduction and casting of medial subluxations and medial swivel dislocations achieved good long-term results. By contrast, the lateral fracture-subluxations had a worse long-term prognosis following closed reduction, as evidenced by the need for isolated calcaneocuboid fusion to achieve pain relief in several instances.

In summary, the seriousness of injury to the midtarsal joint has not been fully appreciated in the past. These injuries are often written off as ankle sprains or entirely overlooked. Often chip fractures of the talus, avulsion fractures of the navicular tuberosity or of the anterior process of the calcaneus, or a compression fracture of the cuboid occur in association with or as a result of subluxation or dislocation of this joint complex. Careful evaluation of the entire joint complex is warranted when these innocuous appearing fractures are noted on radiographs. Closed reduction, if completely achieved and held with plaster (or percutaneous wires) combined with non-weight bearing for 4 to 6 weeks will usually produce a good result when the patient is seen promptly after injury. Persistent subluxation, particularly laterally with an associated flatfoot deformity, will often result in a painful gait and necessitate arthrodesis of the calcaneocuboid joint or the entire midtarsal joint complex to achieve satisfactory alignment and painless function of the midpart of the foot.

Navicular Fractures

Avulsion Fracture of the Navicular Tuberosity

The navicular tuberosity serves as a point of insertion of the posterior tibial tendon and also for a portion of the deltoid ligament. The size of the tuberosity is quite variable, and it often articulates with the variably sized accessory navicular bone. Fracture of the tuberosity may be caused by a direct blow, but most commonly it is an avulsion frac-

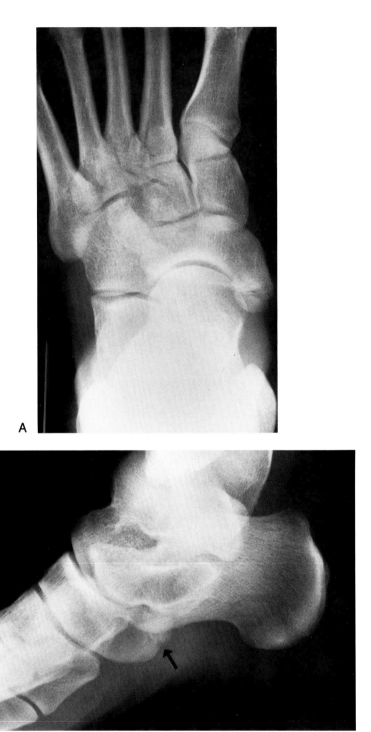

Fig. 158-2. (A,B) An isolated, minimally displaced avulsion fracture of the navicular tuberosity. Note the roughened fractured surface. On clinical examination, the patient had discrete point tenderness at the fracture site.

ture caused by abduction of the forefoot and/or strong contraction of the posterior tibial tendon.[4] The presence of an avulsion fracture of the navicular tuberosity should make the clinician wary of a subluxation of the midtarsal joint with associated impaction fracture of the cuboid or calcaneus.

The isolated avulsion fracture of the navicular tuberosity is rarely displaced significantly (Fig. 158-2). In this situation, it is often difficult to distinguish a fresh fracture from a preexisting accessory navicular. Comparison radiographs of the opposite foot will help distinguish the difference, as the accessory navicular occurs bilaterally two-thirds of the time,[13] and usually the two are quite symmetric. In addition, as with other accessory ossicles, a true accessory navicular will have smooth rounded edges with a thin layer of subchondral bone throughout its entire circumference, while the avulsed fracture fragment will have a jagged fracture surface without the thin line of dense subchondral bone beneath it.

A patient who has a minimally displaced fracture of the navicular tuberosity should be checked carefully to confirm that the function of the posterior tibial tendon is intact by demonstrating active inversion of the foot. When such is the case, treatment in a below-knee weight-bearing cast for 4 to 6 weeks with the foot in a neutral position will usually result in healing of the fracture with no residual loss of posterior tibial tendon function.

Often, moderate prominence of the healed fracture persists, occasionally resulting in irritation from the pressure of the shoe. Rarely, the minimally displaced avulsion fracture fails to unite and remains painful with weight bearing. In both cases, the prominent tuberosity or the nonunited fragment can be excised, much as an accessory navicular is removed. The fragment is removed from the attachments of the posterior tibial tendon, the excision bed is freshened to bleeding bone, and the tendon is sutured back to the bed to maintain its effective insertion. Following excision, a protective cast should be worn for 4 to 6 weeks.

On rare occasions, severe displacement of an avulsed navicular tuberosity occurs (Fig. 158-3). This degree of displacement can only occur as a result of contraction of the posterior tibial tendon and, if untreated, persistent incompetence (hence flatfoot) of the posterior tibial tendon can be antici-

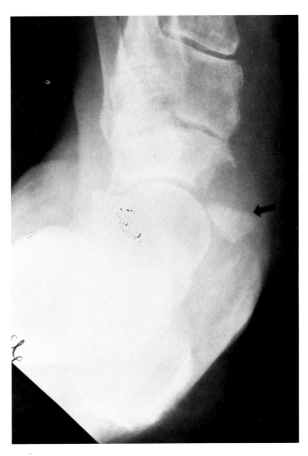

Fig. 158-3. Markedly displaced avulsion fracture of the navicular tuberosity in a 62-year-old patient with diabetes mellitus. Note the subluxation of the forepart of the foot laterally as a result of loss of the stabilizing influence of the posterior tibial tendon.

pated. When seen acutely, avulsion fractures that are displaced by more than 1 cm should be repaired surgically to restore the functional length of the posterior tibial tendon. When seen late, a severe fixed pes planus deformity may be present. When this deformity is present, it can only be corrected effectively by triple arthrodesis.

Cortical Avulsion Fracture

Avulsion fractures of the dorsal lip of the navicular account for almost one-half of all isolated navicular fractures[4] (Fig. 158-4). The dorsal medial cortex of the navicular serves as one point of insertion of the deltoid ligament, reinforcing the capsule of

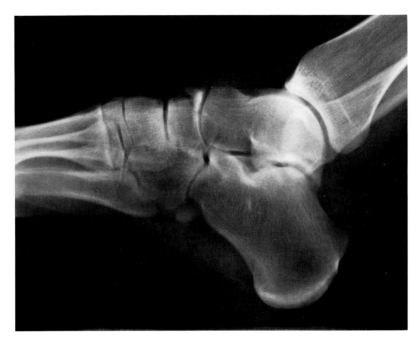

Fig. 158-4. Avulsion fracture of the dorsal lip of the navicular resulting from forced plantar flexion of the forepart of the foot.

the talonavicular joint. Forced plantar flexion or abduction of the foot may result in avulsion of a variably sized fragment. Most of the fracture fragments are small and can be treated by a 3- to 4-week period of cast immobilization. On rare occasions, the fragment may comprise 20 percent or more of the articular surface of the navicular. These large fragments are often displaced, and open reduction and internal fixation with Kirschner wires should be undertaken to ensure congruous reduction of the articular surface, minimizing the risk of later posttraumatic arthritis of the talonavicular joint.

Fractures of the Body of the Navicular

Fractures extending through the body of the navicular will involve two articular surfaces: the talonavicular as well as the naviculocuneiform. Persistent displacement of the fracture often leads to posttraumatic arthritis of one or both of these articulations. While these fractures are uncommon, several different mechanisms have been described by which they may occur: crushing, longitudinally applied forces, and repetitive stress.

With a crushing injury, comminution is frequent and may be severe. Often, there is minimal displacement of the many fracture fragments. In this case, plaster immobilization with careful molding of the arch of the foot in the cast will result in healing of the fracture, but later arthritis may develop in one or both of the injured joints.

Main and Jowett[8] describe the patterns of fracture that may occur in the navicular when longitudinal forces are suddenly applied to the forepart of the foot. If differential forces are transmitted along the medial rays, lines of stress will be created along the intercuneiform lines in the navicular, resulting in a longitudinal fracture (Fig. 158-5). These fractures are frequently displaced, yet are difficult to identify on routine radiographs. Persistent displacement led to fair or poor results in 18 of 24 patients reviewed by Main and Jowett, who recommended open reduction and internal fixation for displaced longitudinal fractures of the navicular.

A variant of the traumatic longitudinal fracture to the navicular is the stress fracture of the body. This pattern of fracture, a vertical fracture in line with the intercuneiform lines, is similar to the frac-

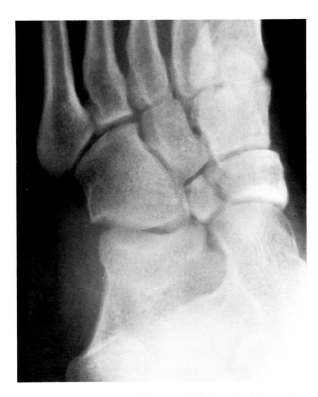

Fig. 158-5. Longitudinal fracture of the body of the navicular in line with the articulation between the middle and lateral cuneiforms.

ture caused by acute longitudinal forces described above. However, the fracture pattern is seen most commonly in young athletes who participate in running and jumping sports, probably resulting from repetitive loading of the plantar-flexed forefoot, with differing forces being applied to the parts of the navicular separated by these intercuneiform lines. These stress fractures are very hard to diagnose, as the patient complains of vague pain in the midpart of the foot and swelling associated with activity, and routine foot radiographs are often normal in appearance.[10] Technetium 99m bone scanning and anteroposterior tomograms are often required to make the correct diagnosis (Fig. 158-6).

In a series of 19 patients with 21 fractures, Torg et al.[15] found that the diagnosis was often delayed for up to 3 years, and the average time from the onset of symptoms until diagnosis was 7 months. In their series, the fracture was complete in 11 pa-

tients and incomplete, involving only the dorsal cortex, in 10. Most of these fractures are nondisplaced and will heal with plaster immobilization combined with non-weight bearing for 6 to 8 weeks. These same investigators have recommended open reduction, internal fixation, and bone grafting to achieve healing of displaced and nonunited stress fractures of this bone.

Cuboid Fractures

A fracture of the cuboid can result from direct crushing injury but more commonly occurs as a result of abduction of the forepart of the foot at the midtarsal joint, as described for the midtarsal joint injuries above. Hermel and Gershon-Cohen[5] aptly described this fracture as the "nutcracker fracture," as the cuboid is compressed against the anterior articulation of the calcaneus by severe abduction of the forepart of the foot. Impaction fractures of the articular surface are accompanied by compression fractures of the trabeculae of this largely cancellous bone (Fig. 158-7). Significant difficulty is encountered when surgical attempts to restore the shape of the cuboid are undertaken, and bone grafting may be necessary to restore adequate length to the impacted bone to support the articular surface in its proper alignment with the calcaneus. Both objectives should be achieved so that satisfactory function of the midtarsal joint can be maintained. Late posttraumatic arthritis of the calcaneocuboid joint as a result of fracture is best treated by arthrodesis.

Displaced fractures of the cuboid may disrupt the groove in which the peroneus longus tendon lies, leading to chronic tendonitis with local pain and swelling, and impairment of normal function of this tendon.[11]

Cuneiform Fractures and Dislocations

The three (medial, middle or intermediate, and lateral) cuneiforms and their articulations are small and relatively well protected from injury. Isolated fractures can obviously occur from direct blows; severe crushing injuries to the midpart of the foot

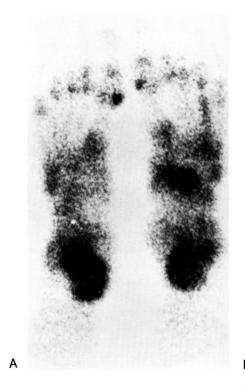

A

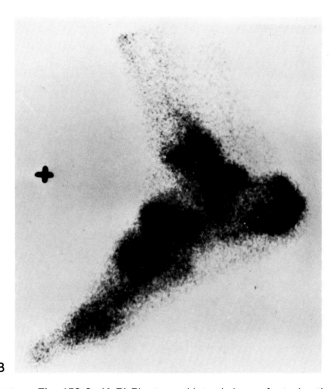

B

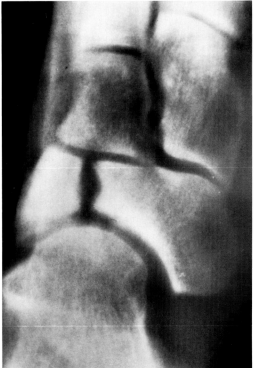

C

Fig. 158-6. (A,B) Plantar and lateral views of a technetium bone scan showing increased nucleotide uptake in the area of the navicular. (Courtesy of H. Pavlov, M.D., New York, New York.) **(C)** Tomogram demonstrating a complete longitudinal stress fracture of the navicular. (Fig. C from Torg,[15] with permission.)

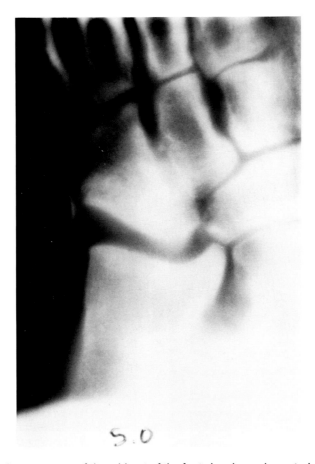

Fig. 158-7. Anteroposterior tomogram of the midpart of the foot showing an impacted compression fracture of the cuboid. Note how the proximal articular surface has been driven into the body of the cuboid by the calcaneus.

will often result in varying degrees of fracture. The cuboid spans the naviculocuneiform articulation, providing stability and resistance to rotational stress in the frontal plane. Thus, most of the cuneiform or intercuneiform dislocations reported have been caused by axial stresses and are associated with, or variants of, tarsometatarsal joint injuries. Indeed, when a dislocation or a fracture-dislocation of a cuneiform bone (particularly the medial one) is diagnosed radiographically, one must carefully inspect the Lisfranc's joint and search for injury there. The most commonly reported cuneiform injury[1,3,12] is an axial dislocation of the entire first ray with the medial cuneiform-first metatarsal articulation remaining intact and the entire first ray displacing proximally and medially. This variant of an isolated first metatarsal base dislocation (Fig. 158-8) can usually be reduced by closed means,

but once an accurate reduction has been achieved, it should be maintained by percutaneous Kirschner wire fixation and a non-weight-bearing cast for 6 weeks to permit satisfactory healing of the disrupted ligaments.

Because each of these cuneiform bones articulates with four other bones in the midpart of the foot, persistent displacement of any fracture, subluxation or dislocation, may result in posttraumatic arthritis. On routine radiographs, it is easy to overlook injuries to these small overlapping bones; when there is a clinical suspicion of injury in this region, magnification views, tomography, or even computed tomography scanning may be indicated. Minimally displaced fractures should be treated in a below-knee weight-bearing cast, but reduction, by open means if necessary, should be undertaken for markedly displaced joint injuries to restore

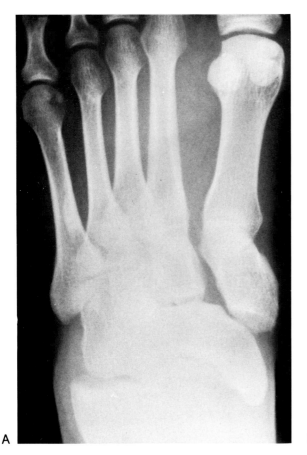

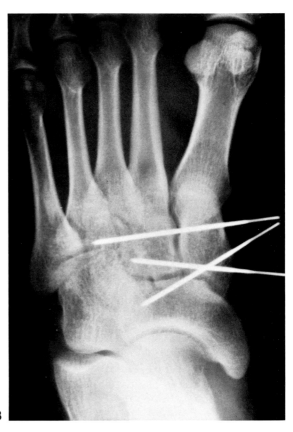

A   B

Fig. 158-8. **(A)** Dislocation of the first ray at the naviculocuneiform joint. This is a variant of an isolated Lisfranc's type injury, where the line of injury passes through the articulation between the medial and middle cuneiforms and out across the naviculocuneiform articulation. **(B)** Satisfactory closed reduction was obtained and then maintained with three percutaneous Kirschner wires.

congruity and minimize the chances of late post-traumatic arthritis.

INJURIES OF THE FOREPART OF THE FOOT

Injury of the Tarsometatarsal Joints

The complex articulation between the tarsals and the metatarsal bases (Lisfranc's joint) is subject to varying patterns of injury depending on the spe-cific mechanism. While injury to Lisfranc's joint is relatively rare,[17] failure to diagnose and treat this injury often leads to arthritis with significant resid-ual symptoms.[33]

The tarsometatarsal joint is intrinsically stable because of the configuration of the bony architec-ture.[42] In the frontal plane, the base of the second metatarsal is recessed proximally, disrupting the confluent alignment of the other four tarsometa-tarsal joints and preventing extreme displacement in abduction or adduction. Further osseous stabil-ity is provided by the trapezoidal cross-sectional shape of the middle three metatarsal bases, which form a modified Roman arch that effectively resists plantar displacement. Plantarly, very strong ligaments reinforce the joint, further stabilizing it. In addition, the bases of the lateral four metatarsals are attached by strong intermetatarsal ligaments, and the base of the second metatarsal is firmly attached to the medial cuneiform by the thick Lisfranc's ligament. By contrast, dorsally the joint capsule is relatively weak, and it is in this direction that the metatarsal bases most often dislocate. Finally, because of the relatively weak ligamentous connection of the first metatarsal to the second, isolated dislocation of the first metatarsal base may occur.

Mechanisms of Injury

Multiple mechanisms ranging in degree of force from mild to severe may cause injury to the Lisfranc's joint complex. These forces can be classified into three general types: twisting, axial loading in hyperextension, and crushing. Twisting forces that produce an abduction moment to the forepart of the foot can result in lateral displacement of all five metatarsals. This mechanism of injury is usually associated with a fracture of the base of the second metatarsal (Fig. 158-9).

Axial loading of the plantar-flexed foot is also a common cause of Lisfranc's joint disruption. While severe forces so applied can produce the injury, apparently trivial stress, such as missing a step and alighting on the ball of the foot, can also result in significant joint injury because of the relative weakness of the dorsal capsule. When an axial load is applied to the plantar-flexed foot, the dorsal capsule cannot withstand the strain and the metatarsal bases dislocate dorsally.

Crushing injuries can produce any configuration of tarsometatarsal joint injury, depending on the direction and severity of the applied force. Plantar dislocations occur almost exclusively with this mechanism following a blow to the dorsum of the foot.[39]

Classification of Injury

While a few common patterns of injury to Lisfranc's joint have been described, the several mechanisms of injury can result in a great variety of injury patterns. Three commonly occurring displacements in the frontal plane were first identified by Quenu and Kuss[40] and are often used to describe injuries to this region:

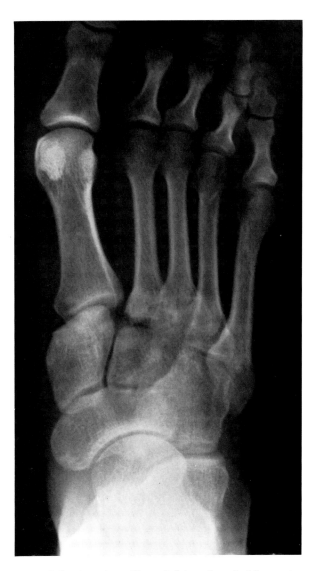

Fig. 158-9. Homolateral lateral dislocation of all five metatarsals at Lisfranc's joint. Note the avulsion fracture at the base of the second metatarsal.

Homolateral: all five metatarsals displaced in the same direction, usually laterally, and usually associated with a fracture of the base of the second metatarsal

Isolated: dislocation of only one or two metatarsals, most often the first

Divergent: medial displacement of the first metatarsal and lateral displacement of the lesser four metatarsals (Fig. 158-10)

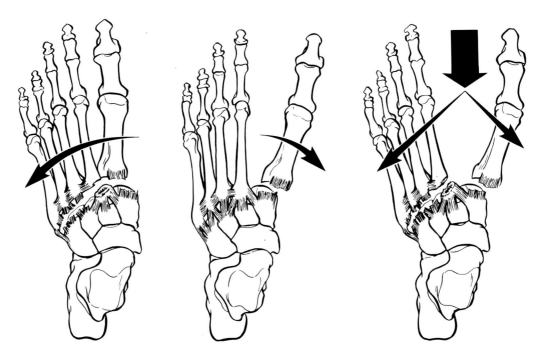

Fig. 158-10.   The three frontal plane displacement patterns that occur frequently with injury to Lisfranc's joint are described as homolateral, isolated, and divergent.

The degree of frontal plane displacement is often difficult to appreciate on radiographs because of overlapping of the metatarsal bases; however, there are certain consistent parameters that may be used to identify even subtle degrees of displacement and should be used to assess the adequacy of reduction. The most consistent radiographic finding with isolated and divergent patterns of injury is an increase in the normal distance between the bases of the first and second metatarsals. The two most consistent bony relationships between the tarsus and the metatarsals in the frontal plane are smooth, unbroken lines extending across the joint: (1) from the medial aspect of the base of the second metatarsal to the medial articular surface of the middle cuneiform, and (2) from the medial aspect of the base of the fourth metatarsal to the medial articular surface of the cuboid.[27] On both the routine anteroposterior and oblique radiographs, inspection of these bony landmarks will identify significant frontal plane displacement.

Displacement can also occur in the sagittal plane with these injuries and is often difficult to appreciate on the lateral radiograph because of overlapping of the metatarsal shafts. The displacement of the metatarsal bases is usually dorsal, except with direct blows to the dorsum of the foot, where plantar displacement can occur.

Diagnosis

Goosens and DeStoop[29] reported that in up to 20 percent of these injuries, the proper diagnosis is overlooked and a high index of suspicion must be present when patients present with complaints of forefoot pain following foot or ankle injury. The wide variety of injury mechanisms makes injury to this joint complex a possibility following virtually any type of foot injury, ranging from a simple twist to a massive crushing injury. While localized tenderness and deformity are sometimes present, marked swelling immediately following the injury may mask the deformity and make precise localization of the point of injury difficult.

Careful inspection of anteroposterior, oblique, and lateral radiographs of the midpart of the foot is essential to the diagnosis in any patient with pain, swelling, or tenderness in the area following injury.

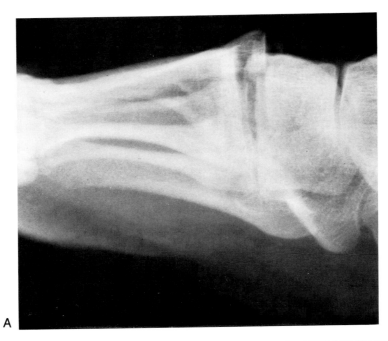

A

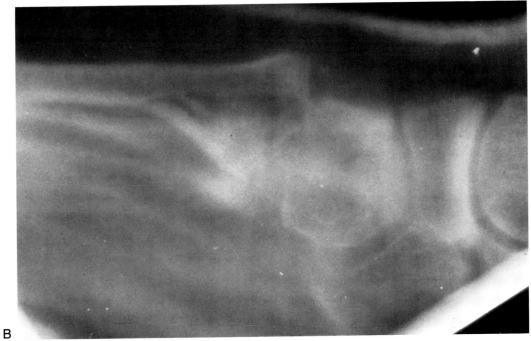

B

Fig. 158-11. (A,B) Plain radiograph and lateral tomogram showing dorsal displacement of the second metatarsal base along with comminution and displacement of the plantar half of its articular surface.

Comparison radiographs of the opposite, uninjured, foot may also help identify disruption of this joint. Small fracture fragments around the metatarsal bases, particularly the second metatarsal, and increased distance between the first and second metatarsal bases, malalignment of the second metatarsal base on the middle cuneiform and of the fourth metatarsal base on the cuboid, and dorsal or plantar displacement of the metatarsal shafts on the lateral view are all certain signs of significant injury to this joint complex (Fig. 158-11).

Careful assessment of the distal circulation should always be made in the patient who has sustained an injury to this region. The dorsalis pedis artery crosses the joint between the bases of the first and second metatarsals and dives between them to create the deep plantar arch. Thus, it is especially vulnerable to injury. While gangrene following this injury is rare, it has been reported,[19] and prompt reduction is indicated if ischemia of the toes is noted on initial examination.

Treatment

Closed Reduction

Most clinical reviews of injuries to Lisfranc's joint indicate that the long-term results are better if an anatomic or near-anatomic reduction can be achieved and maintained. This conclusion is contradicted, however, by Brunet and Wiley,[21] who, when reviewing 34 Lisfranc injuries at 15 years postinjury, found that (1) despite the type of treatment or degree of reduction achieved initially, foot discomfort improved to a stable level by 1½ years after injury; (2) residual deformity was not uncommon; (3) neither the initial fracture pattern nor the method of treatment (including no treatment in some cases) had any apparent bearing on long-term function; and (4) while 80 percent of the patients had some degree of arthrosis on follow-up radiographs, there was little or no relationship of these findings to functional impairment. However, they did note that most of the functionally unsatisfactory results included patients with injury to the medial column (the first metatarsal and its articulations). Despite these disconcerting findings, they recommend accurate and stable reduction of injuries to the Lisfranc's joint. Nondisplaced (sprain) injuries of this joint should be immobilized in a cast for 6

weeks to permit full healing of the injured ligaments. Weight bearing may be allowed in the cast if it is painless. Radiographs should be repeated several days after the injury to be certain that late displacement does not occur as the swelling subsides.

Technique   An accurate closed reduction of displaced fracture-dislocations can usually be achieved, although it is often difficult to maintain the reduction by closed means. A closed reduction under adequate general or regional anesthesia can usually be achieved by applying longitudinal traction to the toes, combined with manual manipulation of the displaced metatarsal bases. Traction is best applied by gravity suspension of the affected toes in wire traps, and full reduction is usually achieved with manual manipulation of the displaced metatarsal bases. If radiographs and traction demonstrate an adequate reduction (realignment of the first, second, and fourth metatarsals with their respective tarsal bones in both anteroposterior and lateral projections and less than 2 mm of diastasis between the first and second metatarsal bases[39] and no significant residual dorsal or plantar displacement), the reduction should be maintained by percutaneous wire fixation. All potentially unstable fragments should be transfixed with 0.625 Kirschner wires or small smooth Steinmann pins passed from the metatarsal base into the tarsus. In most cases, at least two pins will be necessary to maintain a stable reduction. In the case of a homolateral fracture-dislocation of all five metatarsals, one medial (through the first metatarsal into the medial cuneiform) and one lateral (through the fifth metatarsal into the cuboid) pin will usually create a stable reduction (Fig. 158-12). Once pinned in the stable position, the foot should be supported in a splint or below-knee non-weight-bearing cast for 6 weeks until healing occurs.

Open Reduction

Occasionally, a satisfactory reduction cannot be achieved by closed means (persistent displacement of greater than 2 mm, or a talometatarsal angle greater than 15 degrees).[39] Most often, obstruction to reduction occurs at the area of the second metatarsal base due to displaced bony fragments (usually from the second metatarsal base) or to soft tis-

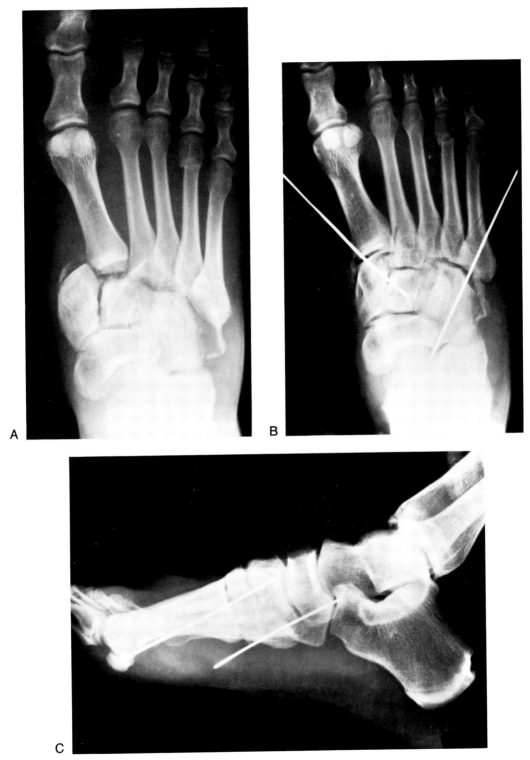

Fig. 158-12. (A) Homolateral fracture-dislocation at Lisfranc's joint. **(B,C)** Satisfactory closed reduction was achieved and maintained by two percutaneous pins.

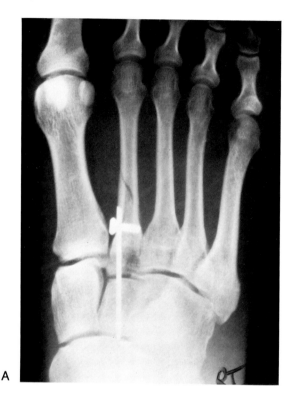

A

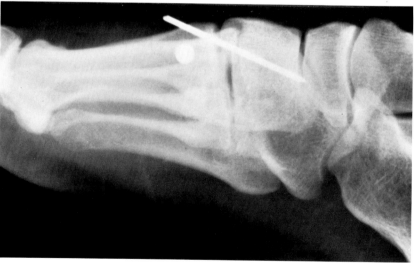

B

Fig. 158-13. (A,B) A displaced isolated fracture-dislocation of the base of the second metatarsal has been reduced and fixed with a screw and percutaneous Kirschner wire.

sue interposition (frequently, part or all of the anterior tibial tendon). When the closed reduction is considered inadequate, open reduction should be undertaken with attention directed to the base of the second metatarsal.

Technique Expose the area through a longitudinal dorsal incision, taking care to protect the dorsalis pedis artery, and remove any loose bone fragments or interposed soft tissue. Replace the second metatarsal base in its proper position with respect to the first metatarsal and the middle cuneiform, and secure it in place with percutaneous pins. Following this part of the reduction, radiographs should be obtained to confirm the anticipated return of the lesser metatarsals to an acceptable position (Fig. 158-13). If persistent displacement of the lateral metatarsals remains, a second longitudinal incision centered over the fourth ray is used to expose and reduce these joints. After satisfactory open reduction has been obtained and stabilized, the foot is

maintained in a non-weight-bearing plaster cast for 6 weeks to permit healing of the injured joint complex.

Arthrodesis

While most patients (80 percent),[21] who sustain an injury to the Lisfranc's joint recover to their previous level of activity by 15 months after injury, some have persistent pain associated with persistent subluxation and posttraumatic arthritis of the Lisfranc joint complex. For these patients, arthrodesis of the affected joint has been recommended. Complete joint resection combined with inlay corticocancellous bone grafts will permit some correction of residual deformity, but in my hands, it has been difficult to achieve and maintain full correction of the deformity and a solid fusion with this technique. Johnson and Johnson[33] described a technique of dowel arthrodesis that was effective in relieving pain in 11 of 13 patients, producing suc-

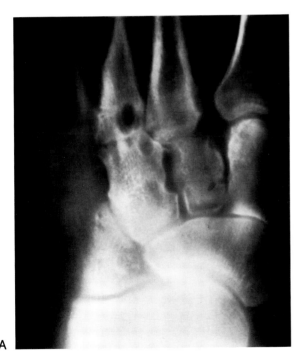

A

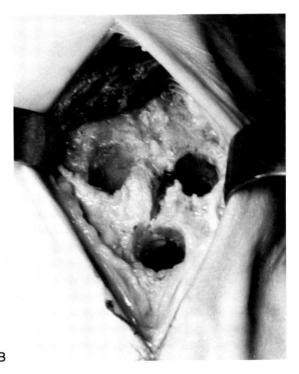

B

Fig. 158-14. Symptomatic degenerative arthritis of Lisfranc's joint should be treated with arthrodesis. **(A)** Anteroposterior tomogram demonstrating posttraumatic degenerative arthritis with cyst formation. **(B)** Technique of dowel arthrodesis is demonstrated. Iliac crest bone grafts of equal size are placed into the trephine defects across the arthritic joints. (From Johnson,[33] with permission.)

cessful fusion in 45 of the 48 individual joints treated.

Technique—Johnson and Johnson   Using a 7.5-mm trephine and a low-powered drill, a bicortical cylindrical bone/joint plug is removed from each affected joint, and a similarly sized core of autogenous iliac crest is harvested and placed into each dowel defect (Fig. 158-14). The arthrodesis site is transfixed with two smooth pins, and the foot is casted for approximately 10 weeks until radiographic signs of graft consolidation appear. This in situ fusion technique makes no attempt to correct residual deformity; however, the good results achieved with this technique indicate that in patients with chronic pain following Lisfranc joint injury, arthrodesis of the affected joints will usually produce good results.

Metatarsal Fractures

Fractures of the metatarsals can be subdivided into four groups: metatarsal shaft, stress fractures, metatarsal head, and fractures of the proximal portion of the fifth metatarsal.

Metatarsal Shaft Fractures

Fractures of the metatarsal shafts can be produced by direct blows or twisting forces applied to the forefoot and also by repetitive bending stresses. Direct blows and twisting forces usually

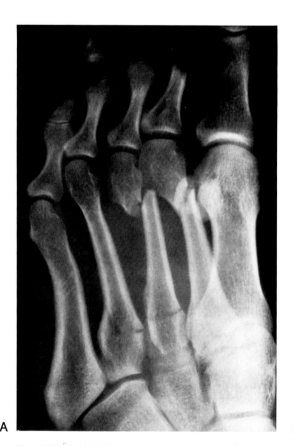
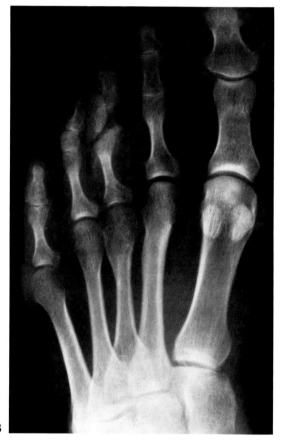

A   B

Fig. 158-15. (A) Nondisplaced fractures of the proximal shafts of the third and fourth metatarsals and moderately displaced fractures of the second and third metatarsals distally. **(B)** Two years following injury, treatment with a below-knee weight-bearing cast for 6 weeks has resulted in satisfactory healing of all four fractures and an asymptomatic foot.

result in minimally displaced metatarsal shaft fractures that should be treated with cast immobilization and early weight bearing as tolerated. Prompt healing in 3 to 4 weeks can be anticipated for the vast majority of these fractures, and minimal long-term disability is seen as fracture treatment in a weight-bearing cast, or even a well-padded stiff-soled shoe can be instituted soon after the injury[18] (Fig. 158-15). On rare occasions, especially after a severe crushing injury to the foot, marked displacement may be present, which requires reduction. Persistent dorsal angulation at the fracture site, best seen on the lateral radiograph, may result in prominence of the metatarsal head on the plantar surface. Malunion of the metatarsal in this position may produce a painful callous because of excessive weight-bearing forces on the bony prominence. As the metatarsals are virtually subcutaneous dorsally, any persistent bony prominence on this surface may be irritated by shoewear, as will residual medial prominence of the first metatarsal or lateral prominence of the fifth metatarsal (Fig. 158-16). Therefore, severe fracture deformities, especially in the directions described above, should be reduced, usually by traction and manual manipulation, and percutaneously pinned to prevent recurrence until healing occurs. Healing usually occurs rapidly, and the pins can be removed in 3 to 4 weeks. The patient should begin weight bearing in a protective cast as soon as the pain of injury subsides, to minimize the risk of reflex sympathetic dystrophy and to maintain motor strength and function.

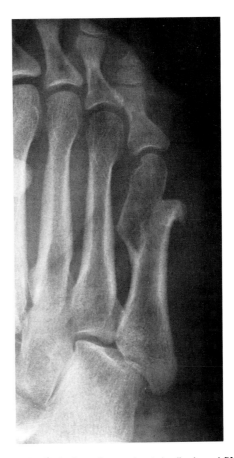

Fig. 158-16. Malunion of a moderately displaced fifth metatarsal shaft fracture with a painful spur on the plantar lateral aspect of the foot. Symptoms were treated by resection of the tender bony prominence.

Stress Fractures

Stress, or fatigue, fractures occur quite commonly in the metatarsals, especially the second and third. In a series of 700 military recruits with stress fractures, Meurman and Elfving identified 140 metatarsal fractures.[37,38] In a series of 54 runners with stress fractures, 10 occurred in the second or third metatarsal,[33] and Ford and Gilula[26] reported four stress fractures of the lesser metatarsals as a complication of the Keller bunionectomy.

In all these circumstances, increased weight-bearing (bending) loads have been applied to the metatarsals, resulting in fatigue failure. Any increase in the amount of walking or running or an alteration in the pattern of weight bearing (even the wearing of a new type of shoe) may be sufficient to cause a metatarsal stress fracture.

The first signs and symptoms of this process are subtle: localized pain, swelling, and point tenderness. When these signs and symptoms have lasted for only a few days, the process can be best described as a stress reaction, as the metatarsal is actively remodeling to accommodate to the newly applied stresses. When the symptoms first appear, radiographs are almost always normal, and technetium bone scanning is required to confirm the diagnosis. If the repetitive loads can be decreased or eliminated during this early stress reaction phase, complete fracture of the bone can be avoided and the symptoms will often resolve within a few days. However, more frequently, the patient presents later in the course of the injury process with pain and swelling that has been present for several days or even weeks. Usually at this point, a complete stress fracture has occurred and, by 2 to 3 weeks, healing callus is usually evident on routine radiographs (Fig. 158-17). With the exception of the proximal diaphyseal fifth metatarsal stress fracture, which is extremely slow to heal (see the section that follows), stress fractures of other metatarsals heal rapidly and will rarely displace. Treatment should include elimination of the excessive bending loads that produced the fracture, and support with a weight-bearing cast or firm well-molded shoe until the pain and point tenderness resolve, usually a period of 4 to 6 weeks.

Fractures of the Metatarsal Head

Fractures of the metatarsal head occur rarely (Fig. 158-18). They most often result from a direct blow to the forefoot, and rarely is marked displacement present. The most common deformity seen is plantar displacement of the distal fragment, which may result in a painful plantar callus if persistent. Markedly displaced fractures can usually be manually reduced but may be unstable and require percutaneous pin fixation for 3 to 4 weeks until bony union begins.

Fractures of the Proximal Fifth Metatarsal

Two specific fracture patterns occur at the base of the fifth metatarsal: avulsion fracture and transverse diaphyseal fracture. Some confusion has ex-

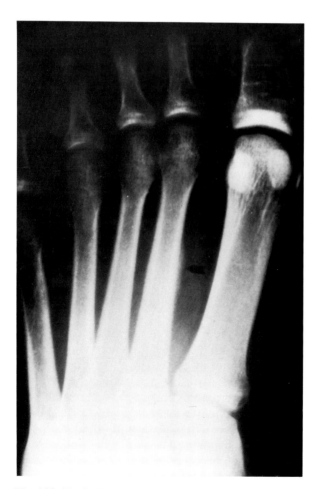

Fig. 158-17. Periosteal new bone formation around a three week old stress fracture of the second metatarsal shaft.

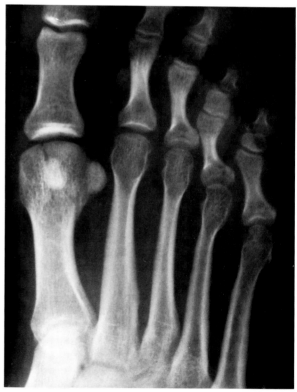

Fig. 158-18. Nondisplaced fracture of the first metatarsal head that resulted from a stubbing injury to the great toe. This fracture healed with cast immobilization for 6 weeks.

isted in the literature because these two distinctly different fractures for a time were both identified as a Jones' fracture following Sir Robert Jones' description in 1902 of six cases (including an injury to his own foot) of a fracture at the base of the fifth metatarsal.[34] All six of his cases were due to sudden inversion stress, and all healed well with 4 to 6 weeks of protection. This clinical course is typical of the common avulsion fracture but is not the characteristic course for the diaphyseal injury.

Avulsion Fracture

The avulsion fracture is extremely common, and results from an inversion stress of the ankle with avulsion of a variably sized portion of the base of the fifth metatarsal at the point of insertion in the peroneus brevis tendon. This injury is often confused with a lateral ankle sprain. Radiographs usually show a slightly displaced fragment representing a variably sized portion of the tuberosity of the metatarsal (Fig. 158-19). These avulsion fractures,

when minimally displaced, heal sufficiently in three to four weeks when immobilized in a cast or supported with an elastic wrap. Occasionally, the avulsed fragment will displace and fail markedly to unite; however, most patients become asymptomatic and do not require further treatment of this nonunion. Persistent symptoms from an nonunited fracture of this type may be treated effectively by excision of the fragment and reattachment of the peroneus brevis to the base of the fifth metatarsal.

Transverse Diaphyseal Fracture

While fracture of the proximal diaphysis of the fifth metatarsal is much less common than the avulsion fracture, it is often slow to heal and painful nonunion is a not uncommon sequel. The pattern of

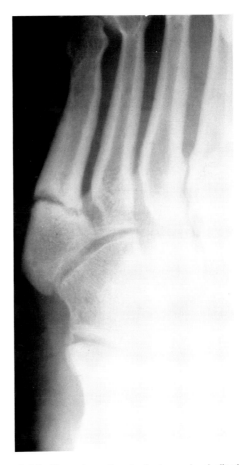

Fig. 158-20. Nonunion of a typical proximal diaphyseal fracture of the fifth metatarsal.

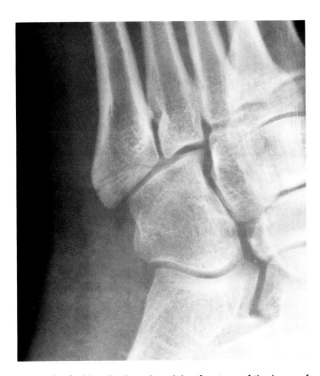

Fig. 158-19. Nondisplaced avulsion fracture of the base of the fifth metatarsal. This fracture healed in 4 weeks with immobilization in a weight-bearing cast.

fracture is quite distinctive: a transverse fracture line occurring about 1.5 cm from the tip of the tuberosity (Fig. 158-20). Many of these fractures occur in competitive athletes, particularly by those competing in jumping sports such as basketball, and some authorities have postulated that it is a stress fracture.[43] Delayed union occurs in as many as two-thirds of cases, and for this reason some investigators recommend surgical treatment, particularly in the young athletic adult. Because the fracture is rarely displaced, surgical treatment using a single compression screw has been recommended by some,[35] while others[24] recommend a sliding cor-

ticocancellous bone graft to bridge the fracture site and facilitate healing.

Closed treatment has its advocates as well, and with this method[16] the key to prompt healing appears to be non-weight-bearing in a below-knee cast for 6 to 8 weeks. While time constraints may sway one's decision toward surgical treatment in certain selected competitive athletes, most patients with this injury should be treated for 6 to 8 weeks in a non-weight-bearing cast. Should there be no evidence of healing at this point (and with this fracture, consolidation gradually progresses from medial to lateral, Fig. 158-21), bone graft-

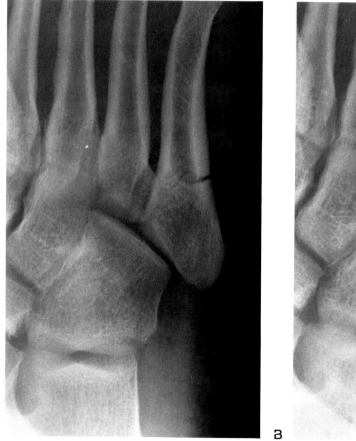
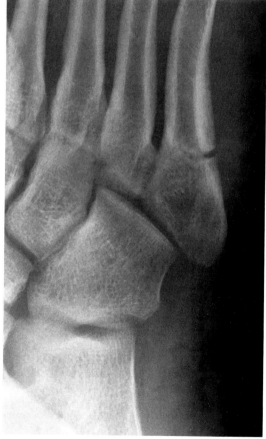

Fig. 158-21. (A) Acute nondisplaced fracture of the proximal diaphysis of the fifth metatarsal in a competitive basketball player. **(B)** Appearance of the fracture after cast immobilization for 2 months (note the early medial consolidation). *(Figure continues.)*

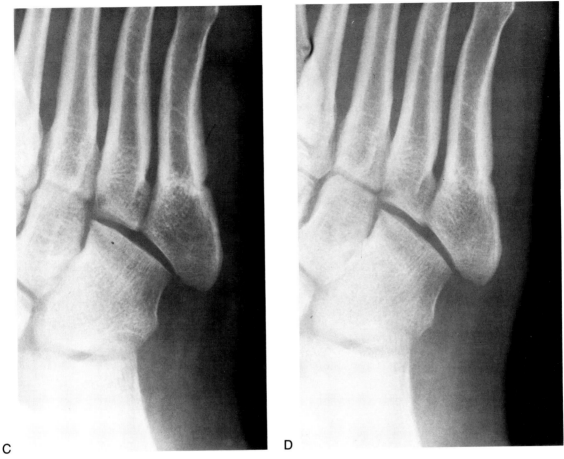

C   D

Fig. 158-21 *(Continued).* **(C)** Appearance of the fracture at 4 months with further healing. **(D)** Full healing of the fracture at 6 months postinjury.

ing or compression screw fixation would be indicated.

Metatarsophalangeal Joint Injuries

Because of their location, the metatarsophalangeal joints are susceptible to injury produced by direct blows and twisting forces applied to the respective toes. Injury to these joints, particularly the first, most often produces a sprain with stretching or tearing of a portion of the supporting ligaments. Sprains can be quite painful and initially may produce significant swelling and joint tenderness. While virtually all sprains will heal with a 3-week period of rest, many patients cannot or will

not limit use of the foot to permit prompt healing, resulting in persistent low-grade pain and swelling of the joint for prolonged periods.

Sprains

Sprain injury to the first metatarsophalangeal joint is especially common among certain groups of athletes and dancers. The term *turf toe*[20] has been used to describe this type of injury in football players who play on artificial surfaces using a flexible-soled soccer-type shoe. The flexible shoe permits greater extension of the first metatarsophalangeal joint, resulting in repeated episodes of hyperextension sprain of the plantar capsule and plate. Repeated episodes of injury lead to chronic pain and significant limitation of performance in the athlete.[22]

Sprains of all the metatarsophalangeal joints will usually heal with 2 to 3 weeks of protection. Some degree of splinting can be achieved by taping the injured toe to the adjacent toe(s) to eliminate the extremes of motion. The use of a stiff-soled shoe during the early phases of healing will also provide protection of the injured joint. Acutely, in the athlete, turf toe injuy should be treated aggressively with rest (no running) until swelling and pain with weight bearing subside and should then be protected from reinjury by taping of the great toe to the second and using a spring steel insert in the sole of the shoe to limit extension of the joint.

Dislocations

Dislocations of the metatarsophalangeal joints are rare because of their relatively stable configuration. Extreme forces may, however, produce a frank dislocation that is frequently associated with fractures or other injuries of the forepart of the foot, and care must be taken not to overlook these associated problems (Fig. 158-22).

Most metatarsophalangeal dislocations are dorsal, with the proximal phalanx displaced dorsally and proximally. Chronic claw toe deformity produces dorsal subluxation or frank dislocation of this joint, and this condition must be distinguished from an acute traumatic dislocation to avoid unnecessary attempts at reduction.

Closed Reduction

Although, on rare occasions, a complex (irreducible by closed means) dislocation, usually of the first metatarsophalangeal joint, may occur, most metatarsophalangeal dislocations can be reduced easily by traction and manual manipulation. Under adequate local digital block anesthesia, longitudinal traction applied to the toe will often reduce the dislocation. If traction fails, the deformity should be exaggerated, usually by hyperextending the joint, and the base of the proximal phalanx pushed distally over the metatarsal head. In most

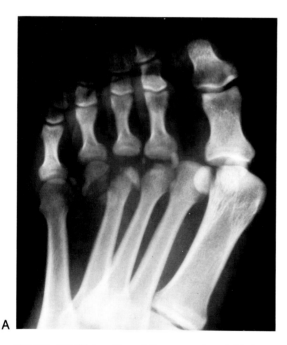
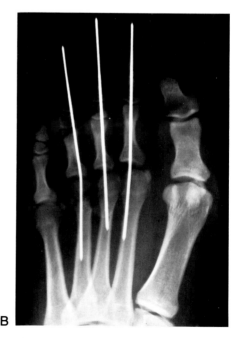

Fig. 158-22. (A) Dislocation of the second and third metatarsophalangeal joints with subluxation of the first metatarsophalangeal joint and fracture-dislocation of the fourth. **(B)** Satisfactory reduction of the three dislocations was achieved with longitudinal traction. The reductions are stabilized with percutaneous Kirschner wires.

cases, one of these two techniques will result in a stable congruous reduction confirmed by repeat radiographs. Once reduced, the joint should be taken through a gentle passive range of motion to test for stability and crepitus. The presence of gross instability, crepitus on motion, incongruity, or intra-articular loose bodies on postreduction radiographs are all indications of an inadequate closed reduction and the need for arthrotomy to relieve any obstruction to full reduction and to remove residual intra-articular fracture fragments.

Open Reduction

On rare occasions, closed reduction may fail. This condition is termed a complex dislocation. In the complex dislocation of the metatarsophalangeal joint of the great toe, as in the corresponding injury of the joints of the hand, the plantar structures of the joint are displaced dorsally, blocking reduction. The metatarsal head is trapped by the medial and lateral tendons of the short flexor and by the plantar plate, which remains attached to the base of the proximal phalanx and is flipped over the top of the metatarsal head. These structures block attempts at manipulative reduction and, indeed, become more constrictive when traction is applied to the great toe. Jahss[31] pointed out that with a complex dislocation of the first metatarsophalangeal joint, the sesamoid mass remains intact. He found that in those dislocations in which there is a fracture of one sesamoid or separation between the two sesamoids, reduction is usually easily achieved, but when this complex is uninjured, it obstructs reduction, producing the complex dislocation.

Technique The complex dislocation of the first metatarsophalangeal joint requires open reduction. While some authorities[28] have recommended a transverse plantar incision over the prominent metatarsal head, I prefer a dorsal incision in the first web space. This approach avoids injury to the displaced neurovascular bundles and provides excellent exposure of the distorted anatomy. Release of the adductor tendon and transection of the intermetatarsal ligament between the first and second metatarsal heads usually frees the plantar plate and sesamoid complex sufficiently so that they can be displaced plantarly out of the joint to make room

for the metatarsal head to return to its articulation with the proximal phalanx.[36] The adductor tendon can then be reattached and a stable joint complex restored. Immobilization in a below-knee weight-bearing cast with toe plate for 3 to 4 weeks will provide protection until soft tissue healing occurs.

Treatment of Dislocations of the Lesser Metatarsophalangeal Joints

On very rare occasions, dislocations of the lesser metatarsophalangeal joints may be irreducible by closed means. While complex dislocations of these joints have been reported,[41] this problem is almost always associated with displaced fractures or fracture-dislocations of the adjacent metatarsals that have resulted in shortening that tethers the dislocated toe and prevents closed reduction. Once the length of the adjacent fractured metatarsal has been restored, tension is released from the extrinsic tendons to the dislocated toe, facilitating closed reduction of the dislocated metatarsophalangeal joint.[25]

Sesamoid Fractures

Direct blows, avulsion forces, and repetitive stress (especially in runners and dancers) can lead to fracture of a sesamoid.[30] The medial sesamoid fractures more frequently. In patients who present with pain over the sesamoid following an acute injury or after repetitive stress, anteroposterior and axial radiographs (the sesamoid view) may show fragmentation of one of these bones. An acute fracture (Fig. 158-23) must be distinguished from a failure of fusion of the centers of ossification, particularly medially, where bipartite or multipartite sesamoids have been found in 8 to 33 percent of the normal population.[32] The bipartite sesamoid is bilaterally symmetric in 85 percent of cases when it is seen. It is generally larger and each segment has smooth sclerotic edges. These findings on radiographs should help distinguish the bipartite sesamoid from an acute fracture, which has rough and irregular fracture edges.

Treatment

Treatment of sesamoid fractures, particularly those caused by repetitive stress, can be very prolonged and frustrating. Authorities generally agree

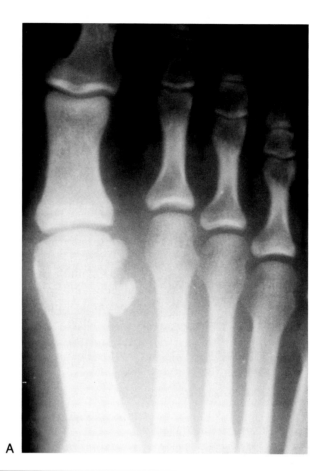

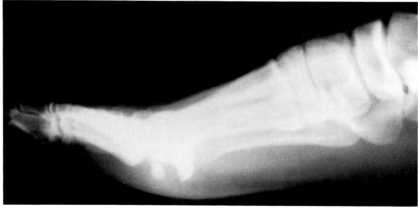

Fig. 158-23. (A,B) Displaced fracture of the lateral sesamoid resulting from severe hyperextension of the first metatarsophalangeal joint.

that nonoperative treatment should be tried first, with the foot immobilized in a below-knee weight-bearing cast with toe plate for 6 weeks followed by the use of a stiff-soled shoe and limitation of running and jumping for an additional 6 weeks. Even with minimally displaced fractures, the nonunion rate is high, and a significant proportion of patients will have persistent pain with weight bearing for as long as 1 year after injury. When persistent disabling pain cannot be relieved by shoe modifications, the painful nonunited sesamoid can be surgically excised. However, it should be very carefully enucleated from the flexor tendon mass, and the tendons should be reconstructed to maintain their dynamic stabilizing function for the first ray. Failure to restore their function may lead to significant deformity of the first metatarsophalangeal joint (hallux valgus, hallux varus, or hyperextension).

Injuries of the Toes

Toe fractures occur frequently, usually as the result of a direct blow. Most are minimally displaced and heal well regardless of the treatment given. However, they are all very painful and create marked temporary disability (limitation of activity and shoe wear) for the patient. Because aggressive treatment is rarely indicated, physicians tend to minimize these injuries and in general are not adequately sympathetic to the problems the fracture creates for the patient. Minimally displaced and nondisplaced fractures of any of the toes should be treated with rest and elevation for 2 to 3 days, followed by buddy-tape splinting to adjacent toes and the use of a stiff-soled shoe for 2 to 3 weeks. The patient should be given an adequate supply of analgesics to minimize discomfort during the healing process, as the fracture hurts and is constantly being irritated during walking. The patient should be advised that the pain and swelling will persist for up to 6 weeks, making shoewear and vigorous activity difficult.

Severely displaced fractures should be reduced by applying longitudinal traction to the toe under adequate local block anesthesia to decrease residual deformity that may produce a bony prominence easily irritated by shoewear. Most displaced fractures, once reduced, can be maintained in satisfac-

tory alignment by buddy-tape splinting to the adjacent toe(s) for 3 weeks until early healing occurs. Care must be taken to place cotton padding between the toes and not to tape them too tightly, to avoid maceration and pressure sores in the web space. On rare occasions, taping may not provide sufficient stability. In these cases, the reduced unstable fracture can be stabilized with an axial Kirschner wire for 3 to 4 weeks until fracture healing occurs.

Intra-articular fractures and dislocations of the interphalangeal joint of the great should be reduced accurately to ensure satisfactory long-term function. Closed reduction of injuries to this joint can usually be achieved but, on occasion, persistent joint incongruity or nonunited avulsion fractures of the joint margin will lead to persistent long-term symptoms. Therefore, persistent intra-articular displacement of fracture fragments should be anatomically reduced and fixed with percutaneous wires to maximize the chances for full recovery of joint function.

REFERENCES

Injuries of the Midpart of the Foot

1. Brown DC, McFarland GB: Dislocation of the medial cuneiform bone in tarsometatarsal fracture-dislocation. A case report. J Bone Joint Surg 57A:858, 1975
2. Dewar FP, Evans DC: Occult fracture-subluxation of the midtarsal joint. J Bone Joint Surg 50B:386, 1968
3. Dines DM, Hershon SJ, Smith N, et al: Isolated dorsomedial dislocation of the first ray at the medial cuneonavicular joint of the foot: a rare injury to the tarsus. A case report. Clin Orthop 186:162, 1984
4. Eichenholtz SN, Levine DB: Fractures of the tarsal navicular bone. Clin Orthop 34:142, 1964
5. Hermel MB, Gershon-Cohen J: The nutcracker fracture of the cuboid by indirect violence. Radiology 60:850, 1953
6. Howie CR, Hooper G, Hughes SPF: Occult midtarsal subluxation. Clin Orthop 209:206, 1986
7. Kenwright J, Taylor RG: Major injuries of the talus. J Bone Joint Surg 52B:36, 1970
8. Main BJ, Jowett RL: Injuries of the midtarsal joint. J Bone Joint Surg 57B:89, 1975

9. Mann R, Inman VT: Phasic activity of intrinsic muscles of the foot. J Bone Joint Surg 46A:469, 1964

10. Pavlov H, Torg JS, Freiberger RH: Tarsal navicular stress fractures: radiographic evaluation. Radiology 148:641, 1983

11. Phillips RD: Dysfunction of the peroneus longus after fracture of the cuboid. J Foot Surg 24(2):99, 1985

12. Schiller MG, Ray RD: Isolated dislocation of the medial cuneiform bone—a rare injury of the tarsus. A case report. J Bone Joint Surg 52A:1632, 1970

13. Shands AR Jr, Wentz IJ: Congenital anomalies, accessory bones, and osteochondritis in the feet of 850 children. Surg Clin North Am 33:1643, 1953

14. Stark WA: Occult fracture-subluxation of the midtarsal joint. Clin Orthop 93:291, 1973

15. Torg JS, Pavlov H, Cooley LH, et al: Stress fractures of the tarsal navicular. A retrospective review of twenty-one cases. J Bone Joint Surg 64A:700, 1982

Injuries of the Forepart of the Foot

16. Acker JH, Drez D Jr: Nonoperative treatment of stress fractures of the proximal shaft of the fifth metatarsal (Jones' fracture). Foot Ankle 7:152, 1986

17. Aitken AP, Poulson D: Dislocations of the tarsometatarsal joint. J Bone Joint Surg 45A:246, 1963

18. Anderson LD: Injuries of the forefoot. Clin Orthop 122:18, 1977

19. Arntz CT, Hansen ST: Dislocations and fracture dislocations of the tarsometatarsal joints. Orthop Clin North Am 18:105, 1987

20. Bowers KD Jr, Martin RB: Turf-toe: a shoe-surface related football injury. Med Sci Sports 8:81, 1976

21. Brunet JA, Wiley JJ: The late results of tarsometatarsal joint injuries. J Bone Joint Surg 69B:437, 1987

22. Coker TP Jr, Arnold JA: Sports injuries to the foot and ankle. p. 1573. In Jahss MH (ed): Disorders of the Foot. Vol. II. WB Saunders, Philadelphia, 1982

23. D'Ambrosia R, Drez D Jr (eds): Prevention and Treatment of Running Injuries. Charles B. Slack, Thorofare, NJ, 1982

24. Dameron TB Jr: Fractures and anatomical variations of the proximal portion of the fifth metatarsal. J Bone Joint Surg 57A:788, 1975

25. English TA: Dislocations of the metatarsal bone and adjacent toe. J Bone Joint Surg 46B:700, 1964

26. Ford LT, Gilula LA: Stress fractures of the middle metatarsals following the Keller operation. J Bone Joint Surg 59A:117, 1977

27. Foster SC, Foster RR: Lisfranc's tarsometatarsal fracture-dislocation. Radiology 120:79, 1976

28. Giannikas AC, Papachristou G, Papavasiliou N, et al: Dorsal dislocation of the first metatarso-phalangeal joint. Report of four cases. J bone Joint Surg 57B:384, 1975

29. Goossens M, DeStoop N: Lisfranc's fracture-dislocations: etiology, radiology, and results of treatment. A review of 20 cases. Clin Orthop 176:154, 1983

30. Hulkko A, Orava S, Pellinen P, et al: Stress fractures of the sesamoid bones of the first metatarsophalangeal joint in athletes. Arch Orthop Trauma Surg 104:113, 1985

31. Jahss MH: Traumatic dislocations of the first metatarsophalangeal joint. Foot Ankle 1:15, 1980

32. Jahss MH: The sesamoids of the hallux. Clin Orthop 157:88, 1981

33. Johnson JE, Johnson KA: Dowel arthrodesis for degenerative arthritis of the tarsometatarsal (Lisfranc) joints. Foot Ankle 6:243, 1986

34. Jones R: Fracture of the base of the fifth metatarsal bone by indirect violence. Ann Surg 35:697, 1902

35. Kavanaugh JH, Brower TD, Mann RV: The Jones fracture revisited. J Bone Joint Surg 60A:776, 1978

36. Lewis AG, DeLee JC: Type-I complex dislocation of the first metatarsophalangeal joint—open reduction through a dorsal approach. A case report. J Bone Joint Surg 66A:1120, 1984

37. Meurman KOA: Less common stress fractures in the foot. Br J Radiol 54:1, 1981

38. Meurman KOA, Elfving S: Stress fracture in soldiers: a multifocal bone disorder. Radiology 134:483, 1980

39. Myerson MS, Fisher RT, Burgess AR, et al: Fracture dislocations of the tarsometatarsal joints: end results correlated with pathology and treatment. Foot Ankle 6:225, 1986

40. Quenu E, Kuss G: Etude sur les luxations du metatarse (luxations metatarso-tarsiennes) du diastasis entre le 1. et le 2. metatarsien. Rev Chir 39:281, 720, 1093, 1909

41. Rao JP, Banzon MT: Irreducible dislocation of the metatarsophalangeal joints of the foot. Clin Orthop 145:224, 1979

42. van der Werf GJIM, Tonino AJ: Tarsometatarsal fracture-dislocation. Acta Orthop Scand 55:647, 1984

43. Zelko RR, Torg JS, Rachun A: Proximal diaphyseal fractures of the fifth metatarsal—treatment of the fractures and their complications in athletes. Am J Sports Med 7:95, 1979

Index

Coccidiodomycosis, 4559, 4578–4579, 4578f
Coccidioides immitis infection
  acute tenosynovitis after immunosuppressive therapy, 1186
  cutaneous manifestation progression, 1186–1187
  upper extremity, 1186
Coccidioidomycosis
  acute synovitis after immunosuppressive therapy, 1186
  upper extremity, 1186
Codman's triangle, 4607
Cold, prior to hand therapy, 1313
Coleman block test, 4017–4018, 4017f
Collagen
  deposition, joint stiffening and, 1298–1299
  flexor tendon healing, 518
  maturation, stiffened hand and, 1304
  production, 95
    fracture healing, 95
Collapsing spine, 2051, 2053f
  surgical treatment, 2059, 2062f
Collateral ligament
  direct primary repair, 3258, 3259f–3261f, 3260–3261
  functional anatomy, 1684, 1684f–1685f
  wrist, 452
Colles' fracture, *see also* Distal radius fracture
  carpal tunnel syndrome, 967–968
  treatment
    osteopenia patient, 193–194, 193f
    unstable, 194
Coloring agents, PMMA, 2962
Comminuted intertrochanteric fracture, *see* Intertrochanteric fracture, comminuted
Comminuted vertebral body fractures, anterior fibular strut stabilization, 2212–2215, 2214f
  graft insertion, 2214–2215, 2214f
  harvesting graft, 2213–2214
  operative technique, 2212–2213
  postoperative management, 2215
  vertebrae preparation, 2213, 2214f
Comminution, distal radius fracture, 354
Compartment syndromes, 605–623
  after intra-arterial drug injection, 600
  anatomy, 605–607, 606f–607f
  definition, 605
  degree of ischemic injury, 605
  diagnosis, 611–613, 612f, 613t, 614f–615f, 616
    clinical approach, 611
    differential, 612
    earliest symptoms, 611
    signs and symptoms of ischemia, 611

tissue pressure, 612f, 613, 613t, 614f–615f, 615–616
    tolerance, 616
  etiology, 610t, 611
  exertional, 622–623
  forearm, 595
  historical aspects, 607–608
  knee
    Maquet barrel-vault tibial osteotomy complication, 3559
    post-realignment, 3453
  late contracture, 621–622, 621f
  lower leg, *see* Lower leg compartment syndrome
  pathophysiology, 608–611, 609f, 610t
    arterial spasm, 608
    arteriovenous gradient degradation, 609–610
    critical closing pressure, 609
    intracompartmental ischemia, 609
    raised pressure, 608
  permanent ischemic injury, 622
  treatment, 616–619, 618f, 620f, 621
    complicated by a fracture, 617
    early, 616
    fasciotomy, *see* Fasciotomy
    forearm, 617–619, 618f
    late contracted state, 621–622
    leg, 619, 620f, 621
    skin grafting, 617
Compensatory arm and shoulder motion, compromised elbow motion, 1759, 1760f
Complement cascade, 4387, 4387f
Component loosening, *see* specific prostheses and procedures
Compression arthrodesis of shoulder, 1557–1558, 1557f–15579
Compression fracture
  cervical spine injuries, 2211f, 2212
  unstable, thoracolumbar spine injuries, 2223
Compression injuries, hand and forearm, 720, 722, 722f–724f, 724
Compression plate
  dynamic, wrist arthrodesis, 781–782, 782f
  hip osteotomy, 2810, 2810f
  tibial nonunions, 3813, 3813f–3814f, 3815
Compression rod, 2265–2266, 2266f
Compression stockings, thromboembolic disease and, 61
Computed tomography, 218, 219f, 220–221, 2399f–2402f, 2402
  above-knee amputation, 5181
  acute herniated lumbar disc, 1889–1890
  arthrography, shoulder, 214f, 215
  avascular necrosis, 220

bilateral calcaneal fractures, 219f, 220
  cartilage tumor diagnosis, 4719
  cervical spine tumors, limitation of, 2409
  closed biopsy, 4639
  congenital hip dysplasia, 220
  diastematomyelia, 2034, 2035f
  distal radioulnar joint injury, 490–491, 491f
  drawbacks, 218
  extent of osteosarcoma, 4858, 4860f
  forequarter amputation, 5185
  giant cell tumor, 4821
  hand tumor, 1200
  head and face injuries, 200
  hemipelvectomy, 5170–5171
  hip and pelvic injuries, 200, 201f
  hip fracture-dislocations, 220
  infections, 220
  ischemic necrosis of femoral head, 2774–2775, 2774t, 2775f–2777f
  isthmic spondylolisthesis, 2102
  local resection of pelvis, 2449
  lumbar fractures, 2239–2240
  versus magnetic resonance imaging, 2773–2774
  malignant fibrous lesions, 4973
  metastatic bone disease, 5023, 5023f
  osteoid osteoma, 4781
  osteomyelitis, 203f, 220
  osteoporosis assessment, 184
  patellofemoral joint evaluation, 3440
  pelvic ring fracture, 2495–2496
  quantitative, 224
  soft tissue tumor, 4611
  spinal injuries, 200
  spinal stenosis, 1895–1896
  thoracolumbar spine injuries, 2223
  three dimensional, supplemental documentation of pelvic ring fracture, 2496
  trauma, 218, 219f, 220
  tumors, 220
Computer-assisted three-dimensional imaging, pelvic osteotomy, 2476
Condylar fracture, 1728
  both medial and lateral, 3480, 3487–3489, 3488f
  classification, 3476–3477, 3476f
  nonunion, 1747
Condylar implant
  failure, 3648
  resurfacing arthroplasty, osteoarthritic hand, 1137f–1138f, 1140
Condylar knee prosthesis
  infected, knee arthrodesis, 3715f–3716f
  prognosis, 3686
Condylocephalic nail

with glenohumeral dislocation, 1449–1450, 1449f
proximal tibial articular fracture-dislocation, 3490, 3490t
tibial and fibular fractures, 3789–3790
Neurovascular island flap
hand skin grafts, 696f–699f, 697, 699
local, 730, 731f–732f
Neurovascular pedicle, transfer, 867, 868f
Neurovascular reflex dystrophy, replantation complication, 665
Neutrophil
chemotaxis, impaired, 4389
phagocytosis and killing of bacteria, 4384, 4384f
Nickel, allergic reactions, 254
Night splint, carpal tunnel syndrome, 968–969
Nocardiosis, 1187–1188, 1189f, 4587
Nodular fasciitis, 4803, 4804f
Nondissociative carpal instability, 485–486
Nonossifying fibroma, 4745–4746, 4746f–4750f, 4750–4751
femoral neck bone cyst and tibial shaft fibroma, 4747f–4750f, 4750–4751
fibrous dysplasia, 4751, 4752f–4754f, 4754
intertrochanteric fibroma, 4746, 4746f, 4750
pathologic fracture, 4745–4746, 4745f
Nonunion, 102–104, 102t; *see also* Bone grafting
ankle fractures, 3857–3858
bone grafting, 107
cervical osteotomy, 2386
clavicle, reconstructive surgery, 1528
elbow fracture, 1745f–1746f, 1747
elephant foot, 3806
external immobilization, 107
factors related to, 102t
femoral neck fracture, 2550
with early weight bearing, 2561
femoral head and neck arthroplasty, 2893f
internal fixation, 2567, 2569f
quality of reduction, 2557–2558, 2558f
timing of surgery, 2557
young adults, 2555–2556
femoral shaft fracture complications, 2725
following spinal surgery, 2313
greater trochanter, total hip reconstruction, 3012
hamate, 364

heavily irradiated bone, 4644
hip arthrodesis, 2875–2876
humerus, *see* Humeral shaft fractures, nonunion
hypothesis, 103–104
infected, *see* Infected nonunion
intracondylar T and Y fractures, 1732, 1733f–1734f
lumbar fractures, prevention, 2268
lumbar osteotomy, 2360
lumbosacral, 2239
metastatic carcinoma, 4667
olecranon fracture, 1727
pelvic ring fracture, 2514
proximal humeral fracture, *see* Proximal humeral fracture
proximal humeral surgical neck, reconstructive surgery, 1529
proximal tibial articular fracture, 3496–3497
scaphoid fracture, 361
sesamoid fracture, 4295
shoulder, *see* Shoulder fractures, nonunion
tibial and fibular fractures, 3786–3787, 3787f–3788f, 3789
tibial shaft, *see* Tibial fractures, nonunion
transverse proximal diaphyseal fracture of fifth metatarsal, 4289, 4289f
treatment effect, 106–107
triple arthrodesis, pes planus, 4048
use of electrical stimulation, 107
Nonvascularized cortical autografts, 118–119, 119f
Norepinephrine, blood flow effects, 84
Notta's node, *see* Trigger finger
Noyes' flexion-rotation drawer test, 3305, 3305f
Nutcracker fracture, 4275, 4277f
Nutrient artery, scaphoid, 76
Nutrition
assessment, infection prevention and, 4314
impaired
immune responses and, 4389
in neuromuscular disorders, 2078
multiply injured patient, 26–27
status, tuberculosis and, 4569

Obesity
cemented total knee arthroplasty and, 3577–3578
femoral head and neck resection arthroplasty contraindication, 2897
knee arthroplasty contraindication, 3625
Oblique metacarpal line, 419

Oblique radiography, local resection of pelvis, 2448
Oblique retinacular ligament, 326
reconstruction, 565, 566f, 567
Obliterative bursitis, *see* Diffuse rotator cuff tendinitis
Occipitoatlantal dislocation, 2177–2179, 2178f–2179f
Occipitoatlantal joint, 2152–2153, 2153f, 2153t, 2175–2179
anatomy, 2152
articulation, 2175–2179
biomechanics, 2152–2153, 2153f, 2153t
flexion and extension limits, 2177
fusion, 2179, 2179f
injury, diagnosis and management, 2177–2179, 2178f–2179f
ligaments of stability, 2175–2176
occiput-condyle fracture, 2177–2179, 2178f–2179f
treatment, 2153
Occipitocervical fusion, cervical spine tumors, 2416
Occiput, posterior approach, 1817–1819, 1818f–1819f
Occiput-atlantoaxial articulation, 2175–2197
atlantoaxial joint, 2181–2191, 2181f–2192f
congenital anomalies, 2185
odontoid fracture, 2185, 2185f
patient positioning, 2187, 2187f
postoperative management, 2189–2191
rotary displacement, 2181, 2182f, 2184
rotary fixation classification, 2181, 2182f, 2184
subluxation and dislocation, 2182–2184, 2183f–2185f
surgical procedure, 2186–2189, 2186f–2189f
wiring methods, 2188–2190, 2188f–2192f
atlas fractures, 2179–2181, 2180f–2181f
burst fracture of atlas, 2180–2181, 2180f–2181f
flexion and extension limits, 2177
Jefferson fracture, 2180–2181, 2180f–2181f
occipitoatlantal joint
injury diagnosis and management, 2177–2179, 2178f–2179f
ligaments of stability, 2175–2176
occipital-condylar fracture, 2177–2179, 2178f
occiput-C2 fusion, 2179f
odontoid fracture, 2185, 2185f
posterior arch fracture, 2180
rotatory fixation, 2181, 2182f